Multiple Sclerosis:
A Comprehensive Text

Commissioning Editor: Michael Parkinson
Development Editor: Janice Urquhart
Project Manager: Joannah Duncan
Design Direction: Sarah Russell
Illustrator: Samantha Elmhurst

Multiple Sclerosis:
A Comprehensive Text

Edited by

Cedric S. Raine PhD DSc FRCPath

Professor, Departments of Pathology (Neuropathology),
Neurology and Neuroscience,
Albert Einstein College of Medicine,
New York, USA

Henry F. McFarland MD

Chief, Neuroimmunology Branch, and Clinical Director,
National Institute of Neurological Disorders and Stroke,
National Institutes of Health, Bethesda,
Maryland, USA

Reinhard Hohlfeld MD

Professor and Director of the Institute for Clinical Neuroimmunology,
Ludwig-Maximilians University, Klinikum Grosshadern,
Institute for Clinical Neuroimmunology,
Munich, Germany

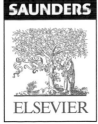

SAUNDERS

ELSEVIER

EDINBURGH LONDON NEW YORK OXFORD PHILADELPHIA ST LOUIS SYDNEY TORONTO 2008

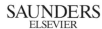

An imprint of Elsevier Limited

© 2008, Elsevier Limited. All rights reserved.

No part of this publication may be reproduced, stored in a retrieval system, or transmitted in any form or by any means, electronic, mechanical, photocopying, recording or otherwise, without the prior permission of the Publishers. Permissions may be sought directly from Elsevier's Health Sciences Rights Department, 1600 John F. Kennedy Boulevard, Suite 1800, Philadelphia, PA 19103-2899, USA: phone: (+1) 215 239 3804; fax: (+1) 215 239 3805; or, e-mail: *healthpermissions@elsevier.com*. You may also complete your request on-line via the Elsevier homepage (http://www.elsevier.com), by selecting 'Support and contact' and then 'Copyright and Permission'.

ISBN 978-0-7020-2811-3

British Library Cataloguing in Publication Data
A catalogue record for this book is available from the British Library

Library of Congress Cataloging in Publication Data
A catalogue record for this book is available from the Library of Congress

Note
Knowledge and best practice in this field are constantly changing. As new research and experience broaden our knowledge, changes in practice, treatment and drug therapy may become necessary or appropriate. Readers are advised to check the most current information provided (i) on procedures featured or (ii) by the manufacturer of each product to be administered, to verify the recommended dose or formula, the method and duration of administration, and contraindications. It is the responsibility of the practitioner, relying on their own experience and knowledge of the patient, to make diagnoses, to determine dosages and the best treatment for each individual patient, and to take all appropriate safety precautions. To the fullest extent of the law, neither the Publisher nor the Editors assume any liability for any injury and/or damage to persons or property arising out of or related to any use of the material contained in this book.

The Publisher

  your source for books,
journals and multimedia
in the health sciences

www.elsevierhealth.com

The
publisher's
policy is to use
paper manufactured
from sustainable forests

Printed in China

Preface

Why another book on multiple sclerosis? To us, the reason was obvious – the terrain of multiple sclerosis (MS) is vast and ever-changing. So much is happening that concepts forged just 2 years ago are already passé. Whether viewed from the platform of the health professional responsible for the day-to-day care of the patient or the scientist working to unravel what makes this a unique disease, MS has over the last decade evolved into a condition necessitating multidisciplinary approaches to both its management and understanding. One needs only to peruse the profiles of the personnel associated with an MS care center (particularly one located in an academic setting) to appreciate the enormous array of skills and treatments now available to the patient. For the scientific investigator, the rapidity of developments in recent years has been quite intimidating as genetics, immunology and molecular biology have assumed center stage, a fact reflected daily in our language, tools and techniques. In short, MS is a moving target and, as a consequence, we need to keep adjusting our sights. This book is the latest adjustment.

Why a 'comprehensive' textbook? In the past, authors of texts on MS have shied away from broad-fronted coverage, with the preface of one renowned 1985 tome announcing 'it is no longer possible even to attempt a comprehensive work on mul-tiple sclerosis'. If that were the case 20-plus years ago when the number of treatments for the MS patient was virtually zero and the diagnostic tools and research options were limited (to say the least), imagine the scope of the endeavor today! We have for certain come a long way since the 1980s – just look how much is out there now for the patient! With more than half-a-dozen approved and effective drugs specifically designed for MS, and dozens in advanced stages of clinical trials and/or awaiting approval, there is a wealth of new information to report. Thus, because the horizon is brighter than ever before for those affected with or involved in the condition, we think the time is ripe for a fresh look at the status of MS as a clinical problem, for the latest coverage on expanding prospects for the patient, and for a state-of-the-art re-evaluation of changes occurring within the nervous system. Since any approach to MS, scientific or care-related, is almost guaranteed to embrace the combined skills of several disciplines, for an individual to embark single-handed upon the preparation of a text on the subject might understandably be deemed over-ambitious. Therefore, fully cognizant of the challenge and somewhat intimidated by recently published excellent works on the subject, the present Anglo-American-German editorial alliance was assembled, each editor having one foot firmly planted in MS and the other in a

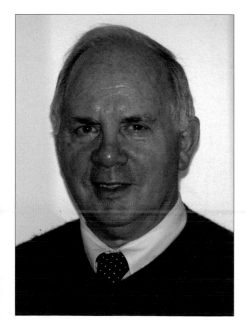

Cedric S. Raine,
New York City, NY, USA

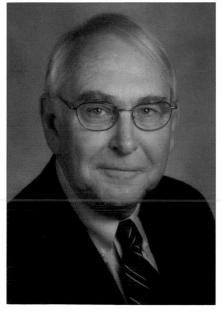

Henry F. McFarland,
Washington, DC, USA

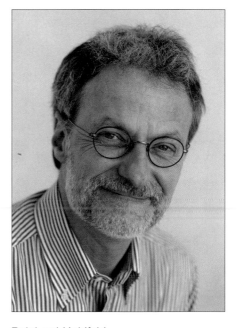

Reinhard Hohlfeld,
Munich, Germany

field different from the other two. Our principal task was to compile a comprehensive Table of Contents replete with outstanding contributors, with long track records in both basic and clinical research. We have invested heavily in the project and are highly satisfied with the result, which is not a dogmatic, subjective treatise reflecting personal viewpoints but rather a series of succinct and interlocking contributions (actually 31 chapters) from a unique team of clinicians and investigators never before assembled whose collective skills traverse the entire landscape of MS.

What will the book achieve? Considering that MS can still be difficult to define both clinically and pathologically, and that not too long ago (to some of us, at least), diagnosis was regarded as proven only after autopsy or biopsy (McDonald & Halliday 1977), we feel that the present coverage more than does justice to the field since it portrays MS as a definable entity and sets what we hope is a new gold-standard for its characterization. Parenthetically, after a long dormancy, it took a lay person (Sylvia Lawry), not a neurologist or a scientist, to bring MS into the limelight and to give it the prominence it deserves. Sylvia was seeking guidance in 1945 to help her brother afflicted with MS when she ran a short announcement in the *New York Times* asking people with MS to contact her, a venture that culminated with the recognition of this as an important disease and the establishment of Multiple Sclerosis Societies around the world. Her efforts were also pivotal in the formation in the USA of what is now known as the National Institute of Neurological Diseases and Stroke. It is largely as a result of her energy and insight that we are where we are today and for this we owe her a debt of gratitude. Thanks in part to work supported by agencies like those Sylvia created, we no longer doubt that the quality of life for the MS patient can be improved, that the clinical course can be beneficially modified, that the immunological assault on the nervous system can be assuaged, that axonal damage can be reduced, and that myelin repair is feasible – the challenge is to correct these anomalies simultaneously in the MS patient. True, many issues still need to be resolved (like whether MS is a single disease or a collection of variants), and we recognize that no book on MS will ever be really complete since, like the canvas of the master painter, details can always be added.

For helping us bring the most recent advances in MS together in one volume, we thank the contributors, each of whom has striven to provide a didactic narrative that is both comprehensive and current. We feel that any reader entering into a dialogue with this book will emerge refreshed, fulfilled and brimming with anticipation about issues such as what the next clinical trial will bring, what triggers this devastating disease and whether more able symptomatic treatments will be uncovered. We are not unaware that this will not be the last word on MS and that it will be the latest for a brief window of time only, but we are confident that it will remain a major source of knowledge for many years to come.

Contributors

Oluf Andersen MD PhD
Professor of Neurology, Institute of Neuroscience and
Physiology, University of Gothenburg, Gothenburg,
Sweden

Brenda L. Banwell MD FRCPC
Assistant Professor of Pediatrics (Neurology) and Associate
Scientist, Research Institute, The Hospital for Sick Children,
University of Toronto, Canada

Ralph H. B. Benedict PhD
Associate Professor of Neurology, Erie County Medical
Center, Buffalo, USA

Jeffrey L. Bennett MD PhD
Associate Professor of Neurology and Ophthalmology,
Departments of Neurology and Ophthalmology, University of
Colorado, Health Sciences Center, Denver, Colorado, USA

Monika Bradl PhD
Head of Cellular Neuroimmunology Group, Medical
University Vienna, Center for Brain Research, Division of
Neuroimmunology, Vienna, Austria

Mark P. Burgoon PhD
Assistant Professor, Department of Neurology, University of
Colorado, Health Sciences Center, Denver, Colorado, USA

Fredric K. Cantor MD
Adjunct Investigator, Neuroimmunology Branch, NINDS,
NIH, Bethesda, Maryland, USA

Stacey S. Cofield PhD
Assistant Professor of Biostatistics, Department of
Biostatistics, University of Alabama at Birmingham, Alabama,
USA

Gary R. Cutter PhD
Professor of Biostatistics, Department of Biostatistics,
University of Alabama at Birmingham, Alabama, USA

Klaus Dornmair PHD
Head of Research Group, Ludwig-Maximilians University,
Klinikum Grosshadern, Institute for Clinical
Neuroimmunology, Munich, Germany

Monique Dubois-Dalcq MD
Honorary Professor, Pasteur Institute, Paris, France; Guest at
National Institute of Neurological Disorders and Stroke Porter
Neuroscience Research Center, Bethesda, Maryland, USA

Halima El-Moslimany MD
Post-doctoral Fellow in Multiple Sclerosis,
The Corinne Goldsmith Dickinson Center for Multiple
Sclerosis, Mount Sinai School of Medicine, New York, USA

Clare J. Fowler FRCP
Professor, Institute of Neurology; Consultant in Uro-
Neurology, National Hospital for Neurology and
Neurosurgery, University College London Hospitals, London,
UK

Claude Genain MD
Associate Professor, California Pacific Medical Center
Research Institute (Neurosciences), San Francisco, California,
USA

Donald H. Gilden MD
Louise Baum Professor and Chairman, Departments of
Neurology and Microbiology, University of Colorado, Health
Sciences Center, Denver, Colorado, USA

Gavin Giovannoni MB ChB PhD FCP FRCP FCPath
Professor of Neurology, Institute of Cell and Molecular
Science, Barts and The London Queen Mary's School of
Medicine and Dentistry, London, UK

Ralf Gold MD
Professor and Chair, Department of Neurology, St Josef-
Hospital, Ruhr-University Bochum, Germany

Douglas S. Goodin MD
Director of the Multiple Sclerosis Center, Department of
Neurology, University of California, San Francisco, California,
USA

Stephen L. Hauser MD PHD
Chair and Robert A. Fishman Distinguished Professor,
Department of Neurology, University of California, San
Francisco, California, USA

Reinhard Hohlfeld MD
Professor and Director of the Institute for Clinical
Neuroimmunology, Ludwig-Maximilians University, Klinikum
Grosshadern, Institute for Clinical Neuroimmunology,
Munich, Germany

Vinay Kalsi MRCS
Registrar in Uro-Neurology, National Hospital for Neurology
and Neurosurgery, University College London Hospitals,
London, UK

Ludwig Kappos MD
Professor of Neurology, Department of Neurology, Universitätsspital Basel, Basel, Switzerland

Jürg Kesselring MD
Professor of Neurology and Neurorehabilitation, Universities of Bern and Zürich, Switzerland; Chair of Neurorehabilitation, Università Vita e Salute, San Raffaele, Milano, Italy

Jeffery D. Kocsis PhD
Professor of Neurology, Department of Neurology, Yale University School of Medicine; Associate Director, Center for Neuroscience and Regeneration Research, VA Medical Center, West Haven Connecticut, USA

Tanya J. Lehky MD
Director, Clinical EMG Laboratory, EMG Branch, NINDS, NIH, Bethesda, Maryland, USA

Catherine Lubetzki MD DSci
Professor of Neurology, Université Pierre et Marie Curie, Faculté de Médecine, Paris; Assistance Publique-Hôpitaux de Paris, Hôpital de la Salpêtrière, Paris, France

Fred D. Lublin MD
Saunders Family Professor of Neurology; Director, The Corinne Goldsmith Dickinson Center for Multiple Sclerosis, Mount Sinai Medical Center, Mount Sinai School of Medicine, New York, USA

Samuel K. Ludwin MB ChB FRCP(C)
Professor of Pathology, Department of Pathology and Molecular Medicine, Queens University and Kingston General Hospital, Kingston, Ontario, Canada

Henry F. McFarland MD
Chief, Neuroimmunology Branch, and Clinical Director, National Institute of Neurological Disorders and Stroke, National Institutes of Health, Bethesda, Maryland, USA

Roland Martin MD
Research Professor, Institute for Neuroimmunology and Clinical MS Research, Center for Molecular Neurobiology Hamburg (ZMNH), University Medical Center Eppendorf, Hamburg, Germany

Aaron E. Miller MD
Medical Director, Corinne Goldsmith Dickinson Center for Multiple Sclerosis; Professor of Neurology, Mount Sinai School of Medicine, New York, USA

David H. Miller MB ChB MD FRACP FRCP
Professor of Clinical Neurology, Department of Neuroinflammation, Institute of Neurology, University College London, London, UK

John H. Noseworthy MD FRCPC
Professor and Chair, Department of Neurology, Mayo Clinic College of Medicine, Rochester, Minnesota, USA

Jorge R. Oksenberg PhD
Professor, Department of Neurology, School of Medicine, University of California at San Francisco, California, USA

Gregory P. Owens PhD
Associate Professor, Department of Neurology, University of Colorado, Health Sciences Center, Denver, Colorado, USA

Trevor Owens PhD
Professor, Medical Biotechnology Centre, Center for Medical Biotechnology, Syddansk Universitet, Odense, Denmark

Chris H. Polman MD PhD
Professor of Neurology, VU Medical Center, Amsterdam, The Netherlands

Maura Pugliatti MD
Research Assistant in Neurology, Institute of Clinical Neurology, Medical Faculty, University of Sassari, Sassari, Italy

Michael K. Racke MD
Professor of Neurology, Department of Neurology, Department of Molecular Virology, Immunology and Medical Genetics, The Ohio State University Medical Center, Columbus, Ohio, USA

Cedric S. Raine PhD DSc FRCPath
Departments of Pathology (Neuropathology), Neurology and Neuroscience, Albert Einstein College of Medicine, New York, USA

Stephen M. Rao PhD
Professor of Neurology, Department of Neurology, Cell Biology, Neurobiology and Anatomy, Medical College of Wisconsin, Milwaukee, Wisconsin, USA

Stephen C. Reingold PhD
Research Counsellor, National Multiple Sclerosis Society, New York City, New York; President Scientific and Clinical Review Associates LLC, Salisbury, Connecticut and New York City, USA

Giulio Rosati MD
Professor of Neurology and Head of Institute of Clinical Neurology; Dean of Medical Faculty, University of Sassari, Sassari, Italy

Randall T. Schapiro MD
Director, The Schapiro Center for Multiple Sclerosis, Minneapolis Clinic of Neurology, Minneapolis; Clinical Professor of Neurology, University of Minnesota, Minneapolis, Minnesota, USA

Neil J. Scolding FRCP PhD
Burden Professor of Clinical Neurosciences, Department of Neurology, University of Bristol, Institute of Clinical Neurosciences, Frenchay Hospital, Bristol, UK

Mireia Sospedra MD
Research Associate Institute for Neuroimmunology and Clinical MS Research, Center for Molecular Neurobiology Hamburg (ZMNH), University Medical Center Eppendorf, Hamburg, Germany

Alan J. Thompson MD FRCP FRCPI
Garfield Weston Professor of Clinical Neurology and Neurorehabilitation, Department of Brain Repair and Rehabilitation, Institute of Neurology, University College London, London, UK

Edward J. Thompson PhD MD DSc FRCPath FRCP
Emeritus Professor of Neurochemistry and Honorary Consultant at the National Hospital for Neurology and Neurosurgery, The Institute of Neurology, London, UK

Bob W. van Oosten MD PhD
Neurologist, VU University Medical Center, Amsterdam, The Netherlands

Stephen G. Waxman MD PhD
Professor and Chairman, Department of Neurology, Yale University Medical School, New Haven, USA; Director, Center for Neuroscience and Regeneration Research, VA Medical Center, West Haven, CT, USA

Brian G. Weinshenker MD FRCP(C)
Consultant in Neurology, Mayo Clinic; Professor of Neurology, Mayo Clinic College of Medicine, Rochester, USA

Dean M. Wingerchuk MD FRCP(C)
Consultant in Neurology, Mayo Clinic; Assistant Professor of Neurology, Mayo Clinic College of Medicine, Scottsdale, USA

Heather A. Wishart PhD
Associate Professor of Psychiatry, Dartmouth Medical School, Lebanon, New Hampshire, USA

Xiaoli Yu PhD
Instructor, Department of Neurology, University of Colorado, Health Sciences Center, Denver, Colorado, USA

Bernard Zalc MD DSci
Directeur de Recherche, Institut National de la Santé et de la Recherche Médicale, and Universîté Pierre et Marie Curie Unit 711, Hôpital de la Salpêtrière, Paris, France

Simone P. Zehntner PHD
Director, Small Animal Imaging Laboratory, Brain Imaging Center, Montreal Neurological Institute, Montreal, Quebec, Canada

Contents

CONTENTS

CHAPTER

1 History of multiple sclerosis

J. Kesselring

The past is always with us, never to be escaped; it alone is enduring; but amidst the changes and chances which succeed one another so rapidly in this life, we are apt to live too much for the present and too much for the future.

Sir William Osler, *Aequanimitas*, 1889

INTRODUCTION

Busy clinicians caring for individuals affected by multiple sclerosis (MS) and researchers interested in the disease as a problem in clinical science might reasonably ask whether it is worthwhile to study historical aspects in detail, and at length, in any medical field, let alone one in which fact and fiction are so inextricably intermingled and the literature so liberally decorated with decoys and distractions on the path to discovery.[1] On May 26, 1789, Friedrich Schiller gave his inaugural lecture as a *Privatdozent* at the University of Jena[2] entitled: 'What does universal history mean and to what end does one study it?' 200 years after the death of this great poet, playwright and philosopher – sometimes called the inventor of German idealism – he is still commemorated and mourned throughout the German-speaking world. In this lecture, Schiller differentiates someone who is merely a professional scholar (*Brotgelehrter*) from the true philosophical mind. While the insights of the former are valuable, these are solely a means of getting rich; gaining attention from the newspapers; securing office, rank, esteem and reputation; and coaxing favours from the nobility. The professional scholar lives from science, not for it. He (or she) lacks dedication. For that person, the development of mental and spiritual attributes and scholarship are the means to an end and not aims in themselves. To Schiller, this type of scholar is immersed in a fortress school system and indifferent to the genuine evolution of knowledge. Constrained from making real progress, understandings offered by the professional scholar soon stagnate, only to become fossilised in dogmatism. Competition evokes fear in the professional scholar and his sterile fiefdom is vigorously defended. Johann Gottlieb Fichte in 1794 and Friedrich Wilhelm Joseph von Schelling in 1799 each drew heavily on Schiller's ideas when themselves referring to the petty individual, the mercenary creature (*Krämerseelen*) who misses the practical usefulness and daily applicability of universal history.[3] Does one sense that, perhaps, Schiller did not altogether hold the professional scholar in high esteem?

Having thus parcelled and reduced the professional scholar, Schiller elevates, and unambiguously admires, the philosophical mind. Here, there is a love of truth more than systems; and the confidence and preparedness to test ideas and be examined are much in evidence. Now the passions are the questions, not the proved and soothed answers. The philosophical mind is open to novelty, longing to search wider horizons; and moved by questions such as: Where are we coming from? Where are we going to? and What purpose does all this serve? Enthusiastically, Friedrich Schiller ends his lecture: 'we have come very far already, and therefore we will be able to go on much farther still'. From this positive and clear understanding of history, Schiller offers his own contribution to the rich legacy of truths, morals and freedoms that make up the imperishable strand fastening our transient participation in the human endeavour. But this clear and bright understanding of history in general is contradicted by Schiller himself in a much less well known piece, written at about the same time. In *Der Geisterseher* (The Ghost Seer)[4] he adopts a much darker, more sceptical and desperate note: only the present exists and the philosophy of history dazzles with the vision of a permanence that can never be sustained:

We are gliding over the ocean of history and forget that we are only a furrow or wrinkle that winds have blown into the surface of the sea. A historical entirety does not exist as an experienced reality but only as a mental construct. We live on the narrow edge of a real presence between the two enormous realities of past and future . . . hanging as dark, impenetrable curtains at each end of one's life. . . . A deep silence reigns behind these covers and no one who ever gets behind them will ever give an answer, the only thing you can hear is a hollow echo of the question as if one had been calling into a vault . . . it is the experience of senselessness. The cover makes a fool of a man who is looking for a secret behind and he can hardly avoid the suspicion that behind it there lies nothing. . . .'[1]

EARLY CASE HISTORIES

Multiple sclerosis is a very conspicuous disease that, when full-blown, has signs that no experienced clinician should fail to recognize. Nevertheless, until the Middle Ages, there are no descriptions in medical texts of any disease that we would recognize and diagnose as MS today. A possible exception to this may be the history of Saint Lidwina von Schiedham (1380–1422), a nun from the Netherlands.[5] Over the course of 37 years, she showed waxing and waning clinical manifestations of symptoms that could be attributed to disorders of various parts of the nervous system. In February 1395 she fell while ice skating and broke several ribs. Over the course of her life several clinical manifestations are described that might be attributed to dysfunctions of the central nervous system: paralysis of both legs and of the right arm and face; blindness with different gradations in both eyes; sensibility disturbances; difficulties in swallowing. It can not be clarified, however, whether these symptoms and signs might not be interpreted as consequences of an abscess in the spinal canal on the one hand and of a hysterical personality trait on the other.[6]

The diary and letters of Augustus Frederick d'Este (1794–1848) (Fig. 1.1), an illegitimate grandson of the English King George III and cousin to Queen Victoria, do provide a record of a case of MS.

In 1822, at the age of 28, he suffered from sudden visual disturbances after having attended the funeral of a close relative: 'Soon after . . . and without anything having been done to my eyes, they completely recovered their strength and distinctness of vision'. Some 5 years later, while in Florence, both his legs became paralyzed: 'I remained in this extreme state of weakness for about 21 days, during which period I fell down about five times (never fainting) from my legs not being strong enough to carry my body.' In the following years he writes of 'very violent pains' and that 'my making water is attended with difficulty'. Then 2 years later: 'while in the act of getting out of bed a considerable portion of stool flowed from me, without my having been made aware of wanting to go to the closed stool'. In a note made in 1830, we can detect a hint of impotence: 'I formed a liaison with a young woman – I find in my acts of connection a deficiency of a wholesome vigour. . . .' Some 13 years later, during which time he had been searching for cures in various

spas and with various physicians, he noticed some sensory disturbances: 'Sitting produces a numbness all down the back part of my thighs and legs, and gives me a curious numb sensation in the lower region of the belly. When standing or walking I cannot keep my balance without a stick.' 3 months after this, he records a feeling of vertigo for the first time: 'For the first time in my life I was attacked by giddiness in the head, sickness, and total abruption of strength in my limbs.' In 1844 Sir Augustus needed a wheelchair, 'with which a "wind cushion", price 10 shillings, was used'. The last entry in his diary was written in 1846, 2 years before his death. His writing is clearly affected by ataxia, the previously fluent, orderly script disintegrating into single letters (Fig. 1.2).

He describes the use of an orthopaedic aid and ends full of hope: 'and I walk without my left foot, which some time ago always turned over outwards at the ankle joint unless supported by a steel upright, showing any disposition so to do. Surely this is a decided improvement! Thanks be to the Almighty!'[7,8]

There can be found in several biographies of poets of that time, for example Heinrich Heine (1797–1856)[9,10] and Eduard Mörike (1804–1875) (HJ Grüsser, personal communication 1987), various signs and symptoms of disease that, in retrospect, might suggest a diagnosis of MS. Despite the paucity of historical examples, however, we may assume that the disease did not exist with the same signs, and certainly not with the same frequency, as it does today.

FIRST DESCRIPTIONS OF MULTIPLE SCLEROSIS

Jean Cruveilhier (1791–1873) (Fig. 1.3A) is usually credited with being the first to have described MS. This assumption (discussed by Compston[11] and de Jong[12]) is based on the first monograph on the disease, which was edited by Charcot's pupil Bourneville in 1869.[13] Cruveilhier was professor of pathological anatomy in Paris and, between the years 1829 and 1842, he published a beautiful atlas with the title *Anatomie pathologique du corps human*.[14] In the second volume there is a description of four disease protocols and an illustration of 'maladies de la moëlle épinière'. The disease is described as 'paraplégie par dégéneration grise des cordons de la moëlle' and Cruveilhier uses expressions such as 'en tâches' and 'en îles' to describe the pathological processes. 'Apart from the scars having encroached, mainly at the cervical enlargement, upon the flanks of the spinal cord, comparable changes extend along the cord's posterior midline. A few smaller scars additionally mark the front of the spinal cord'. In the spinal cord cross-section, the typical wedge shape of lateral and posterior spinal patches is shown (Fig. 1.3B).

Cruveilhier draws attention to the firm consistency of these spots and was not able to compare them to any tissue in the body known to him. In his opinion, this disease was, like rheumatism, the sequel to suppressed sweating.

At about the same time, Robert Carswell (1793–1857) (Fig. 1.4A, B), later to become professor of pathology in London, was working as a student in Paris when he produced nearly 2000 watercolors and drawings of normal and pathological tissues. These later formed the basis of his work *Pathological anatomy: illustrations of elementary forms of disease*, which appeared in 1838.[14a] Carswell describes what we today would call MS as 'a peculiar disease state of the cord and pons Varolii, accompanied by atrophy of the discoloured portions' (Fig. 1.4C). One of his figures mirrors one from Cruveilhier's atlas so closely that it is tempting to assume that both authors had used the same preparation as a model. However, careful research into the years of these publications shows that the relevant figures in Cruveilhi-

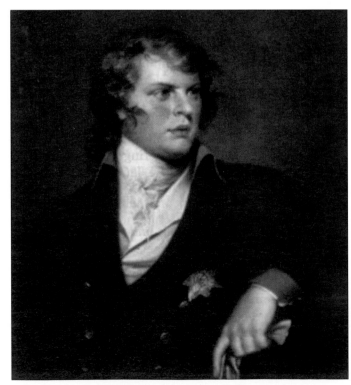

FIG. 1.1 Augustus Frederick d'Esté (1794–1848).

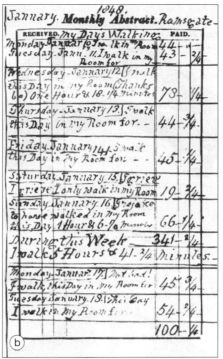

FIG. 1.2 A. The first page of 'The Case of Augustus d'Esté'. **B.** Page from the diary of Augustus d'Esté, showing record of time spent in 'walking' and characteristic alterations in writing after 18 years of disease.

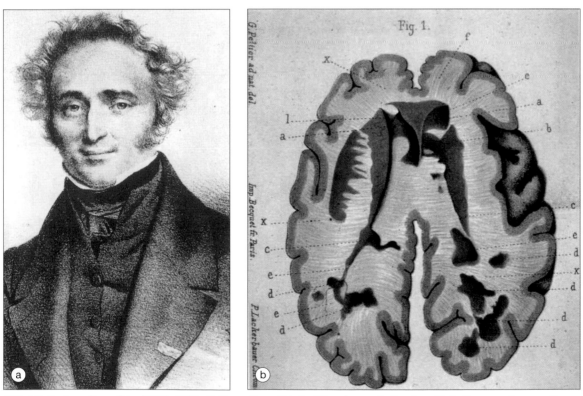

FIG. 1.3 A. Jean Cruveilhier (1791–1874). **B.** From Cruveilhier's *Atlas*, demonstrating beautifully the grey degeneration in the white matter around the ventricles by way of a reddish or grey transformation in the form of 'islands'.

er's atlas, which was produced in 40 'livraisons', cannot have appeared before 1841, whereas Carswell' s work was finished and published in 1838. Thus, the first patient whose disease was diagnosed as MS was French but the lesions that formed the basis of the disease were depicted for the first time by a Scotsman.[15]

It has been debated whether the dispute as to who was the first to describe MS might be resolved by the atlas *The morbid anatomy of the human brain, illustrated by coloured engravings of the most frequent and important organic diseases to which that viscus is subject*, by Robert Hooper (1773–1835), which was published in 1828 in London by Longman, Rees, Orme,

Brown & Green.[16] Hooper was a pathologist and practicing physician in London and he based his atlas on his experiences, gained over 30 years, of more than 4000 autopsies that he performed at the St Mary-le-bone Infirmary.[17] He describes:

Diseased structures, and unnatural appearances without tumefaction: Morbid firmness, hardness, or induration . . . is not uncommon in the substance of the brain. . . . It is mostly accompanied by a dark hue. . . . With this preternaturally great cohesion of its particles, the brain feels not merely firm, but morbidly hard, and the cut surface does not show the natural number of blood vessels in the medullary substance, nor does it receive the impression of the finger readily: and when the finger is removed, it quickly rises to its level. . . .

and later: 'The delicate colour of the medullary substance frequently undergoes a change. I have seen it of palestone or albine colour . . .'. Certainty as to a firm diagnosis is always difficult in retrospect, however, and this description by Hooper does not firmly enough establish his cases as MS in order to be recognized as the first description of the disease.

The same is probably true of an interesting description by Karl Marx (not the philosopher!) that has been proposed as to being an early description of MS (Fig. 1.5):[18] A 45-year-old noble woman (*Aegra femina nobilis MDCCCXXIV erat agens annum quadragesimum quantum*) with spasms in the lower limbs (*Extremitates inferiores saepe spasmis contractae*); not able to sit (*sedere non poterat*); with ascending paralysis (*paralyseos ascension*) with sensory disturbances and pain in the lower limbs and face (*In cruribus sensum percipiebat similem gustui menthae piperitae; doloribus in plantis pedum; dolori faciali*); paralysis of the right hand, forcing her to write with the left hand (*Praesertim in dextro debilitatem, sinistra manu scribere instituit*); psychologically completely unaffected (*Animus ipse ab omni turbatione liberrimus constitit (illibato ingenio, acri iudicio, fida memoria)*); visited all the German spas, including the one in Eilsen (*1826/7 ad itinera per quasidam Germaniae regiones facienda et aquis salubribus in vico Eilsen*); no remedies were really helpful (*Nullum autem remedium tam praesens certumque auxilium attulit*); died peacefully after seven years of illness in 1830 (*Viribus tenerae vitae consumtis anno MDCCCXXX post septem morbi graves annos placide animam expiravit, dormienti similis*). Describing the pathological anatomy findings after this patient had died, Marx was convinced that some pressure was exerted over the lower part of the spinal cord (*Pressionem aliquam ad*

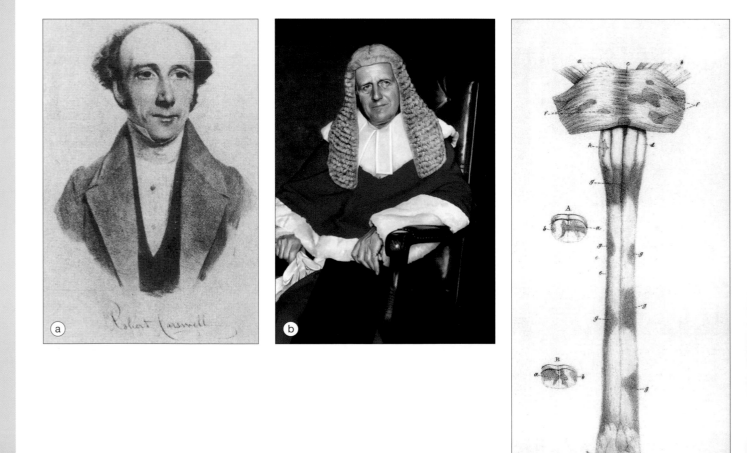

FIG. 1.4 A, **B**. Robert Carswell (1793–1857). **C**. Carswell's *Pathological anatomy: illustrations on elementary forms of disease*, Longman: London, 1838 – plate, 'a peculiar disease state of the cord and Pons Varolii, accompanied by atrophy of the discoloured portions.

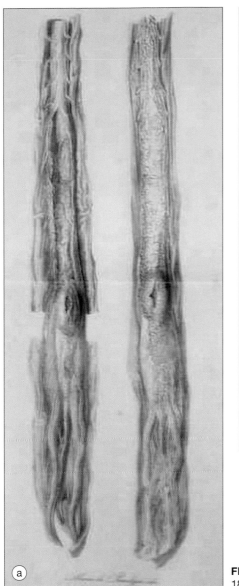

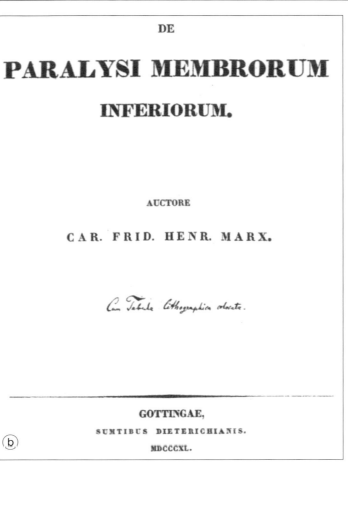

DE

PARALYSI MEMBRORUM

INFERIORUM.

AUCTORE

C A R. F R I D. H E N R. M A R X.

Cum Tabula lithographica colorata.

GOTTINGAE,

SUMTIBUS DIETERICHIANIS.

MDCCCXL.

FIG. 1.5 Figure (**A**) and title page (**B**) from Marx CFH. *On paralysis of the lower limbs*, Göttingen, 1840.

inferiorem medullae spinalis partem adesse extra omne mihi dubium est); There was some vascular congestion (*Piae matris vasa sanguine tumebant. Medullae vasa numerosa . . . redundabant*); the white and grey matter were partly indistinguishable (*Substantia alba et grisea nullo modo inter se distingui et internosci poterant . . . in unum confluxit*); in the spinal cord itself there was reddishness and there were indurations (*In medulla ipsa, totum spinae canalem implente ideoque amplificata . . . conspicui erant rubicundiores et reliquia massa duriores . . . inspissationem et indurationem substantiae*). This is not a proven case of MS but rather a chronic inflammation of the spinal cord.[19]

The first clinical descriptions of MS were by Frerichs in Göttingen, Germany,[20] and appeared in the middle of the 19th century (Fig. 1.6). Frerichs's clinical reports mention for the first time transient remissions as a characteristic feature of MS; he describes nystagmus in detail and provides the first medical description of mental disturbances in MS ('*Psychische Störungen höheren Grades . . . fast regelmässig*').

Frerichs's clinical diagnosis of '*Hirnsclerose*' was challenged until, in 1856, his pupil Valentiner reported pathological findings from patients who had died and pronounced his master's clinical diagnosis to be 'so brilliantly confirmed by postmortem examination'. Treatment was very limited at his time: 'Without sanguine hope of success he ordered the use of iodine potassium'.

Rindfleisch (Fig. 1.7), in Zurich in 1863, first identified the pathological changes of the blood vessels: 'their wall is enormously thickened by the aggregation of nuclei and cells in the adventitia'.[20a] He considered 'often recurring or persistent irritations of the entire central organs' to be primary events and changes in the parenchyma to be secondary phenomena: 'The neuroglia undergoes a series of metamorphoses in continuation of the formative irritations from the vessel walls to the neighbourhood. This process carries throughout the mark of scantiness.' Rindfleisch draw the conclusion that *ein elementarer Entzündungzustand* ('an elementary inflammatory reaction') was responsible for demyelination.[20a]

A vascular theory of MS was adhered to for several decades.[21] It was based on the observation that plaques develop mainly in the neighbourhood of small veins in which, from time to time, organized thrombi can be found. This theory led to several

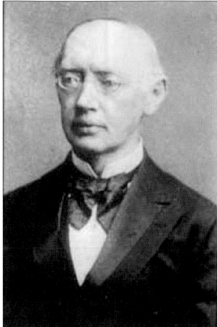

FIG. 1.6 Friedrich von Frerichs (1819–1885).

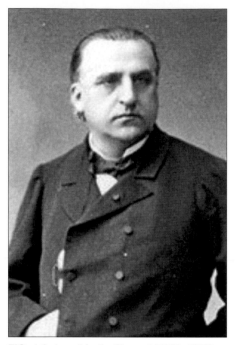

FIG. 1.8 Jean-Martin Charcot (1825–1893).

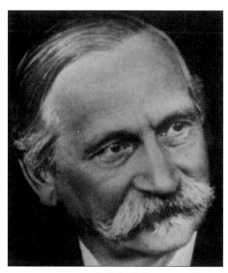

FIG. 1.7 Eduard Rindfleisch (1836–1908).

therapeutic trials with vasoactive substances and anticoagulants, but without success.

In 1863 Leyden[22] summarized the state of knowledge related to MS of that time as follows:

- Women are affected much more often than men (25 : 1)
- The onset of the disease is usually between the 20th and 25th year
- There had been only a single hereditary case
- There are two main etiological factors: exposure to cold and wet, and trauma
- Psychological events are important in triggering the disease.

Jean Marie Charcot (1825–1893) (Fig. 1.8) gave the first comprehensive description of MS, describing its clinical peculiarities in his famous lectures at the Salpêtrière in Paris.[23–25] He distinguished myatrophic lateral sclerosis from MS and evaluated tremor not as a disease but as a symptom. He clearly distinguished intention tremor from tremor with Parkinson's disease. The classical symptom triad of nystagmus, intention tremor and scanning speech that is named after him was not considered important by Charcot himself, and he stressed repeatedly that the lack of one, or even of all three, of these symptoms could not preclude the diagnosis. He also drew attention to benign cases of the disease.[26] As a successor to Vulpian in the chair of pathology, and possibly in collaboration with him, he elaborated the histology of MS and produced drawings of myelin loss and preservation of axon cylinders, proliferation of glia, and perivascular phagocytes containing fatty deposits[27] (Fig. 1.9). He gave the first comprehensive histological description of MS lesions with destruction of myelin and accumulation of nuclei.

ETIOLOGICAL THEORIES

Charcot maintained that the cause of the disease was unknown. He assumed it to have some connection with acute infection and described cases in which it had been preceded by infections such as typhus, smallpox or cholera. He also mentioned an association with exposure to cold and with emotional factors such as shock or trauma, and speculated that grief, vexation and adverse changes in social circumstances were related to the onset of MS.

Babinski demonstrated in his doctoral thesis all-important elements of the histological features of MS that were known in his time (Fig. 1.10).[27a]

In 1906, Marburg described an acute form of MS that is still named after him. He postulated a myelinolytic toxin as a causal factor. This toxin theory was supported for

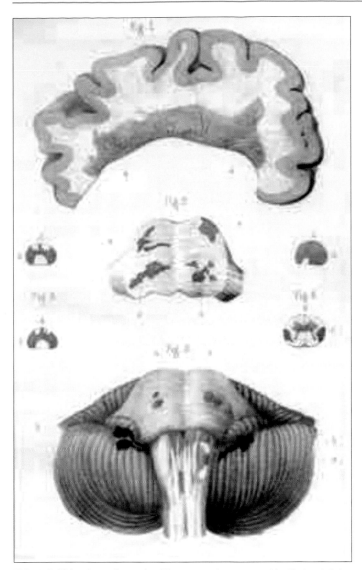

FIG. 1.9 This plate, drawn by Charcot and presented in Ordenstein's 1867 Parisian thesis, was the first to display specific ventricle-based lesion expansions into the cerebral hemispheres. It forms the earliest and still unmatched synopsis of the specific postmortem findings of multiple sclerosis of brain and spinal cord.

several decades and received particular attention in the work of Baasch,[28] who thought the disease was caused by chronic mercury intoxication from amalgam fillings in the teeth. Despite his elegant arguments (which led to the removing of thousands of amalgam-filled teeth), his conclusions were not confirmed.

The theory that MS is an infectious disease has had its supporters for more than a century, since Charcot and Pierre Marie[29] (Fig. 1.11).[30]

In his lectures on the diseases of the spinal cord (*Leçons sur les maladies de la moëlle*) Pierre Marie clearly stated that 'the irritating agent in the blood vessels is of an infectious nature' and that 'the time of its isolation will come beyond any doubt' (*'l'agent irritant circulant dans les vaisseaux est, avons-nous dit, manifestement de nature infectieuse. Quel est-il au juste? Nul jusqu'ici n'a pu l'isoler, mais cela viendra, n'en doutez pas'*) and he strikes a note of caution regarding the

therapies available and advises his listeners and readers to retain their doubts in this regard (*'D'après ce que Vous connaissez, Messieurs, de la nature et des lesions de cette affection, vous devez éprouver quelque doutes sur l'efficacité des agents thérapeutiques dont nous disposons actuellement. Ces doutes, conservez-les précieusement'*).

In the 1930s, the theory of MS as an infectious disease gained new impetus following the observation that the histological picture of perivenous demyelination in postinfectious and post-vaccination encephalomyelitis could not be distinguished from that seen in MS.[31] On many occasions, specific organisms were isolated and considered as etiological factors. The search for viruses that could be responsible for MS is always accompanied by the same hope and confidence that, in the case of poliomyelitis, were rewarded by vaccination against poliomyelitis viruses. Various viral diseases in humans and animals may lead to changes in the central nervous system (CNS) that, histologically and otherwise, resemble MS. In viral disease, there may be focal inflammation as well as primary demyelination. The recognition of virus persistence in the CNS gave an important impetus to the search for a viral etiology for MS. Several chronic CNS diseases in animals (visna, scrapie, mink encephalopathy) and in humans (Creutzfeldt–Jakob disease, kuru) may be associated with transmissible agents. However, conventional viruses such as measles are also able to persist within the CNS under certain immunological conditions, such as in the case of subacute sclerosing panencephalitis. Since the early 1960s, the measles virus has often been implicated in MS,[32] following the discovery on several occasions of elevated antibody titers against measles in some MS patients and the detection of the measles viral genome in the brains of some people suffering from this disease.[33,34] The fact that positive findings have not been found in all brains and body fluids examined does not exclude the possibility of an etiological connection. However, in the case of the measles hypothesis, definitive proof up until now is still lacking. If there were a causal relationship, vaccination against measles, which has been practiced for over 20 years in the USA, should lead to a significant reduction in the incidence of MS in the near future. An association between MS and other viruses, such as rabies, parainfluenza, cytomegalovirus, corona, herpes simplex, etc., has been suggested on several occasions. Some of these have been dismissed as artifacts or laboratory infections, and further extensive research has failed to prove any connection with others.

A relationship between MS and particular forms of spirochete (*Spirochaeta myelophthora*), which was postulated by Gabriel Steiner during more than 50 years of scientific work,[35] could not be proved in numerous other studies. Similarly, a prematurely postulated causal relationship between MS and viruses of the group to which the human immunodeficiency virus (HIV) belongs[36] was refuted in numerous controlled studies.

The observation of perivenous infiltrates of lymphocytes stimulated great interest in the autoimmune theory of MS. It was possible in animal experiments to induce autoimmune disease following sensitization to myelin basic protein[37] – the so-called experimental allergic (autoimmune) encephalomyelitis, which, in several respects, is similar to MS. Interest in this animal model has continued and has been stimulated by numerous further experiments.

Over the last century, interest in the various theories concerning the etiology of the disease has waxed and waned in a way that is reminiscent of the courses of the clinical signs of the disease. It is interesting to read the old literature and to compare what was understood about MS with the state of our knowledge today. Various conference volumes and review

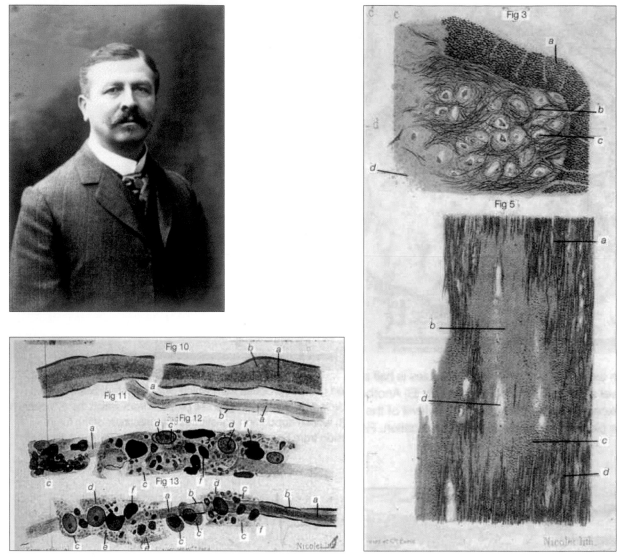

FIG. 1.10 Babinski JM. Recherche sur l'anatomie pathologique de la sclérose en plaque et etude comparative des divers variétés de seclérose de la moëlle. *Archives de physiologie normale et pathologique* 1885; 2: 186–207.

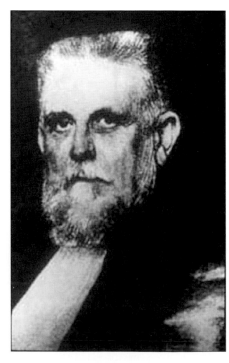

FIG. 1.11 Pierre Marie (1853–1940).

articles made history when they were published and have been consulted by thousands of researchers over the years. They form the landmarks from which an overview may be gained of research past and present, and they contain many discussions that are worth reading, for example: the *Research Publications of the Association for Research in Nervous and Mental Diseases*, Volume 2 (1921) and Volume 28 (1950); *Annals of the New York Academy of Sciences*, Volume 122 (1965) and Volume 436 (1984); *Handbook of Clinical Neurology*, Volume 9 (1970) and Volume 47 (1986). Most recent and most comprehensive texts on the history of MS are Jock Murray's 600-page volume[6] and Alastair Compston's unsurpassed introductory chapter 'The story of multiple sclerosis' to the 4th edition of *McAlpine's Multiple Sclerosis*.[11]

REFERENCES

1. Kesselring J. The history of multiple sclerosis. Oral communication at the 7th State of the Art Meeting MS of the Swiss Multiple Sclerosis Society, Lucerne, January 2005.
2. Schiller F. Was heisst und zu welchem Ende studiert man Universalgeschichte? Eine akademische Antrittsrede. In: Friedrich Schiller: Sämtliche Werke. Vierter Band. Historische Schriften. Wissenschaftliche Buchgesellschaft Darmstadt; 1989a: 749–767.
3. Safranski R. Friedrich Schiller oder die Erfindung des Deutschen Idealismus. Wissenschaftliche Buchgesellschaft Darmstadt; 2005: 312.
4. Schiller F. Der Geisterseher. Aus den Memoiren des Grafen von O**. In: Friedrich Schiller: Sämtliche Werke. Fünfter Band. Erzählungen/Theoretische Schriften. Wissenschaftliche Buchgesellschaft Darmstadt; 1989b: 48–182.
5. Medaer R. Does the history of multiple sclerosis go back as far as the 14th century? Acta Neurol Scand 1979; 60: 189–192.
6. Murray TJ. Multiple Sclerosis: The history of the disease. New York: Demos; 2005.
7. Firth D. The case of Augustus d'Este. At the University Press, Cambridge 1948.
8. McDonald WI. Doyne lecture: The significance of optic neuritis. Trans ophthal Soc UK 1983; 103: 230–246.
9. Jellinek EH. Heine's illness: the case for multiple sclerosis. J R Soc Med 1990; 83: 516–519.
10. Stenager E. The course of Heinrich Heine's illness: diagnostic considerations. J Med Biogr 1996; 5: 197–199.
11. Compston A. The story of Multiple Sclerosis. In: Compston A, ed. McAlpine's multiple sclerosis, 4th ed. Edinburgh: Churchill Livingstone; 2005: 1–68.
12. De Jong RN. Multiple sclerosis. History, definition and general considerations. In: Vinken PJ, Bruyn GW (eds): Multiple sclerosis and other demyelinating diseases. Handbook of Clinical Neurology, Vol. 9. Amsterdam: North Holland; 1970: 45–62.
13. Bourneville DM, Guérard I. De la sclérose en plaques disséminées. Paris: A. Delahaye; 1869.
14. Cruveilhier J. Anatomie pathologique du corps humam. Paris: J. B. Bailliére; 1829–1842.
14a. Carswell R. Pathological anatomy: illustrations on elementary forms of disease. London: Longman; 1838.
15. Compston A. The 150th anniversary of the depiction of the lesions of multiple sclerosis. J Neurol Neurosurg Psychiat 1988; 51: 1249–1252.
16. Hooper R. The morbid anatomy of the human brain, illustrated by colored engravings of the most frequent and important organic diseases to which that viscus is subject. London: Longman, Orme, Brown & Green; 1828.
17. McHenry LC. Garrinson's History of Neurology. Charles C Thomas Publisher; 1969.
18. Keppel Hesselink JM. Een monografie van K.F.H. Marx uit 1838; mogelijk de eerste klinisch-pathologische beschrijving van multipele sclerose. Ned Tijdschr Geneeskd 1991; 135(51): 2439–43. (A monograph by Karl Friedrich Heinrich Marx from 1838; possibly the first clinicopathological description of multiple sclerosis).
19. Kesselring J. What means, and to what end does one study history? Multiple sclerosis: the history of a disease. By T. Jock Murray 2005. New York: Demos. Brain 2005; 128: 1466–1468 [Book review].
20. Frerichs FT. Über Hirnsklerose. Arch Ges Med 1849; 10: 334–337.
20a. Rindfleisch E. Histologisches Detail zu der grauen Degeneration von Gehirn und Rückenmark. Arch Pathol Anat Physiol 1863; 26: 474–483.
21. Putnam TJ. The pathogenesis of multiple sclerosis: a possible vascular factor. N Engl J Med 1993; 209: 786–790.
22. Leyden E. Über graue Degeneration des Rückenmarks. Dtsch Klin 1863; 15: 121–128.
23. Charcot JM. Lessons sur les maladies du Système nerveux faites à la Salpêtrière. A. Delahaye, Paris (1872–1873).
24. McDonald WI. The dynamics of multiple sclerosis. The Charcot lecture. J Neurol 1993; 240: 28–36.
25. McDonald I. Multiple sclerosis in its European matrix. Mult Scler 2002; 8(3): 181–191.
26. Charcot JM. Diagnostic des formes frustes de la sclérose en plaques. Progr Méd 1879; 7: 97–99.
27. Charcot JM. Histologie de la sclérose en plaques. Gaz Hôp 1868; 41: 554–555, 557–558, 566.
27a. Babinski JM. Recherche sur l'anatomie pathologique de la sclérose en plaque et étude comparative des divers variétés de sclérose de la moëlle. Archives de physiologie normale et pathologique 1885; 2: 186–207.
28. Baasch E. Theoretische Überlegungen zur Aetiologie der Sclerosis multiplex. Schweiz Arch Neurol Neurochir Psychiat 1966; 98: 1–19.
29. Marie P. Leçons sur les maladies de la moëlle. Paris G Masson, Editeur 1892.
30. Larner AJ. Aetiological role of viruses in multiple sclerosis: a review. J R Soc Med 1986; 79: 412–417.
31. Brain WR. Critical review: disseminated sclerosis. Quart J Med 1930; 23: 343–391.
32. Adams JM, Imagawa DT. Measles antibody in multiple sclerosis. Proc Soc exp Biol 1962; 111: 562–566.
33. Haase AT, Ventura P, Gibbs CJ, Tourtellotte WW. Measles virus nucleotide sequences: detection by hybridization in situ. Science 1981; 212: 672–675.
34. Haase AT, Pagano J, Waksman BH, Nathanson N. Detection of viral genes and their products in chronic neurologic diseases. Ann Neurol 1984; 15: 119–121.
35. Steiner G. Regionale Verteilung der Entmarkungsherde in ihrer Bedeutung für die Pathogenese der multiplen Sklerose. In: Krankheitserreger und Gewebsbefund bei Multipler Sklerose. Berlin: Springer-Verlag; 1931: 108–120.
36. Koprowski H, Defreitas EC, Harper ME, Sandberg-Wollheim M, Sheremata WA, Robert-Guroff M, Saxinger CW, Feinberg MB, Wong-Staal F, Gallo RC. Multiple sclerosis and human T-cell lymphotropic viruses. Nature 1985; 318: 154–160.
37. Rivers TM, Sprunt DH, Berry GP. Observations on attempts to produce acute disseminated encephalomyelitis in monkeys. J Exp Med 1933; 58: 39–53.

Clinical features in multiple sclerosis

H. El-Moslimany and F. D. Lublin

INTRODUCTION

Despite the advent of magnetic resonance imaging (MRI), the use of evoked potentials and cerebrospinal fluid (CSF) studies that can be suggestive of the disease, multiple sclerosis (MS) remains a clinical diagnosis in the absence of a definitive diagnostic test.[1] An issue, as you will read in the rest of the chapter, is that multiple neurological symptoms and signs can be seen in both MS and other disorders. Some of these symptoms and signs can be very unusual and are atypical of MS. The myriad number of symptoms and signs are due to the location of damage in the brain, optic nerves and spinal cord resulting from the pathological process of MS, which includes inflammatory demyelination, axonal loss and gliosis.[2]

Prior to the advent of disease-modifying therapy, diagnosis of MS was not as crucial as it is today. As the CHAMPS and ETOMS study have illustrated, treatment with an interferon can delay the occurrence of a second relapse of a neurological deficit in a patient with a history of a clinically isolated syndrome, thereby delaying the official diagnosis of MS.[3,4] Therefore, prompt diagnosis of a demyelinating disease that is either MS or could possibly become MS, and initiation of therapy may improve the patient's quality of life by limiting the number of relapses and delaying the onset of more severe disease.

CLINICAL COURSE OF MULTIPLE SCLEROSIS

Multiple sclerosis has several forms of presentation, including episodic acute periods of worsening (the most common, initially), gradual progressive deterioration of neurologic function or combinations of both.[5] These different presentations have been given standardized names, which are relapsing–remitting, secondary progressive, primary progressive, and progressive relapsing.[5] These terms describe the clinical phenotype of the disease. Unfortunately, we do not yet have reliable biomarkers, either laboratory or imaging, that predict the clinical course. Further, the clinical course for any given individual is rather unpredictable, although group predictive elements exist. The different types of presentation are important to ascertain, because treatment options differ between the different types. While the interferons, glatiramer acetate, mitoxantrone and natalizumab are available for relapsing forms of MS, there is nothing that is proven to be efficacious in the primary progressive form of the illness.[6–10]

Relapsing–remitting MS is defined as clearly defined disease relapses with either full recovery or sequelae and residual deficit upon recovery; periods between disease relapses are characterized by a lack of disease progression.[5] Primary progressive MS is a gradual, nearly continuously worsening baseline (progressive from onset) with minor fluctuations but no distinct relapses.[5] Secondary progressive MS is an initial relapsing–remitting disease course followed by progression with or without occasional relapses, minor remissions and/or plateaus.[5] While most patients begin with relapsing–remitting MS, many patients switch to secondary progressive MS when they begin to progressively worsen between relapses.[5] Progressive–relapsing MS is the disease course in which there is progressive disease from onset, with distinct acute relapses occurring later in the disease, with or without full recovery. The periods between relapses are characterized by continuing progression[5] (Figs 2.1–2.4).

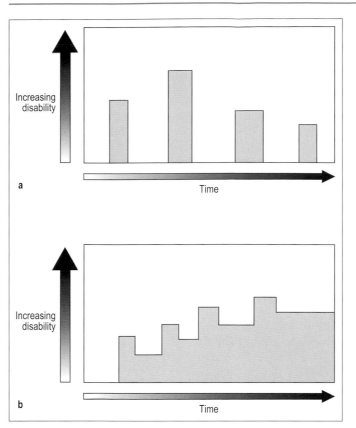

FIG. 2.1 Relapsing–remitting MS is characterized by clearly defined acute attacks with full recovery (A) or with sequelae and residual deficit upon recovery (B). Periods between disease relapses are characterized by lack of disease progression. Redrawn from Lublin and Reingold 1996.[5]

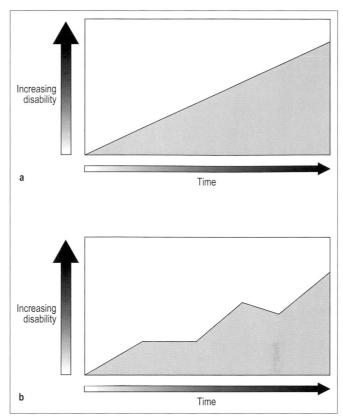

FIG. 2.2 Primary progressive MS is characterized by disease showing progression of disability from onset, without plateaus or remissions (A) or with occasional plateaus and temporary minor improvements (B). Redrawn from Lublin and Reingold 1996.[5]

Approximately 85% of patients start out with relapsing–remitting MS.[11] A relapse occurs when symptoms of neurological deficit develop in an acute or subacute manner.[2] As per the McDonald diagnostic criteria, an attack is an episode of neurological disturbance of the kind seen in MS, lasting for at least 24 hours and not associated with a fever or infection.[12] A repeat relapse has to occur at least 30 days after the initial relapse to be considered a separate event.[12] For a relapse to be considered a true event, it should not be a recurrence of old symptoms associated with an accompanying metabolic or toxic change, which resolve upon correction of the aggravating metabolic alteration.[2] In the case of elevated temperature, there is a reversible conduction alteration that causes a temporary recurrence of old symptoms, or the development of new symptoms, from lesions that were subclinical.[2] Relapses are unpredictable in frequency and in the length of time between relapses.[2] Also unpredictable is the extent of recovery after a specific exacerbation. A meta-analysis of several clinical trials studying MS demonstrates that residual deficit from exacerbations occurs after approximately 50% of attacks, leading to stepwise accrual of disability.[13] Possible precipitating factors for relapses in MS include the postpartum period and viral infections.[14–16] Sibley's and Poser's retrospective studies on the increased relapse rate in the postpartum period were corroborated by prospective studies.[17,18] In the more recent prospective study, which followed 254 MS patients, the postpartum exacerbation rate was 1.2 ± 0.2, compared to 0.7 ± 0.9 which was the exacerbation rate prior to pregnancy.[17] Sibley's retrospective study on the risk of relapses from a viral infection was corroborated by a

prospective study done by Sibley 20 years after the first study.[18] In this study, 9% of infections were temporally related to exacerbations.[18] Some 27% of exacerbations were related to infections.[18]

About 30% of patients have secondary progressive disease.[11] Natural history studies have indicated that at least 50% of patients with relapsing–remitting disease will transition to secondary progressive disease.[11] The burden of disease gets progressively worse as time goes on, possibly because of axonal loss.[11] The less common form of progressive disease is primary progressive MS, which accounts for about 10% of patients. The patients tend to be older and often present with spinal cord dysfunction without as much brain involvement.[11] The least common form of MS is progressive relapsing disease, which accounts for only 5% of the MS population.[11] These patients are similar to either primary progressive patients or secondary progressive patients.[11,20]

As mentioned above, diagnosis is crucial because of the availability of disease-modifying agents in the prevention of relapses, which may be beneficial in delaying the severity of disease in patients treated early. Accurate diagnosis is essential, because treatable disorders should be discovered and treated, and patients who don't have MS should not be treated with an annoying therapy for a disease that they do not have.

Many different signs and symptoms can be seen in the course of the disease; however, some of the signs and symptoms occur more frequently in patients with MS compared to others. The following pages list the signs and symptoms seen in MS, from most frequently encountered to least (Table 2.1).

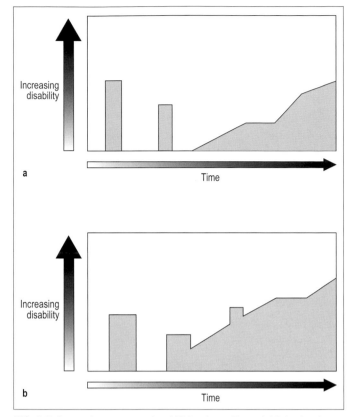

FIG. 2.3 Secondary progressive MS begins with an initial relapsing–remitting course, followed by progression of variable rate (**A**), which may also include occasional relapses and minor remissions (**B**). Redrawn from Lublin and Reingold 1996.[5]

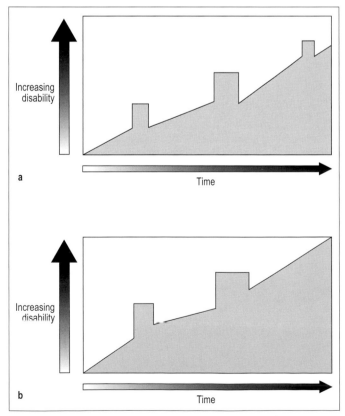

FIG. 2.4 Progressive–relapsing MS shows progression from onset but with clear acute relapses with (**A**) or without (**B**) full recovery. Redrawn from Lublin and Reingold 1996.[5]

SENSORY SYMPTOMS

The most common sensory symptom, initially, is the onset of numbness and paresthesias in one or more limbs.[1] Usually, the patient will have acute onset of distal limb paresthesias, which travel proximally, increasing in intensity, perhaps even involving other limbs.[1] The sensory symptoms can be due to a myelopathy, which can produce a spinal sensory level. The sensory symptoms can also be in a hemibody distribution, either involving or not involving the face, resulting from one or more brain lesions. A crossed face–body hemisensory deficit would place the lesion in the brainstem. Patients may also have radicular symptoms due to a lesion at the dorsal root entry zone of the spinal cord or the brainstem.[1] The sensory symptoms may be numbness, paresthesias, dysesthesias, itching or pain. The loss of sensation can be quite disabling. With the loss of proprioception and two-point discrimination, the patient's hand can be functionally impaired. Without proprioception and sensory feedback of movement, the patient's limb is essentially useless. This is usually due to a lesion in the dorsal root entry zone, posterior column or medial lemniscus, in either the high cervical or brainstem areas.[1] This phenomenon is seen more in hands than legs but when present in the lower extremities can make walking extremely difficult.

MOTOR SYMPTOMS

Weakness can occur in any extremity, singly or in combination.[1] The weakness is usually pyramidal in distribution.[2] The most dramatic of the acute motor syndromes is an acute transverse myelitis.[1] Damage to descending motor pathways causes weakness.[20] While myelitis is a common manifestation of MS, a complete acute transverse myelitis is not a common presenting symptom.[1,22]

Slowly progressive weakness of the lower extremities can be seen in MS as a chronic progressive myelopathy.[1] One does need to rule out spinal cord and dural arteriovenous malformations, herniated thoracic disks, intramedullary tumors, Arnold–Chiari malformations and syringomyelia.[23] Tropic spastic paraparesis is another possibility that needs to be ruled out, as well as other infections (such as Lyme disease, tuberculosis, syphilis), rheumatological etiologies, toxic agents, vitamin deficiencies (B_{12}), traumatic lesions, paraneoplastic causes (anti Hu) and electrical injury.[24–27]

While uncommon, patients with MS can present with a motor radiculopathy.[28] Lower motor neuron facial palsy was recognized as a presenting symptom in MS in the early part of the 20th century.[29] The patients do recover, but the disability can recur.[30]

SPASTICITY

Spasticity is a common complication in MS and can be potentially disabling.[31–33] It can consist of spasms or constant stiffness.[34] The spasms are a particular problem overnight, disturbing sleep and contributing to fatigue.[34] Spasms can either be extensor or flexor. In extensor spasm there is exaggeration of extensor tone, which can cause forceful activation of leg muscles inducing plantar flexion of the ankle, together with hip and knee joint extension.[21] The spasms can be so severe so as to eject a seated patient from a chair.[21] With flexor spasms, there is a generalized flexion of muscles at the ankle, knee and hip, giving rise to limb withdrawal and retraction.[21] Spasms are a problem for maintenance of posture, interference in ambulation and, in bedridden patients, interfering with hygiene and nursing care.[34] However, spasticity can aid in walking, standing and transferring.[34] This dichotomy makes it difficult to treat patients with antispasticity

TABLE 2.1 Symptoms and signs throughout the course of the illness

Symptom/sign	%	Symptom/sign	%
Sensory loss	90	Depression	25–54
Leg weakness	90	Decreased sensation	25
Spasticity	90	Arm weakness	22
Nystagmus	85	Decreased vaginal lubrication	21
Sensory level (posterior column of lower limbs)	85	Retinal perivenous sheathing	20
Bladder frequency	80	Titubation	20
Bladder urgency	80	Paroxysmal sensory	20
Nocturia	80	Diffuse pain	20
Fatigue	80	Paroxysmal motor	15
Retinal nerve fiber loss	80	Bipolar disorder	13–40
Optic atrophy	77	Euphoria	10–60
Cognitive changes	70	Trigeminal neuralgia	10–30
Constipation	70	Trigeminal sensory decrease	10
Optic neuritis	65	Sensory level (pain and temp)	10
Erectile dysfunction	63	Action tremor	10
Mixed urgency and retention	60	VIth nerve palsy	10
Ataxia of gait and trunk	50–80	Dysphagia	10
Incontinence	50	Radicular pain	10
Spasms	50	Hemiplegia	9
Cramps	50	Deafness	5–17
Dysarthria	50	Vertigo	5–50
Intention tremor	50	Useless hand syndrome	5
Amyotrophy	50	Seizures	5
Decreased libido	40	Primary position nystagmus	5
Pain	40	Facial palsy	4–16
Ejaculatory dysfunction	37	Paroxysmal dysarthria	<5
Headache	30	Hypothermia	Rare
Sensory level (posterior columns upper limbs)	30	Peripheral neuropathy	Rare
Sensory level (pain and temp lower limbs)	30	IIIrd nerve palsy	Rare
Lhermitte's phenomenon	30	IVth nerve palsy	Rare
Internuclear ophthalmoplegia	30	Parinaud's phenomenon	Rare

Adapted from Paty DW, Hashimoto SA, Ebers GC. Management of multiple sclerosis and interpretation of clinical trials. In: Paty D, Ebers G, eds. Multiple sclerosis. Philadelphia, PA: FA Davis; 1998: 427–519; Poser S. Multiple sclerosis: an analysis of 812 cases by means of electronic data processing. New York: Springer; 1978; and Studney D, Lublin F, Marcucci L et al. MS COSTAR: a computerized record for use in clinical research in multiple sclerosis. J Neurol Rehab 1993; 7: 145–152.

drugs, for an overdose of antispasticity medications in this case is a dose that can unmask or even increase weakness.[34]

Spasticity is a form of hypertonia due to a velocity-dependent increase in tonic stretch reflexes, which results from abnormal spinal processing of proprioceptive input.[35] In a patient with spasticity, there is a considerable amount of muscle activity with stretch with a fairly good linear relationship. It is mediated by Ia afferents in the muscle spindle. Passive stretch of the muscle excites the muscle spindle, sending sensory input back to the spinal cord through largely monosynaptic but also oligo and polysynaptic reflexes, which in turn send an efferent impulse to the muscle, causing it to contract.[35]

In MS, spasticity occurs as a result of a demyelinating lesion in the upper motor pathways, which travel closely with pyramidal fibers. The demyelinating lesion enhances the reflex within the spinal cord, causing increased excitability within the spinal

fibers, resulting in a greater muscle contraction than is normally experienced.[35] In a study of MS patients enrolled in the NARCOMS patient registry, Rizzo et al found that 84% of the patients in the registry had spasticity.[33] They found that patients with more severe spasticity were more likely to be male, disabled, unemployed, with a longer duration of disease, more relapses and worsening MS symptoms in the time leading up to the study.[33] Patients with more severe spasticity tended to have secondary progressive MS, and tended to have poorer quality of life scores.[33]

BLADDER AND SEXUAL FUNCTION

Brain and spinal cord lesions caused by MS can produce bladder dysfunction, through detrusor hyperreflexia, detrusor–sphincter dyssynergia or detrusor areflexia.[36–38] The most common cystometric finding in MS patients is detrusor overactivity.[39] This produces the sensation of urgency despite low bladder volume.[38] Urge incontinence occurs if high intravesical pressures result in the loss of some urine.[39] In two studies evaluating bladder symptoms in patients with MS, more than 70% of the female patients had complaints of incontinence or urgency.[40,41]

Detrusor-sphincter dyssynergia is characterized by contraction of the internal urethral sphincter during an involuntary detrusor contraction.[39] This is due to the loss of synchronization between the detrusor and the internal urethral sphincter.[39] In this case, patients could have an interrupted urinary flow, as well as incomplete bladder emptying and hesitancy.[39]

Urinary tract infections are common in MS, particularly in patients with high residual bladder volumes.[34] One always needs to be on the alert for urinary tract infections, because they could present with low-grade fever and fatigue without any urological symptoms.[34] Any obstacle to urine flow needs to be removed.[34] Another issue with urinary tract infections is that their presence can cause neurological symptoms to appear or get worse in an MS patient.

There is a correlation between bladder and sexual dysfunction in MS.[39,41,42] The sexual response is under the control of nerves from the S2, S3 and S4 spinal levels, while detrusor overactivity is due to suprasacral lesions.[39] Male patients with MS can have erectile dysfunction, ejaculatory disorders and difficulty reaching orgasm, which can be compounded by reduced sensation and fatigue.[39] Erectile dysfunction often follows the development of urinary symptoms.[43] Depression, fatigue, anxiety and drug effects also contribute considerably to sexual dysfunction.[34] Female patients complain of decreased sexual desire, diminished vaginal lubrication, vaginal spasms and diminished orgasmic capacity.[44–46] Female patients' sexual function is affected by abnormal genital sensation, pelvic floor muscle weakness, fatigue, muscle spasms and loss of coordination, as well as depression and high levels of disability.[41,46,47] Psychological issues are another issue in terms of impact on sexual function. Patients who have a negative self-image and less confidence about their sexuality can have potential for sexual dysfunction.[48] Despite this, the majority of patients in one study were sexually active, were capable of feeling arousal, experienced orgasm and enjoyed sexual activities.[41]

FATIGUE

Multiple studies indicate that more than half of patients with MS suffer from fatigue.[49–55] Females are more likely to report fatigue than males.[56–58] Level of fatigue can be measured using the Fatigue Severity Scale.[53]

Fatigue is difficult to define but it is considered to be a subjective experience or feeling.[59] A common definition is that fatigue is a 'sense of physical tiredness and lack of energy, distinct from sadness or weakness'.[49] There is no statistically significant correlation between age and fatigue.[60–62] There are conflicting studies about the relationship between disease course and fatigue among patients with MS; however most studies have found that individuals with primary progressive and secondary progressive MS report higher levels of fatigue than patients with relapsing–remitting MS.[51,63–68] There is no correlation found between fatigue and disease activity seen on MRI, but disease activity assessed by functional MRI did correlate with fatigue measured by the Fatigue Severity Scale.[67–70]

BOWEL SYMPTOMS

Constipation is the most common bowel symptom in MS.[34] It is a feature in around 50% of all cases of MS.[71,72] Rarely, constipation can be a presenting symptom of MS.[73] It is due, in part, to paradoxical contraction of the puborectalis muscle during defecation.[74,75] The other bowel symptom is bowel urgency and incontinence.[34] When a person has fecal incontinence, one needs to rule out an impaction, because incontinence can occur around an impaction, requiring removal by either enema or manually.[33] Also, patients with MS could have primary bowel disorders such as colitis, gluten enteropathy or celiac disease.[34] Patients with MS can have abnormal bowel transit time.[76]

COGNITIVE IMPAIRMENT

Cognitive impairments in attention and memory have been reported in a majority of patients with MS.[77,78] This is thought to be due to the multiple lesions and diffuse axonal pathology interrupting the networks in place for different cognitive functions.[79] It was initially believed that cognitive impairment is more prevalent in the later stages of the disease; however, more recent studies have found cognitive impairment detectable at initial presentation and during the early phase of the disease.[80–85]

Preliminary studies using magnetization transfer imaging have shown a consistent correlation between diffuse tissue damage within the brain and cognitive impairment.[86–89] Brochet and colleagues found that cognitive impairment is common in the early stages of MS, mainly affecting attention, working memory, information processing speed and conceptualization. However, it is subtle and does not significantly affect quality of life at this stage.[90] Lyon-Caen and colleagues also found that patients with early clinically definite MS had cognitive impairment.[91] Pelosi and colleagues studied patients with isolated spinal cord syndromes suspected to be due to MS and found objective evidence of subclinical working memory dysfunction at an early stage of demyelinating disease, before they have developed symptoms of cognitive or memory dysfunction.[81] Patients can present with cognitive or neuropsychiatric symptoms as the first indication of MS.[92–95]

MS has been considered to be a subcortical dementia.[92] Subcortical dementia is characterized by early psychomotor retardation and mood disturbance, with relative perseveration of language, calculation and object recognition.[96] However there are patients with MS who have a marked impairment of abstract–conceptual reasoning, impaired language, and memory impairment suggesting cortical dysfunction.[96–98] Recent MRI studies demonstrate considerable pathology in the cortical gray matter.[99] Because of the evidence pointing to symptoms of cortical dysfunction being present in MS, one should consider demyelinating disease as an etiology for depression or early-onset dementia, particularly in younger people with cognitive abnormalities.[100]

OPTIC NEURITIS

Many patients with MS will have some form of optic neuritis during the course of their disease.[101] Inflammation of the optic nerve can lead to the acute or subacute onset of monocular visual blurring or loss, particularly in the central visual field.[102] Patients usually have decreased visual acuity; however, patients can have optic neuritis with no change in their visual acuity.[103] They can have eye pain and photopsias (flashes of light).[1]

The pain can precede, accompany or follow the loss of vision.[104] The pain is usually periorbital and increases with eye movements.[105] Some 92% of patients in the Optic Neuritis Treatment Trial (ONTT) had pain.[106] Patients with eye pain and blurred vision should be ruled out for uveitis, which can also been seen in patients with MS.[107] The pain of optic neuritis is thought to be due to dural distention by a swollen nerve, or inflammation involving the dural sheath.[1] It could also be secondary to traction on the optic nerve sheath by the rectus muscles.[105] Scotomas can be temporal, nasal, hemianopic or even altitudinal but are most commonly central.[1] An afferent papillary defect can be seen in optic neuritis.[108,109] Visual loss tends to be proportional to the apparent length of the involved segment of optic nerve in optic neuritis.[110,111] Some patients with optic neuritis can have a loss of the retinal nerve fiber layer.[112] Patients with optic neuritis also complain about impairment of color vision.[101] Ishihara plate testing was abnormal in 88.2% of patients in the ONTT.[106] The disk can be normal in the acute setting, with development of optic pallor later.[101] Some patients with MS can have subacute or chronic forms of optic neuritis in which the patient notices a gradual decline in vision, often associated with papillary abnormalities, disk pallor and nerve fiber bundle defects.[113]

Optic neuritis is a consideration in cases of optic neuropathy but needs to be distinguished from other etiologies, including Lyme disease, sarcoidosis, Leber's optic neuropathy and acute ischemic optic neuropathy. Optic neuritis tends to produce vision loss evolving over days but not usually more than 2 weeks.[101] The absence of pain is also a concern, as 90% of the patients in the ONTT had pain associated with their visual symptoms.[106] Patients should begin to have visual recovery within 30 days of onset.[101] When comparing optic neuritis to acute ischemic optic neuropathy, patients with optic neuritis tend to be younger, more likely female, less likely to have disk swelling, more likely to have associated pain and less likely to have an altitudinal defect, and usually have good return of vision.[101] There is also a greater likelihood of optic nerve enhancement of the orbits on MRI with contrast in patients with optic neuritis.[114] Rizzo and Lessell found that the rate of visual deterioration and range of acuities were similar in optic neuritis and acute ischemic optic neuropathy.[115]

Not everyone with optic neuritis will get MS. Some patients who have first-degree relatives with MS have only one episode of optic neuritis in their life.[116] Other causes of optic neuritis include sarcoidosis,[117] systemic lupus erythematosus,[1] Sjögren's syndrome,[118] syphilis,[1] Lyme disease[119] and human immunodeficiency virus (HIV),[120] all of which need to be ruled out in order to better predict the likelihood that a patient will develop MS after an episode of optic neuritis.

While most patients develop MS within a few years of their episode of optic neuritis, the development of MS can occur any time in a patient's lifetime.[1] Studies analyzing this found that there were certain factors associated with an increased risk of MS.[121–128] Factors that increase the risk for MS include younger age, female gender, previous nonspecific sensory symptoms, multiple MRI lesions, the presence of HLA-DR2 and the presence of oligoclonal bands in CSF.[123]

DYSARTHRIA

Patients with MS can have different forms of dysarthria. Dysarthria of the cerebellar type results in scanning speech. Scanning speech is monotonous speech interspersed with explosive consonants, resulting in irregular volume and indistinct articulation[2]. Many patients with cerebellar involvement develop an intention tremor of the voice. The tremor can be reproduced by having a patient sustain a vowel sound for at least 10 seconds. There is a variation in the intensity and pitch of the sound, oscillating at about 5–7 Hz.[2]

Pseudobulbar dysarthria is caused by spastic vocal cords, which causes a high-pitched, low-volume speech with slurred consonants.[2] There is no explosive variability of speech seen in

a patient with a pure pseudobulbar dysarthria; however, there are patients who have elements of both types of dysarthria.[2]

TREMORS AND OTHER MOVEMENT DISORDERS

Tremors in MS are usually seen in action or intention.[34] Charcot noted that rest tremor was not a sign of MS;[129] however, in severe cases the tremor can be apparent at rest.[34] The tremor that is apparent at rest is thought to be due to an intense intention tremor that allows the tremor to appear even with merely the intention to move the limb in question.[34] Tremor is thought to be due to damage to the cerebellum, or to its connections.[130]

The most common location for the tremor is in the upper extremities, while the head is the least common location.[131] Gender, age and duration of MS had no significant effect on presence or severity of tremor.[131] However, the presence of tremor was strongly associated with higher scores on the Expanded Disability Status Scale (EDSS), the Incapacity Status Scale and the Environmental Status Scale, all measures of disability or impairment.[131] Therefore, tremor in MS is associated with greater impairment, disability and handicap.[131]

While tremor is the most common extrapyramidal syndrome seen in MS, there are other extrapyramidal manifestations of the disease. Paroxysmal dystonia can be the presenting symptom in patients with MS.[132] Patients rarely develop movements like hemiballismus, chorea or choreoathetosis.[2] Parkinsonian features in MS patients, such as a rest tremor, could be due to either lesions in the basal ganglia and their connections or the coincidental occurrence of both MS and Parkinson's disease.[2]

Intention tremor is one of the many manifestations of disease in the cerebellum. Patients could also have titubation, gait ataxia and cerebellar dysarthria, depending on the location of the cerebellar lesion(s).[2]

PAIN

A significant number of patients with MS have pain, which may be due to many factors.[133–135] Patients can have musculoskeletal pain due to weakness, spasticity, imbalance, osteoporosis, compression fractures or osteoarthritis. All these processes are due to the disease or to immobility secondary to the disease.[134]

Headaches are more frequent in patients with MS.[136] Migraine was the most frequent primary headache among patients with relapsing–remitting MS in one study, while tension-type headache was more prevalent among patients with secondary progressive MS. However, those with and without headache did not differ in terms of type of MS, disease duration or severity. While the association could be due to the fact that similar patient populations get both disorders, the authors did speculate whether demyelination of brainstem structures could lead to headaches similar to migraine.[136]

The most common pain syndrome seen in MS is neuropathic pain. The pain is burning in quality and difficult to manage. Ebers and Paty believe that the mechanism could be spontaneous activity in deafferented neurons, ephaptic transmission or sympathetic activation.[34] Transmission of abnormal electrical discharges laterally across a demyelinated plaque might produce painful symptoms.[34] In the survey done by Moulin, the patients with this pain syndrome had evidence of posterior column demyelination but not spinothalamic demyelination.[134] The pain is more common in females than males and does not correlate with disease duration.[34]

Trigeminal neuralgia is the best known of the pain syndromes.[134] It is indistinguishable from the facial pain associated with idiopathic trigeminal neuralgia, except that it tends to occur at a younger age and is more often bilateral.[137] The pain is described as stabbing, electric shock-like, in the maxillary or mandibular branches of the trigeminal nerve.[134] The pain is triggered by non-noxious stimuli when applied to the involved area of the face; however, there is little if any sensory loss.[134] Demyelinating disease is always a diagnostic consideration in a patient who has trigeminal neuralgia under the age of 50.[134]

Patients with spasticity can develop severe leg spasms. These can be exacerbated by the presence of bedsores, urinary tract infections, constipation, ingrown toenails and urinary retention. These problems need to be managed in order to limit the number of spasms.

Patients can have acute pain episodes characterized by stereotyped paroxysmal attacks.[134] The pain can last from seconds to minutes, one to multiple times a day, for weeks, months or even years. Sometimes such episodes are the initial symptom of the disease.[138] The symptoms are difficult to manage, because of the brevity of the episodes and the type of pain experienced by these patients.

Other areas affected by paroxysmal pain include the extremities, whether the pain occurs spontaneously or in response to hyperventilation, tactile stimulation or movement of the involved limb.[134] Some patients with MS develop paroxysmal or chronic pains in a radicular distribution. The pain can mimic root compression syndromes such as occur with disk protrusion.[34] However, even though the pain could be purely due to MS, one must look for root entrapment secondary to disk protrusion or spondylosis.

There are times when acute radicular pain can be a presenting symptom. In the work by Ramirez-Lassepas et al, over a 15-year period, 11 patients presented with acute radicular pain as a first symptom of MS, in whom radicular compression was ruled out by imaging. Acute radicular pain accounted for 3.9% of the 282 newly diagnosed patients.[139] In the patients diagnosed after the advent of MRI, two were found to have demyelinating plaques within the spinal cord in the appropriate location to explain the symptoms.[139]

LHERMITTE'S PHENOMENON

A specific sensory symptom seen in patients with myelopathic processes is Lhermitte's phenomenon. It was first described by Babinski and Dubois in 1891.[140] They defined it as a sensation of electric shock in the back and legs of patients with traumatic disease of the cervical spinal cord, occurring during neck flexion. Lhermitte noted that the symptom was most frequently seen in patients with MS.[141] In patients with MS, Lhermitte's phenomenon can be produced by flexion of the neck, twisting of the dorsal spine or a jolt to the spine when the patient is walking on uneven ground. It can be spontaneous.[1] The symptom usually remits quickly but can persist, and it commonly fatigues. The sensation will extend from the neck to the base of the spine, or occasionally down one limb, or both.[1] While Lhermitte's phenomenon is seen frequently in MS, it can also be seen in many different etiologies of myelopathy including subacute combined degeneration of the spinal cord, cervical spondylosis, arachnoiditis, cervical disk protrusion, radiation myelitis, syringomyelia, combined systems disease, and tumor. A useful question to ask is whether the sensation occurs with neck extension, which is seen in cervical spondylosis but not in MS.[1]

VISUAL SIGNS AND SYMPTOMS

Patients with MS can have a variety of field defects depending on which part of the cortex is affected by a demyelinated lesion.[113]

There is an increased risk of inflammation of the eye itself in patients with MS, including uveitis, both anterior and posterior, pars planitis and periphlebitis.[101] Uveitis is ten times more common in patients with MS than in the general population.[113] The most common form of anterior uveitis is granulomatous uveitis, which can be a presenting symptom of the disease.[113] However, MS is not the only possibility in patients with granulomatous uveitis. One must also exclude sarcoid, Lyme disease, syphilis, tuberculosis, rheumatological disorders and Behçet's disease.

Periphlebitis is due to sheathing of the retinal veins by lymphocytes and plasma cells, which has been demonstrated to be associated with MS.[142-145] The changes are usually asymptomatic and do not typically cause complications.

MS is the most common cause of internuclear ophthalmoplegia.[101,146] Internuclear ophthalmoplegia (INO) is due to a demyelinating plaque in the medial longitudinal fasciculus, which causes an ipsilateral adduction deficit, with abducting nystagmus in the contralateral eye.[101,146] A subtle INO can be seen with slowing of saccadic adducting movements or may be elicited with the optokinetic nystagmus strip.[101] Bilateral INO will cause vertical gaze holding defects and upbeat nystagmus and may also be associated in skew deviation, with the higher eye on the side of the medial longitudinal fasciculus lesion.[101,146] The vertical gaze disorders may be due to disruption of connections with the rostral interstitial nucleus of the medial longitudinal fasciculus.[146] Occasionally patients with a bilateral INO may appear to be 'wall-eyed' because of associated exotropia.[101] Patients can either be asymptomatic or complain of diplopia on lateral eye movements. An INO can also be seen in a brainstem infarction, gliomas and anticonvulsant activity.

Usually ocular motor palsies are associated with other deficits, particularly nystagmus or an INO.[146] However when an isolated ocular motor palsy occurs, a demyelinating lesion is found to be in the fascicular portion of the nerve or the nucleus.[146] Partial or complete oculomotor deficits can occur due to brainstem lesions. Patients may have pupillary involvement with a nuclear third nerve lesion. Ptosis usually occurs only with a bilateral third nerve lesion, because the central caudal nucleus of the oculomotor complex innervates bilateral levator palpebrae muscles.[101] An isolated oculomotor nerve palsy can be a presenting symptom of MS as well.[148,149] Trochlear nuclear lesions occur contralateral to the lesion, resulting in the eye being deviated up and out.[101] One can tell that a patient has a trochlear lesion by the tilt of the patient's head to the opposite side, in order for the patient to not experience diplopia due to a torsional defect.

Abducens lesions can cause smooth pursuit, and saccadic eye movement impairment on horizontal gaze.[101] An abducens palsy is the most common ocular motor nerve palsy.[150] Trochlear nerve palsies are the least common.[151] Horizontal gaze palsies can be due to lesions of either the ipsilateral paramedian pontine reticular formation rostral to the abducens nucleus and/or the abducens nucleus.[152] Horizontal gaze palsy could also be due to a lesion in both the VIth nerve fascicle and contralateral medial longitudinal fasciculus.[147] To distinguish between complete gaze palsies due to a paramedian pontine reticular formation (PPRF) lesion and ocular motor nuclear lesions, oculocephalic stimulation is done. If there is a gaze palsy, the eyes will not move when oculocephalic stimulation is done. However, if there is a lesion in the PPRF, the eyes will move when oculocephalic stimulation is done, because the oculovestibular response does not require the PPRF to function.[146] Usually ocular motor palsies are associated with other deficits, particularly nystagmus.[147] Disturbances of conjugate gaze are one of the most common eye movement abnormalities found in MS.[146] Reulen et al found that MS patients have a high incidence of saccadic and pursuit eye movement defects,[153] which has been confirmed in other studies.[153,154]

Patients could also have a lesion in the dorsal midbrain resulting in inability to look up, eyelid retraction, near-light dissociation of the pupils, accommodation paralysis, convergence paralysis, convergence-retraction nystagmus, skew deviation and paresis of downgaze, commonly know as Parinaud's syndrome.[146]

The most common form of nystagmus is associated with INO.[101] Pathological gaze-evoked nystagmus may result from vestibular pathway lesions. Downbeat nystagmus could be due to demyelinating lesions involving the cervicomedullary junction or the cerebellum but is uncommon. Upbeat nystagmus is often seen with bilateral INOs.[101]

A lesion to Mollaret's triangle can produce oculopalatal myoclonus and hypertrophy of the inferior olivary nucleus, as well as pendular nystagmus.[101,146]

Vertical nystagmus can also be seen. Patients may also have saccadic overshoot or undershoot dysmetria, pendular nystagmus and fixation instability due to cerebellar lesions.[146] Vestibulocerebellar lesion can cause gaze-paretic and rebound nystagmus.[146]

PSYCHIATRIC SYMPTOMS – DEPRESSION

Charcot noted that mood disturbances were a common feature of MS.[155] However, it is difficult to ascertain how much of the depression is secondary to the fact that the patient has an unpredictable, chronic illness and how much is actually due to the neurobiological changes engendered by the disease itself.[156] There is conflicting data about the risk of depression in MS, with most studies supporting the idea of depression being more prevalent in MS than in other chronic conditions.[157–161] Major depression may occur in almost half of the MS population.[162] It is an important determinant of quality of life in MS.[163–165] Suicide appears also to be more common in the MS population than in the general population.[166,167] Factors that predict suicidal intent include living alone, severe depression and alcohol problems.[168]

Feinstein and colleagues used brain MRI to compare MS patients with major depression with nondepressed MS patients.[169] The patients all met the DSM-IV criteria for major depression.[170] The depressed MS patients had more lesions in the left inferior medial frontal regions and greater atrophy of the left anterior temporal regions.[169]

While fatigue is a common symptom in both depression and MS, there has been little evidence to relate the high incidence of depression with fatigue.[170] Krupp et al found no significant correlation between clinical depression and fatigue in a group of MS patients.[49] However, one study did correlate depression and fatigue in patients with MS.[171] This study examined fatigue by separating it into three different categories, mental, physical and total fatigue.[171] Depression was more strongly related to mental fatigue than physical fatigue.[171]

Cognitive impairment is found in both patients with MS and depression.[172,173] However, no association has been found between depression and cognitive impairment in MS.[172,174,175] Depressed MS patients are more likely to have effortful than automatic information processing compromised by the disease.[176,177] Arnett and his colleagues have also reported that cognitive impairments in patients with MS seem to be closely related with mood and negative self-evaluations, but less so with the vegetative symptoms of depression.[177]

SLEEP

Approximately half of all patients with MS report sleep-related problems.[178] Contributions to sleep disruption include pain, depression, sleep-disordered breathing and disease severity.[179] Patients with MS may have disorders including insomnia, sleep apnea, restless leg syndrome (RLS), narcolepsy and rapid-eye-movement sleep behavior disorder.[179]

Most patients who have sleep-related problems and MS have insomnia, with difficulty either initiating or maintaining sleep.[178] This is influenced by factors such as pain associated with muscle spasms, periodic limb movement syndrome (PLMS), RLS, nocturia, medication effect and psychiatric illness such as depression.[179]

The incidence of PLMS and RLS is higher in patients with MS than in the general population.[179] RLS is characterized by an urge to move the legs, usually accompanied or caused by uncomfortable and unpleasant sensations in the legs. The sensations are exacerbated by periods of rest or inactivity and are partially or totally relieved by movement. The sensations are worse in the evening or at night.[180] RLS is described as an uncomfortable, aching, crawling feeling in the legs, which can often interfere with sleep onset.[179]

PLMS causes flexion of both lower extremities during sleep with the potential of disrupting sleep by causing frequent arousals.[181] The incidence of PLMS has been reported to be as high as 36%.[182] The majority of patients with RLS also have PLMS when asleep.[183,184] Nocturnal hypopnea and apnea occur as a result of a collapse of the tissues and muscles in the pharynx or a failure of the medullary respiratory signal, in the case of MS, from a demyelinating lesion.[179] Patients with daytime somnolence and increased fatigue should be evaluated for central sleep apnea, paroxysmal hyperventilation, hypoventilation, respiratory muscle weakness and respiratory arrest.[185,186]

Narcolepsy can appear before or after other symptoms of MS but is uncommon.[187] Both narcolepsy and MS are strongly linked to similar human leukocyte antigen (HLA) expression.[188]

Rapid-eye-movement behavior disorder is characterized by complex motor behaviors during rapid-eye-movement sleep, seen in MS, in one instance as a presenting symptom.[189]

PAROXYSMAL SYMPTOMS

While an attack has been determined to be a period of neurological dysfunction lasting for 24 hours,[11] patients with MS can have brief episodes of neurological dysfunction without signs indicative of structural damage.[190] These episodes could be motor,[191–193] visual,[194] sensory, dysarthria and ataxia.[195] These symptoms are brief, occur frequently (from 1–2 times per day to hundreds of times a day) and occur in an ephaptic fashion.[196] One hypothesis as to the cause of paroxysmal symptoms is that nerve fibers within a partially demyelinated lesion spread the neuronal conduction and create paroxysmal attacks by activating adjacent anatomical structures. One retrospective study in an MS center in Istanbul looked at the locations of lesions that could cause certain paroxysmal symptoms.[196] Paroxysmal tonic spasms appeared to be due to lesions in any level of the motor pathway, including the posterior limb of the internal capsule, centrum semiovale and anterior portion of the pons.[196] Paroxysmal dysarthria and ataxia are related to the upper pons and midbrain.[195] Paroxysmal diplopia could be due to a midbrain or pontine lesion.[196]

In one case report, paroxysmal hemidystonia occurred in a patient with a demyelinating lesion in the subthalamic region involving the posterior arm of the internal capsule and extending to the subthalamic nucleus and mesencephalon.[197] The patient presented with a 6-week history of painful tonic spasms affecting his right side. De Seze et al described a

16-year-old patient with paroxysmal kinesogenic choreoathetosis as the presenting symptom of MS, with demyelinating lesions at the posterior part of the globus pallidus, posterior part of the internal capsule and lateral anterior part of the thalamus.[198]

A Japanese patient had paroxysmal urinary incontinence that was characterized by sudden onset, short duration and frequent repetition.[199] A urodynamic study done during the paroxysmal attacks revealed uninhibited detrusor contractions with coordinated relaxation of external urethral sphincter muscle, occurring only during the period of the attack. The patient had a demyelinating lesion in the right rostral pons, the location of which was similar to the pontine micturition center reported in previous animal experiments. Treatment with carbamazepine suppressed the attacks, including the associated urinary incontinence.[199]

Patients may have facial myokymia.[195] McAlpine and Compston found several cases of facial spasm, even as a presenting symptom, preceding the onset of paralysis or following an attack of facial paresis that had recovered.[193] Andermann found in his review of facial myokymia in MS that the myokymia usually starts in the orbicularis oculi and spreads to involve all facial muscles.[200] Hemifacial spasm is also seen uncommonly in MS.[200] If an ectatic vertebrobasilar vessel, aneurysm or mass lesion is ruled out, one can presume an MS plaque in the brainstem, corticobulbar tract or cranial nerve VII fascicle.[201]

DYSPHAGIA

Bronchopneumonia is a common cause of death and morbidity in late MS that can be secondary to dysphagia leading to aspiration.[202] Potential mechanisms of dysphagia include disruption of the corticobulbar tracts, cerebellar dysfunction, brainstem and lower cranial nerve involvement, and abnormal respiratory control and capacity.[202]

The symptoms of dysphagia include an alteration in eating habits such as eating pureed foods or avoiding certain foods, coughing or choking while eating, and associated dysphonia and dysarthria.[203] The frequency of dysphagia increases with increasing disability.

One group analyzed their MS population for dysphagia.[203] They found that the pharyngeal phase of swallowing was the most commonly affected. Dysphagia is most commonly connected to brainstem dysfunction. The ventromedial reticular formation and the nucleus tractus solitarius appear to play a central role in the control of deglutition and its coordination with respiration.

VERTIGO

Vertigo occurs in about 20% of patients during the illness and can be the presenting manifestation of MS in up to 5%.[204–206] Vertigo is usually due to lesions in the medial vestibular nucleus and the root entry zone of cranial nerve VIII.[207–211] However, vertigo in patients with MS is not necessarily due to an active demyelinating lesion.[210] The most common cause of vertigo is benign positional vertigo in the MS population, which is not an MS exacerbation.[213] Episodes of vertigo lasting only seconds and provoked by head movement often reflect benign positional vertigo.[212] Paroxysmal vertiginous events are characterized by the abrupt onset of spontaneous vertigo that lasts for seconds to minutes, not necessarily associated with positional factors, recurrent and stereotypic in nature.[212] Vertigo caused by a brainstem lesion is usually chronic and is usually associated with other brainstem findings.[1]

HEARING LOSS

Hearing loss in MS is rather uncommon. The magnitude and type of hearing deficit present can vary quite considerably.[214] Hearing loss is usually attributed to lesions of the central auditory pathways of the brainstem.[214] The hearing loss is sensorineural and there are rare cases of sudden deafness.[215]

EPILEPSY

Multiple studies have explored the frequency of epilepsy in MS but, because the accuracy of the diagnosis of MS could not be established, particularly in the studies containing pediatric populations, one must be cautious in the interpretation of the results.[216] The concern over diagnostic accuracy is warranted because the most common condition confused with MS is a postinfectious or postvaccinal encephalomyelitis, in which epileptiform seizures can occur.[216] The other issue is the determination of whether the patient's event was epileptiform or simply a nonepileptiform paroxysmal manifestation of MS.[216] Despite the caveats mentioned above, epilepsy is more common among patients with MS than in the general population.[216]

All types of seizures have been reported in association with MS.[216] Most seizures in MS had a focal component.[216] There have been rare episodes of epilepsia partialis continua and status epilepticus.[217–219] Epilepsy can rarely be the initial clinical manifestation of MS.[218] In some cases the onset of seizure activity could be the sole representation of an acute relapse; however, a seizure may not necessarily represent new activity.[218,220,221] There are conflicting reports as to whether seizures are more likely to occur during a relapse.[218,221–226] In MRI studies examining MS and epilepsy, it has not been determined whether there is an anatomical/clinical correlation between a demyelinating lesion and a seizure.[216] In the work of Striano et al, seizure recurrence and status epilepticus were more common in cases with severe neurological and cognitive impairment and a secondary progressive course.[227] Prognosis of epilepsy during the course of MS is usually favorable.[216]

RESPIRATORY SYMPTOMS

Among patients with MS who die from complications of the disease, pneumonia is the most frequent underlying cause.[228–230] Respiratory muscles may be affected by demyelination of the central nervous system, resulting in acute[231–234] or chronic ventilatory failure,[235–237] although this is a less common event in MS than in other chronic, progressive neurological conditions.

Patients with respiratory involvement tend to have high cervical cord lesions or bulbar lesions, which could lead to acute respiratory insufficiency.[238] Bulbar dysfunction increases the risk of aspiration and lower respiratory tract infection.[239]

Carter and Noseworthy observed that progressive breathlessness, orthopnea and sleep disturbances were signs of impending respiratory failure, due to diaphragmatic weakness causing a drop in vital capacity while in the supine position.[238,240] In order to recognize respiratory symptoms, one needs to ask the patient about difficulty in clearing pulmonary secretions, and strength of cough. The examiner must also observe the cough and listen to the patient count in a single exhalation.[231]

AUTONOMIC SYMPTOMS

Bladder and bowel dysfunction are common autonomic symptoms, each requiring a separate section for discussion[241] (see above). Orthostatic hypotension and cardiac disorders due to autonomic dysfunction are not uncommon.[242–246] Most studies have failed to find any correlation between autonomic dysfunction and brain or brainstem lesions; however, there are two studies that did find a correlation between autonomic dysfunction and brainstem lesions on MRI.[243,245–249] There is evidence of autonomic dysfunction in patients with primary progressive forms of the disease.[250] The frequency of dysfunction correlates with a reduction in spinal cord area, not with the presence of hyperintensities, suggesting that autonomic dysfunction is secondary to axonal loss and not to demyelination.[250] The cardiovascular autonomic regulation failure manifests itself in both the heart rate response to deep breathing and the heart rate and blood pressure response during the tilt table test.[251]

SYNDROME OF INAPPROPRIATE SECRETION OF ANTIDIURETIC HORMONE

The syndrome of inappropriate secretion of antidiuretic hormone (SIADH) has only been reported a few times in cases of MS.[252–255] In each of these cases, the syndrome occurred during an exacerbation. The hypothesis is that a lesion in the hypothalamic pathways can lead to SIADH.[255]

CONCLUSION

The chapter illustrates that patients with MS can present with a variety of different signs and symptoms, most if not all of which are nonspecific for MS but are localizable to the CNS and reflect primarily, but not exclusively, white matter involvement. Some are more common than others, as seen in the list above. While optic neuritis or an internuclear ophthalmoplegia makes most if not all neurologists consider MS as a diagnosis, some symptoms, such as the autonomic symptoms, are rarely found in MS and would require an experienced clinician to think of MS as a possible etiology when other etiologies are ruled out. Particularly in the patients with unusual symptoms, ancillary studies, such as MRI, would be helpful in the diagnosis of MS. While prior to the early 1990s rushing to diagnose a patient with MS was not a priority for neurologists, the discovery of disease-modifying therapy has changed that. As mentioned at the beginning of the chapter, prompt diagnosis of MS or what could possibly become MS could result in prompt initiation of disease-modifying therapy, which could potentially lead to improved quality of life. This highlights the need for the diagnosis of MS to be made by experienced neurologists who are aware of the numerous ways that the disease may present, as well as the likelihood that the patient's complaints are due to MS and not another etiology. Once the diagnosis is made, however, because of the plethora of manifestations of the disease, neurologists who take care of patients with MS need to master the management of the many different symptoms associated with the condition. As regards the clinical course of MS, we would hope to have more biologically based markers of disease course and activity that improve on our ability to accurately predict an individual patient's prognosis. This will probably involve a composite assessment of clinical features, MRI metrics and biomarkers. Such knowledge would allow for better risk/benefit judgments for new therapeutic agents.

REFERENCES

1. Paty DW, Noseworthy J, Ebers GC. Diagnosis of multiple sclerosis. In: Paty D, Ebers G, eds. Multiple sclerosis. Philadelphia, PA: FA Davis; 1998: 48–134.

2. Paty DW, Ebers GC. Clinical features. In: Paty D, Ebers G, eds. Multiple sclerosis. Philadelphia, PA: FA Davis; 1998: 135–192.

3. Jacobs LD, Beck RW, Simon JH et al. Intramuscular interferon beta-1a therapy initiated during a first demyelinating event in multiple sclerosis. N Engl J Med 2000; 343: 898–904.

4. Filippi M, Rovaris M, Inglese M et al. Interferon beta-1a for brain tissue loss in patients at presentation with syndromes suggestive of multiple sclerosis: a randomised, double-blind, placebo-controlled trial. Lancet 2004; 364: 1489–1496.

5. Lublin FD, Reingold SC. Defining the clinical course of multiple sclerosis: results of an international survey. National Multiple Sclerosis Society (USA) Advisory Committee on Clinical Trials of New Agents in Multiple Sclerosis. Neurology 1996; 46: 907–911.

6. IFNB Multiple Sclerosis Study Group. Interferon beta-1b is effective in relapsing–remitting multiple sclerosis. I. Clinical results of a multicenter, randomized, double-blind, placebo-controlled trial. The IFNB Multiple Sclerosis Study Group. Neurology 1993; 43: 655–661.

7. PRISMS Study Group. Randomised double-blind placebo-controlled study of interferon beta-1a in relapsing/remitting multiple sclerosis. PRISMS (Prevention of Relapses and Disability by Interferon beta-1a Subcutaneously in Multiple Sclerosis) Study Group. Lancet 1998; 352: 1498–1504.

8. Johnson KP, Brooks BR, Cohen JA et al. Copolymer 1 reduces relapse rate and improves disability in relapsing-remitting multiple sclerosis: results of a phase III multicenter, double-blind placebo-controlled trial. The Copolymer 1 Multiple Sclerosis Study Group. Neurology 1995; 45: 1268–1276.

9. Leary SM, Thompson AJ. Primary progressive multiple sclerosis: current and future treatment options. CNS Drugs 2005; 19: 369–376.

10. Polman CH, O'Connor PW, Havrova E et al. A randomized, placebo-controlled trial of natalizumab for relapsing multiple sclerosis. N Engl J Med 2006; 354(9): 899–910.

11. Committee on Multiple Sclerosis. Clinical and biological features. In: Joy JE, Johnston RB Jr, eds. Multiple sclerosis status and strategies for the future. Washington, DC: National Academies Press; 2001: 30.

12. McDonald WI, Compston A, Edan G et al. Recommended diagnostic criteria for multiple sclerosis: guidelines from the international panel on the diagnosis of multiple sclerosis. Ann Neurol 2001; 50: 121–127.

13. Lublin FD, Baier M, Cutter G. Effect of relapses on development of residual deficit in multiple sclerosis. Neurology 2003; 61: 1528–1532.

14. Sibley WA, Paty DW. A comparison of multiple sclerosis in Arizona (USA) and Ontario (Canada): preliminary report. Acta Neurol Scand 1981; 64(suppl 87): 60–65.

15. Poser S, Poser W. Multiple sclerosis and gestation. Neurology 1983; 33: 1422–1427.

16. Sibley WA, Foley JM. Infection and immunization in multiple sclerosis. Ann NY Acad Sci 1965; 122: 457–468.

17. Worthington J, Jones R, Crawford M et al. Pregnancy and multiple sclerosis: a three year prospective study. J Neurol 1994; 241: 228–233.

18. Confavreux C, Hutchinson M, Hours MM et al. Rate of pregnancy-related relapse in multiple sclerosis. N Engl J Med 1998; 339: 285–291.

19. Sibley WA, Bamford CR, Clark K. Clinical viral infections and multiple sclerosis. Lancet 1985; 1: 1313–1315.

20. Tullman MJ, Oshinsky RY, Lublin FD et al. Clinical characteristics of progressive relapsing multiple sclerosis. Mult Scler 2004; 10: 451–454.

21. Committee on Multiple Sclerosis. Characteristics and management of major symptoms. In: Joy JE, Johnston RB Jr, eds. Multiple sclerosis status and strategies for the future. Washington, DC: National Academies Press; 2001: 118–181.

22. Altrocchi PH. Acute transverse myelopathy. Arch Neurol 1963; 9: 21–29.

23. Ransohoff RM, Whitman GJ, Weinstein MA. Noncommunicating syringomyelia in multiple sclerosis: detection by magnetic resonance imaging. Neurology 1990; 40: 718–721.

24. Gessain A, Barin F, Vernant JC. Antibodies to human T-lymphotropic virus type-I in

patients with tropical spastic paraparesis. Lancet 1985; 2: 407–410.

25. Gessain A, Gout O. Chronic myelopathy associated with human T-lymphotropic virus type I (HTLV-I). Ann Intern Med 1992; 117: 913–914.

26. Rudge P, Ali A, Cruickshank JK. Multiple sclerosis, tropical spastic paraparesis and HTLV-1 infection in Afro-Caribbean patients in the United Kingdom. J Neurol Neurosurg Psychiatr 1991; 54: 689–694.

27. Ghezzi A, Baldini SM, Zaffaroni M. Differential diagnosis of acute myelopathies. J Neurol Sci 2001; 22: S60–S64.

28. Noseworthy JH, Heffernan LPH. Motor radiculopathy–an unusual presentation of multiple sclerosis. Can J Neurol Sci 1980; 1: 207–209.

29. Oppenheim H. Jahresber Leistungen und Fortschr Geb Neurol Psychiat 1916; 20: xiv.

30. Nonne M. Multiple Sclerose und Faziälisahmung. Deutsch Z Nervenheilk 1918; 60: 201.

31. Barnes MP, Kent RM, Semlyen JK et al. Spasticity in multiple sclerosis. Neurorehabil Neural Repair 2003; 17: 66–70.

32. Kesselring J, Thompson AJ. Spasticity, ataxia and fatigue in multiple sclerosis. Baillières Clin Neurol 1997; 6: 429–445.

33. Rizzo MA, Hadjimichael OC, Preiningerova J et al. Prevalence and treatment of spasticity reported by multiple sclerosis patients. Mult Scler 2004; 10: 589–595.

34. Paty DW, Hashimoto SA, Ebers GC. Management of multiple sclerosis and interpretation of clinical trials. In: Paty D, Ebers G, eds. Multiple sclerosis. Philadelphia, PA: FA Davis; 1998: 427–519.

35. Sheean G. The pathophysiology of spasticity. Eur J Neurol 2002; 9(suppl 1): 3–9.

36. Hinson JL, Boone TB. Urodynamics and multiple sclerosis. Urol Clin North Am 1996; 23: 475–481.

37. Yang S, Chancellor M. Neurological disorders. In: Cardozo L, Staskin D, eds. Textbook of female urology and urogynaecology. London: ISIS; 2001: 837–855.

38. Blaivis J, Chaikin D, Chancellor M et al. Pathophysiology of the neurogenic bladder. In: Mancall E, Munsat T, eds. Continuum: lifelong learning in neurology–neurourology. Baltimore, MD: Williams & Wilkins; 1998.

39. DasGupta R, Fowler CJ. Sexual and urological dysfunction in multiple sclerosis: better understanding and improved therapies. Curr Opin Neurol 2002; 25: 271–278.

40. Mayo ME, Chetner MP. Lower urinary tract dysfunction in multiple sclerosis. Urology 1992; 39: 67–70.

41. Borello-France D, Leng W, Xavier M et al. Bladder and sexual function among women with multiple sclerosis. Mult Scler 2004; 20: 455–461.

42. Zivadinov R, Zorzon M, Bosco A et al. Sexual dysfunction in multiple sclerosis: II. Correlation analysis. Mult Scler 1999; 5: 428–431.

43. Vas CJ. Sexual impotence and some autonomic disturbances in men with multiple sclerosis. Acta Neurol Scand 1969; 45: 166–184.

44. Zorzon M, Zivadinov R, Bosco A et al. Sexual dysfunction in multiple sclerosis: a case control study. I. Frequency and comparison of groups. Mult Scler 1999; 5: 418–427.

45. Zorzon M, Zivadinov R, Bosco A et al. Sexual dysfunction in multiple sclerosis: a 2-year follow-up study. J Neurol Sci 2001; 187: 1–5.

46. Hulter BM, Lundborg PO. Sexual function in women with advanced multiple sclerosis. J Neurol Neurosurg Psychiatr 1995; 59: 83–86.

47. Nortvedt MW, Riise T, Myhr KM et al. Reduced quality of life among multiple sclerosis patients with sexual disturbance and bladder dysfunction. Mult Scler 2001; 7: 231–235.

48. Aisen ML, Sanders AS. Sexual dysfunction in neurologic disease: mechanisms of disease and counseling approaches. AUA Update Series Lesson 35, Volume XVII; 1998.

49. Krupp LB, Alvarez LA, LaRocca NG et al. Fatigue in multiple sclerosis. Arch Neurol 1988; 45: 435–437.

50. Chen MK. The epidemiology of self-perceived fatigue among adults. Prev Med 1986; 15: 74–81.

51. Fisk JD, Pontefract A, Ritvo PG et al. The impact of fatigue on patients with multiple sclerosis. Can J Neurol Sci 1994; 21: 9–14.

52. Freal JE, Kraft GH, Coryell JK. Symptomatic fatigue in multiple sclerosis. Arch Phys Med Rehabil 1984; 65: 135–138.

53. Krupp LB, LaRocca NG, Muir-Nash J et al. The fatigue severity scale. Application to patients with multiple sclerosis and systemic lupus erythematosus. Arch Neurol 1989; 46: 1121–1123.

54. Midgard R, Riise T, Nyland H. Impairment, disability, and handicap in multiple sclerosis. A cross-sectional study in an incident cohort in More and Romsdal County, Norway. J Neurol 1996; 243: 337–344.

55. Murray TJ. Amantadine therapy for fatigue in multiple sclerosis. Can J Neurol Sci 1985; 12: 251–254.

56. Loge JH, Ekeberg O, Kaasa S. Fatigue in the general Norwegian population: normative data and associations. J Psychosom Res 1998; 45: 53–65.

57. Pawlikowska T, Chalder T, Hirsch SR et al. Population based study of fatigue and psychological distress. Br Med J 1994; 308: 763–766.

58. Watt T, Groenvold M, Bjorner JB. Fatigue in the Danish general population. Influence of sociodemographic factors and disease. J Epidemiol Community Health 2000; 54: 827–833.

59. Lerdal A, Celius EG, Moum T. Fatigue and its association with sociodemographic variables among multiple sclerosis patients. Mult Scler 2003; 9: 509–514.

60. Krupp LB, Pollina DA. Mechanisms and management of fatigue in progressive neurological disorders. Psychosocial correlates of fatigue in multiple sclerosis. Curr Opin Neurol 1996; 9: 456–460.

61. Schwartz CE, Coulthard-Morris L, Zeng Q. Psychosocial correlates of fatigue in multiple sclerosis. Arch Phys Med Rehabil 1996; 977: 165–170.

62. Bakshi R, Miletch RS, Henschel K et al. Fatigue in multiple sclerosis: cross-sectional correlation with brain MRI findings in 71 patients. Neurology 1999; 53: 1151–1153.

63. Flachenecker P, Kumpfel T, Kallmann B et al. Fatigue in multiple sclerosis: a comparison of different rating scales and correlation to clinical parameters. Mult Scler 2002; 8: 523–526.

64. Colosimo C, Millefiorni E, Graso MG et al. Fatigue in MS is associated with specific clinical features. Acta Neurol Scand 1995; 92: 353–355.

65. Grossman M, Armstrong C, Onishi K et al. Patterns of cognitive impairment in relapsing–remitting and chronic progressive multiple sclerosis. Neuropsychiatry Neuropsychol Behav Neurol 1994; 7: 194–210.

66. Kroencke DC, Lynch SG, Denney DR. Fatigue in multiple sclerosis: relationship to depression, disability, and disease pattern. Mult Scler 2000; 6: 131–136.

67. Van der Werf SP, Jongen PJ, Nijeholt GJ et al. Fatigue in multiple sclerosis: interrelations between fatigue complaints, cerebral MRI abnormalities and neurological disability. J Neurol Sci 1998; 160: 164–170.

68. Vercoulen JH, Hommes OR, Swanink CM et al. The measurement of fatigue in patients with multiple sclerosis. A multidimensional comparison with patients with chronic fatigue syndrome and healthy subjects. Arch Neurol 1996; 53: 642–649.

69. Colombo B, Martinelli Boneschi FM, Rossi P et al. MRI and motor evoked potential findings in nondisabled multiple sclerosis patients with and without symptoms of fatigue. J Neurol 2000; 247: 506–509.

70. Filippi M, Rocca MA, Colombo B et al. Functional magnetic resonance imaging correlates of fatigue in multiple sclerosis. Neuroimage 2002; 15: 559–567.

71. Hinds JP, Eidelman BH, Wald A. Prevalence of bowel dysfunction in multiple sclerosis. A population survey. Gastroenterology 1990; 98: 1538–1542.

72. Sullivan SN, Ebers GC. Gastrointestinal dysfunction in multiple sclerosis. Gastroenterology 1983; 84: 1640–1646.

73. Lawthorn C, Durdey P, Hughes T. Constipation as a presenting symptom. Lancet 2003; 362: 958.

74. Chia YW, Gill KP, Jameson JS et al. Paradoxical puborectalis contraction is a feature of constipation in patients with multiple sclerosis. J Neurol Neurosurg Psychiatr 1996; 60: 31–35.

75. Mathers SE, Ingram DA, Swash M. Electrophysiology of motor pathways for sphincter control in multiple sclerosis. J Neurol Neurosurg Psychiatr 1990; 53: 955–960.

76. Hinds JP, Wald A. Colonic and anorectal dysfunction associated with multiple sclerosis. Am J Gastroenterol 1989; 84: 587–595.

77. Rao SM, Leo GJ, Bernardin L et al. Cognitive dysfunction in multiple sclerosis. I. Frequency, patterns, and prediction. Neurology 1991; 41: 685–691.

78. Ron MA, Callanan MM, Warrington EK. Cognitive abnormalities in multiple sclerosis: a psychometric and MRI study. Psychol Med 1991; 21: 59–68.

79. Mesulam MM. Large-scale neurocognitive networks and distributed processing for attention, language, and memory. Ann Neurol 1990; 28: 597–613.

80. Feinstein A, Kartsounis LD, Miller DH et al. Clinically isolated lesions of the type seen in multiple sclerosis: a cognitive, psychiatric, and MRI follow up study. J Neurol Neurosurg Psychiatr 1992; 55: 869–876.

81. Pelosi L, Geesken JM, Holly M et al. Working memory impairment in early multiple sclerosis. Evidence from an event-related potential study of patients with clinically isolated myelopathy. Brain 1997; 120: 2039–2058.

82. Achiron A, Barak Y. Cognitive impairment in probable multiple sclerosis. J Neurol Neurosurg Psychiatr 2003; 74: 443–446.

83. Grant I, McDonald WI, Trimble MR et al. Deficient learning and memory in early and middle phases of multiple sclerosis. J Neurol Neurosurg Psychiatr 1984; 47: 250–255.

84. Lyon-Caen O, Jouvent R, Hauser S et al. Cognitive function in recent-onset demyelinating diseases. Arch Neurol 1986; 43: 1138–1141.

85. Amato MP, Ponziani G, Pracucci G et al. Cognitive impairment in early-onset multiple sclerosis. Pattern, predictors, and impact on everyday life in a 4-year follow-up. Arch Neurol 1995; 52: 168–172.

86. Zivadinov R, De Masi R, Nasuelli D, et al. MRI techniques and cognitive impairment in the early phase of relapsing–remitting multiple sclerosis. Neuroradiology 2001; 43: 272–278.

87. Rovaris M, Filippi M, Falautano M et al. Relation between MR abnormalities and patterns of cognitive impairment in multiple sclerosis. Neurology 1998; 50: 1601–1608.

88. Rovaris M, Filippi M, Minicucci L et al. Cortical/subcortical disease burden and cognitive impairment in patients with multiple sclerosis. Am J Neuroradiol 2000; 21: 402–408.

89. Filippi M, Tortorella C, Rovaris M et al. Changes in the normal appearing brain tissue and cognitive impairment in multiple sclerosis. J Neurol Neurosurg Psychiatr 2000; 68: 157–161.

90. Deloire MSA, Salort E, Bonnet M et al. Cognitive impairment as marker of diffuse brain abnormalities in early relapsing remitting multiple sclerosis. J Neurol Neurosurg Psychiatr 2005; 76: 519–526.

91. Lyon-Caen O, Jouvent R, Hauser S et al. Cognitive function in recent-onset demyelinating diseases. Arch Neurol 1986; 43: 1138–1141.

92. Zarei M, Chandran S, Compston A et al. Cognitive presentation of multiple sclerosis: evidence for a cortical variant. J Neurol Neurosurg Psychiatr 2003; 74: 872–877.

93. Skegg K. Multiple sclerosis presenting as a pure psychiatric disorder. Psychol Med 1993; 23: 909–914.

94. Matthews WB. Multiple sclerosis presenting with acute remitting psychiatric symptoms. J Neurol Neurosurg Psychiatr 1979; 42: 859–863.

95. Young AC, Saunders JM, Ponsford JR. J Neurol Neurosurg Psychiatr 1976; 39: 1008–1013.

96. Rao SM, Multiple sclerosis. In: Cumming JL, ed. Subcortical dementias. Oxford: Oxford University Press; 1990: 164–180.

97. Salmon DP, Hodges JP. Neuropsychological assessment of early onset dementia. In: Hodges JR, ed. Early onset dementia. Oxford: Oxford University Press; 2001: 47–73.

98. Peyser JM, Rao SM, LaRocca NG et al. Guidelines for neuropsychological research in multiple sclerosis. Arch Neurol 1990; 47: 94–97.

99. Valsasina P, Benedetti B, Rovaris M et al. Evidence for progressive gray matter loss in patients with relapsing–remitting MS. Neurology 2005; 65: 1126–1268.

100. Benedict RH, Bakshi R, Simon JH et al. Frontal cortex atrophy predicts cognitive impairment in multiple sclerosis. J Neuropsychiatr Clin Neurosci 2002; 14: 44–51.

101. Jacobs DA, Galetta SL. Multiple sclerosis and the visual system. Ophthalmol Clin North Am 2004; 17: 265–273.

102. Nikoskelainen E, Riekkinen P. Optic neuritis: a sign of multiple sclerosis or other diseases of the central nervous system. Acta Neurol Scand 1974; 50: 690–718.

103. Fredriksen JL, Larsson HB, Ottovay E et al. Acute optic neuritis with normal visual acuity. Acta Ophthalmol Suppl 1991; 69: 357–366.

104. Perkin GD, Rose FC. Optic neuritis and its differential diagnosis. Oxford: Oxford University Press; 1979: 19–31.

105. Lepore FE. The origin of pain in optic neuritis. Determinants of pain in eyes with optic neuritis. Arch Neurol 1991; 48: 748–749.

106. Optic Neuritis Study Group. The clinical profile of optic neuritis. Experience of the Optic Neuritis Treatment Trial. Arch Ophthalmol 1991; 109: 1673–1678.

107. Bachman DM, Rosenthal AR, Beckingsale AB. Granulomatous uveitis in neurological disease. Br J Ophthalmol 1985; 69: 192–196.

108. Cox TA. Relative afferent pupillary defects in multiple sclerosis. Can J Ophthalmol 1989; 24: 207–210.

109. Cox TA. Pupillary escape. Neurology 1992; 42: 1271–1273.

110. Johnson G, Miller DH, MacManus D et al. STIR sequences in NMR images of the optic nerve. Neuroradiology 1987; 29: 238–245.

111. Miller DH, MR Newton MR, van der Poel JC et al. Magnetic resonance imaging of the optic nerve in optic neuritis. Neurology 1988; 38: 175–179.

112. MacFadyen DJ, Drance SM, Douglas GR et al. The retinal nerve fiber layer, neuroretinal rim area, and visual evoked potentials in MS. Neurology 1988; 38: 1353–1358.

113. Newman NJ. Multiple sclerosis and related demyelinating diseases. In: Miller NR, Newman NJ, eds. Walsh and Hoyt's clinical neuro-ophthalmology, 5th ed. Baltimore, MD: Williams & Wilkins; 1998: 5539–5676.

114. Rizzo JF, Andreoli CM, Rabinov JD. Use of magnetic resonance imaging to differentiate optic neuritis and nonarteritic anterior ischemic optic neuropathy. Ophthalmology 2002; 109: 1679–1684.

115. Rizzo JF, Lessell S. Risk of developing multiple sclerosis after uncomplicated optic neuritis: a long-term prospective study. Arch Ophthalmol 1991; 109: 1668–1672.

116. Ebers GC, Cousin HK, Feasby TE et al. Optic neuritis in familial MS. Neurology 1981; 31: 1138–1142.

117. Engelken JD, Yuh WT, Carter KD et al. Optic nerve sarcoidosis: MR findings. J Neuroradiol 1992; 13: 228–230.

118. Tesar JT, McMillan V, Molina R et al. Optic neuropathy and central nervous system disease associated with primary Sjögren's syndrome. Am J Med 92: 686–692.

119. Jacobsen DM, Marx JJ, Dlesk A. Frequency and clinical significance of Lyme seropositivity in patients with isolated optic neuritis. Neurology 1991; 41: 706–711.

120. Sweeney BJ, Manji H, Gilson RJ et al. Optic neuritis and HIV-1 infection. J Neurol Neurosurg Psychiatr 1993; 56: 705–707.

121. Nikoskelainen E, Riekkinen P. Optic neuritis – a sign of multiple sclerosis or other diseases of the central nervous system. Acta Neurol Scand 1974; 50: 690–718.

122. Compston DAS, Batchelor JR, Earl CJ et al. Factors influencing the risk of multiple sclerosis developing in patients with optic neuritis. Brain 1978; 101: 495–511.

123. Landy PJ, Innis M, Boyle R et al. Factors likely to affect the development of multiple sclerosis in patients presenting with optic neuritis in a tropical and subtropical area. Clin Exp Neurol 1979; 16: 175–182.

124. Cohen MM, Lessell S, Wolf PA. A prospective study of the risk of developing multiple sclerosis in uncomplicated optic neuritis. Neurology 1979; 29: 208–213.

125. Kinnunen E. The incidence of optic neuritis and its prognosis for multiple sclerosis. Acta Neurol Scand 1983; 68: 371–377.

126. Parkin, PJ, Hierons R, McDonald WI. Bilateral optic neuritis. A long-term follow-up. Brain 1984; 107: 951–964.

127. Hely, MA, McManis PG, Doran TJ, et al. Acute optic neuritis: a prospective study of risk factors for multiple sclerosis. J Neurol Neurosurg Psychiatr 1986; 49: 1125–1130.

128. Francis DA, Compston DA, Batchelor JR et al. A reassessment of the risk of multiple sclerosis developing in patients with optic neuritis after extended follow-up. J Neurol Neurosurg Psychiatr 1987; 50: 758–765.

129. Charcot JM. Leçons sur les maladies du system nerveux faites à la Salpêtrière, 2nd edn. Paris: A Delahaye; 1875.

130. Alusi, SH, Worthington J, Glickman S et al. A study of tremor in multiple sclerosis. Brain 2001; 124: 720–730.

131. Pittock SJ, McClelland RL, Mayr WT et al. Prevalence of tremor in multiple sclerosis and associated disability in the Olmsted County population. Movement Dis 2004; 19: 1482–1485.

132. Berger JR, Sheremata WA, Melamed E. Paroxysmal dystonia as the initial manifestation of multiple sclerosis. Arch Neurol 1984; 41: 747–750.

133. Clifford DB, Trotter JL. Pain in multiple sclerosis. Arch Neurol 1984; 41: 1270–1272.

134. Moulin DE. Pain in multiple sclerosis. Neurol Clin 1989; 7: 321–331.

135. Beiske AG, Pedersen ED, Czujko B et al. Pain and sensory complaints in multiple sclerosis. Eur J Neurol 2004; 11: 479–482.

136. D'Amico D, La Mantia L, Rigamonti A et al. Prevalence of primary headaches in people

with multiple sclerosis. Cephalalgia 2004; 24: 980–984.

137. Rushton JG, Olafson RA. Trigeminal neuralgia associated with multiple sclerosis. A case report. Arch Neurol 1965; 13: 383–386.

138. Twomey JA, Espir ML. Paroxysmal symptoms as the first manifestations of multiple sclerosis. J Neurol Neurosurg Psychiatr 1980; 43: 296–304.

139. Ramirez-Lassepas M, Tulloch JW, Quinones MR et al. Acute radicular pain as a presenting symptom in multiple sclerosis. Arch Neurol 1992; 49: 255–258.

140. Babinski J, Dubois R. Douleurs à forme de décharge electrique, consecutive aux tramatismes de la nuque. Presse Med 26: 64; 1891.

141. Lhermitte J, Bollak G, Nicholas M. Les douleurs a type de décharge electrique consecutives à la flexion céphalique dans la sclerose en plaques. Rev Neurol 1924; 42: 56–62.

142. Hornsten G. The relation of retinal periphlebitis to multiple sclerosis and other neurological disorders. Acta Neurol Scand 1971; 47: 413–425.

143. Rucker CW. Sheathing of the retinal veins in multiple sclerosis. Mayo Clinic Proc 1944; 19: 176–178.

144. Arnold AC, Pepose JS, Hepler RS et al. Retinal periphlebitis and retinitis in multiple sclerosis. I. Pathologic characteristics. Ophthalmology 1984; 91: 255–262.

145. Shaw PJ, Smith NM, Ince PG et al. Chronic periphlebitis retinae in multiple sclerosis: a histopathological study. J Neurol Sci 1987; 77: 147–152.

146. Barnes, D, McDonald WI. The ocular manifestations of multiple sclerosis. 2. Abnormalities of eye movements. J Neurol Neurosurg Psychiatr 1992; 55: 863–868.

147. Bronstein AM, Rudge P, Gresty MA, et al. Abnormalities of horizontal gaze. Clinical, oculographic and magnetic resonance imaging findings. II. Gaze palsy and internuclear ophthalmoplegia. J Neurol Neurosurg Psychiatr 1990; 53: 200–207.

148. Uitti RJ, Rajput AH. Multiple sclerosis presenting as isolated oculomotor nerve palsy. Can J Neurol Sci 1986; 13: 270–272.

149. Newman NJ, Lessell S. Isolated pupil-sparing third-nerve palsy as the presenting sign of multiple sclerosis. Arch Neurol 1990; 47: 817–818.

150. Peters GB, Bakri SJ, Krohel GB. Cause and prognosis of nontraumatic sixth nerve palsies in young adults. Ophthalmology 2002; 109: 1925–1928.

151. Jacobson DM, Moster ML, Eggenberger ER et al. Isolated trochlear nerve palsy in patients with multiple sclerosis. Neurology 1999; 53: 877–879.

152. Reulen JPH, Sanders EACM, Hogenhuis LAH. Eye movement disorders in multiple sclerosis and optic neuritis. Brain 1983; 106: 121–140.

153. Grenman R. Involvement of the audiovestibular system in multiple sclerosis. An otoneurologic and audiologic study. Acta Otolaryngol Suppl 1985; 420: 1–95.

154. Tedeschi G, Allocca S, Di Constanzo A et al. Role of saccadic analysis in the diagnosis of multiple sclerosis in the era of magnetic resonance imaging. J Neurol Neurosurg Psychiatr 1989; 52: 967–969.

155. Charcot JM. Lectures on the diseases of the nervous system. Philadelphia: Henry C Lea, 1879.

156. Dalton EJ, Heinrichs RW. Depression in multiple sclerosis: a quantitative review of the evidence. Neuropsychology 2005, 19: 152–158.

157. Joffe R, Lippert GP, Gray TA et al. Mood disorder and multiple sclerosis. Arch Neurol 1987; 44: 376–378.

158. Ron MA, Logsdail SJ. Psychiatric morbidity in multiple sclerosis: a clinical and MRI study. Psychol Med 1989; 19: 887–895.

159. Silverstone PH. Prevalence of psychiatric disorders in medical inpatients. J Nerv Ment Dis 1996; 184: 43–51.

160. Rabins PV, Brooks BR, O'Connell P et al. Structural brain correlates of emotional disorder in multiple sclerosis. Brain 1986; 109: 585–597.

161. Taillefer SS, Kirmayer LJ, Robbins JM et al. Correlates of illness worry in chronic fatigue syndrome. J Psychosom Res 2003; 54: 331–337.

162. Feinstein A. The neuropsychiatry of multiple sclerosis. Can J Psychiatr 2004; 49: 157–163.

163. Janardhan V, Bakshi R. Quality of life in patients with multiple sclerosis: the impact of fatigue and depression. J Neurol Sci 2002; 205: 51–58.

164. Janssens ACJW, van Doorn PA, de Boer JB et al. Impact of recently diagnosed multiple sclerosis on quality of life, anxiety, depression and distress of patients and partners. Acta Neurol Scand 2003; 108: 389–395.

165. Lobentanz IS, Asenbaum S, Vass K et al. Factors influencing quality of life in multiple sclerosis patients: disability, depressive mood, fatigue and sleep quality. Acta Neurol Scand 2004; 110: 6–13.

166. Sadovnick AD, Eisen K, Ebers GC et al. Cause of death in patients attending multiple sclerosis clinics. Neurology 1991; 42: 1193–1196.

167. Stenager EN, Stenager E, Kock-Henricksen N et al. Suicide and multiple sclerosis: an epidemiological investigation. J Neurol Neurosurg Psychiatr 1992; 55: 542–545.

168. Feinstein A. An examination of suicidal intent in patients with multiple sclerosis. Neurology 2002; 59: 674–678.

169. Feinstein A, Roy P, Labaugh N et al. Structural brain abnormalities in multiple sclerosis patients with major depression. Neurology 2004; 62: 586–590.

170. Mohr DC, Hart SL, Goldberg A. Effects of treatment for depression on fatigue in multiple sclerosis. Psychosom Med 2003; 65: 542–547.

171. Ford H, Trigwell P, Johnson M. The nature of fatigue in multiple sclerosis. J Psychosom Res 1998; 45: 33–38.

172. Siegert RJ, Abernethy DA. Depression in multiple sclerosis: a review. J Neurol Neurosurg Psychiatr 2005; 76: 469–475.

173. Elliott R. The neuropsychological profile in unipolar depression. Trends Cogn Sci 1998; 2: 447–454.

174. Rao SM. Neuropsychology of multiple sclerosis. Curr Opin Neurol 1995; 8: 216–220.

175. Rao SM. Neuropsychology of multiple sclerosis: a critical review. J Clin Exp Neuropsychol 1986; 8: 503–542.

176. Arnett PA, Higginson CI, Voss WD et al. Depression in multiple sclerosis:

relationship to working memory capacity. Neuropsychology 1999; 13: 434–446.

177. Arnett PA, Higginson CI, Randolph JJ. Depression in multiple sclerosis: relationship to planning ability. J Int Neuropsychol Soc 2001; 7: 665–674.

178. Tachibana N, Howard RS, Hirsch NP et al. Sleep problems in multiple sclerosis. Eur Neurol 1994; 34: 320–323.

179. Fleming WE, Pollak CP. Sleep disorders in multiple sclerosis. Sem Neurol 2005; 25: 64–68.

180. Stiasny-Kolster K, Trenkwalder C, Fogel W et al. Restless legs syndrome – new insights into clinical characteristics, pathophysiology, and treatment options. J Neurol 2004; 251(suppl 6): VI39–VI43.

181. Coleman RM, Pollak CP, Weitzman ED. Periodic movements in sleep (nocturnal myoclonus): relation to sleep disorders. Ann Neurol 1980; 8: 416–421.

182. Ferini-Strambi L, Filippi M, Martinelli V et al. Nocturnal sleep study in multiple sclerosis: correlations with clinical and brain magnetic resonance imaging findings. J Neurol Sci 1994; 125: 194–197.

183. Montplaisir J, Lapierre O, Warnes H et al. The treatment of the restless leg syndrome with or without periodic leg movements in sleep. Sleep 1992; 15: 391–395.

184. Lugaresi E, Cirignotta F, Coccagna G et al. Nocturnal myoclonus and restless legs syndrome. Adv Neurol 1986; 43: 295–307.

185. Auer RN, Rowlands CG, Perry SF et al. Multiple sclerosis with medullary plaques and fatal sleep apnea (Ondine's curse). Clin Neuropathol 1996; 15: 101–105.

186. Howard RS, Wiles CM, Hirsch NP et al. Respiratory involvement in multiple sclerosis. Brain 1992; 115: 479–494.

187. Bonduelle M, Degos C. Symptomatic narcolepsies: a critical study. In: Guilleminault C, Dement WC, Passouant P, eds. Narcolepsy. New York: Spectrum; 1976: 322–325.

188. Younger DS, Pedley TA, Thorpy MJ. Multiple sclerosis and narcolepsy: possible similar genetic susceptibility. Neurology 1991; 41: 447–448.

189. Plazzi G, Montagna P. Remitting REM sleep behavior disorder as the initial sign of multiple sclerosis. Sleep Med 2002; 3: 437–439.

190. Zeldowicz L. Paroxysmal motor episodes as early manifestations of multiple sclerosis. Can Med Assoc J 1961; 84: 937–941.

191. Von Hoesslin R. Über multiple Sklerose. Exogene Aetiologie, Pathogenese und Verlauf. Munich: JF Lehmanns Verlag; 1934.

192. McAlpine D, Compston N, Some aspects of the natural history of disseminated sclerosis. Q J Med 1952; 21: 135.

193. McAlpine D Compston N, Lumsden CE. Multiple sclerosis. Edinburgh: E & S Livingstone; 1955.

194. Franklin CR, Brickner RM. Vasospasm associated with multiple sclerosis. Arch Neurol Psychiat 1947; 58: 125–162.

195. Andermann, F, Cosgrove JBR, Lloyd-Smith D et al. Paroxysmal dysarthria and ataxia in multiple sclerosis; a report of 2 unusual cases. Neurology 1959; 9: 211–215.

196. Tüzün E, Akmain-Demir G, Eraksoy M. Paroxysmal attacks in multiple sclerosis. Mult Scler 2001; 7: 402–404.

197. Fontoura P, Vale J, Guimarâres. Symptomatic paroxysmal hemidystonia due to a demyelinating subthalamic lesion. Eur J Neurol 2000; 7: 559–562.

198. De Seze J, Stojkovic T, Destée M et al. Paroxysmal kinesigenic choreoathetosis as a presenting symptom of multiple sclerosis. J Neurol 2000; 247: 478–480.

199. Yoshimura N, Nagahama Y, Ueda T et al. Paroxysmal urinary incontinence associated with multiple sclerosis. Urol Int 1997; 59: 197–199.

200. Andermann F, Cosgrove JBR, Lloyd-Smith DL et al. Facial myokymia in multiple sclerosis. Brain 1961; 64: 31–44.

201. Telischi FF, Grobman LR, Sheremata WA et al. Hemifacial spasm. Occurrence in multiple sclerosis. Arch Otolaryngol Head Neck Surg 1991; 117: 554–556.

202. Thomas FJ, Wiles CM. Dysphagia and nutritional status in multiple sclerosis. J Neurol 1999; 246: 677–682.

203. Calcagno P, Ruoppolo G, Grasso MG et al. Dysphagia in multiple sclerosis – prevalence and prognostic factors. Acta Neurol Scand 2002; 105: 40–43.

204. Herrera WG, Vestibular and other balance disorders in multiple sclerosis. Diagn Neurol 1990; 8: 407–420.

205. McAlpine D, Lumsden CE, Ancherson ED. Multiple sclerosis: a reappraisal, 2nd ed. Edinburgh: Churchill Livingstone; 1972: 83–307.

206. Muller R. Studies on disseminated sclerosis with special reference to symptomatology, course and prognosis. Acta Med Scand 1949; 133(suppl): 1–124.

207. Francis D, Bronstein AM, Rudge P et al. The site of brainstem lesions causing semicircular canal paresis: an MRI study. J Neurol Neurosurg Psychiatr 1992; 55: 446–449.

208. Brandt T, Dieterich M. Preliminary classification of vestibular brainstem disorders. In Caplan LR, Hopf HC, eds. Brainstem localization and function. Berlin: Springer; 1993: 79–91.

209. Lawden MC, Bronstein AM, Kennard C. Repetitive paroxysmal nystagmus and vertigo. Neurology 1995; 45: 276–280.

210. Gass A, Steinke W, Schwartz A et al. High resolution magnetic resonance imaging in peripheral vestibular dysfunction in multiple sclerosis. J Neurol Neurosurg Psychiatr 1998; 65: 945.

211. Thomke F, Hopf HC. Pontine lesions mimicking acute peripheral vestibulopathy. J Neurol Neurosurg Psychiatr 1999; 66: 340–349.

212. Frohman EM, Kramer PD, Dewey RB et al. Benign paroxysmal positioning vertigo in multiple sclerosis: diagnosis, pathophysiology and therapeutic techniques. Mult Scler 2003; 9: 250–255.

213. Frohman EM, Zhang H, Dewey RB, Hawker K. Vertigo in MS: utility of positional and particle repositioning maneuvers. Neurology 2000; 55: 1566–1568.

214. Boucher RM, Hendrix RA. The otolaryngic manifestations of multiple sclerosis. Ear Nose Throat J 1991; 70: 224–233.

215. Daugherty WT, Lederman RJ, Nodar RH et al. Hearing loss in multiple sclerosis. Arch Neurol 1983; 40: 33–35.

216. Poser CM, Brinar VV. Epilepsy and multiple sclerosis. Epilepsy Behav 2003; 4: 6–12.

217. Bau-Prussak S, Prussak L. Über epileptische Anfale bei der multipler Sklerose. Z Ges Neurol Psychiatr 1929; 122: 510.

218. Drake W, Macrae D. Epilepsy in multiple sclerosis. Neurology 1961; 11: 810–816.

219. Engelsen B, Gronning M. Epileptic seizures in patients with multiple sclerosis. Is the prognosis of epilepsy underestimated? Seizure 1997; 6: 377–382.

220. Thompson A, Kermode A, Moseley I et al. Seizures due to multiple sclerosis: seven patients with MRI correlations. J Neurol Neurosurg Psychiatr 1993; 56: 1317–1320.

221. Fuglsang-Frederiksen V, Thygesen P. Seizures and psychopathology in multiple sclerosis. Acta Psychiat Neurol Scand 1952; 27: 17–41.

222. Zavalishin I, Nevskaia O. Epileptic seizures in multiple sclerosis patients. Zh Nevropatol Psikhiat 1984; 84: 868–871.

223. Buttner T, Hornig C, Dorndorf W. Multiple sclerosis and epilepsy. An analysis of 14 case histories Nervenarzt 1989; 60: 262–267.

224. Sokic D, Stojsavljevic N, Drulovic J et al. Seizures in multiple sclerosis. Epilepsia 1999; 40: 745–747.

225. Kinnunen E, Wikstrom J. Prevalence and prognosis of epilepsy in patients with multiple sclerosis. Epilepsia 1986; 27: 729–733.

226. Ghezzi A, Montanini R, Basso P et al. Epilepsy in multiple sclerosis. Eur Neurol 1990; 30: 218–223.

227. Striano P, Orefice G, Brescia et al. Epileptic seizures in multiple sclerosis: clinical and EEG correlations. Neurol Sci 2003; 24: 322–328.

228. Sadovnick AD, Eisen K, Ebers GC et al. Cause of death in patients attending multiple sclerosis clinics. Neurology 1991; 41: 1193–1196.

229. Phadke JG. Survival pattern and cause of death in patients with multiple sclerosis: results from an epidemiological survey in north east Scotland. J Neurol Neurosurg Psychiatr 1987; 50: 523–531.

230. Midgard R, Riise T, Kvale G et al. Disability and mortality in multiple sclerosis in western Norway. Acta Neurol Scand 1996; 93: 307–314.

231. Smeltzer SC, Utell MJ, Rudic RA et al. Pulmonary function and dysfunction in multiple sclerosis. Arch Neurol 1988; 45: 1245–1249.

232. Foglio K, Clini E, Facchetti D et al. Respiratory muscle function and exercise capacity in multiple sclerosis. Eur Respir J 1994; 7: 23–28.

233. Smeltzer SC, Skurnick JH, Troiano R. Pulmonary function and dysfunction in multiple sclerosis. Chest 1992; 101: 479–484.

234. Buyse B, Demedts M, Meekers J et al. Respiratory dysfunction in multiple sclerosis: a prospective analysis of 60 patients. Eur Respir J 1997; 10: 139–145.

235. De Troyer A, Borenstein S, Cordier R. Analysis of lung volume restriction in patients with respiratory muscle weakness. Thorax 1980; 35: 603–610.

236. Baydur A. Respiratory muscle strength and control of ventilation in patients with neuromuscular disease. Chest 1991; 99: 330–338.

237. Vincken W, Elleker MG, Cosio MG. Determinants of respiratory muscle weakness in stable chronic neuromuscular disorders. Am J Med 1987; 82: 53–58.

238. Gosselink R, Kovacs L, Decramer, M. Respiratory muscle involvement in multiple sclerosis. Eur Respir J 1999; 13: 449–454.

239. Howard RS, Wiles CM, Hirsch NP et al. Respiratory involvement in multiple sclerosis. Brain 1992; 115: 479–494.

240. Carter JL, Noseworthy JH. Ventilatory dysfunction in multiple sclerosis. Clin Chest Med 1994; 15: 693–703.

241. Hennessy A, Robertson NP, Swingler R et al. Urinary, faecal and sexual dysfunction in patients with multiple sclerosis. J Neurol 1999; 246: 1027–1032.

242. Drory VE, Nisipeanu PF, Kroczyn AD. Tests of autonomic dysfunction in patients with multiple sclerosis. Acta Neurol Scand 1995; 92: 356–360.

243. Ferrini-Strambi L, Rovaris M, Oldani A et al. Cardiac autonomic function during sleep and wakefulness in multiple sclerosis. J Neurol 1995; 42: 639–643.

244. Flachenecker P, Wolf A, Krauser M et al. Cardiovascular autonomic dysfunction in multiple sclerosis: correlation with orthostatic intolerance. J Neurol 1999; 246: 578–586.

245. Linden D, Diehl RR, Berlit P. Subclinical autonomic disturbances in multiple sclerosis. J Neurol 1995; 242: 374–378.

246. Vita G, Fazio MC, Milone S et al. Cardiovascular autonomic dysfunction in multiple sclerosis is likely related to brainstem lesions. J Neurol Sci 1993; 120: 82–86.

247. Anema JR, Heijenbrok MW, Faes TJC et al. Cardiovascular autonomic function in multiple sclerosis. J Neurol Sci 1991; 104: 129–134.

248. Giubilei F, Vitale A, Urani C et al. Cardiac autonomic dysfunction in relapsing–remitting multiple sclerosis during a stable phase. Eur Neurol 1996; 36: 211–214.

249. Acevedo AR, Nava C, Arriada N et al. Cardiovascular dysfunction in multiple sclerosis. Acta Neurol Scand 2000; 101: 85–88.

250. De Seze J, Stojkovic T, Gauvrit J-Y et al. Autonomic dysfunction in multiple sclerosis: cervical spinal cord atrophy correlates. J Neurol 2001; 248: 297–303.

251. Saari A, Tolonen U, Pääkkö E et al. Cardiovascular autonomic dysfunction correlates with brain MRI lesion load in MS. Clin Neurophysiol 2004; 115: 1473–1478.

252. Apple D, Kreines K, Biechl JP. The syndrome of inappropriate antidiuretic hormone secretion in multiple sclerosis. Arch Intern Med 1978; 138: 1713–1714.

253. Sakai N, Miyajima H, Shimizu T et al. Syndrome of inappropriate secretion of antidiuretic hormone associated with multiple sclerosis. Intern Med 1992; 31: 463–466.

254. Ishikawa E, Ohgo S, Nakatsuru K et al. Syndrome of inappropriate secretion of antidiuretic hormone (SIADH) in a patient with multiple sclerosis. Jpn J Med 1989; 28: 75–79.

255. Liamis G, Elisaf M. Syndrome of inappropriate antidiuresis associated with multiple sclerosis. J Neurol Sci 2000; 172: 38–40.

Unusual presentations and variants of idiopathic central nervous system demyelinating diseases

D. M. Wingerchuk and B. G. Weinshenker

Multiple sclerosis (MS) and other central nervous system (CNS) demyelinating syndromes have been described using the umbrella term 'idiopathic inflammatory demyelinating diseases' (IIDDs).[1] We will explore acute, typically monophasic forms of CNS demyelination including acute disseminated encephalomyelitis (ADEM), tumefactive presentations, the Marburg variant and Baló's concentric sclerosis (BCS). Typical MS, including relapsing–remitting and primary and secondary progressive courses, is discussed elsewhere. Clinically isolated syndromes that often herald typical MS, such as optic neuritis (ON) and transverse myelitis (TM), are also reviewed in a separate chapter but we will discuss the recurrent forms of ON and TM as part of the neuromyelitis optica (NMO) spectrum of disorders. After reviewing the distinguishing clinical and pathological features of each syndrome, we will discuss their distinction from typical MS and recent advances in diagnosis and management. The differential diagnosis and approach to acute leukoencephalopathies is beyond the scope of this chapter; for a concise review, see Weinshenker and Lucchinetti.[2]

OVERVIEW AND NOSOLOGY

There are several potential methods for classifying IIDDs. The most recent diagnostic guidelines for MS, best known as the McDonald criteria, focus on establishing that CNS white matter disease is disseminated in time and space.[3] Such criteria have limited utility when applied to the diagnosis of acute, tumor-like clinical presentations, acute monophasic leukoencephalopathies or progressive entities. One might categorize them by acuity of clinical onset, clinical severity, course (monophasic, relapsing or progressive), rate of progression, topographic distribution within the CNS (focal, site-restricted or disseminated) and pathological features. Table 3.1 outlines one schema based on clinical severity, distribution and progression rate. The early establishment of a firm diagnosis may, in some instances, require a tissue biopsy or observation of the clinical response to corticosteroid therapy. In many circumstances, a period of observation to determine whether disease relapses occur is essential for classification. For example, clinical behavior over time determines the level of confidence in a diagnosis of mono-phasic ADEM, the evolution of ON or TM from monophasic to recurrent disease, or conversion to NMO.

MONOPHASIC FOCAL CEREBRAL EVENTS: 'TUMEFACTIVE' DEMYELINATING LESIONS

'Tumefactive (tumor-like) MS', unlike the pathologically based BCS, is a descriptive clinical diagnosis. The adjective 'tumefactive' has been applied to situations involving multiple large cerebral lesions with mass effect or a single large lesion in the context of known MS.[4–9] However, the most vexing clinical situation is a first-ever, solitary white matter lesion that causes uncertainty because of its similarity to a primary brain neoplasm on both clinical and neuroimaging grounds.[7,9–11] Any of these scenarios may require diagnostic biopsy; this has been an important source of pathological material for sophisticated immunohistochemical studies such as the MS Lesion Project. The natural history of these disorders is quite variable since they can occur in the context of typical MS. In at least some cases of solitary tumefactive lesions, the clinical course remains monophasic for 5 years or longer.[8]

There has been a recent proliferation of reports describing advanced imaging techniques that may discriminate focal demyelinating disease from neoplasm. On conventional brain magnetic resonance imaging (MRI), demyelinating lesions are more likely than tumors or abscesses to exhibit large size yet little mass effect or edema, an 'open-ring' pattern of gadolinium enhancement (confined to the side of the lesion facing white matter) (Fig. 3.1B), and more rapid improvement after therapy.[12–15] Nonconventional techniques such as contrast-enhanced T2*-weighted MRI,[16] proton magnetic resonance spectroscopy (MRS),[15,17–20] diffusion and perfusion imaging,[17,21] and magnetization transfer imaging[12,15,17] have been explored. The enhanced T2*-weighted technique allows measurement of cerebral blood volume that complement standard anatomical MRI data. Therefore, it may be useful for detecting relatively lower vascularity of demyelinating lesions compared to neoplasms; in one study, this technique was also able to demonstrate multiple linear vascular structures in tumefactive lesions that were not present in neoplasms.[16] Reduced magnetization ratio has been noted in

TABLE 3.1 Spectrum of idiopathic inflammatory demyelinating diseases of the central nervous system

Disorder	Recognition method	Spatial distribution	Typical severity	Course	Duration	Attack-related impairment
Tumefactive lesions	Clinical, MRI	Focal, cerebral	+ to +++	Monophasic	Days to weeks	None to severe
Marburg's MS	Clinical, MRI	Multifocal, cerebral	++++	Monophasic	Days to weeks	Severe to death
Baló's concentric sclerosis	MRI, pathology	Focal/multifocal, cerebral	++++	Monophasic or relapsing	Days to weeks	Moderate to death
ADEM	Clinical, MRI	Multifocal/diffuse, cerebral, cord, ON	++ to +++	Monophasic or oligophasic	Days to weeks	Mild-severe
NMO	Clinical, MRI, NMO-IgG	ON, spinal cord	+++	80% relapsing 20% monopasic	Usually chronic	Moderate to severe
Recurrent ON	Clinical, MRI, NMO-IgG	ON	++ to +++	Relapsing	Chronic	Moderate
Recurrent TM	Clinical, MRI, NMO-IgG	Spinal cord	+++	Relapsing	Chronic	Moderate to severe
RRMS	Clinical, MRI, CSF	Cerebral, ON, cord	+ to +++	Relapsing, >60% SP	Chronic	None to moderate
PPMS	Clinical, MRI, CSF	Spinal cord, cerebral	++	Progressive from onset	Chronic	N/A

ADEM, acute disseminated encephalomyelitis; CSF, cerebrospinal fluid; MRI, magnetic resonance imaging; MS, multiple sclerosis; NMO, neuromyelitis optica; ON, optic neuritis; PPMS, primary progressive multiple sclerosis; RRMS, relapsing–remitting multiple sclerosis; TM, transverse myelitis; SP, secondary progressive.

demyelinating lesions, a gradient of reduction that is maximal at the lesion center may suggest demyelination rather than neoplasm.[12,17] Reduced or normal perfusion in a lesion, especially in an area of gadolinium enhancement, favors demyelination, since malignancies are usually associated with hypervascularity and increased regional blood flow.[17,21] Proton MRS findings have been advocated in differentiating these lesions but there is substantial overlap in spectral findings.[15,18–20]

The usual approach to these syndromes includes a search for secondary causes of white matter disease, determining the likelihood of an IIDD based on prior clinical history and diagnosis and current neuroimaging and cerebrospinal fluid (CSF) results, and then proceeding with either biopsy or empiric corticosteroid therapy with observation of post-treatment response.[2] The mainstays of treatment for mass-like demyelinating lesions are intravenous corticosteroids; if there is no clinical response, plasmapheresis (a total of seven exchanges performed every other day for 2 weeks) may be beneficial.[22–24] Plasmapheresis appears beneficial for patients with immunopathological evidence suggesting a humoral contribution to their lesion,[25] a feature currently identifiable only by procuring CNS tissue.

MONOPHASIC MULTIFOCAL/ DISSEMINATED DISORDERS

These include the Marburg and Baló forms of CNS demyelinating disease and the various forms of perivenous encephalomyelitis, including ADEM.

MARBURG'S ACUTE MULTIPLE SCLEROSIS

The term 'Marburg multiple sclerosis' denotes an acute, monophasic demyelinating syndrome that rapidly worsens and typically leads to death from a herniation syndrome or brain stem dysfunction. Otto Marburg's original case description from 1906 details the clinical course of a 30-year-old woman who developed

acute confusion, headache, vomiting, left hemiparesis and gait disorder progressing to death 26 days after onset.[26] Very few cases were reported until Mendez and Pogacar described a case quite similar to Marburg's in 1988;[27] theirs was a previously healthy 25-year-old man who experienced vertigo, nausea, vomiting, ataxia, confusion, and left hemiparesis and sensory impairment. Computed tomography (CT) imaging showed bilateral white matter hypodensities and focal contrast enhancement and CSF revealed a moderate pleocytosis (25 white blood cells (WBC); 88% lymphocytes, 6% monocytes and 6% polymorphonuclear leukocytes) with elevated myelin basic protein and IgG but negative oligoclonal banding. Despite high-dose intravenous methylprednisolone and dexamethasone, adrenocorticotropic hormone (ACTH) and azathioprine, he developed decerebrate posturing and coma with focal seizures and died 19 days after disease onset. Autopsy showed brain swelling with uncal and cerebellar tonsil herniation and 'abundant' demyelinating plaques in the cerebral white matter (including periventricular lesions), pontine tegmentum and cerebellar peduncle. A few lesions demonstrated a 'concentric demyelination–myelination pattern' (as did Marburg's original case; see section on BSC below). Individual lesions showed myelin loss with relative axonal preservation, numerous macrophages and myelin breakdown products, and some perivascular lymphocytic and plasma cell infiltration (although perivenous demyelination was rare).

Most cases reported over the last two decades describe remarkably similar findings, although some reports have noted CSF oligoclonal banding.[28–31] Widespread, destructive plaques consisting of either large individual lesions, multiple small foci that coalesce as the disorder progresses, or both, affect the cerebral white matter and may also involve the brain stem, spinal cord and optic nerves. Confluent lesions, often associated with gadolinium enhancement in an 'open-ring' pattern, are readily seen on brain MRI (Fig. 3.1). Microscopically, some lesions demonstrate necrosis in the context of severe macrophage infiltration along with astrogliosis.[29] One detailed pathological study of lesions from a patient who died 6 weeks from clinical onset

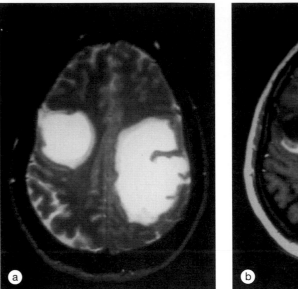

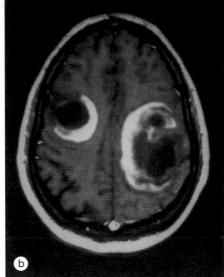

FIG. 3.1 A. T2-weighted axial brain MRI study demonstrating Marburg MS lesions. **B.** Post-gadolinium T1-weighted images demonstrating an open-ring pattern of enhancement.

suggested that a developmentally immature form of myelin basic protein (MBP) is associated with the Marburg variant.[28] MBP derived from uninvolved white matter from an autopsy specimen was slightly larger (accounted for, in part, by the deimination of 18 of 19 arginyl residues to citrulline) and much less cationic than normal MBP. The authors interpreted this as being consistent with a genetic influence and with the concept that the less cationic MBP could not normally compact multi-layered myelin. More recent immunopathological studies suggest that immunoglobulin binding (especially IgG) and complement activation occur in regions of active demyelination, and that antibodies mediate some or all of the demyelinating process at those sites.[32,33]

There have been case reports of 'Marburg' variant MS in which the course was polyphasic or in which acute, severe, multifocal white matter lesions evolved in the course of what had otherwise behaved as typical MS.[34] These cases introduce heterogeneity to the diagnostic term that may or may not be valid; however, to date, there have been no convincing pathological or immunological differences reported between Marburg disease and MS.

The Marburg form of MS is typically refractory to treatment with corticosteroids but there have been case reports indicating clinical response to plasmapheresis (including one patient in a controlled trial of true versus sham procedures)[22,23,35] and to mitoxantrone in combination with repeated intravenous methylprednisolone courses.[30,36]

BALÓ'S CONCENTRIC SCLEROSIS

Baló's concentric sclerosis is considered to be an MS variant but the term is reserved for cases in which there is pathological evidence of large lesions with a concentric pattern of alternating layers of preserved and destroyed myelin.[37] It is usually associated with acute, severe clinical events, similar to Marburg's acute MS. As noted above, Marburg's original report described this pattern. Baló, more than 20 years later, reported a patient with large hemispheric white matter lesions consisting entirely of the alternating layers that thereafter carried his eponymous designation.[38,39] The first antemortem diagnosis was reported in 1986, based on biopsy results.[40] In 1988, the first report of

a case with both MRI and pathological confirmation appeared.[41] Brain MRI has allowed identification of the concentric lesion pattern in cases that later developed a more favorable course than expected[42-44] and even in the context of rather typical MS.[26,45] Therefore, BCS and Baló-like lesions represent a recognizable radiological and pathological lesion pattern rather than a clinical entity with a predictable outcome.

The MRI characteristics of BCS lesions using standard T2-weighted or fluid-attenuated inversion-recovery (FLAIR) techniques are hyperintense rings (associated with myelin destruction) alternating with normal-appearing white matter.[40,43-51] The demyelinated lamellae appear hypointense on T1-weighted imaging. Pathologically, the alternating rings surround the so-called 'storm center', may appear quite regular or irregular, with lamellae of various thicknesses, and can occur in the spinal cord as well as the brain.[52] All BCS lesions seem to conform to 'pattern III' pathology as described by Lucchinetti and colleagues.[53] This pattern is associated with oligodendrocyte apoptosis and 'dying back' and does not contain either immunoglobulin deposition or activated complement, although one report did suggest coexisting complement reactivity in a single case.[54]

The pathophysiogical explanation for concentric demyelination in BCS is unknown. Hypotheses have included precipitation of an unknown toxin or lecithinolytic factor (H-Spatz), hypoxia and cyanide-like mechanisms. One report indicated that the rings might be accounted for by substantial remyelination occurring within plaques.[52] Two subsequent case series, however, have demonstrated either minimal remyelination or that remyelinating oligodendrocytes are detectable in both the demyelinated and preserved areas.[55,56] A recent summary of immunopathological findings from 14 BCS cases revealed that active concentric lesions show a pattern of demyelination that resembles hypoxia-like tissue injury with increased expression of inducible nitric oxide synthase in macrophages and microglia. At the lesion edges, and sometimes in the outermost layer of preserved myelin, proteins implicated in tissue preconditioning, such as hypoxia-inducible factor 1α and heat-shock protein 70, were expressed in oligodendrocytes and to some degree in astrocytes and macrophages. The investigators hypothesized that the initial inflammatory reaction causes excessive local production of substances that induce 'histotoxic hypoxia', which, in turn, causes myelin and axonal destruction. Sublethal tissue injury at the lesion edge may induce tissue preconditioning, a physiological response, but the severe and rapidly progressive lesion overruns this preconditioned edge, causing a new layer of demyelination and the process repeats itself, resulting in the concentric ring pattern.

ACUTE DISSEMINATED ENCEPHALOMYELITIS AND VARIANTS

The ADEM spectrum of disorders includes several monophasic clinical syndromes linked by the common pathological thread of perivenous demyelination. These include idiopathic ADEM, postinfectious encephalomyelitis, postvaccinial encephalomyelitis and acute hemorrhagic leukoencephalomyelitis (AHLE).[57] We will summarize the clinical, laboratory and pathological evidence supporting the existence of various ADEM subtypes and features that assist in differentiating ADEM from MS. Clinicians must appreciate that it is impossible to confidently distinguish ADEM from MS at presentation due to overlap of these syndromes. The relationship of ADEM syndromes to MS is not clear, as evidenced by so-called 'multiphasic' ADEM (MDEM) and 'relapsing' ADEM, as well as pathological 'transitional' forms with features of both ADEM and MS.

There are no validated clinical diagnostic criteria for ADEM.[57,58] Described cases are typically children (especially infants) or young adults with focal or multifocal neurological symptoms and signs coinciding with an acute meningoencephalitic syndrome.[59–63] Childhood cases are usually preceded by a febrile illness or exanthem (postinfectious ADEM) or an immunization (postvaccinial ADEM).[57,59–61,63] However, an antecedent event is not necessary to establish the diagnosis and objective evidence implicating a specific causative agent is often absent. Table 3.2 lists several infection, vaccine and other associations;

many of these associations emerge from single case reports or small case series and their respective agents are not proven as being causative rather than coincidental.[64] However, the association of ADEM with measles, rubella, mumps, varicella and vaccinia appears to be quite firm.[65,66] Prior to measles, varicella and rubella vaccination programs, ADEM was estimated to account for up to 30% of all encephalitis cases.[67] Lethal cases of ADEM have followed measles and smallpox vaccinations. Recent case reports or series have expanded the spectrum of ADEM triggered by infections (parainfluenza virus, Pontiac fever, *Chlamydophila* (formerly *Chlamydia*) *pneumoniae*, *Legionella pneumophila*, dengue fever, *Pasteurella multocida*, *Leptospira* spp. and *Campylobacter* spp.),[68–75] immunizations (vaccinia, hepatitis B, tetanus and meningococcus A and C immunizations)[76–79] and a variety of miscellaneous causes (bee sting, parenteral use of herbal extracts, snake bite, liver transplantation).[80–83] The sporadic nature of ADEM makes epidemiological studies challenging; one group estimated the incidence in a California county as 0.4 cases per 100 000 population annually.[84]

The cause of ADEM syndromes is not known. Attempts to demonstrate the presence of virus, viral antigens or viral nucleic acid in affected neural tissue have failed, and the absence of pathological findings of viral infection suggests that CNS infection is not the direct cause.[37] A latent interval between infection or immunization and the onset of the neurological illness and the presence of pathological changes similar to those observed in acute experimental autoimmune encephalomyelitis induced by immunization with white matter or myelin support an autoimmune etiology.[85–87] Autoimmunity may be triggered by several mechanisms, including molecular mimicry, bystander activation, epitope spreading and mistaken self.[88,89]

The diagnosis of ADEM remains primarily clinical and has not been standardized. Recent retrospective case series[59–62] and one prospective study[63] used quite varied ADEM case definitions (Table 3.3), none of which required a prodromal or triggering illness. The most loosely defined criteria required acute neurological symptoms in association with undefined brain MRI white matter abnormalities 'compatible with ADEM' or no MRI at all.[59,60] More recent series in children and adults specifically required first-ever neurological events with white matter lesions and no evidence of prior white matter involvement (although this is not well-defined). The results of these studies suggest that the broad spectrum of clinical and MRI findings in ADEM and their overlap with MS may hinder the development of any more precise diagnostic criteria until the discovery of a biological marker for either entity.

The diagnosis of ADEM is more commonly considered in children than in adults. About two-thirds of children experience an infectious illness during the month preceding neurological symptoms, often in the form of a typical exanthem, and there may be a slight male preponderance (Table 3.4).[59–61,63] The clinical and laboratory features are summarized in Table 3.5. Symptoms and signs depend upon lesion number, distribution and severity but generally evolve over several days.[59–63,90,91] Focal or multifocal pyramidal signs, ataxia, cranial neuropathies and unilateral or bilateral optic neuritis are common while myelitis is clinically evident in about one-quarter of cases. Less common features include aphasia and involuntary movements. The most common meningoencephalitic presentation is impairment of consciousness, sometimes progressing to coma often accompanied by headache, fever and seizures. Behavioral and sleep disturbances may occur, including psychosis (which may lead to an incorrect diagnosis of conversion disorder), hypersomnia and narcolepsy.[92–98] Respiratory failure secondary to suppressed level of consciousness or cervical myelitis occurs in 11–16%. Cumulative data from most case series suggest that adult ADEM

TABLE 3.2 Infections and immunizations associated with acute disseminated encephalomyelitis

Viral infections	
Measles	Hepatitis A or B
Mumps	Herpes simplex
Rubella	Human herpes virus-6
Varicella	Epstein–Barr virus
Influenza A or B	Cytomegalovirus
Rocky mountain spotted fever	Vaccinia
HTLV-1	Parainfluenza
Dengue fever	
Bacterial or spirochetal infections	
Mycoplasma pneumoniae	*Campylobacter*
Chlamydophila	*Streptococcus*
Legionella	*Pasteurella multocida*
Pontiac fever	*Leptospira*
Immunizations	
Rabies	Measles
Diphtheria–tetanus–polio	Japanese B encephalitis
Smallpox	Hog vaccine
Vaccinia	Hepatitis B
Meningococcus A and C	Tetanus

TABLE 3.3 Definitions of acute disseminated encephalomyelitis in recent case series

	Dale et al 2000	Hynson et al 2001	Murthy et al 2002	Tenembaum et al 2002	Schwarz et al 2001
Study sample age	Pediatric	Pediatric	Pediatric	Pediatric	Adult
Clinical inclusion	Monophasic event of disseminated CNS demyelination	Acute neurological disturbance	Acute neurological signs and symptoms	Presumed inflammatory demyelinating event with acute or subacute onset affecting multifocal areas of the CNS; polysymptomatic	Acute neurological symptoms
Clinical exclusion	Preceding neurological abnormality Isolated ON or TM Infection/other inflammatory disease	Not stated	Not stated	History of symptoms suggesting earlier demyelinating episode Isolated acute ON or TM	Preceding unexplained neurological symptoms Isolated TM or unilateral ON
MRI inclusion	None	Brain MRI white matter changes in a distribution consistent with ADEM	MRI evidence of multifocal, hyperintense lesions on FLAIR and T2-weighted MRI	White matter changes on brain-spinal imaging without radiological evidence of a previous destructive white matter process	One or multiple supra- or infratentorial demyelinating lesions and absence of T1 black holes
Laboratory	None	None	None	None	CSF analysis excludes infection, vasculitis, autoimmune disease

ADEM, acute disseminated encephalomyelitis; CSF, cerebrospinal fluid; CNS, central nervous system; ON, optic neuritis; TM, transverse myelitis; MRI, magnetic resonance imaging; FLAIR, fluid-attenuated inversion recovery (MRI technique).
Source: with permission from Wingerchuk 2003.[57]

TABLE 3.4 Study and patient sample features from five acute disseminated encephalomyelitis series

	Dale et al 2000	Hynson et al 2001	Murthy et al 2002	Tenembaum et al 2002	Schwarz et al 2001
Study sample	Pediatric	Pediatric	Pediatric	Pediatric	Adult
Country of origin	UK	Australia	USA	Argentina	Germany
Patients, n	35	31	18	84	26
Age range, years	3–15	2–16	2.5–22	0.4–16	19–61
Female sex, n (%)	16 (46)	18 (58)	7 (39)	30 (36)	17 (65)
Antecedent infection, n (%)	22 (63)	24 (77)	13 (72)	52 (62)	12 (46)
Antecedent vaccination, n (%)	2 (6)	2 (6)	0	10 (12)	0
Mean (range) days prodrome to onset of ADEM	13 (2–31)	Not stated	10 (range not stated)	12 (2–30)	Not stated
Seasonal occurrence	Winter	No	Winter and spring	Not stated	Not stated
Mean (range), days ADEM onset to nadir	7.1 (1–31)	4.2 (1–42)	<1 week from hospitalization	4.5 (1–45)	4* (0–14)

*Value represents median time from prodrome until hospital admission.
ADEM, acute disseminated encephalomyelitis.
Source: with permission from Wingerchuk 2003.[57]

generally parallels that of children (Tables 3.4 and 3.5). Some differences include preponderance of females (65%), lower frequency of clinically evident antecedent infection (46% versus 62–77% in children) and less frequent coinciding acute meningoencephalitic syndrome. Notably, these features are also more characteristic of typical MS.

The preceding infectious agent or vaccination does not seem to cause a recognizable discrete syndrome in most cases. Recently, however, group A β-hemolytic streptococcal pharyngitis has been linked to the presence of elevated antibasal ganglia antibody titers and a syndrome, distinct from rheumatic fever or Sydenham's chorea, of impaired consciousness or pyramidal

TABLE 3.5 Clinical and laboratory features from five acute disseminated encephalomyelitis series

	Dale et al 2000	Hynson et al 2001	Murthy et al 2002	Tenembaum et al 2002	Schwarz et al 2001
Study sample	Pediatric	Pediatric	Pediatric	Pediatric	Adult
Meningoencephalitic features, %					
Fever	43	52	39	Not stated	15
Headache	58	45	23	32	Not stated
Meningism	31	26	6	43	15
Alteration of consciousness	69	74	45	69	19 (loss of consciousness)
Focal neurological features, %					
ON	23 (all bilateral)	13	Unclear	23	Not stated
Cranial neuropathy	51	45	23 (includes ON)	44	Not stated
Pyramidal/focal motor signs	71	23	39	85	77
Sensory deficit	17	3	28	Unclear	65
Aphasia/language disturbance	0	26	6	21	8
Seizure	17	13	17	35	4
Ataxia	49	65	39	50	38
Movement disorder	3	Not stated	Not stated	12	Not stated
Spinal cord syndrome	23	Not stated	Unclear	24	15
Cerebrospinal fluid, %					
Pleocytosis	64	62	39	28 (combined with protein)	81
Elevated protein level	60	48	55	28 (combined with pleocytosis)	Not stated
Oligoclonal bands present	29	3	13	4	58

Source: with permission from Wingerchuk 2003.[57]

weakness with a prominent dystonic/extrapyramidal syndrome (70%) or behavioral disorder such as emotional lability or inappropriate speech (50%).[99]

Cerebrospinal fluid results are summarized in Table 3.5. Most often, a lymphocytic pleocytosis of several hundred cells is detected in conjunction with an elevated total protein level. The frequency of unique CSF oligoclonal bands is generally low in children (3–29%) but more common in adult ADEM even after prolonged follow-up (58%) and those who have their diagnosis revised to clinically definite MS (80%).[59–63]

Early descriptions of brain MRI abnormalities in ADEM emphasized the presence of large, reasonably symmetric, multifocal, primarily subcortical cerebral white matter lesions that uniformly enhanced after gadolinium administration. Recent large clinical case series clarify the relative frequency of various MRI characteristics (Table 3.6). First, there is significant overlap between ADEM and MS, with up to 60% of ADEM cases revealing periventricular lesions and up to 29% demonstrating callosal abnormalities on follow-up examinations.[59–63] Approximately half of cases present with no gadolinium-enhancing lesions. Bilateral symmetric thalamic or basal ganglia lesions (Fig. 3.2), present in about 15% of patients, are more suggestive of ADEM than of MS or AHLE and are even more common (80%) in those children with the group A streptococcus-associated subtype.[99,100] Serial brain MRI studies performed several months after clinical improvement may reveal partial or complete lesion resolution without new lesion development in monophasic cases.[101] Exceptional case reports describe unusual imaging characteristics such as normal initial brain scan,[102] normal scan followed by the development of lesions during clinical

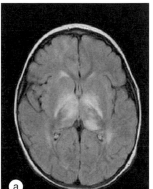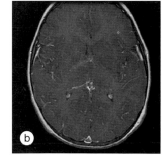

FIG. 3.2 A. T2-weighted axial brain MRI demonstrating deep gray lesions in a child with ADEM. **B**. Post-gadolinium T1-weighted images revealing mild enhancement.

recovery,[103] lesions in the deep gray matter[104] or thalami,[105,106] a solitary lesion restricted to an area such as the brainstem,[107,108] or the presence of multiple cystic lesions[109] or ring-enhancing lesions with mass effect.[110,111]

Preliminary and limited MRS, diffusion- and perfusion-weighted MRI and positron emission tomography findings have been reported in ADEM cases. Diffusion tensor MR studies confirm that the basal ganglia are affected in ADEM but not MS and that 'normal appearing' white matter in ADEM is indeed spared.[112–118] It is unclear whether any of these imaging

TABLE 3.6 Magnetic resonance imaging characteristics of acute disseminated encephalomyelitis

	Dale et al 2000	Hynson et al 2001	Murthy et al 2002	Tenembaum et al 2002	Schwarz et al 2001
No. with MRI (% of total)	32 (91)	31 (100)	15 (83)	79 (94)	26 (100)
Lesion site, % of those with MRI					
White matter	91	90	93	Not stated	100
Periventricular	44	29	60	Not stated	54
Corpus callosum	Not stated	29	7 (splenium)	Not stated	23
Subcortical/deep	91	80	93	Not stated	38
Cortical gray matter	12	Not stated	80	Not stated	8
Brainstem	56	42	47	Not stated	57
Cerebellum	31	Not stated	13	Not stated	31
Thalamus	41	32	27	13 (bilateral, symmetric)	15 (includes basal ganglia)
Basal ganglia	28	39	20	Not stated	15 (includes thalamus)
Spinal cord	*n* not stated (28)	4/6 (67)	5/7 (71)	Not stated	Not stated
Gadolinium enhancement (%)	Not stated	8/28 (29)	7/15 (47)	10/27 (37)	20/21 (95)
Follow-up brain MRI (%)	19/32 (59)	8/31 (26)	14/15 (93)	Not stated	20/26 (77)
Mean MRI follow-up, years (range)	1.5 (0.2–9)	0.2–2 (range only)	0.04–1.5 (range only)	Not stated	Not stated
Original brain lesion change (%)					
Complete resolution	37	Unclear	7	Not stated	30
Partial resolution	53	*n* = 6	57	Not stated	55
No change	10	Unclear	21	Not stated	0
New lesions	0	*n* = 3 (all relapsed clinically)	14 (all within 8 weeks)	0 (denominator not stated)	15 (no clinical relapses)

MRI, magnetic resonance imaging.
Source: with permission from Wingerchuk 2003.[57]

techniques will prove useful in discriminating ADEM from MS and other idiopathic demyelinating syndromes.

It is desirable to differentiate ADEM from MS early in the disease course, ideally at onset. 35 children with either ADEM or MDEM (multiphasic disease; still considered a form of ADEM but with early relapse within 8 weeks of discontinuing corticosteroid treatment)[57–59,119] more commonly experienced an antecedent infection, polysymptomatic presentation, pyramidal signs and encephalopathy than did 13 children with MS.[59] Seizures, bilateral optic neuritis and CSF pleocytosis were also more common but the rate difference was not statistically significant. Unilateral ON occurred only in the MS group. Periventricular brain MRI lesions were common in the MS group but present in 44% of the ADEM/MDEM patients. Therefore, some clinical features appear to be more suggestive of ADEM but the clinical phenotypes still overlap significantly.[59,90,91]

Many adult cases with ADEM like presentation will ultimately evolve into typical MS. Although some cases do remain monophasic for many years, both clinically and by neuroimaging criteria,[101] this does not confirm an ADEM diagnosis. Schwarz et al reported that 14/40 (35%) adults with ADEM developed clinically definite MS during a mean follow-up period of 38 months.[62] There were no helpful clinical or laboratory predictors of disease course. Nearly half of the monophasic ADEM group had periventricular or callosal MRI lesions compatible with MS and some developed new, asymptomatic lesions

in early follow-up, thus raising serious doubts about the diagnosis of ADEM and the utility of MRI for ADEM diagnosis. Table 3.7 outlines features that favor ADEM or MS, with the caveat that, due to overlap, it seems sensible to apply the diagnosis of ADEM with caution and to follow patients with serial clinical and MRI examinations.

The clinical outcome of ADEM is highly variable. Persistent and serious neurological abnormalities occur in 15–33% of children, including motor dysfunction (17%; half of these severe), cognitive impairment (11%), visual loss (11%) and behavioral problems (11%).[59] Adults with monophasic ADEM have more severe initial symptoms but better overall recovery than those ultimately diagnosed with MS.[62] At last follow-up, a greater proportion of ADEM patients were asymptomatic (46% versus 14% in the MS group). Moderate neurological deficits persisted in 12% of ADEM patients whereas 43% of the MS group accrued moderate to severe deficits after mean follow-up of 38 months. MRI normalization predicts a better outcome,[120,121] although subtle cognitive impairment may persist[121] and is more likely in patients who contract ADEM before age 5 years.[122]

The concept of ADEM as a monophasic disease is generally accepted but there are several descriptions of 'relapsing' or 'recurrent' forms that appear to lack features of typical MS.[123–126] One series reported that 10% of cases had biphasic disease with a single relapse occurring between 2 months and 8 years (median 2 years) after ADEM onset; all were oligoclonal-band-negative.[63]

TABLE 3.7 Features useful in discriminating acute disseminated encephalomyelitis from multiple sclerosis

	Favors ADEM	Favors MS
Age	Pediatric, especially infant	Adult
Symptom and signs		
Antecedent infection	Yes	No
Antecedent immunization	Yes	No
Onset	Fulminant/acute	Subacute
Severity	More severe	Less severe
Presentation	Polysymptomatic	Monosymptomatic
Type	Fever Headache/meningism Alteration of consciousness Aphasia, seizures Bilateral optic neuritis	Unilateral optic neuritis
CSF		
Cell count	>50 WBC/mm^3	<50 WBC/mm^3
Total protein	Increased	Normal
Oligoclonal bands	Absent	Present
Brain MRI		
Lesion size	Larger	Small to medium
Lesion distribution (predominant)	± Symmetric; subcortical	Asymmetric; periventricular
Mass effect and edema	Present	Absent
Grey matter involvement	Present	Absent
Gadolinium enhancement	Uniform (all lesions)	Heterogeneous (some lesions)
T1 'black holes'	Absent	Present
Serial MRI scanning	No new lesions	New lesions

ADEM, acute disseminated encephalomyelitis; CSF, cerebrospinal fluid; MRI, magnetic resonance imaging; MS, multiple sclerosis; WBC, white blood cells.

The patients who relapsed early (within the first 2 months) might have been considered by some to have MDEM, whereas others might have diagnosed MS. One potential differentiating factor that was not clarified was whether the recurrence was at the same site as the original event. Cohen et al found that 5/21(24%) of ADEM patients developed between two and four relapses.[124] These relapses occurred in the same brain region in 6/9 recurrences in 3/5 patients. Some of the relapses were recurrent events of large, tumor-like lesions and most were corticosteroid-responsive. The investigators confirmed the diagnosis of ADEM using brain biopsy, which demonstrated diffuse demyelination and perivascular mononuclear cell infiltration, loss of white matter, and foamy macrophages. Therefore, it seems that ADEM may rarely become polyphasic but still lack features characteristic of typical MS.

Pathologically, fulminant ADEM causes brain swelling and congestion, and may cause signs of herniation. The freshly sliced brain may reveal only swelling and scattered petechial hemorrhages whereas acute MS lesions are usually visible to the unaided eye. Lesions may involve the deeper layers of the cerebral cortex, thalamus, hypothalamus and basal ganglia as well

as the vasculature within the walls of the lateral and third ventricle, prompting synonyms such as 'perivenous encephalomyelitis' and 'acute perivascular myelinoclasis'.

The hallmark of ADEM is a perivenous 'sleeve-like' pattern of demyelination associated with reactive microglial infiltrates.[127] Lymphocytes, and to a lesser degree neutrophils, are present outside the Virchow–Robin spaces, and there is vessel wall invasion by inflammatory cells, perivascular edema, petechial hemorrhage and endothelial swelling. Axons are relatively preserved but those affected are often tortuous and swollen. Narrow zones of subpial demyelination in spinal cord and brainstem may be present. Lymphocytic meningitis is almost always present. There is no convincing evidence of inflammatory cells in spinal roots, ganglia or peripheral nerves.

Acute hemorrhagic leukoencephalitis (AHLE), also known as Hurst's disease, appears to be a hyperacute and particularly severe form of ADEM.[128] It is often fatal, although successful recovery has been described.[129–131] It is characterized by predominantly neutrophilic infiltrates with pericapillary ball or ring hemorrhages surrounding necrotic venules. Occasionally, fibrinous exudates may be seen within the vessel or extending into adjacent tissue. Perivenous demyelinating lesions identical to those seen in ADEM may also be present. Brain MRI may not distinguish AHLE from ADEM but in the former lesions tend to be larger, exhibit 'mass effects' and spare the basal ganglia.[132] Hemorrhagic lesions may or may not be detectable by MRI.[132,133]

The pattern of ADEM pathology differs notably from that of MS, allowing more precise diagnosis in cases where biopsy has been obtained. It should be noted that some individuals have lesions with overlapping immunopathological features, suggesting a continuum of IIDDs and possibly common pathogenesis. This is especially important when considering cases of so-called 'relapsing ADEM' that lack pathological verification. It is important to reliably distinguish MS from ADEM to initiate appropriate long-term therapy for those at risk of relapse. Because the clinical, laboratory and imaging features are so often similar, pathology remains the gold standard for diagnosis of ADEM. Since biopsies are obtained in a minority of cases, ADEM is probably overdiagnosed. The term is at times used to describe patients with a first-ever demyelinating syndrome with moderate to severe, multifocal neurological symptoms and signs but many of these cases, especially in adults, will probably relapse and satisfy criteria for MS. Better clinicopathological, neuroimaging and immune biomarker correlations will advance diagnostic accuracy. Until that time, ADEM will remain a clinical construct, at least for clinicians who elect not to biopsy affected nervous tissue.

There have been no controlled clinical therapeutic trials for ADEM. Most children are treated empirically for infectious meningoencephalitis until the diagnosis of ADEM is established, whereupon the mainstay of treatment is high-dose corticosteroids. In one study, neurological status was better (Expanded Disability Status Scale score 1 versus 3; $p=0.029$) in a group of 21 children who received pulsed intravenous methylprednisolone compared with 25 others treated with intravenous dexamethasone.[134] Plasma exchange is second-line or rescue therapy indicated in the scenario of deterioration or failure to improve from severe deficits despite corticosteroid therapy.[23,135–137] In refractory or severe cases, improvement has been reported with use of intravenous immune globulin,[138–145] intravenous cyclophosphamide[62] and hypothermia.[146] The utility of long-term immunosuppressive therapy for rare relapsing cases is not known.

TOPOGRAPHICALLY-RESTRICTED IDIOPATHIC INFLAMMATORY DEMYELINATING DISEASES: THE NEUROMYELITIS OPTICA SPECTRUM

This category encompasses disorders we term 'the neuromyelitis optica spectrum'. They include both monophasic (NMO) and relapsing (recurrent ON, recurrent TM, relapsing NMO) clinical syndromes of the optic nerve and spinal cord.

Neuromyelitis optica (also known as Devic's syndrome or Devic's disease) is an inflammatory disorder that preferentially affects the optic nerves and spinal cord with relative sparing of the brain.[147–149] Albutt, in 1870, was the first to associate visual loss with an acute episode of myelitis.[150] Achard and Guinon presented the first pathological account of NMO in 1889 and described complete loss of the myelin sheath from the optic nerves.[151] In 1894, Devic described cases of either papillitis or retrobulbar neuritis in conjunction with acute myelitis after studying a case and reviewing 16 others from the literature.[152] His student Gault summarized these cases using the term *neuromyélite optic aiguë* (acute optic neuromyelitis) for the disorder

thereafter named for Devic.[153] Throughout the 20th century, investigators published case reports and series, with or without pathological data, and debated the relationship of NMO to MS.[154] Major advances in the understanding of the underlying immunopathology, neuroimaging characteristics and identification of a serum autoantibody (NMO-IgG)[155] and its target antigen (aquaporin-4, a water channel)[156] have provided strong support for the hypothesis that NMO is a distinct disease. The presence of NMO-IgG in the serum of patients with isolated recurrent ON or recurrent, longitudinally extensive myelitis and Japanese 'optic-spinal MS' – but not typical MS – suggests that these disorders are either incompletely developed NMO or NMO variants.[155,157] In this section, we review new clinical, imaging, pathological and immunological developments relevant to these syndromes.

EPIDEMIOLOGY AND GENETICS

Neuromyelitis optica has a predilection for women.[158] The relapsing form, which affects more than 80% of people with NMO, has a female to male ratio of 4 : 1 whereas the sex ratio is approximately 1 : 1 in monophasic cases. The median onset age is late in the fourth decade, about 10 years later than for typical MS, but new-onset NMO has been reported in infants and octogenarians.[158,159]

The role of genetic factors in NMO is not clear. Most patients do not have a family history of demyelinating disease of any type. There are reports of familial cases, including a set of identical twins with a similar age of disease onset.[160–163] In Japan, where Asian-type 'optic-spinal MS' is a common phenotype, fewer than 1% of families contained more than one affected individual.[164] Neuromyelitis optica may differ genetically from typical MS in that most studies do not find an association with the HLA-DRB1*1501 allele that is associated with typical MS, while in Japan it has been associated with DPB1*0501.[165–167]

The incidence and prevalence of NMO are unknown; although it has certainly been under-recognized, it probably represents less than 2% of CNS demyelinating disease in Caucasians. However, even in North American patients, the rate is clearly much higher in people with Japanese and other Asian backgrounds and people of African, Hispanic and Native American lineage.[157,158,164,168–173] The Japanese 'optic-spinal' form of MS is clinically identical to NMO and may be the same disease, since both demonstrate frequent NMO-IgG seropositivity whereas 'classical' or 'Western' MS does not.

DIAGNOSTIC CRITERIA AND CLINICAL PRESENTATION

Diagnostic criteria are outlined in Table 3.8; they include clinical, neuroimaging and laboratory rules that attempt to increase specificity and have been periodically refined.[158,174–176] The absolute requirement for a clinical diagnosis of NMO is coexistence of ON and myelitis. However, this clinical combination may occur in typical MS, in association with systemic autoimmune disorders (e.g., systemic lupus erythematosus; Sjögren syndrome), as a parainfectious phenomenon similar to ADEM, and in association with infectious diseases (pulmonary tuberculosis and a myriad of viral illnesses) and immunizations. Disease associations, including connective tissue disorders, are summarized in Table 3.9.[148,149] The additional clinical factors that differentiate most cases of NMO from MS and other disorders that it may mimic are the severity of individual clinical attacks, tendency to a relapsing course and its persistent predilection, over the course of the disease, for the optic nerves and spinal cord. These findings have generally been replicated throughout the world.[177–179] Table 3.10 summarizes the clinical, imaging and laboratory features relevant to judging the likelihood of NMO versus MS.

Optic neuritis attacks are usually severe and may be unilateral or bilateral. Roughly 20% of patients experience bilateral simultaneous ON, somewhat more often if the course is monophasic. Asymptomatic optic nerve involvement detectable by visual evoked responses can rarely be detected in patients with early disease or at autopsy. The first episode of ON carries a 40% risk of complete blindness (no light perception) at its nadir but most patients experience some visual recovery, especially if their disease course is monophasic.[158] Relapsing cases accumulate visual impairment with successive recurrences of ON.[158,159]

Acute myelitis attacks typically cause 'complete transverse myelitis', defined as severe, bilateral, possibly symmetric, motor, sensory and sphincter dysfunction evolving over hours to days.[158] As with ON, the NMO myelitis attacks are more severe than spinal cord exacerbations in MS, frequently causing paraplegia

---

TABLE 3.8 Proposed diagnostic criteria for neuromyelitis optica (1999)

Diagnosis requires:

All absolute criteria AND
   One major supportive criterion OR
   Two minor supportive criteria

Absolute criteria:

1. Optic neuritis
2. Acute myelitis
3. No clinical disease outside of the optic nerves and spinal cord

Major supportive criteria:

1. Negative brain MRI at disease onset (normal or not meeting radiological diagnostic criteria for MS)
2. Spinal cord MRI with T2 signal abnormality extending over >3 vertebral segments
3. CSF pleocytosis (>50 WBC/mm³) OR >5 neutrophils/mm³

Minor supportive criteria:

1. Bilateral optic neuritis
2. Severe ON with fixed visual acuity worse than 20/200 in at least one eye
3. Severe, fixed, attack-related weakness (MRC grade 2 or less) in one or more limbs

---

TABLE 3.9 Infectious agents and diseases associated with neuromyelitis optica

Infections and Immunizations	Other diseases
Varicella	Systemic lupus erythematosus
Infectious mononucleosis	Autoimmune thyroid disease
Influenza A	Sjögren's syndrome
Streptococcal pharyngitis	Pernicious anemia
Human herpes virus types 6 and 8	Behçet's disease
Human immunodeficiency virus	Mixed connective tissue disease
Mycobacterium tuberculosis	Disseminated cholesterol emboli
Chlamydophila pneumoniae	Ulcerative colitis
Rubella vaccine	Primary sclerosing cholangitis
Smallpox vaccine	Idiopathic thrombocytopenic purpura

TABLE 3.10 Characteristics that help distinguish neuromyelitis optica from multiple sclerosis

	Favors NMO	Favors MS
Age of onset	Median: late 30s	Median: 29
Clinical features		
Optic neuritis	More severe/poor recovery Sometimes bilateral and simultaneous	Less severe/better recovery Rarely bilateral and simultaneous
Brain or brain stem	Not clinically involved	Usually involved
MRI		
Brain	Normal or nonspecific at onset Nonspecific abnormalities not meeting MS criteria	Usually abnormal at onset Increasing number of typical MS lesions
Spinal cord: acute lesions	Cord expansion Lesion(s) extend over three or more vertebral segments	Rarely cord expansion Lesion(s) less than one vertebral segment
Spinal cord: chronic lesions	Long segment of atrophy common	Atrophy less common or only over a short segment
CSF		
Pleocytosis	Sometimes >50 WBC/mm³	Rarely >50 WBC/mm³
Cell differential	Sometimes neutrophilic	Lymphocytic
Oligoclonal banding	About 30%	About 85%
Associated autoimmunity		
Clinical disease	Substantial minority	Uncommon except hypothyroidism
Autoimmune serology	Common, multiple autoantibodies	Minority, usually low titer autoantibody
NMO-IgG assay	Positive (>70%)	Negative

CSF, cerebrospinal fluid; MRI, magnetic resonance imaging; MS, multiple sclerosis; NMO, neuromyelitis optica; WBC, white blood cells.

or quadriplegia and occasionally 'spinal shock'. Lhermitte's symptom, paroxysmal tonic spasms and radicular pain are common occurrences in patients with relapsing disease. 78–88% of patients improved by one or more levels on a seven-point ordinal scale of motor function regardless of eventual disease course, but recovery is usually incomplete.[158,159] Acute cervical myelitis may ascend and cause respiratory failure and death, especially in relapsing disease.[158,180]

Standard NMO diagnostic criteria exclude patients with clinical disease outside the optic nerves and spinal cord. However, many cases have been noted in which an otherwise typical course is associated with minor or subjective features such as vertigo, facial numbness, nystagmus and postural tremor.[158] Occasionally, a cervical cord lesion will extend into the brain stem, resulting in ataxia, bulbar symptoms, vomiting or ophthalmoparesis. Rare cases expressing seizures, ataxia, dysarthria, encephalopathy, dysautonomia or peripheral neuropathy have been reported.[181,182] Clinically based criteria are always susceptible to exceptions and we have identified a number of patients with cerebral or brain stem symptoms at some time during the disease course, even at onset; however, other clinical features seemed highly compatible with NMO and met other components of the diagnostic criteria. Some of these cases are NMO-IgG-seropositive, suggesting (but not establishing) that they are NMO with exceptional clinical features.

NEUROIMAGING AND LABORATORY EVALUATION

Spinal cord MRI is the single most useful diagnostic procedure. Almost all NMO patients have a contiguous, longitudinally extensive, central cord lesion spanning three or more vertebral segments when scans are performed during the acute phase of myelitis.[158] During acute myelitis, the cord is usually expanded and swollen, and may enhance with gadolinium (Fig. 3.3a). In contrast, partial myelitis attacks in MS are associated with MRI lesions that measure one vertebral segment or less in length.[183,184] Although the optic nerve lesions tend to occur over longer segments of the optic nerves than in patients with MS, the optic nerve lesions may not be detectable with standard MR brain techniques or, when present, indistinguishable from MS (Fig. 3.3b). Brain MRI is otherwise normal or reveals only nonspecific white matter lesions that do not meet MS MRI criteria.[158,175,178] Some patients with relapsing disease accumulate white matter lesions over time but these lesions tend to be nonspecific punctate foci that fail to meet radiological criteria for MS.[158] A recent series described brain MRI findings in 60 patients, 70% of

whom were NMO-IgG positive, who met the diagnostic criteria outlined in Table 3.8 except allowing for symptoms or signs outside the optic nerve and spinal cord if the patient had a longitudinally extensive myelitis (longer than three vertebral segments).[185] 50% had brain MRI lesions and 10% met Barkhof criteria for MS. Three children had unusual lesions in the diencephalon with variable extension into the midbrain and cerebellar peduncles. Two patients had extensive white matter disease, one with gadolinium enhancement, associated with coma. Otherwise, cerebral lesions were typically silent or caused only mild symptoms. Therefore, the presence of MS-like cerebral or brain stem lesions should not negate the possibility of NMO in an otherwise typical case.

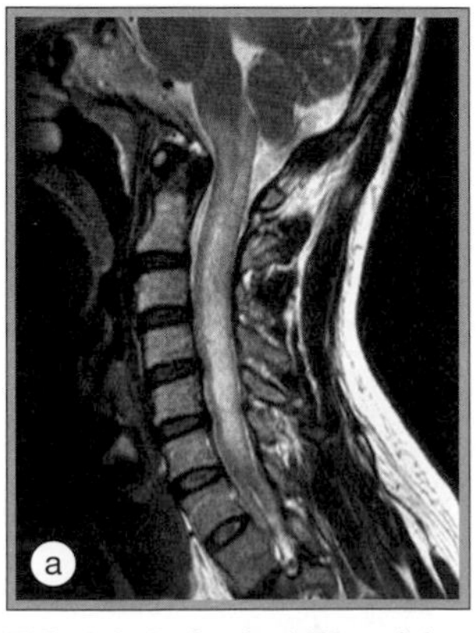

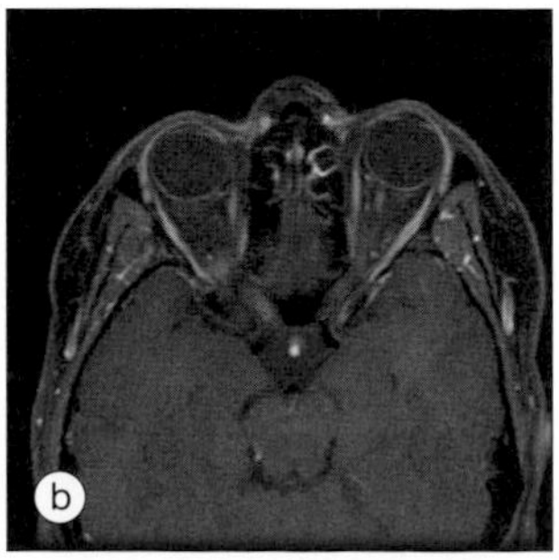

Research imaging tools, such as magnetization transfer ratio (MTR) brain and spinal cord imaging, detect abnormalities in brain tissue that appears normal by conventional MRI techniques. In NMO, Filippi et al demonstrated that MTR brain images were not different from controls.[186] Furthermore, despite the more longitudinally extensive cord lesions in NMO, MTR imaging characteristics of spinal lesions were similar in NMO and MS. Recently, however, Rocca et al used MTR and diffusion tensor imaging to study MTR of white and gray matter separately in NMO patients and healthy controls. White matter results were normal, but gray matter was not.[187] This unexpected finding is of uncertain significance and worthy of further study.

Cerebrospinal fluid analysis reveals that about one-third of patients will have a pleocytosis of more than $50\,WBC/mm^3$ in the setting of an acute myelitis exacerbation and the differential may contain neutrophils.[158,174,175] This degree of pleocytosis and the presence of neutrophils are very rare findings in typical MS. Approximately 85% of patients with MS have unique CSF oligoclonal bands[188,189] whereas the rate in NMO ranges from 20–40%.[158,174,175,178,190] The protein level is variably elevated in NMO. None of the CSF findings appear to correlate with clinical features, with the exception that detection of pleocytosis is more likely if lumbar puncture is performed during a clinical myelitis attack.[158]

Other 'minor criteria' within the original NMO diagnostic algorithm emphasize some of its common but less unique clinical features. Bilateral simultaneous optic neuritis occurs in about one-third of patients with monophasic NMO and 15% of those with relapsing disease but may also occur in MS.[158] The criteria detailing fixed postexacerbation visual loss and weakness reflect the fact that attacks and their residual effects are more severe in NMO than MS.

Although not part of the Mayo Clinic NMO diagnostic criteria, the presence of one or more serum autoantibodies, such as antinuclear antibody, anti-double-stranded-DNA antibody, extractable nuclear antigen or antithyroid antibodies, occurs in about half of NMO patients.[158] Frequently, an individual patient will have multiple positive autoantibodies. The rate of seropositivity appears significantly higher than in typical MS and suggests a predilection to develop multiple autoimmune diseases, even in patients not symptomatic of the illness defined by the corresponding antibody.

Lennon et al. recently reported the discovery of a novel serum autoantibody, termed 'NMO-IgG', that appears to discriminate NMO from typical MS.[155] The assay was sensitive (73%; 95% confidence interval=60–86%) and highly specific (91%; 95% confidence interval=79–100%) for NMO in 45 North American patients when the Mayo Clinic diagnostic criteria were used as the gold standard. It was also present in about half of people deemed to have a syndrome at 'high risk' for NMO, such as idiopathic, isolated recurrent ON or recurrent longitudinally extensive myelitis. Furthermore, 7/12 (58%) Japanese opticospinal MS patients were seropositive and all Japanese patients with

FIG. 3.3 A. Sagittal T2-weighted cervical spinal cord MRI demonstrating a lesion extending from the cervicomedullary junction to the C4 vertebral level. **B.** Post-gadolinium T1-weighted orbital MRI revealing unilateral left optic nerve enhancement.

'Western-type' MS were seronegative. This finding represents the first specific biological marker for NMO, strongly suggests that Asian opticospinal MS and NMO are the same entity, and expands the spectrum of NMO to include some cases of idiopathic recurrent optic neuritis[191,192] or recurrent myelitis[193–195] that may represent incompletely evolved NMO or an NMO variant.

NMO-IgG may have prognostic utility. A follow-up study showed that about half of NMO-IgG-seropositive patients with a first-ever event of longitudinally extensive myelitis experienced recurrent myelitis or optic neuritis within 1 year.[196] In contrast, none of the NMO-IgG-seronegative patients relapsed.

Experience with NMO spectrum disorders over the past decade, together with the NMO-IgG discovery, has prompted reconsideration of NMO diagnostic criteria. The very high individual specificity of NMO-IgG seropositive status or presence of a longitudinally extensive spinal cord lesion led us to propose revised NMO diagnostic criteria in 2006 (Table 3.11). These criteria are 99% sensitive and 90% specific for NMO in patients presenting with an optic–spinal clinical syndrome.[197]

NATURAL HISTORY OF NEUROMYELITIS OPTICA: DISEASE COURSE

Several revisions to historical concepts about NMO have gained general acceptance. These include:

- The interval between the initial events of ON and myelitis is quite variable (occasionally decades)
- Some patients experience unilateral rather than bilateral optic neuritis
- The course may be monophasic or relapsing.[158]

Although the diagnostic criteria have not been formally validated in the strictest sense (no 'gold standard' for the diagnosis exists), they have clearly improved the ability to define a relatively homogeneous group of patients whose natural history differs significantly from those with typical forms of MS and are consistent with results obtained by independent investigators.

Patients who meet NMO diagnostic criteria proceed along either a monophasic or a relapsing course.[158,159] A *monophasic* course, which probably accounts for fewer than 20% of all NMO cases, is defined by co-occurrence of either unilateral or bilateral ON and a single episode of myelitis and extended follow-up (several years) during which no further exacerbations emerge. In contrast, most patients experience *relapsing* disease, in which the index events of ON and myelitis may be many weeks or even years apart but attacks of ON, myelitis or both recur over the next months to years. The relapsing course is usually established quite early. After fulfilling diagnostic criteria, the cumulative proportion of patients who experience another attack that defines relapsing disease is 55% at 1 year, 78% at 3 years and 90% at 5 years. The relapsing nature of NMO was recognized earlier in Japan, where such cases were diagnosed as 'opticospinal' or 'Asian' variants of MS, distinguishing it clearly from 'Western' or typical MS.[157] This form appears to have the same demographic, clinical, neuroimaging and pathological characteristics as cases of relapsing NMO reported from North America, with the exception that coexisting systemic autoimmunity is noted more commonly in the West. The characteristics of a 'pure' subgroup of opticospinal MS (clinical opticospinal disease, normal head MRI except for optic nerve abnormalities, and more than 5 years of clinical follow-up) are virtually identical to cases of relapsing NMO.[167]

Clinical and laboratory features that predict the development of NMO after a first attack or a relapsing disease course would be very useful for prognosis and treatment planning. The best clinical predictor of a relapsing course is a long first interattack interval.[159] Patients who present with ON and myelitis attacks several weeks or months apart are highly likely to have relapsing disease whereas simultaneous ON and myelitis occurrence at onset suggests that a monophasic course is still possible. Additional independent predictors of a relapsing course include female sex (relative risk=10.0 female versus male) and less severe motor impairment with the initial myelitis event. Complete paraplegia occurs with the first myelitis attack in 70% of monophasic patients compared with only 31% of those who later develop relapsing disease. Initial ON attack severity was not an independent risk factor for disease course prediction. MRI and CSF variables did not predict disease course or severity. Recently, it was shown that NMO-IgG seropositivity after a first attack of idiopathic longitudinally extensive myelitis predicts a 50% risk of another myelitis or ON attack (confirmed NMO) at 1 year.[196] These prognostic variables may be useful when considering the use of preventative immunosuppressant therapies early in the disease course and in planning epidemiological and therapeutic studies.

In long-term follow-up, people with monophasic NMO develop less impairment than those with relapsing disease; although their index attacks tend to be more severe than those with relapsing disease, they do not experience recurrences.[158,159] Approximately 22% of patients with monophasic disease remain functionally blind (20/200 vision or worse) in at least one affected eye but more than 50% of ON episodes recover visual acuity to a level of 20/30 or better. Myelitis attacks do not recover quite as well. Most patients have at least moderate permanent limb weakness and bladder or bowel dysfunction and residual monoplegia or paraplegia occurs in 31%. The 5-year survival of patients with monophasic NMO is approximately 90%.

Relapsing NMO often manifests as clusters of attacks months or years apart. Relapse frequency in NMO is highly variable, with remissions lasting weeks or more than a decade. In one patient cohort followed over a median of 16.9 years, the median number of relapses was five (range 1–18).[158] When attack severity and cumulative disability are considered, the natural history of relapsing NMO is markedly different from that of a typical MS cohort. A majority of people with relapsing NMO have permanent and severe visual impairment in at least one eye or are nonambulatory as a result of attack-related paraplegia or quadriplegia within 5 years of NMO onset. This compares unfavorably to MS, in which most patients recover well (or completely) from early attacks and experience relatively mild impairment until evolution of the secondary progressive phase of the disease. Progressive disease is an uncommon feature of NMO, although this may be because the severe deficits as a result of attack precludes appreciation of progressive weakness and ataxia, which are the hallmarks of secondary progressive MS.

Relapsing NMO reduces survival. In one longitudinal series, 5-year survival was 68%, with all deaths secondary to

TABLE 3.11 Proposed diagnostic criteria for definite neuromyelitis optica (2006)
1. Optic neuritis
2. Acute myelitis
3. At least two of three supportive criteria: • Contiguous spinal cord MRI lesion extending over ≥3 vertebral segments   • Brain MRI not meeting diagnostic criteria for MS   • NMO-IgG seropositive status

myelitis-related respiratory failure.[158,159] The true incidence of myelitis-associated respiratory failure is probably lower, since referral bias may have influenced these results. Predictors of mortality in relapsing NMO include a history of systemic autoimmune disease (relative risk = 4.15), greater exacerbation frequency during the first 2 years of disease (relative risk = 1.21 per attack) and better motor recovery following the first myelitis attack.

When bilateral ON and myelitis occur simultaneously or in rapid succession, it usually predicts a monophasic course; such instances may indicate that the NMO syndrome can occur as a 'restricted form of ADEM' if ADEM is broadly defined as any monophasic demyelinating illness. More commonly, however, the sentinel events occur weeks or months apart and consist of unilateral or bilateral ON, myelitis or a combination. In one series, the initial presentation was an isolated event of either ON or myelitis in 90% of patients destined for a relapsing course compared with only 48% of those who had a monophasic illness.[158] Patients with unilateral ON pursue a course indistinguishable from those with bilateral ON.

PATHOLOGY AND IMMUNOPATHOLOGY

Optic nerve tissue demonstrates demyelination with variable inflammatory infiltrates that are typically more extensive than seen in MS. Brain parenchyma is usually normal or reveals small areas of patchy demyelination, gliosis, or perivascular infiltrates.

Acute spinal cord lesions may reveal tissue expansion, softening and cavitation. Microscopic findings range from perivascular inflammatory demyelination to necrotic destruction of both gray and white matter. In many cases, large numbers of neutrophils and eosinophils are present.[198] The polymorphonuclear pattern of inflammation is very different from the macrophage and lymphocyte-dominated lesions found in typical MS. The contribution of eosinophils in NMO is unknown; their presence may be a primary response or reflect secondary recruitment by chemotactic factors generated by complement activation. Medium-sized spinal cord arteries may have a distinctive hyalinized appearance that is associated with tissue necrosis and a mild macrophage-predominant infiltrate.[198–200] The cause and significance of this vascular pathology is unknown.

Recent immunopathological scrutiny of spinal cord material obtained through biopsy and autopsy strongly implicates humoral pathogenic mechanisms in NMO. Lucchinetti et al detected prominent IgG and C9 neoantigen (a marker of complement activation) deposition in areas of active myelin destruction.[198] These deposits were also present in vessel walls accompanying vascular proliferation and fibrosis. Parallel findings from patients with 'optic–spinal MS' were described by investigators in Japan, further linking these two entities.[201]

There are limited but increasing numbers of immunological studies of NMO. A recent peripheral blood and CSF study provided further evidence for humoral mechanisms in NMO by comparing immune responses in NMO patients with age- and sex-matched MS controls.[202] The NMO patients demonstrated a measurable humoral response (especially antimyelin oligodendrocyte glycoprotein IgM and eosinophil activation) exclusively in the CSF. A CSF study followed up on the observations that oligoclonal banding is less prevalent in Japanese opticospinal MS, an association apparent even when consecutive MS patients in Japan were compared based on their oligoclonal banding status; of those who were band-negative, 50% had opticospinal MS and 78% had no or few MRI lesions.[203] Nakashima et al recently found that both NMO and MS patients have higher CSF IgG concentrations than controls; the proportion of IgG that is IgG1 and the IgG1 index were elevated only in the MS

cases.[204] The investigators speculated that lack of IgG1 response might explain the absence of oligoclonal banding in NMO. Furthermore, since IgG1 is associated with T-helper (Th)1 autoimmunity, these findings are congruent with hypotheses that Th2 mechanisms are operative in NMO.

Immunological or biochemical CSF biomarkers that correlate with clinical outcome would be clinically useful. The degree of pleocytosis, total protein level and presence or absence of CSF oligoclonal bands are not independent predictors of disease course or outcome.[158,159] The level of 14-3-3 protein was associated with disability and other CSF abnormalities suggestive of severe CNS tissue injury in Japanese opticospinal MS and myelitis patients,[205] similar to what was found in studies of patients with isolated transverse myelitis and MS.[206,207] Further study of such markers is an area of active study in all CNS demyelinating syndromes.

NMO-IgG AND AQUAPORIN-4

In 2005, Lennon and colleagues reported that aquaporin-4 is the target antigen of NMO-IgG.[156] In a series of experiments, they demonstrated that NMO-IgG and anti-aquaporin-4 colocalize, that NMO-IgG binds specifically to cell membranes transfected with aquaporin-4-expressing reporter constructs but not with control vectors, and that both NMO-IgG and anti-aquaporin-4 antibodies fail to bind to brain tissue of aquaporin-4 knockout animals. Furthermore, Roemer and colleagues recently showed selective loss of aquaporin-4 immunostaining in NMO lesions whereas there was no comparable loss in MS lesions; these findings are also reported by Misu and colleagues and Sinclair and colleagues.[208,209,210]

Aquaporins are water channels that play a major role in fluid homeostasis.[211] Most aquaporins exclusively transmit water but some allow passage of solutes such as glycerol or urea. Suspected to exist for decades, they were discovered by Peter Agre in 1992. He shared the 2003 Nobel Prize for Chemistry for his research with Roderick MacKinnon, an ion channel researcher.

There are now more than a dozen known members of the aquaporin family, each with a distinct distribution in body organs and cells. Aquaporin types 1, 4 and 9 exist in the CNS. In rats, aquaporin-4 is present on astrocytic foot processes along endothelial tight junctions, on the abluminal side of cerebral microvessels, within the cerebellar Purkinje cell layer and in the hypothalamus.[212] Aquaporin-4 is not expressed in neurons, oligodendrocytes or microglia. It has been implicated in control of mechanisms related to cytotoxic edema and is a potential therapeutic target in brain trauma, stroke and epilepsy; many other potential disease associations are likely.[213]

This exciting discovery represents the first known specific autoantibody marker of a CNS inflammatory demyelinating disease and may be the first of a new class of autoimmune channelopathy. If NMO-IgG is the fundamental cause of NMO, it is postulated that peripheral antibody must somehow access the CNS – either through regions of absent blood–brain barrier (e.g. circumventricular organs), susceptible barrier (e.g. possibly the spinal cord) or at sites of barrier damage. Lennon et al postulate that NMO-IgG might cause complement activation, a fundamental pathological finding in NMO, by one of two mechanisms.[156] The homotetrameric structure of aquaporin-4 might directly induce complement activation after NMO-IgG binding. Alternatively, NMO-IgG may interfere with aquaporin fluid homeostatic mechanisms, resulting in endothelial leakage and secondary complement activation. There are now many opportunities for basic and clinical research into the relationship of this antibody and its target antigen with NMO disease mechanisms.

THERAPY

Treatment of acute exacerbations

Acute ON and myelitis exacerbations are typically treated with intravenous methylprednisolone 1000 mg/d for 5 consecutive days or an equivalent dose of a glucocorticoid medication. Clinical observation suggests that corticosteroids enhance the rate of attack recovery, as has been documented in MS, but it is unclear if long-term clinical outcome is altered; a substantial proportion of patients with severe attacks have poor results following corticosteroid therapy. An oral prednisone taper is optional but temporary oral maintenance therapy is often started after the parenteral course is complete if an attack prevention strategy is necessary for relapsing NMO (see below).

For severe, steroid-refractory exacerbations, a frequent occurrence in NMO, plasmapheresis is the treatment of choice. Plasmapheresis seems to be especially useful in patients with NMO; a recent report of uncontrolled experience at the Mayo Clinic described moderate or marked improvement associated with plasmapheresis in 6/10 patients and patients with NMO showed the best response in a double-blind crossover study of plasmapheresis versus sham exchanges.[23,25] Early treatment initiation, male sex and preserved muscle stretch reflexes are associated with a favorable response; therefore, plasmapheresis should be considered in cases where severe attacks either worsen or fail to improve substantially within a few days of steroid initiation.

Prevention and treatment of medical complications has probably contributed to improved survival, especially for patients who have suffered respiratory failure due to ascending, severe cervical myelitis.[158,159] Patients at risk for this complication require intensive care unit observation with frequent evaluation of respiratory and bulbar status to determine the need for ventilatory support. Medical measures to prevent thromboembolic complications, aspiration pneumonia, decubiti and urinary tract infections are also necessary for patients who become immobile.

Preventative immunotherapy

Patients with relapsing NMO accrue disability in a stepwise fashion as a direct result of attacks and a secondary progressive disease course seems to be a rare phenomenon. Therefore, successful attack prevention strategies can be expected to significantly improve the natural history of the disease; unfortunately, therapeutic decisions must still be made based on anecdotal evidence and case series.

Standard MS immunomodulatory therapies, such as interferon β or glatiramer acetate, appear to be ineffective or minimally effective in NMO, based on North American clinical experience. A recent randomized controlled trial suggested that high-dose interferon β-1b was efficacious in reducing the relapse rate for Japanese relapsing–remitting MS compared to a low dose of the same drug.[214] The study was not designed to assess benefit in the opticospinal and Western forms of MS separately, and the result in the opticospinal subset was not statistically significant when this subgroup was analyzed separately; however, the trend favored improvement in the opticospinal group and the overall result in both groups combined showed significant reduction in attacks and MRI lesions. Subsequent studies have challenged the benefits claimed for interferon β in NMO.[215,216]

There have been no controlled trials of current immunomodulatory or immunosuppressive drugs for NMO. Most specialists consider the combination of oral prednisone and azathioprine to be the standard therapy for NMO attack prevention.[217] This is based on a prospective study of seven newly diagnosed NMO patients treated with the combination for at least 18 months.[218] After an initial course of intravenous methylprednisolone, oral prednisone (1 mg/kg/d) was started; 3 weeks later, patients received azathioprine (2 mg/kg/d). At 2 months, the prednisone dose was gradually tapered (by 10 mg every 3 weeks to 20 mg/d, then an even slower reduction to a maintenance dose of 10 mg/d). Most patients were maintained on prednisone 10 mg/d and azathioprine 75–100 mg/d. During the 18 month follow-up period, no exacerbations occurred and disability scores improved modestly. In practice, azathioprine is typically initiated at 50 mg/d and the dose is increased in 50 mg increments over several weeks to a target of 3 mg/kg/d. Prednisone, at doses of 60–80 mg/d, is continued for 3–6 months when there has been evidence of recent disease activity or until there is laboratory evidence of azathioprine effect (persistent mild reduction in leukocyte count and elevation in mean corpuscular volume). It is then gradually tapered over several months. We have observed that ongoing low-dose prednisone (5–15 mg daily or every other day) may be necessary for some patients because when they attempt to taper the dose further they experience breakthrough attacks. In this instance, use of the lowest possible dose on alternate days may help to limit adverse effects. Combination prednisone/azathioprine requires ongoing monitoring of CBC and liver function, surveillance for infection, interventions to limit secondary osteopenia, and avoidance of live vaccinations.

Rituximab, a chimeric anti-CD20 monoclonal antibody that depletes B cells, is a new therapeutic option.[219] The rationale is that rituximab therapy results in persistent B cell clearance and may reduce the antigen-presenting function of B cells. Eight worsening relapsing NMO patients, including four who had experienced treatment failure with azathioprine (n = 3) and mitoxantrone (n = 1) were treated with rituximab 375 mg/m² infusions, once per week for 4 consecutive weeks, in an open-label study.[220] They were retreated with two doses of 1000 mg/m² 2 weeks apart when their B cells became detectable again 6–12 months later. There were no serious adverse effects and 6/8 patients were attack-free for a mean of 12 months (range 6–18 months). 7/8 patients recovered some neurological function compared to their pretreatment status. Rituximab appears to be quite well tolerated but does carry a risk of infusion or allergic reaction and cardiopulmonary side effects. It represents an option for a second-line agent in patients who continue to experience objective breakthrough disease activity despite immunosuppression. Its rapid onset of action also suggests that it may be appropriate as a first-line agent in some patients with very severe and active disease, but experience to date remains quite limited.

Anecdotes indicate occasional success with various other immunosuppressive drugs. Mycophenolate mofetil (1000 mg b.i.d. orally) is not associated with the idiosyncratic gastrointestinal symptoms that can occur with azathioprine but its onset of action may be no more rapid. Two patients, one having failed azathioprine therapy, remained attack-free for at least 1 year using monthly infusions of intravenous immunoglobulin, which could be expected to benefit a B-cell-mediated disorder.[221] The chemotherapeutic agents mitoxantrone (approved for use in rapidly worsening secondary progressive or relapsing–remitting MS)[222,223] and cyclophosphamide have B cell effects and are reasonable to consider in situations where other therapies have failed.[224] The emergence of the data supporting humoral mechanisms may allow more focused interventions and clinical investigations in future studies of this uncommon disorder.

CONCLUSION

The unusual and variant forms of IIDDs represent a varied collection of disorders that may be classified according to their clinical presentation, imaging features, severity, course and tendency to relapse. Serial clinical, neuroimaging and laboratory evaluations can usually achieve the correct diagnosis but in certain instances CNS biopsy is required. Tissue obtained from such biopsies, or from unfortunate instances where autopsy material is available, will advance the current inquiry into pathological heterogeneity and its relevance to clinical disease expression and treatment response. The discovery that NMO is associated with an antibody that targets the water channel aquaporin-4 opens up a new and exciting research area. From the clinician's point of view, the discovery of this biological marker has provided insight into the spectrum of NMO, a diagnosis that may be broadened to include clinical disorders unified by the tendency to experience severe attacks of myelitis and optic neuritis and includes limited forms (e.g. relapsing myelitis), Japanese 'optic–spinal MS', and myelitis and optic neuritis that occur in the context of underlying connective tissue diseases. Future studies aimed at early noninvasive diagnosis, better prediction of disease course and improved understanding of IIDD natural history will facilitate eventual understanding of the genetic and environmental determinants of these disorders and development of focused therapies.

REFERENCES

1. Siva A, Kantarci O. An introduction to the clinical spectrum of inflammatory demyelinating disorders of the central nervous system In: Siva A, Kesselring J, Thompson A, eds. Frontiers in multiple sclerosis, vol II. London: Martin Dunitz; 1999: 1–9.
2. Weinshenker B, Lucchinetti C. Acute leukoencephalopathies: differential diagnosis and investigation. Neurologist 1998; 4: 148–166.
3. McDonald WI, Compston A, Edan G et al. Recommended diagnostic criteria for multiple sclerosis: guidelines from the international panel on the diagnosis of multiple sclerosis. Ann Neurol 2001; 50: 121–127.
4. Sagar HJ, Warlow CP, Sheldon PWE, Esiri MM. Multiple sclerosis with clinical and radiological features of cerebral brain tumor. J Neurol Neurosurg Psychiatry 1982; 45: 802–808.
5. Nesbit GM, Forbes GS, Scheithauer BW et al. Multiple sclerosis: histopathologic and MR and/or CT correlation in 37 cases at biopsy and three cases at autopsy. Radiology 1991; 180: 467–474.
6. Kepes JJ. Large focal tumor-like demyelinating lesions of the brain: intermediate entity between multiple sclerosis and acute disseminated encephalomyelitis? A study of 31 patients. Ann Neurol 1993; 33: 18–27.
7. Dagher AP, Smirniotopoulos J. Tumefactive demyelinating lesions. Neuroradiol 1996; 38: 560–565.
8. Yapici Z, Eraksoy M. Bilateral demyelinating tumefactive lesions in three children with hemiparesis. J Child Neurol 2002; 17: 655–660.
9. McAdam LC, Blaser SI, Banwell BL. Pediatric tumefactive demyelination: case series and review of the literature. Pediatr Neurol 2002; 26: 18–25.
10. Tan HM, Chan LL, Chuah KL et al. Monophasic, solitary tumefactive demyelinating lesion: neuroimaging features and neuropathological diagnosis. Br J Radiol 2004; 77: 153–156.
11. Khoshyomn S, Braff SP, Penar PL. Tumefactive multiple sclerosis plaque. J Neurol Neurosurg Psychiatry 2002; 73: 85.
12. Metafratzi Z, Argyropoulou MI, Tzoufi M et al. Conventional MRI and magnetisation transfer imaging of tumour-like multiple sclerosis in a child. Neuroradiol 2002; 44: 97–99.
13. Masdeu JC, Moreira J, Tasi S et al. The open-ring sign: a new imaging sign in demyelinating disease. J Neuroimaging 1996; 6: 104–107.
14. Given CA II, Stevens BS, Lee C. The MRI appearance of tumefactive demyelinating lesions. AJR 2004; 182: 195–199.
15. Enzinger C, Strasser-Fuchs S, Ropele S et al. Tumefactive demyelinating lesions: conventional and advanced magnetic resonance imaging. Mult Scler 2005; 11: 135–139.
16. Cha S, Pierce S, Knopp EA et al. Dynamic contrast-enhanced T2*-weighted MR imaging of tumefactive demyelinating lesions. Am J Neuroradiol 2001; 22: 1109–1116.
17. Ernst T, Chang L, Walot I, Huff K. Physiologic MRI of a tumefactive multiple sclerosis lesion. Neurology 1998; 51: 1486–1488.
18. Law M, Meltzer DE, Cha S. Spectroscopic magnetic resonance imaging of a tumefactive demyelinating lesion. Neuroradiology 2002; 44: 986–989.
19. Saindane AM, Cha S, Law M et al. Proton MR spectroscopy of tumefactive demyelinating lesions. Am J Neuroradiol 2002; 23: 1378–1386.
20. Butteriss DJ, Ismail A, Ellison DW, Birchall D. Use of serial proton magnetic resonance spectroscopy to differentiate low grade glioma from tumefactive plaque in a patient with multiple sclerosis. Br J Radiol 2003; 76: 662–665.
21. Tsui EY, Leung WH, Chan JH et al. Tumefactive demyelinating lesions by combined perfusion-weighted and diffusion weighted imaging. Comput Med Imaging Graph 2002; 26: 343–346.
22. Rodriguez M, Karnes WE, Bartleson JD, Pineda AA. Plasmapheresis in acute episodes of fulminant CNS inflammatory demyelination. Neurology 1993; 43: 1100–1104.
23. Weinshenker BG, O'Brien PC, Petterson TM et al. A randomized trial of plasma exchange in acute central nervous system inflammatory demyelinating disease. Ann Neurol 1999; 46: 878–886.
24. Mao-Draayer Y, Braff S, Pendlebury W, Panitch H. Treatment of steroid-unresponsive tumefactive demyelinating disease with plasma exchange. Neurology 2002; 59: 1074–1077.
25. Keegan M, König F, McClelland R et al. Relation between humoral pathological changes in multiple sclerosis and response to therapeutic plasma exchange. Lancet 2005; 366: 579–582.
26. Marburg O. Die sogenannte 'akute multiple Sklerose' (Encephalomyelitis periaxalis scleroticans). J Neurol Psychiatr 1906; 27: 213–312.
27. Mendez MF, Pogacar S. Malignant monophasic multiple sclerosis or 'Marburg's disease'. Neurology 1988; 38: 1153–1155.
28. Wood DD, Bilbao JM, O'Connors P, Moscarello MA. Acute multiple sclerosis (Marburg type) is associated with developmentally immature myelin basic protein. Ann Neurol 1996; 40: 18–24.
29. Schwarz U, Marino S, Hess K. Marburg's encephalitis in a young woman. Eur Neurol 2002; 48: 42–44.
30. Jeffery DR, Lefkowitz DS, Crittenden JP. Treatment of Marburg variant multiple sclerosis with mitoxantrone. J Neuroimaging 2004; 14: 58–62.
31. Capello E, Mancardi GL. Marburg type and Balo's concentric sclerosis: rare and acute variants of multiple sclerosis. Neurol Sci 2004; 25(Suppl 4): S361–S363.
32. Storch MK, Piddlesden S, Haltia M et al. Multiple sclerosis: in situ evidence for antibody and complement-mediated demyelination. Ann Neurol 2000; 47: 707–717.
33. Genain CP, Cannella B, Hauser SL et al. Identification of autoantibodies associated with myelin damage in multiple sclerosis. Nat Med 1999; 5: 170–175.
34. Giubilei F, Sarrantonio A, Tisei P et al. Four-year follow-up of a case of acute multiple sclerosis of the Marburg type. Ital J Neurol Sci 1997; 18: 163–166.
35. Jacquerye P, Osseman H, Laloux P et al. Acute fulminant multiple sclerosis and plasma exchange. Eur Neurol 1999; 41: 174–175.
36. Monaca C, Stojkovic T, De Seze J et al. Fulminant multiple sclerosis. Rev Neurol (Paris) 2000; 156: 180–181.
37. Lucchinetti CF, Parisi J, Bruck W. The pathology of multiple sclerosis. Neurol Clin 2005; 23: 77–105.
38. Baló J. A leukoenkephalitis periaxialis concentricaról. Magy Orvosi Arch 1927; 28: 108–24.
39. Baló J. Encephalitis periaxialis concentrica. Arch Neurol Psychiatr 1928; 19: 242–64.
40. Garbern J, Spence AM, Alvord EC. Balo's concentric demyelination diagnosed premortem. Neurology 1986; 36: 1610–1614.
41. Gharagozloo AM, Poe LB, Collins GH. Antemortem diagnosis of Balo concentric sclerosis: correlative MR imaging and pathologic features. Radiology 1994; 191: 817–819.
42. Revel MP, Valiente E, Gray F et al. Concentric MR patterns in multiple sclerosis. Report of two cases. J Neuroradiol 1993; 20: 252–257.
43. Korte JH, Bom EP, Vos LD et al. Balo concentric sclerosis: MR diagnosis. Am J Neuroradiol 1994; 15: 1284–1285.

44. Ng SH, Ko SF, Cheung YC et al. MRI features of Baló's concentric sclerosis. Br J Radiol 1999; 72: 400–403.

45. Iannucci G, Mascalchi M, Salvi F, Filippi M. Vanishing Balo-like lesions in multiple sclerosis. J Neurol Neurosurg Psychiatry 2000; 69: 399–400.

46. Spiegel M, Krüger H, Hofmann E, Kappos L. MRI study of Baló's concentric sclerosis before and after immunosuppressive therapy. J Neurol 1989; 236: 487–488.

47. Hanemann CO, Kleinschmidt A, Reifenberger G et al. Baló's concentric sclerosis followed by MRI and positron emission tomography. Neuroradiology 1993; 35: 578–580.

48. Chen CJ, Chu NS, Lu CS, Sung CY. Serial magnetic resonance imaging in patients with Baló's concentric sclerosis: natural history of lesion development. Ann Neurol 1999; 46: 651–656.

49. Karaarslan E, Altintas A, Senol U et al. Baló's concentric sclerosis: clinical and radiological features of five cases. Am J Neuroradiol 2001; 22: 1362–1367.

50. Chen CJ. Serial proton magnetic resonance spectroscopy in lesions of Balo concentric sclerosis. J Comp Assist Tomogr 2001; 25: 713–718.

51. Caracciolo JT, Murtagh RD, Rojiani AM, Murtagh FR. Pathognomonic MR imaging findings in Balo concentric sclerosis. Am J Neuroradiol 2001; 22: 292–293.

52. Moore GR, Neumann PE, Suzuki K et al. Balo's concentric sclerosis: new observations on lesion development. Ann Neurol 1985; 17: 604–611.

53. Lucchinetti CF, Brück W, Parisi J et al. Heterogeneity of multiple sclerosis lesions: implications for the pathogenesis of demyelination. Ann Neurol 2000; 47: 707–717.

54. Barnett MH, Prineas JW. Relapsing and remitting multiple sclerosis: pathology of the newly-forming lesion. Ann Neurol 2004; 55: 458–468.

55. Yao DL, Webster HD, Hudson LD et al. Concentric sclerosis (Balo): morphometric and in situ hybridization study of lesions in six patients. Ann Neurol 1994; 35: 18–30.

56. Stadelmann C, Ludwin S, Tabira T et al. Tissue preconditioning may explain concentric lesions in Balo's type of multiple sclerosis. Brain 2005; 128: 979–987.

57. Wingerchuk DM. Postinfectious encephalomyelitis. Curr Neurol Neurosci Rep 2003; 3: 256–264.

58. Bennetto L, Scolding N. Inflammatory/post-infectious encephalomyelitis. J Neurol Neurosurg Psychiatry 2004; 75(suppl I): i22–i28.

59. Dale RC, de Sousa C, Chong WK et al. Acute disseminated encephalomyelitis, multiphasic encephalomyelitis and multiple sclerosis in children. Brain 2000; 123: 2407–2422.

60. Hynson JL, Kornberg AJ, Coleman LT et al. Clinical and neuroradiologic features of acute disseminated encephalomyelitis in children. Neurology 2001; 56: 1308–1312.

61. Murthy SN, Faden HS, Cohen ME, Bakshi R. Acute disseminated encephalomyelitis in children. Pediatrics 2002; 110: e21.

62. Schwarz S, Mohr A, Knauth M et al. Acute disseminated encephalomyelitis. A follow-up study of 40 adult patients. Neurology 2001; 56: 1313–1318.

63. Tenembaum S, Chamoles N, Fejerman N. Acute disseminated encephalomyelitis. A long-term follow-up study of 84 pediatric patients. Neurology 2002; 59: 1224–1231.

64. Pittock SJ, Wingerchuk DM. Acute disseminated encephalomyelitis. In: Minegar A, Livingstone JS, eds. Inflammatory diseases of the nervous system. Totowa, NJ: Humana Press; 2005: 147–162.

65. Miller HG, Evans MJL. Prognosis in acute disseminated encephalomyelitis; with a note on neuromyelitis optica. Q J Med 1953; 22: 347–349.

66. Litvak AM, Sands IJ, Gibel H. Encephalitis complicating measles: report of 56 cases with follow-up studies in 32. Am J Dis Child 1943; 65: 265–295.

67. Scott TFM. Post infectious and vaccinal encephalitis. Med Clin North Am 1867; 51: 701–716.

68. Spieker S, Petersen D, Rolfs A et al. Acute disseminated encephalomyelitis following Pontiac fever. Eur Neurol 1998; 40: 169–172.

69. Heick A, Skriver E. Chlamydia pneumoniae-associated ADEM. Eur J Neurol 2000; 7: 435–438.

70. Sommer JB, Erbguth FJ, Neundorfer B. Acute disseminated encephalomyelitis following Legionella pneumophila infection. Eur Neurol 2000; 44: 182–184.

71. Alonso-Valle H, Munoz R, Hernandez JL, Matorras P. Acute disseminated encephalomyelitis following Leptospira infection. Eur Neurol 2001; 46: 104–105.

72. Yamamoto Y, Takasaki T, Yamada K et al. Acute disseminated encephalomyelitis following dengue fever. J Infect Chemother 2002; 8: 175–177.

73. Au WY, Lie AK, Cheung RT et al. Acute disseminated encephalomyelitis after para-influenza infection post bone marrow transplantation. Leuk Lymphoma 2002; 43: 455–457.

74. Proulx NL, Freedman MS, Chan JW et al. Acute disseminated encephalomyelitis associated with Pasteurella multocida meningitis. Can J Neurol Sci 2003; 30: 155–158.

75. Orr D, McKendrick MW, Sharrack B. Acute disseminated encephalomyelitis temporally associated with Campylobacter gastroenteritis. J Neurol Neurosurg Psychiatry 2005; 75: 792–793.

76. Py MO, Andre C. Acute disseminated encephalomyelitis and meningococcal A and C vaccine: case report. Arq Neuro-Psiquiatr 1997; 55: 632–635.

77. Bolukbasi O, Ozemenoglu M. Acute disseminated encephalomyelitis associated with tetanus vaccination. Eur Neurol 1999; 41: 231–232.

78. Ascherio A, Zhang SM, Hernan MA et al. Hepatitis B vaccination and the risk of multiple sclerosis. N Engl J Med 2001; 344: 327–332.

79. Centers for Disease Control and Prevention. Vaccinia (smallpox) vaccine: recommendations of the Advisory Committee on Immunization Practices 2001. Morb Mortal Wkly Rep 2001; 50: 1–24.

80. Schwarz S, Knauth M, Schwab S et al. Acute disseminated encephalomyelitis after parenteral therapy with herbal extracts: report of two cases. J Neurol Neurosurg Psychiatry 2000; 69: 516–518.

81. Boz C, Velioglu S, Ozmenoglu M. Acute disseminated encephalomyelitis after bee sting. Neurol Sci 2003; 23: 313–315.

82. Malhotra P, Sharma N, Awasthi A, Vasishta RK. Fatal acute disseminated encephalomyelitis following treated snake bite in India. Emerg Med J 2005; 22: 308–309.

83. Lindzen E, Gilani A, Markovic-Plese S, Mann D. Acute disseminated encephalomyelitis after liver transplantation. Arch Neurol 2005; 62: 650–652.

84. Leake JA, Albani S, Kao AS et al. Acute disseminated encephalomyelitis in childhood: epidemiologic, clinical and laboratory features. Ped Infect Dis J 2004; 23: 756–764.

85. Johnson RT. Pathogenesis of acute viral encephalitis and post infectious encephalomyelitis. J Infect Dis 1987; 155: 359–364.

86. Johnson RT. Postinfectious demyelinating diseases. In: Johnson RT. Viral infections of the nervous system, 2nd ed. Philadelphia: Lippincott-Raven; 1998: 181–210.

87. Cherry JD, Shields WD. Encephalitis and meningoencephalitis. In: Feigin RD, Cherry JD, eds. Textbook of pediatric infectious diseases. Philadelphia: WB Saunders; 1992: 445–454.

88. Stocks M. Genetics of childhood disorders: XXIX. Autoimmune disorders, part 2: molecular mimicry. J Am Acad Child Adolesc Psychiatry 2001; 40: 977–980.

89. Miller SD, Vanderlugt CL, Begolka WS et al. Persistent infection with Theiler's virus leads to autoimmunity via epitope spreading. Nat Med 1997; 3: 1133–1136.

90. Anlar B, Basaran C, Kose G et al. Acute disseminated encephalomyelitis in children: outcome and prognosis. Neuropediatrics 2003; 34: 194–199.

91. Brass SD, Caramanos Z, Santos C et al. Multiple sclerosis vs acute disseminated encephalomyelitis in childhood. Ped Neurol 2003; 29: 227–231.

92. Patel SP, Friedman RS. Neuropsychiatric features of acute disseminated encephalomyelitis: a review. J Neuropsychiatr Clin Neurosci 1997; 9: 534–540.

93. Moscovich DG, Singh MB, Eva FJ, Puri BK. Acute disseminated encephalomyelitis presenting as an acute psychotic state. J Nerv Ment Dis 1995; 183: 116–117.

94. Wang PN, Fuh JL, Liu HC, Wang S-J. Acute disseminated encephalomyelitis in middle-aged or elderly patients. Eur Neurol 1996; 36: 219–223.

95. Nasr JT, Andriola MR, Coyle PK. ADEM: literature review and case report of acute psychosis presentation. Pediatr Neurol 2000; 22: 8–18.

96. Abay E, Balci K, Ates I. Acute disseminated encephalomyelitis presenting as conversion disorder. J Neuropsychiatry Clin Neurosci 2005; 17: 259–260.

97. Kubota H, Kanbayashi T, Tanabe Y et al. A case of acute disseminated encephalomyelitis presenting hypersomnia with decreased hypocretin level in cerebrospinal fluid. J Child Neurol 2002; 17: 537–539.

98. Gledhill RF, Bartel PR, Yoshida Y et al. Narcolepsy caused by acute disseminated

encephalomyelitis. Arch Neurol 2004; 61: 758–760.

99. Dale RC, Church AJ, Cardoso F et al. Poststreptococcal acute disseminated encephalomyelitis with basal ganglia involvement and auto-reactive antibasal ganglia antibodies. Ann Neurol 2001; 50: 588–595.

100. Kuperan S, Ostrow P, Landi MK, Bakshi R. Acute hemorrhagic leukoencephalitis vs ADEM: FLAIR MRI and neuropathology findings. Neurology 2003; 60: 721–722.

101. O'Riordan JI, Gomez-Anson B, Moseley IF, Miller DH. Long term MRI follow-up of patients with post infectious encephalomyelitis: evidence for a monophasic disease. J Neurol Sci 1999; 167: 132–136.

102. Murray BJ, Apetauerova D, Scammell TE. Severe acute disseminated encephalomyelitis with normal MRI at presentation. Neurology 2000; 55: 1237–1238.

103. Honkaniemi J, Dastidar P, Kähärä V, Haapasalo H. Delayed MR imaging changes in acute disseminated encephalomyelitis. Am J Neuroradiol 2001; 22: 1117–1124.

104. Baum PA, Barkovich AJ, Koch TK, Berg BO. Deep gray matter involvement in children with acute disseminated encephalomyelitis. Am J Neuroradiol 1994; 15: 1275–1283.

105. Olivero WC, Deshmukh P, Gujrati M. Bilateral enhancing thalamic lesions in a 10 year old boy: case report. J Neurol Neurosurg Psychiatry 1999; 66: 633–635.

106. Hamed LM, Silbiger J, Guy J et al. Parainfectious optic neuritis and encephalomyelitis. A report of two cases with thalamic involvment. J Clin Neuro-ophthalmol 1993; 13: 18–23.

107. Miller DH, Scaravilli F, Thomas DCT et al. Acute disseminated encephalomyelitis presenting as a solitary brainstem mass. J Neurol Neurosurg Psychiatry 1993; 56: 920–922.

108. Firat AK, Karakas HM, Yakinci C et al. An unusual case of acute disseminated encephalomyelitis confined to brainstem. Magn Reson Imaging 2004; 22: 1329–1332.

109. De Recondo A, Guichard JP. Acute disseminated encephalomyelitis presenting as multiple cystic lesions. J Neurol Neurosurg Psychiatry 1997; 63: 15.

110. Van der Meyden CH, de Villiers JFK, Middlecote BD, Terblanche J. Gadolinium ring enhancement and mass effect in acute disseminated encephalomyelitis. Neuroradiol 1994; 36: 221–223.

111. Lim KE, Hsu YY, Hsu WC, Chan CY. Multiple complete ring-shaped enhanced MRI lesions in acute disseminated encephalomyelitis. Clin Imaging 2003; 27: 281–284.

112. Bizzi A, Ulug AM, Crawford TO et al. Quantitative proton MR spectroscopic imaging in acute disseminated encephalomyelitis. Am J Neuroradiol 2001; 22: 1125–1130.

113. Harada M, Hisaoka S, Mori K et al. Differences in water diffusion and lactate production in two different types of postinfectious encephalopathy. J Magn Res Imag 2000; 11: 559–563.

114. Bernarding J, Braun J, Koennecke H-C. Diffusion- and perfusion-weighted MR

imaging in a patient with acute disseminated encephalomyelitis (ADEM). J Magn Res Imag 2002; 15: 96–100.

115. Holtmannspotter M, Inglese M, Rovaris M et al. A diffusion tensor MRI study of basal ganglia from patients with ADEM. J Neurol Sci 2003; 206: 27–30.

116. Inglese M, Salvi F, Iannucci G et al. Magnetization transfer and diffusion tensor MR imaging of acute disseminated encephalomyelitis. Am J Neuroradiol 2002; 23: 267–272.

117. Tan TXL, Spigos DG, Mueller CF. Abnormal cortical metabolism in acute disseminated encephalomyelitis. Clin Nucl Med 1998; 23: 629–630.

118. Axer H, Ragoschke-Schumm A, Bottcher J et al. Initial DWI and ADC imaging may predict outcome in acute disseminated encephalomyelitis: report of two cases of brain stem encephalitis. J Neurol Neurosurg Psychiatry 2005; 76: 996–998.

119. Dale RC, Branson JA. Acute disseminated encephalomyelitis or multiple sclerosis: can the initial presentation help in establishing a correct diagnosis? Arch Dis Child 2005; 90: 636–639.

120. Richer LP, Sinclair DB, Bhargava R. Neuroimaging features of acute disseminated encephalomyelitis in childhood. Pediatr Neurol 2005; 32: 30–36.

121. Hahn CD, Miles BS, MacGregor DL et al. Neurocognitive outcome after acute disseminated encephalomyelitis. Pediatr Neurol 2003; 29: 117–123.

122. Jacobs RK, Anderson VA, Neale JL et al. Neuropsychological outcome after acute disseminated encephalomyelitis: impact of age at illness onset. Pediatr Neurol 2004; 31: 191–197.

123. Durston JHJ, Milnes JN. Relapsing encephalomyelitis. Brain 1970; 93: 715–730.

124. Cohen O, Steiner-Birmanns B, Biran I et al. Recurrence of acute disseminated encephalomyelitis at the previously affected brain site. Arch Neurol 2001; 58: 797–801.

125. Hartel C, Schilling S, Gottschalk S, Sperner J. Multiphasic disseminated encephalomyelitis associated with streptococcal infection. Eur J Paed Neurol 2002; 6: 327–329.

126. Mariotti P, Batocchi AP, Colosimo C et al. Multiphasic demyelinating disease involving central and peripheral nervous system in a child. Neurology 2003; 60: 348–349.

127. Prineas JW, McDonald WI, Franklin RJM. Demyelinating diseases. In: Graham DI, Lantos PL, eds. Greenfield's neuropathology, 7th ed. London: Arnold; 2002: 471–535.

128. Hurst EW. Acute hemorrhagic leukoencephalitis: a previously undefined entity. Med J Aust 1941; 1: 1–6.

129. Klein C, Wijdicks EFM, Earnest IVF. Full recovery after acute hemorrhagic leukoencephalitis (Hurst's disease). J Neurol 2000; 247: 977–979.

130. Rosman NP, Gottlieb SM, Bernstein CA. Acute hemorrhagic leukoencephalitis: recovery and reversal of magnetic resonance imaging findings in a child. J Child Neurol 1997; 12: 448–454.

131. Seales D, Greer M. Acute hemorrhagic leukoencephalitis: a successful recovery. Arch Neurol 1991; 48: 1086–1088.

132. Kuperan S, Ostrow P, Landi MK, Bakshi R. Acute hemorrhagic leukoencephalitis vs ADEM: FLAIR MRI and neuropathology findings. Neurology 2003; 60: 721–722.

133. Friedman DP. Neuroradiology case of the day. Radiographics 1998; 18: 246–250.

134. Straub J, Chofflon M, Delavelle J. Early high-dose intravenous methylprednisolone in acute disseminated encephalomyelitis: a successful recovery. Neurology 1997; 49: 1145–1147.

135. Kanter DS, Horensky D, Sperling RA et al. Plasmapheresis in fulminant acute disseminated encephalomyelitis. Neurology 1995; 45: 824–827.

136. Balestri P, Grosso S, Acquaviva A, Bernini M. Plasmapheresis in a child affected by acute disseminated encephalomyelitis. Brain Devel 2000; 22: 123–126.

137. Miyazawa R, Hikima A, Takano Y et al. Plasmapheresis in fulminant acute disseminated encephalomyelitis. Brain Dev 2001; 23: 424–426.

138. Kleiman M, Brunquell P. Acute disseminated encephalomyelitis: response to intravenous immunoglobulin? J Child Neurol 1995; 10: 481–483.

139. Hahn JS, Siegler DJ, Enzmann D. Intravenous gammaglobulin therapy in recurrent acute disseminated encephalomyelitis. Neurology 1996; 46: 1173–1174.

140. Pradhan S, Gupta RP, Shashank S, Pandey N. Intravenous immunoglobulin therapy in acute disseminated encephalomyelitis. J Neurol Sci 1999; 165: 56–61.

141. Apak RA, Anlar B, Saatci I. A case of relapsing acute disseminated encephalomyelitis with high dose corticosteroid treatment. Brain Dev 1999; 21: 279–282.

142. Sahlas DJ, Miller SP, Guerin M et al. Treatment of acute disseminated encephalomyelitis with intravenous immunoglobulin. Neurology 2000; 54: 1370–1372.

143. Marchioni E, Marinou-Aktipi K, Uggetti C et al. Effectiveness of intravenous immunoglobulin treatment in adult patients with steroid-resistant monophasic or recurrent acute disseminated encephalomyelitis. J Neurol 2002; 249: 100–104.

144. Andersen JB, Rasmussen LH, Herning M, Paerregaard A. Dramatic improvement of severe acute disseminated encephalomyelitis after treatment with intravenous immunoglobulin in a three-year-old boy. Dev Med Child Neurol 2001; 43: 136–138.

145. Unay B, Sarici SU, Bulakbasi N et al. Intravenous immunoglobulin therapy in acute disseminated encephalomyelitis associated with hepatitis A infection. Pediatr Int 2004; 46: 171–173.

146. Takata T, Hirakawa M, Sakurai M, Kanazawa I. Fulminant form of acute disseminated encephalomyelitis: successful treatment with hypothermia. J Neurol Sci 1999; 165: 94–97.

147. Weinshenker BG, Miller D. MS: one disease or many? In: Siva A, Kesselring J, Thompson A, eds. Frontiers in multiple sclerosis. London: Martin Dunitz; 1999: 37–46.

148. Cree BA, Goodin DS, Hauser SL. Neuromyelitis optica. Semin Neurol 2002; 22: 105–122.

149. Wingerchuk DM, Lennon VA, Lucchinetti CF et al. The spectrum of neuromyelitis optica. Lancet Neurol 2007; 6: 805–815.

150. Allbutt TC. On the ophthalmoscopic signs of spinal disease. Lancet 1870; 1: 76–78.

151. Devic E. Myélite subaiguë compliquée de néurite optique. Bull Med 1894; 8.

152. Gault F. De la neuromyélite optique aiguë. Lyon: thesis, 1894.

153. De Seze J. Neuromyelitis optica. Arch Neurol 2003; 60: 1336–1338.

154. Weinshenker BG. Neuromyelitis optica: what it is and what it might be. Lancet 2003; 361: 889–890.

155. Lennon VA, Wingerchuk DM, Kryzer TJ et al. A serum autoantibody marker of neuromyelitis optica: distinction from multiple sclerosis. Lancet 2004; 364: 2106–2112.

156. Lennon VA, Kryzer TJ, Pittock SJ et al. IgG marker of optic-spinal multiple sclerosis binds to the aquaporin-4 water channel. J Exp Med 2005; 202: 473–477.

157. Kira J. Multiple sclerosis in the Japanese population. Lancet Neurol 2003; 2: 117–127.

158. Wingerchuk DM, Hogancamp WF, O'Brien PC, Weinshenker BG. The clinical course of neuromyelitis optica (Devic's syndrome). Neurology 1999; 53: 1107–1114.

159. Wingerchuk DM, Weinshenker BG. Neuromyelitis optica: clinical predictors of a relapsing course and survival. Neurology 2003; 60: 848–853.

160. McAlpine D. Familial neuromyelitis optica: its occurrence in identical twins. Brain 1938; 61: 430–438.

161. Ch'ien LT, Medeiros MO, Belluomini JJ et al. Neuromyelitis optica (Devic's syndrome) in two sisters. Clin Electroencephalogr 1982; 13: 36–39.

162. Keegan BM, Weinshenker B. Familial Devic's disease. Can J Neurol Sci 2000; 27(suppl 2): S57–S58.

163. Yamakawa K, Kuroda H, Fujihara K et al. Familial neuromyelitis optica (Devic's syndrome) with late onset in Japan. Neurology 2000; 55: 318–320.

164. Kuroiwa Y, Igata A, Itahara K et al. Nationwide survey of multiple sclerosis in Japan: clinical analysis of 1,084 cases. Neurology 1975; 25: 845–851.

165. Ono T, Zambenedetti MR, Yamasaki K et al. Molecular analysis of HLA class (HLA-A and -B) and HLA class II (HLA-DRB1) genes in Japanese patients with multiple sclerosis (Western type and Asian type). Tiss Antigens 1998; 52: 539–542.

166. Yamasaki K, Horiuchi I, Minohara M et al. HLA-DPB1*0501-associated opticospinal multiple sclerosis: clinical, neuroimaging and immunogenetic studies. Brain 1999; 122: 1689–1696.

167. Misu T, Fujihara K, Nakashima I et al. Pure optico-spinal form of multiple sclerosis in Japan. Brain 2002; 125: 2460–2468.

168. Okinaka S, Tsubaki K Kuroiwa Y et al. Multiple sclerosis and allied diseases in Japan: clinical characteristics. Neurology 1958; 8: 756–763.

169. Osuntokun BO. The pattern of neurological illness in tropical Africa: experience at Ibadan, Nigeria. J Neurol Sci 1971; 12: 417–442.

170. Jain S, Maheshwari MC. Multiple sclerosis: Indian experience in the last thirty years. Neuroepidemiology 1985; 4: 96–107.

171. Phillips PH, Newman NJ, Lynn MJ. Optic neuritis in African Americans. Arch Neurol 1998; 55: 186–192.

172. Mirsattari SM, Johnston JB, McKenna R et al. Aboriginals with multiple sclerosis: HLA types and predominance of neuromyelitis optica. Neurology 2001; 56: 317–323.

173. Cabre P, Heinzlef O, Merle H et al. MS and neuromyelitis optica in Martinique (French West Indies). Neurology 2001; 56: 507–514.

174. Mandler RN, Davis LE, Jeffery DR, Kornfeld M. Devic's neuromyelitis optica: a clinicopathological study of 8 patients. Ann Neurol 1993; 34: 162–168.

175. O'Riordan JI, Gallagher HL, Thompson AJ et al. Clinical, CSF, and MRI findings in Devic's neuromyelitis optica. J Neurol Neurosurg Psychiatry 1996; 60: 382–387.

176. Wingerchuk DM. Neuromyelitis optica: current concepts. Front Biosci 2004; 9: 834–840.

177. Papais-Alvarenga, RM, Miranda-Santos CM, Puccioni-Sohler M et al. Optic neuromyelitis syndrome in Brazilian patients. J Neurol Neurosurg Psychiatry 2002; 73: 429–435.

178. De Seze J, Stojkovic T, Ferriby D et al. Devic's neuromyelitis optica: clinical, laboratory, MRI and outcome profile. J Neurol Sci 2002; 197: 57–61.

179. De Seze J, Lebrun C, Stojkovic T et al. Is Devic's neuromyelitis optica a separate disease? A comparative study with multiple sclerosis. Mult Scler 2003; 9: 521–525.

180. Pittock SJ, Weinshenker BG, Wijdicks EF. Mechanical ventilation and tracheostomy in multiple sclerosis. J Neurol Neurosurg Psychiatry 2004; 75: 1331–1333.

181. Baudoin D, Gambarelli D, Gayraud D et al. Devic's neuromyelitis optica: a clinicopathological review of the literature in connection with a case showing fatal dysautonomia. Clin Neuropathol 1998; 17: 175–183.

182. Aimoto Y, Ito K, Moriwaka F et al. Demyelinating peripheral neuropathy in Devic disease. Jpn J Psychiatr Neurol 1991; 45: 861–864.

183. Thielen KR, Miller GM. Multiple sclerosis of the spinal cord: magnetic resonance appearance. J Comput Assist Tomogr 1996; 20: 434–438.

184. Bot JC, Barkhof F, Polman CH et al. Spinal cord abnormalities in recently diagnosed MS patients: added value of spinal MRI examination. Neurology 2004; 62: 226–233.

185. Pittock SJ, Lennon VA, Krecke K et al. Brain MRI abnormalities in neuromyelitis optica. Arch Neurol 2006; 63: 390–396.

186. Filippi M, Rocca MA, Moiola L et al. MRI and magnetization transfer imaging changes in the brain and cervical cord of patients with Devic's neuromyelitis optica. Neurology 1999; 53: 1705–1710.

187. Rocca MA, Agosta F, Mezzapesa DM et al. Magnetization transfer and diffusion tensor MRI show gray matter damage in neuromyelitis optica. Neurology 2004; 62: 476–478.

188. Andersson M, Alvarez-Cermeno J, Bernardi G et al. Cerebrospinal fluid in the diagnosis of multiple sclerosis: a consensus report. J Neurol Neurosurg Psychiatry 1994; 57: 897–902.

189. Rudick RA, Cookfair DL, Simonian NA et al. Cerebrospinal fluid abnormalities in a phase III trial of Avonex (IFNbeta-1a) for relapsing multiple sclerosis. The Multiple Sclerosis Collaborative Research Group. J Neuroimmunol 1999; 93: 8–14.

190. Bergamaschi RS, Tonietti S, Franciotta D et al. Oligoclonal bands in Devic's neuromyelitis optica and multiple sclerosis: differences in repeated cerebrospinal fluid abnormalities. Mult Scler 2004; 10: 2–4.

191. Kidd D, Burton B, Plant, GT, Graham EM. Chronic relapsing idiopathic optic neuropathy. Brain 2003; 126: 276–284.

192. Pirko I, Blauwet LK, Lesnick TG, Weinshenker BG. The natural history of recurrent optic neuritis. Arch Neurol 2004; 61: 1401–1405.

193. Tippett DS, Fishman PS, Panitch HS. Relapsing transverse myelitis. Neurology 1991; 41: 703–706.

194. Pandit L, Rao S. Recurrent myelitis. J Neurol Neurosurg Psychiatry 1996; 60: 336–338.

195. Hummers LK, Krishnan C, Casciola-Rosen L et al. Recurrent transverse myelitis associated with anti-Ro (SSA) antibodies. Neurology 2004; 13: 147–149.

196. Weinshenker BG, Wingerchuk DM, Vukusic S et al. NMO-IgG predicts relapse following longitudinally extensive transverse myelitis. Ann Neurol 2006; 59: 566–569.

197. Wingerchuk DM, Lennon VA, Pittock SJ et al. Revised diagnostic criteria for neuromyelitis optica. Neurology 2006; 66: 1485–1489.

198. Lucchinetti CF, Mandler RN, McGavern D et al. A role for humoral mechanisms in the pathogenesis of Devic's neuromyelitis optica. Brain 2002; 125: 1450–1461.

199. Ortiz de Zarate JC, Tamaroff L, Sica RE, Rodriguez JA. Neuromyelitis optica versus subacute necrotic myelitis. II. Anatomical study of two cases. J Neurol Neurosurg Psychiatry 1968; 31: 641–645.

200. Lefkowitz D, Angelo JN. Neuromyelitis optica with unusual vascular changes. Arch Neurol 1984; 41: 1103–1105.

201. Misu T, Kakita A, Fujihara K et al. A comparative neuropathological analysis of Japanese cases of neuromyelitis optica and multiple sclerosis. Neurology 2005; 64: A39.

202. Correale J, Fiol M. Activation of humoral immunity and eosinophils in neuromyelitis optica. Neurology 2004; 63: 2363–2370.

203. Nakashima I, Fujihara K, Misu T et al. A comparative study of Japanese multiple sclerosis patients with and without oligoclonal IgG bands. Mult Scler 2002; 8: 459–462.

204. Nakashima I, Fujihara K, Fujimori J et al. Absence of IgG1 response in the cerebrospinal fluid of relapsing neuromyelitis optica. Neurology 2004; 62: 144–146.

205. Satoh J, Yukitake M, Kurohara K et al. Detection of the 14-3-3 protein in the cerebrospinal fluid of Japanese multiple sclerosis patients presenting with severe myelitis. J Neurol Sci 2003; 212: 11–20.

206. Irani DN, Kerr DA. 14-3-3 protein in the cerebrospinal fluid of patients with acute myelitis. Lancet 2000; 355: 901.

207. Martinez-Yelamos A, Saiz A, Sanchez-Valle R et al. 14-3-3 protein in the CSF as a

prognostic marker in early multiple sclerosis. Neurology 2001; 57: 722–724.

208. Roemer SF, Parisi JE, Lennon VE et al. Pattern specific loss of aquaporin 4 immunoreactivity distinguishes neuromyelitis optica from multiple sclerosis. Brain 2007; 130: 1194–1205.

209. Misu T, Fujihara K, Kakita A et al. Loss of aquaporin 4 in lesions in neuromyelitis optica: distinction from multiple sclerosis. Brain 2007; 130: 1224–1234.

210. Sinclair C, Kirk J, Herron B et al. Absence of aquaporin 4 expression in lesions of neuromyelitis optica but increased expression in multiple sclerosis lesions and normal-appearing white matter. Acta Neuropathol 2007; 113: 187–194.

211. Agre P, Kozono D. Aquaporin water channels: molecular mechanisms of human disease. FEBS Lett 2003; 555: 72–78.

212. Nielsen S, Nagelhus EA, Amiry-Moghaddam M et al. Specialized membrane domains for water transport in glial cells: high-resolution immunogold cytochemistry of aquaporin-4 in rat brain. J Neurosci 1997; 17: 171–180.

213. Castle NA. Aquaporins as targets for drug discovery. Drug Discov Today 2005; 10: 485–493.

214. Saida T, Tashiro K, Itoyama Y et al, Interferon-beta Multiple Sclerosis Study Group of Japan. Interferon beta-1b is effective in Japanese RRMS patients: a randomized multicenter study. Neurology 2005; 64: 621–630.

215. Papeix C, Vidal JS, de Seze J et al. Immunosuppressive therapy is more effective than interferon in neuromyelitis optica. Mult Scler 2007; 13: 256–259.

216. Warabi Y, Matsumoto Y, Hayashi H. Interferon beta-1b exacerbates multiple sclerosis with severe optic nerve and spinal cord demyelination. J Neurol Sci 2007; 252: 257–261.

217. Wingerchuk DM, Weinshenker BG. Neuromyelitis optica. Curr Treat Options Neurol 2005; 7: 173–182.

218. Mandler RN, Ahmed W, Dencoff JE. Devic's neuromyelitis optica: a prospective study of seven patients treated with prednisone and azathioprine. Neurology 1998; 51: 1219–1220.

219. Silverman GJ, Weisman S. Rituximab therapy and autoimmune disorders. Prospects for anti-B cell therapy. Arthritis Rheum 2003; 48: 1484–1492.

220. Cree BAC, Lamb S, Morgan K et al. An open label study of the effects of rituximab in neuromyelitis optica. Neurology 2005; 64: 1270–1272.

221. Bakker J, Metz L. Devic's neuromyelitis optica treated with intravenous gamma globulin (IVIG). Can J Neurol Sci 2004; 31: 265–267.

222. Hartung HP, Gonsette R, Konig N et al. Mitoxantrone in progressive multiple sclerosis: a placebo-controlled, double-blind, randomized, multicenter trial. Lancet 2002; 360: 2018–2025.

223. Goodin DS, Arnason BG, Coyle PK et al. The use of mitoxantrone (Novantrone) for the treatment of multiple sclerosis: Report of the Therapeutic and Technology Assessment Subcommittee of the American Academy of Neurology. Neurology 2003; 61: 1332–1338.

224. Weinstock-Guttman B, Ramanathan M, Lincoff N et al. Study of mitoxantrone for the treatment of recurrent neuromyelitis optica (Devic disease). Arch Neurol 2006; 63; 957–963.

Pediatric multiple sclerosis

B. L. Banwell

INTRODUCTION

The onset of multiple sclerosis (MS) in childhood has captured increased attention over the last few years. Pediatric health care practitioners are now more likely to consider MS in the differential of acute relapsing neurological dysfunction in children, and are more vigilant in the long term observation and care of children who have experienced an initial acute demyelinating event. The advent of magnetic resonance imaging (MRI) technology has contributed to increased confidence in MS diagnosis in children, although formal MRI criteria for pediatric MS are not yet available.

Children with MS, who by virtue of their young age have a limited time for subclinical disease activity, are uniquely close to the biological onset of the MS disease process. Study of the environmental exposures, immunological responses, and MRI parameters in these very young MS patients may lead to novel insights into the inciting events in MS pathobiology.

The present chapter will review the clinical presentation and natural history, MRI features, management, and environmental and immunological aspects of MS in children.

CLINICAL FEATURES OF ACUTE DEMYELINATION

There are several clinical phenotypes of acute demyelination, which relate to the location and extent of the white matter lesions in the optic nerve, spinal cord or brain. Figure 4.1 represents the relative frequency of clinical demyelinating phenotypes at presentation in published cohorts of children subsequently diagnosed with MS. The term 'clinically isolated syndrome' (CIS) is commonly used in adults with an initial isolated demyelinating event. Monolesional CIS refers to an acute demyelinating presentation that is localizable to a single location in the central nervous system (CNS) – typical examples include optic neuritis, transverse myelitis, intranuclear ophthalmoplegia, hemisensory loss or hemimotor weakness. Polylesional CIS refers to a demyelinating presentation in which the clinical symptoms must be localized to more than one site in the CNS. It is important to note that, although the term 'lesional' is used, the delineation of 'mono-' versus 'poly-' is based on clinical localization, not on MRI features. MRI find-

ings of multiple clinically silent white matter lesions in a patient with a clinical demyelinating phenotype localized to a single CNS site (e.g. optic neuritis) does not change the diagnosis to polylesional CIS. The implications of multiple MRI findings in patients with CIS are discussed further in the section on MRI below.

OPTIC NEURITIS

Optic neuritis (ON) is a relatively common demyelinating phenotype in children. Pain with ocular movement (often described as headache) and reduced visual acuity are the most common expressed symptoms. Examination typically reveals markedly reduced visual acuity, attenuated color perception, centrocecal scotoma and papillitis (in approximately 50%). It has been stated that acute ON in childhood differs from adult onset ON in that visual recovery is more complete, the risk of subsequent diagnosis of MS is less and bilateral ON is more common than unilateral ON.[1,2] However, it is possible that some children with unilateral ON may not report visual loss if they have full function of the other eye.

The risk of MS following childhood ON has been variably reported as being from 6–56%.[1,3,4] In a study of 36 children presenting with optic neuritis to our institution, 17 had one or more clinically silent white matter lesions on MRI and 13 of these children have been diagnosed with MS to date. None of the 17 children with normal brain MRI (exclusive of the optic nerves) have evidence of ongoing demyelination to date,[5] although many years of clinical observation are required to truly evaluate MS risk in these children. In one series of 79 childhood ON patients, a second MS-defining event occurred in 13% by 10 years and in 26% more than 40 years after the initial ON.[4]

TRANSVERSE MYELITIS

Transverse myelitis (TM) in children typically presents with acute neurological deficits below the level of spinal cord involvement, Lhermitte's sign (a sudden vibrating or painful sensation mediated by flexion of the spine) and occasionally back pain. Bladder and bowel dysfunction are often present. The MRI appearance varies from discrete longitudinally-restricted lesions to longitudinally extensive lesions spanning multiple cord

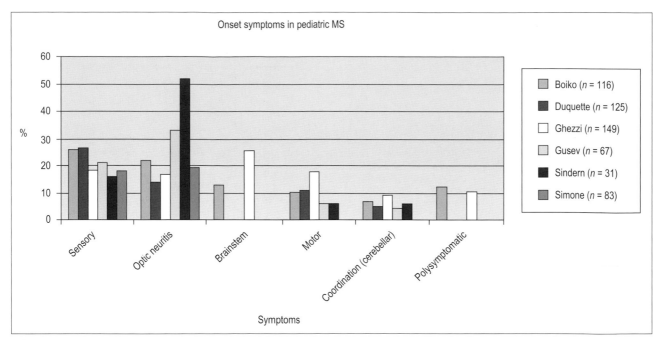

FIG. 4.1 Presenting features of acute demyelination in children.

levels. Oval-shaped discrete spinal cord lesion patterns are felt to be characteristic of adult MS[6] while longitudinally extensive lesions are more characteristic of Devic's neuromyelitis optica (NMO),[7] vasculitis of the cord or vascular ischemia.[6] Detailed review of the MRI appearance of TM in children has not been published but longitudinally extensive lesions appear to be relatively common both in isolated TM and in children with MS (as demonstrated in Fig. 4.2). Inflammatory lesions of the spinal cord, often with involvement of the proximal nerve roots, can be associated with CNS Lyme disease and with infection with West Nile Virus,[6] and thus these diagnoses must be specifically excluded in patients presenting in endemic regions.

DEVIC'S NEUROMYELITIS OPTICA

Neuromyelitis optica is a demyelinating syndrome characterized by recurrent demyelination of the optic nerves and spinal cord.[7,8] MRI of the spine demonstrates longitudinally extensive lesions, and spinal fluid analyses often demonstrate pleocytosis and absence of oligoclonal banding.[7] In adults, relapsing NMO is associated with severe disability within 5 years of onset.[7] The outcome in children appears to be more favorable. In a study of nine children with NMO followed for a mean of 5.3 years, full recovery of visual and motor function was achieved in all nine, despite severe initial demyelinating episodes.[9] Recently, an antibody has been identified in serum that appears to be highly specific for NMO and allows NMO to be distinguished from typical adult-onset MS.[10] The antibody (termed NMO-IgG) outlines CNS microvessels, pia, subpia and Virchow–Robin spaces. The pathogenicity of this antibody has yet to be determined. The target antigen has recently been identified to be aquaporin-4 water channel and may represent a completely novel autoimmune target.[11] Whether children with NMO harbor this antibody has to be evaluated.

MONOLESIONAL CLINICALLY ISOLATED SYNDROME – OTHER

Young children tend to under-report hemisensory symptoms, either because they lack the vocabulary to adequately describe them or because the symptoms are not of a severity as to limit play or other activities. Isolated hemimotor weakness can be the first manifestation of MS. Focal neurological deficits, particularly those associated with rapid onset, appropriately lead to investigations for vascular etiologies.

POLYLESIONAL CLINICALLY ISOLATED SYNDROME

The first attack of demyelination in children often involves multiple concurrent symptoms. If the patient exhibits altered mental function, particularly in conjunction with headache, fever and meningism and accompanied by cerebrospinal fluid (CSF) pleocytosis, the term polysymptomatic CIS is replaced by the term acute disseminated encephalomyelitis (ADEM). ADEM is discussed in more detail below. Polysymptomatic CIS with preserved consciousness (e.g. a child with unilateral ON, hemimotor weakness and ataxia) occurs with relative frequency in children, although the exact prevalence of this demyelinating phenotype is difficult to glean from the literature because of the fact that some clinicians use the term ADEM in these patients. Whether children with polylesional CIS are at particularly high risk for subsequent MS diagnosis remains to be determined.

DIAGNOSIS OF MULTIPLE SCLEROSIS IN CHILDREN

Pediatric onset of MS has been the subject of several retrospective studies,[12–25] longitudinal studies[26,27] and reviews.[28,29] As in adult MS, the cornerstone of MS diagnosis in children is confirmation of recurrent or progressive demyelination over time involving multiple areas of the CNS.[30,31] Recently, criteria for the diagnosis of MS in children have been proposed by an international working group.[32]

The vast majority of children will manifest with the relapsing remitting form of MS.[12,15,19,20,22–24,27,33,34] The time from first presentation to second MS-defining attack is short, typically less than 1 year.[29] Primary progressive MS is exceptionally rare in children, representing 0–2% of children reported in recent

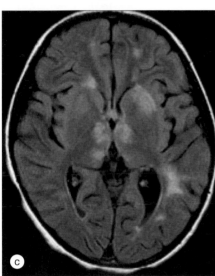

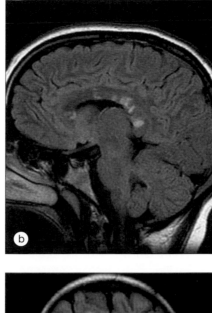

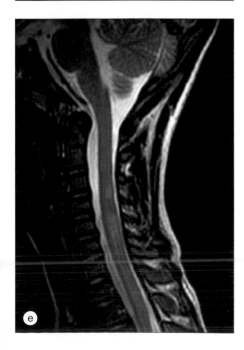

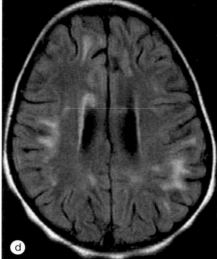

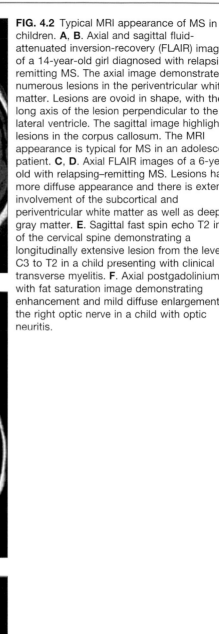

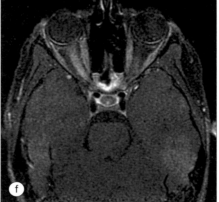

FIG. 4.2 Typical MRI appearance of MS in children. **A, B**. Axial and sagittal fluid-attenuated inversion-recovery (FLAIR) images of a 14-year-old girl diagnosed with relapsing–remitting MS. The axial image demonstrates numerous lesions in the periventricular white matter. Lesions are ovoid in shape, with the long axis of the lesion perpendicular to the lateral ventricle. The sagittal image highlights lesions in the corpus callosum. The MRI appearance is typical for MS in an adolescent patient. **C, D**. Axial FLAIR images of a 6-year-old with relapsing–remitting MS. Lesions have a more diffuse appearance and there is extensive involvement of the subcortical and periventricular white matter as well as deep gray matter. **E**. Sagittal fast spin echo T2 image of the cervical spine demonstrating a longitudinally extensive lesion from the level of C3 to T2 in a child presenting with clinical transverse myelitis. **F**. Axial postgadolinium T1 with fat saturation image demonstrating enhancement and mild diffuse enlargement of the right optic nerve in a child with optic neuritis.

series.[29,35] The available data on the features and management of primary progressive MS is insufficient for further discussion in this chapter.

CEREBROSPINAL FLUID ANALYSIS

Children presenting with acute demyelination often have spinal fluid analysis performed to exclude infection, and CSF examinations are more valuable in the exclusion of other diseases than as a means of confirmation of MS diagnosis.[35] CNS demyelination has been well documented to occur in the context of acute CNS infection with Epstein–Barr virus (EBV), *Mycoplasma* spp., enteroviruses and other pathogens.[36] However, in the vast majority of MS patients, no acute infection is documented. Mild CSF pleocytosis, defined as CSF white blood cell counts below 30 cells/μl, occurs in approximately 60% of children.[37]

Spinal fluid analysis for the presence of oligoclonal banding (OCB) was positive in 92% of 136 pediatric MS reported in one series.[37] The yield of OCB may vary depending on the age of the child at the time of procurement and on the timing of CSF analysis relative to disease duration. In one series, CSF OCB positivity was present in only 8% of very young children (less than 10 years of age) at the time of first attack but rose to 60–70% if sampled after five or more relapses and was positive at all time points in over 70–80% of older children and adolescents.[35] The technique of CSF analysis probably contributes significantly to the detection of positive results. Isoelectric focusing is considered the 'gold standard' and requires less than 200 μl of CSF. CSF protein electrophoresis, a technique still used in some laboratories, is less sensitive and requires a volume of CSF (often >5 ml) that may be more than is typically available from spinal fluid samples obtained in young children. Finally, pediatric health care practitioners unfamiliar with OCB analyses may fail to send a matched serum sample with the CSF as required to determine the intrathecal origin of immunoglobulin.

MAGNETIC RESONANCE IMAGING FEATURES

Application of the McDonald criteria for MS diagnosis,[30] particularly with respect to the use of MRI evidence of subclinical disease activity, remains controversial in children both with respect to lesion 'distribution in space' and to lesion 'evolution over time'. Relative to adults, the MRI appearance of lesion distribution in children presenting with the first attack is less likely to conform to the MRI criteria for dissemination in space.[38] Children tend to have fewer lesions at the time of first presentation (and thus do not meet the '9 T2 lesion' aspect of the criteria), and seem to be less likely than adults to have lesions centered around the periventricular region. It is possible that the regional proclivity for lesion development differs in the children in whom primary myelination is not yet complete. Pediatric MS MRI criteria are under development.

Application of the MRI lesion dissemination in time aspect of the McDonald criteria may also be problematic. There are few longitudinal MRI studies in children recovering from an initial demyelinating event, and thus the natural history of lesion evolution on MRI in the first few months is relatively unknown. Analysis of MRI data obtained at the time of initial acute CNS demyelination in 116 children found that the rate of a second MS-defining attack was highest in children with corpus callosum long axis perpendicular lesions and/or the sole presence of well defined lesions.[39] Detailed studies of the predictive application of serial MRI analyses are in progress (funded by the Canadian Multiple Sclerosis Scientific Research Foundation). In the absence of such data, the diagnostic significance of clinically silent new lesions in the first few months after initial demyelination must be cautiously interpreted.

Figure 4.2 demonstrates the varied appearances of white matter lesion pattern and distribution in adolescents and children with MS. Overall, the MRI appearance of MS in most pediatric patients does not differ from that in adults.[35] Posterior fossa lesions, large lesions with ill-defined margins and tumefactive lesions appear to be more common in children, particularly those less than 10 years of age. Multiple ring-enhancing lesions have been reported in pediatric MS[40] and must be distinguished from infections such as cysticercosis.

Magnetic resonance spectroscopy (MRS) studies of lesions and normal-appearing white matter (NAWM) in small cohorts of children with MS have shown decreased N-acetyl aspartate and choline, and increased myoinositol in lesions.[41] One small study suggested that the MRS of NAWM appears not to differ from spectra obtained from healthy age-matched children,[41] suggesting that changes in NAWM occur later in the MS disease process. Magnetization transfer and diffusion tensor imaging studies of normal-appearing brain tissue in 13 children with recently diagnosed MS (mean 17 months, range 8–36 months) revealed only a slight increase in diffusivity.[42] Larger studies are required to determine whether abnormalities in NAWM can be detected in young children with MS, or whether NAWM involvement is truly a secondary consequence of the MS disease process.

In adults, quantification of MRI lesion burden on T2-weighted scans and the number of enhancing lesions on T1-weighted images obtained after administration of gadolinium have been used as metrics in studies of clinical outcome and particularly in studies of treatment efficacy.[43,44] However, the T2 lesion burden is a poor correlate for clinical disability.[45] Measures of regional or global brain atrophy appear to more accurately associate with clinical findings on physical and neuropsychological examination.[46] One small study of four children with MS failed to demonstrate brain atrophy over a time period of 6–8 years.[47] However, as is highlighted in Figure 4.3, rapidly progressive atrophy can occur in children with MS. Further studies in this area are clearly required, particularly in light of the neurocognitive issues discussed below.

CHARACTERISTICS OF MULTIPLE SCLEROSIS IN CHILDREN

PREVALENCE

There are no prospective population-based studies of the incidence of MS in children and adolescents to date, although such a study is now under way in Canadian children. Data from a recent population-based database survey found that 3.3% of all MS patients presented under age 16 years,[48] which is consistent with published estimates stating that 3–5% of all MS cases begin prior to 16 years of age.[16,18] The onset of MS under age 10 years occurs in only 0.2–0.7% of all MS cases.[25,28,49]

DEMOGRAPHICS

The female to male ratio in pediatric MS has been reported variably as being from 0.42–7.6 (reviewed in reference 35). Children less than 10 years of age appear to have either an equal representation of females and males or a male predominance.[28,50] The F:M ratio in children between age 10 and 16 in most series is 1.3–2.0,[35] with an increasing female preponderance noted with increasing age. The absence of a female preponderance in MS prior to age 10 years supports the role of sex hormones in MS.

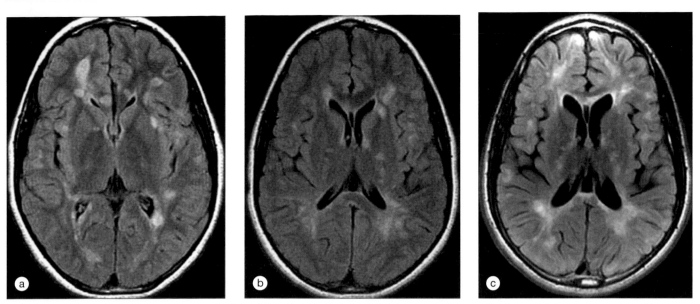

FIG. 4.3 Rapidly progressive cerebral atrophy in a child with MS. **A.** Axial FLAIR image obtained at the time of clinical presentation with isolated optic neuritis in a 12-year-old boy subsequently diagnosed with MS (based on further clinical attacks). **B.** Axial FLAIR image of the same patient 1 year later. Note increase in the number of lesions, with new lesions visible in the peritrigonal white matter and in the region of the corticospinal tract. Ventricular size is more prominent. **C.** Axial FLAIR image of the same patient 2 years from initial presentation. New lesions are visible. The most striking finding is rapid progression of the ventricular enlargement and increased cerebrospinal fluid overlying the convexities. These findings are consistent with progressive cerebral atrophy. The patient was on treatment with interferon beta-1b but was not receiving corticosteroid therapy.

RELAPSES AND CLINICAL COURSE

Clinical features of MS relapses in children are similar to those experienced by adults. The annualized relapse rate in the first 2–3 years after clinical disease onset typically ranges from 0.3–1.3.[35] Headache is present in approximately 30% of relapses (personal data) and seizures have been reported in as many as 20% of children in some series.[35] Seizures and headache are particularly prominent features in children with tumefactive demyelination, a demyelinating phenotype characterized by one or more large areas of demyelination, perilesional edema with mass-effect, and often ring-enhancement.[51] Despite the dramatic appearance of these tumor-like plaques, clinical and MRI response to corticosteroid therapy can be rapid and recovery from the acute episode can be complete. Children with onset of MS under age 6 years are more likely to present with ataxia (61%) and seizures (22%), and appear to have a poorer prognosis.[28]

OUTCOME

Recovery from attacks
Recovery from acute demyelinating attacks typically occurs over a period of 4–8 weeks.[35] Recovery may be particularly poor in children with longitudinally extensive transverse myelitis. Lhermitte's sign can persist for several months following spinal cord lesions.

Progression to sustained disability
The clinical course of MS in children has been reported as being more favorable than that of adults based on comparison of the time from disease onset to sustained clinical disability.[12,28] In a study of 296 children with acute demyelination, 57% of whom were diagnosed with MS during the study period (mean 2.9 years of observation), sustained disability for more than 6 months with an Expanded Disability Status Scale (EDSS) score greater than 4 (limited walking ability but able to walk unaided for more than 500 m) occurred in 10% of patients, and an EDSS of 6 (ability to walk with unilateral support no more than 100 m) in 5%.[34] Studies with a longer duration of clinical observation have demonstrated that the mean time to sustained disability in pediatric-onset MS is approximately 20 years.[12] Although the time to SPMS is longer in children, the mean age at permanent disability is considerably younger in the pediatric-onset MS population.[24,52] In a retrospective series involving 83 pediatric-onset MS patients, the time from disease onset to EDSS of 4 was 20.22 years, compared to 10.79 years for a cohort of adult-onset MS patients followed at the same institution.[24] Overall, sustained disability occurs in approximately 10% of children within a few years of disease onset and in approximately 38% by 30 years.[12] The impact of sustained disability on vocational and social achievement is likely to be profound, although published data on the long-term quality of life of pediatric-onset MS patients has yet to be documented.

Cognitive impact of multiple sclerosis in children
The onset of MS during childhood occurs during the key formative years of academic education. The impact of the MS disease process on cognition in children has been the subject of a few small series.[53–55] Cognitive deficits in working memory, executive function and processing speed were prominent in children with earlier age at MS onset and longer duration of disease.[53] Cognitive deficits may occur independent of physical disability,[53] although some children with advanced MS show particularly dramatic cognitive impairment.[55] Further studies are required, but these preliminary studies strongly suggest that cognitive impairment is one of the major sequelae of childhood-onset MS.

TABLE 4.1 Disorders to be considered in the differential of acute central nervous system demyelination in children

Disorder	Distinguishing feature(s)	Diagnostic tests
Monophasic demyelination	Absence of sustained CNS autoimmune activity over time	No diagnostic test to distinguish acute monophasic demyelination from MS Absence of new lesions on MRI is supportive
CNS lupus	Headache Neuropsychiatric features	Serological evidence for antibodies directed against nuclear antigens
CNS vasculopathy	Stroke-like episodes Lesion pattern consistent with vascular distribution	CNS angiography
CNS infection	High fever (if present) May have systemic illness Rash	Lyme antibody titres West Nile virus serology and Western blot Serum serology and CSF PCR assays for neurotrophic viruses
Mitochondrial disease	Presence or family history of: –short stature –deafness –myopathy	Serum and CSF lactate MRS analysis of lactate in CNS DNA testing for MELAS, MERRF, NARP Muscle and skin biopsies for biochemical analyses of respiratory chain function
Leukodystrophies: –MLD –ALD –Pelizaeus–Merzbacher disease (PMD) –Alexander's disease	Typically progressive CNS decline Cognitive or neuropsychiatric manifestations early in the disease Evidence of peripheral nerve involvement (MLD, PMD)	Serum very long chain fatty acids (ALD) Analysis of arylsulfatase A activity in white blood cells and fibroblasts (MLD) DNA analysis of *PMP20* gene (PMD) DNA analysis of *GFAP* gene (Alexander's)
Macrophage-activating syndromes	Typically associated with rheumatological disease	White blood cell and platelet counts Bone marrow aspirate
Sarcoidosis	Exceptionally rare in children	Serum ACE level Chest X-ray
Vitamin B_{12} deficiency	Consider in patients with myelopathy History of short gut syndrome, malnutrition or extreme diets	Serum vitamin B_{12} homocysteine and folate levels

ACE, angiotensin converting enzyme; ALD, adrenoleukodystrophy; CNS, central nervous system; CSF, cerebrospinal fluid; GFAP, glial fibrillary acidic protein; MELAS, mitochondrial encephalopathy and lactic acidosis with stroke-like episodes; MERRF, mitochondrial encephalopathy with ragged red fibers; MLD, metachromatic leukodystrophy; NARP, neuropathy, ataxia and retinitis pigmentosa; PCR, polymerase chain reaction.

DIFFERENTIAL DIAGNOSES

Table 4.1 lists the major conditions to be considered in the differential of acute CNS demyelination in children.

MONOPHASIC DEMYELINATION WITHOUT ENCEPHALOPATHY

Acute CNS demyelination represents a time of great uncertainty. There are currently no diagnostic tests that can reliably predict whether the current demyelinating event represents a monophasic or transiently multiphasic illness, or whether it represents the first clinical manifestation of MS.

The likelihood that a clinically isolated demyelinating event represents the first attack of MS is strengthened by MRI or neurophysiological evidence of clinically silent lesion dissemination in the brain, optic nerves, or spinal cord.

ACUTE DISSEMINATED ENCEPHALOMYELITIS

The term ADEM is typically reserved for children with isolated acute polysymptomatic neurological dysfunction accompanied by encephalopathy.[15,34] Seizures, meningism and cerebrospinal fluid (CSF) pleocytosis may also be present. Most definitions of ADEM include MRI findings of multifocal, bilateral, asymmet-

ric hyperintense lesions of T2-weighted images scattered diffusely in the CNS white matter, often associated with increased signal in the deep grey nuclei.[34,56] The results of cerebrospinal fluid analysis for oligoclonal bands has been reported as positive in 3–10% of children.[15,57] Antecedent infection with a variety of infectious organisms, including varicella, rubella and influenza, occurs much more frequently in ADEM than in other demyelinating phenotypes.[58] ADEM has also been temporally linked to immunization with rabies, smallpox, measles and Japanese encephalitis vaccines (reviewed in reference 59). Vaccination-related demyelination is reportable in Canada and appears to be exceptionally rare.

Although ADEM is typically considered a monophasic illness, some children may experience one or more recurrences as the corticosteroid therapy is reduced (steroid-dependent ADEM), may experience a re-emergence of the same clinical and radiographic features within 6 months of their acute illness (relapsing ADEM) or may experience two episodes of demyelination that fulfill the criteria for ADEM, although the second episode may include new clinical or radiographic disease (multiphasic ADEM). These definitions are based on the clinical definitions proposed by the International Pediatric Multiple Sclerosis Working Group of the National Multiple Sclerosis Society.[32]

An ADEM phenotype can also represent the first attack of MS.[59–62] In a recent review of 296 children with acute demyelination, 34 of 119 children (29%) initially diagnosed with ADEM were ultimately diagnosed with MS based on evidence of recurrent demyelination.[63] In comparison, a longitudinal study of 84 children with ADEM followed for a mean of 6.6 years found that, although the disease was biphasic in 10% of children, none met the criteria for MS.[57] These two studies highlight the discrepancies in outcome reported in pediatric ADEM. The use of MRI is unlikely to resolve these discrepancies (reviewed in reference 64). MRI findings of bilaterally extensive white and often deep gray involvement, with multiple areas of enhancement, are characteristic of ADEM but can evolve into an MRI picture of 'typical' MS over time, and children with an ADEM clinical phenotype can have an MRI appearance characteristic of MS.[65] In a study of adults with ADEM, 15 of 40 patients (38%) were ultimately diagnosed with MS. Careful analysis of this adult ADEM cohort failed to identify a clinical, MRI or CSF finding that was reliably associated with an MS outcome.[61]

Thus, the debate as to whether ADEM is a distinct, ultimately transient, clinical demyelinating syndrome distinct from MS will not be resolved in the absence of a distinguishing biological marker. It is important to note that the most important determinant of outcome is time. Consistent longitudinal surveillance of all children with a history of acute CNS demyelination of any phenotype is critical if the true risk of MS in these children is to be fully appreciated.

CENTRAL NERVOUS SYSTEM VASCULOPATHY

Vasculitis of the CNS is typically associated with systemic as well as neurological symptoms. Recurrent fever, weight loss and dermatological and multiorgan involvement are features that distinguish vasculitis from MS in most patients. However, fatigue, sensory disturbance and headache may be the presenting features of both vasculitis and demyelination. MRI images of CNS vasculitis may reveal small, punctuate white matter changes that at first glance may appear similar to demyelination. Laboratory evidence of anemia and leukocytosis, persistent elevation of erythrocyte sedimentation rates and the presence of antinuclear and antineutrophil antibodies are more consistent with vasculitis. MRI angiography or conventional angiograms are required but can be normal even in biopsy-proven disease. CSF analysis for oligoclonal bands is negative in CNS vasculitis.

MACROPHAGE ACTIVATION SYNDROMES

Macrophage activation syndrome (MAS) can present with CNS demyelination, or with fulminant necrotizing encephalitis. MAS is most commonly associated with rheumatological diseases. Persistent fever and decreased platelet and white blood cell counts, hepatosplenomegaly, lymphadenopathy and evidence of hemophagocytosis in bone marrow aspirates lead to a diagnosis of MAS.[66,67] In patients in whom the initial manifestations of MAS are neurological, differentiation from acute demyelination may be difficult.[63]

GENETIC AND METABOLIC DISEASES INVOLVING CENTRAL NERVOUS SYSTEM WHITE MATTER

Detailed reviews of the clinical and MRI features of pediatric-onset mitochondrial disease and the leukodystrophies have been published elsewhere.[68–72] In addition to neurological symptoms, children with mitochondrial disease may also show restricted somatic growth, sensorineural hearing loss, myopathy

or cardiomyopathy. Acute neurological deficits occur, particularly in MELAS syndrome. When these acute deteriorations occur prior to, or in the absence of, chronic systemic features of mitochondrial disease, distinction from MS may be difficult. Analysis of serum, CSF and MRS evidence of lactate, DNA studies for the more common mitochondrial disease mutations and even muscle biopsy for biochemical analysis of respiratory chain function may be required.

The clinical features of progressive spasticity and neurocognitive decline characteristic of X-linked adrenoleukodystrophy, metachromatic leukodystrophy and Krabbe's disease are rarely confused with MS. These diagnoses are more often raised by the radiologist viewing the MRI appearance of confluent white matter lesions in a child with MS in whom previously discrete white matter lesions have progressed to a more confluent appearance. It is important to note that the MRI appearance of juvenile-onset Alexander's disease may include discrete white matter lesions quite similar to those of MS.[73] Although juvenile Alexander's disease is characterized by progressive ataxia and spasticity that may have a similarity to MS, the prominent features of seizures, cognitive decline, parkinsonism, palatal myoclonus and pseudobulbar dysfunction would be atypical of childhood-onset MS.[74]

MANAGEMENT

ACUTE DEMYELINATION

Management of acute demyelination is determined by the clinical severity. Mild symptoms do not require pharmacological intervention. However, counseling of the child and family regarding the diagnosis and possible future risk of MS is a key aspect of care (see General care, below).

Children with acute demyelinating symptoms that are sufficiently severe to interfere with function or that cause discomfort are treated with corticosteroids. Although there have been no formal studies of corticosteroid therapy for acute demyelination in children, most clinicians commence therapy with intravenous Solu-Medrol at 20–30 mg/kg/day for 3–5 days.[75] The decision to offer a tapering schedule for prednisone depends on the initial response. If the symptoms have resolved completely, a tapering dose of prednisone is not required. For children with partial but not yet complete recovery, a tapering schedule of prednisone starting at a dose of 1 mg/kg/day tapered by 5 mg every 2–3 days is offered.

Not all children will respond to corticosteroids and some children will respond initially but will have a recurrence of their symptoms as soon as the corticosteroid dose is lowered. Case-report- and case-series-level evidence exists for the use of intravenous immune globulin (IVIg) in such patients.[76–79] A total of 12 papers in which one to three children with ADEM were treated with IVIg have reported complete recovery from clinical symptoms in 10 of the 12 children treated. IVIg has also been shown to be of benefit in adults with ADEM.[80,81] In our clinic, we use 2 g/kg IVIg divided over 2 days in children under 50 kg, and divided over 4–5 days in children who are more than 50 kg in weight.[75]

RELAPSING-REMITTING MULTIPLE SCLEROSIS

General care

There are many aspects of management of children with MS. A multidisciplinary team approach, with care by a neurologist with expertise in childhood MS, nurses familiar with MS care, physiotherapy, occupational therapy and social work, as well as collaboration with pediatric neuroophthalmology, psychiatry and urology, is optimal.

Conveying the diagnosis of MS to the child and the family invariably leads to shock and disbelief. Coping with the diagnosis is aided by timely education and support. Several resources are available for children and their families through the multiple sclerosis societies in North America (http://www.mssociety.ca/en/help/YoungPersonsMS.htm, http://www.nationalmssociety.org/peds_network.asp), and we have designed a website discussing acute CNS demyelination for children and families (http://pedsdemyelination.ccb.sickkids.ca).

Immunomodulatory therapies

There are now four immunomodulatory medications approved in relapsing–remitting MS: three forms of interferon (IFN)-β and glatiramer acetate. The use of these medications in children with MS is increasing, particularly in light of emerging evidence that initiation of therapy early in the MS disease course improves long-term outcome.[82–84]

Two of the interferon-β preparations are administered by subcutaneous injection, IFNβ-1b (Betaseron) 8 MIU every second day and IFNβ-1a (Rebif) 22 μg or 44 μg three times weekly. IFNβ-1a (Avonex) is administered by intramuscular injection once weekly. Glatiramer acetate is administered at a dose of 20 mg daily by subcutaneous injection.

A key issue in the initiation of treatment and in the selection of which preparation is best for an individual child is patient and parent acceptance and education. In our clinic, a teaching puppet is used to demonstrate injection technique, which is practiced by both parents and the child (even if the child will not be the one to administer the injection). We encourage the entire family to attend these teaching sessions, including siblings, so that they have a better appreciation of what their brother or sister is experiencing. The selection of subcutaneous or intramuscularly administered IFN or glatiramer acetate depends on the clinician's impression of the best choice for the child, but equally on which preparation is most acceptable to the child and family. Some children strongly favor infrequent injections over all other factors – for these children once weekly therapy is likely to be associated with the best compliance. For other children, smaller needles and the option of the use of an autoinjector may be the most important criteria. Younger children seem to find the springload effect of the autoinjector – the sound and the rapid force in which it injects the needle – frightening and often prefer manual injection. The family-centered, patient-focused approach to medication choice and the education and support provided by our pediatric-MS-certified nurses has led to a compliance and acceptability rate of over 90% in our patients.

The mechanism of action and biological rationale for the interferons and glatiramer acetate has been reviewed elsewhere.[75,85–87] The efficacy of these preparations and the pivotal trials that led to their approval for use in adults with MS have also been published.[88–91]

Interferon-β in children with multiple sclerosis To date, there have been no formal treatment trials of interferon-β (IFNβ) in children with MS. Case reports and case series of treatment tolerability have been reported.[92–95] There are no published guidelines of the dosing or titration of IFN-β in pediatric MS. Discussions with other pediatric MS specialists, combined with the experience in our clinic in managing over 50 children on MS therapies, indicates that the doses recommended in adults can be applied to children. We start with one-quarter dose, and increase gradually to full dose depending on patient tolerability

and on liver function studies. Other centers start with full dose and have not found tolerability to be problematic.[94]

Pohl et al published the safety and tolerability of subcutaneous IFNβ-1a in a cohort of 51 children and adolescents with MS.[94] IFNβ-1a was commenced at 22 μg subcutaneously three times weekly in 46 of the children; five children were commenced on 44 μg subcutaneously three times weekly. Of the 46 children treated with the lower dose, 22 were switched to the 44 μg subcutaneously three times weekly schedule because of ongoing MS disease activity. Mild leukopenia was noted in 27% and elevated liver enzymes in 35%. In none of the children were the laboratory abnormalities of sufficient concern to alter therapy. At the end of the study observation period of 1.8 years (range 1 month to 4.4 years) 42 of the children (82%) continued on therapy.

The safety and tolerability of IFNβ-1a by intramuscular injection was reviewed in a survey of nine children.[96] Initiation of therapy varied from doses of 10 μg to the full dose of 30 μg intramuscular injection weekly. Flu-like side effects were experienced by half of the children but none of them discontinued therapy because of adverse events. The impact of IFNβ-1a by intramuscular injection on laboratory values was not reported.

An international working group retrospectively reviewed safety and tolerability of IFNβ-1b in a cohort of 43 children and adolescents treated for a mean of 29.2 months.[97] Elevated liver enzymes occurred in 26% and mild flu-like symptoms in 35%. No serious adverse events were reported.

Glatiramer acetate There are no guidelines for administration of glatiramer acetate in children, but it can be commenced and maintained at the same dose as in adults (20 mg subcutaneous injection daily).[75]

The most significant side effect reported in children (as in adults) is a systemic flushing reaction associated with tachycardia. This reaction typically occurs once or twice, often within the first weeks of therapy. Liver function and leukocyte counts are not significantly impacted by glatiramer acetate and routine monitoring is not required. Frequent subcutaneous injections in young children require rotation of injection sites and careful monitoring to avoid regional lipoatrophy.

Intravenous immunoglobulin as a treatment to prevent relapses and disability Intravenous immunoglobulin has been studied in adult MS (reviewed in a meta-analysis[98]) and found to reduce relapse rate with a trend toward reduced disability. The strongest evidence of efficacy of IVIg in MS was demonstrated in a 2-year randomized control trial of 0.15–0.20 g/kg per month in which relapse rate and proportion of relapse-free patients significantly favored the treated group.[99] Monthly IVIg, in a randomized placebo-controlled double-blind study in patients with a first attack of demyelination, led to a reduced incidence of a second MS-defining attack and led to reduced MRI evidence of disease.[100] There are no data on the use of regularly scheduled IVIg in pediatric MS patients.

Immunosuppressive therapies

Mitoxantrone is an antineoplastic agent that intercalates with DNA, inhibiting DNA synthesis, and provides its immunosuppressive activity by reducing the circulating T-cell population, inhibiting B-cell antibody production, and inhibition of helper-, but not suppressor-T-cell function.[101] Although mitoxantrone has been approved for use in adults with aggressive (enhancing lesions on MRI, and frequent MS relapses) relapsing–remitting MS, the use of mitoxantrone in children with MS is extremely limited. Side effects reported in adults, including amenorrhea and a cumulative dose-dependent risk of cardiac toxicity, make mitoxantrone a less attractive therapeutic option in children.

Cyclophosphamide is an alkylating agent with potent immunosuppressive properties. The use of cyclophosphamide in MS is controversial. Cyclophosphamide in combination with corticosteroid therapy led to clinical stabilization of disease in a cohort of MS patients with highly active disease,[102] and many specialists use cyclophosphamide for young adult MS patients with highly active MS disease. Cyclophosphamide has been used in children with frequent relapses (typically children who have continued to experience MS relapses despite use of immunomodulatory therapies). In this highly selected population, cyclophosphamide reduces acute relapse disability, reduces relapse frequency, and improves fatigue in children with aggressive MS. This data is anecdotal, and clearly needs validation in a controlled study. All families must be counseled on the long-term risks of infertility, bladder carcinoma or other malignancies, and short term risks of alopecia, immune suppression, hemorrhagic cystitis, and nausea.

SECONDARY PROGRESSIVE MULTIPLE SCLEROSIS

The management of secondary progressive MS remains largely symptomatic and supportive. Few children reach this stage of the MS disease process during their childhood.

Symptomatic management

Fatigue Generalized fatigue of sufficient severity as to interfere with daily functioning is reported by approximately 30% of pediatric MS patients. Fatigue may be pervasive or may occur only in close temporal proximity to clinical relapses. Management requires a careful history of daily activity. Carrying heavy backpacks to school, repeated trips up and down school stairs and extensive homework assignments are a few examples of modifiable activities that can be reduced to allow a more meaningful expenditure of a child's energy. If lifestyle modification alone is insufficient, we have found medications such as modafinil or amantadine to be of benefit.[75]

Spasticity The management of spasticity in children with severe MS is similar to the management of spasticity in other pediatric neurological disorders. Localized injection of botulinum toxin,[103] and oral medications such as tizanidine (reviewed in reference 104) and benzodiazepines, may be effective.

STUDIES OF MULTIPLE SCLEROSIS PATHOBIOLOGY IN CHILDREN

The pathobiology of MS is considered to relate to a complex interaction between genetic predisposition, environmental triggers and host immunological responses.

GENETIC PREDISPOSITION

Approximately 3–10% of children with MS report a history of MS in first-degree relatives.[35] There does not appear to be a heightened familial aggregation of MS in families with affected children; however, many first-degree relatives of these children are themselves still under the age of 40 and may yet develop MS. An increased frequency of HLA-DR2 alleles was demonstrated in pediatric MS patients in Russia.[33] Studies of myelin–oligodendroglial gene[105] or tumor necrosis factor alpha gene[106] mutations or polymorphisms have failed to find a specific association with pediatric MS.

ENVIRONMENTAL TRIGGERS

Exposure to environmental agents such as viruses triggers an obligatory host immunological response. While the vast majority of these responses are adaptive, aberrant host responses have been well documented to lead to autoimmune diseases.[107] Association between MS and a variety of common infective agents such as EBV, *Chlamydophila* (formerly *Chlamydia*) *pneumoniae* and human herpes virus (HHV)-6, among others, have been described in cohorts of adult-onset MS.[108–112]

EBV is a virus of particular interest in MS because of its biological properties of lifelong B-cell infection, ongoing T-cell surveillance of infected B cells and genetic homology between EBV nuclear antigen and myelin basic protein.

If viral infection plays a role in the MS disease process, it may be that infection must occur at a key age, during a period of immunological vulnerability, or even that the order of viral exposures influences the host immune system in such a manner as to lead to heightened immunological activation only in selected situations. Evaluation of the viral repertoire in young pediatric MS patients provides the unique advantage of a limited lifetime of irrelevant viral exposure, and an increased likelihood of detection of relevant viral exposures as compared to age-matched healthy children who are destined to experience infection at a 'less vulnerable' age. In a study of 30 children with MS and 90 age-matched controls, we found that 83% of the MS cohort had serological evidence of prior infection with EBV, compared to only 42% of controls.[113] The association of EBV in childhood MS is further strengthened by data from a single center study from Germany, and from a multinational pediatric MS project.[114,115] In both of these studies, over 85% of children with MS are seropositive for remote EBV infection, which differs significantly from the seroprevalence of healthy age-matched children living in the same regions. There was no difference in seropositivity rate to other common childhood viruses.

Further studies of viral and other environmental exposures in pediatric MS will be aided by international collaborations. Sunlight and vitamin D, diet, exposure to cow's milk antigens and other environmental experiences are all worthy of further evaluation, and children with MS manifest with their disease in unique proximity to these putative exposures.

FUTURE DIRECTIONS

Immunological features of MS in children in both the serum and CSF are currently the subject of several research studies. It has been suggested that the immunological response to key CNS targets expands over time in MS as damage to myelin proteins and axons leads to access of the immune system to novel antigens. If so, and if this process requires time to occur, then the earliest targets of the immunological process in MS will be most apparent in the youngest MS populations. Understanding the key events involved early in the disease may provide novel therapeutic opportunities.

Future research in pediatric MS will require not only laboratory studies, but also detailed prospective collaborative data on the impact of the MS disease process on accrual of disability, on cognitive sequelae, on vocational and social achievement, and on quality of life. As MS-targeted therapies evolve, application of these therapies and the inherent safety monitoring required will require collaborative studies specifically designed for the pediatric MS patient.

ACKNOWLEDGMENT

The author wishes to thank Dr XingChang Wei for his expert assistance on the production of the figures.

REFERENCES

1. Morales DS, Siatkowski RM, Howard CW, Warman R. Optic neuritis in children. J Pediatr Ophthalmol Strabismus 2000; 37: 254–259.

2. Lana-Peixoto MA, Andrade GC. The clinical profile of childhood optic neuritis. Arq Neuropsiquiatr 2001; 59: 311–317.

3. Riikonen R, Donner M, Erkkila H. Optic neuritis in children and its relationship to multiple sclerosis: a clinical study of 21 children. Dev Med Child Neurol 1988; 30: 349–359.

4. Lucchinetti CF, Kiers L, O'Duffy A et al. Risk factors for developing multiple sclerosis after childhood optic neuritis. Neurology 1997; 49: 1413–1418.

5. Brown VE, Pilkington CA, Feldman BM, Davidson JE. An international consensus survey of the diagnostic criteria for juvenile dermatomyositis (JDM). Rheumatology (Oxford) 2006; 45: 990–993.

6. Scotti G, Gerevini S. Diagnosis and differential diagnosis of acute transverse myelopathy. The role of neuroradiological investigations and review of the literature. Neurol Sci 2001; 22(suppl 2): S69–S73.

7. Wingerchuk DM, Weinshenker BG. Neuromyelitis optica: clinical predictors of a relapsing course and survival. Neurology 2003; 60: 848–853.

8. Mandler RN, Davis LE, Jeffery DR, Kornfeld M. Devic's neuromyelitis optica: a clinicopathological study of 8 patients. Ann Neurol 1993; 34: 162–168.

9. Jeffery AR, Buncic JR. Pediatric Devic's neuromyelitis optica. J Pediatr Ophthalmol Strabismus 1996; 33: 223–229.

10. Lennon VA, Wingerchuk DM, Kryzer TJ et al. A serum autoantibody marker of neuromyelitis optica: distinction from multiple sclerosis. Lancet 2004; 364: 2106–2112.

11. Lennon VA, Kryzer TJ, Pittock SJ et al. IgG marker of optic-spinal multiple sclerosis binds to the aquaporin-4 water channel. J Exp Med 2005; 202: 473–477.

12. Boiko A, Vorobeychik G, Paty D et al. Early onset multiple sclerosis: a longitudinal study. Neurology 2002; 59: 1006–1010.

13. Boutin B, Esquivel E, Mayer M et al. Multiple sclerosis in children: report of clinical and paraclinical features of 19 cases. Neuropediatrics 1988; 19: 118–123.

14. Cole GF, Stuart CA. A long perspective on childhood multiple sclerosis. Dev Med Child Neurol 1995; 37: 661–666.

15. Dale RC, de Sousa C, Chong WK et al. Acute disseminated encephalomyelitis, multiphasic disseminated encephalomyelitis and multiple sclerosis in children. Brain 2000; 123: 2407–2422.

16. Duquette P, Murray TJ, Pleines J et al. Multiple sclerosis in childhood: clinical profile in 125 patients. J Pediatr 1987; 111: 359–363.

17. Gall J, Hayles A, Siekert R, Keith H. Multiple sclerosis in children: a clinical study of 40 cases with onset in childhood. Pediatrics 1958; 21: 703–709.

18. Ghezzi A, Deplano V, Faroni J et al. Multiple sclerosis in childhood: clinical features of 149 cases. Mult Scler 1997; 3: 43–46.

19. Guilhoto LM, Osorio CA, Machado LR et al. Pediatric multiple sclerosis report of 14 cases. Brain Dev 1995; 17: 9–12.

20. Gusev E, Boiko A, Bikova O et al. The natural history of early onset multiple sclerosis: comparison of data from Moscow and Vancouver. Clin Neurol Neurosurg 2002; 104: 203–207.

21. Pinhas-Hamiel O, Barak Y, Siev-Ner I, Achiron A. Juvenile multiple sclerosis: clinical features and prognostic characteristics. J Pediatr 1998; 132: 735–737.

22. Ozakbas S, Idiman E, Baklan B, Yulug B. Childhood and juvenile onset multiple sclerosis: clinical and paraclinical features. Brain Dev 2003; 25: 233–236.

23. Selcen D, Anlar B, Renda Y. Multiple sclerosis in childhood: report of 16 cases. Eur Neurol 1996; 36: 79–84.

24. Simone IL, Carrara D, Tortorella C et al. Course and prognosis in early-onset MS: comparison with adult-onset forms. Neurology 2002; 59: 1922–1928.

25. Sindern E, Haas J, Stark E, Wurster U. Early onset MS under the age of 16: clinical and paraclinical features. Acta Neurol Scand 1992; 86: 280–284.

26. Hanefeld F, Bauer HJ, Christen HJ et al. Multiple sclerosis in childhood: report of 15 cases. Brain Dev 1991; 13: 410–416.

27. Ghezzi A, Pozzilli C, Liguori M et al. Prospective study of multiple sclerosis with early onset. Mult Scler 2002; 8: 115–118.

28. Ruggieri M, Polizzi A, Pavone L, Grimaldi LM. Multiple sclerosis in children under 6 years of age. Neurology 1999; 53: 478–484.

29. Banwell BL. Pediatric multiple sclerosis. Curr Neurol Neurosci Rep 2004; 4: 245–252.

30. McDonald WI, Compston A, Edan G et al. Recommended diagnostic criteria for multiple sclerosis: guidelines from the International Panel on the diagnosis of multiple sclerosis. Ann Neurol 2001; 50: 121–127.

31. Poser CM, Paty DW, Scheinberg L et al. New diagnostic criteria for multiple sclerosis: guidelines for research protocols. Ann Neurol 1983; 13: 227–231.

32. Krupp L, Banwell B, Tenembaum S, for the International Pediatric MS Study Group. Consensus definitions proposed for pediatric multiple sclerosis. Neurology 2007; 68, S7–S12.

33. Boiko AN, Guseva ME, Guseva MR et al. Clinico-immunogenetic characteristics of multiple sclerosis with optic neuritis in children. J Neurovirol 2000; 6(suppl 2): S152–S155.

34. Mikaeloff Y, Suissa S, Vallee L et al. First episode of acute CNS inflammatory demyelination in childhood: prognostic factors for multiple sclerosis and disability. J Pediatr 2004; 144: 246–252.

35. Huggieri M, Iannetti P, Polizzi A et al. Multiple sclerosis in children under 10 years of age. Neurol Sci 2004; 25(suppl 4): S326–S335.

36. Sriram S, Steinman L. Postinfectious and postvaccinial encephalomyelitis. Neurol Clin 1984; 2: 341–353.

37. Pohl D, Rostasy K, Reiber H, Hanefeld F. CSF characteristics in early-onset multiple sclerosis. Neurology 2004; 63: 1966–1967.

38. Hahn CD, Shroff MM, Blaser S, Banwell BL. MRI criteria for multiple sclerosis: Evaluation in a pediatric cohort. Neurology 2004; 62: 806–808.

39. Mikaeloff Y, Adamsbaum C, Husson B et al. MRI prognostic factors for relapse after acute CNS inflammatory demyelination in childhood. Brain 2004; 127: 1942–1947.

40. Wang CH, Walsh K. Multiple ring-enhancing lesions in a child with relapsing multiple sclerosis. J Child Neurol 2002; 17: 69–72.

41. Bruhn H, Frahm J, Merboldt KD et al. Multiple sclerosis in children: cerebral metabolic alterations monitored by localized proton magnetic resonance spectroscopy in vivo. Ann Neurol 1992; 32: 140–150.

42. Mezzapesa DM, Rocca MA, Falini A et al. A preliminary diffusion tensor and magnetization transfer magnetic resonance imaging study of early-onset multiple sclerosis. Arch Neurol 2004; 61: 366–368.

43. Calabresi PA, Stone LA, Bash CN et al. Interferon beta results in immediate reduction of contrast-enhanced MRI lesions in multiple sclerosis patients followed by weekly MRI. Neurology 1997; 48: 1446–1448.

44. Li DK, Paty DW. Magnetic resonance imaging results of the PRISMS trial: a randomized, double-blind, placebo-controlled study of interferon-beta1a in relapsing-remitting multiple sclerosis. Prevention of relapses and disability by interferon-beta1a subcutaneously in multiple sclerosis. Ann Neurol 1999; 46: 197–206.

45. Kappos L, Moeri D, Radue EW et al. Predictive value of gadolinium-enhanced magnetic resonance imaging for relapse rate and changes in disability or impairment in multiple sclerosis: a meta-analysis. Gadolinium MRI Meta-analysis Group. Lancet 1999; 353: 964–969.

46. Kalkers NF, Bergers E, Castelijns JA et al. Optimizing the association between disability and biological markers in MS. Neurology 2001; 57: 1253–1258.

47. Balassy C, Bernert G, Wober-Bingol C et al. Long-term MRI observations of childhood-onset relapsing-remitting multiple sclerosis. Neuropediatrics 2001; 32: 28–37.

48. Knox K, Hader W. Paediatric multiple sclerosis: a population based study (Abstract). Neurology 2004; 62: A230.

49. Cole GF, Auchterlonie LA, Best PV. Very early onset multiple sclerosis. Dev Med Child Neurol 1995; 37: 667–672.

50. Haliloglu G, Anlar B, Aysun S et al. Gender prevalence in childhood multiple sclerosis and myasthenia gravis. J Child Neurol 2002; 17: 390–392.

51. McAdam L, Blaser S, Banwell B. Pediatric tumefactive demyelination: case series and review of the literature. Pediatr Neurol 2002; 26: 18–25.

52. Trojano M, Liguori M, Bosco ZG et al. Age-related disability in multiple sclerosis. Ann Neurol 2002; 51: 475–480.

53. Banwell BL, Anderson PE. The cognitive burden of multiple sclerosis in children. Neurology 2005; 64: 891–894.

54. Kalb RC, DiLorenzo TA, LaRocca NA et al. The impact of early onset multiple sclerosis

on cognitive and social indices. Int J Mult Scler Care 1999; 1: 2–17.

55. MacAllister WS, Belman AL, Milazzo M et al. Cognitive functioning in children and adolescents with multiple sclerosis. Neurology 2005; 64: 1422–1425.

56. Alper G, Schor NF. Toward the definition of acute disseminated encephalitis of childhood. Curr Opin Pediatr 2004; 16: 637–640.

57. Tenembaum S, Chamoles N, Fejerman N. Acute disseminated encephalomyelitis: a long-term follow-up study of 84 pediatric patients. Neurology 2002; 59: 1224–1231.

58. Idrissova Z, Boldyreva MN, Dekonenko EP et al. Acute disseminated encephalomyelitis in children: clinical features and HLA-DR linkage. Eur J Neurol 2003; 10: 537–546.

59. Hartung HP, Grossman RI. ADEM: distinct disease or part of the MS spectrum? Neurology 2001; 56: 1257–1260.

60. Wingerchuk DM. Postinfectious encephalomyelitis. Curr Neurol Neurosci Rep 2003; 3: 256–264.

61. Schwarz S, Mohr A, Knauth M et al. Acute disseminated encephalomyelitis: a follow-up study of 40 adult patients. Neurology 2001; 56: 1313–1318.

62. Leake JA, Albani S, Kao AS et al. Acute disseminated encephalomyelitis in childhood: epidemiologic, clinical and laboratory features. Pediatr Infect Dis J 2004; 23: 756–764.

63. Tardieu M, Mikaeloff Y. What is acute disseminated encephalomyelitis (ADEM)? Eur J Paediatr Neurol 2004; 8: 239–242.

64. Tenenbaum S, Martin S, Fejeman N. Disease-modifying therapies in childhood and juvenile multiple sclerosis. Mult Scler 2001; 7: S57.

65. Hynson JL, Kornberg AJ, Coleman LT et al. Clinical and neuroradiologic features of acute disseminated encephalomyelitis in children. Neurology 2001; 56: 1308–1312.

66. Kounami S, Yoshiyama M, Nakayama K et al. Macrophage activation syndrome in children with systemic-onset juvenile chronic arthritis. Acta Haematol 2005; 113: 124–129.

67. Sawhney S, Woo P, Murray KJ. Macrophage activation syndrome: a potentially fatal complication of rheumatic disorders. Arch Dis Child 2001; 85: 421–426.

68. Vanderver A. Tools for diagnosis of leukodystrophies and other disorders presenting with white matter disease. Curr Neurol Neurosci Rep 2005; 5: 110–118.

69. Schiffmann R, van der Knaap MS. The latest on leukodystrophies. Curr Opin Neurol 2004; 17: 187–192.

70. Lerman-Sagie T, Leshinsky-Silver E, Watemberg N et al. White matter involvement in mitochondrial diseases. Mol Genet Metab 2005; 84: 127–136.

71. Moroni I, Bugiani M, Bizzi A et al. Cerebral white matter involvement in children with mitochondrial encephalopathies. Neuropediatrics 2002; 33: 79–85.

72. Kolodny EH. Dysmyelinating and demyelinating conditions in infancy. Curr Opin Neurol Neurosurg 1993; 6: 379–386.

73. Van der Knaap MS, Salomons GS, Li R et al. Unusual variants of Alexander's disease. Ann Neurol 2005; 57: 327–338.

74. Li R, Johnson AB, Salomons G et al. Glial fibrillary acidic protein mutations in infantile, juvenile, and adult forms of Alexander disease. Ann Neurol 2005; 57: 310–326.

75. Banwell B. Treatment of children and adolescents with multiple sclerosis. Expert Rev Neurother 2005; 5: 391–401.

76. Hahn JS, Siegler DJ, Enzmann D. Intravenous gammaglobulin therapy in recurrent acute disseminated encephalomyelitis. Neurology 1996; 46: 1173–1174.

77. Nishikawa M, Ichiyama T, Hayashi T et al. Intravenous immunoglobulin therapy in acute disseminated encephalomyelitis. Pediatr Neurol 1999; 21: 583–586.

78. Pradhan S, Gupta RP, Shashank S, Pandey N. Intravenous immunoglobulin therapy in acute disseminated encephalomyelitis. J Neurol Sci 1999; 165: 56–61.

79. Apak RA, Anlar B, Saatci I. A case of relapsing acute disseminated encephalomyelitis with high dose corticosteroid treatment. Brain Dev 1999; 21: 279–282.

80. Finsterer J, Grass R, Stollberger C, Mamoli B. Immunoglobulins in acute, parainfectious, disseminated encephalomyelitis. Clin Neuropharmacol 1998; 21: 258–261.

81. Sahlas DJ, Miller SP, Guerin M et al. Treatment of acute disseminated encephalomyelitis with intravenous immunoglobulin. Neurology 2000; 54: 1370–1372.

82. PRISMS-4: Long-term efficacy of interferon-beta-1a in relapsing MS. Neurology 2001; 56: 1628–1636.

83. Jacobs LD, Beck RW, Simon JH et al. Intramuscular interferon beta-1a therapy initiated during a first demyelinating event in multiple sclerosis. CHAMPS Study Group. N Engl J Med 2000; 343: 898–904.

84. Comi G. Why treat early multiple sclerosis patients? Curr Opin Neurol 2000; 13: 235–240.

85. O'Connor P. Key issues in the diagnosis and treatment of multiple sclerosis. An overview. Neurology 2002; 59(6 suppl 3): S1–S33.

86. Yong VW, Chabot S, Stuve O, Williams G. Interferon beta in the treatment of multiple sclerosis: mechanisms of action. Neurology 1998; 51: 682–689.

87. Yong VW. Differential mechanisms of action of interferon-beta and glatiramer aetate in MS. Neurology 2002; 59: 802–808.

88. PRISMS. Randomised double-blind placebo-controlled study of interferon beta-1a in relapsing–remitting MS. Lancet 2000; 352: 1498–1504.

89. Interferon beta-1b is effective in relapsing-remitting multiple sclerosis. I. Clinical results of a multicenter, randomized, double-blind, placebo-controlled trial. The IFNB Multiple Sclerosis Study Group. Neurology 1993; 43: 655–661.

90. Johnson KP, Brooks BR, Cohen JA et al. Copolymer 1 reduces relapse rate and improves disability in relapsing-remitting multiple sclerosis: results of a phase III multicenter, double-blind placebo-controlled trial. The Copolymer 1 Multiple Sclerosis Study Group. Neurology 1995; 45: 1268–1276.

91. Jacobs LD, Cookfair DL, Rudick RA et al. Intramuscular interferon beta-1a for disease progression in relapsing multiple sclerosis. The Multiple Sclerosis Collaborative Research Grou. Ann Neurol 1996; 39: 285–294.

92. Adams AB, Tyor WR, Holden KR. Interferon beta-1b and childhood multiple sclerosis. Pediatr Neurol 1999; 21: 481–483.

93. Etheridge LJ, Beverley DW, Ferrie C, McManus E. The use of interferon beta in relapsing–remitting multiple sclerosis. Arch Dis Child 2004; 89: 789–791.

94. Pohl D, Rostasy K, Gartner J, Hanefeld F. Treatment of early onset multiple sclerosis with subcutaneous interferon beta-1a. Neurology 2005; 64: 888–890.

95. Mikaeloff Y, Moreau T, Debouverie M et al. Interferon-beta treatment in patients with childhood-onset multiple sclerosis. J Pediatr 2001; 139: 443–446.

96. Waubant E, Hietpas J, Stewart T et al. Interferon beta-1a in children with multiple sclerosis is well tolerated. Neuropediatrics 2001; 32: 211–213.

97. Banwell B, Reder AT, Krupp L et al. Safety and tolerability of interferon beta-1b in pediatric multiple sclerosis. Neurology 2006; 66: 472–476.

98. Sorensen PS, Fazekas F, Lee M. Intravenous immunoglobulin G for the treatment of relapsing-remitting multiple sclerosis: a meta-analysis. Eur J Neurol 2002; 9: 557–563.

99. Fazekas F, Deisenhammer F, Strasser-Fuchs S et al. Randomised placebo-controlled trial of monthly intravenous immunoglobulin therapy in relapsing-remitting multiple sclerosis. Austrian Immunoglobulin in Multiple Sclerosis Study Group. Lancet 1997; 349: 589–593.

100. Achiron A, Pras E, Gilad R et al. Open controlled therapeutic trial of intravenous immune globulin in relapsing-remitting multiple sclerosis. Arch Neurol 1992; 49: 1233–1236.

101. Millefiorini E, Gasperini C, Pozzilli C et al. Randomized placebo-controlled trial of mitoxantrone in relapsing-remitting multiple sclerosis: 24-month clinical and MRI outcome. J Neurol 1997; 244: 153–159.

102. Hauser SL, Dawson DM, Lehrich JR et al. Intensive immunosuppression in progressive multiple sclerosis. A randomized, three-arm study of high-dose intravenous cyclophosphamide, plasma exchange, and ACTH. N Engl J Med 1983; 308: 173–180.

103. Hyman N, Barnes M, Bhakta B et al. Botulinum toxin (Dysport) treatment of hip adductor spasticity in multiple sclerosis: a prospective, randomised, double blind, placebo controlled, dose ranging study. J Neurol Neurosurg Psychiatry 2000; 68: 707–712.

104. Weinstock-Guttman B, Cohen JA. Emerging therapies for multiple sclerosis. Neurologist 1996; 2: 342–355.

105. Ohlenbusch A, Pohl D, Hanefeld F. Myelin oligodendrocyte gene polymorphisms and childhood multiple sclerosis. Pediatr Res 2002; 52: 175–179.

106. Anlar B, Alikasifoglu M, Kose G et al. Tumor necrosis factor-alpha gene polymorphisms in children with multiple sclerosis. Neuropediatrics 2001; 32: 214–216.

107. Misko IS, Cross SM, Khanna R et al. Crossreactive recognition of viral, self, and bacterial peptide ligands by human class I-restricted cytotoxic T lymphocyte clonotypes: implications for molecular mimicry in autoimmune disease. Proc Natl Acad Sci USA 1999; 96: 2279–2284.

108. Marrie RA, Wolfson C. Multiple sclerosis and Epstein–Barr virus. Can J Infect Dis 2002; 13: 111–118.

109. Ascherio A, Munch M. Epstein–Barr virus and multiple sclerosis. Epidemiology 2000; 11: 220–224.

110. Ascherio A, Munger KL, Lennette ET et al. Epstein-Barr virus antibodies and risk of multiple sclerosis: a prospective study. JAMA 2001; 286: 3083–3088.

111. Swanborg RH, Whittum-Hudson JA, Hudson AP. Human herpesvirus 6 and *Chlamydia pneumoniae* as etiologic agents in multiple sclerosis. Microbes Infect 2002; 4: 1327–1333.

112. Munger KL, Peeling RW, Hernan MA et al. Infection with *Chlamydia pneumoniae* and risk of multiple sclerosis. Epidemiology 2003; 14: 141–147.

113. Alotaibi S, Kennedy J, Tellier R et al. Epstein-Barr virus in pediatric multiple sclerosis. JAMA 2004; 291: 1875–1879.

114. Banwell B, Krupp L, Kennedy J et al. Clinical features and viral serologies in children with multiple sclerosis: a multinational observational study. Lancet Neurol 2007; 6: 773–781.

115. Pohl D, Krone B, Rostasy K et al. High seroprevalence of Epstein-Barr virus in children with multiple sclerosis. Neurology 2006; 67(11): 2063–2065.

C. H. Polman and B. W. van Oosten

INTRODUCTION

The diagnosis of multiple sclerosis (MS) is currently based on both clinical parameters, such as medical history and neurological examination, and paraclinical measures, such as magnetic resonance imaging (MRI), cerebrospinal fluid (CSF) examination and evoked potential testing. There is no MS-specific diagnostic test and the intermittent nature of the disease and high variability in presenting symptoms make diagnosis difficult. The presentation of MS can be monosymptomatic or have multifocal signs and symptoms, and many neurological disorders can be similar to MS in their initial presentation.

Traditionally, diagnostic criteria for MS state that a diagnosis of 'clinically definite' MS requires clinical evidence of two or more white matter lesions on at least two occasions.[1] In 1983, these criteria were expanded by Poser et al to include the use of paraclinical parameters, and they have been the standard MS diagnostic criteria for about 20 years.[2] In 2001, an international panel further revised the criteria, in particular to make MRI information a more integral component.[3] Commonly referred to as the 'McDonald criteria', in recognition of the panel's distinguished chair, W. Ian McDonald of the Institute of Neurology, Queen Square and the Royal College of Physicians, the criteria have been widely disseminated and discussed since their original publication. Because these were the first full MS diagnostic criteria to rely heavily on MRI, the panel provided a rather conservative interpretation of what constitutes a positive MRI scan, focusing on high specificity rather than high sensitivity.

In the absence of a specific diagnostic test, elimination of alternative conditions that might 'mimic' the disease remains an essential requirement for diagnosing MS.

BACKGROUND

Multiple sclerosis is a chronic disabling disease of the central nervous system (CNS), characterized by the disease manifestations disseminated in time and in space. Pathologically the disease manifests with recurrent acute focal inflammatory demyelination and with variable remyelination, culminating in chronic multifocal sclerotic plaques that are scattered throughout the brain, spinal cord and optic nerves. Traditionally, the diagnosis depends on the demonstration of at least two necessarily separate sites of CNS damage in an individual with a history of at least two episodes of focal neurological dysfunction consistent with the inflammatory pathology. It is not difficult to demonstrate this in the established case but considerable problems can arise early in the course of the disease.

To facilitate the diagnostic evaluation of a patient, MS diagnostic criteria have included results from investigations assessing aspects of CNS physiology or markers of inflammation.[2] The Poser criteria give specific guidelines as to how to classify abnormalities found with evoked potential techniques and how to interpret CSF immunological abnormalities but specific recommendations on how to use MRI findings were not given.

In recent years MRI has been shown to be the single most informative diagnostic procedure. Areas of abnormality on T2-weighted or proton-density-weighted images in a pattern highly characteristic for MS occur in more than 95% of patients with clinically definite disease and even in approximately two-thirds of patients presenting with a clinically isolated syndrome (CIS) suggestive of demyelination (e.g. optic neuritis or subacute myelopathy). MRI is also a powerful method for excluding other diseases that might simulate MS, a critical additional diagnostic step.

In 2001, an international panel published new guidelines for the diagnosis of MS. These rely, as did the previous Poser criteria, on objective evidence of dissemination in time and space. However, these revised criteria include MRI evidence of dissemination in time and space. In presenting what have become the McDonald criteria, the international panel stressed the traditional requirement for demonstration of lesions suggestive of inflammatory demyelinating disease separated in both time and space to confirm an MS diagnosis. The diagnostic scheme was presented as a series of possible (and quite typical) clinical presentation scenarios and the steps – including clinical assessment, paraclinical laboratory studies and imaging – that should be taken in each scenario to make a diagnosis (Table 5.1).

Even though the panel also tried to streamline and simplify certain definitions, the main change compared to the 'old' Poser

TABLE 5.1 Steps in making a diagnosis of multiple sclerosis using 'McDonald criteria'

Clinical presentation	Additional data needed
2 or more attacks 2 or more objective clinical lesions	None; clinical evidence will suffice (additional evidence desirable but must be consistent with MS)
2 or more attacks 1 objective clinical lesion	Dissemination in space, demonstrated by: MRI *or* a positive CSF and 2 or more MRI lesions consistent with MS *or* further clinical attack involving different site
1 attack 2 or more objective clinical lesions	Dissemination in time, demonstrated by: MRI *or* second clinical attack
1 attack 1 objective clinical lesion (monosymptomatic presentation)	Dissemination in space, demonstrated by: MRI *or* positive CSF and 2 or more MRI lesions consistent with MS *and* Dissemination in time, demonstrated by: MRI *or* second clinical attack
Insidious neurological progression suggestive of MS (primary progressive MS)	One year of disease progression (retrospectively or prospectively determined) *and* two of the following: a. Positive brain MRI (nine T2 lesions or four or more T2 lesions with positive visual evoked potential) b. Positive spinal cord MRI (two focal T2 lesions) c. Positive CSF

Source: adapted from Polman et al.[25]

criteria was the integration of MRI. In allowing MRI to play a role in diagnosis, the panel concluded that, because high specificity is important, stringent criteria for MRI abnormalities should be followed with respect to dissemination both in space and in time.

POSITIONING OF THE McDONALD CRITERIA

The McDonald criteria introduce a new concept in the diagnostic criteria for MS. They represent the first constructive effort to address how to use noninvasive pathological observations in conjunction with clinical findings. MRI measures of T2 hyperintense or gadolinium-enhancing lesions would not be regarded as surrogates but rather as markers of pathological change. Biopsy and autopsy studies have clearly shown that changes on MRI do reflect the underlying pathology of the disease, even though there is no direct and invariant mapping of histopathological measures of disease (e.g. inflammation, demyelination/remyelination, axonal damage).[4,5] Widespread recognition of the particular value of MRI in this context had already led to widespread usage of MRI as a diagnostic tool, in the absence of testable guidelines for implementation, and therefore the criteria presented by the international panel were very timely.

These criteria have the potential to enable an earlier diagnosis, especially in patients presenting with a CIS. This is clearly demonstrated in some studies that specifically addressed the ability of the new McDonald criteria to predict which CIS patients will develop clinically definite MS. Dalton et al found that, at 3 months, 20 of 95 (21%) patients had MS with the McDonald criteria, whereas only 7 of 95 (7%) had developed clinically definite MS. After 1 year, the corresponding figures were 38 of 79 (48%) and 16 of 79 (20%), and after 3 years, they were 29 of 50 (58%) and 19 of 50 (38%).[6] Tintoré et al found that in 12 months the new criteria more than tripled the frequency of diagnosis of MS: 40 vs. 11%.[7]

Early diagnosis of MS is now important. Some currently available treatments have demonstrated ability to delay the next relapse. Greater inflammation and demyelination early in the disease course may lead to greater later axonal loss. An additional motivation for establishing an accurate and early diagnosis is to allow for the provision of information and discussion of prognosis. Previously, clinicians have been hesitant to pursue a definite diagnosis at the presentation of first symptoms as they considered the benefit to the patient limited. Therefore, they were reluctant to discuss the possibility of MS at the presentation of first symptoms and deferred further diagnostic investigations to prevent psychological harm to patients. The impact of an MS diagnosis was believed to lead to a substantial loss of quality of life, even in the absence of any physical disability. However, considerable recent work indicates that patients themselves prefer to know the diagnosis at a very early stage and that they generally benefit from an earlier diagnosis.[8,9]

The McDonald criteria combine a high information content: MRI of the brain, and also of the spinal cord, is not only able to provide evidence of temporal and spatial resolution supportive of MS, it also is a powerful tool to exclude other disease that might mimic MS.

Concerns about the McDonald criteria include that the MRI criteria have been derived from only very limited and selected data: they were based on studies that only included small numbers of patients recruited from specialized secondary or tertiary referral centers who had been carefully selected as having a 'typical' CIS. Based on the studies they were derived from, the McDonald criteria could also be perceived as prognostic rather than diagnostic. This issue was particularly stressed in a report of the Therapeutics and Technology Assessment Subcommittee of the American Academy of Neurology (AAN) on the utility of MRI in suspected MS.[10] The subcommittee argued that the MRI criteria proposed in the McDonald criteria are not concerned with the diagnosis of MS but rather with the time required to convert to clinically definite MS, which is a different, although related, issue.

DISSEMINATION IN SPACE

To demonstrate dissemination in space on imaging, the panel relied upon a definition of a 'positive MRI' for MS that is based on criteria developed by Barkhof et al,[11] which have been shown to be more specific than previous criteria. These refer to the presence or absence of enhancing lesions and to lesion location (juxtacortical, infratentorial and periventricular) to provide a cumulative chance model. The panel recommended implementing these criteria as modified by Tintoré et al,[12] in which a threshold of at least three positive criteria is required, with the possibility of substituting a single gadolinium-enhancing lesion with nine or more T2 lesions (Table 5.2). In addition, one spinal cord lesion was accepted as having equivalent diagnostic significance to one brain lesion. While these criteria for a positive MRI are rather stringent, if CSF findings are characteristic of MS (oligoclonal IgG bands or raised IgG index), MRI criteria are relaxed somewhat – simply to the presence of two or more MS-characteristic lesions.

Since their publication, the initial experience in implementation of the McDonald criteria generally supports their use with respect to predicting which CIS patients will develop clinically definite MS in the future. Dalton et al examined the value of MRI findings in predicting which patients who presented with CIS would develop clinically definite MS within 3 years.[6] With their patient population drawn from a specialist referral clinic, they found a sensitivity of 83%, a specificity of 83% and an accuracy (based on progression to clinically definite MS within 3 years) of 83%. Tintoré et al reported similar findings in a separate specialist referral population followed for a median of 3 years with a sensitivity of 74%, a specificity of 86% and an accuracy of 80%.[7] Both studies suffer from a relatively short follow-up, which could tend to underestimate sensitivity and accuracy.

Experience with implementation of the criteria also has suggested several conceptual and/or practical issues.

The MRI criteria for dissemination in space specifically limit sensitivity for greater specificity. A report of the Therapeutics and Technology Assessment Subcommittee of the AAN addressed the utility of MRI in suspected MS and argued that the MRI characteristics proposed in the McDonald criteria are overly restrictive. The subcommittee argued that in patients with CIS the finding of even a few (three, perhaps even one) white matter lesions on a T2-weighted MRI scan is a more sensitive and appropriate predictor of the subsequent development of clinically definite MS within the next 7–10 years (assuming other possible diagnoses have been excluded) than the fulfillment of the more stringent criteria proposed by the McDonald panel. The study with the longest follow-up of patients with CIS so far was performed by Brex et al,[13] who

found that in CIS patients with abnormalities on MRI at baseline, 98% exhibited either clinical or radiological evidence of multiphasic disease during (14 years) follow-up, which confirms that white matter lesions on MRI in young adults with isolated syndromes, irrespective of number or location, are in almost all instances associated with MS.

In the absence of any clear data on spinal cord imaging, the international panel decided to allow for substitution of one brain lesion by one spinal cord lesion. Since publication of the international panel criteria, two studies have addressed the role of spinal cord imaging in MS diagnosis according to the McDonald criteria. Bot et al investigated the prevalence and characteristics of spinal cord lesions in 104 patients with a recent (within 6 months) clinical diagnosis of MS according to the Poser criteria and assessed their potential impact on the diagnostic classification according to the McDonald criteria.[14] They found that in 34% of newly diagnosed patients with clinically definite MS the McDonald criteria for dissemination in space on the basis of brain MRI only were not fulfilled. Substituting one spinal lesion for one brain lesion, an option recommended in the McDonald criteria, decreased this percentage to 15%. This thus supports the important role of spinal cord MRI in the diagnostic work-up of MS, not only in excluding other diseases but also in facilitating an early diagnosis of MS.[15] Strikingly, these data are not in line with those by Dalton et al,[16] who could not find much additional yield of spinal cord imaging. In their study in patients with clinically isolated optic neuritis, a positive spinal cord MRI contributed to the diagnosis in only one or two patients. It is not clear whether the discrepancies between these conclusions are due to different phases of the disease being studied (clinically definite MS versus isolated optic neuritis) or to differences in the topographical distribution of the presenting symptom (optic neuritis being only a minority of the patients in the study by Bot et al).

Very recently a re-analysis of the spinal cord imaging data in the Bot et al cohort was performed,[17] testing three different interpretations of the original criterion that one spinal cord lesion can be substituted for one brain lesion: spinal cord lesions can only be used to reach the criterion of nine T2 lesions (A); spinal cord lesions can be used to fulfill one of the four brain criteria if not yet fulfilled, e.g. the criterion requiring at least one infratentorial lesion (B); or spinal cord lesions can be used to fulfill more than one criterion if not yet fulfilled, e.g. the criterion of at least one infratentorial lesion, as well as that of one juxtacortical lesion, if appropriate (C). The number of patients that fulfilled the criteria for dissemination in space rose from 79 if only the brain scan was analyzed, to 82 using the most restrictive interpretation (A), 93 with interpretation B and 98 with the most liberal interpretation (C), clearly showing that current implementation of spinal cord MR in the McDonald criteria is ambiguous.

In addition, the McDonald MRI criteria may not have equal sensitivity and specificity for all clinical presentations. Sastre et al confirmed that also in patients with brainstem CIS the modified Barkhof criteria have greater specificity in predicting conversion to MS than other published criteria (Paty's and Fazekas's criteria) but that the accuracy is lower than was reported previously for mixed cohorts of CIS patients.[18]

DISSEMINATION IN TIME

Dissemination in time determined from imaging was defined in the McDonald criteria as a new T2- or gadolinium-enhancing lesion appearing at least 3 months after the onset of the clinical event. However, in patients with a CIS suggestive of MS, this may require three MRI scans if the first scan is performed less

---

TABLE 5.2 What constitutes a positive MRI?

Three out of four*:

- 1 gadolinium-enhancing lesion *or* 9 T2-hyperintense lesions if no gadolinium-enhancing lesion
- 1 or more infratentorial lesions
- 1 or more juxtacortical lesions
- 3 or more periventricular lesions

*A spinal cord lesion can be considered equivalent to a brain infratentorial lesion: an enhancing spinal cord lesion is considered to be equivalent to an enhancing brain lesion and individual spinal cord lesions can contribute together with individual brain lesions to reach the required number of T2 lesions.
Source: adapted from Polman et al.[25]

than 3 months after the onset of the clinical event, depending on the appearance of sequential scans. At the 3-month follow-up a new gadolinium-enhancing lesion is required. If this is not present, then a gadolinium-enhancing lesion or T2-hyperintense lesion is necessary on a further scan acquired at least 3 months later. These criteria may be overly restrictive. Preliminary results suggest that, when evaluating dissemination in time, the appearance of just new T2 lesions at least 3 months after presentation with a CIS is a powerful predictor for clinically definite MS and does not result in reduced specificity.

In a study of 56 CIS patients followed for at least 3 years, Dalton et al specifically addressed the issue of how many scans are required to reliably show early MRI dissemination in time. They focused in particular on whether a new T2 lesion at the 3-month scan is sufficient, instead of a new enhancing lesion as proposed by the criteria, and found that, if new T2 lesions at 3 month follow-up MRI scans were allowed as an alternative for dissemination in time, sensitivity increased (from 58% to 74%) with maintained specificity (92%), enabling a more accurate diagnosis of MS in more patients.[19] Therefore, these authors proposed that, in adults aged 16–50 years presenting with CIS, the McDonald MRI criteria for dissemination in time should be relaxed to allow diagnosis simply if new T2 lesions are seen on a 3-month follow-up scan, as long as the baseline scan is obtained within 3 months of CIS onset. However, the broad utility of this suggested modification is unclear, for two reasons. In the first place, it is unknown how often in a general radiological practice (as opposed to a specialized MRI reading center) 'new' T2 lesions can be an artifact of repositioning error or lack of radiological expertise. In the second place, it is important to recognize the possibility that a new T2 lesion at 3 months has resulted from the index episode but was not (yet) visible as such on the first scan. This issue is especially relevant because baseline MRI investigations in the study by Dalton et al were performed relatively long (5 weeks median) after the onset of the episode, which in most cases was an optic neuritis. It is unclear whether the same results would have been obtained in patients with a brainstem or spinal cord syndrome, in whom MRI scanning is much more likely to occur within the first few days or weeks after the onset of symptomatology.

CEREBROSPINAL FLUID

Results of CSF examination continue to play an important role, both in patients with relapse-onset and in patients with primary progressive onset of disease.

Tintoré et al compared the diagnostic accuracy of the full MRI criteria for dissemination in space to that of the less stringent criteria (two lesions or more) in the presence of typical CSF abnormalities.[7]

For patients with relapse-onset disease, neither the Poser nor the McDonald criteria for MS have an absolute dependence on the documentation of CSF abnormalities consistent with MS – intrathecal synthesis of immunoglobulins, either indicated by an increased immunoglobulin gamma (IgG) index or synthetic rate or the presence of oligoclonal bands not found in the serum. However, the international panel criteria do allow for some loosening of MRI criteria in patients who have abnormal CSF immune markers: the presence of two or more lesions is sufficient to demonstrate dissemination in space in these patients. In CIS patients, CSF data were analyzed in this way by Tintoré et al and by Calabrese et al.[7,20] Both groups reported that inclusion of CSF analyses increased diagnostic sensitivity (because less restrictive MRI criteria were required). However, Tintoré et al also found that the inclusion of CSF findings lowered specificity (and accuracy) of the diagnostic criteria as compared

to MRI only. Calabrese et al reported the presence of CSF oligoclonal bands to be a slightly better predictor of conversion to MS than the presence of MRI dissemination in space.

In patients with primary progressive clinical history, to improve diagnostic certainty, the McDonald criteria mandate the presence of CSF abnormalities. In a study of treatment for primary progressive MS, patients were enrolled whether or not they had a positive CSF finding at time of screening, as long as other entry criteria consistent with primary progressive MS were fulfilled.[21] Follow-up analysis of these patients suggested that there was no difference in MRI or clinical patterns between those patients who were CSF-positive (≈80%) and those who were CSF-negative (≈20%) at study enrollment. However, when stratified for disability at enrollment (based on Expanded Disability Status Scale (EDSS)), those with the higher EDSS (more disabled) were more often CSF positive and had more MRI-defined inflammatory disease than those with lower EDSS (less disabled).

These data suggest that CSF status may not be an absolute requirement for the diagnosis of MS in patients presenting with a primary progressive disease course. However, it appears that CSF status (along with baseline disability and inflammatory disease burden) may indicate the relative 'aggressiveness' of disease and its potential for progression over time.

IMPLEMENTATION

Unfortunately, no study has addressed the 'true' specificity of the new criteria, which requires analysis of the important issue of a false-positive diagnosis. This would necessitate testing the criteria in a setting including diseases different from MS although clinically 'mimicking' it. While the theoretical strength of the modified Barkhof criteria used in the McDonald criteria is their potential to decrease misdiagnosis, since they include specific MS-like lesion characteristics that are less likely to occur in conditions mimicking MS, it is unknown how many patients who fulfill the criteria still do not have MS. A first approach to address this issue was recently presented by Nielsen et al.[22] These authors compared MRI features of 28 MS patients to 28 patients from the same cohort (377 patients consecutively referred for confirmation of diagnosis) and center who were initially suspected to have MS but afterwards turned out to have another diagnosis. In this analysis, the (more restrictive) criteria for dissemination in space as incorporated in the McDonald criteria turned out to have superior specificity (89% vs 29%) when compared to the more liberal criteria as proposed by the AAN subcommittee.

Even though the original description of the McDonald international panel explicitly warned against this, the impact of MRI on the diagnostic process and the increasing dependence on it might come at the expense of a detailed history and neurological examination. It cannot be stressed enough that the international panel criteria add value only when the MRI evidence is interpreted in the context of a careful clinical history and physical examination. In fact, the McDonald criteria cannot even be applied without an associated careful clinical evaluation of the patient. Classification of presenting symptoms and signs as either monofocal or multifocal (evidenced respectively by a single lesion or by more than one lesion) is fundamental to knowing whether a second event has occurred (either clinically or seen with MRI), which is required to constitute a diagnosis of MS. In this regard, a standardized approach to the interpretation of clinical symptoms and signs in patients with clinically isolated syndrome in the context of a clinical trial was recently published by Uitdehaag et al.[23] These authors demonstrated that, in the absence of such a standardized approach, interpretation of clinical symptoms and signs is highly variable, even when performed by skilled, MS-interested neurologists.

IMPLEMENTATION OF THE McDONALD CRITERIA IN A CLINICALLY ISOLATED SYNDROME

Miller and colleagues provided guidance on how the approach to investigation of patients who present with a typical CIS should now take in to account the McDonald diagnostic criteria.[24] The following approach to management could be implemented:

1. At the time of diagnosis of CIS MRI scanning of the brain is performed, and scanning of the spinal cord in cases of myelitis. Additional investigations are performed to exclude other diseases.
2. In the absence of other pathology, brain MRI provides a more accurate prediction of likelihood of developing MS: an abnormal scan predicts a 60–80% likelihood of having the disease whereas a normal scan implies a 20% likelihood.
3. Repeat MRI can add additional diagnostic information. In those who opt to be scanned and in whom initial scanning took place within the first month of onset of CIS, a reference T2 scan should be arranged at least 1 month after onset.
4. T2-weighted and gadolinium-enhanced brain scanning more than 3 months after the attack can fulfill the McDonald criteria for dissemination in space and time, in which case MS is diagnosed.
5. If significant diagnostic doubt exists at any stage, but inflammatory demyelination is suspected, spinal cord scanning and CSF examination for oligoclonal bands can be very helpful.

Obviously, at all stages, MRI should be performed to a high standard consistent with modern neuroradiological practice and should be reported by a clinician with extensive experience of the imaging appearances in MS and other white matter disorders. In addition, investigation of a patient with CIS should always also include consideration of other potential diagnoses.

IMPLEMENTATION IN LESS TYPICAL CASES

This represents the group of patients who pose the greatest clinical diagnostic challenge and for whom, in general, criteria are potentially most useful. It has to be recognized that in these patients the McDonald criteria have not been validated and, therefore, should only be used with great caution. Confirmation that the criteria reliably predict the development of MS in these patients by the use of traditional, largely clinical, assessment is necessary to confirm their clinical relevance in this situation.

In patients with a less typical presentation it is recommended to perform MRI, to seek for alternative diagnosis or find features suggestive of MS. Under these circumstances, high specificity in a test is even more important than high sensitivity. In these patients gadolinium-enhancing lesions represent a very specific finding; spinal cord MRI may also be considered because this adds specificity, also in cases that are 'lookalikes'.[15] In addition, CSF examination and visual evoked potential should be considered. In these patients it might be appropriate to focus on clinical follow-up rather than on new MRI examinations to prove dissemination in space or time.

THE 2005 REVISION OF THE McDONALD CRITERIA

The international panel re-convened in March 2005 in Amsterdam, nearly 5 years after the original panel convened in London, to review progress since the original criteria were developed, to evaluate whether the global framework of the criteria continued to be appropriate and to determine if revisions to the original criteria should be recommended.

The goal of these revisions was to incorporate new evidence where available, develop refined consensus where evidence from research studies is scarce and to simplify and clarify original definitions and concepts that users thought were confusing or difficult to implement.

The international panel evaluated all available published research relating to the original criteria and input provided from the MS clinical community and determined that the criteria provided reasonably good utility for 'classical' MS seen in a typical adult Caucasian population of western European ethnic origin. Data collected to date suggest that the criteria, although imperfect, provide a good mix of specificity and sensitivity to allow for an early diagnosis of MS.

However, in order to incorporate evidence-based data obtained since the publication of the original criteria, to present revised consensus and to simplify and clarify issues that have caused confusion and misinterpretation, the international panel proposed some changes in the criteria, in particular for imaging and CSF findings.[25]

I. With respect to demonstrating dissemination in time using imaging, two (new) ways have been defined, replacing the previous ones:
   a. Detecting gadolinium enhancement at least 3 months after the onset of the initial clinical event, if not at the site corresponding to the initial event
   b. Detecting a *new* T2 lesion if it appears at any time compared to a reference scan done at least 30 days after the onset of the initial clinical event.
II. For dissemination in space, the role of spinal cord lesions has been redefined, so that a spinal cord lesion is equivalent to, and can substitute for, a brain infratentorial lesion but *not* for a periventricular or juxtacortical lesion; an enhancing spinal cord lesion can 'count' doubly in fulfilling the criteria; and individual spinal cord lesions can contribute along with individual brain lesions to reach the required nine T2 lesions to satisfy the Barkhof criteria as modified by Tintoré.
III. For diagnosing primary progressive MS, CSF abnormalities are no longer an absolute requirement. A diagnosis of primary progressive MS can now be made on the basis of the following:
   1. One year of disease progression (retrospectively or prospectively determined)
   2. *plus* two of the following:
      a. Positive brain MRI (nine T2 lesions or four or more T2 lesions with + visual evoked potential)
      b. Positive spinal cord MRI (two focal T2 lesions)
      c. Positive CSF (isoelectric focusing evidence of oligoclonal bands and/or elevated IgG index).

Despite these changes, the core features of the original McDonald Criteria are retained in the 2005 Revisions: emphasis on objective clinical findings; dependence upon evidence of dissemination of lesions in time and space; use of supportive and confirmatory paraclinical examination to speed the process and help eliminate false negative and false positive diagnoses; and focus on specificity rather than sensitivity.

ELIMINATION OF ALTERNATIVE CONDITIONS

Using the diagnostic criteria discussed in the previous section, the diagnosis of MS will be fairly straightforward in many cases. Nevertheless, it is wise to realize that these criteria are probably not definitive and have never been (and cannot be) a 'gold standard'. In general, an awareness that many diseases can present in a MS-like manner may prevent erroneous diagnoses. There are several situations in which a diagnosis of MS has to be considered, each situation bringing about its own differential diagnostic considerations and difficulties. Since one of the most diagnostic hallmarks of MS is the relapsing and remitting disease course, diagnostic problems are most likely to occur in patients with a slowly progressive neurological deficit, in patients with only one episode of neurological dysfunction ('clinically isolated syndrome' or CIS) or in patients with no episodes of MS-like symptoms at all but who have MS-like abnormalities on radiological (MRI) examinations done for another reason. However, even in patients who have an apparently typical relapsing–remitting disease course, many differential diagnostic possibilities have to be considered.

PATIENTS WITH A SLOWLY PROGRESSIVE NEUROLOGICAL DEFICIT

A slowly progressive neurological deficit with pyramidal and sensory symptoms and signs can be seen in patients with primary progressive MS. In most patients this will present as a myelopathy, with the legs affected more than the arms. However, a slowly progressive hemiparesis or cerebellar syndrome might also occur.[26] The mean age of disease onset is approximately 40 years,[27,28] which is about 10 years later than in relapse-onset MS. Because of the absence of typical relapses, primary progressive MS can pose considerable diagnostic problems. The generally older age of these patients may further add to diagnostic difficulties, especially when MRI studies reveal cerebral white matter lesions, which could be interpreted as areas of demyelination, or as age-related vasculopathic changes. Moreover, cerebral white matter lesions in primary progressive MS are generally less in number than in relapse-onset MS with equal disease duration and disability. To prevent an erroneous diagnosis of MS in patients with a slowly progressive disease course, the current diagnostic criteria therefore put strong emphasis on the role of positive CSF findings and/or stringent imaging criteria.

Since the great majority of primary progressive MS patients present with a slowly progressive myelopathy, all possible other causes of this will have to be included in the differential diagnosis. Generally, MRI-studies of brain and spinal cord as well as examination of the CSF are necessary.

Compressive myelopathy

The most important cause of myelopathy to exclude is compression. This can be the result of congenital malformations (Chiari malformations), tumor (meningioma, schwannoma, metastatic) and degenerative disease (intervertebral disc herniation, cervical spondylosis) as well as rare diseases such as epidural lipomatosis.[29] MRI studies of the spinal cord can easily detect spinal cord compression and should be performed in every patient with unexplained myelopathy.

A special situation occurs in MS patients who develop symptoms of myelopathy in the course of the disease. Although in many cases this is the result of spinal cord demyelination, one should always be alert for other causes. A well known example is cervical spondylosis.[30] In case of doubt, patients with established MS who develop symptoms of myelopathy might therefore benefit from spinal cord MRI.

Vascular myelopathy

Other potentially treatable causes of a slowly progressive myelopathy are dural arteriovenous fistulas and spinal arteriovenous malformations. Symptoms are the result of venous hypertensive myelopathy or ischaemia.[31] The diagnosis can be suspected on the basis of MRI studies, which usually show diffuse high signal on T2 images, less consistently flow voids from dilated veins. Angiography is the gold standard in demonstrating abnormal vascular anatomy. Endovascular treatment is possible in many cases.

Hereditary myelopathy

Slowly progressive pyramidal and mild vibration sense disturbances of the legs are the major symptoms of hereditary spastic paraplegia.[32] The disease is clinically and genetically heterogeneous and can start at any age. MRI studies usually reveal spinal cord atrophy but cerebral white matter abnormalities suggestive of MS are not found. In the CSF a high protein may be present but there are no signs of intrathecal immunoglobulin synthesis. In most cases the usually autosomal dominant heredity will prevent confusion with progressive MS. However, rare autosomal recessive and X-linked variants are reported. Here, MRI and CSF studies will usually prevent confusion with MS.

Metabolic diseases – peroxisomal

The metabolic disease that is most likely to produce a slowly progressive myelopathy mimicking MS is X-adrenoleukodystrophy (X-ALD). Although the childhood-onset cerebral phenotype is very distinct from MS, the adult-onset adrenomyeloneuropathy phenotype usually presents in the third or fourth decade with a spastic paraplegia, loss of vibration sense and disorders of micturition.[33] Some of these patients are initially diagnosed as MS. Diagnostic clues indicating X-ALD are the axonal sensorimotor neuropathy, which can often be found by nerve conduction studies, a positive family history, the absence of oligoclonal bands in the cerebrospinal fluid of most, but not all X-ALD patients, adrenocortical dysfunction and MRI studies, which do not show the characteristic lesions of MS in the majority of patients. The diagnosis of X-ALD can be confirmed by finding high levels of very-long-chain fatty acids in plasma. There is no cure but there are many treatment options, ranging from dietary measures to bone marrow transplants. Although the disease is X-linked, female carriers with a relatively mild adrenomyeloneuropathy phenotype are not exceptional.[34] Usually, onset is a little bit later (fourth decade).

Metabolic diseases – lysosomal

Metachromatic leukodystrophy and Krabbe's disease are autosomal recessive lysosomal storage diseases that mostly present in infants or juveniles. Rare adolescent and adult forms exist, which may cause confusion with MS. Adult-onset metachromatic leukodystrophy usually presents with dementia, behavioral disorder and polyneuropathy but there are reports of a primary-progressive-MS-like presentation.[35] Krabbe's disease may present as a spastic paraplegia with[36] or without[37] MRI abnormalities. In these leukodystrophies, MRI usually shows more or less symmetrical and diffuse white matter signal abnormalities.[38] There are very few reports of CSF findings in these adult forms but, apart from high protein levels, no other abnormalities such as oligoclonal bands seem to be present. The positive family history and MRI findings should alert the clinician of a possible hereditary metabolic disease, which can be confirmed by further metabolic tests.

Deficiencies

Subacute combined degeneration of the spinal cord leads to a gradually progressive spastic paraparesis, symmetric dysaesthesia and disturbance of position sense. It is caused by deficiency of vitamin B$_{12}$, which can lead to neurological disease without overt megaloblastic anemia. At risk are patients with malabsorption syndromes (pernicious anemia, Crohn's disease). Nitrous oxide anesthesia can provoke subacute combined degeneration in patients with marginal vitamin B$_{12}$ levels.[39] MRI studies reveal signal abnormalities in the spinal cord posterior columns in some, but not all patients. Rarely, cerebral lesions are visible. The spinal cord abnormalities appeared to be reversible after treatment.[40] Subacute combined degeneration should be considered in all patients with progressive myelopathy, especially in patients with malabsorption syndromes, anemia or onset of symptoms following surgery with nitrous oxide anesthesia.

Infection

Human immunodeficiency virus (HIV)-related vacuolar myelopathy is invariably progressive and leads to severe paralysis of the lower limbs, with loss of the ability to walk and of sphincter control.[41] It is a disease of advanced HIV infection. Therefore, differentiation from MS will only lead to difficulty in undiagnosed HIV infection.

The human T-cell lymphotropic virus type I (HTLV-I) results in HTLV-I-associated myelopathy, also known as tropical spastic paraparesis, in approximately 1–2% of infected patients.[42] Most infections are in tropical regions, such as South America, the Caribbean, southern and central parts of Africa and southern Japan. Apart from pyramidal and sensory disturbances, many patients complain of low back pain. MRI studies reveal spinal cord atrophy and cerebral subcortical and periventricular white matter lesions, which can however be differentiated from MS lesions with reasonable accuracy in, at least, Japanese MS.[43] In the CSF one can find oligoclonal bands in most patients. HTLV-1 serology should be done in patients with progressive myelopathy (with or without low back pain) living in or originating from high prevalence regions.

Bacterial (*Treponema pallidum*, *Borrelia burgdorferi*, *Mycobacterium tuberculosis*) and fungal (*Histoplasma* spp.) infections can rarely produce a slowly progressive myelopathy. In many, but not all, cases this is associated with fever and pain. MRI and CSF studies will usually enable differentiation from MS.

The rare Whipple's disease is caused by *Tropheryma whipplei* and can lead to neurological symptoms in patients with weight loss, diarrhea, abdominal pain and arthropathy. The most reported neurological symptoms are personality change and dementia, but cranial nerve palsies, ophthalmoplegia, nystagmus, myoclonus, ataxia, myelopathy and the very specific but less sensitive symptom of oculomasticatory myorhythmia can all occur.[44] Diagnosis is by polymerase chain reaction (PCR) of duodenal biopsy and/or CSF. Antibiotic treatment is possible with trimethoprim–sulfamethoxazole or ceftriaxone.

Radiation-induced myelopathy

Early myelopathy following irradiation of the spinal cord will usually not cause diagnostic problems, since this occurs within months after irradiation. Diagnostic problems could however occur in delayed radiation myelopathy, which is thought to be of vasculopathic origin. This usually has a latency of one to four years, but longer latencies have been reported. In these patients the connection with radiotherapy is less clear. Here, it is important to see if the myelopathic area is within the irradiated area. MRI and CSF studies can be necessary to make a correct diagnosis.

Motor neuron disease

Motor neuron disease, of which amyotrophic lateral sclerosis is the most prevalent expression, is a degenerative disease of both central and peripheral motor neurons. It usually presents with gradually progressive paresis of one or more limbs, accompanied by pyramidal signs, muscular atrophy and fasciculations. Some patients with early motor neuron disease are wrongly diagnosed as (primary progressive) MS, sometimes after the erroneous attribution of age-related cerebral white-matter lesions to demyelinating disease. The early muscular atrophy, fasciculations and the absence of sensory symptoms are clinical clues to the correct diagnosis. A critical appraisal of MRI studies will help to prevent incorrect classification.

PATIENTS WITH ACUTE OR SUBACUTE PRESENTATIONS OF NEUROLOGICAL SYMPTOMS SUGGESTIVE OF DEMYELINATION

In patients with one episode of neurological deficit suggestive of MS, the diagnosis of MS can usually not be made because dissociation in time is lacking. On the basis of the clinical presentation and the results of radiological and laboratory studies many of these patients are diagnosed as 'possible MS' or as 'CIS'. However, in some of these patients the diagnosis of acute disseminated encephalomyelitis (ADEM) is suspected on clinical and radiological grounds.

Patients with multiple episodes of typical MS nature will not cause nearly the same amount of diagnostic problems as can be seen in the primary progressive patients. Still, even in these patients other causes than MS have to be considered. This also includes MS 'variants', of which neuromyelitis optica (NMO) or Devic's disease is the most important.

Acute disseminated encephalomyelitis

Formal diagnostic criteria for ADEM have never been formulated. Nevertheless, a common notion of the distinguishing features of ADEM exists: ADEM is widely regarded as a monophasic postinfectious or postvaccination disease, although many cases are seen without obvious preceding infection. In typical cases, rapidly progressive polysymptomatic neurological deficits are seen in patients with fever, meningism and impaired consciousness. Hemiparesis, paraparesis, ataxia, transverse myelitis and cranial nerve dysfunction (often with (bilateral) optic neuritis) are commonly seen. However, in clinical practice many patients without fever, meningism or altered state of consciousness are diagnosed with ADEM.

MRI studies reveal cerebral and spinal cord white matter lesions, which often enhance. Although it is sometimes claimed that in ADEM patients (nearly) all lesions are enhancing simultaneously, this is not a universal finding. Some MRI abnormalities are suggestive of ADEM (extensive symmetric abnormalities in the cerebral or cerebellar white matter or basal ganglia) but in many cases MRI lesions are indistinguishable from those seen in MS.[45] CSF findings will also usually not separate ADEM in the acute phase from MS, since in both conditions oligoclonal bands can be found. Contrary to the findings in MS, where oligoclonal bands are stable and present throughout the disease, they will disappear in ADEM patients.

A sobering illustration of diagnostic problems in the acute phase can be found in a recent publication, where, after a follow-up of 38 months, 35% of 26 patients initially classified as ADEM had eventually been diagnosed as MS.[46] Only the presence of fever or meningism seemed to be reliably predictive of ADEM but these were rarely present.

The conclusion that can be derived from this would then be that in some typical cases ADEM can be reliably diagnosed but that in many other cases only a probability diagnosis is possible and that careful clinical and radiological follow-up will lead to a definitive conclusion. Table 5.3 summarizes the most important distinguishing features of ADEM and MS.

TABLE 5.3 Differentiation of acute disseminated encephalomyelitis and multiple sclerosis

⟵ ADEM more probable	MS more probable ⟶
Clinical presentation	
Children, adolescents	Adults
Postinfectious, postvaccination	May occur after fever (!)
Fever, meningism	No fever, no meningism
Impaired consciousness	Normal consciousness
Clinically disseminated	Clinically isolated
Hospitalization within days	No/later hospitalization
Bilateral optic neuritis	Unilateral optic neuritis
Complete transverse myelitis	Partial myelopathy
MRI features	
Diffuse symmetrical lesions	Asymmetrical, demarcated lesions
Lesions in basal ganglia	Lesions in corpus callosum
(Partial) resolution at follow-up	Progression at follow-up
CSF	
Pleocytosis, high protein	Normal cell count and protein
No/temporary intrathecal IgG production	Persistent intrathecal IgG production

No formal criteria exist. Indications of higher or lower probability are given, as found in relevant literature.[46,47]
ADEM, acute disseminated encephalomyelitis; CSF, cerebrospinal fluid; MRI, magnetic resonance imaging; MS, multiple sclerosis.

TABLE 5.4 Proposed diagnostic criteria for neuromyelitis optica*

Optic neuritis
Acute myelitis
At least two of three supportive criteria:

1. Contiguous spinal cord MRI lesion extending over 3 vertebral segments
2. Brain MRI not meeting diagnostic criteria for multiple sclerosis
3. NMO-IgG seropositive status

* Revised criteria (2006).[48]
MRI, magnetic resonance imaging; NMO-IgG, neuromyelitis optica immunoglobulin G.

Neuromyelitis optica or Devic's disease

In the past, NMO was considered to be a monophasic illness, with severe unilateral or bilateral optic neuritis (loss of visual acuity) and severe acute myelopathy (tetraparesis, loss of bladder control). Recent research has found evidence that relapsing forms of NMO exist. Relapses can be composed of both optic neuritis and myelopathy but these elements can also occur separately.

MRI studies do not show typical cerebral and spinal cord MS-like lesions. However, longitudinally extending spinal cord lesions spanning three or more vertebral segments can be seen. In the acute phase CSF pleocytosis is present but there is no evidence of intrathecal immunoglobulin synthesis.

New diagnostic criteria have been formulated (Table 5.4), incorporating a serum test aimed at distinguishing MS and NMO; sensitivity and specificity were 99% and 90%.[48] This serum autoantibody marker was recently shown to bind to the aquaporin-4 waterchannel[49] and will probably become an important diagnostic instrument if these results are validated in a separate patient sample. Once a diagnosis of NMO has been made, it is important to realize that, whereas in some cases NMO is a primary idiopathic disease, it will occur in others as a secondary disease; important to consider here are systemic lupus erythematosus (SLE), sarcoidosis, Sjögren's syndrome and Behçet's disease. NMO patients have a prognosis that is worse than that of MS patients. There are no known evidence-based treatments. Probably the most reasonable treatment option for NMO is azathioprine and prednisone,[50] but similar results were recently published with the anti-B-cell antibody rituximab.[51]

Asian opticospinal multiple sclerosis variant

In Asian countries MS is much less prevalent than in Europe and North America. A high proportion of these patients are suffering from an opticospinal MS variant, which in many ways shows resemblance to NMO. In the autoantibody assay that was already mentioned in the NMO section above, Japanese opticospinal MS patients behaved similarly to American NMO patients. Although the Asian opticospinal MS variant has been documented most extensively in Japan,[52] it has also been reported in other Asian countries.[53]

Neuropsychiatric systemic lupus erythematosus

Neurological manifestations in the course of SLE are frequent, but since most of these are headaches, mononeuropathies, strokes and cognitive or psychiatric symptoms, they do not usually mimic MS.[54] The only probable exceptions are transverse myelitis and optic neuritis, which in some patients occur simultaneously.[55] Transverse myelitis occurs in approximately 1–2% of SLE patients and may present with monoparesis or paraparesis of the legs in some patients and with paresthesias in others. Optic neuritis in SLE often presents bilaterally.[56] Transverse myelitis and optic neuritis can be the presenting SLE manifestation, so that diagnoses such as idiopathic NMO or ADEM are considered initially. It depends on concomitant symptoms (arthritis, nephritis, Raynaud's, hematological abnormalities) and serological studies whether SLE will be suspected in this stage.

In SLE patients with neurological symptoms (stroke, headache, cognitive decline) MRI studies will often demonstrate cerebral white and gray matter lesions[57] that on superficial inspection could simulate MS lesions. However, the distribution of the lesions is generally subcortical as opposed to the mainly periventricular MS lesions. Apart from abnormalities consistent with transverse myelitis, no focal or diffuse spinal cord lesions as seen in MS are found.[15] CSF studies are not sufficient to distinguish SLE and MS, intrathecal immunoglobulin production can be found in both conditions.[58] Serological studies for SLE should be done in patients presenting with bilateral optic neuritis, transverse myelitis or NMO.

Sjögren's syndrome

Sjögren's syndrome is an autoimmune disease that leads to dysfunction of exocrine glands by lymphocytic infiltration. Primary and secondary forms exist, the latter in the course of other diseases, such as SLE. Sjögren's syndrome is thought to be one of the more prevalent autoimmune diseases, with reported prevalences varying from 0.1–5%. Older studies reported 20–60% neurological manifestations in Sjögren's syndrome, more recent studies generally report about 10–20%.[59] Neurological complaints can at times precede very mild dryness of mouth and eyes, so that Sjögren's syndrome is not always suspected. Even if it is suspected, serological tests (SS-A, SS-B) can be negative, and minor salivary gland biopsy and scintigraphy would have to be done for confirmation. A sensorimotor axonal polyneuropathy is most commonly found. Central nervous system pathology consists of 'diffuse' symptoms, such as cognitive complaints, and focal manifestations such as sub-acute transverse myelitis, recurrent optic neuritis, a motor neuron syndrome, aseptic meningitis and a 'MS-like syndrome'.[59,60] Disease courses mimicking both relapsing–remitting MS and primary progressive MS are seen.[61]

Various patterns of MRI abnormalities have been reported in Sjögren's syndrome, some of them indistinguishable from MS. In general, MRI lesions tend to be more discrete than in SLE and MS, and spinal cord lesions are rare.[15,62] Oligoclonal bands are present in the CSF of about 30% of patients with Sjögren's syndrome, which tend to be patients with CNS involvement.[61]

In the past few years there has been some discussion concerning a possible high prevalence of Sjögren's syndrome in primary progressive MS patients.[63–65] So far, the question whether some primary progressive MS patients have to be reclassified as Sjögren's syndrome with neurological symptoms, or whether they are not different from other primary progressive MS patients but have secondary Sjögren's syndrome as is seen in many other autoimmune diseases, cannot be answered conclusively.

In general, differentiation of MS and Sjögren's syndrome should not be difficult in typical relapsing–remitting disease types. In primary progressive disease courses, differentiation relies more heavily on results of CSF and MRI studies and could become difficult if oligoclonal bands are lacking and cerebral MRI is not typical of MS. Spinal cord MRI will then be a useful investigation.[15]

Behçet's disease

Behçet's disease can be diagnosed in patients with recurrent oral and genital aphthae, uveitis and dermatological symptoms such as folliculitis, erythema nodosum and a positive pathergy skin reaction.[66] Most authors report a male preponderance. High prevalences are found in Mediterranean countries and Japan. The central nervous system involvement in Behçet's disease will occur after several years' disease duration in most patients but can occur simultaneously with or before other organ involvement as well. Neuro-Behçet's can present in various temporal patterns, mimicking relapsing–remitting, primary progressive and secondary progressive courses as seen with MS.[67] A distinction can be made between parenchymal involvement, causing pyramidal (hemiparesis), cognitive, brainstem and, rarely, sensory symptoms and nonparenchymal involvement, which is mainly vasculopathic, e.g. dural sinus thrombosis.

In neuro-Behçet's, MRI scans are abnormal in 70% and most often show lesions in basal ganglia, brainstem and diencephalic structures, some of which are contrast-enhancing (Fig. 5.1). Small scattered lesions in cerebral hemispheric white matter can also be found, some of which are periventricular. CSF shows a mild pleocytosis and high protein in about 50% of the patients. An elevated IgG index is found in 73% and oligoclonal bands in 16%. However, no patient had more than two bands.

Differentiation from MS should be possible on the basis of clinical findings, which are more severe than usually is the case in MS, combined with results of MRI and CSF studies (Table 5.5).[68]

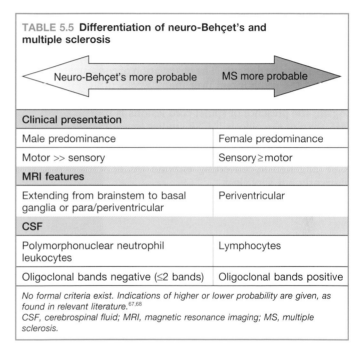

TABLE 5.5 Differentiation of neuro-Behçet's and multiple sclerosis

← Neuro-Behçet's more probable	MS more probable →
Clinical presentation	
Male predominance	Female predominance
Motor >> sensory	Sensory ≥ motor
MRI features	
Extending from brainstem to basal ganglia or para/periventricular	Periventricular
CSF	
Polymorphonuclear neutrophil leukocytes	Lymphocytes
Oligoclonal bands negative (≤2 bands)	Oligoclonal bands positive

No formal criteria exist. Indications of higher or lower probability are given, as found in relevant literature.[67,68]
CSF, cerebrospinal fluid; MRI, magnetic resonance imaging; MS, multiple sclerosis.

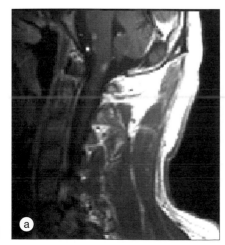

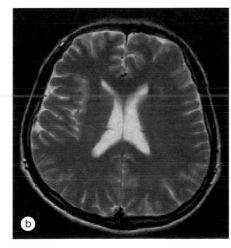

FIG. 5.1 A. T1-weighted MRI of the spine. Gadolinium-enhancing lesions in brainstem and cervicomedullary junction in a 23-year-old man of Turkish descent with a progressive right-sided pyramidal syndrome. In the recent past he had recovered from a left-sided pyramidal syndrome. He also suffered from recurrent oral and genital aphthae and uveitis. In the CSF there was an elevated protein content, normal cell counts and glucose; oligoclonal bands were not found. A diagnosis of neuro-Behçet's was made. **B.** T2-weighted cerebral MRI of the same patient. No supratentorial abnormalities.

Neurosyphilis

Neurosyphilis is traditionally subdivided into an early stage, during which meningeal infection and meningovascular symptoms may occur, and a late stage during which the so-called 'general paresis' with neuropsychiatric symptoms and the well known tabes dorsalis are mostly seen. During the early stage symptoms mimicking MS could occur, such as cranial nerve palsies and episodes of transient neurological dysfunction as a result of focal ischaemia. The late-stage neuropsychiatric symptoms are less likely to result in diagnostic confusion and tabes dorsalis has become very rare.[81,82]

Cranial MRI is usually nonspecific. MS-like white matter lesions may be seen. Serological and CSF studies have to be done to come to a correct diagnosis. Although one will find signs of intrathecal immunoglobulin synthesis in most neurosyphilis patients, the elevated protein content and results of serological studies are clearly different from what is found in MS patients.

PATIENTS WITHOUT MULTIPLE SCLEROSIS SYMPTOMS BUT WITH MULTIPLE-SCLEROSIS-LIKE MRI-ABNORMALITIES

From autopsy studies it was already known that in some patients MS lesions were found that had apparently not caused symptoms.[83] More recently, a few patients were reported who underwent MRI scans for various reasons and appeared to have typical MS lesions.[84,85] Only after several years did these patients start to have clinical symptoms suggestive of MS. With the ever-increasing use of diagnostic MRI, it is not hard to predict that more similar cases will be found. Repeat MRI could give some idea of lesional activity in these patients. However, treatment should only be started if symptoms occur, according to existing criteria.

It is important to be aware that accidentally found white-matter lesions on cerebral MRI in patients without a clinical suspicion of MS are no reason to consider MS in the overwhelming majority of cases. Certainly, in patients above 50, ischemic vasculopathy is a much more likely diagnosis. In younger patients many other causes of white-matter lesions can be summed up, such as migraine[86,87] and scuba diving,[88] to mention but a few.

CONCLUSION

In the absence of tests that can diagnose MS with 100% accuracy, doctors have to rely on the skillful combination of clinical and paraclinical evidence. One of the most important aims is to exclude other diseases that 'mimic' MS. Since there are many potential 'mimics', it is not possible nor desirable to exclude all of them in every patient. One has to have knowledge of potential 'mimics' and know when to investigate them; Table 5.7 might be of help. Even in the time of MRI, a well taken patient history remains paramount in this respect. Part of this is a certain vigilance concerning potential alternative diagnoses. For instance, a positive family history of neurological complaints will greatly change the differential diagnosis, influence which diagnostic tests will be asked for and also influence the interpretation of these tests, e.g. MRI results. Interpretation of MRI, CSF and other tests has to be done bearing in mind the clinical presentation. Not all cerebral white-matter lesions in young adults are MS lesions, nor are CSF oligoclonal bands always the result of MS.

TABLE 5.7 Warning signs and symptoms raising doubt concerning multiple sclerosis

Sign/symptom	Possible diagnosis
History	
Age >40 Stroke-like presentation	Vasculopathy
Positive family history	HSP, X-ALD, MLD, Krabbe's disease, LHON, CADASIL
Malabsorption	SCD, Whipple's disease
Recent anesthesia	SCD
Living in tropics Originating from tropics	TSP/HAM
Preceding infection/vaccination	ADEM
Migraine with aura	CADASIL
Arthropathy, ulcers, rash, uveitis	SLE, Behçet's disease, sarcoidosis, Whipple's disease
Neurological features	
Fever, meningism	ADEM
Pure motor signs	MND, Behçet's disease
Bilateral optic neuritis Optic neuritis not recovering	ADEM, NMO, SLE, sarcoidosis, LHON
Bilateral facial palsy Facial palsy not recovering	Sarcoidosis, borreliosis
Transverse myelitis Optic neuritis and transverse myelitis	ADEM, NMO, SLE
Polyneuropathy	X-ALD, MLD, Krabbe's disease, SLE
MRI features	
Normal	Psychosomatic
Symmetrical, diffuse	MLD, Krabbe's disease
Subcortical lesions	Vasculopathy
Meningeal enhancement Persistent enhancement	Sarcoidosis, Behçet's disease
No spinal cord lesions	Vasculopathy, SLE, Sjögren's syndrome
CSF features	
Normal	No specific disease; reconsider diagnosis
Pleocytosis	ADEM, NMO, SLE, sarcoidosis, Behçet's disease, borreliosis, syphilis
Elevated CSF protein	Compressive myelopathy, HSP, MLD, Krabbe's disease, LHON, Behçet's disease, sarcoidosis, borreliosis, syphilis

ADEM, acute disseminated encephalomyelitis; CADASIL, cerebral autosomal dominant arteriopathy with subcortical infarcts and leukoencephalopathy; HSP, hereditary spastic paraplegia; LHON, Leber's hereditary optic neuritis; MLD, metachromatic leukodystrophy; MND, motor neuron disease; NMO, neuromyelitis optica; SCD, subacute combined degeneration; SLE, systemic lupus erythematosus; TSP/HAM, tropical spastic paraparesis/HTLV-I associated myelopathy; X-ALD, X-linked adrenoleukodystrophy.

REFERENCES

1. Schumacher GA, Beebe G, Kibler RF et al. Problems of experimental trials of therapy in multiple sclerosis: report by the panel on the evaluation of experimental trials of therapy in multiple sclerosis. Ann NY Acad Med 1965; 122: 552–568.

2. Poser CM, Paty DW, Scheinberg L et al. New diagnostic criteria for multiple sclerosis: guidelines for research protocols. Ann Neurol 1983; 13: 227–231.

3. McDonald WI, Compston A, Edan G et al. Recommended diagnostic criteria for multiple sclerosis: guidelines from the International Panel on the diagnosis of multiple sclerosis. Ann Neurol 2001; 50: 121–127.

4. Van Waesberghe JH, Kamphorst W, De Groot CJ et al. Axonal loss in multiple sclerosis lesions: magnetic resonance imaging insights into substrates of disability. Ann Neurol 1999; 46: 747–754.

5. Lycklama a Nijeholt GJ, Bergers E, Kamphorst W et al. Post-mortem high-resolution MRI of the spinal cord in multiple sclerosis: a correlative study with conventional MRI, histopathology and clinical phenotype. Brain 2001; 124: 154–166.

6. Dalton CM, Brex PA, Miszkiel KA et al. Application of the new McDonald criteria to patients with clinically isolated syndromes suggestive of multiple sclerosis. Ann Neurol 2002; 52: 47–53.

7. Tintoré M, Rovira A, Rio J et al. New diagnostic criteria for multiple sclerosis. Application in first demyelinating episode. Neurology 2003; 60: 27–30.

8. Mushlin AI, Mooney C, Grow V et al. The value of diagnostic information to patients with suspected multiple sclerosis. Arch Neurol 1994; 51: 67–72.

9. Heesen C, Kolbeck J, Gold SM et al. Delivering the diagnosis of MS – results of a survey among patients and neurologists. Acta Neurol Scand 2003; 107: 363–368.

10. Frohman E, Goodin DS, Calabresi PA et al. The utility of MRI in suspected MS. Report of the Therapeutics and Technology Assessment Subcommittee of the American Academy of Neurology. Neurology 2003; 61: 602–611.

11. Barkhof F, Filippi M, Miller DH et al. Comparison of MR imaging criteria at first presentation to predict conversion to clinically definite multiple sclerosis. Brain 1997; 120: 2059–2069.

12. Tintoré M, Rovira A, Martinez M et al. Isolated demyelinating syndromes: comparison of different MR imaging criteria to predict conversion to clinically definite MS. Am J Neuroradiol 2000; 21: 702–706.

13. Brex PA, Ciccarelli O, O'Riordan JI et al. A longitudinal study of abnormalities on MRI and disability from multiple sclerosis. N Engl J Med 2002; 346: 158–164.

14. Bot JCJ, Barkhof F, Polman CH et al. Spinal cord abnormalities in newly diagnosed MS patients: added value of spinal MRI examination. Neurology 2004; 62: 226–233.

15. Bot JCJ, Barkhof F, Lycklama a Nijeholt G et al. Differentiation of multiple sclerosis from other inflammatory disorders and cerebrovascular disease: value of spinal MR imaging. Radiology 2002; 223: 46–56.

16. Dalton CM, Brex PS, Miszkiel KA et al. Spinal cord MRI in clinically isolated optic neuritis. J Neurol Neurosurg Psychiatry 2003; 74: 1577–1580.

17. Korteweg T, Barkhof F, Uitdehaag BMJ et al. How to use spinal cord magnetic resonance imaging in the McDonald diagnostic criteria for MS. Ann Neurol 2005; 57: 606–607.

18. Sastre-Garriga J, Tintore M, Rovira A et al. Conversion to multiple sclerosis after a clinically isolated syndrome of the brainstem: cranial magnetic resonance imaging, cerebrospinal fluid and neurophysiological findings. Mult Scler 2003; 9: 39–43.

19. Dalton CM, Brex PA, Miszkiel KA et al. New T2 lesions enable an earlier diagnosis of multiple sclerosis in clinically isolated syndromes. Ann Neurol 2003; 53: 673–676.

20. Calabrese M, Ranzato F, Tiberio M et al. The early MRI-based diagnosis of multiple sclerosis (McDonald Criteria): a prospective study in an homogeneous cohort of clinically isolated syndromes. Neurology 2004; 62(suppl 5): A293.

21. Wolinsky JS, the PROMiSe Study Group. The diagnosis of primary progressive MS. J Neurol Sci 2003; 206: 45–152.

22. Nielsen JM, Korteweg T, Barkhof F et al. Specificity of the modified Barkhof criteria. Mult Scler 2004; 10(suppl 2): S186.

23. Uitdehaag BMJ, Kappos L, Bauer L et al. Discrepancies in the interpretation of clinical symptoms and signs in the diagnosis of MS: a proposal for standardization. Mult Scler 2005; 11: 227–231.

24. Miller DH, Filippi M, Fazekas F et al. The role of MRI within diagnostic criteria for MS: a critique. Ann Neurol 2004; 56: 273–278.

25. Polman CH, Reingold SC, Edan G et al. Diagnostic criteria for multiple sclerosis: 2005 revisions to the 'McDonald Criteria'. Ann Neurol 2005; 58: 840–846.

26. Thompson A. Overview of primary progressive multiple sclerosis (PPMS): similarities and differences from other forms of MS, diagnostic criteria, pros and cons of progressive diagnosis. Mult Scler 2004; 10(suppl 1): S2–S7.

27. Andersson PB, Waubant E, Gee L et al. Multiple sclerosis that is progressive from the time of onset: clinical characteristics and progression of disability. Arch Neurol 1999; 56: 1138–1142.

28. Stevenson VL, Miller DH, Rovaris M et al. Primary and transitional progressive MS: a clinical and MRI cross-sectional study. Neurology 1999; 52: 839–845.

29. Dar MS, Daoud S. Images in clinical medicine. Epidural lipomatosis causing spinal cord compression. N Engl J Med. 2003; 349: e14.

30. Bashir K, Hadley MN, Whitaker JN. Surgery for spinal cord compression in multiple sclerosis. Curr Opin Neurol 2001; 14: 765–769.

31. Ferch RD, Morgan MK, Sears WR. Spinal arteriovenous malformations: a review with case illustrations. J Clin Neurosci 2001; 8: 299–304.

32. McDermott C, White K, Bushby K et al. Hereditary spastic paraparesis: a review of new developments. J Neurol Neurosurg Psychiatry 2000; 69: 150–160.

33. Moser HW. Adrenoleukodystrophy: phenotype, genetics, pathogenesis and therapy. Brain 1997; 120: 1485–1508.

34. Van Geel BM. [Carrier state of x-linked adrenoleukodystrophy] Ned Tijdschr Geneeskd 2000; 144: 1764–1768.

35. Kazibutowska Z, Bal A, Golba A et al. [Metachromatic leukodystrophy in adult patient initially diagnosed as multiple sclerosis] Neurol Neurochir Pol 2002; 36: 1209–1219.

36. Farina L, Bizzi A, Finocchiaro G et al. MR imaging and proton MR spectroscopy in adult Krabbe disease. Am J Neuroradiol 2000; 21: 1478–1482.

37. Bajaj NP, Waldman A, Orrell R et al. Familial adult onset of Krabbe's disease resembling hereditary spastic paraplegia with normal neuroimaging. J Neurol Neurosurg Psychiatry 2002; 72: 635–638.

38. Barkhof F, Scheltens P. Imaging of white matter lesions. Cerebrovasc Dis 2002; 13(suppl 2): 21–30.

39. Layzer RB. Myeloneuropathy after prolonged exposure to nitrous oxide. Lancet 1978; 2: 1227–1230.

40. Hemmer B, Glocker FX, Schumacher M et al. Subacute combined degeneration: clinical, electrophysiological, and magnetic resonance imaging findings. J Neurol Neurosurg Psychiatry 1998; 65: 822–827.

41. Di Rocco A, Simpson DM. AIDS-associated vacuolar myelopathy. AIDS Patient Care STDS 1998; 12: 457–461.

42. Manns A, Hisada M, La Grenade L. Human T-lymphotropic virus type I infection. Lancet 1999; 353: 1951–1958.

43. Kuroda Y, Matsui M, Yukitake M et al. Assessment of MRI criteria for MS in Japanese MS and HAM/TSP. Neurology 1995; 45: 30–33.

44. Marth T, Raoult D. Whipple's disease. Lancet 2003; 361: 239–246.

45. Kesselring J, Miller DH, Robb SA et al. Acute disseminated encephalomyelitis. MRI findings and the distinction from multiple sclerosis. Brain 1990; 113: 291–302.

46. Schwarz S, Mohr A, Knauth M et al. Acute disseminated encephalomyelitis: a follow-up study of 40 adult patients. Neurology 2001; 56: 1313–1318.

47. O'Riordan JI, Gomez-Anson B, Moseley IF et al. Long term MRI follow-up of patients with post infectious encephalomyelitis: evidence for a monophasic disease. J Neurol Sci 1999; 167: 132–136.

48. Wingerchuk DM, Lennon VA, Pittock SJ et al. Revised diagnostic criteria for neuromyelitis optica. Neurology 2006; 66: 1485–1489.

49. Lennon VA, Kryzer TJ, Pittock SJ et al. IgG marker of optic-spinal multiple sclerosis binds to the aquaporin-4 water channel. J Exp Med 2005; 202: 473–477.

50. Mandler RN, Ahmed W, Dencoff JE. Devic's neuromyelitis optica: a prospective study of seven patients treated with prednisone and azathioprine. Neurology 1998; 51: 1219–1220.

51. Cree BA, Lamb S, Morgan K et al. An open label study of the effects of rituximab in neuromyelitis optica. Neurology 2005; 64: 1270–1272.

study and also in another cohort of 74 patients.[11] While these study findings are intriguing – and ultrasonography is relatively cheap – the limited depiction of intracranial anatomy in what is a multifocal and diffuse disorder of the CNS is a drawback.

MYELOGRAPHY

Prior to the advent of MRI, myelography using intrathecal injection of radiographic contrast media was the only means of identifying compressive lesions involving the spinal cord. This invasive and often uncomfortable investigation is now virtually obsolete: it is occasionally required when cord compression must be ruled out and MRI is not possible, e.g. patients with cardiac pacemakers or extreme obesity that precludes MRI.

RETINAL NERVE FIBER LAYER IMAGING

The retinal nerve fiber layer is a region of potential interest in MS since it contains axons that are more directly accessible to noninvasive imaging than elsewhere in the CNS and because optic nerve and retinal axonal loss occurs after optic neuritis due to MS. The thickness of the retinal nerve fiber layer can be measured using optical coherence tomography (OCT). This modality enables cross-sectional imaging of internal tissue microstructure by measuring the echo time delay of back-scattered infrared light using an interferometer and a low-coherence light source. An early study reported retinal nerve fiber layer atrophy in MS patients who had a previous episode of optic neuritis.[12] OCT methodology has improved and, in glaucoma, robust correlations between sector-specific visual field deficits and corresponding thinning of the retinal nerve fiber layer have been reported, suggesting that it is possible to detect functionally important axonal loss. Similar observations have recently been made in subjects who experienced incomplete visual recovery following an episode of optic neuritis.[13] Thinning of the retinal nerve fiber layer has also been reported in a cohort of 90 MS patients with mainly relapsing–remitting disease;[14] while atrophy was most marked in eyes previously affected by optic neuritis, it was also lower in MS non-optic-neuritis eyes than in healthy control eyes, and the extent of thinning in the MS cohort was correlated with impairment of low-contrast visual acuity and contrast sensitivity. OCT should have a future role in evaluating neuroprotective treatments in optic neuritis and MS.[15,16]

MAGNETIC RESONANCE IMAGING AND SPECTROSCOPY

The key principle underlying MRI is the ability to harness nuclear magnetic resonance (NMR) signals from nuclei that contain an uneven number of protons and neutrons. Such nuclei have tiny magnetic fields and when placed in a MR scanner – which is a powerful magnet – they are aligned along the direction of the strong magnetic field. A radiofrequency pulse can then tip the spinning nuclei out of their alignment and in so doing generate a small NMR signal. Using a variety of additional pulses – known as read, phase encoding and slice select – and Fourier transformation, it is possible to localize the NMR signals into two- or three-dimensional space, thus producing MR images.

Because hydrogen-1 nuclei are by far the most abundant MR-accessible nuclei in the body, conventional MRI is based on hydrogen-1 imaging. These are predominantly water protons, although significant signals arise from protons in fat in some sequences. The signal contrast depends on the concentration of water protons and also on the rate at which NMR signals are lost after the radiofrequency pulse is discontinued. The latter process is determined by two relaxation rate constants: longitudinal (T1) and transverse (T2) to the external magnetic field. Thus, three main types of contrast are employed in conventional MRI scans that are used in routine diagnosis: proton density, T1- and T2-weighted. However, additional MR measures can also be acquired that employ less conventional or more complex pulse sequences with different contrast mechanisms. Table 6.1 provides a range of MR measures that has been used to study MS and indicates their actual or suggested correlation to pathology and functional effects. These are discussed in greater detail in a later section that has MS pathology as the starting point for understanding what can be learnt from MR measures in vivo. In the present section, a brief account is provided of the range of MR methods available.

T2-weighted images have proved especially sensitive in detecting MS lesions in cerebral hemisphere white matter, posterior fossa and spinal cord. Such sequences are in standard use during diagnostic examination. While a conventional spin echo or fast spin echo sequence is very successful in detecting high-signal T2 lesions in MS, the signal from cerebrospinal fluid (CSF) is also high and this may obscure the detection of lesions adjacent to the ventricles or subarachnoid spaces. Fluid-attenuated inversion-recovery (FLAIR) sequences suppress CSF signal but retain MS lesion hyperintensity and improve sensitivity in detecting supratentorial lesions, especially those in a juxtacortical location. FLAIR sequences are less sensitive in the posterior fossa and spinal cord.

A minority (20–30%) of T2 lesions are seen as areas of hypointensity on two-dimensional T1-weighted spin echo images. These lesions have longer T1 relaxation times than T1-isointense lesions. This could be due to extracellular edema or to loss of tissue matrix with an expanded extracellular space. On three-dimensional T1-weighted gradient echo sequences, almost all lesions appear as areas of T1 hypointensity and these likely have lower pathological specificity when compared with the hypointense lesions observed on two-dimensional T1-weighted spin echo.

Routine MRI studies often employ an intravenous contrast agent, which is a chelate of gadolinium. Gadolinium is a paramagnetic element and it causes enhanced T1 and T2 relaxation in regions where it accumulates. This is seen as contrast enhancement (high signal) on T1-weighted sequences. Gadolinium chelates do not cross a normal blood–brain barrier but in new and inflammatory MS lesions there is a breakdown of the blood–brain barrier and thus gadolinium enhancement.

Protons contained in macromolecules are relatively immobile and hence not accessible using conventional MR sequences but the addition of a radiofrequency pulse that selectively saturates macromolecular and adjacent water protons allows an indirect assessment of this proton pool since its normal exchange of magnetization with mobile water protons is modified. Such an approach is called magnetization transfer imaging. The magnetization transfer ratio (MTR) is higher in normal white matter than in gray matter and is substantially influenced by myelin.

Additional sequences have been developed for evaluating diffusion and perfusion of water protons. Abnormalities of directional diffusion in white matter tracts can be assessed using a measure called fractional anisotropy. Size and connectivity of white matter pathways can also be assessed using a number of diffusion tractography algorithms that link neighboring voxels in which there is a similar directionality of diffusion.[17] These methods have potential to detect structural disruption of white matter tracts. Reduced perfusion may reflect decreased metabolic activity secondary to neuroaxonal damage.

TABLE 6.1 **MRI measure, pathology and functional effect**

MRI measure		Pathology	Functional effect
White matter lesions	T2	Sensitive to focal lesions but nonspecific: inflammation, demyelination, remyelination, variable axonal loss, gliosis, microglial clusters without demyelination	T2 load moderately predicts disability early on in relapse-onset MS but little or no correlation or prediction otherwise
	Gadolinium	Blood–brain barrier breakdown, perivenular lymphocytes, macrophage infiltrates, active myelin breakdown	Acute relapse
	T1 hypointensity	Demyelinated, axonal loss (if persistent) Edema (if acute and reversible)	Slightly stronger correlation with disability than T2
	MTR	Demyelination (marked decrease) and remyelination (mild decrease)	Relapse and recovery
Normal-appearing white matter	MTR	Nonspecific: diffuse inflammation, glial proliferation, edema, axonal loss	Increasing abnormality with increasing disability
	NAA	Axonal dysfunction and loss (reduced NAA)	Contribute to disability
	T1	Nonspecific but sensitive measure of abnormality (increased T1)	?
	Diffusivity	Nonspecific (increased diffusivity)	?
	Fractional anisotropy	Axonal fiber tract integrity (decreased FA)	Disability
	Myoinositol	Glial proliferation and activity	Relapse and disability
	Perfusion	Inflammation (increased perfusion)	?
Normal appearing gray matter	MTR	Cortical demyelinating lesions	Disability and cognitive impairment
	T1	Nonspecific	?
	Diffusivity	Nonspecific	Disability in primary progressive MS
	NAA	Neuroaxonal loss	Disability and cognitive impairment
	Perfusion	Neuronal loss and altered metabolism (reduced perfusion)	Dysfunction in primary progressive MS
Functional MRI	Decreased activation in primary cortical region of relevance	Damage to subcortical networks or cortex	Loss of function
	Increased activation beyond primary cortical region of relevance	Adaptive response but also indicating increased neuronal stress	Short term maintenance of function; longer term poorer prognosis

Loss of tissue in the brain and spinal cord is often found in MS and can be measured using sensitive and reproducible segmentation or registration methods. Such atrophy is probably in a large part due to neuroaxonal loss, although loss myelin per se will contribute. Fluctuations in brain volume may also be caused by inflammation, glial proliferation and edema (increase), dehydration and anti-inflammatory treatment (decrease) (Table 6.2).

Activation of regional cortical neurons results in an increase in local cerebral blood flow and a transient decrease in the proportion of deoxy- to oxyhemoglobin in blood. Since deoxyhemoglobin is paramagnetic, this process causes a change in MR signal. In functional MRI (fMRI), a stimulus algorithm is applied to elicit a focal change in blood oxygenation. Because the signal changes occur within seconds of onset of the stimulus, and detection of local cortical fMRI response requires subtraction of the active from resting state, rapid echo planar imaging sequences are acquired. Visual, motor and cognitive algorithms have been established that characterize a consistent pattern of response from healthy controls, which in the case of the former two stimuli is predominantly in the primary visual cortex and contralateral primary motor cortex respectively. In MS and other neurological disorders, abnormal responses are seen both within and beyond the areas activated in healthy controls.

TABLE 6.2 Potential influences on brain volume measurements

Factors causing brain volume increases	Factors causing brain volume decreases
Edema	Axonal loss (45% of white matter bulk)
Inflammation	Resolution of inflammation and edema
Gliosis (tissue bulk)	Gliosis (retraction scar)
Remyelination	Demyelination
Fluid retention e.g. renal failure	Dehydration
Therapies causing cerebral edema	Anti-inflammatory therapies
Learning (focal gray matter increase)	Aging

Proton (hydrogen-1) spectroscopy investigates proton-containing metabolites and molecules other than water from which it is possible to generate a signal in the brain. These include N-acetyl aspartate (NAA, an amino acid that is almost entirely confined to neurons and axons in the adult CNS), choline-containing compounds (Cho, which reflects membrane turnover), creatine/phosphocreatine (Cr, which may reflect overall cellular activity), myoinositol (Ins, which is produced by glial cells) and glutamate/glutamine (these cannot be separated in a standard spectroscopic examination but it is possible to do so at high field using editing techniques[18]). These metabolites are present in millimolar concentrations (compared with water which is in molar amounts) and a large voxel of interest – typically 1–4 ml – is required in order to reliably measure the signals. The spectroscopic examination may be of a single small or large voxel; multivoxel and single slice; multivoxel and multislice;[19] or – in the case of NAA – a whole-brain measure.[20] More widespread anatomical coverage has the merit of more completely surveying what is a widespread disease process, although it is easier to obtain high-quality spectra from smaller regions of interest.

DIAGNOSIS AND DIFFERENTIAL DIAGNOSIS

In routine clinical practice, the major indication for neuroimaging investigation – and specifically MRI – is within the framework of diagnostic work-up. In patients with clinically definite MS, brain MRI reveals multifocal cerebral white matter lesions in more then 95% of patients and in 75–85% there are focal spinal cord lesions. When both investigations are combined, probably fewer than 1–2% of patients who are thought to definitely have MS on clinical grounds will have normal imaging: the rarity of completely normal CNS imaging should lead to careful re-evaluation of diagnosis in subjects who have previously been told they have MS.

EVOLUTION OF MAGNETIC RESONANCE IMAGING WITHIN DIAGNOSTIC CRITERIA

About two thirds of patients experiencing a single episode of suspected demyelination (called clinically isolated syndrome (CIS)) have cerebral white matter lesions indistinguishable from those seen in definite MS. After numerous studies from the late 1980s onwards showed that the presence of such lesions increases the likelihood of developing clinically definite MS, it was not surprising that MRI features for dissemination in space and time were formally incorporated within the diagnostic criteria for MS by an international panel in 2001[21] (Table 6.3). These now allow a diagnosis of MS after a CIS. The criteria for primary progressive MS also included abnormalities on both cranial and spinal cord MRI, although the presence of CSF oligoclonal bands was a mandatory requirement.

Subsequent application of the 2001 criteria in several natural history or treatment trial cohorts indicated that they enabled an earlier diagnosis and predicted conversion to clinically definite MS in CIS patients.[22–25] Specificity for clinically definite MS was high when MRI dissemination in time was present: dissemination in space per se was less specific. The requirement for a gadolinium-enhancing lesion to fulfill dissemination in time after 3 months had poor sensitivity but allowing a new T2 lesion instead overcame this limitation.[26]

In the light of subsequent studies, and in view of a number of criticisms – most notably from a Therapeutics and Technology Assessment Subcommittee of the American Academy of Neurology, which recommended 1–3 lesions per se as sufficient evidence for diagnosing MS[27] – the 2001 criteria were reviewed and revised by a re-convened international panel during 2005.[28] The summary MRI criteria of the 2001 and 2005 panels are provided in Table 6.3.

A constant feature in both 2001 and 2005 criteria is use of the Barkhof–Tintoré brain criteria for dissemination in space (Fig. 6.1(A–C)). These require three of the following four features to be present: 1) nine T2 lesions or a gadolinium-enhancing lesion; 2) three periventricular lesions; 3) one juxtacortical lesion; 4) one infratentorial lesion. They differ in the extent to which a spinal cord lesion (Fig. 6.1(D)) can also assist with fulfillment of dissemination in space: in 2001 only one cord lesion could substitute for one brain lesion whereas in 2005 any number of cord lesions can substitute for brain lesions and a cord lesion is also assigned the same status as an infratentorial lesion. The greater incorporation of cord lesions may have been based on a study in 107 early but definite MS patients, where cord lesions substantially increased the proportions with dissemination in space from 67% using brain MRI alone to 94% using all available cord lesions to complement brain lesions.[29] However, in a series of 115 patients with isolated optic neuritis, although 27% had clinically silent cord lesions these were present in only four (3.5%) subjects with normal brain MRI, and the inclusion of cord lesions only increased the proportion of patients fulfilling the dissemination in space criteria from 36% to 38%, whether including one or all cord lesions.[30] These findings raise doubt that the modifications to the dissemination in space criteria will have much impact on the time at which MS can be diagnosed. On the other hand, cord MRI has additional benefits, which include the exclusion of alternative pathology in patients with cord syndromes and the higher specificity for MS than brain MRI findings when comparison is made with other neurological disorders and with older healthy controls, who frequently have white matter lesions due to small vessel disease.[31,32] It is also useful in diagnosis of the small minority of patients who have MS in spite of normal brain imaging: the presence of cord lesions along with CSF oligoclonal bands and/or delayed visual evoked responses may be decisive.[33]

The 2005 criteria for dissemination in time were more substantially revised to include a new T2 lesion occurring more than 1 month after clinical onset (Fig. 6.2). This should increase the sensitivity while retaining specificity in making an earlier diagnosis of MS in CIS patients.[34] In primary progressive MS, the presence of CSF oligoclonal bands is no longer required, although in their absence it is necessary to have at least two spinal cord lesions and either nine brain lesions or four to eight brain lesions plus abnormal visual evoked potentials (Table 6.3). The least specific of these criteria – especially in an older age group – is the presence of brain lesions. Areas of spinal cord signal abnormality may also be seen in association with cord

TABLE 6.3 2001 and 2005 diagnostic criteria for multiple sclerosis: magnetic resonance imaging features for dissemination in space and time

	2001 criteria*	2005 criteria†
MRI dissemination in space: relapse onset disease	Three of the following four: 1. ≥1 gadolinium enhancing lesions or ≥9 T2 lesions if there is no gadolinium enhancing lesion 2. ≥1 infratentorial lesion 3. ≥1 juxtacortical lesion 4. ≥3 periventricular lesions Note: (i) One spinal cord lesion can substitute for one brain lesion	Three of the following four: 5. ≥1 gadolinium enhancing lesions or ≥9 T2 lesions if there is no gadolinium enhancing lesion 6. ≥1 infratentorial lesion 7. ≥1 juxtacortical lesion 8. ≥3 periventricular lesions Note: (i) A spinal cord lesion can be considered equivalent to a brain infratentorial lesion; (ii) an enhancing spinal cord lesion is considered to be equivalent to an enhancing brain lesion; (iii) individual spinal cord lesions can contribute along with individual brain lesions to reach the required number of T2 lesions
MRI dissemination in time: relapse onset disease	1. If a scan first occurs 3 months or more after the onset of the clinical event, the presence of a gadolinium enhancing lesion is sufficient evidence for dissemination in time provided that it is not at the site implicated in the initial event. If there is no enhancing lesion at this time, a follow up scan is required. The timing of this follow-up scan is not crucial but 3 months is recommended. A new T2- or gadolinium enhancing lesion at this time then fulfils the criterion for dissemination in time 2. If the first scan is performed less than 3 months after the onset of the clinical event, a second scan done 3 months or more after the clinical event showing a new gadolinium-enhancing lesion provides sufficient evidence for dissemination in time. However, if no gadolinium enhancing lesion is seen at this second scan, a further scan not less than 3 months after the first scan that shows a new T2 lesion or an enhancing lesion will suffice	There are two ways to show dissemination in time using imaging: 1. Detecting gadolinium enhancement at least 3 months after the onset of the initial clinical event, if not at the site corresponding to the initial event 2. Detecting a NEW T2 lesion if it appears at any time compared to a reference scan done at least 30 days after the onset of the initial clinical event

Diagnosis of multiple sclerosis in disease with progression from onset	1. Positive CSF
	AND
	2. Dissemination in space by MRI evidence of 9 or more T2 brain lesions
	Or 2 or more cord lesions
	Or 4–8 brain lesions and 1 cord lesion
	Or positive VEP with 4–8 brain lesions
	Or positive VEP with less than 4 brain lesions and 1 cord lesion
	AND
	3. Dissemination in time by MRI
	Or continued progression for 1 year
		1. One year of disease progression (retrospectively or prospectively determined)
		2. PLUS two of the following three:
		  a. Positive brain MRI (≥9 T2 lesions or ≥4 T2 lesions with abnormal visual evoked potentials)
		  b. Positive spinal cord MRI (≥2 T2 lesions)
		  c. Positive cerebrospinal fluid (isoelectric focusing evidence of oligoclonal bands and/or elevated IgG index)

*McDonald et al 2001.[21]
†Polman et al 2005.[28]

compression in cervical spondylosis. Prospective studies of patients with suspected progressive-onset MS – especially those with progressive myelopathy – should clarify the performance of these criteria.

Some anomalies and limitations are apparent in the 2005 revised criteria. First, although a new T2 lesion is allowed after 1 month from clinical onset, a gadolinium-enhancing lesion is not allowed until 3 months have elapsed: there seems no rationale for not allowing a new gadolinium-enhancing lesion that first appears more than 1 month but less than 3 months after onset. Secondly, gadolinium enhancement is a feature of lesion state not location and thus it is not logical to include it in the dissemination in space criteria. Thirdly, the dissemination in space criteria are complex, not easy to remember in routine clinical work, reduce diagnostic sensitivity and on their own –

i.e. without requiring dissemination in time – have limited specificity for early MS diagnosis, especially in patients with isolated brainstem syndromes.[35]

Simplified dissemination in space criteria, when combined with mandatory evidence for dissemination in time, may allow a more specific and sensitive early diagnosis. Swanton et al[36] evaluated a simplified criterion for dissemination in space that required only one lesion in two of the following locations: periventricular, juxtacortical, infratentorial and spinal cord. When combined with requiring a new T2 lesion after 3 months for dissemination in time and applied in 90 patients with a CIS, they gave a sensitivity of 77% and specificity of 92% for development of clinically definite MS within 3 years, compared with 46% and 94% respectively for the 2001 McDonald criteria.[36]

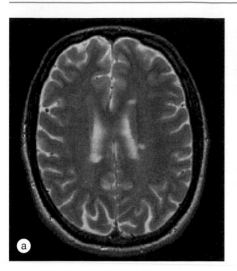

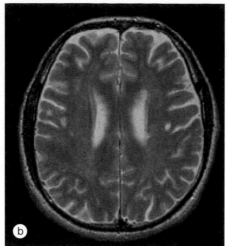

FIG. 6.1 Lesions are seen in the four regions defined in the McDonald criteria[21] and the 2005 revision[28] for dissemination in space: (A) periventricular; (B) juxtacortical; (C) infratentorial; (D) spinal cord.

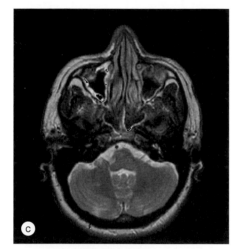

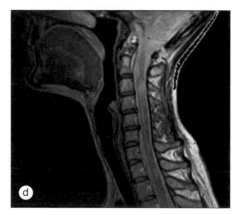

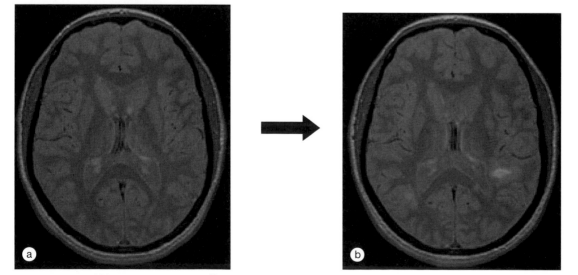

FIG. 6.2 Revised McDonald 2005 criteria[28] for dissemination in time – any new T2 lesion that appears more than 1 month after clinical onset. **A.** Baseline. **B.** 3 months later.

MAGNETIC RESONANCE IMAGING AND LONG-TERM PROGNOSIS

Whereas MRI findings are often decisive in confirming a diagnosis when there is a high level of clinical suspicion, prediction of long-term outcome in established disease is more problematic. One early study showed that T2 lesion load was smaller in disabled patients with primary progressive MS than in other cohorts and that patients with benign disease had a similar lesion load to those with secondary progressive MS in spite of less disability.[37] Longitudinal studies over 1–3 years have repeatedly shown significant but weak correlations between change in disability and increase in T2 lesion volume.

Stronger correlations have emerged when patients have been followed up for prolonged periods from onset with a CIS. Brex et al[38] reported on 71 patients followed up 14 years after presentation with a CIS of the optic nerves, brainstem or spinal cord. At follow up, 44/50 with an abnormal initial T2 brain MRI had developed clinically definite MS while only 4/21 with a normal scan did so. There was a correlation between T2 lesion volume at baseline and 14-year Expanded Disability Status Scale (EDSS) ($r=0.48$). A stronger correlation was seen between the increase in T2 volume during the first 5 years of follow up and EDSS at year 14 ($r=0.60$). T2 volume measures at later time points revealed a weaker correlation with disability.

Minneboo et al[39] reported the 8-year follow-up of 41 patients scanned when they presented with a CIS and reported that baseline total brain and infratentorial T2 lesion loads were correlated with subsequent disability. Tintoré et al[40] have followed up 156 CIS patients for 5 years and found a correlation between baseline T2 number and disability at follow up ($r=0.43$).[40] In contrast the Optic Neuritis Treatment Trial 10-year follow-up report of 388 patients found that, although MRI findings influenced the likelihood of developing MS (56% with abnormal MRI versus 22% with a normal scan),[41] they were only marginally correlated with disability (of those developing clinically definite MS, 38% with an abnormal scan had an EDSS of 3 or more compared with 29% who had a normal scan[42]). This negative finding partly reflects the exclusion of CIS patients who did not develop MS, many of whom had normal baseline MRI.

One can conclude from the available evidence that long-term prediction using MRI is limited and largely confined to T2 lesion load measures at first presentation with relapse-onset MS or within the next few years.

MAGNETIC RESONANCE IMAGING, PATHOLOGY AND CLINICAL EFFECTS

The limited correlation between routine lesion load measures and disability exposes a major limitation of T2-weighted MRI: its low pathological specificity (Table 6.1). A T2 lesion that is otherwise indistinguishable to the eye may contain little or much axonal loss, complete demyelination or remyelination; prominent or no inflammation; and variable amounts of gliosis. T2-weighted imaging also provides no information on alterations in the cellular components of MS lesions (e.g. reduced oligodendrocytes and axons, increased microglia, macrophages and astrocytes) that may have an important impact of tissue damage and prognosis. Thus a need has emerged to develop MR measures that are more specific when investigated in focal white matter lesions, whether they occur in the brain, spinal cord or optic nerves.

A second limitation of T2-weighted MRI is that it does not detect pathological abnormalities that exist in the normal appearing white and gray matter. Both old and more recent neuropathological studies indicate an abundance of pathology in both regions and – by implication – the potential to account for an important component of MS-related dysfunction, both physical and cognitive.

LESIONS

Acute inflammatory lesions

The development of new lesions in relapse-onset MS is associated with breakdown of the blood–brain barrier, an event detected on gadolinium-enhanced T1-weighted scans.[43] Biopsy and post mortem studies have correlated gadolinium enhancement with histopathological features of active inflammation – perivascular cuffs of lymphocytes and extensive macrophage infiltrates – in association with active myelin degradation.[44,45] Enhancement usually lasts 2–6 weeks but may be shorter or longer. Most new lesions are small (typically 1–5 mm diameter) and show homogeneous enhancement, compatible with the foci of perivenular inflammation and demyelination that characterize most acute inflammatory lesions seen at post-mortem. Larger new lesions, which are seen less often, display ring enhancement as they expand outwards. The ring itself displays lower signal on T2-weighted scan, which may reflect T2 and/or T2* shortening due to dense cellular infiltrates with lipid breakdown products. Beyond the gadolinium-enhancing ring there is often an irregular area of high signal that may reflect periplaque edema, although a more pathogenically specific cellular process in periplaque white matter is not excluded.

Not all acute lesions display gadolinium enhancement, especially in primary progressive MS.[46] Lucchinetti and colleagues have reported ring enhancement in type I and II lesions classified according to the criteria of Lucchinetti et al[47] but such enhancement was not observed in type III lesions.[48]

The acute T2 lesion normally waxes and wanes in association with the appearance and then disappearance of gadolinium enhancement. There is usually a permanent residual T2 abnormality and this may be smaller in size than the maximum focus of enhancement. Edema and inflammation probably account for the reversible component of T2 lesions; remyelination is not the explanation since the new myelin is morphologically abnormal and completely remyelinated lesions are observed on T2-weighted scans.[49,50]

Gadolinium enhancement per se need not be accompanied by inflammation – it is seen in other pathologies, e.g. vascular malformations, tumors. More specific imaging of the cellular components of inflammation may be achieved by using superparamagnetic ultrasmall particles of iron oxide (USPIO). USPIO is taken up in phagocytic cells and in the CNS this implies macrophages and activated microglia, as has been confirmed in experimental allergic encephalomyelitis.[51] USPIO-enhanced MRI has been evaluated in 10 MS patients: there were a total of 55 gadolinium-enhancing lesions, of which 31 also displayed USPIO enhancement. Two additional lesions displayed USPIO enhancement only.[52] This preliminary study suggests that, while not all gadolinium-enhancing lesions contain significant amounts of macrophage activity, such cellular activity may be present without gadolinium-enhancement.

Demyelination and remyelination

It would be valuable to have reliable imaging measures for both demyelination and remyelination. The former causes acute conduction block and if it persists may predispose to reduced axonal survival. The latter may restore nerve conduction (and hence clinical function) in postacute lesions and may also promote long-term axonal survival. MTR was significantly higher in remyelinated than demyelinated lesions in two recent studies with post-mortem correlation.[49,50] However, in an earlier study, MTR reduction was correlated with axonal loss,[53] although a confound of this observation is that in post-mortem MS tissue there is a strong correlation between myelin content and axonal density.[54] In order to determine whether these two pathological features have differential effects on MTR, Schmierer et al[50] regressed both measures on MTR in co-registered post mortem tissue and found that there was a robust correlation of MTR with myelin content alone ($r=0.74$). This suggests that MTR is influenced by myelin and could be used to monitor potential remyelination treatments in selected white matter lesions.

Another proposed MR marker for myelin is the short T2 component measured from a multiecho T2 decay sequence.[55]

Normal white matter has a short T2 component (T2 <50 ms) and loss of this component has been reported in MS lesions in vivo and also in a post-mortem study where there was evidence for demyelination in the corresponding tissue section.[56] Recent development of a multislice acquisition from which to measure short T2 will improve the applicability of this approach in MS studies.[57] Most recently, Song et al[58] have proposed based on an experimental model in mouse corpus callosum that increase in radial diffusivity followed by normalization is due to sequential demyelination and remyelination.

Axonal loss

Approximately 20–30% of chronic T2 lesions exhibit T1 hypointensity on two-dimensional T1-weighted spin echo MRI. The latter subgroups of lesions have exhibited a greater amount of tissue matrix destruction and axonal loss in post mortem studies,[59] although the difference from T1-isointense lesion has not been significant in all studies.[50] Such lesions – colloquially known as 'black holes' – have been regarded as markers for axonal loss.[43] This is a useful concept but is limited by the reversibility of such lesions seen during acute evolution. Features of the acute lesion that are more likely to result in persistent T1 hypointensity are large size, ring enhancement, prolonged enhancement and acute T1 hypointensity.[60] Notably, remyelinated lesions are usually T1-isointense (although visible on T2-weighted MRI).

A limitation of using T1-hypointense lesions as surrogate measures for axonal loss is that they are largely confined to supratentorial regions; they are relatively infrequent in the posterior fossa[61] (although they correlate with disability when present[62]) and almost never occur in the spinal cord. Most of the pathology that accounts for physical disability in MS is within the posterior fossa or spinal cord.

Other approaches that have been proposed for quantifying axonal loss or damage in lesions are the measurement of NAA or abnormalities of diffusion, including increased diffusivity, reduced fractional anisotropy and altered ratios of perpendicular to longitudinal diffusion values along a fiber pathway. A limitation of measuring NAA is that it can only be done in large lesions and it may be transiently reduced in acute lesions,[63] implying that it measures sublethal dysfunction, not simply loss of axons. Experimental work suggests that reduced longitudinal diffusion with preserved (restricted) perpendicular diffusion is relatively specific for axonal destruction in fiber pathways.[64] However, a study of MS post-mortem brain showed that mean diffusivity and fractional anisotropy were correlated with axonal density, myelin content and gliosis but not with any of these features selectively.[65] Interpretation of diffusion measures in human in vivo studies is impeded by the confounding effects of crossing fiber tracts and limitations in resolution for diffusion tensor imaging. There is potential for more specific correlations to emerge with high field scanners, multichannel coils, parallel imaging and more refined tractography algorithms.

NORMAL APPEARING WHITE MATTER

Pathological abnormalities of macroscopically normal appearing white matter (NAWM) include astrocytic proliferation, microglial activation, perivascular inflammatory cuffs, reduced axonal density and small foci of demyelination.[66,67] Such abnormalities appear more extensive in subjects with progressive MS[68] and may have an important role in determining the clinical progression of the disease.

Quantitative abnormalities of a variety of MR measures have been consistently reported from NAWM of MS subjects since the late 1980s.[69,70] Early studies reported the findings from small regions of interest whereas more recent studies have used segmentation algorithms and histogram analysis to investigate the global white matter or indeed whole brain.[71,72]

The abnormalities seen on MTR are quantitatively small and, unlike the larger changes seen in lesions, are likely to be less specific for variations in myelin content per se. There is experimental evidence that inflammation alone slightly reduces MTR[73] and axonal degeneration will also contribute. MTR is perhaps the most robust quantitative measure of NAWM abnormality: reduced MTR is already present in patients with clinically isolated syndromes,[74] increases progressively in subjects with early relapsing–remitting MS[75] (Fig. 6.3) and is most abnormal in patients with secondary progressive disease.[76] MTR histograms are also abnormal in primary progressive MS.[77] In a cohort of 73 MS patients with various clinical subtypes, whole-brain MTR histograms were related to development of disability over the next 4.5 years.[78]

Diffusion tractography analysis of subjects with isolated optic neuritis has revealed decreased connectivity within the optic radiations that was unrelated to the presence of occipital radiation lesions.[79] Such connectivity measures have potential to detect and quantify wallerian or trans-synaptic degeneration.

On MR spectroscopy, reduced NAWM NAA is observed in established MS. This implies diffuse axonal dysfunction or loss and may partly reflect wallerian degeneration secondary to white matter lesions, although it can be reversible.[80] NAA reduction is greater in secondary progressive than relapsing–remitting MS[81] and has been correlated with disability.[82,83] How early NAA decreases is uncertain: normal concentrations were seen in single-voxel spectrum from NAWM of 94 CIS patients,[84] although another CIS cohort were reported to have a 22% reduction in whole brain NAA.[85]

On short TE spectroscopy, myoinositol is increased in MS NAWM[86] and also in patients with CIS.[84] It has been correlated with clinical impairment and disability in early and late MS, both relapse onset and primary progressive.[87–89] Myoinositol is produced by glial cells and may indicate the extent of astrocytic or microglial proliferation or other inflammatory events. A TE-averaged PRESS sequence has been applied on a 3 T scanner and successfully identified and quantified the peak arising from glutamate: an increase was observed in NAWM as well as gadolinium-enhancing lesions.[90] Similar approaches in future could explore the role of glutamate excitotoxicity in MS pathogenesis and tissue damage.

NORMAL APPEARING GRAY MATTER

Both old[91,92] and recent[93,94] pathological studies have demonstrated that cortical demyelinating lesions occur in MS and indeed are abundant and sometimes seen in the relative absence of white matter pathology.[95] It has proved very difficult to visualize cortical lesions on MRI. They are less inflammatory than white matter lesions, which will reduce their T1 and T2 contrast with surrounding tissue. Furthermore, normal cortex has a longer T1 and T2 than white matter, which further diminishes contrast with lesions contained within. Additional difficulty arises because the cortical ribbon is thin and often contaminated by signal from adjacent CSF. In a post-mortem study, suppression of CSF using a three-dimensional FLAIR sequence only marginally increased the detection rate of pathologically confirmed intracortical lesions from 3% (for conventional T2-weighted scans) to 5%.[96] Partial success in detecting cortical lesions in vivo has been achieved with application of a three-dimensional, double inversion recovery sequence, which provides high resolution images with CSF suppression and enhanced gray matter–white matter contrast: in 10 patients, 80 intracortical lesions were detected on double inversion recovery compared with only 31 on three-dimensional FLAIR.[97] Cortical

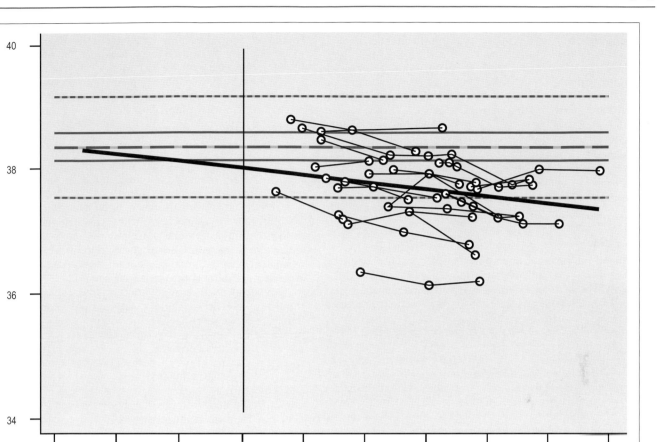

FIG. 6.3 MTR of normal appearing white matter (NAWM) in early relapsing remitting MS. All patients had first MTR study within 3 years of clinical onset and were followed up annually for two years. Extrapolation backwards assuming linear rate of change suggests that the NAWM abnormality appears before clinical onset. Redrawn from Davies et al 2005[75] with permission from the *Journal of Neurology*.

lesions are also detected on three-dimensional inversion recovery T1-weighted sequences with high signal-to-noise ratio.[98] High field scanning (3 T and above) and multichannel coils will improve signal to noise in cortex and should improve lesion detection in future.[99]

Demyelinating lesions also occur in deep gray matter structures and are sometimes visible on MRI, although it is likely that some lesions are missed, as in the cortex.

Gray matter abnormalities are found by segmenting whole or regional gray matter and quantifying a variety of MR parameters, including MTR, diffusivity and T1 and T2 hypointensity.[77,100–104] Reduced NAA is reported from cortical and deep gray matter.[88,105,106] Reduced thalamic MTR has been identified as an early feature of relapse-onset MS using voxel-based morphometry to localize gray matter abnormality.[107] T2 hypointensity in deep gray matter may reflect an increase in iron content and decreased T2 signal in the dentate nucleus has been correlated with ambulatory impairment.[108] Basal ganglia T2 hypointensity is also associated with accelerated brain atrophy.[109] Reduced gray matter diffusivity is most apparent in patients with primary and secondary progressive MS.[101] Reduced gray matter MTR is seen in CIS patients[74] and progressively increases in early relapsing–remitting MS.[75] These findings suggest that early gray matter abnormalities are more common than is thought from neuropathological studies that usually study patients with late progressive disease.[95]

SPINAL CORD

Much of the locomotor disability in MS comes from spinal cord pathology but, as in the brain, there is a poor correlation between the number of spinal cord T2 lesions and disability.[31] On the other hand there is a correlation between atrophy in the upper cervical cord and disability.[110] Abnormal cord MTR and diffusivity measures have also been associated with functional impairment.[111,112] Post-mortem studies have shown both focal and diffuse regions of demyelination and axonal loss in MS spinal cord.[113–115] with involvement of both gray[54,116] and white matter. While routine T2-weighted images detect foci of demyelination, they are insensitive to the extent of axonal loss;[117] probably the global measures of atrophy or MTR better reflect diffuse pathology and axonal loss. Diffuse hyperintensity may be seen on proton density-weighted images of the cord, especially in primary progressive MS, but this is difficult to recognize consistently. In vivo studies of the cord at high field have potential to improve clinical–MRI correlations.

OPTIC NERVES

Optic nerve imaging is challenging because of the small size of the nerve, confounding signals from surrounding CSF in the nerve sheath and orbital fat, and the potential for motion artifacts. Nevertheless, high-resolution fat-suppressed sequences reveal the symptomatic lesion of optic neuritis as a hyperintense T2 lesion and acute lesions display gadolinium enhancement.[118] The cross-sectional area of the nerve can be measured, and atrophy with a mean loss of 12% area occurs following an attack of optic neuritis.[119] Optic nerve MTR has been measured on two- and three-dimensional sequences[120] and a correlation made with visual evoked potential latency suggesting that it reflects myelination within the nerve.[121] Serial in vivo MRI of the optic nerve when combined with retinal nerve fiber layer imaging, visual function assessment and visual evoked potentials, provides considerable information on the structure–function relationships of an evolving inflammatory/demyelinating lesion and also provides a template for evaluating anti-inflammatory or neuroprotective treatments that as yet have not been utilized.

ATROPHY

Permanent and progressive disability in MS is probably due to loss of axons in clinically eloquent locations in the CNS. Measurement of brain tissue volume loss is a plausible global measure of neuroaxonal loss.[122] Sensitive and largely automated methods are available for quantifying small amounts of tissue loss: in MS typically 0.5–1% of brain volume is lost per year, which is 3–5 times the normal age-related rate of atrophy. However, tissue volumes are also made up of myelin, glial connective tissue and blood vessels and in MS inflammation and associated edema may cause temporary tissue swelling whereas anti-inflammatory therapies can decrease tissue bulk (Table 6.2).

Several techniques have been applied to study MS atrophy in natural history studies or clinical trials. Both two- and three-dimensional images can be analyzed; the latter yield greater precision but the former also prove adequate in detecting change. Brain segmentation algorithms have been developed that are largely automated, although expert interaction is needed to optimize the threshold for separation of brain from nonbrain tissue and to edit tissue misclassification errors. The techniques are most often applied to T1-weighted scans but some methods are also effective when applied to FLAIR or T2-weighted spin echo images.[123] Registration of serial scans provides a sensitive measure of change over time: two such approaches that have been used in MS are structural image evaluation using normalisation of atrophy (SIENA)[124,125] and brain boundary shift integral (BBSI).[126,127] Both these measures are more sensitive and consistent in demonstrating change in a pair of scans obtained 1 year apart when compared with segmentation of each scan separately and subtraction of the second from the first[128] (Fig. 6.4).

Regional measures that have been applied include ventricular volume,[127] central cerebral slice volumes,[129] gray and white matter volumes[130] and thalamic volume.[105] Although atrophy has been observed globally and on all of the regional measures, proportionately greater change over time has been reported in gray matter versus white matter[131] and in ventricles and central cerebral slices rather than whole brain.[127,132] The distribution of regional atrophy changes has been reported to affect predominantly periventricular regions in relapsing–remitting MS and to occur more globally, including cortical involvement, in secondary progressive MS.[133] On the other hand, reductions in gray matter fraction, neocortical volume and cortical thickness have been reported in relapsing–remitting MS.[130,134,135]

Although correlation between brain volume measures and disability has not always been strong, this may reflect variations in the location and extent of atrophy that are not captured in a single global measure. Better correlations have been observed when neuropsychological measures have been incorporated[136,137] and when there has been long term follow-up.[138]

Accelerated brain atrophy occurs from onset with a CIS through to advanced secondary and primary progressive MS. It is uncertain whether the rate of atrophy varies over time and between clinical subgroups as long-term follow-up studies have not directly addressed this issue. Short-term evaluation of ventricular enlargement over 1 year reported greater change in secondary progressive compared with relapsing–remitting MS,[139] and a trend for secondary progressive patients to have a higher rate of whole brain atrophy has been reported.[140] At all stages of disease the correlations between T2 lesion load and extent of atrophy are weak and the latter measure provides complementary information about disease evolution.

Tissue volume measures do not study the integrity of the remaining tissue. Such tissue is also abnormal in MS as seen by alterations in MTR, diffusion and other measures, including reductions in NAA that suggest reduced axonal density or function. Thus, the measurement of atrophy underestimates the full extent of neuroaxonal loss.[105,141]

PERFUSION AND FUNCTIONAL MAGNETIC RESONANCE IMAGING

While structural imaging has provided much insight into the pathology and its evolution during the course of MS, MR can also assess tissue perfusion and – using functional MRI – the response of brain regions to a variety of sensory, motor or cognitive activation paradigms.

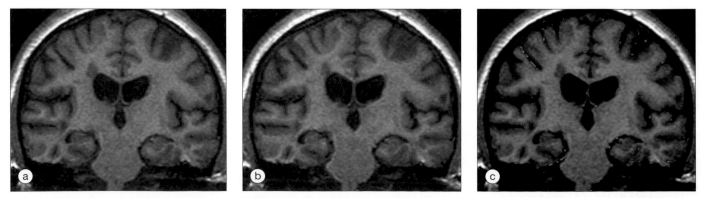

FIG. 6.4 Three-dimensional T1-weighted coronal MRI scans (**A**) at baseline and (**B**) 1 year later in a patient with early relapsing–remitting multiple sclerosis. **C**. The images have been registered using the brain boundary shift integral and areas of difference (i.e. loss of brain tissue) are shown in red.

Perfusion

Perfusion and/or regional cerebral blood volume measures can be obtained by injecting a bolus of gadolinium chelate and following the time course and extent of signal change over the next minute. Alternatively, arterial spin tagging methods allow selective detection of flowing protons and provide a measure of perfusion without the need for a contrast injection but with lower signal-to-noise. Bolus methods have identified a reduction in perfusion in prelesional NAWM[142] and both increased and decreased perfusion in relapsing–remitting MS white matter lesions.[143] Arterial spin tagging has identified a decrease in perfusion in gray matter in subjects with progressive MS: the most striking decreases were in deep gray matter in primary progressive patients.[144] These changes may reflect more extensive neuronal loss or dysfunction in progressive disease. In a segmented map of whole white matter (including lesions), perfusion was increased in relapsing–remitting MS, which may reflect an increased metabolic rate secondary to inflammation.[144]

Functional magnetic resonance imaging

There are well defined paradigms for the normal pattern of activation of contralateral primary motor cortex with finger tapping and primary visual cortex activation in response to a flashing light stimulus. These and other algorithms (including cognitive and lower limb motor) have been applied in MS patients at all stages of disease from CIS onwards. Abnormal activation patterns in response to finger tapping have been elicited in all MS patient subgroups: relapsing or progressive, disabled or nondisabled and early or late.[145–147] Significant correlations with lesion load and abnormalities in normal-appearing brain tissue have been interpreted as evidence that the fMRI responses are adaptive. A cross-sectional study of fMRI response to a simple motor task involving three cohorts with CIS, relapsing–remitting and secondary progressive MS reported abnormal activation mainly within motor areas at the early disease stage but more extensive and bilateral in secondary progressive disease.[148]

MS patients exhibit abnormal responses to several cognitive paradigms[149] and activation following optic neuritis is reduced within the visual cortex but increased beyond it. An effort to combine both optic nerve lesion size (seen on structural MRI) and the fMRI response to better explain visual function at various stages following optic neuritis met with limited success: the positive relationship at presentation when abnormal activation was seen in lateral occipital cortex suggested that the fMRI response could be adaptive, whereas the lack of relationship at later time points did not support the still altered fMRI response being adaptive.[150]

Interpretation of the functional significance of altered fMRI responses is complex. One view is that the activation of new regions helps to maintain function in the presence of structural pathology. A second hypothesis is that such activation reflects already stressed neural networks that are liable to fail completely: there is evidence that abnormal fMRI responses in the medial temporal cortex in patients with minimal cognitive impairment are associated with a greater likelihood of developing Alzheimer's disease at follow-up.[151] A third possibility is that some of the new activations are redundant epiphenomena manifesting when there has been damage to the primary pathway of interest.

MONITORING TREATMENT

MRI is a regular component of evaluation in randomized and controlled clinical trials in MS (Table 6.4). Serial T2-weighted scans in the late 1980s by Paty and coworkers revealed many clinically silent new or enlarging lesions that exhibited a waxing and waning pattern over several weeks in relapsing–remitting and chronic progressive MS.[152–154] A short time later, serial studies with gadolinium-enhanced T1-weighted sequences also revealed numerous clinically silent lesions in both relapsing–remitting and secondary progressive MS.[46,155–157] In parallel with natural history studies in the early 1990s, Paty and his group led the way in applying serial T2-weighted MRI in a placebo-controlled trial of β-interferon-1b in relapsing–remitting MS.[158] In addition to this pivotal trial showing a decrease in relapse rate, there was a dramatic 75% decrease in the number of new T2 lesions and total T2 volume was also reduced by β-interferon. This trial set the standard for all subsequent controlled MS trials in which MRI is an outcome measure but also identified a discordance in the extent of treatment effect on clinical (modest) and MRI (marked) outcomes.

PHASE II PROOF-OF-CONCEPT EXPLORATORY TRIALS

Studies of monthly MRI in relapsing–remitting MS show that gadolinium enhancement is twice as sensitive as T2 scans alone in detecting new disease activity[159] and proof-of-concept trials are feasible using frequent MRI.[160,161] In the mid 1990s, the National MS Society (USA) asked a Task Force to develop recommendations for use of MRI in treatment trials. A central focus was the design of proof-of-concept phase II exploratory studies using MRI to determine efficacy.[162] Parallel-group, placebo-controlled trial designs provide robust efficacy assessment: if 50–60 relapsing-remitting MS patients per arm undergo serial monthly MRI for 6 months, it is possible to detect a 50% reduction in the frequency of new MRI lesions. Because inter-patient variation in lesion activity is greater than that seen within patients over time, smaller sample sizes are required to detect a decrease in MRI activity when comparing a baseline pretreatment phase with a subsequent treatment phase in the same patients using baseline-crossover design. A disadvantage of the latter trial design is the potential confound of regression to the mean.

Numerous therapies have decreased MRI lesion activity in MS trials (Table 6.4) and in most instances there has been a concomitant decrease in relapse rate. While gadolinium-enhancing lesions have been associated with relapse rate in several individual studies and in a meta-analysis of several cohorts,[163] it has not been consistently correlated with disability either concurrently or in the future. There is consensus that phase III studies are required to determine clinical efficacy, especially the extent of relapse suppression and whether the accumulation of disability is slowed. Relatively short-term phase II studies using MRI outcomes will also not be adequate to identify rare but serious side effects: as seen recently with natalizumab, these may only emerge later.[164,165]

While phase II MRI outcome trials are widely used to screen new therapies, several issues need to be considered in planning them. First, compared to 10 years ago when such studies were novel, fewer patients nowadays are prepared or available to receive a placebo – this is more problematic for long-term phase III trials but can be an issue in phase II. Secondly, the control arm may be on active treatment that reduces the amount of MRI activity. This will necessitate an increase in sample size, although such a study is still feasible if the effect of the active comparator on MRI is modest.[166] Thirdly, with experimental therapies, one must be alert to the possibility that there will be an unanticipated increase in disease activity – seen as an

TABLE 6.4 Therapies evaluated on magnetic resonance imaging in phase II or III multiple sclerosis trials

Drug	Study design	MS group	MRI activity	Relapses	Disability	Reference
β-interferon-1b	Parallel groups, PC	RR	↓↓	↓	(↓)	Paty et al 1993[158]
β-interferon-1a (IM)	Parallel groups, PC	RR	↓↓	↓	↓	Simon et al 1998[188]
β-interferon-1a (SC)	Parallel groups, PC	RR	↓↓	↓	↓	Li et al 1999[189]
β-interferon-1a (IM)	Parallel groups, PC	CIS	↓↓	↓	?	Jacobs et al 2000[190]
β-interferon-1a (SC)	Parallel groups, PC	CIS	↓↓	↓	?	Comi et al 2001a[191]
β-interferon-1b	Parallel groups, PC	SP	↓↓	↓	↓	Miller et al 1999[192]
β-interferon-1b	Parallel groups, PC	SP	↓↓	↓	↔	Panitch et al 2004[168]
β-interferon-1a (SC)	Parallel groups, PC	SP	↓↓	↓	↔	Li et al 2001[193]
β-interferon-1a (IM)	Parallel groups, PC	SP	↓↓	↓	↔	Cohen et al 2002[194]
β-interferon-1a (IM)	Parallel groups, PC	PP	↓↓	N/A	↔	Leary et al 2003[195]
Glatiramer acetate	Parallel groups, PC	RR	↓	↓	?	Comi et al 2001b[167]
Mitoxantrone	Parallel groups, steroid control	RR/SP	↓↓↓	↓↓	↓↓	Edan et al 1997[196]
Mitoxantrone	Parallel groups, PC	RR/SP	↓↓↓	↓↓	↓	Hartung et al 2002[197]
Natalizumab	Parallel groups, PC	RR/SP	↓↓↓	↓↓	?	Miller et al 2003[198]
Natalizumab	Parallel groups, PC	RR	↓↓↓	↓↓	↓↓	Polman et al 2006[174]
Campath-1H	Crossover, open	SP	↓↓↓	↓↓	?	Coles et al 1999[169]
Campath-1H	Parallel groups, β-interferon control	RR	↓↓↓	↓↓	↓↓	Genzyme website statement September 2005
Laquinimod	Parallel groups, PC	RR/SP	↓	?	?	Polman et al 2005b[199]
Daclizumab	Crossover, open	RR/SP	↓↓	?	?	Bielekova et al 2004[200]
TNF receptor fusion protein	Parallel groups, PC	RR	↑	↑		Lenercept study group 1999[201]
Anti-TNF antibody	Crossover, open	SP	↑	↑	?	Van Oosten et al 1996[202]
Anti-CD4 antibody	Parallel groups, PC	RR/SP	↔	↓	?	Van Oosten et al 1997[203]
CC chemokine receptor 1 antagonist	Parallel groups, PC	RR	↔	↔	?	Zipp et al 2005[204]
Anti-TcR-Vβ5.2	Parallel groups, PC	RR	↔	↔	?	Killestein et al 2002[205]
Rosiglitazone	Crossover, PC	RR	↔	↔	?	Miller et al 2005[206]
FTY720	Parallel groups, PC	RR/SP	↓↓	↓↓	?	Kappos et al 2006[207]
CTLA4Ig	Parallel groups, PC	RR	↑	?	?	Fieschi et al 2005[208]
Cladribine	Parallel groups, PC	SP/PP	↓↓↓	N/A	↔	Rice et al 2000[170]
Simvastatin	Crossover, open	RR	↓	↔	?	Vollmer et al 2004[209]

↓, mild decrease (<50%); ↓↓, moderate decrease (50–75%); ↓↓↓, marked decrease (>75%); ↔, no effect; ↑increase; ?, not known (usually because phase 2 data only). CIS, clinically isolated syndrome; N/A, not applicable; PC, placebo-controlled; PP, primary progressive multiple sclerosis; MRI, magnetic resonance imaging; MS, multiple sclerosis; RR, relapsing–remitting multiple sclerosis; SP, secondary progressive multiple sclerosis.

increase in new MRI lesions – that may necessitate an early termination of study. It is good clinical practice for central MRI analysis in phase II trials to take place shortly after the scans are acquired and for the data to be available to an independent data safety monitoring board. Fourthly, the latency to onset of treatment effect should be considered: if it is 3 months or more – as was apparently the case with glatiramer acetate[167] – the monitoring period should be extended accordingly. Finally, if a treatment is thought to be effective not by preventing new inflammatory lesions but rather by another mechanism (e.g. neuroprotection, remyelination, cortical adaptation), gadolinium-enhancing lesions are not appropriate as the primary outcome measure.

PHASE III TRIALS

Lesions

Magnetic resonance imaging measures of gadolinium-enhancing, T2- and T1-hypointense lesions are used as supportive outcome measures in phase III trials of potential disease-modifying treatments. The number of new lesions and total lesion volumes are evaluated, usually at annual intervals over 2 years. More frequent scanning will add little unless non-linearity is anticipated in the temporal dynamics of the outcome measures. These outcome measures are not well correlated with disability – a fact most graphically demonstrated in progressive MS. The North American trial of β-interferon-1b in secondary progressive MS showed almost compete stabilization of T2 volume but no slowing of disability accumulation.[168] Similar observations were made in an open-label, baseline-crossover study of Campath-1H in secondary progressive MS[169] and in a trial of cladribine in a mixed primary/secondary MS cohort.[170]

The conversion of gadolinium-enhancing lesions to regions of persistent T1 hypointensity has been evaluated within both phase II and III designs: the proportion of lesions becoming T1 hypointense is lowered by natalizumab[171] and glatiramer acetate[172] but not by β-interferon-1b.[173]

While most studies have shown concordance of effect on relapses and new MRI lesions – i.e. both reduced or both unaltered – the magnitude of treatment effects has not been the same. All the β-interferons and glatiramer acetate reduce relapse rate by ≈30% but reduce MRI activity by amounts varying between 30% and 75%. Natalizumab reduces relapse rate by 67% and gadolinium-enhancing lesions by 90%.[174] Several factors probably contribute to this discrepancy, including the location of new lesions, the extent of demyelination and conduction block in new lesions (not measurable on gadolinium-enhanced or T2-weighed images), and the potential for some clinical relapses to have pathophysiological mechanisms unrelated to new inflammatory lesions, e.g. conduction block in pre-existing lesions.

Atrophy

Because irreversible and progressive disability are not inevitably related to either new lesions or relapses, other MRI measures that are more directly related to neuroaxonal loss should be more reliable in determining whether therapies have a reasonable prospect of delaying disability. Measures of atrophy are most favored at present, partly because of their robustness in detecting small changes. However, measurement of brain atrophy may be confounded by factors other than axonal loss alone (Table 6.2). Anti-inflammatory treatments may reduce brain volume, at least in the short term. A short course of pulsed intravenous methylprednisolone had this effect for up to 2 months[175] and accelerated atrophy in the first year of trials of β-interferon and natalizumab has been ascribed to such a mechanism.[123,176] In the latter trials, slowing of atrophy in the second year of treatment supported the notion that there is delayed protection against ongoing tissue loss from treatments that are partially effective in preventing new lesions and relapses. In a placebo-controlled trial of intravenous immunoglobulin, the significant reduction in atrophy in the treatment arm was seen mainly in the first year and the discussants of the study acknowledge the possibility that a relative increase in brain volume due to therapy has not been excluded.[177]

Several placebo-controlled trials of β-interferon have reported either absent or modest (30%) slowing in the rate of brain tissue loss in early and late MS.[123,125,175,179] Comparison of individual drug effects and the stage of disease at which treatment is initiated are complicated by differences in the analysis methods used and limitations in the number of cases that could be analyzed because of technical problems with the scans. These problems should lessen as acquisition and analysis protocols are prospectively designed that optimize the measurement of atrophy in multicenter trials.

The sample sizes required for using brain atrophy as a primary outcome measure are likely to be considerable because the absolute changes in brain volume are small and there is intersubject variation in the rate of atrophy. Using central cerebral slice volume as the outcome measure from the placebo arm of a secondary progressive MS trial in which measurements were made at 6 monthly intervals for 3 years, we have calculated that 60 patients per arm will be sufficient to detect a 50–60% slowing in the rate of atrophy over 2 years (D. Altmann, personal communication). These calculations have been used to power an exploratory trial of lamotrigine in secondary progressive MS – an approach based on the hypothesis that sodium channel blockade promotes the survival of demyelinated axons and following the encouraging results of sodium channel blockade in experimental allergic encephalomyelitis.[180] Another calculation in a primary progressive cohort showed slightly smaller sample size requirements for measurement of percentage whole brain volume change using SIENA versus a central cerebral slices volume measure.[132] Although cord atrophy is likely to be more relevant to evolution of disability, the measurement of small changes in an already small structure (average ≈1% decrease in cross-sectional area per annum but with considerable interpatient variation[181,182]) will probably require large sample sizes for demonstration of therapeutic efficacy.

There are still unanswered questions when optimizing sample sizes using atrophy as the outcome measure: How often should scans be performed? Is there value in repeat scanning at the same visit and taking the average measure? Should an early follow-up scan be performed in controlled trials to allow for decrease in brain volume due to anti-inflammatory treatment? Should whole brain or a region be studied (e.g. gray matter, central slices)? Should three-dimensional or two-dimensional acquisitions be used? Which of the many available analysis methods is to be preferred?

Measures of normal appearing brain tissue

Measurement of abnormalities in the normal-appearing white and gray matter should complement atrophy measures as an indication of the overall extent of tissue damage occurring outside of focal white matter lesions. However, measurement is more challenging in a multicenter setting, where the acquisition sequences required for outcomes such as MTR, T1 relaxation, diffusion and metabolite concentrations are more complex. MR physics expertise may be needed to standardize acquisitions across centers.

MTR is perhaps the most robust of the currently available measures.[183] Personal experience suggests that reproducible and stable measures can be obtained on the same scanner over many years even across major hardware upgrades.[184] MTR measurements of whole brain have been reported from multicenter trials of β-interferon and intravenous immunoglobulin and in both there was no evidence for significant treatment-related modification.[185,186] A single center study also showed no obvious alterations in whole brain MTR following the introduction of β-interferon.[187]

EVALUATION OF REPAIR THERAPIES

When effective treatments arrive that promote remyelination, it would be desirable to directly demonstrate the process of repair by imaging. In lesions, MTR provides an indication of myelination[49,50] and one could envisage a placebo-controlled clinical trial of a systemic remyelination therapy in which brain lesions of patients are identified at baseline by virtue of having a stable MTR below a predefined threshold for demyelination. Determination of stability would require exclusion of acute enhancing or early postacute lesions in which MTR is changing. During follow-up, remyelination would be inferred by an increase in MTR to a predefined threshold for remyelination within individual lesions. Careful serial scanning would be needed, with accurate patient repositioning, and automated image registration of a high-resolution – possibly three-dimensional – MTR acquisition sequence would be preferable. A positive study outcome would be a significant increase in the proportion of patients in the actively treated arm with lesions reaching the threshold for remyelination.

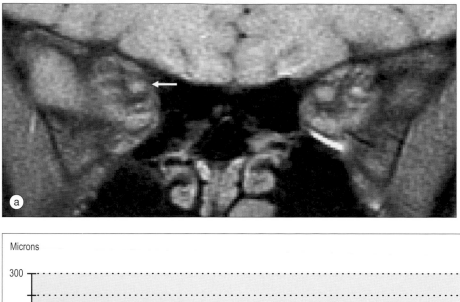

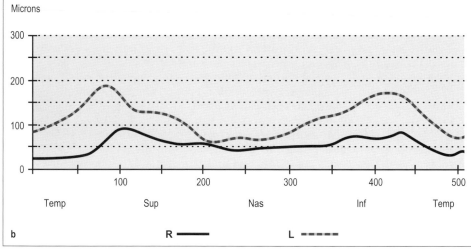

FIG. 6.5 A patient with a previous episode of right optic neuritis. **A.** Coronal fat-suppressed fast fluid-attenuated inversion-recovery (FLAIR) sequence demonstrating right optic nerve atrophy (arrow). **B.** Circular arc measurement of retinal nerve fibre layer on optical coherence tomography, showing thinning on the right.

To investigate treatments to enable recovery of individual symptomatic lesions that have resulted in a fixed deficit, optic neuritis is a particularly suitable syndrome for investigation. Imaging of both anterior and posterior visual pathways can be combined with sensitive clinical and electrophysiological measures to provide a comprehensive readout of functional response and its structural basis. In particular, optic nerve MTR and atrophy[119,121] and retinal nerve fiber layer thickness are measures that investigate remyelination and neuroprotection (Fig. 6.5).

MAGNETIC RESONANCE IMAGING IN MANAGEMENT OF INDIVIDUAL PATIENTS

Magnetic resonance imaging clearly has a valuable role in supporting the clinical diagnosis of MS and excluding other conditions. Repeat scanning may be needed where there is diagnostic doubt and when the criterion of dissemination in time is not fulfilled. The indications for MRI in starting, continuing or changing disease-modifying treatments is less clear. Clinical evaluation is clearly more important but in some circumstances imaging findings may help. For example, gadolinium-enhancing lesions, when associated with clinical activity and deterioration, strengthen the case for more aggressive immunomodulation. It is, however, unwise to make hasty changes in treatment when patients are clinically stable but show activity on MRI: neurologists should remember that the correlations between MRI lesion activity and the clinical course of MS are modest. Although for now it is not practical to monitor changes in brain volume or MTR in individual patients, these measures have greater potential for future assessment of the course of MS in the longer term.

REFERENCES

1. Cala LA, Mastaglia FL. Computerised axial tomography in multiple sclerosis. Lancet 1976; 7961: 689.
2. Vinuela FV, Fox AJ, Debrun GM et al. New perspectives in computed tomography of multiple sclerosis. Am J Radiol 1982; 139: 123–127.
3. Young IR, Hall AS, Pallis CA et al. Nuclear magnetic resonance imaging of the brain in multiple sclerosis. Lancet 1981; 8255: 1063–1066.
4. Brooks DJ, Leenders KL, Head G et al. Studies on regional cerebral oxygen utilisation and cognitive function in multiple sclerosis. J Neurol Neurosurg Psychiatr 1984; 47: 1182–191.
5. Blinkenberg M, Rune K, Jensen CV et al. Cortical cerebral metabolism correlates with MRI lesion load and cognitive dysfunction in MS. Neurology 2000; 54: 558–564.
6. Pozzilli C, Passafiume D, Bernardi S et al. SPECT, MRI and cognitive functions in multiple sclerosis. J Neurol Neurosurg Psychiatr 1991; 54: 110–115.
7. Lycke J, Wikkelso C, Bergh AC et al. Regional cerebral blood flow in multiple sclerosis measured by single photon emission tomography with technetium-99m hexamethylpropyleneamine oxime. Eur Neurol 1993; 33: 163–167.

8. Banati RB, Newcombe J, Gunn RN et al. The peripheral benzodiazepine binding site in the brain in multiple sclerosis. Quantitative in vivo imaging of microglia as a measure of disease activity. Brain 2000; 123: 2321–2337.

9. Debruyne JC, Versijpt J, van Laere KJ et al. PET visualisation of microglia in multiple sclerosis patients using [11C]PK11195. Eur J Neurol 2003; 10: 257–264.

10. Kallmann BA, Sauer J, Schliesser M et al. Determination of ventricular diameters in multiple sclerosis patients with transcranial sonography (TCS) – a two year follow-up study. J Neurol 2004; 251: 30–34.

11. Berg D, Maurer M, Warmuth-Metz M et al. The correlation between ventricular diameter measured by transcranial sonography and clinical disability and cognitive dysfunction in patients with multiple sclerosis. Arch Neurol 2000; 57: 1289–1292.

12. Parisi V, Manni G, Spadaro M et al. Correlation between morphological and functional retinal impairment in multiple sclerosis patients. Invest Ophthalmol Vis Sci 1999; 40: 2520–2527.

13. Trip SA, Schlottmann PG, Jones SJ et al. Retinal nerve fiber layer axonal loss and visual dysfunction in optic neuritis. Ann Neurol 2005; 58: 383–391.

14. Fisher JB, Jacobs DA, Markowitz CE et al. Relation of visual function to retinal nerve fiber layer thickness in multiple sclerosis. Ophthalmology 2006; 113: 324–332.

15. Costello F, Coupland S, Hodge W et al. Quantifying axonal loss after optic neuritis with optical coherence tomography. Ann Neurol 2006; 59: 963–969.

16. Sepulcre J, Murie-Fernandez M, Salinas-Alaman A et al. Diagnostic accuracy of retinal abnormalities in predicting disease activity in MS. Neurology 2007; 68: 1488–1494.

17. Parker GJ, Wheeler-Kingshott CA, Barker GJ. Estimating distributed anatomical brain connectivity using fast marching methods and diffusion tensor imaging. IEEE Trans Med Imaging 2002; 21: 505–512.

18. Hurd R, Napapon S, Srinivasan R et al. Measurement of brain glutamate using TE-averaged PRESS at 3 T. Magn Reson Med 2004; 51: 435–446.

19. Inglese M, Li BSY, Rusinek H et al. Diffusely elevated cerebral choline and creatine in relapsing-remitting multiple sclerosis. Magn Reson Med 2003; 50: 190–195.

20. Gonen O, Catalaa I, Babb JS et al. Total brain N-acetylaspartate: a new measure of disease load in MS. Neurology 2000; 54: 15–19.

21. McDonald WI, Compston A, Edan G et al. Recommended diagnostic criteria for multiple sclerosis: guidelines from the international panel on the diagnosis of multiple sclerosis. Ann Neurol 2001; 50: 121–127.

22. Dalton CM, Brex PA, Miszkiel KA et al. Application of the new McDonald criteria in patients with clinically isolated syndromes suggestive of multiple sclerosis. Ann Neurol 2002; 52: 47–53.

23. Tintoré M, Rovira A, Rio J et al. New diagnostic criteria for multiple sclerosis: application in first demyelinating episode. Neurology 2003; 60: 27–30.

24. Barkhof F, Rocca M, Francis G et al. Validation of diagnostic magnetic resonance imaging criteria for multiple sclerosis and response to interferon beta1a. Ann Neurol 2003; 53: 718–724.

25. CHAMPS Study Group. MRI predictors of early conversion to clinically definite MS in the CHAMPS placebo group. Neurology 2002; 59: 998–1005.

26. Dalton CM, Brex PA, Miszkiel KA et al. New T2 lesions to enable an earlier diagnosis of multiple sclerosis in clinically isolated syndromes. Ann Neurol 2003; 53: 673–676.

27. Frohman EE, Goodin DS, Calabrese PA et al. The utility of MRI in suspected MS: report of the Therapeutics and Technology Assessment Subcommittee of the American Academy of Neurology. Neurology 2003; 61: 602–611.

28. Polman CH, Reingold SC, Edan G et al. Diagnostic criteria for multiple sclerosis: 2005 revisions of the McDonald criteria. Ann Neurol 2005; 58: 840–846.

29. Bot JC, Barkhof F, Polman C et al. Spinal cord abnormalities in recently diagnosed MS patients: added value of spinal MRI examination. Neurology 2004; 62: 226–233.

30. Dalton CM, Brex PS, Miszkiel KM et al. Spinal cord MRI in clinically isolated optic neuritis. J Neurol Neurosurg Psychiatr 2003; 74: 1577–1580.

31. Kidd D, Thorpe JW, Thompson AJ et al. Spinal cord MRI using multi-array coils and fast spin echo. II: Findings in multiple sclerosis. Neurology 1993; 43: 2632–2637.

32. Bot JC, Barkhof F, Lycklama a Nijeholt G et al. Differentiation of multiple sclerosis from other inflammatory disorders and cerebrovascular disease: value of spinal MR imaging. Radiology 2002; 223: 46–56.

33. Thorpe JW, Kidd D, Moseley IF et al. Spinal MRI in patients with suspected multiple sclerosis and negative brain MRI. Brain 1996; 119: 709–714.

34. Swanton JK, Rovira A, Tintore M et al. MRI criteria for multiple sclerosis in patients presenting with clinically isolated syndromes: a multicentre retrospective study. Lancet Neurol 2007; 6: 677–686.

35. Sastre-Garriga J, Tintoré M, Rovira A et al. Specificity of Barkhof criteria in predicting conversion to multiple sclerosis when applied to clinically isolated brainstem syndromes. Arch Neurol 2004; 61: 222–224.

36. Swanton JK, Fernando K, Dalton CM et al. Modification of MRI criteria for multiple sclerosis in patients with clinically isolated syndromes. J Neurol Neurosurg Psychiatr 2006; 77: 830–833.

37. Thompson AJ, Kermode AG, MacManus DG et al. Patterns of disease activity in multiple sclerosis: clinical and magnetic resonance imaging study. Br Med J 1990; 300: 631–634.

38. Brex PA, Ciccarelli O, O'Riordan JI et al. A longitudinal study of abnormalities on MRI and disability from multiple sclerosis. New Engl J Med 2002; 346: 158–164.

39. Minneboo A, Barkhof F, Polman CH et al. Infratentorial lesions predict long-term disability in patients with initial findings suggestive of multiple sclerosis. Arch Neurol 2004; 61: 217–221.

40. Tintoré M, Rovira A, Rio J et al. Baseline MRI predicts future attacks and disability in clinically isolated syndromes. Neurology 2006; 67: 968–972.

41. Beck RW, Trobe JD, Moke PS et al. High and low risk profiles for the development of multiple sclerosis within 10 years after optic neuritis: experience of the optic neuritis treatment trial. Arch Ophthalmol 2003; 121: 944–949.

42. Beck RW, Smith CH, Gal RL et al. Neurologic impairment 10 years after optic neuritis. Arch Neurol 2004; 61: 1386–1389.

43. Frohman EM, Racke MK, Raine CS. Multiple sclerosis: the plaque and its pathogenesis. N Engl J Med 2006; 354: 942–955.

44. Katz D, Taubenberger J, Cannella B et al. Correlation between magnetic resonance imaging findings and lesion development in multiple sclerosis. Ann Neurol 1993; 34: 661–669.

45. Bruck W, Bitsch A, Kolenda H et al. Inflammatory central nervous system demyelination: correlation of magnetic resonance imaging findings with lesion pathology. Ann Neurol 1997; 42: 783–793.

46. Thompson A, Kermode A, MacManus D et al. Major differences in the dynamics of primary and secondary progressive multiple sclerosis. Ann Neurol 1991; 29: 53–62.

47. Lucchinetti C, Bruck W, Parisi J et al. Heterogeneity of multiple sclerosis lesions: implications for the pathogenesis of demyelination. Ann Neurol 2000; 47: 707–717.

48. Lucchinetti CF, Bruck W, Lassmann H. Evidence for pathogenic heterogeneity in multiple sclerosis. Ann Neurol 2004; 56: 308.

49. Barkhof F, Bruck W, de Groot JC et al. Remyelinated lesions in multiple sclerosis: magnetic resonance image appearance. Arch Neurol 2003; 60: 1073–1081.

50. Schmierer K, Scaravilli F, Altmann DR et al. Magnetization transfer ratio and myelin in post-mortem multiple sclerosis brain. Ann Neurol 2004; 56: 407–415.

51. Dousset V, Dellalande C, Ballarino L et al. In vivo macrophage activity imaging in the central nervous system detected by magnetic resonance. Magn Reson Med 1999; 41: 329–333.

52. Dousset V, Brochet B, Deloire MS et al. MR imaging of relapsing multiple sclerosis patients using ultra-small-particle iron oxide and compared with gadolinium. Am J Neuroradiol 2006; 27: 1000–1005.

53. Van Waesberghe JH, Kamphorst W, de Groot CJ et al. Axonal loss in multiple sclerosis lesions: magnetic resonance imaging insights into substrates of disability. Ann Neurol 1999; 46: 747–754.

54. Mottershead JP, Schmierer K, Clemence M et al. High field MRI correlates of myelin content and axonal density in multiple sclerosis: a post-mortem study of the spinal cord. J Neurol 2003; 250: 1293–1301.

55. Whittal KP, MacKay AL, Graeb DA et al. In vivo measurement of T2 distributions and water contents in normal human brain. Magn Reson Med 1997; 37: 34–43.

56. Moore GR, Leung E, MacKay AL et al. A pathology-MRI study of the short-T2 component in formalin-fixed multiple sclerosis brain. Neurology 2000; 55: 1506–1510.

57. Pelletier D, Han ET, Nelson SJ, Oh J. Multi-slice myelin water measurements at

3T in multiple sclerosis. Mult Scler 2005; 11(suppl 1): S15.

58. Song SK, Yoshino J, Le TQ et al. Demyelination increases radial diffusivity in corpus callosum of mouse brain. NeuroImage 2005; 26: 132–140.

59. Van Walderveen MA, Kamphorst W, Scheltens P et al. Histopathological correlate of hypointense lesions on T1-weighted spin echo MRI in multiple sclerosis. Neurology 1998; 50: 1282–1288.

60. Minneboo A, Uitdehaag BM, Ader HJ et al. Patterns of enhancing lesion evolution in multiple sclerosis are uniform within patients. Neurology 2005; 65: 56–61.

61. Gass A, Filippi M, Rodegher ME et al. Characteristics of chronic MS lesions in the cerebrum, brainstem, spinal cord, and optic nerve on T1-weighted MRI. Neurology 1998; 50: 548–550.

62. Hickman SJ, Brierley CMH, Silver NC et al. Infratentorial hypointense lesion volume on T1-weighted magnetic resonance imaging correlates with disability in patients with chronic cerebellar ataxia due to multiple sclerosis. J Neurol Sci 2001; 187: 35–39.

63. Davie C, Hawkins CP, Barker GJ et al. Serial proton magnetic resonance spectroscopy of multiple sclerosis lesions. Brain 1994; 117: 49–58.

64. Song SK, Sun SW, Ju WK et al. Diffusion tensor imaging detects and differentiates axon and myelin degeneration in mouse optic nerve after retinal ischemia. NeuroImage 2003; 1714–1722.

65. Schmierer K, Scaravilli F, Boulby P et al. Pathological correlates of diffusion tensor imaging (DTI) in post mortem MS brain. Mult Scler 2004; 10(suppl 2): S229.

66. Allen IV, McKeown SR. A histological, histochemical and biochemical study of the macroscopically normal white matter in multiple sclerosis. J Neurol Sci 1979; 41: 81–89.

67. Evangelou N, Esiri MM, Smith S et al. Quantitative pathological evidence for axonal loss in normal appearing white matter in multiple sclerosis. Ann Neurol 2000; 47: 391–395.

68. Kutzelnigg AE, Luchhinetti CF, Stadelmann C et al. Brain damage outside demyelinated white matter plaques in multiple sclerosis. Mult Scler 2005; 11(suppl 1): S5.

69. Lacomis D, Osbakken M, Gross G. Spin-lattice (T1) relaxation times of cerebral white matter in multiple sclerosis. Magn Reson Med 1986; 3: 194–202.

70. Miller DH, Johnson G, Tofts PS et al. Precise relaxation time measurements of normal appearing white matter in inflammatory central nervous system disease. Magn Reson Med 1989; 7: 331–336.

71. Van Buchem MA, Udupa JK, McGowan JC et al. Global volumetric estimation of disease burden in multiple sclerosis based on magnetization transfer imaging. Am J Neuroradiol 1997; 18: 1287–1290.

72. Filippi M, Iannucci G, Tortorella C et al. Comparison of MS clinical phenotypes using conventional and magnetization transfer MRI. Neurology 1999; 52: 588–594.

73. Dousset V, Grossman RI, Ramer KN et al. Experimental allergic encephalomyelitis and multiple sclerosis: lesion characterization with magnetization transfer imaging. Radiology 1992; 182: 483–491.

74. Fernando KTM, Tozer DJ, Miszkiel KA et al. Magnetization transfer histograms in clinically isolated syndromes suggestive of multiple sclerosis. Brain 2005; 128: 2911–2925.

75. Davies GR, Altmann DR, Hadjiprocopis A et al. Increasing normal appearing grey and white matter magnetisation transfer ratio abnormality in early relapsing remitting MS. J Neurol 2005; 252: 1037–1044.

76. Filippi M, Campi A, Dousset V et al. A magnetization transfer imaging study of normal-appearing white matter in multiple sclerosis. Neurology 1995; 45: 478–482.

77. Dehmeshki J, Chard DT, Leary SM et al. The normal appearing grey matter in primary progressive multiple sclerosis. A magnetisation transfer imaging study. J Neurol 2003; 250: 67–74.

78. Rovaris M, Agosta F, Sormani MP et al. Conventional and magnetization transfer MRI predictors of clinical multiple sclerosis evolution: a medium-term follow-up study. Brain 2003; 126: 2323–2332.

79. Ciccarelli O, Toosy AT, Hickman SJ et al. Optic radiation changes after optic neuritis detected by tractography-based group mapping. Hum Brain Mapp 2005; 25: 308–316.

80. De Stefano N, Narayanan S, Matthews PM et al. In vivo evidence for axonal dysfunction remote from focal cerebral demyelination of the type seen in multiple sclerosis. Brain 1999; 122: 1933–1939.

81. Fu L, Matthews PM, De Stefano N et al. Imaging axonal damage of normal-appearing white matter in multiple sclerosis. Brain 1998; 121: 103–113.

82. Davie C, Barker GJ, Webb S et al. Persistent functional deficit in multiple sclerosis and autosomal dominant cerebellar ataxia is associated with axon loss. Brain 1995; 118: 1583–1592.

83. Sarchielli P, Presciutti O, Pelliciolli GP et al. Absolute quantification of brain metabolites by proton magnetic spectroscopy of normal appearing white matter of patients with multiple sclerosis. Brain 1999; 122: 513–522.

84. Fernando KT, McLean MA, Chard DT et al. Elevated white matter myoinositol in clinically isolated syndromes suggestive of multiple sclerosis. Brain 2004; 127: 1361–1369.

85. Filippi M, Bozzali M, Rovaris M et al. Evidence for widespread axonal damage at the earliest clinical stage of multiple sclerosis. Brain 2003; 126: 433–437.

86. Vrenken H, Barkhof F, Uitdehaag BM et al. MR spectroscopic evidence for glial increase but not for neuro-axonal damage in MS normal-appearing white matter. Magn Reson Med 2005; 53: 256–266.

87. Kapeller P, Brex PA, Chard D et al. Quantitative ^{1}H-MR spectroscopic imaging 14 years after presenting with a clinically isolated syndrome suggestive of MS. Mult Scler 2002; 8: 207–210.

88. Chard D, Griffin CM, McLean MA et al. Brain metabolite changes in cortical grey matter and normal appearing white matter in clinically early relapsing remitting multiple sclerosis. Brain 2002; 125: 2342–2352.

89. Sastre-Garriga J, Ingle GT, Chard DT et al. Metabolite changes in normal appearing grey and white matter are linked with disability in early primary progressive multiple sclerosis. Arch Neurol 2005; 62: 569–573.

90. Srinivasan R, Sailasuta N, Hurd R et al. Evidence of elevated glutamate in multiple sclerosis using magnetic resonance spectroscopy at 3T. Brain 2005; 128: 1016–1025.

91. Brownell B, Hughes JT. The distribution of plaques in the cerebrum in multiple sclerosis. J Neurol Neurosurg Psychiatr 1962: 315–320.

92. Lumsden CE. The neuropathology of multiple sclerosis. In: Vinken PJ, Bruyn GW, eds. Handbook of clinical neurology, vol. 9. Amsterdam: Elsevier; 1970: 217–309.

93. Kidd D, Barkhof F, McConnell R et al. Cortical lesions in multiple sclerosis. Brain 1999; 122: 17–26.

94. Peterson JW, Bo L, Mork S et al. Transected neuritis, apoptotic neurons, and reduced inflammation in cortical multiple sclerosis lesions. Ann Neurol 2001; 50: 389–400.

95. Kutzelnigg A, Lassmann H. Cortical lesions and brain atrophy in MS. J Neurol Sci 2005; 233: 55–59.

96. Geurts JJ, Pouwels PJ, Bo L et al. Cortical lesions in multiple sclerosis: combined postmortem MR imaging and histopathology. Am J Neuroradiol 2005; 26: 572–577.

97. Geurts JJ, Pouwels PJ, Uitdehaag BM et al. Intracortical lesions in multiple sclerosis: improved detection with 3D double inversion-recovery MR imaging. Radiology 2005; 236: 254–260.

98. Bagnato F, Talagala L, Calabrese A et al. In vivo visualisation of cortical lesions by 3 Tesla magnetic resonance imaging in patients with multiple sclerosis. Mult Scler 2005; 11(suppl 1): S178.

99. Wattjes MP, Lutterbey GG, Gieseke J et al. Double inversion recovery brain imaging at 3T: diagnostic value in the detection of multiple sclerosis lesions. Am J Neuroradiol 2007; 28: 54–59.

100. Cercignani M, Bozzali M, Iannucci G et al. Magnetisation transfer ratio and mean diffusivity of normal appearing white and grey matter from patients with multiple sclerosis. J Neurol Neurosurg Psychiatr 2001; 70: 311–317.

101. Bozzali M, Cercignani M, Sormani MP et al. Quantification of brain gray matter damage in different MS phenotypes by use of diffusion tensor MR imaging. Am J Neuroradiol 2002; 23: 985–988.

102. Griffin CM, Chard DT, Parker GJM et al. The relationship between lesion and normal appearing brain tissue abnormalities in early relapsing remitting MS. J Neurol 2002; 249: 193–199.

103. Bakshi R, Benedict RH, Bermel RA et al. T2 hypointensity in the deep gray matter of patients with multiple sclerosis: a quantitative magnetic resonance imaging study. Arch Neurol 2002; 59: 62–68.

104. Khaleeli Z, Cercignani M, Audoin B et al. Localized grey matter damage in early primary progressive multiple sclerosis contributes to disability. Neuroimage 2007; 37: 253–261.

105. Cifelli A, Arridge M, Jezzard P et al. Thalamic neurodegeneration in multiple sclerosis. Ann Neurol 2002; 52: 650–653.

106. Wylezinska M, Cifelli A, Jezzard P et al. Thalamic neurodegeneration in relapsing-remitting multiple sclerosis. Neurology 2003; 60: 1949–1954.

107. Audoin B, Ranjeva JP, Au Duong MV et al. Voxel-based analysis of MTR images: a method to locate gray matter abnormalities in patients at the earliest stage of multiple sclerosis. J Magn Reson Imaging 2004; 20: 765–771.

108. Tjoa CW, Benedict RH, Weinstock-Guttman B et al. MRI T2 hypointensity of the dentate nucleus is related to ambulatory impairment in multiple sclerosis. J Neurol Sci 2005; 234: 17–24.

109. Bermel RA, Puli SR, Rudick RA et al. Prediction of longitudinal brain atrophy in multiple sclerosis by gray matter magnetic resonance imaging T2 hypointensity. Arch Neurol 2005; 62: 1371–1376.

110. Losseff NA, Webb SL, O'Riordan JI et al. Spinal cord atrophy and disability in multiple sclerosis. A new reproducible and sensitive MRI method with potential to monitor disease progression. Brain 1996; 119: 701–708.

111. Filippi M, Bozzali M, Horsfield MA et al. A conventional and magnetization transfer MRI study of the cervical cord in patients with MS. Neurology 2000; 54: 207–213.

112. Valsasina P, Rocca MA, Agosta F et al. Mean diffusivity and fractional anisotropy histogram analysis of the cervical cord in MS patients. NeuroImage 2005; 26: 822–828.

113. Ganter P, Prince C, Esiri MM. Spinal cord axonal loss in multiple sclerosis: a post-mortem study. Neuropathol Appl Neurobiol 1999; 25: 459–467.

114. Lovas G, Szilagyi N, Majtenyi K et al. Axonal changes in chronic demyelinated cervical spinal cord plaques. Brain 2000; 123: 308–317.

115. Berger E, Bot JCJ, van der Valk P et al. Diffuse signal abnormalities in the spinal cord in multiple sclerosis: direct postmortem in situ magnetic resonance imaging correlated with in vitro high-resolution magnetic resonance imaging and histopathology. Ann Neurol 2002; 51: 652–656.

116. Gilmore CP, Bo L, Owens T et al. Extensive grey matter demyelination occurs in the spinal cord in multiple sclerosis. Mult Scler 2005; 11(suppl 1): S179.

117. Bot JC, Blezer EL, Kamphorst W et al. The spinal cord in multiple sclerosis: relationship of high-spatial-resolution quantitative MR imaging findings to histopathologic results. Radiology 2004; 233: 531–540.

118. Kupersmith MJ, Alban T, Zieffer B, Lefton D. Contrast-enhanced MRI in acute optic neuritis: relationship to visual performance. Brain 2002; 125: 812–822.

119. Hickman SJ. Toosy AT, Jones SJ et al. A serial MRI study following optic nerve mean area in acute optic neuritis. Brain 2004; 127: 2498–2505.

120. Inglese M, Ghezzi A, Bianchi S et al. Irreversible disability and tissue loss in multiple sclerosis: a conventional and magnetization transfer magnetic resonance imaging study of the optic nerves. Arch Neurol 2002; 59: 250–255.

121. Hickman SJ, Toosy AT, Jones SJ et al. Serial magnetization transfer imaging in acute optic neuritis. Brain 2004; 127: 692–700.

122. Anderson VM, Fox NC, Miller DH. Magnetic resonance imaging measures of brain atrophy in multiple sclerosis. J Magn Reson Imaging 2006; 23: 605–618.

123. Rudick RA, Fischer E, Lee J-C et al. Use of brain parencyhmal fraction to measure whole brain atrophy in relapsing-remitting MS. Neurology 1999; 53: 1698–1704.

124. Smith S, de Stefano N, Jenkinson M, Matthews P. Normalised accurate measurement of longitudinal brain change. J Comput Assist Tomog 2001; 25: 466–475.

125. Filippi M, Rovaris M, Inglese M et al. Interferon beta-1a for brain tissue loss in patients at presentation with syndromes suggestive of multiple sclerosis: a randomised, double-blind, placebo-controlled trial. Lancet 2004; 364: 1489–1496.

126. Freeborough PA, Fox NC. The boundary shift integral: An accurate and robust measure of cerebral volume changes from registered repeat MRI. IEEE Trans Med Imag 1997; 16: 623–629.

127. Fox NC, Jenkins R, Leary SM et al. Progressive cerebral atrophy in MS: a serial study using registered, volumetric MRI. Neurology 2000; 54: 807–812.

128. Anderson VM, Fernando KT, Davies GR et al. Cerebral atrophy measurement in clinically isolated syndromes and relapsing remitting multiple sclerosis: a comparison of registration-based methods. J Neuroimaging 2007; 17: 61–68.

129. Losseff NA, Wang L, Lai HM et al. Progressive cerebral atrophy in multiple sclerosis. A serial study. Brain 1996; 119: 2009–2019.

130. Chard DT, Griffin CM, Parker GJM et al. Brain atrophy in clinically early relapsing-remitting multiple sclerosis. Brain 2002; 125: 327–337.

131. Tiberio M, Chard DT, Altmann DR et al. Gray and white matter volume changes in early RRMS: A 2-year longitudinal study. Neurology 2005; 64: 1001–1007.

132. Stevenson VL, Smith SM, Matthews PM et al. Monitoring disease activity and progression in primary progressive multiple sclerosis using MRI: sub-voxel registration to identify lesion changes and to detect cerebral atrophy. J Neurol 2002; 294: 171–177.

133. Pagani E, Rocca MA, Gallo A et al. Regional brain atrophy evolves differently in patients with multiple sclerosis according to clinical phenotype. Am J Neuroradiol 2005; 26: 341–346.

134. De Stefano N, Matthews PM, Filippi M et al. Evidence of early cortical atrophy in MS: relevance to white matter changes and disability. Neurology 2003; 60: 1157–1162.

135. Sailer M, Fischl B, Salat D et al. Focal thinning of the cerebral cortex in multiple sclerosis. Brain 2003; 126: 1734–1744.

136. Benedict RH, Weinstock-Guttman B, Fishman I et al. Prediction of neuropsychological impairment in multiple sclerosis: comparison of conventional magnetic resonance imaging measures of atrophy and lesion burden. Arch Neurol 2004; 61: 226–230.

137. Benedict RH, Carone DA, Bakshi R. Correlating brain atrophy with cognitive dysfunction, mood disturbances, and personality disorder in multiple sclerosis. J Neuroimaging 2004; 14(3 suppl): 36S–45S.

138. Fisher E, Rudick RA, Simon JH et al. Eight year follow up study of brain atrophy in patients with MS. Neurology 2002; 59: 1412–1420.

139. Dalton CM, Miszkiel KA, O'Connor PW et al. Ventricular enlargement in MS: one year change at various stages of disease. Neurology 2006; 66: 693–698.

140. Ge Y, Grossman RI, Udupa JK et al. Brain atrophy in relapsing-remitting multiple sclerosis and secondary progressive multiple sclerosis: longitudinal data analysis. Radiology 2000; 214: 665–670.

141. Rovaris M, Gallo A, Falini A et al. Axonal injury and overall tissue loss are not related in primary progressive multiple sclerosis. Arch Neurol 2005; 62: 898–902.

142. Wuerfel J, Bellmann-Strobl J, Brunecker P et al. Changes in cerebral perfusion precede plaque formation in multiple sclerosis: a longitudinal perfusion MRI study. Brain 2004; 127: 111–119.

143. Ge Y, Law M, Johnson G et al. Dynamic susceptibility contrast perfusion MR imaging of multiple sclerosis lesions: characterizing hemodynamic impairment and inflammatory activity. Am J Neuroradiol 2005; 26: 1539–1547.

144. Rashid W, Parkes LM, Ingle GT et al. Abnormalities of cerebral perfusion in multiple sclerosis. J Neurol Neurosurg Psychiatry 2004; 75: 1288–1293.

145. Lee M, Reddy H, Johansen-Berg H et al. The motor cortex shows adaptive functional changes to brain injury from multiple sclerosis. Ann Neurol 2000; 47: 606–613.

146. Reddy H, Narayanan S, Arnoutelis R et al. Evidence for adaptive functional changes in the cerebral cortex with axonal injury from multiple sclerosis. Brain 2000; 123: 2314–2320.

147. Rocca M, Falini A, Colombo B et al. Adaptive functional changes in the cerebral cortex of patients with nondisabling multiple sclerosis correlate with the extent of brain structural damage. Ann Neurol 2002; 51: 330–339.

148. Rocca M, Colombo B, Falini A et al. Cortical adaptation in patients with MS: a cross-sectional functional MRI study of disease phenotypes. Lancet Neurol 2005; 4: 618–626.

149. Penner IK, Rausch M, Kappos L et al. Analysis of impairment related functional architecture in MS patients during performance of different attention tasks. J Neurol 2003; 250: 461–472.

150. Toosy AT, Hickman SJ, Miszkiel KA et al. Adaptive cortical plasticity in higher visual areas after acute optic neuritis. Ann Neurol 2005; 57: 622–633.

151. Dickerson B, Salat DH, Bates JH et al. Medial temporal lobe function and structure in mild cognitive impairment. Ann Neurol 2005; 56: 27–35.

152. Isaac C, Li DK, Genton M et al. Multiple sclerosis: a serial study using MRI in relapsing patients. Neurology 1988; 38: 1511–1515.

153. Willoughby EW, Grochowski E, Li DK et al. Serial magnetic resonance scanning in multiple sclerosis: a second prospective

study in relapsing patients. Ann Neurol 1989; 25: 43–49.

154. Koopmans RA, Li DK, Oger JJ et al. Chronic progressive multiple sclerosis: serial magnetic resonance brain imaging over six months. Ann Neurol 1989; 26: 248–256.

155. Thompson AJ, Miller DH, Youl B et al. Serial gadolinium enhanced MRI in relapsing remitting multiple sclerosis of varying disease duration. Neurology 1992; 42: 60–63.

156. Harris JO, Frank JA, Patronas N et al. Serial gadolinium-enhanced magnetic resonance imaging scans in patients with early, relapsing-remitting multiple sclerosis: implications for clinical trials and natural history. Ann Neurol 1991; 29: 548–555.

157. Barkhof F, Scheltens P, Frequin ST et al. Relapsing-remitting multiple sclerosis: sequential enhanced MR imaging vs. clinical findings in determining disease activity. AJR 1992; 159: 1041–1047.

158. Paty DW, Li DKB, the UBC MS/MRI Study Group and the IFNB Mult Scler Study Group. Interferon-1b is effective in relapsing-remitting multiple sclerosis. II. MRI analysis result of a multicentre, randomized, double-blind, placebo-controlled trial. Neurology 1993; 43: 662–667.

159. Miller DH, Barkhof F, Nauta JJP. Gadolinium enhancement increases the sensitivity of MRI in detecting disease activity in multiple sclerosis. Brain 1993; 116: 1077–1094.

160. McFarland HF, Frank J, Albert P et al. Using gadolinium-enhanced magnetic resonance imaging lesions to monitor disease activity in multiple sclerosis. Ann Neurol 1992; 32: 758–766.

161. Tubridy N, Ader HJ, Barkhof F et al. Exploratory treatment trials in multiple sclerosis using MRI: sample size calculations for relapsing remitting and secondary progressive subgroups using placebo controlled parallel groups. J Neurol Neurosurg Psychiatr 1998; 64: 50–55.

162. Miller DH, Albert PS, Barkhof F et al. Guidelines for using magnetic resonance techniques in monitoring the treatment of multiple sclerosis. Ann Neurol 1996; 39: 6–16.

163. Kappos L, Moeri D, Radue EW et al. Predictive value of gadolinium-enhanced magnetic resonance imaging for relapse rate and changes in disability or impairment in multiple sclerosis: a meta-analysis. Lancet 1999; 353: 964–969.

164. Langer-Gould A, Atlas SW, Green AJ et al. Progressive multifocal leukoencephalopathy in a patient treated with natalizumab. N Engl J Med 2005; 353: 375–381.

165. Yousry TA, Major EO, Ryschkewitsch C et al. Evaluation of patients treated with natalizumab for progressive multifocal leukoencephalopathy. N Engl J Med 2006; 354: 924–933.

166. Sormani MP, Rovaris M, Bagnato F et al. Sample size estimations for MRI monitored trials of MS comparing new vs. standard treatments. Neurology 2001; 57: 1883–1885.

167. Comi G, Filippi M, Wolinsky JS. European/Canadian multicenter, double-blind, randomized, placebo-controlled study of the effects of glatiramer acetate on magnetic resonance imaging–measured disease activity and burden in patients with relapsing multiple sclerosis. European/Canadian Glatiramer Acetate Study Group. Ann Neurol 2001; 49: 290–297.

168. Panitch H, Miller A, Paty D et al. Interferon beta-1b in secondary progressive MS: results from a 3-year controlled study. Neurology 2004; 63: 1788–1795.

169. Coles AJ, Wing MG, Molyneux P et al. Monoclonal antibody treatment exposes three mechanisms underlying the clinical course of multiple sclerosis. Ann Neurol 1999; 46: 296–304.

170. Rice GP, Filippi M, Comi G. Cladribine and progressive MS: clinical and MRI outcomes of a multicenter controlled trial. Cladribine MRI Study Group. Neurology 2000; 54: 1145–1155.

171. Dalton CM, Miszkiel KA, Barker GJ et al. Effect of natalizumab on conversion of gadolinium enhancing lesions to T1 hypointense lesions in relapsing multiple sclerosis. J Neurol 2004; 251: 407–413.

172. Filippi M, Rovaris M, Rocca MA et al. Glatiramer acetate reduces the proportion of new MS lesions evolving in to 'black holes'. Neurology 2001; 57: 731–733.

173. Brex PA, Molyneux PD, Smiddy P et al. The effect of interferon beta-1b on the size and evolution of enhancing lesions in secondary progressive MS. Neurology 2001; 57: 2185–2190.

174. Polman CH, O'Connor PW, Havrdova E et al. A randomized, placebo-controlled trial of natalizumab for relapsing multiple sclerosis. N Engl J Med 2006; 354: 899–910.

175. Rao AB, Richert N, Howard T et al. Methylprednisolone effect on brain volume and enhancing lesions in MS before and during IFNβ-1b. Neurology 2002; 59: 688–694.

176. Miller DH, Soon D, Fernando KT et al. MRI outcomes in a placebo-controlled trial of natalizumab in relapsing MS. Neurology 2007; 68: 1390–1401.

177. Fazekas F, Sorensen PS, Filippi M et al. MRI results from the European Study on Intravenous Immunoglobulin in Secondary Progressive Multiple Sclerosis (ESIMS). Mult Scler 2005; 11: 433–440.

178. Molyneux PD, Kappos L, Polman C et al. The effect of interferon beta-1b treatment on MRI measures of cerebral atrophy in secondary progressive multiple sclerosis. Brain 2000; 123: 2256–2263.

179. Jones CK, Riddehough A, Li DKB et al. MRI cerebral atrophy in relapsing remitting MS: results of the PRISMS trial. Neurology 2001; 56(suppl 3): A379.

180. Bechtold DA, Kapoor R, Smith KJ. Axonal protection using flecainide in experimental autoimmune encephalomyelitis. Ann Neurol 2004; 55: 607–616.

181. Stevenson VL, Leary SM, Losseff NA et al. Spinal cord atrophy and disability in MS. A longitudinal study. Neurology 1998; 51: 234–238.

182. Rashid W, Davies GR, Chard DT et al. Increasing cord atrophy in early relapsing-remitting multiple sclerosis: a three year study. J Neurol Neurosurg Psychiatry 2006; 77: 51–55.

183. Ropele S, Filippi M, Valsasina P et al. Assessment and correction of B1-induced errors in magnetization transfer ratio measurements. Magn Reson Med 2005; 53: 134–140.

184. Silver NC, Barker GJ, Miller DH. Standardization of magnetization transfer imaging for multicentre studies. Neurology 1999; 53(suppl 3): S33–S39.

185. Inglese M, van Waesberghe JHTM, Rovaris M et al. The effect of interferon B-1b on quantities derived from MT MRI in secondary progressive MS. Neurology 2003; 60: 853–860.

186. Filippi M, Rocca M, Pagani E et al. European study on intravenous immunoglobulin in multiple sclerosis: results of magnetization transfer magnetic resonance imaging analysis. Arch Neurol 2004; 61: 1409–1412.

187. Richert ND, Ostuni JL, Bash CN et al. Serial whole-brain magnetization transfer imaging in patients with relapsing-remitting multiple sclerosis at baseline and during treatment with interferon beta-1b. Am J Neuroradiol 1998; 19: 1705–1713.

188. Simon JH, Jacobs LD, Campion M et al. Magnetic resonance studies of intramuscular interferon beta-1a for relapsing multiple sclerosis. The Multiple Sclerosis Collaborative Research Group. Ann Neurol 1998; 43: 79–87.

189. Li DK, Paty DW. Magnetic resonance imaging results of the PRISMS trial: a randomized, double-blind, placebo-controlled study of interferon-beta1a in relapsing-remitting multiple sclerosis. Prevention of Relapses and Disability by Interferon-β1a Subcutaneously in Multiple Sclerosis. Ann Neurol 1999; 46: 197–206.

190. Jacobs LD, Beck RW, Simon JH et al. Intramuscular interferon beta-1a therapy initiated during a first demyelinating event in multiple sclerosis. CHAMPS Study Group. N Engl J Med 2000; 343: 898–904.

191. Comi G, Filippi M, Barkhof F et al. Effect of early interferon treatment on conversion to definite multiple sclerosis: a randomised study. Lancet 2001; 357: 1576–1582.

192. Miller DH, Molyneux PD, Barker GJ et al. Effect of Interferon Beta1b on magnetic resonance imaging outcomes in secondary progressive multiple sclerosis: results of a European multicenter, randomised, double-blind, placebo-controlled trial. Ann Neurol 1999; 46: 850–859.

193. Li DK, Zhao GJ, Paty DW et al. Randomized controlled trial of interferon-beta-1a in secondary progressive MS: MRI results. Neurology 2001; 56: 1505–1513.

194. Cohen JA, Cutter GR, Fischer JS et al. Benefit of interferon beta-1a on MSFC progression in secondary progressive MS. Neurology 2002; 59: 679–687.

195. Leary SM, Miller DH, Stevenson VL et al. Interferon beta-1a in primary progressive MS: an exploratory, randomized, controlled trial. Neurology 2003; 60: 44–51.

196. Edan G, Miller D, Clanet M et al. Therapeutic effect of mitoxantrone combined with methylprednisolone in multiple sclerosis: a randomised multicentre study of active disease using MRI and clinical criteria. J Neurol Neurosurg Psychiatr 1997; 62: 112–118.

197. Hartung HP, Gonsette R, Konig N et al. Mitoxantrone in progressive multiple sclerosis: a placebo-controlled, double-blind, randomised, multicentre trial. Lancet 2002; 360: 2018–2025.

198. Miller DH, Khan OA, Sheremata WA et al. A controlled trial of natalizumab for relapsing multiple sclerosis. N Engl J Med 2003; 348: 15–23.

199. Polman C, Barkhof F, Sandberg-Wollheim M et al. Treatment with laquinimod reduces development of active MRI lesions in relapsing MS. Neurology 2005; 64: 987–991.

200. Bielekova B, Richert N, Howard T et al. Humanized anti-CD25 (daclizumab) inhibits disease activity in multiple sclerosis patients failing to respond to interferon beta. Proc Natl Acad Sci USA 2004; 101: 8705–8708.

201. Lenercept Multiple Sclerosis Study Group and University of British Columbia MS/MRI Analysis Group. TNF neutralization in MS: results of a randomized, placebo-controlled multicenter study. Neurology 1999; 53: 457–465.

202. Van Oosten BW, Barkhof F, Truyen L et al. Increased MRI activity and immune activation in two multiple sclerosis patients treated with the monoclonal anti-tumor necrosis factor antibody cA2. Neurology 1996; 47: 1531–1534.

203. Van Oosten BW, Lai M, Hodgkinson S et al. Treatment of multiple sclerosis with the monoclonal anti-CD4 antibody cM-T412: results of a randomized, double-blind, placebo-controlled, MR-monitored phase II trial. Neurology 1997; 49: 351–357.

204. Zipp F, Hartung HP, Hillert J et al. Blockade of chemokine receptor in multiple sclerosis. Mult Scler 2005: 11(suppl 1): S13.

205. Killestein J, Olsson T, Wallstrom E et al. Antibody-mediated suppression of Vβ5.2/5.3$^+$ T cells in multiple sclerosis: results from an MRI-monitored phase II clinical trial. Ann Neurol 2002; 51: 467–474.

206. Miller DH, MacManus DG, Miszkiel KA et al. Efficacy of six months' therapy with oral rosiglitazone maleate in relapsing-remitting multiple sclerosis. Mult Scler 2005; 11(suppl 1): S164.

207. Kappos L et al. Oral fingolimod (FTY720) for relapsing multiple sclerosis. N Engl J Med 2006; 355: 1124–1140.

208. Fieschi C, Andersen O, Markowitz C et al. A phase II, randomised, placebo-controlled study to evaluate the preliminary efficacy and safety of abatacept, a selective costimulation molecule, in relapsing-remitting MS. J Neurol 2005; 252(suppl 2): II/41.

209. Vollmer T, Key L, Durkalski V et al. Oral simvastatin treatment in relapsing-remitting multiple sclerosis. Lancet 2004; 363: 1607–1608.

showed that MS plaques contained higher amounts of IgG than could be found in the corresponding CSF compared with parallel serum.[20,21] These two observations led to the seminal notion of local synthesis of IgG within the brain of subjects with MS. Tourtellotte also used the Laurell rocket technique[22] to estimate both albumin and IgG on the same agar dish and was one of the first to recognize the importance of immunofixation for the study of CSF proteins in MS.[23] Klaus Felgenhauer showed that high-molecular-weight haptoglobin oligomers were not present in normal CSF.[24] Hans Link then showed that the bands in the gamma region on CSF electrophoresis were IgG.[25] Magnhild Sandberg-Wollheim showed that CSF lymphocytes from patients with MS synthesized radiolabeled proteins that migrated in the gamma region after incubation of the CSF cells in tissue culture.[26] Christian Laterre undertook an extensive survey of abnormalities of CSF proteins in several diseases, including MS, giving the differential diagnosis for the presence of oligoclonal bands;[27] it was he who coined the term 'oligoclonal'.

DIAGNOSTIC TESTING

The detection of intrathecal synthesis of oligoclonal immunoglobulins can be very helpful in making a diagnosis of MS. The Polman or 'revised McDonald' criteria[18] were formulated to simplify the McDonald criteria[17] while maintaining diagnostic sensitivity and specificity. The McDonald and Polman criteria specifically focused on the use of MRI to demonstrate dissemination of the disease process in time and space. With regard to CSF analysis, the Polman criteria differ from McDonald criteria in that they do not require a positive CSF analysis as an absolute requirement for a diagnosis of primary progressive MS.[18] The latter change is based on the findings of a large multicenter primary progressive MS study.[28] Unfortunately, the methods of CSF analyses performed in this study were not standardized and allowed the use of quantitative indices to determine intrathecal synthesis of IgG. Quantitative indices are less sensitive than the recommended qualitative methods.[2] This may explain why only 79% of subjects with primary progressive MS had intrathecal synthesis of IgG in this study.[28] Had the earlier criteria for diagnosing primary progressive MS been used,[17,29] this figure would have needed to be 100%. With isoelectric focusing and immunofixation 95–98% of subjects with clinically definite MS[16] have intrathecal synthesis of oligoclonal IgG.[1,2] This is therefore an invariable feature of MS and remains a useful diagnostic aid, particularly where there is some doubt about the clinical diagnosis. A negative result suggests an alternative diagnosis whereas a positive one strongly supports a diagnosis of MS.

B CELL IMMUNOLOGY

The humoral response to a specific antigenic challenge is a complex process involving antigen recognition and the initial production of IgM. This IgM-producing step may be T-cell-independent but it is then followed by a process of immunoglobulin isotype switching and affinity maturation that requires T-cell help. T-cell help involves crosstalk between T and B cells via cell surface molecules and cytokines. The production of immunoglobulins can be divided into the stages activation, proliferation and differentiation of B cells. The activation of B cells occurs via antigen-specific surface IgM receptors in the presence of the B-cell-activating cytokines (see reference 30 for review). The antigen bound to the IgM receptors is then internalized, processed and presented in the context of major histocompatibility complex (MHC) class II molecules. Proliferation now needs antigen-specific T-cell help in the form of cytokines interleukin (IL)-2, IL-4, IL-5 and BAFF. This step requires the antigen-specific interactions of T and B cells via the TCR-MHC

II receptor complex, and important non-antigen-specific costimulatory signals via other receptor ligand pairs such as LFA1–ICAM1, LFA3–CD2 and CD28–B7. This results in T-cell activation and the production of the T-cell cytokines, which induce B-cell proliferation and differentiation with isotype switching and affinity maturation. At this stage the type of T-cell help influences the immunoglobulin isotype and subclass switching that occurs. In general the T helper (Th)2-like cytokines result in the production of IgE, IgG2 and IgG4, whereas Th1-like cytokines IL-12 and interferon (INF)γ induce IgG1 and IgG3 production. The net result of these processes is the formation of mature clones of plasma cells, each producing a specific antibody. This antibody is characterized by the combination of a single class of light and heavy chain having unique variable and hypervariable regions defining the molecule's antigen specificity. The microenvironment that exists in the inflamed CNS supports the survival of long-lived plasma cells and explains why the oligoclonal IgG bands (OCBs) persist in the CSF of subjects with MS.[30]

ANTIBODY SPECIFICITY AND AFFINITY

Antibody specificity can either be viewed as a measure of the goodness of fit between the antibody-combining site (paratope) and the corresponding antigenic determinant (epitope) or the ability of the antibody to discriminate between similar or even dissimilar antigens. This binding specificity is associated with particular functional consequences, which are due to the properties conferred on the immunoglobulin molecule by its non-antigen-binding sites, e.g. the ability to activate complement. The biological functions are isotype- and subclass-dependent. In comparison with specificity, affinity of an antibody is a measure of the strength of the binding between antibody and antigen, such that a low-affinity antibody binds weakly and high-affinity antibody binds firmly. The process of affinity maturation preferentially selects for survival of B cells and subsequently plasma cells that produce high-affinity antibodies rather than those producing low-affinity antibodies. High-affinity antibodies to a specific antigen are a good indicator that the antigen is directly involved in driving the humoral response. Conversely, the presence of low-affinity antibodies usually represents cross-reactivity or an anamnestic response.

TYPE OF HUMORAL RESPONSE

Using electrophoresis it is possible to classify a humoral response according to the number of antibody clones produced: a monoclonal antibody results from a single plasma cell clone; oligoclonal antibodies are due to several clones; and a polyclonal antibody response represents a general increase in immunoglobulin production with no specific discernible clones noted above the background.

Monoclonal

A monoclonal response can represent the initial stage of an oligoclonal response, before the other antibody clones become visible, or, more commonly, a single abnormal clone of plasma cells associated with a B-cell or plasma-cell dyscrasia. Methods such as isoelectric focusing (IEF), which is more sensitive than standard agarose gel electrophoresis, often detect bands invisible by methods with a lower resolution. The clinical significance of a monoclonal gammopathy detected by IEF but not by agarose electrophoresis is currently unknown.

Oligoclonal

An oligoclonal response represents an immunological response to a specific antigen or set of antigens and is associated with

TABLE 7.2 Inflammatory diseases of the central nervous system associated with cerebrospinal fluid oligoclonal IgG bands

Disorder	Approximate incidence of oligoclonal bands (%)
Multiple sclerosis	95
Autoimmune	
Neuro-SLE	50
Neuro-Behçet's	20
Neurosarcoid	<5
Harada's meningitis–uveitis	60
Infectious	
Acute viral encephalitis (<7 days)	<5
Acute bacterial meningitis (<7 days)	<5
Subacute sclerosing panencephalitis	100
Progressive rubella panencephalitis	100
Neurosyphilis	95
Neuro-AIDS	80
Neuroborreliosis	80
Tumor	<5
Hereditary	
Ataxia–telangiectasia	60
Adrenoleukodystrophy	100

AIDS, acquired immunodeficiency syndrome; SLE, systemic lupus erythematosus.

infections and several putative autoimmune and inflammatory conditions (Table 7.2). The oligoclonal response to a set of known antigens can be used as a specific diagnostic tool, e.g. viral encephalitis.[31] When the eliciting antigens are unknown, as in MS for example, the presence of an oligoclonal pattern is presumed to be nonspecific, representing a local humoral response. Although 'nonspecific', it is helpful as a diagnostic aid provided other known causes of local synthesis of oligoclonal bands have been excluded.

Polyclonal

This is a nonspecific increase in immunoglobulin synthesis and is commonly associated with systemic diseases with an immunological response to numerous antigens, e.g. in subjects with chronic liver disease. This is not a pattern associated with MS.

MODERN METHODS OF DETECTION

Quantitative methods

An increase in CSF immunoglobulin was initially detected using the Lange colloidal gold curve.[32–34] This was replaced by a number of different techniques, which measured the amount of Ig present within the CSF and serum and determined whether the immunoglobulin was synthesized intrathecally or diffused passively from the systemic compartment via the blood–CSF barrier. Linear,[35] exponential[36] and hyperbolic[37] formulae were developed to assess intrathecal Ig synthesis in relation to the integrity of the blood–CSF barrier; the exponential and hyperbolic formulae have theoretical advantages over the linear model.[36] However, all three formulae lack sensitivity. Quantitative IgG analyses are only abnormal in 75% of subjects with clinically definite MS[38] and have now been superseded by qualitative methods.[1,2]

Qualitative methods

Isoelectric focusing on agarose gels followed by immunoblotting is now the accepted 'gold standard' for detecting the presence of oligoclonal Ig bands.[2,39] This technique uses a pH gradient to separate IgG populations on the basis of charge. These are then transferred on to a nitrocellulose membrane and immunostained using an antihuman immunoglobulin (Fig. 7.2). Problems with interpretation can arise when inhomogeneities in the ampholytes used in establishing the pH gradients cause artifactual bands. As this is a qualitative test and subject to observer bias, it should ideally be read by an observer blinded to the other clinical information. Polyacrylamide gel electrophoresis and IEF combined with silver staining of proteins is still being used but lacks the specificity provided by immunodetection.

Dual staining for kappa and lambda light chains (both free and bound) improves the sensitivity of IEF. Staining using an antiserum that recognizes a specific light chain reduces the polyclonal background staining substantially. For example, kappa staining will not detect polyclonal lambda-associated immunoglobulin, which makes faint kappa-associated bands easier to see against a polyclonal background. Free kappa and lambda light chain oligoclonal bands can be detected in the CSF from MS patients.[40–44] The sensitivity of IEF with immunoblotting to detect locally synthesized oligoclonal Ig bands is in excess of 95% (Table 7.3). The presence of intrathecal oligoclonal bands is an almost invariable feature of MS (>95%) and is therefore a very useful paraclinical test to help one make a diagnosis of MS.

The observation that CSF oligoclonal bands are such an unvarying feature of MS questions whether or not subjects who fulfill contemporary diagnostic criteria for having MS but do not have oligoclonal bands have the same disease. An obvious explanation is that IEF with immunoblotting is not 100% sensitive. Using a new immunoaffinity technique followed by immunoblotting to detect oligoclonal free kappa light chains, Goffette et al found that 18 out of 33 patients (54%) with clinical signs and symptoms suggestive of MS but without CSF oligoclonal IgG had oligoclonal kappa chains in their CSF.[44] All the subjects in this study with a positive MRI according to Barkhof's criteria[45] had free kappa bands in their CSF.[44] The authors conclude that the presence of free kappa bands in the CSF may be a suitable substitute for oligoclonal IgG in the diagnosis of MS.[44] In another series 34 cases of oligoclonal band negative MS were restudied;[46] only three subjects with clinically definite MS were found to be oligoclonal band negative.[46] A negative result, after using a sensitive method, is more likely to indicate another disease than to be a false-negative result. The specificity of the diagnosis varies depending on how sure one is that there is no other reason for intrathecal inflammation. In typical populations in which the prevalence of MS is high the sensitivity is more than 86% (Table 7.3). It is rare for one of the quantitative IgG indices to be elevated in the absence of locally synthesized oligoclonal bands when using IEF with immunoblotting. Several laboratories have therefore stopped using quantitative tests and rely solely on the results of the superior method of IEF with immunoblotting.

ISOELECTRIC FOCUSING PATTERNS

As CSF is an ultrafiltrate of plasma, it contains immunoglobulins that are passively transferred from the plasma, as well as any immunoglobulins synthesized locally. Any systemic pattern of immunoglobulin production seen in serum will therefore be seen or mirrored in the CSF. Any CSF analysis for oligoclonal bands therefore has to be accompanied by a paired blood analysis to be interpreted. Figure 7.3 represents the various

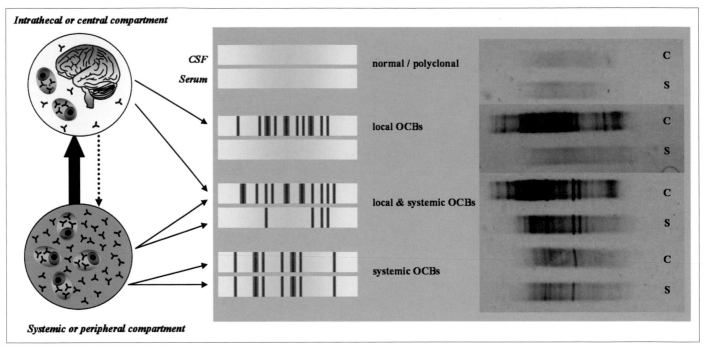

FIG. 7.2 Cerebrospinal fluid (CSF) and serum isoelectric focusing (IEF). On the left is a diagram depicting the contribution of systemically and intrathecally synthesized IgG on the CSF IEF focusing patterns. On the right are examples of actual immunoblots of cerebrospinal fluid and serum isoelectric focusing. Paired CSF and serum analysis allows one to determine in which compartment the oligoclonal IgG bands (OCBs) are synthesized. OCBs produced in the intrathecal or central nervous system (CNS) compartment are only detected in the CSF as too little IgG enters the systemic compartment to be detected. However, OCBs detected in the systemic compartment are produced in greater quantity and are always detected in the CSF. As the systemic OCBs are identical to those in the CSF, they mirror each other. **A**. Normal CSF and serum IEF, with a polyclonal IgG response in both compartments (C⁻,S⁻). **B**. OCBs present in the CSF with no apparent corresponding abnormality in serum, i.e. intrathecal or a local synthesis pattern (C⁺,S⁻). **C**. There are OCBs in both the CSF and serum, but with additional bands present in the CSF, i.e. a 'greater than' pattern (C⁺⁺,S⁺). The oligoclonal bands which are common to both CSF and serum imply a systemic B cell response, whilst the bands which are restricted to the CNS represent a CNS-only B cell response. **D**. There are oligoclonal bands present in the CSF, which are identical to those in serum, i.e. a 'mirror' pattern (C⁺,S⁺). This is not indicative of local synthesis, but rather, the pattern is consistent with passive transfer of oligoclonal IgG from a systemic B cell response. Patterns **B** and **C** are typically found in MS.

TABLE 7.3 Sensitivity and specificity of isoelectric focusing for multiple sclerosis

Reference	Total no. of cases	Number of multiple sclerosis cases	Sensitivity (%)	Specificity (%)
Kostulas et al[103]	1114	58	100	–
McLean et al[49]	1007	82	95	–
Ohman et al[36]	558	112	96	–
Beer et al[104]	189	98	–	87
Paolino et al[105]	44	26	–	86

combinations of patterns found in the CSF and serum, together with our current interpretation (Table 7.4).

Pattern type 1 is negative (i.e. no specific CSF bands) whereas types 2 and 3 show specific bands present only in the CSF, not the serum. Pattern 4 is a mirror pattern and indicates a systemic oligoclonal B-cell immune response. Pattern 5 indicates the presence of a monoclonal gammopathy; other electrophoretic techniques resolve a single band on isoelectric focusing into multiple bands differing by one unit of charge. This peculiarity is probably due to post-translational modifications such as glycosylation and/or number of disulfide bonds. The latter rarely occurs with intrathecal synthesis (pattern 6). Pattern 6 is a singlet or intrathecally derived monoclonal band, which does not display the same post-translation modifications.

Subjects with an isolated CSF monoclonal band (pattern 6) need careful consideration. In a group of subjects with such a

pattern who underwent subsequent follow-up lumbar puncture, approximately one-third converted to an oligoclonal band pattern within 6 months;[47] these cases typically had early disease (i.e. clinically isolated syndromes) or progressive disease. Many of the nonconverters were diagnosed with alternative disorders. Importantly, one had a CNS mantle cell lymphoma.[47,48] Therefore, although negative by definition, a single CSF band is an indication for repeating a CSF analysis, unless other criteria clearly point to a diagnosis of MS, and considering an alternative diagnosis.

DIFFERENTIAL DIAGNOSIS

Several inflammatory neurological diseases characterized by an intrathecal inflammatory response can produce an oligoclonal

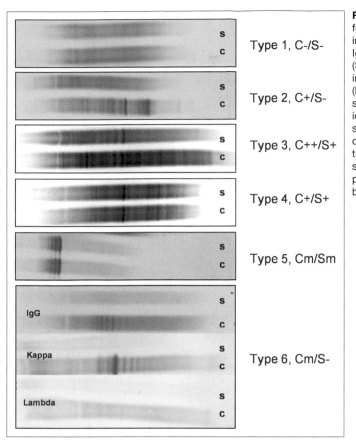

Type 1, C-/S-

Type 2, C+/S-

Type 3, C++/S+

Type 4, C+/S+

Type 5, Cm/Sm

Type 6, Cm/S-

FIG. 7.3 The six cerebrospinal fluid (CSF) and serum isoelectric focusing (IEF) patterns. Isoelectric focusing on agarose gels with immunoblotting. Note that all the oligoclonal bands present are due to IgG. There are 6 classic patterns: type 1: no bands in CSF and serum (S) sample; type 2: oligoclonal IgG bands in CSF, not in the S sample, indicative of intrathecal IgG synthesis; type 3: oligoclonal bands in CSF (like type 2) and additional identical oligoclonal bands in CSF and the S sample (like type 4), still indicative of intrathecal IgG synthesis; type 4: identical oligoclonal bands in CSF and the S sample illustrative of a systemic rather than intrathecal immune reaction, with a leaky or normal or abnormal blood–CSF barrier and oligoclonal bands passively transferred in the CSF; type 5: monoclonal bands in CSF and the S sample; this is the pattern seen owing to the presence of a paraprotein (monoclonal IgG component); and type 6; a monoclonal band in the CSF.

TABLE 7.4 Interpretation of isoelectric focusing patterns

Pattern	Interpretation	Examples
Type 1	Normal	
Type 2	Oligoclonal IgG is present in the CSF with no apparent corresponding abnormality in serum, indicating local intrathecal synthesis of IgG.	Multiple sclerosis
Type 3 (or 'greater than' pattern)	There are IgG bands in both the CSF and serum, with additional bands present in the CSF. The oligoclonal bands which are common to both CSF and serum imply a systemic inflammatory response, whilst the bands which are restricted to the CNS suggest that there is an additional CNS-only response.	Multiple sclerosis, SLE, etc.
Type 4 (or 'mirror' pattern)	There are oligoclonal bands present in the CSF, which are identical to those in serum. This is not indicative of local synthesis, but rather, the pattern is consistent with passive transfer of oligoclonal IgG from a systemic inflammatory response.	Guillain–Barré syndrome
Type 5	There is a monoclonal IgG pattern in both CSF and serum, the source of which lies outside the CNS.	Myeloma, monoclonal gammopathy of undetermined significance (MGUS)
Type 6	There is a monoclonal IgG pattern in the CSF with no apparent corresponding abnormality in serum, indicating local intrathecal synthesis of a monoclonal IgG.	Dominant or early clone in the evolution of an intrathecal oligoclonal response. Rarely due to an intrathecal B cell lymphoma

See also Figure 7.2.

IgG response.[49] Table 7.2 provides a list, with an approximate proportion of cases having oligoclonal bands. In general intrathecal oligoclonal IgG bands are found in CNS infections, paraneoplastic CNS disorders and putative CNS autoimmune diseases such as MS and CNS lupus.

PREDICTIVE TESTING

Cerebrospinal fluid analysis is helpful in predicting the subsequent development of MS in subjects presenting with a clinically isolated syndrome compatible with demyelination (CIS) (Table

TABLE 7.5 Predictive value of cerebrospinal fluid oligoclonal bands versus magnetic resonance imaging in clinically isolated symptom (CIS)

Study	No. of patients	Duration of follow-up	Progression to MS			
			MRI +ve (%)	MRI −ve (%)	OCB +ve (%)	OCB −ve (%)
Paolino et al[105]	44	7 years	18/22 (82)	12/22 (55)	24/26 (92)	6/18 (33)
Rolak et al[51]	83	2 years	11/37 (30)	2/39 (5)	11/38 (29)	2/38 (5)
Sharief et al[50]	45	18 months	17/24 (71)	5/21 (24)	18/22 (82)	4/23 (17)
Söderström et al[106]	60	2 years	14/38 (37)	3/22 (14)	16/41 (39)	1/19 (5)
Tintore et al[107]	112	31 months	17/43* (40)	4/45 (9)	21/70 (30)	5/42 (11)
Total	232	18 months–7 years	77/164 (47)	26/149 (17)	90/197 (46)	18/140 (13)

*Barkhof criteria.[45]

7.5).[50–54] The probability of MS developing in subjects presenting with a CIS with both a normal MRI and CSF analysis is very low (<5%).[54] In subjects presenting with a CIS where the MRI is either negative or shows only nonspecific lesions, the CSF analysis is positive in more than 25% of individuals and is predictive of the subsequent development of MS (Table 7.5).[52–54] In this context CSF analysis is helpful in interpreting the pathological significance of nonspecific lesions. If CSF analysis is positive, only two lesions are required on MRI to satisfy the new diagnostic criteria for dissemination in space,[17] i.e. CSF analysis adds diagnostic specificity to white matter lesions detected on MRI.

THE REMAINDER OF THE CEREBROSPINAL FLUID PROFILE

The CSF in MS is typically clear. In rare cases of transverse myelitis, cord swelling may be of sufficient severity to cause a spinal block. In this situation the CSF may appear straw-colored because of a high total protein content. This situation is usually associated with a low CSF pressure or, rarely, a dry CSF tap. The CSF pressure is normal in subjects with MS, the exception being the rare cases presenting with large pseudotumoral lesions.[55] A total leukocyte count of more than 5 cells/mm^3 is found in approximately a third of subjects with MS.[2] This is more likely to occur in cases with acute spinal cord lesions. A CSF cell count greater than 50 cells/mm^3 is very rare in MS and should alert one to an alternative diagnosis. CSF glucose, CSF-to-plasma glucose ratio and CSF lactate levels are typically normal in subjects with MS. A raised total CSF protein is found in approximately a quarter of subjects with MS, although levels above 1 g/l are very rare[56] and indicate an alternative or additional diagnosis.

PATHOGENETIC STUDIES AND MONITORING DISEASE PROCESSES

There are literally hundreds of hypothesis-driven CSF studies that have investigated various aspects of the pathogenesis of MS.[57] A detailed review of this body of work is beyond the scope of this chapter. The majority of these CSF studies have focused on studying potential immunological mechanisms; these include studies measuring levels of cytokines, chemokines, inflammatory mediators, soluble adhesion molecules, metalloproteases and cellular changes in the CSF in comparison to control groups of subjects. Other CSF studies have focused on infectious agents with the hope of implicating a specific agent as the cause of MS.[58] More recently, investigators have focused on trying to monitor specific MS-related pathological processes (Fig. 7.1),[59] e.g. myelin basic protein as a marker of demyelination, tau and

neurofilament levels for axonal damage and glial fibrillary acid protein as a marker of gliosis.[59] Positive studies of potential CSF biomarkers in MS are seldom reproducible, mainly because of methodological problems, underpowering and insufficient duration of follow-up. Similarly, the majority of studies are not reported in a standardized way and published results lack sufficient detail to allow a critical review of the studies or their reproduction.[57]

DEFINING PROGNOSIS

A clinical endpoint is 'a characteristic or variable that reflects how a patient feels, functions or survives'.[3] A surrogate endpoint 'is a biomarker that is intended to substitute for a clinical endpoint; it is expected to predict clinical benefit (or harm, or lack of benefit or harm) based on epidemiologic, therapeutic, pathophysiologic or other scientific evidence'.[3] At present no CSF parameters can be used as a surrogate endpoint,[57] i.e. a substitute for a clinical endpoint. However several potential CSF biomarkers are worth mentioning as they may turn out to be good surrogate endpoints after further studies.

CEREBROSPINAL FLUID OLIGOCLONAL IgG BANDS

Some patients with MS have been found to be oligoclonal-negative at their initial presentation but become oligoclonal-positive later on in their disease course.[46] Similarly, patients with MS of relatively recent onset are more likely to develop increased numbers of CSF bands as their disease progresses. This is in contrast to the stable pattern found in patients with disease of long duration.[60] These observations suggest that the number of antigenic epitopes inducing the oligoclonal response increases over time. The oligoclonal response not only has temporal variability but has also been elegantly shown to vary spatially, with the elutes from individual MS plaques of the same patient demonstrating different banding patterns.[61] These findings suggest that different antigens are driving the immunological response in MS at a focal rather than a systemic level and that the phenomenon of antigenic spread occurs in MS.

It has been reported that subjects with MS who do not have local synthesis of OCBs have a more benign course.[46,62] However this has not been confirmed by other investigators.[63]

CEREBROSPINAL FLUID OLIGOCLONAL IgM

The intrathecal synthesis of IgM in early MS may predict a worse prognosis. In a small study of 29 subjects with relapsing–remitting MS, the majority of those who had oligoclonal

IgM bands subsequently converted to secondary progressive MS, compared to none of the subjects without intrathecal IgM OCBs.[64] At the end of the study, 60% of subjects with intrathecal IgM OCBs had reached Expanded Disability Status Scale (EDSS) 6, whereas none of the patients lacking intrathecal IgM OCBs had an EDSS of more than 3.[64] In this study, the majority of subjects (80%) with benign MS lacked intrathecal IgM OCBs.[64] In an earlier study intrathecal production of IgM was shown to correlate with MS relapse activity, the time interval between the last relapse and lumbar puncture, and disease duration.[65]

CEREBROSPINAL FLUID NEUROFILAMENT LEVELS AND ANTINEUROFILAMENT ANTIBODIES

Neurofilaments (NFs) are structural proteins that form the internal scaffolding of neuronal processes. NFs play an important role in determining the size and stability of axons. There are three neurofilament proteins: light, medium and heavy NF chains. They are synthesized as nonphosphorylated proteins but become phosphorylated as they are incorporated into the exoskeleton. The extent of NF phosphorylation correlates with size of the axon. When axons are damaged, e.g. in MS by focal areas of inflammation, NF proteins are partially dephosphorylated. This property is used as an immunohistochemical surrogate to detect damaged axons in histological sections.[66] Soluble NF can be detected in the CSF of healthy subjects and tends to be of the hyperphosphorylated form, indicating that it is probably being released by healthy axons.[67] In contrast, in diseases characterized by neuroaxonal pathology, less phosphorylated or hypophosphorylated NF isoforms are released.[67] The ratio of the NF phosphoforms in the CSF could potentially be used as an axonal health index. In other words, acute damage of healthy axons is reflected in increased CSF levels of hyper- or extensively phosphorylated NF and acute-on-chronic damage increases levels of both NF phosphoforms.

Neurofilament light chain

Increased CSF neurofilament light chain (NfL) levels reflect axonal degeneration in MS. In a longitudinal study, Lycke and colleagues showed that median baseline CSF NfL concentrations were significantly higher in patients with relapsing MS ($n=60$) than in healthy controls ($n=11$) ($p<0.001$), with 78% of MS patients having levels above the limit of detection.[68] NfL concentrations and EDSS scores correlated weakly at study entry ($r=0.27$, $p<0.05$) and after 2 years ($r=0.34$, $p<0.01$). NfL levels also correlated weakly with relapse rates over the 2 years of the study ($r=0.38$, $p<0.01$) and moderately correlated with relapse rates during the 2 years prior to study entry ($r=0.56$, $p<0.001$).[68] Importantly, NfL concentrations were highest in the 2–3-month period after a relapse and gradually declined thereafter, indicating that NfL levels are an intermittent marker and are released in response to acute axonal injury.

Neurofilament heavy chain

Different isoforms or phosphoforms of neurofilament heavy chain (NfH) can be defined using Sternberg's panel of monoclonal antibodies (SM=Sternberg monoclonal antibody). These monoclonals recognize different phosphorylation states of NF: a hyperphosphorylated form (NfHSMI34) that is characteristic of healthy axons and a less phosphorylated form (NfHSMI35) that predominates in damaged axons.[67] Several recent studies have investigated the association between CSF NfH levels and disease progression.

In a 3-year follow-up study of 34 patients with MS and controls with other noninflammatory neurological diseases, baseline CSF concentrations of NfHSMI35 correlated with three clinical scales after 3 years' follow-up: EDSS score ($r=0.54$,

$p<0.01$), ambulation index ($r=0.42$, $p<0.05$) and the nine-hole peg test ($r=0.59$, $p<0.01$).[69] More severely disabled MS patients, based on the global Multiple Sclerosis Severity Score (MSSS),[70] had an increased ratio of NfHSMI35:NfHSMI34 compared with mildly disabled MS patients.[71] The degree of neurofilament phosphorylation (ratio of NfHSMI34 to NfHSMI35) was eightfold higher in patients with severe (median MSSS 6.5) as opposed to mild (MSSS 3.2) disability (7.3 versus 0.9, $p=0.03$). The correlation coefficient between CSF NfHSMI35 and global MSSS in this study was 0.44 ($p=0.016$).[71]

In a study by Lim and colleagues, median CSF NfHSMI35 levels in 41 patients with recent optic neuritis did not differ from those of 17 controls with other neurological diseases.[72] This finding is not unexpected because the subjects with optic neuritis were monosymptomatic and had no evidence of previous spinal cord damage. In contrast, median CSF NfHSMI34 concentrations were higher in patients with optic neuritis than in controls ($p<0.05$), suggesting that healthy neurofilament is released from optic nerves undergoing acute damage during a first demyelinating event.[72]

In another study by Lim and colleagues, CSF NfH levels were measured in two cohorts of patients receiving a 15-day course of either oral methylprednisolone or placebo for acute monosymptomatic optic neuritis ($n=18$) or clinical attacks of MS ($n=32$).[73] Clinical disability, as assessed by EDSS, was evaluated before treatment and at 1, 3, 8 and 52 weeks post-treatment. CSF was sampled before treatment and at week 3 (1 week after completing treatment). In the MS cohort, the absolute concentration of NfHSMI35 (i.e. NF from damaged axons) at week 3 predicted greater worsening of EDSS from week 0 to week 8 (odds ratio=4.24, $p=0.044$). Also, an increased release of NfHSMI34 from baseline to week 3 predicted a worsening of disability over 1 year (odds ratio=1.76, $p=0.035$) and from week 8 to week 52 (odds ratio=2.24, $p=0.030$). In this study, no relationship between the NfHSMI34:NfHSMI35 ratio and disability was found.[73] Steroid treatment had no effect on CSF NfH levels.[73] Baseline CSF NfHSMI34 and NfHSMI35 concentrations both correlated positively with baseline gadolinium-enhanced lesion volume ($r=0.50$ ($p=0.005$) and $r=0.53$ ($p<0.01$) respectively).[73] NfH SMI35 levels at week 3 also correlated positively with this baseline MRI endpoint ($r=0.65$, $p<0.01$).[73] The correlation of both phosphoforms of NfH with gadolinium enhancement suggests that, during acute relapse, higher concentrations of neurofilaments are released into the CSF as a result of focal inflammation. Lim and colleagues also reported that CSF NfHSMI35 levels at baseline and week 3 correlated positively with baseline CSF myelin basic protein concentrations ($r=0.56$ ($p=0.006$) and $r=0.77$ ($p<0.001$) respectively).[73] Myelin basic protein is a marker of acute demyelination. In addition, there was a positive correlation between NfHSMI34 and myelin basic protein levels at week 3 ($r=0.58$, $p=0.004$).[73]

Antineurofilament antibodies

Antineurofilament IgG and IgM antibodies are found in both the serum and CSF of subjects with MS.[74] An anti-NF-L index correlated with brain parenchymal fraction, T2 and T1 lesion loads and MRI markers of tissue damage in a cohort of subjects with MS.[75] In another study serum anti-NF-L IgG antibodies were significantly elevated in subjects with primary progressive MS.[76] This indicates that anti-NF-L antibodies may serve as a marker of tissue damage in MS.

CEREBROSPINAL FLUID MYELIN BASIC PROTEIN

Myelin basic protein (MBP) is a unique protein found in the inner myelin layer. During demyelination, MBP and/or its fragments are released into the CSF and can be used as an index of active demyelination.[77] During clinical attacks CSF MBP levels are raised in approximately 80% of subjects. In comparison they are only raised in approximately 40% of subjects with nonrelapsing progressive disease and in a minority of subjects with clinically stable disease. CSF levels remain raised for a period of 5–6 weeks after the onset of a clinical attack. Raised CSF MBP levels are associated with MRI activity and are reduced by corticosteroid therapy. Levels of CSF MBP correlate weakly with clinical disability and are associated with other markers of intrathecal inflammation.[78] MBP levels in the lumbar CSF are rarely raised in acute optic neuritis, presumably because the pathology is too distal to the CSF outflow path of the fourth ventricle.[79]

CEREBROSPINAL FLUID TAU

Tau or microtubule-associated phosphoprotein is found predominantly within axons. Tau promotes the assembly and stabilization of microtubules.[80] A number of neurological diseases or tauopathies are associated with abnormal tau metabolism. A raised CSF tau level is nonspecific and has been described in many neurological diseases. In a small study of 35 subjects with MS and 28 control subjects, tau levels were increased in MS compared to controls and were higher in subjects with progressive disease.[81] This has not been confirmed in another study.[82]

CEREBROSPINAL FLUID 14-3-3

14-3-3 is a highly conserved protein that is not brain-specific and is present in most mammalian tissues. It exists mainly as a soluble cytoplasmic protein with small amounts bound to synaptic membranes. Different isoforms of 14-3-3 are associated with different neuron types and/or membrane compartments. 14-3-3 exists in different phosphorylated states and has several functions.[83,84] Raised CSF 14-3-3 levels are useful diagnostically in Creutzfeldt–Jakob disease. In one study, 5/38 (13%) subjects with CIS had detectable 14-3-3 protein in the CSF; the presence of 14-3-3 in the CSF was an independent predictor for a shorter time to conversion to definite MS (RR=4.1; 95% CI 1.1–15) and to reach an EDSS ≥2 at the end of follow-up (OR 14.8; 95% CI 2.86–76.8).[85] This was not confirmed by another group.[86] A separate group detected 14-3-3 in the CSF in 38% subjects with either a CIS or MS; in this study the presence of CSF 14-3-3 correlated with disease severity.[84] The latter has been confirmed in a larger cohort of subjects.[87]

CEREBROSPINAL FLUID S100b

S-100b is an acidic calcium-binding protein located in the cytoplasm of astrocytes and Schwann cells. Raised CSF S-100b is found in all conditions associated with astrocytosis or gliosis. CSF and serum levels of S-100b are raised in a proportion of subjects with MS, particularly during clinical relapse.[88–90] Raised CSF levels are found from day 5 after the onset of the attack and reach a maximum after a period of 2–3 weeks.[90] CSF S100b levels are raised in a greater proportion of chronic progressive than relapsing–remitting patients.[90] Levels of CSF S100b are higher in subjects with primary progressive compared to subjects with secondary progressive or relapsing–remitting disease.[91]

CEREBROSPINAL FLUID GLIAL FIBRILLARY ACIDIC PROTEIN

Glial fibrillary acidic protein (GFAP) is the major structural protein of the glial intermediate filament of astrocytes and its level in CSF increases in association with astrocytosis. GFAP was first isolated from chronic MS plaques, which have a high concentration of fibrous astrocytes.[92] CSF concentrations of GFAP are increased in a varying proportion (9–39%) of patients with MS.[93] A longitudinal study that measured CSF GFAP concentrations in 13 patients with relapsing–remitting MS found that CSF levels were raised compared to controls and that levels increased over the study period of 24 months from a baseline.[94] The latter increase correlated strongly with the increase in clinical deficit scores and was not associated with clinical relapse.[94] Subjects with MS with severe disability have significantly higher CSF GFAP levels than less disabled subjects, with a moderate correlation between CSF GFAP levels and ambulation in subjects with secondary progressive MS.[91] These findings imply that CSF GFAP levels may be used as a bulk marker of astrocytosis but this clearly needs to be confirmed.

MONITORING EFFECTS OF THERAPEUTIC INTERVENTIONS

Although CSF analysis provides useful information on the impact of therapeutic interventions in MS, it has been studied relatively infrequently. The following examples provide some insights that can be obtained from studying the effect of treatments on CSF parameters.

CICLOSPORIN A

In a double-blind placebo-controlled trial of ciclosporin A, CSF free light chain analysis was performed pre- and post-treatment in 19 patients; nine received ciclosporin A and 10 placebo.[95] The placebo-treated subjects had continued evidence of B- or plasma-cell activity, as evidenced by an increase in both free kappa and lambda chains. In comparison ciclosporin A treatment resulted in no change or an improvement in the light chain response, suggesting that it partially suppressed B or plasma cell activity.[95]

AUTOLOGOUS BONE MARROW TRANSPLANTATION

Intense immunosuppression in subjects with active MS, e.g. with autologous bone marrow transplantation[96] and anti-CD52 (Campath-1h or alemtuzumab, personal observations), does not result in the disappearance of the intrathecal oligoclonal IgG bands. This implies that long-lived plasma cells are probably resistant to systemic immunosuppression. This may have implications for the treatment of MS, particularly if intrathecal oligoclonal immunoglobulin plays a direct role in the pathogenesis of MS.

RITUXIMAB

Cerebrospinal fluid B cells were not depleted in four subjects with primary progressive MS treated with rituximab, a B cell depleting anti-CD20 monoclonal antibody.[97] Rituximab did, however, temporarily suppress the activation state of B cells in cerebrospinal fluid.[97] In comparison, B lymphocytes were depleted in both the CSF and peripheral blood in a single subject with relapsing-remitting MS treated with rituximab.[98]

NATALIZUMAB

In subjects with MS treated with natalizumab, a human monoclonal antibody that recognizes very-late-activating antigen (VLA)-4 and acts as a selective adhesion molecule inhibitor, there is a dramatic reduction in CSF total leukocyte counts,

CD4[+] and CD8[+] T cells, CD19[+] B cells and CD138[+] plasma cells compared to subjects with untreated MS.[99] This indicates that natalizumab probably has a profound effect on CNS immunosurveillance and explains why treated cases developed progressive multifocal leukoencephalopathy, a rare but usually fatal opportunistic infection of the CNS.[100–102]

CONCLUSIONS

The detection of a CSF oligoclonal IgG response by IEF is a nonspecific but sensitive aid in the diagnosis of MS. It should be used in parallel with evoked potentials and MRI in aiding the clinical diagnosis of MS, as each set of investigations provides different information about the pathogenesis of the condition. Importantly, the CSF oligoclonal IgG response is not only a diagnostic but a predictive test, allowing one to assess the risk of developing MS to a person presenting with a clinically isolated syndrome compatible with demyelination. The standard CSF profile is also useful in identifying potential MS mimics. Currently no CSF biomarkers hitherto studied in subjects with MS can be used as surrogate endpoints. The main reasons for this are methodological: in general studies have been too small, cross-sectional in design or have had insufficient follow-up to allow meaningful conclusions to be drawn about their utility.

REFERENCES

1. Andersson M, Alvarez-Cermeno J, Bernardi G et al. Cerebrospinal fluid in the diagnosis of multiple sclerosis: a consensus report. J Neurol Neurosurg Psychiatr 1994; 57: 897–902.
2. Freedman MS, Thompson EJ, Deisenhammer F et al. Recommended standard of cerebrospinal fluid analysis in the diagnosis of multiple sclerosis: a consensus statement. Arch Neurol 2005; 62: 865–870.
3. Floyd E, McShane TM. Development and use of biomarkers in oncology drug development. Toxicol Pathol 2004; 32(suppl 1): 106–115.
4. Nilsson C, Stahlberg F, Thomsen C et al. Circadian variation in human cerebrospinal fluid production measured by magnetic resonance imaging. Am J Physiol 1992; 262: R20–R24.
5. Thompson EJ. CSF proteins: a biochemical approach. Edinburgh: Churchill Livingstone; 1988: 172.
6. Reiber H. Flow rate of cerebrospinal fluid (CSF) – a concept common to normal blood–CSF barrier function and to dysfunction in neurological diseases. J Neurol Sci 1994; 122: 189–203.
7. Blennow K, Fredman P, Wallin A et al. Formulas for the quantitation of intrathecal IgG production. Their validity in the presence of blood–brain barrier damage and their utility in multiple sclerosis. J Neurol Sci 1994; 121: 90–96.
8. Statz A, Felgenhauer K. Development of the blood–CSF barrier. Dev Med Child Neurol 1983; 25: 152–161.
9. Eeg-Olofsson O, Link H, Wigertz A. Concentrations of CSF proteins as a measure of blood brain barrier function and synthesis of IgG within the CNS in 'normal' subjects from the age of 6 months to 30 years. Acta Paediatr Scand 1981; 70: 167–170.
10. Seyfert S, Kunzmann V, Schwertfeger N et al. Determinants of lumbar CSF protein concentration. J Neurol 2002; 249: 1021–1026.
11. Jacobi C, Reiber H, Felgenhauer K. The clinical relevance of locally produced carcinoembryonic antigen in cerebrospinal fluid. J Neurol 1986; 233: 358–361.
12. Flier FJ, de Vries Robbe PF. Nosology and causal necessity; the relation between defining a disease and discovering its necessary cause. Theor Med Bioeth 1999; 20: 577–488.

13. Lassmann H, Raine CS, Antel J, Prineas JW. Immunopathology of multiple sclerosis: report on an international meeting held at the Institute of Neurology of the University of Vienna. J Neuroimmunol 1998; 86: 213–217.
14. Engell T. A clinico-pathoanatomical study of multiple sclerosis diagnosis. Acta Neurol Scand 1988; 78: 39–44.
15. Schumacker GA, Beebe G, Kibler RF et al. Problems of experimental trials of therapy in multiple sclerosis: report by the Panel on the Evaluation of Experimental Trials of Therapy in Multiple Sclerosis. Ann NY Acad Sci 1965; 122: 552–568.
16. Poser CM, Paty DW, Scheinberg L et al. New diagnostic criteria for multiple sclerosis: guidelines for research protocols. Ann Neurol 1983; 13: 227–231.
17. McDonald WI, Compston A, Edan G et al. Recommended diagnostic criteria for multiple sclerosis: guidelines from the International Panel on the diagnosis of multiple sclerosis. Ann Neurol 2001; 50: 121–127.
18. Polman CH, Reingold SC, Edan G et al. Diagnostic criteria for multiple sclerosis: 2005 revisions to the 'McDonald Criteria'. Ann Neurol 2005; 58: 840–846.
19. Lowenthal A, Vansande M, Karcher D. The differential diagnosis of neurological diseases by fractionating electrophoretically the CSF gamma-globulins. J New Drugs 1960; 6: 51–56.
20. Tourtellotte WW, Parker JA. Multiple sclerosis: brain immunoglobulin-G and albumin. Nature 1967; 214: 683–686.
21. Tourtellotte WW, Parker JA. Multiple sclerosis: correlation between immunoglobulin-G in cerebrospinal fluid and brain. Science 1966; 154: 1044–1045.
22. Tourtellotte WW, Tavolato B, Parker JA, Comiso P. Cerebrospinal fluid electroimmunodiffusion. An easy, rapid, sensitive, reliable, and valid method for the simultaneous determination of immunoglobulin-G and albumin. Arch Neurol 1971; 25: 345–350.
23. Cawley LP, Minard BJ, Tourtellotte WW et al. Immunofixation electrophoretic techniques applied to identification of proteins in serum and cerebrospinal fluid. Clin Chem 1976; 22: 1262–1268.
24. Felgenhauer K. Quantitation and specific detection methods after disc electrophoresis of serum proteins. Clin Chim Acta 1970; 27: 305–312.

25. Link H. Qualitative changes in immunoglobulin G in multiple sclerosis-cerebrospinal fluid. Acta Neurol Scand 1967; 43(suppl 31): 180.
26. Sandberg–Wollheim M. Immunoglobulin synthesis in vitro by cerebrospinal fluid cells in patients with multiple sclerosis. Scand J Immunol 1974; 3: 717–730.
27. Laterre EC, Callewaert A, Heremans JF, Sfaello Z. Electrophoretic morphology of gamma globulins in cerebrospinal fluid of multiple sclerosis and other diseases of the nervous system. Neurology 1970; 20: 982–990.
28. Wolinsky JS. The diagnosis of primary progressive multiple sclerosis. J Neurol Sci 2003; 206: 145–152.
29. Thompson AJ, Montalban X, Barkhof F et al. Diagnostic criteria for primary progressive multiple sclerosis: a position paper. Ann Neurol 2000; 47: 831–835.
30. Meinl E, Krumbholz M, Hohlfeld R. B lineage cells in the inflammatory central nervous system environment: migration, maintenance, local antibody production, and therapeutic modulation. Ann Neurol 2006; 59: 880–892.
31. Morris P, Davies NW, Keir G. A screening assay to detect antigen-specific antibodies within cerebrospinal fluid. J Immunol Methods 2006; 311: 81–86.
32. Von Storch TJ, Lawyer T Jr, Harris AH. Colloidal gold reaction in multiple sclerosis. AMA Arch Neurol Psychiatr 1950; 64: 668–675.
33. Foley JM, Donovan AM, Moloney WC. Correlation of the zinc sulfate precipitation test with the colloidal gold test in neurosyphilis, multiple sclerosis, and cerebral vascular disease. J Neuropathol Exp Neurol 1951; 10: 89–91.
34. Cosgrove JB, Agius P. Studies in multiple sclerosis. II. Comparison of the beta-gamma globulin ratio, gamma globulin elevation, and first-zone colloidal gold curve in the cerebrospinal fluid. Neurology 1966; 16: 197–204.
35. Lefvert AK, Link H. IgG production within the central nervous system: a critical review of proposed formulae. Ann Neurol 1985; 17: 13–20.
36. Ohman S, Ernerudh J, Forsberg P et al. Comparison of seven formulae and isoelectrofocusing for determination of intrathecally produced IgG in neurological diseases. Ann Clin Biochem 1992; 29: 405–410.

37. Reiber H, Felgenhauer K. Protein transfer at the blood cerebrospinal fluid barrier and the quantitation of the humoral immune response within the central nervous system. Clin Chim Acta 1987; 163: 319–328.

38. Sindic CJ, Van Antwerpen MP, Goffette S. The intrathecal humoral immune response: laboratory analysis and clinical relevance. Clin Chem Lab Med 2001; 39: 333–340.

39. Keir G, Luxton RW, Thompson EJ. Isoelectric focusing of cerebrospinal fluid immunoglobulin G: an annotated update. Ann Clin Biochem 1990; 27: 436–443.

40. Rudick RA, Peter DR, Bidlack JM, Knutson DW. Multiple sclerosis: free light chains in cerebrospinal fluid. Neurology 1985; 35: 1443–1449.

41. Rudick RA, Pallant A, Bidlack JM, Herndon RM. Free kappa light chains in multiple sclerosis spinal fluid. Ann Neurol 1986; 20: 63–69.

42. Sindic CJ, Laterre EC. Oligoclonal free kappa and lambda bands in the cerebrospinal fluid of patients with multiple sclerosis and other neurological diseases. An immunoaffinity-mediated capillary blot study. J Neuroimmunol 1991; 33: 63–72.

43. Krakauer M, Schaldemose Nielsen H, Jensen J, Sellebjerg F. Intrathecal synthesis of free immunoglobulin light chains in multiple sclerosis. Acta Neurol Scand 1998; 98: 161–165.

44. Goffette, S et al. Detection of oligoclonal free kappa chains in the absence of oligoclonal IgG in the CSF of patients with suspected multiple sclerosis. J Neurol Neurosurg Psychiatry 2004; 75: 308–310.

45. Barkhof F, Filippi M, Miller DH et al. Comparison of MRI criteria at first presentation to predict conversion to clinically definite multiple sclerosis. Brain 1997; 120: 2059–2069.

46. Zeman AZ, Kidd D, McLean BN et al. A study of oligoclonal band negative multiple sclerosis. J Neurol Neurosurg Psychiatr 1996; 60: 27–30.

47. Davies G, Keir G, Thompson EJ, Giovannoni G. The clinical significance of an intrathecal monoclonal immunoglobulin band: a follow-up study. Neurology 2003; 60: 1163–1166.

48. Trip SA, Wroe SJ, Davies G, Giovannoni G. Primary CNS mantle cell lymphoma associated with an isolated CSF monoclonal IgG band. Eur Neurol 2003; 49: 187–188.

49. McLean BN, Luxton RW, Thompson EJ. A study of immunoglobulin G in the cerebrospinal fluid of 1007 patients with suspected neurological disease using isoelectric focusing and the Log IgG-Index. A comparison and diagnostic applications. Brain 1990; 113: 1269–1289.

50. Sharief MK, Thompson EJ. The predictive value of intrathecal immunoglobulin synthesis and magnetic resonance imaging in acute isolated syndromes for subsequent development of multiple sclerosis. Ann Neurol 1991; 29: 147–151.

51. Rolak LA, Beck RW, Paty DW et al. Cerebrospinal fluid in acute optic neuritis: experience of the optic neuritis treatment trial. Neurology 1996; 46: 368–372.

52. Tumani H, Tourtellotte WW, Peter JB, Felgenhauer K. Acute optic neuritis: combined immunological markers and magnetic resonance imaging predict subsequent development of multiple sclerosis. The Optic Neuritis Study Group. J Neurol Sci 1998; 155: 44–49.

53. Jin YP, de Pedro-Cuesta J, Huang YH, Soderstrom M. Predicting multiple sclerosis at optic neuritis onset. Mult Scler 2003; 9: 135–141.

54. Soderstrom M, Ya-Ping J, Hillert J, Link H. Optic neuritis: prognosis for multiple sclerosis from MRI, CSF, and HLA findings. Neurology 1998; 50: 708–714.

55. Poser CM. Pseudo-tumoral multiple sclerosis. Clin Neurol Neurosurg 2005; 107: 535.

56. Tourtellotte WW. Cerebrospinal fluid in multiple sclerosis. In: Vinken P, Bruyn G, eds. Handbook of clinical neurology, vol. 9. Amsterdam: North Holland; 1970: 324–382.

57. Bielekova B, Martin R. Development of biomarkers in multiple sclerosis. Brain 2004; 127: 1463–1478.

58. Gilden DH. Infectious causes of multiple sclerosis. Lancet Neurol 2005; 4: 195–202.

59. Teunissen CE, Dijkstra C, Polman C. Biological markers in CSF and blood for axonal degeneration in multiple sclerosis. Lancet Neurol 2005; 4: 32–41.

60. Thompson EJ, Kaufmann P, Rudge P. Sequential changes in oligoclonal patterns during the course of multiple sclerosis. J Neurol Neurosurg Psychiatr 1983; 46: 115–118.

61. Mattson DH, Roos RP, Arnason BG. Isoelectric focusing of IgG eluted from multiple sclerosis and subacute sclerosing panencephalitis brains. Nature 1980; 287: 335–337.

62. Sa MJ, Sequeira L, Rio ME, Thompson EJ. [Oligoclonal IgG bands in the cerebrospinal fluid of portuguese patients with multiple sclerosis: negative results indicate benign disease.]. Arq Neuropsiquiatr 2005; 63(2B): 375–379.

63. Vilisaar J, Wilson M, Niepel G et al. A comparative audit of anticardiolipin antibodies in oligoclonal band negative and positive multiple sclerosis. Mult Scler 2005; 11: 378–380.

64. Villar LM, Masjuan J, Gonzalez-Porque P et al. Intrathecal IgM synthesis is a prognostic factor in multiple sclerosis. Ann Neurol 2003; 53: 222–226.

65. Sharief MK, Thompson EJ. Intrathecal immunoglobulin M synthesis in multiple sclerosis. Relationship with clinical and cerebrospinal fluid parameters. Brain 1991; 114: 181–195.

66. Trapp BD, Peterson J, Ransohoff RM et al. Axonal transection in the lesions of multiple sclerosis. N Engl J Med 1998; 338: 278–285.

67. Petzold A. Neurofilament phosphoforms: surrogate markers for axonal injury, degeneration and loss. J Neurol Sci 2005; 233: 183–198.

68. Lycke JN, Karlsson JE, Andersen O, Rosengren LE. Neurofilament protein in cerebrospinal fluid: a potential marker of activity in multiple sclerosis. J Neurol Neurosurg Psychiatr 1998; 64: 402–404.

69. Petzold A, Eikelenboom MJ, Keir G et al. Axonal damage accumulates in the progressive phase of multiple sclerosis: three year follow up study. J Neurol Neurosurg Psychiatry 2005; 76: 206–211.

70. Roxburgh RH, Seaman SR, Masterman T et al. Multiple Sclerosis Severity Score: using disability and disease duration to rate disease severity. Neurology 2005; 64: 1144–1151.

71. Petzold A, Eikelenboom MI, Keir G et al. The new global multiple sclerosis severity score (MSSS) correlates with axonal but not glial biomarkers. Mult Scler 2006; 12: 325–328.

72. Lim ET, Grant D, Pashenkov M et al. Cerebrospinal fluid levels of brain specific proteins in optic neuritis. Mult Scler 2004; 10: 261–265.

73. Lim ET, Sellebjerg F, Jensen CV et al. Acute axonal damage predicts clinical outcome in patients with multiple sclerosis. Mult Scler 2005; 11: 532–536.

74. Silber E, Sharief MK. Axonal degeneration in the pathogenesis of multiple sclerosis. J Neurol Sci 1999; 170: 11–18.

75. Eikelenboom MJ, Petzold A, Lazeron RH et al. Multiple sclerosis: Neurofilament light chain antibodies are correlated to cerebral atrophy. Neurology 2003; 60: 219–223.

76. Ehling R, Lutterotti A, Wanschitz J et al. Increased frequencies of serum antibodies to neurofilament light in patients with primary chronic progressive multiple sclerosis. Mult Scler 2004; 10: 601–606.

77. Cohen SR, Brooks BR, Herndon RM, McKhann GM. A diagnostic index of active demyelination: myelin basic protein in cerebrospinal fluid. Ann Neurol 1980; 8: 25–31.

78. Whitaker JN. Myelin basic protein in cerebrospinal fluid and other body fluids. Mult Scler 1998; 4: 16–21.

79. Sellebjerg F, Christiansen M, Nielsen PM, Frederiksen JL. Cerebrospinal fluid measures of disease activity in patients with multiple sclerosis. Mult Scler 1998; 4: 475–479.

80. Goedert M, Spillantini MG, Crowther RA. Tau proteins and neurofibrillary degeneration. Brain Pathol 1991; 1: 279–286.

81. Jimenez-Jimenez FJ, Zurdo JM, Hernanz A et al. Tau protein concentrations in cerebrospinal fluid of patients with multiple sclerosis. Acta Neurol Scand 2002; 106: 351–354.

82. Colucci M, Roccatagliata L, Capello E et al. The 14-3-3 protein in multiple sclerosis: a marker of disease severity. Mult Scler 2004; 10: 477–481.

83. Bridges D, Moorhead GB. 14-3-3 proteins: a number of functions for a numbered protein. Sci STKE 2004; 2004(242): re10.

84. Boston PF, Jackson P, Thompson RJ. Human 14-3-3 protein: radioimmunoassay, tissue distribution, and cerebrospinal fluid levels in patients with neurological disorders. J Neurochem 1982; 38: 1475–1482.

85. Martinez-Yelamos A, Saiz A, Sanchez-Valle R et al. 14-3-3 protein in the CSF as prognostic marker in early multiple sclerosis. Neurology 2001; 57: 722–724.

86. De Seze J, Peoc'h K, Ferriby D et al. 14-3-3 Protein in the cerebrospinal fluid of patients with acute transverse myelitis and multiple sclerosis. J Neurol 2002; 249: 626–627.

87. Martinez-Yelamos A, Rovira A, Sanchez-Valle R et al. CSF 14-3-3 protein assay and MRI as prognostic markers in patients with a clinically isolated syndrome suggestive of MS. J Neurol 2004; 251: 1278–1279.

88. Lamers KJ, van Engelen BG, Gabreels FJ et al. Cerebrospinal neuron-specific enolase, S-100 and myelin basic protein in neurological disorders. Acta Neurol Scand 1995; 92: 247–251.

89. Michetti F, Massaro A, Murazio M. The nervous system-specific S-100 antigen in cerebrospinal fluid of multiple sclerosis patients. Neurosci Lett 1979; 11: 171–175.

90. Michetti F, Massaro A, Russo G, Rigon G. The S-100 antigen in cerebrospinal fluid as a possible index of cell injury in the nervous system. J Neurol Sci 1980; 44: 259–263.

91. Petzold A, Eikelenboom MJ, Gveric D et al. Markers for different glial cell responses in multiple sclerosis: clinical and pathological correlations. Brain 2002; 125: 1462–1473.

92. Eng LF. Glial fibrillary acidic protein (GFAP): the major protein of glial intermediate filaments in differentiated astrocytes. J Neuroimmunol 1985; 8: 203–214.

93. Noppe M, Crols R, Andries D, Lowenthal A. Determination in human cerebrospinal fluid of glial fibrillary acidic protein, S-100 and myelin basic protein as indices of non-specific or specific central nervous tissue pathology. Clin Chim Acta 1986; 155: 143–150.

94. Rosengren LE, Lycke J, Andersen O. Glial fibrillary acidic protein in CSF of multiple sclerosis patients: relation to neurological deficit. J Neurol Sci 1995; 133: 61–65.

95. McLean BN, Rudge P, Thompson EJ. Cyclosporin A curtails the progression of free light chain synthesis in the CSF of patients with multiple sclerosis. J Neurol Neurosurg Psychiatry 1989; 52: 529–531.

96. Samijn JP, te Boekhorst PA, Mondria T et al. Intense T cell depletion followed by autologous bone marrow transplantation for severe multiple sclerosis. J Neurol Neurosurg Psychiatry 2006; 77: 46–50.

97. Monson NL, Cravens PD, Frohman EM et al. Effect of rituximab on the peripheral blood and cerebrospinal fluid B cells in patients with primary progressive multiple sclerosis. Arch Neurol 2005; 62: 258–264.

98. Stuve O, Cepok S, Elias B et al. Clinical stabilization and effective B-lymphocyte depletion in the cerebrospinal fluid and peripheral blood of a patient with fulminant relapsing-remitting multiple sclerosis. Arch Neurol 2005; 62: 1620–1623.

99. Stuve O, Marra CM, Jerome KR et al. Immune surveillance in multiple sclerosis patients treated with natalizumab. Ann Neurol 2006; 59: 743–747.

100. Van Assche G, Van Ranst M, Sciot R et al. Progressive multifocal leukoencephalopathy after natalizumab therapy for Crohn's disease. N Engl J Med 2005; 353: 362–368.

101. Kleinschmidt-DeMasters BK, Tyler KL. Progressive multifocal leukoencephalopathy complicating treatment with natalizumab and interferon beta-1a for multiple sclerosis. N Engl J Med 2005; 353: 369–374.

102. Langer-Gould A, Atlas SW, Green AJ et al. Progressive multifocal leukoencephalopathy in a patient treated with natalizumab. N Engl J Med 2005; 353: 375–381.

103. Kostulas VK, Link H, Lefvert AK. Oligoclonal IgG bands in cerebrospinal fluid. Principles for demonstration and interpretation based on findings in 1114 neurological patients. Arch Neurol 1987; 44: 1041–1044.

104. Beer S, Rosler KM, Hess CW. Diagnostic value of paraclinical tests in multiple sclerosis: relative sensitivities and specificities for reclassification according to the Poser committee criteria. J Neurol Neurosurg Psychiatr 1995; 59: 152–159.

105. Paolino E, Fainardi E, Ruppi P et al. A prospective study on the predictive value of CSF oligoclonal bands and MRI in acute isolated neurological syndromes for subsequent progression to multiple sclerosis. J Neurol Neurosurg Psychiatry 1996; 60: 572–575.

106. Soderstrom M. The clinical and paraclinical profile of optic neuritis: a prospective study. Ital J Neurol Sci 1995; 16: 167–176.

107. Tintore M, Rovira A, Brieva L et al. Isolated demyelinating syndromes: comparison of CSF oligoclonal bands and different MR imaging criteria to predict conversion to CDMS. Mult Scler 2001; 7: 359–363.

Natural history of multiple sclerosis

O. Andersen

INTRODUCTION

The natural history of multiple sclerosis (MS) has probably been more thoroughly described than the course of any other chronic autoimmune disorder. The prognosis of MS has been uniquely delineated by population-based longitudinal follow-up studies.[1-3] The results of such longitudinal studies are dependent on the selection of cases and the population base, and were corroborated by studies from areas where prevalence and repeat incidence studies were performed.[4-7] The relatively late introduction of effective immunomodulatory treatment for MS contributed to the validity of these natural history studies. Azathioprine, the first widely used immunosuppressive agent in MS, was, although it suppresses magnetic resonance imaging (MRI) activity,[8] never proved beyond doubt to have a significant disease-modifying effect.[9-11] In contrast, in systemic lupus erythematosus effective disease-modifying drugs have been in general use since the 1980s. However, even in Scandinavia, with its conservative therapeutic tradition, a large proportion of MS patients are now treated by immunomodulatory drugs (or participating in clinical trials), barring new population-based long-term natural history studies.

FORESHADOWING SYMPTOMS AND SUBCLINICAL DYSFUNCTION BEFORE THE FIRST EPISODE OF UNEQUIVOCAL SYMPTOMS

It is uncontroversial that cerebrospinal fluid (CSF) and MRI data are suggestive of an immunological process of a much longer duration than the neurological episodes. A CSF analysis obtained during the first days after onset already reveals an intrathecal oligoclonal immunological reaction in almost the same proportion of cases as in later stages of MS[12] and CSF cytology will often show small lymphocytes with an unreactive appearance. Casuistic CSF analysis obtained in family studies (unpublished follow-up after Andersen and Lindholm 1976[13]) have set the possible limits for the presymptomatic onset of this immunopathy to be at least 15 years before clinical onset. Such immunopathy may be presymptomatic to MS or remain asymptomatic.[14] Intracerebral or spinal lesions demonstrated by MRI in 61–87% of patients in the very first stages of the disease send the same message.[15,16]

In addition to immunological dysfunction preceding the unequivocal onset episode, several types of more or less subtle neurological dysfunction may occur before the onset episode. It is not unusual – although open for recall bias – that MS patients report symptoms highly suggestive of a neurological episode, e.g. transient leg weakness, during childhood or adolescence. Thus, latency may be protracted far beyond the time intervals usually reported between attacks. Optic neuritis in childhood progressed to MS after a long latency. In 19% of the cases the latency was 20 years and in 26% it was 40 years.[17] Furthermore, in the study on 'monosymptomatic optic neuritis' a finding of 'fellow eye abnormalities' with visual field defects was reported in 48% of contralateral eyes.[18] At the time of the first episode in an adult – notably also when it was located in a region other than the optic nerve – there was already approximately 20% loss of channels in the visual tracts, as evaluated by high-resolution perimetry (the rationale for evaluation of loss of channels in the visual tracts from the results of high resolution perimetry is provided by Frisén[19]). As this asymptomatic loss of visual function progresses slowly[20] during the subsequent years after clinical onset, a considerable loss of visual channels probably develops insidiously during a stage considered asymptomatic by conventional wisdom.

PREMONITORY SYMPTOMS AS PART OF THE GENERAL MULTIPLE SCLEROSIS SYMPTOMATOLOGY

Periodic symptoms of suspected neuropsychiatric nature, or periods of excessive tiredness, may occur before the focal neurological episode which is the unambiguous onset of MS.

Preceding depression was shown to occur significantly more often (35%, $n=45$) than in a control group with a pain syndrome. The depression occurred before the onset of focal neurological symptoms.[21] Several uncontrolled studies describe a similar sequence of events.[22–24] The clinical course in these reports usually suggests that depression was a premonitory part of the MS symptomatology and does not support a hypothetical link between bipolar affective disorder and MS. Moreover, a transition may occur from symptoms presenting as convincingly functional (as shown by their neurological incongruence and inconsistency, classical signs of psychogenesis) to incontestable multifocal symptomatology.

CASE REPORT 1

A female patient was referred to our clinic because of recurring short periods of incapacitating fatigue. A diagnosis of a chronic fatigue syndrome was contemplated. At age 30, coincident with the fourth of these episodes, a transient internuclear ophthalmoplegia was noted. After further episodes of oculomotor disturbance and sensory myelopathy, a diagnosis of remitting–relapsing MS was established, with fatigue becoming a chronic symptom.

CASE REPORT 2

A female patient presented, during a 10-year period, symptoms of astasia–abasia with dramatic disequilibrium at examination but perfectly normal gait when occasionally observed at home. However, during the subsequent 5-year period she insidiously developed a cerebellar tetra-ataxia and a diagnosis of MS was established from progressive polyfocal lesions.

THE FIRST UNAMBIGUOUS MULTIPLE SCLEROSIS SYMPTOMS: THE 'CLINICALLY ISOLATED SYNDROME' OR INSIDIOUS PROGRESSION

The first strong dichotomy, usually obvious for the patient and the neurologist within a few months (but with some fallacies to be discussed) is between 1) a subacute episode developing over days or weeks with complete or incomplete remission over weeks or months or 2) an insidious and steadily progressive course from onset. The experienced neurologist who encounters the first type of onset will call it a 'clinically isolated syndrome' (CIS) if it is sufficiently typical to be prospectively recognized as MS and investigations confirm or at least do not disprove it. Such an acute episode usually heralds a relapsing–remitting course, which tends to be benign for several years but ultimately may change into a secondary progressive course. On the contrary, the second type of onset usually heralds a continued insidious progression, termed a primary progressive course. There is a dramatic difference in prognosis as expressed in time to disability grade 6 (gait with support) according to the Disability Status Scale (DSS)[25] between onset with a bout (a subacute episode) or with insidious progression (Fig. 8.1). Insidious motor involvement or limb ataxia indicated a shorter time to disability milestones. This was revealed in a multifactorial analysis of initial symptoms where prognostic coefficients indicated an increased risk with these symptoms.[26] Some even contend that this dichotomy is between two different diseases; however, they constitute a genetic and clinical continuum.

THE 'CLINICALLY ISOLATED SYNDROME'

The consensus definition of the CIS is indirect: An episode typical for MS, in which the initial diagnostic investigation

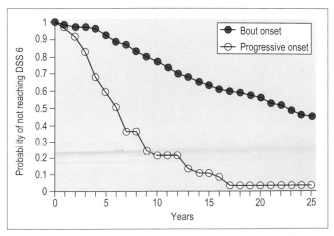

FIG. 8.1 Life-table analysis with endpoint Disability Status Score (DSS) 6. The probability of reaching DSS 6 is markedly higher in the group with progressive onset than with bout (attack) onset. Redrawn from Runmarker and Andersen 1993,[2] with permission from Oxford University Press.

supports MS but without dissemination in time and therefore not fulfilling the Poser diagnostic criteria[27] (clinical criteria in McDonald et al[28]) for MS. The definition of the CIS is more distinct if restricted to three broad topographical categories, the three central nervous system (CNS) regions most susceptible to initial MS attacks, the optic nerve, the brainstem and the spinal cord.[29] This term was used for monofocal attacks only in one trial[30] and included polyfocal episodes in another.[31] In real life, the CIS is sufficiently disturbing to alert the patient to seek advice. Importantly, this concept did not exist in the large natural history studies[1,3,32,33] which used the Poser diagnostic criteria,[27] postponing the diagnosis of MS until a further episode had occurred (and for clinically definite MS, until a new episode with evidence for a new focus had occurred). They cannot, therefore, be used for unbiased prediction of the risk of second and later episodes after an isolated episode suggestive of MS. A second event will, by definition, always occur in these studies. Patients with the CIS are 1) the source for patients 'seen from onset' and developing clinically definite MS and 2) the only source for the 'possible MS' group that does not fulfill the Poser criteria. 'Possible MS' patients constituted about 20% (45/220) of patients in a repeat incidence study associated with a long-term follow-up study keeping track of CISs.[34,35] This is slightly lower than the proportion remaining possible after the CIS in recent prospective MRI supported natural history studies (cited below); however, these are still short-term.

With its chronic course, MS provides ample opportunities for retrospective re-evaluation of the onset episode, revealing that the disease may indeed present with symptoms from any site in the CNS, more diverse than the three categories of the CIS suggest. A list of diverse onset symptoms has been provided.[36] In the young age at onset (20–30 years) categories, cranial (optic neuritis, brainstem) lesions constitute approximately 50% of onset attacks. The remaining 50% are spinal, hemispheric, polyfocal, unlocalizable and a group of rare symptoms such as sudden deafness. The proportion of onset attacks presenting with spinal focal lesions increases with age, reaching the same frequency as the cranial lesions in the 40–44 years onset age group.[37] However, with increasingly atypical symptoms, the background frequency of the particular symptom in other disorders is increasingly important. As an example, only a small fraction of cases of peripheral facial palsy turned out to herald MS.[38,39] There is support for the argument that a short (few years) interval between atypical premonitory symptoms and subsequent unambiguous MS symptoms is in favour of a relationship. As a comparison, this interval was only rarely more than a few years after optic neuritis.[40]

INSIDIOUS PROGRESSION

In approximately 15% of cases, the course is insidiously progressive from onset, implying that the patient belongs to the primary progressive or progressive–relapsing category.[2,41] While the major division of course between progressive and remitting course is usually straightforward for the clinical neurologist, borderland cases exist. Thus, in a few cases the pace of initial symptoms is intermediate between that of bouts (with an evolution over days or a few weeks) and that of primary progression (over several months), with subsequent slow, partial regression. However, the long-term course after this type of subacute initial episode was found to be similar to that of primary progressive cases, so these intermediate cases are best classified into the progressive category.[2] There is also a continuum between primary and secondary progression. Transient minor sensory symptoms, suggestive of a spinal level, may be embedded in the very first stages of an otherwise progressive paraparesis. When such subtle information is added to the history retrospectively,

the clinical category may be changed from primary to secondary progression rather arbitrarily, however with far-reaching consequences for therapy.

THE SECOND ATTACK IN RELAPSING–REMITTING MULTIPLE SCLEROSIS

New diagnostic criteria[28,42,43] rely on dissemination of lesions not only in clinical topography but also in MRI, and may be supplemented by results from the CSF analysis. As these criteria are essentially prognostic rather than diagnostic, yet provide the basis for decisions on early therapy (while the ultimate diagnosis is by autopsy), median time from onset to a second attack may be studied in several steps: from the CIS to the McDonald diagnosis (confirmed by MRI or by a second attack) and from the McDonald diagnosis to the Poser diagnosis (second attack). The two year risk of reaching the MS diagnosis after CIS in patients given a placebo was 85% according to McDonald, and 45% according to Poser.[44]

However, we shall restrict the present discussion to prediction of robust clinical endpoints and consider studies that 1) use only the (essentially prospective) information that a CIS occurred (If and when does conversion to MS occur?) or 2) perform a follow-up in a Poser clinically definite MS epidemiological material, which by definition contains a second attack (When does conversion occur?). The calculated median time to the second attack is expected to be longer (if reached at all) in the first type of analysis. The median time from the first to the second episode was 2 years in a 'when' study[45] and 3.25 years in an 'if and when' study.[34]

'IF AND WHEN' STUDIES OF A SECOND ATTACK AFTER OPTIC NEURITIS

Several predictive studies explored the prognosis of optic neuritis. This is a distinct entity in which it is feasible to obtain incidence-based material (a quality criterion for a random sample) for inclusion. Serial brain MRI was performed in 53 patients with clinically isolated optic neuritis. Multiple focal lesions were found in 34 patients. After a mean of 12 months follow-up, five of these 34 patients had developed both clinical and MRI relapses, while clinical relapse only was seen in seven and MRI recurrence in another seven. In 19 patients with normal MRI at presentation, three patients had new MRI lesions and none had a clinical relapse.[46] In a prospective study of a 6-year incidence cohort of optic neuritis ($n=147$), 36% developed clinically definite MS within 5 years. In this study, the presence of cerebral MRI lesions fulfilling the Paty criteria for 'MRI strongly suggestive of MS'[47] was associated with the development of MS with a sensitivity of 85% and a specificity of 65%, indicating a significant proportion of false positives. A CSF oligoclonal immunopathy was also associated with the development of MS within the 5-year follow-up period, with a sensitivity of 96% but a modest specificity of 42%, implicating that many patients remained in the possible category with an intrathecal oligoclonal reaction. Only four patients with an MRI strongly suggestive of MS were negative for oligoclonal bands, and two of these converted to positive at a subsequent CSF examination, implicating that a positive finding with MRI essentially predicted an oligoclonal reaction, while 31% of optic neuritis patients with oligoclonal bands at baseline did not fulfil the Paty criteria. The most distinct prediction comes from the negative findings: With a normal MRI study and normal CSF studies no patient converted to clinically definite MS within the 5-year interval[48] and this high negative predictive value was confirmed in other studies.[49]

In a 10-year follow-up study after a trial of high-dose corticosteroids in optic neuritis the risk of MS was 56%, with at least one lesion in the baseline MRI, whereas the risk was 22% with a normal baseline MRI study.[50] Still longer follow-up information was achieved by actuarial analyses indicating that the probability of developing clinically definite MS within 15 years was 75%.[51] However, a population based study with more complete long-term follow-up after optic neuritis found that 40% developed MS.[52] The latter study was recently extended to 19–31 years before a single follow-up examination was performed in 43 of 50 patients with previous optic neuritis. With the survival technique used, events (transition to MS) are expected to be less frequent with time; however, the distribution was highly skewed: 60% of the events indicating MS had developed within 3 years after the episode of optic neuritis and only one patient developed MS during the extension study. The proportion developing MS was similar to those found in a large clinical trial in optic neuritis.[50] MRI was not available at the onset; however, in their extension study, MRI data revealed cerebral lesions in 20/30 patients with optic neuritis only, and nine of these fulfilled the Barkhof–Tintoré criteria,[53] which were used in the recommended criteria for MS.[28] Repeat MRI was performed in 19 patients and in three of these the second examination showed new lesions while the clinical diagnosis was still isolated optic neuritis. The study confirmed that young age, initial CSF oligoclonal immunopathy and recurrent optic neuritis are risk factors for MS.[40]

In a population-based study using a strict criterion of a diagnosis of monosymptomatic optic neuritis the risk of a subsequent MS diagnosis continued to increase: The risk in a survival analysis was 39% after 10 years, 49% after 20 years and 54% after 30 years.[54]

'IF AND WHEN' STUDIES ON A SECOND ATTACK AFTER THE OTHER MAIN TYPES OF 'CLINICALLY ISOLATED SYNDROME'

Compared with the relative abundance of follow-up data in optic neuritis, only a small number of studies with limited follow-up time are devoted to the prognosis after a CIS presenting as a focal myelopathy or a brainstem lesion. The risk for subsequent MS is low after severe transverse myelitis, which however is known to have an etiological spectrum beyond MS. That said, when MS began with a mild to moderate focal, predominantly sensory myelopathy, the short-term outcome was positive with no further attacks in 88% of the cases; however, the follow-up was only 12 months on average.[55]

Prospective studies with successively longer follow-up after the CIS were performed at the National Hospital in London. They showed considerable predictive value of baseline MRI for the second episode and further, although some were possibly biased by moderate loss of follow-up. In a short-term follow-up study of the CIS, 23 patients with an isolated brainstem syndrome and 33 patients with an acute noncompressive spinal syndrome were followed for a mean of 14–15 months. At follow-up eight of the 23 brainstem patients had a second relapse (and new MRI lesions), all belonging to the group (17/23) with multifocal cerebral lesions at the initial MRI scan. Similarly, the follow-up of spinal onset syndromes showed a second relapse above foramen magnum in seven patients, all belonging to the group (18/33) with multifocal cerebral lesions at the initial MRI scan.[56] In a study with longer follow-up, consecutive CIS cases (n=89) were included during 7 years. Conversion to clinically definite MS was observed within 5 years in 65% of the patients (n=57), with at least one baseline MRI lesion compatible with MS, compared with only two of 32 cases with normal MRI.[57] For the 81 patients still followed at 10 years, the corresponding values were 83% and 11%.[58] At follow-up until 14 years, the proportion was 88% and 19% for the 71 patients remaining

under study.[29] Thus, the negative predictive value of a normal baseline MRI is somewhat weaker after longer follow-up.

Also the total lesion volume in MRI had predictive value. This was assessed in 58 patients 5 and 10 years after a CIS. All patients (n=11) with a high lesion volume (>3 ml) had developed MS before the 5-year follow-up, and 45% had a disability score greater than 6. In contrast, 22% (n=34) with the low volume had not developed clinically definite MS after 10 years, and only 15% had a disability score greater than 6. However, the predictive value of the total lesion volume became weaker as the disease progressed.[16] Generally, the predictive value of the first MRI study mirrors lesions from a long presymptomatic course, probably decades, while a repeat MRI study at 5 years of follow-up only produces additional information on the limited number of events that occurred in that interval. Integration with long-term prediction from clinical data is an important future task.

For short-term follow-up (2 years), the placebo arm of therapeutic trials, although a nonrandom patient selection, provided prospective data that may be used for prediction in similar cases. The cumulative probability of developing a second episode after 2 years, qualifying for a Poser diagnosis of clinically definite MS, was 38% in the placebo group of a trial of intramuscular interferon (IFN)β1a[30] and 45% in a trial of subcutaneous IFNβ1a.[31] The relative prognostic power of clinical versus MRI factors was not settled. In the first trial mentioned, the presence of enhancing lesions on the baseline MRI proved to be the strongest predictor for development of a second episode but this was not predictive in the second trial. The conversion rate from the CIS to clinically definite MS was double for multifocal compared with monofocal CIS in the second trial. Recently prediction of disability scores from a large database of cumulated placebo data with a median of 5.6 years of follow-up was presented from the Sylvia Lawry center in Munich.[59]

RISK OF A SECOND ATTACK IN MULTIPLE SCLEROSIS INCIDENCE STUDIES

These results were corroborated in 'if and when' studies based on MS incidence materials believed to have a complete ascertainment of the CIS events, combining neurology and ophthalmology. In a study based on the Danish national register, the mean delay from the first manifestation of MS to the final diagnosis of MS was longer in optic neuritis (6.1 years) than in other first attacks (4.2 years).[60] In the Gothenburg cohort, where different CISs were ascertained during the incidence period, the median delay from the CIS to clinically definite or probable MS was also significantly longer for optic neuritis (6.9 years) than for brainstem (2.7 years) and spinal cord (2.1 years) lesions. The elimination of topography as a prognostic factor by the Cox regression analysis in this study does not eliminate optic neuritis that was part of the 'system' analysis where 'afferent' remained significant in the final Cox analysis.[34] Figure 8.2 illustrates a 25-year follow-up after the CIS, showing the different prognosis after an onset attack with pure afferent or other (efferent and combined) symptomatology.[34]

COMPOSITE PREDICTIVE PARAMETERS

Comparison of several studies[16,34] with a common endpoint, the second episode indicating clinically probable or definite MS, demonstrates that MRI data have stronger short-term discriminating capacity from onset than the clinical predictors. However, the opposite conclusion, on the superiority of the clinical versus MRI predictors, was reached from studies somewhat later, yet still early in the course, from a database of placebo patients, a nonrandom sample, as discussed below.[61] The integration of

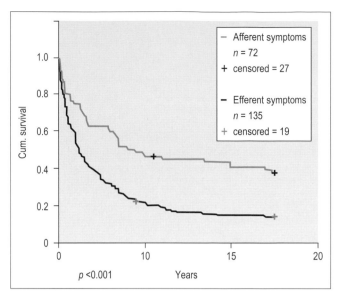

FIG. 8.2 Probability of a second attack after a CIS with pure afferent or including efferent symptom. 'Cum. survival' is the probability of not reaching the second attack. Redrawn from Eriksson et al 2003,[34] with permission from Sage Publications.

databases with short- and medium term prognostic MRI studies and long-term clinical studies is a challenge for future studies. Arbitrary integrated scores of MRI and clinical parameters, but not the clinical or MRI scores alone, were predictive in a short-term study of 98 consecutive cases seen at the time of the CIS or clinically definite MS (first attack could then be by history). Their endpoint was a sustained increase by 1 point in a disability score, a less intuitive and potentially erroneous endpoint,[62] yet widely utilized in clinical trials. 84% had MRI lesions suggestive of MS at the time of clinically definite MS. Based on previous experience, six prognostic factors were recorded: 1) age at onset, 2) symptoms at onset, 3) MRI status, 4) the interval between first and second attack, 5) attack frequency during the first 2 years and 6) the severity and completeness of recovery from the first attack (postattack Expanded Disability Status Scale (EDSS) score 1.5 or lower, or 2.0 and higher). Higher initial disability score or MRI status alone did not significantly predict final EDSS. However, time to sustained increase by 1 disability score point was 87 months for the existence of none to three of these combined prognostic factors, as compared to 34 months for more than three risk factors.[63]

PREDICTION INTEGRATING CLINICAL AND IMMUNOLOGICAL DATA

In addition to MRI parameters, some investigators claimed potential for biochemical parameters observed with the CIS to predict clinically definite MS with up to 3 years of follow-up, in addition to the CSF enriched oligoclonal IgG reaction discussed above. Myelin oligodendrocyte glycoprotein and myelin basic protein antibodies in the serum[64] were reported to predict the conversion to clinically definite MS. However, in three subsequent studies, one essentially confined to optic neuritis, prediction of clinically definite MS by these antibodies was not confirmed.[65] Other potential predictors identified in single studies were intrathecal IgM synthesis[66] and the 14-3-3 protein in the CSF.[67] In a study of 52 CIS patients, the sensitivity predicting conversion from the CIS to clinically definite MS was higher for tau protein level in the CSF (40%) than for MRI with

the Barkhof criteria (34%)[68] but increased to 60% when these two criteria were combined.[69]

THE PHASE OF RELAPSING–REMITTING MULTIPLE SCLEROSIS

The course after the first episode may be latent or stationary but new episodes usually supervene. The term stationary describes a latent state with residual symptoms. This latency may be lifelong, which is particularly liable to occur directly after the onset attack. When the 25-year follow-up of 100 patients from the Gothenburg incidence material was segmented into 2-year periods, it was found that the patients were in a progressive phase in 54% of the periods, in a latent or stationary phase in 30% and in a relapsing–remitting phase 16% of these periods.[70] The general symptomatology of subsequent relapses does not deviate significantly from that of the onset bout. There is an increased risk for each attack to localize in the same region as the previous episode. There is no systematic, craniocaudal or other topographic gradient. In a substantial proportion (131/837), attacks were migrating within a region (within the 1-month interval defining an attack) or were polyfocal (35/837 attacks) with a rapid series of recrudescences from new foci. There is no significant tendency for old lesions to flare up in conjunction with new distinct lesions, as might be expected if the main mechanism was epitope spread.[37] There is a distinct individual factor of good or worse capacity for recovery from attacks, documented by a significant ($p < 0.001$) tendency for the second attack to repeat the degree of remission (complete or incomplete) from the onset episode (unpublished data from the Gothenburg incidence cohort). The risk of incomplete recovery after bouts does not increase with time.[71]

The relapse frequency decreases spontaneously with time as evaluated in successive 5-year periods.[72] The risk of a relapse is largest immediately after a preceding relapse, and tapers with time. Expected relapse frequencies may be calculated from natural course databases, for power calculations. The relapse frequency during a subsequent year is on average lower than that observed during the present year. For instance, the risk of a further relapse during the subsequent year following a year with two attacks was estimated to be 56%.[73] In a recent study using placebo data compiled at the Sylvia Lawry Center, relapse frequency during the on-study period was predicted from the relapse frequency prior to the study together with the duration of the disease. In a multifactorial analysis, MRI gadolinium enhancement status, given the clinical covariates, had no independent influence on the on-study relapse rate.[61] These data may apply to a similar active patient population to the patients eligible for the trials; however, they cannot be generalized.

PSEUDORELAPSES

Pseudorelapses may be elicited by transient factors influencing the function of the diseased CNS, mainly increase in the body temperature or exhaustion. They mirror neurophysiological events in partially demyelinated areas and are not an essential part of the long-term course, nor of the immunopathology. Nevertheless, they are influenced by the ongoing type of course. Pseudorelapses tend to be echoes of recent relapses when they occur in the remitting–relapsing phase, while they tend to anticipate future progressive deficit when they appear, during the development of irreversible handicap, in the progressive phases (unpublished data from the Gothenburg incidence cohort). For instance, the development of a later persistent internuclear ophthalmoplegia or tetraparesis in a progressive phase may be anticipated during a transient pseudorelapse.

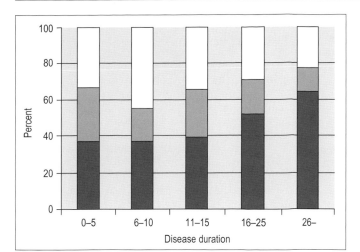

FIG. 8.3 Vocational status by disease duration in 5-year periods in prevalent patients aged 18–64 years. White fields, not sick listed; shaded fields, partially sick listed; black fields, sick listed. Proportion of patients on half and full sick leave correlates only vaguely to duration of MS. Redrawn from Sundström et al 2003,[74] with permission from Sage Publications.

EVOLUTION OF COGNITIVE SYMPTOMS AND FATIGUE

A large proportion of MS patients in the remitting–relapsing phase are on half- or full-time sick leave. This proportion was only vaguely related to the duration of the disease as evaluated in a multifactorial analysis[74] (Fig. 8.3). Although sick leave was correlated to disability as evaluated by the EDSS and age, the lack of correlation with duration strongly suggests the impact of an independent early MS-related factor on work ability. This factor probably includes cognitive symptoms, fatigue or a combination of both, and may even be decisive for the individual's working capacity in the presence of a considerable motor deficit. The fatigue score was higher in primary progressive ($n=20$) and secondary progressive ($n=70$) than in the relapsing–remitting course ($n=147$) but no correlation to disease course remained after correction for disability.[75] In a recent study, 80 patients were examined by a neuropsychological test battery showing cognitive impairment in 44–48%. 3-yearly re-examinations showed no deterioration.[76] In a study with relapsing–remitting ($n=42$) and progressive ($n=43$) patients it was found that the disease type, remitting or progressive, contributed to the prediction of performance in only three out of 15 cognitive variables measured.[77] In a 3-year longitudinal study, MS patients were divided into those cognitively preserved ($n=20$) and those who were cognitively mildly impaired ($n=22$). The first group was essentially stable whereas the second group showed continued progressive cognitive decline in several tests. There was no significant correlation with the EDSS.[78] In a series of mainly remitting patients a poor correlation was found between the extent of cognitive decline and clinical characteristics of the disease. However, both physical disability level and cognitive impairment were found to be independent predictors of working capacity.[79] Aspects of cognitive decline were described to occur sequentially in several studies. In one study, based on a cross-sectional analysis, it occurred at first in visuospatial learning. This was followed by delayed recall and then by delayed attention and information processing speed. Fatigue in MS persisted without relation to physical disability.[80] Cognitive percentile curves were claimed to be useful in evaluating the pattern of progression and identifying patients at increased risk of cognitive decline.[81]

PAIN AND PAROXYSMAL SYMPTOMS AND THE COURSE OF MULTIPLE SCLEROSIS

Several types of pain occur in MS. Painful paresthesia of different modalities may be associated with sensory relapses, with segmental or pseudoradicular distribution, and tend to remit. However, occasionally they persist stubbornly after a relapse. A few patients accumulate several areas of persisting unpleasant paresthesia. In contrast, the chronic deep-seated bilateral pain in back and legs called medullary pain is usually associated with a progressive parasyndrome.

Cranial neuralgia and paroxysmal symptoms appear to be evenly distributed between the relapsing–remitting and progressive phases. A few solitary epileptic attacks, mostly focal, occur in the relapsing–remitting phase, while the frequency of generalized attacks increases cumulatively to over 10% in the later progressive phase, associated with cognitive symptoms and higher disability.[82]

STATE AT THE ONSET OF SECONDARY PROGRESSION

The onset of secondary progression of neurological dysfunction is a milestone in the impact of the disease, which may or may not coincide with a point of incipient dissemination over the seven functional systems.[25] The secondary progression is characterized by a slow, generally nonremitting development of new symptoms, which may start subtly but almost invariably results in successive development of disability. At the stage of onset of the secondary progression, some residual symptoms from previous relapses have regularly accumulated; however, the patient may have made a complete recovery from previous relapses. Time to disability milestones such as EDSS 6 was similar in three categories selected to facilitate determination of time to onset of secondary progression:

- Cases of primary progressive disease
- Attack-onset disease where only a single attack had occurred before onset of progression ('single attack progressive')
- Secondary progressive disease in which substantial recovery from previous relapses allowed recognition of the earliest clinical stages when progression began, defined as DSS score less than 3.

There was no difference in the time to disability milestones between these three categories. The authors concluded that the progressive course is independent of relapses preceding or during the progression. It was suggested that the early remitting stages and the progressive phase have different pathogenesis.[83] Time of onset of secondary progression is often easy to determine when a hitherto unlimited normal walking capacity fails and an insidious pyramidal parasyndrome is observed. The range of uncertainty is then typically a few months up to 1–2 years. However, the time of onset is often identified retrospectively[84] and in many trials progression did not ensue as expected in the placebo group, although this was a basic criterion for eligibility.[85] In a few cases where two episodes occur, each with a course suggestive of incipient progression, the range of uncertainty may be a decade.[37]

TIME TO THE ONSET OF PROGRESSION

Total cohort studies are distinct from relapsing–remitting MS onset studies. Studies encompassing a cohort with progressive course as an endpoint will have a starting-point of the

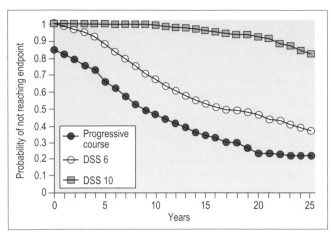

FIG. 8.4 Total cohort study. All patients with clinically definite or probable multiple sclerosis from the Gothenburg incidence cohort included. Endpoints are progressive course, or Disability Status Score (DSS) 6 (gait with support) and 10 (death from MS) according to the DSS. Individuals who died from other causes were censored to the right. The survival curve for progression does not start from probability 1.0, as primary progressive cases (approximately 15%) were included. Redrawn from Runmarker and Andersen 1993,[2] with permission from Oxford University Press.

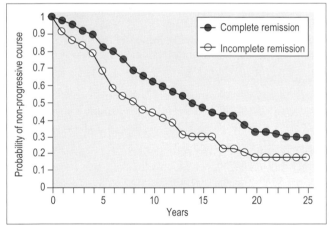

FIG. 8.5 Attack onset study in clinically probable or definite multiple sclerosis, not strictly prospective from the clinically isolated symptom. Time to secondary progression predicted from complete or incomplete remission of the onset attack. Lower risk after onset attack with complete remission. Redrawn from Runmarker and Andersen 1993,[2] with permission from Oxford University Press.

Kaplan–Meier curve at approximately 85% (allowing for approximately 15% primary progressive cases with endpoint year 0), while studies selecting for a relapsing–remitting initial course will start from 100% (Figs 8.4 and 8.5). The median time to progression in whole cohort studies was 11 years,[86] 9 years[2,34] or 6 years,[3,41] the latter containing a higher proportion of primary progressive cases. Approximately 80% of initially relapsing–remitting cases converted to secondary progression within two decades.[83]

In a hierarchical analysis where significant predictors were separated in a stepwise manner, the first step was demographic factors and the next step contained several factors (motor, insidious course) able to exclude primary progressive cases from the whole cohort. The following step revealed a significant effect of complete remission of the first attack, and thereafter the last attack was analysed.[26] However, an experienced neurologist, aware of the type of onset course, would probably want to start

with the third step, arguing that it is more relevant to study the time to secondary progression separately (and outcome in primary progressive MS cases separately). The median time to secondary progression among 1565 patients with an exacerbating-remitting onset in the Lyon series was 19 years, with 49% of patients having received immunomodulating treatment (mainly azathioprine with unproven but possible disease-modifying effect) at any time.[45] The corresponding median time in the Gothenburg series[2] was 16 years and in the Canadian series[3] between 11 and 15 years. Utilizing the availability of an incidence cohort with an allegedly complete retrieval of CIS only cases, and recomputing the 'if and when' prognosis from the CIS to the second attack in 220 patients, the median time to secondary progression was 19 years.[34]

THE COURSE OF SECONDARY PROGRESSION

The secondary progression is characterized by a slow, generally nonremitting development of new symptoms. The symptoms have, in contrast to the many distinctly focal lesions in the relapsing–remitting phase, a more symmetrical neurological topography, usually impossible to localize precisely by clinical topographical analysis, resulting from a cumulative effect of multiple lesions. In approximately 90% the initially dominating symptom is a progressive central paraparesis, often associated with bladder paresis, which may progress to a central tetraparesis. In approximately two-thirds of cases (unpublished data from Gothenburg incidence cohort) different degrees of cerebellar ataxia supervene. However, dissemination may reach all seven functional systems and all regions. Long-term follow-up reveals a slowly progressive optic neuropathy in approximately 20% of clinically probable and definite cases. A bilateral internuclear ophthalmoplegia is an important transient component of many brainstem attacks but frequently develops insidiously during secondary progression as part of a multisystem dissemination. Usually, sensory dysfunction occurs earlier in the posterior cord qualities (vibration, position sense) than in the spinothalamic qualities (pain),[2] which may, however, be explained by a higher safety factor in the spinothalamic system.

After 5 years of progression, 39 patients (out of 119 reaching that stage) had involvement of only one functional system,[25] 47 patients had two or three functional systems involved and 33 patients had involvement of four or more systems.[34] As a general rule, once progression has started it continues for a lifetime. However, it continues at very different paces. 30% of patients with chronic progressive disease (and 20% with progressive–relapsing disease) were considered stable.[87] Evaluated with a scoring system sensitive for small changes, stability may not be absolute, yet ultimate near-leveling out of the later progressive course was confirmed in one-third of the secondary progressive cases (unpublished data from Gothenburg incidence database). A more dramatic reversal of the progressive course, after years of incapacitating steady progression, occurs in a few cases initially dominated by cerebellar ataxia, with considerable improvement of neurological deficit during subsequent years, only to ultimately resume the insidiously progressive course now with a central para- or tetraparesis (unpublished data, Gothenburg incidence cohort). It has been speculated that this striking phenomenon is due to new focal lesions in the thalamic area counteracting the cerebellar symptomatology.

SUPERIMPOSED RELAPSES

Superimposed relapses are more numerous and important in secondary progression than in primary progression. One type of superimposed relapse supervenes separately, without interfering with the course and symptomatology of the ongoing steady progression. For instance, a tetrahypesthesia, with a sensory level indicating an acute focal cervical myelopathy, develops subacutely and remits, with symptoms indistinguishable from a typical relapse with acute myelopathy in the relapsing–remitting phase, independent of the ongoing insidious paraparesis (which usually has no distinct sensory level). Another type of superimposed relapse imitates and expands the progressive symptomatology, usually a parasyndrome. These superimposed attacks may be difficult to distinguish from fatigue-related pseudoattacks. A false impression of an acute deterioration, which may be termed an 'incompensation artifact', occurs when the patient does not pay attention to a slowly increasing disability and crosses the threshold to exhaustion. However, in secondary progression, superimposed attacks may also heal with residual symptoms. Nevertheless, superimposed attacks are generally not associated with an increase in the long-term EDSS accrual. The time between EDSS 4 and EDSS 6 was reported to be essentially the same with and without superimposed relapses.[32]

PRIMARY PROGRESSIVE AND PROGRESSIVE–RELAPSING COURSE

Insidious progression at onset regularly implicates the onset of a steadily progressive course. This type of course is, at that stage, termed primary progressive. In longitudinal series, primary progressive MS occurred in 14%,[2] 15%[1] or 20%[88] of patients. However, some of these cases will sooner or later have a superimposed relapse. After reclassification, the progressive–relapsing course was introduced as a fourth type of course.[89] The superimposed relapse activity is not severe, usually consisting of only a single mild and remitting relapse (often optic neuritis), which may sporadically occur even two to three decades after onset.[90] In the Canadian series, later relapses occurred in 28% of patients with a progressive onset. Time to long-term outcomes of disability, DSS 6, 8 and 10,[25] were not different between the primary progressive and the progressive–relapsing course.[91] (Kremenchutzky et al 1999).

MEDIAN TIME TO A DEFINED DISABILITY SCORE IN PRIMARY PROGRESSIVE MULTIPLE SCLEROSIS

While some therapeutic trials require objective gait and other performance tests for the higher scores of the disability scale, many epidemiological studies use a simplified schedule for the EDSS.[25] Thus, EDSS score 4 was used when ambulation starts to be restricted, score 6 when the patient needs gait support and score 7 when the patient becomes essentially confined to a wheelchair.[1] In the present chapter the terms 'DSS' and 'EDSS' are cited as used by the authors but no essential distinction is made between these two terms and the scales are referred to as the 'disability score'. However, score 10 must uncompromisingly be restricted to death from MS. In a Kaplan–Meier analysis, death from other causes must be accounted for by censoring to the right.

A primary progressive type of course is more frequent with onset at higher age and in males – two factors that are interrelated. The time from onset to sustained EDSS 6 in longitudinal databases was 6 years,[2] 7 years[1] or 8.5 years.[88] From the Canadian material of 1099 patients recruited between 1972 and 1984, and followed on an annual or biannual basis, 216 patients were finally identified with primary progressive MS. Reliable prediction was possible only from the time after the onset of progression. Patients with early progression, defined as time to

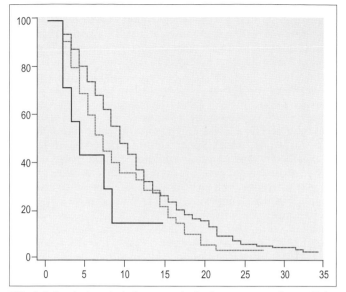

FIG. 8.6 Survival analysis from onset of primary progressive multiple sclerosis to Disability Status Score (DSS) 6. A total of 162 patients had one system involved at onset (long-dashed lines), 47 had two (short-dashed lines) and seven had three or more (continuous lines). 100 on the vertical axis is 1.00 probability. The prognosis was worse with more systems involved at onset of secondary progression. Redrawn from Cottrell et al 1999,[88] with permission from Oxford University Press.

DSS 3 2 years or less, reached level 8 of the DSS 10 years faster than those with slower initial progression, defined as 3 or more years to EDSS 3. Also, the number of functional systems involved influenced the prognosis (Fig. 8.6). Involvement of three or more neurological systems at onset of progression resulted in a median time to DSS 10 (death from MS) of 13.5 years. In contrast, primary progressive MS patients with one system involved at onset had a median time to DSS 10 of 33 years.[88] The predictor 'number of functional systems involved' is similar between primary and secondary progression.[34]

The findings in the three longitudinal databases were challenged by recent findings of a more benign course. A primary progressive MS study was terminated early, partly because of unexpectedly slow progression of the placebo group.[92] From their graphs the median time from diagnosis to EDSS 8 was 25 years (n=11).[93] However, as recognized by the authors, this is a transversal sample and it is therefore difficult to generalize. A recent study from British Columbia reported a longer median time of 13.3 years to EDSS 6 in primary progressive (including progressive–relapsing) MS, however with much variation. The authors found few predictors other than age at onset in the youngest group and time to EDSS 6, which predicted time for EDSS 8, expressed as 'sooner to cane, sooner to wheelchair'.[94] They did not claim to have an inception cohort and report a disability score (EDSS) of 4.9 at first assessment.

Several studies concluded that the speed of progression, as assessed by the time to disability milestones, was essentially similar in primary and secondary progressive MS.[7,32,83]

MEDIAN TIME FROM ONSET TO A DEFINED DISABILITY SCORE IN ATTACK ONSET AND SECONDARY PROGRESSIVE MULTIPLE SCLEROSIS

The median time to progression or to a defined handicap is dependent on the characteristics of the patients recruited to (and the patients missed from) the targeted cohort. Cohorts have different aims. Generally, the median time to a disability endpoint is shortest for the whole cohort, longer for the group of definite MS with attack onset and still longer in materials starting from a CIS. In the Lyon cohort, median time from the onset of MS to the assignment of EDSS score 6 was 20.1 years in the whole cohort and 23.1 years in patients with a relapsing–remitting initial course.[45] The median time to EDSS 6 was 24 years in the year 2000 prevalence cohort from Olmsted County.[7] In the Gothenburg incidence cohort, the median time from onset to EDSS 6 was 16 years in the whole cohort and 22 years with attack onset.[2] The time from attack onset to secondary progression was 12 years, while the 'if and when' median time to secondary progression from the CIS was 19 years.[34] In a Norwegian series from an area where MS prevalence had been thoroughly studied, improving the preconditions for a complete ascertainment, the interval to EDSS 6 was 20 years.[5] In the Canadian series, the time to EDSS 6 in the original cohort, including 30% primary progressive cases, was 15 years (Fig. 8.7).[3] A large study based on four MS clinics in British Columbia and utilizing a large common database found a much longer time to disability milestones, challenging the previous studies. The time to EDSS 6 was 27.9 years in the whole study and 30.3 years in the group with relapsing–remitting initial course. However, inclusion was dependent on contact with the MS clinics at specified times, and was not defined by onset during a specified period (an incidence period). In a subsequent study the proportion of benign cases at 10 years who were 'no longer benign' at 20 years was almost 50% suggesting a transition to a progressive course similar to other natural history studies.

THE CLUSTER OF PREDICTORS IN THE RELAPSING–REMITTING COURSE

There is a cluster of clinical predictors that are useful throughout the relapsing–remitting phase,[34] although they were more extensively analyzed in the initial stage of the disease. These factors are: 1) constitutional, e.g. sex; 2) probably subtle aspects of an individual constitution, e.g. the capacity for complete remission (Figs 8.5 and 8.8); and 3) symptoms that subtly probe and reveal the intensity and the progressive potential of the process already at an early stage.

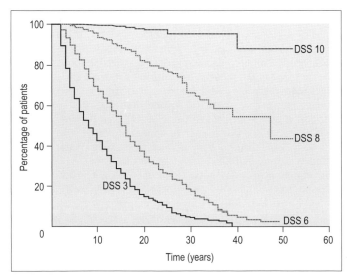

FIG. 8.7 Survival analysis to disability endpoints Disability Status Score (DSS) 3, 6, 8 and 10 according to the DSS. Total cohort study. The graph shows never ending activity of the disease during decennia but unexpected low mortality (DSS 10). Redrawn from Weinshenker et al 1989,[3] with permission from Oxford University Press.

One cluster predicts a benign course and the complementary features predict a more severe course. These predictive features in each cluster are partially but not completely interrelated. Generally the course will be increasingly benign with an increasing number of predictors from the benign cluster[96] (Fig. 8.9). Coefficients for prediction of future disability in a large natural history study were provided for optic neuritis, sensory symptoms, acute motor symptoms, diplopia and vertigo, all

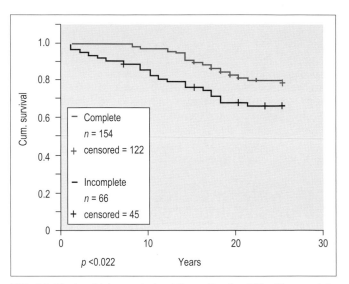

FIG. 8.8 Kaplan–Meier analysis of time after the CIS with complete or incomplete remission to Extended Disability Status Score (EDSS) 7 in CIS. Redrawn from Eriksson et al 2003,[34] with permission from Sage Publications.

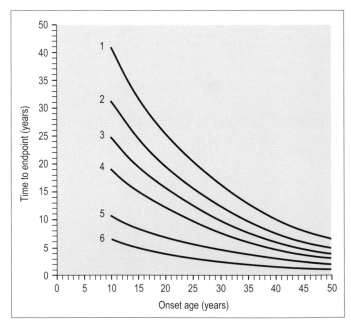
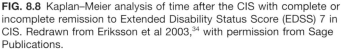

FIG. 8.9 Predicted median time (vertical axis) to onset of progressive course for males with different combinations of onset characteristics, calculated from coefficients in a multifactorial model. Increasingly benign course predicted from increasing number of predictors from benign cluster. 1) Complete remission of the onset attack, monoregional, pure afferent tracts. 2) As (1) but incomplete remission. 3) As (1) but symptoms from efferent and combined tracts. 4) Incomplete remission, and efferent and combined fibres. 5) Incomplete remission, polyregional but only afferent tracts. 6) As (5) but symptoms from efferent and combined tracts. Redrawn from Runmarker et al 1994,[96] with kind permission of Springer Science and Business Media.

associated with a relapsing–remitting course.[26] These coefficients may be recalculated as the ratio between the risk to reach an endpoint (e.g. DSS 6) in the presence of the benign or severe character of each variable. They may be included in models together with other coefficients, demographic and neurological, to estimate absolute time to a certain disability level (Fig. 8.9). A formula can predict time to a disability endpoint.[96] Ideally, this formula should be verified in other clinical materials but differences in variables and definitions have delayed reproduction of the studies to validate the model. However, this cluster of predictors in the early relapsing–remitting course was established in a large body of data evaluating the prognosis reaching to, but not encompassing, the progressive phase[34,86,97] (see Fig. 8.13).

DEMOGRAPHIC PARAMETERS

Older age at onset entails a worse prognosis in several studies with different techniques. Male sex is a negative prognostic factor. These two negative factors were observed in several studies and confirmed in long-term longitudinal studies.[1–3] They were synergistic in the Gothenburg series.[96]

THE INDIVIDUAL CAPACITY FOR REMISSION AS A PREDICTOR

The degree of remission from the first attack was a powerful predictor in several studies[2,26,34,45] (Figs 8.5 and 8.8). Later attacks in the relapsing–remitting phase had the same predictive capacity as the onset attack (Fig. 8.10). These results were obtained despite divergent definitions of the term 'complete' remission. In the Lyon series incomplete recovery was defined as the persistence of at least a minimum ambulation-related problem qualifying for a disability score (DSS) of 3 or more after the first neurological episode, indicating persistence of a substantial deficit. 18% of 1562 patients with relapsing–remitting course matched this definition of incomplete recovery after their first episode. The prediction from complete or incomplete recovery from the first relapse was forceful in the course after disability score 4, which was otherwise 'amnesic' or unpredictable.[45]

The Gothenburg incidence cohort used a far more sensitive criterion for incomplete recovery. This was fulfilled if any constant residual symptom persisted in the appropriate functional system[25] 1 year after the acute phase of the relapse.[2] The number of patients with complete recovery after the CIS was 154/220 and the number of patients with incomplete recovery was 66/220. The corresponding numbers after an early bout (arbitrarily selected as the last attack in the first 5-year period) was 69 and 66.[34] The individual tendency to remit tends to be repeated in the subsequent relapses (unpublished data from the Gothenburg incidence cohort), although an exceptional attack may leave severe residual symptoms between several attacks with good remission. A minority of patients accumulate residual symptoms from repeated relapses and their course may be classified as 'stepwise progression'. Some databases contain a number of patients in the relapsing–remitting phase with a high disability score (4–7).[45] However, the most dramatic cases previously reported as evidence of 'stepwise progression' in MS may instead show serology supporting a diagnosis of Devic's disease and post-mortem histological findings of subnecrotic lesions.[98]

THE CONTROVERSIAL ATTACK FREQUENCY

Whether attack frequency acts as a predictor remains controversial. Essentially negative results were produced in some studies,[99] including a study with a limited follow-up of 15 years.[100] However, several studies found that long first remission was significantly associated with a good prognosis,[101] and similarly a shorter interval between the first two attacks was associated with a higher risk for DSS 6 (essentially meaning need of support for gait). Patients who had one attack in the first 2 years had a median time of 20 years to requirement of a cane, while in patients with five or more attacks this duration

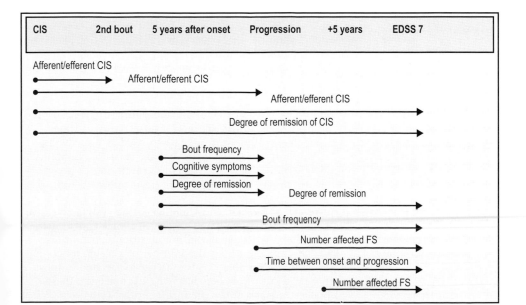

FIG. 8.10 Arrows indicate individual predictors that remained significant after Kaplan–Meier analysis followed by multivariate Cox analysis, as described in text. Predictors from: CIS, from a point in time 5 years after onset, from the onset of progression and from a point in time 5 years after the onset of secondary progression. Prediction of: time to the second relapse, time to the time of onset of secondary progression and to Extended Disability Status Score (EDSS) 7. Redrawn from Eriksson et al 2003,[34] with permission from Sage Publications.

was reduced to 7 years.[41,102] In the Gothenburg incidence cohort[2] attack number was without predictive capacity when examined as a continuous variable. Also, no predictive power was gained by dichotomizing the material in approximately equal halves (≤ 2 or ≥ 3 relapses/5 years). However, prognostic variables are often skewed against a smaller subgroup with a serious prognosis.[96] Further analysis of the Gothenburg incidence cohort[34] showed that the prognostic capacity of relapse frequency was linked to a high frequency subgroup (≥ 5 attacks/5 years), which is close to the predictive attack frequency in the Canadian series. The interaction between relapse frequency and remission is complex, with complete remission as a stronger positive factor overriding the negative effect of a high relapse frequency (unpublished results from the Gothenburg incidence cohort).

EARLY SYMPTOMS 'PROBING' AND PREDICTING THE SEVERITY OF THE DISEASE PROCESS

The functional systems[25] are not prognostically neutral. There is a higher 'safety factor' in the motor than in the sensory systems, which are symptomatically more eloquent.[37,103] When symptoms occur from less eloquent motor systems in any phase of the disease they indicate a more profound lesion related to a more severe prognosis.

Several studies unanimously describe that **sensory symptoms** in the first attack predict a favourable prognosis, largely independent of the method. In a hierarchical analysis based on the complete material, sensory symptoms at onset were a predictor for longer time to disability, while motor symptoms were negative both from onset and from the last visit.[26] The favourable prognosis associated with sensory symptoms remained significant in an attack onset sample[2] and in an 'if and when' analysis starting from the CIS.[34]

Optic neuritis generally predicts a longer time to a second attack, as discussed above, and also to later disability milestones.[1,4,6,41] However, in a direct comparison with the two other main CNS regions (spine and brainstem) the long-term prognosis for optic neuritis was more favourable only when possible cases (CISs only) were included, suggesting that the prediction is most important for the second bout.[2] There is no constant relationship between optic neuritis in the relapsing–remitting phase (often unilateral) and the later occurrence of optic nerve atrophy (often bilateral and part of a multisystem involvement) in the progressive phase.

Brainstem symptoms predict a favourable prognosis in some studies.[4] They must be separated from cerebellar syndromes, which are associated with progression. Brainstem symptoms were found to have a better prognosis than a cerebellar syndrome.[26] In the Gothenburg incidence cohort, there was a shorter interval to the second bout after an initial brainstem or spinal cord attack than after an optic neuritis, but this prediction was only significant for the transition to clinically definite MS, not for the time to secondary progression or later disability.[34]

Mono- or polyfocal symptomatology. Most authors found a better prognosis after an initial monofocal lesion.[2] A worse prognosis was found with a higher number of functional systems involved in both a total study and in a relapsing–remitting subgroup.[100] In a transversal study based on a prevalence study with a 24.5-year follow-up a better prognosis was found with monosymptomatic lesions.[6]

Each of these factors (or the complementary negative factors) has moderate independent predictive power, generally with risk ratios in the range of 2–3.[97] Multifactorial analysis using models (GLIM analysis)[96] reveals that the yearly risk of progression increases with an increasing number of the negative factors (Fig.

8.9). This model is based on multiplication, and in addition an interaction factor was identified between higher age and male sex, meaning that this combination has a particularly bad prognosis. However, the independence within the cluster is not absolute. Models that multiply these risk factors may exaggerate the predictive potential. Several studies tested the predictive power of early characteristics one by one in dichotomous Kaplan–Meier analysis (afferent yes/no, optic neuritis yes/no). Thereafter significant factors (often defined by $p < 0.1$) were selected for further testing with a Cox proportional hazards analysis for independent prediction. A matrix shows factors that were independently predictive in different stages of the disease. Some of the predictors are valid from the onset only, from the CIS only, or from an early relapse (arbitrarily, the last attack during the first 5-year period was chosen), and some are valid from a set of clinical predictors at the start of secondary progression, or 5 years after the onset of progression[34] (Fig. 8.10).

Not every study confirmed this cluster of predictors. A possible explanation for such negative results may be that mainly relapses requiring hospitalization were included, or relapse frequency was lower with longer (retrospective) duration in the study,[5] reducing the span of symptomatic variation constituting the source of prediction.

HOW WELL DOES THE CURRENT IMPAIRMENT LEVEL PREDICT SUBSEQUENT IMPAIRMENT LEVELS?

If the individual neurological deficit or impairment score at one stage could predict deficit or impairment score at any later stage of the disease, this would immensely facilitate prediction and provide convenient virtual placebo data for therapeutic trials in MS. A unique study provided evidence that each patient's course follows a given, seemingly predetermined path. The progression was described graphically from a scoring system and a formula calculating deficit scores for the continued course. The individual accumulation of neurological deficit smoothly followed a curve described by this formula, and in some cases extrapolation backwards to the time of onset was successful. However, the scoring system was redundant, which may have contributed to the smoothness of the curves. The formulas used by the authors to describe the curves included polynomia that are not biologically interpretable. As the material was based on data from a rehabilitation center, there may have been a selection of steadily progressive cases.[104]

Prediction from the present disability level can use different approaches:

- **Input: The patient's score at one point in time. Desired output: the disability score at a later point in time.** Although disability score was often used as a predictor, the endpoint was usually the average time to a disability endpoint rather than the patient's condition at a given time after onset. In the Gothenburg incidence cohort, the deficit at year 5 was predictive for the time to EDSS 6. However, at that point in time, a scoring system sensitive for multi-system involvement (the Regional Functional Systems Score (RFSS)[105]) did not contribute significantly more to prediction than the number of affected functional systems. The number of systems was correlated to most other prognostic variables but, when considering these variables one at a time, the number of systems was still independently significant.[2] A strict evaluation method widely used in clinical trials, the MS functional composite (MSFC), was found to predict later disability.[106] However, a severe limitation of early prognostic factors is their restriction to the relapsing–remitting phase. The rate of the subsequent progression was reported to be unpredictable, impossible to predict from the previous course.[34,45] On the other hand, it was reported that the time between later disability milestones was relatively constant between patients.[45] If a patient has reached score 4 of the EDSS and we want to know when she will reach score 7, could we just add the time interval reported to lapse between score 4 and 7 in a large sample? The time from assignment of score 4 to 7 was 10 years for males and 13 years for females.[45] The reported 95% confidence intervals of 4 years in males and 3 years in females were relatively narrow, which seem reasonable for a progressive course, although still too wide for a precise prognosis.

- **Input: A 'progression index' based on disability scores at two points in time. Desired output: Disability score at a later point in time.** The actuarial analysis revealed that the time (short, intermediate or long) from onset to disability score 3 significantly predicted the time from disability score 3 to 6.[41] However, the scatterplots revealed marked interindividual variation, precluding a precise individual prognosis. Furthermore, this relationship was only marginally confirmed.[93]

- **Input: The patient is assigned at one point to a severity percentile from a large reference study[107,108] and the output is the prognosis in terms of the same percentile throughout the disease.** In a recent study, a set of percentile curves (reminiscent of growth curves) was provided from the EDSS scores for consecutive years 1–10 in a large reference material with frequent observations, describing the average deterioration of the patient cohort. However, for patients assigned to the 25% percentile there was only a 75% probability of remaining within this percentile at 10 years of follow-up, while patients assigned to the 50th percentile retained an 88% probability of remaining in this percentile.[107] Thus, there was a considerable tendency for individual patients to cross between percentile tiers, limiting its usefulness for prediction. Nevertheless, as emphasized by the authors, the recording method may be useful to detect particularly devastating change or therapy failure. A similarly structured study was based on a transverse multicenter study. For each of 25 years after onset, available patients were ranked in deciles from the lowest to the highest EDSS score in a very large European reference sample. This effectively normalized the EDSS by converting it to a decile score, termed the Multiple Sclerosis Severity Score (MSSS), which is more informative than a crude 'EDSS index' (EDSS score/disease duration). The MSSS allows for a comparison of disease progression from single assessments in patients. However, there was also in this study a considerable tendency for patients to cross between percentile tiers, which according to the authors precluded its use as a predictor of future disability in an individual.[108]

LIMITATION OF PREDICTORS TO THE CURRENT PHASE

As described in the previous sections, MRI data in the initial stages are powerfully predictive of the risk of a second episode[68] and also seem to be predictive of the course as examined up to 14 years after onset.[29] For longer prediction, the cluster of predictors in the relapsing–remitting stage, as described above, are moderately strong predictors of the onset of secondary progression and the only existing predictor for later disability. However, there is now consensus that prediction from the onset attack is

limited to the relapsing–remitting phase. The rate or speed of secondary progression cannot be predicted from onset or early relapse phase characteristics. With a shorter range, the average rate of progression can be predicted by factors present at the time of onset of secondary progression, with similar predictors to those for primary progression. Why then, can average time to disability score 7 be predicted from the characteristics of the onset attack?[34] The prediction of time to these late disability milestones may conceivably be a consequence of the power to predict the time to a progressive course, combined with a more invariant time interval spanning the initial progressive phase. This was confirmed in a series of recent studies from the Lyon group. The median times from score 4 to 6 or 7, observed to be 5.7 and 12.1 years, were not influenced by any potential predictor in their study, nor by gender, age at onset of MS, or early features. Their conclusion was astute: progression of irreversible disability is 'amnesic' (unpredictable) for the clinical characteristics of the relapses that occurred during the initial stages of the disease.[32] In the recent British Columbia study the time from disability score 3 to 6 was shorter only for a subgroup with very rapid progression to disability score 3 (<5 years) but otherwise independent of the time to disability score 3.[95] In the year 2000 prevalence material from Olmsted County, the rate of progression from onset to EDSS 3 did not influence the time from EDSS 3 to EDSS 6.[93] In the Gothenburg incidence material, the time from MS onset to the start of the progressive phase showed only negligible correlation with the rate of progression. The other early prognostic factors were unable to predict the rate of secondary progression. This conclusion was maintained with progression speed either measured as time to DSS 6 from start of progression[2] or as increment of deficit during the progressive phase with a scoring system sensitive for multi-system dissemination.[34]

However, if the patient reaches the onset phase of secondary progression, new predictors become available at that stage. Like the corresponding early predictors, these are essentially components of the course. At the start of progression a higher number of functional systems involved, or a higher deficit score with a system sensitive for multisystem dissemination (RFSS),[105] increased the risk of reaching EDSS 7. The risk of reaching EDSS 7 was doubled with two to three Kurtzke functional systems[25] involved and was 17 times higher with lesions in four or more functional systems. In a confirmatory analysis, a higher number of Kurtzke functional systems was associated with a higher rate of progression evaluated as an increment in deficit with the Regional Functional Systems Score[34] (Fig. 8.11). This is similar to the prediction from the number of Kurtzke functional systems in primary progressive MS discussed above.[88]

Long-standing apparently benign relapsing/remitting disease can occasionally terminate in very disabling progressive disease. In contrast, after a protracted relapsing–remitting phase with benign relapses, a progressive phase may ensue almost imperceptibly, with continued insidious and extremely slow progression, which may appear to arrest for several years in terms of the EDSS.

CASE REPORT 3

A woman with a severe and well documented central vestibular episode at age 25 developed, after 30 years of latency with complete freedom from symptoms, parahypesthesia, which remitted. Thereafter she developed within a few months an encephalopathy with multifocal progression, including moderate dementia and internuclear ophthalmoplegia. Extensive investigations were negative for degenerative and infectious processes but revealed clinical, cerebrospinal and MRI findings typical of MS.

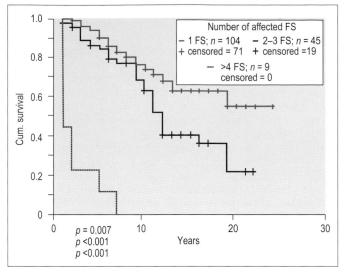

FIG. 8.11 Prediction from number of Kurtzke functional systems involved during the year of onset of secondary progression, one, two to three or four or more systems. Kaplan–Meier analysis of the risk to reach Disability Status Score (DSS) 7 after the onset of secondary progression. Redrawn from Eriksson et al 2003,[34] with permission from Sage Publications.

ONE EXTREME OF THE COURSE: THE ISSUE OF 'BENIGN' CASES

'Benign' may be an ambiguous term without information on follow-up time, but historically it is important. Charcot described in his lectures how diplopia often remitted and paraparesis often progressed. He described *formes frustes*, where the disease activity seemed to cease.[109] (Charcot 1875). Initial series of so-called benign MS had limited follow-up, approximately 10 years. Nevertheless they defined the set of positive predictors used today.[101,110] In a 37–50 year follow-up of the Gothenburg incidence cohort (n=308) the proportions of benign cases of clinically definite or probable MS (excluding possible cases), defined as patients with freedom from progression and a maximum EDSS of 4.0, was 36% after 30 years and 21% after 40 years.[111]

The indirect evidence from unsuspected MS revealed at autopsy may be considered to be of limited value, as late-life medical records retrieved in order to document freedom from MS were usually completely dedicated to other health problems.[112] However, a bold attempt was made, from frequencies of unsuspected MS at neuropathological examinations and total frequencies of neuropathological examinations performed in Denmark, to estimate 'clinically silent' MS, which was found to correspond to one-quarter of the mortality with in vivo diagnosis of MS.[113] During the ascertainment phase for the Gothenburg incidence cohort, unsuspected MS was found at autopsy in a case with schizophrenia and sequel after poliomyelitis that could obviously have concealed the MS. In a case of optic neuritis and a slight sensory episode, disseminated demyelinating lesions were detected at autopsy performed when the patient died from an unrelated cause many years later.[114] Such findings are less astonishing in the MRI era.

Another important group of patients with a benign course are those who suffer one clinical episode only, the possible MS cases who experience no new symptoms after the CIS. The proportion of patients who are asymptomatic after a CIS is difficult to ascertain since such studies demand a complete 'seen from onset' case retrieval (an 'if and when' study is required).

An optic neuritis study that fulfilled these criteria and had a complete follow-up reported a 55% probability of escaping a second bout after 15 years.[52] In the Gothenburg incidence cohort, claiming a reasonable coverage of all types of the CIS during the incidence period, 20% remained free from symptoms after 25 years of follow-up. The lower proportion as compared with optic neuritis may be explained partly by the higher propensity for the non-optic-neuritis CISs to progress to MS, and admittedly by the difficulty to ascertain all acute central vestibular syndromes and focal myelopathies (as compared to optic neuritis cases).[34]

THE SKEWED SPECTRUM OF RISK

A spectrum of risk scores based on yearly risk for transition to the secondary progressive phase was described in the relapsing–remitting phase. The distribution in a model according to severity was inhomogeneous, with about 80% showing a moderate risk score for the transition to progression rate, while approximately 20% showed a considerable deviation with much higher risk scores.[96] A similar distribution of the crude progression index (EDSS change/year) in the progressive phase was reported,[3] with a relatively even distribution of patients between progression index 0.0–1.2, and a small subgroup with much higher index of 1.4–2.0.

THE ISSUE OF 'MARBURG MULTIPLE SCLEROSIS'

Marburg MS is a variant with extremely fast progression, with a relentless series of prolonged and hardly remitting bouts leading to death in between a few months and 1–2 years.[115] In the Gothenburg 15-year incidence material (1950–64), there were 2/308 patients who belonged to this category. In one additional patient the disease process surprisingly stopped after the Marburg-like phase, providing an extreme example of the phenomenon of levelling-out.

We did not observe any further Marburg cases after 1964. However, two personal cases had an acute-disseminated-encephalomyelitis-like initial phase, with weeks of impaired consciousness and with a moderate sequel succeeded by a series of slight to moderate relapses. Initial high-dose corticosteroid therapy may have influenced the course.

> ### CASE REPORT 4
>
> A previously healthy male experienced at age 24 problems with gait and coordination. A steadily progressive cerebellar tetra-ataxia developed, associated with cognitive deterioration and incipient deficit in all functional systems. Apart from a short period of improvement the progression was swift and relentless. After 2 years the patient was in a helpless state, with dementia, ataxia described as almost ballistic, and vision below Snellen 0.1. His CSF showed an oligoclonal immunological reaction. After 5 years he was paralytic and responseless. He had spontaneous respiration but needed continuous respiratory care with suction. At that stage the disease activity seemed to stop and the patient remained in this vegetative state until he died at age 46. Histological examination confirmed a diagnosis of MS, of unusual severity with almost total demyelination of the brain and spinal cord, axon loss in severely involved areas but relatively conserved in the cortex and basal ganglia, and a perivascular lymphoplasmacytic inflammatory reaction close to the ventricles.

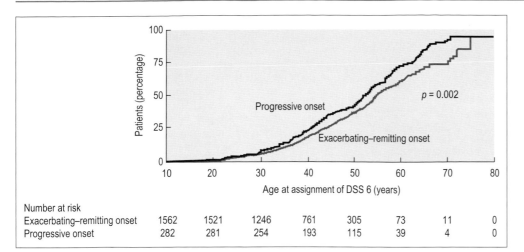

FIG. 8.12 Similar distribution of age at assignment of Disability Status Score (DSS) 6 for exacerbating-remitting and progressive onset. Redrawn from Confavreux and Vukusic 2006,[32] with permission from Oxford University Press.

DISABILITY AS A FUNCTION OF AGE: THE HAZARD FUNCTION FOR TRANSITION TO PROGRESSION

After updating their comprehensive long-term Lyon database, Confavreux and co-workers found that important milestones of disability, EDSS scores 4, 6 and 7, occur at similar ages in primary and secondary progression, independently of initial predictors. Similar results were obtained in two other studies, suggesting that the two types of progressive phase have a similar pathogenesis.[34,83] However, the Lyon group goes beyond the common median age for primary and secondary progression disability checkpoints, contending that age universally determines the evolution of disability in MS. As mentioned in the section on the progression of irreversible disability from EDSS 4 to EDSS 6 and EDSS 7 was the same in the total relapsing–remitting material as in the cases selected to be secondary progressive. They found that all categories, relapsing–remitting, primary and secondary progressive MS have a roughly similar age for the disability milestones.[1] Thus, they find a final common path for all MS patients, regardless of any conceived predictor (Fig. 8.12).[32] Their confidence intervals on the median are narrow, which does not exclude substantial and important variability. Indeed, their presentation of percentiles is more instructive. Furthermore, cases are mainly expected to be informative concerning higher disability after transition to secondary progression, and patients remaining in the relapsing–remitting course in the Lyon cohort had indeed a shorter duration, so a more benign subgroup may escape from the presentation. Ages at which successive age at onset cohorts reach milestone disability are at increasingly close intervals, suggesting that the hazard function is increasing with increasing age at onset.[32] In the Gothenburg incidence cohort, a maximum in the hazard function was distinctly seen around age 45 when the hazard function for secondary progression at each age of onset is considered separately (Fig. 8.13).[96]

RELATIVE CONTRIBUTION FROM RELAPSES VERSUS PROGRESSION TO THE ULTIMATE DEFICIT

There is a consensus that the main component of the handicap associated with MS accumulates during the progressive phases while the contribution from the attacks is slight to moderate.

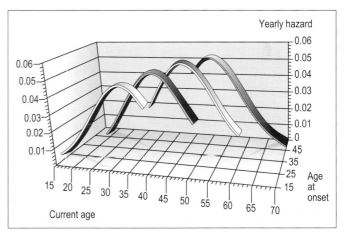

FIG. 8.13 The predicted risk of a progressive course was calculated for different onset age groups as a function of current age in the group of patients with complete remission of the onset episode. The risk has a maximum based on the subdivision of the cohort into four age groups. Redrawn from Runmarker et al 1994,[96] with permission from Sage Publications.

Graphic reconstructions of the course (deficit/time) with a scoring system sensitive for multisystem dissemination of neurological deficit (RFSS)[105] allowed for measurements of the relative contribution from relapses and progression to the ultimate neurological deficit in a subgroup ($n=20$) of the Gothenburg incidence cohort. In patients with a relapsing–remitting course, this deficit score after 25 years was mainly attributable to residual symptoms after relapses (average deficit score approximately 1/100). On the contrary, after a course with transition to a secondary progressive phase the accumulated deficit after 25 years was mainly attributable to steady progression (average RFSS deficit score approximately 16/100), and less than 10% to residual symptoms after relapses (average RFSS deficit score approximately 2/100).[70] The major part of severe disability accumulates during the progressive phases, although relapses may remit with partial or discrete residual symptoms, which nevertheless may be focal and distinct enough to be traced back to specific relapses. Neurological deficit does not mirror the cumulative impact of relapses: Cerebrospinal fluid markers reveal axonal disintegration during relapses,[116] which is probably irreversible, while neurological deficit is compensated by several mechanisms.

MORTALITY

The proportion of survivors in the Gothenburg MS incidence cohort was 75% after 25 years, compared to 88% in the general Swedish population. The cause of death was MS in 20/49 cases and a combination including MS in 10/49 cases.[72] In a study on survival based on the Danish Multiple Sclerosis Registry, the average time from onset to death was estimated to be 28 years for men and 33 years for women. Their survival curves indicate that the median time from onset to death is about 10 years shorter for the MS patients than for the general population. MS was associated with an almost threefold increase in mortality. According to death certificates, 56% of the patients died from MS. However the patients also had excess mortality from vascular and infectious diseases, but not from cancer. Death from infections may represent combinations with MS. A secular trend of decreasing mortality was ascertained, plausibly interpreted as an effect of improved general medical care over time. Thus, the 10-year excess mortality was almost halved at the end of observation by 1996, as compared with the first included patients from 1949 (Fig. 8.14).[117] In a study devoted to the cause of death in patients attending MS clinics, the cause could be determined in 82%. Of these, 47% were directly attributed to the effects of MS.[118] Mean age at death from MS in the Canadian series of primary progressive MS was 58.8±12.0 years and from other causes 66.8±9.9 years. Approximately two-thirds of patients who developed primary progressive MS died as a direct result of the complications of MS.[88]

PREGNANCY AND THE COURSE OF MULTIPLE SCLEROSIS

After several studies suggested that the relapse rate diminishes during pregnancy, the multicenter Pregnancy in Multiple Sclerosis Study confirmed this association in a prospective study of 227 women with pregnancy as an inclusion criterion, and prospective follow-up. The average retrospective prepregnancy rate was 0.7±0.9/year, which diminished to 0.2±1.0 in the third trimester of pregnancy and rebounded to 1.2±2.0 per year in the 3-month postpartum period. During the following 21 months, the relapse rate fell slightly but did not differ from the rate in the prepregnancy year. During the total 45 months period on study there was a 0.9 point increase in the EDSS, close to the expected increment over time.[119] Few studies addressed the question of whether pregnancy leaves an imprint, immunological or other, on the disease process. One study revealed no impact of pregnancy on subsequent long-term disability.[120] However, a study based on the Gothenburg cohort demonstrated a 3.2 times diminished yearly risk for transition to the progressive phase after pregnancy compared with non-pregnant controls in the same cohort. The internal case-control procedure arbitrarily matched previously pregnant and never-pregnant women with less than 2 years difference in duration, less than 5 years difference in age and a minimal difference in deficit score. Possibly, a confounding factor (undetermined, but conceivably representing an aspect of vitality favouring the decision to become pregnant) in the case-control procedure was associated with both pregnancy and a favourable course. Therefore no conclusion is warranted on any causal interaction between the pregnant state and the long-term outcome of MS. Nevertheless, pregnancy may disclose (or be a marker for) otherwise elusive predictors for a favourable course.[121]

INFECTIONS AND THE COURSE OF MULTIPLE SCLEROSIS

Previous studies demonstrated a moderately increased risk of MS relapses during intervals, termed 4 or 7 weeks 'at risk' periods[122] encompassing the onset of upper respiratory infections. The increased risk, expressed as a risk ratio between bouts during and outside these 'at risk' periods, differed between studies. The ratio was 2.8 in the next extensive prospective study.[123] However, in a subsequent study using strictly prospective methodology with controlled monthly reports, it was only 1.3 for the 4 weeks 'at risk' period, and nonsignificant for the 7 weeks 'at risk' period.[124] Two subsequent studies, part of IFNβ

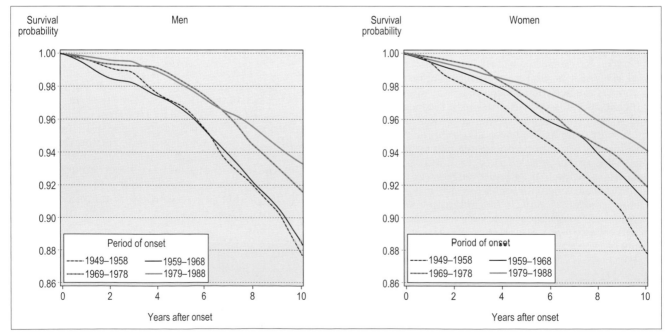

FIG. 8.14 10-year survival probability for 1949–58, 1959–68, 1969–78 and 1979–88 of men and women with MS aged 35 years at onset, by period of onset. Reduced mortality over decades probably due to general improved medical care. Redrawn from Brønnum-Hansen et al 2004,[117] with permission from Oxford University Press.

trials, showed a maximum risk 1–2 weeks after the infection when reporting weekly relapse frequencies.[125,126] In a recent prospective study with a strict follow-up schedule, this risk ratio was 2.1, and 3.8 for a subgroup of major relapses.[127] While a moderate surplus risk for relapses seems to exist in the 'at risk' interval, the etiology of a specific trigger infection, if any, remains to be determined. A relationship between adenovirus complement fixation titer increases and 'at risk' relapses was reported.[124] In another prospective study, Epstein–Barr virus antibodies (in particular the antibodies against the viral capsid antigen) were stated to increase with attacks, while influenza, parainfluenza and adenovirus antibodies fluctuated. The Epstein–Barr virus finding was dismissed as unspecific activation.[125] In a case-control study, influenza and other vaccinations did not increase the risk of relapse in MS.[128] A recent study using polymerase chain reaction on nasal swab specimens for picorna- and coronaviruses, and culture for other upper respiratory tract infection viruses, showed that 7/9 MS relapses were associated with picornavirus, most probably human rhinovirus infections. Relapses were retrospectively identified[129] and confirmation is needed.

Two studies failed to show any relationship between upper respiratory tract infections and cerebral MRI activity.[126,127] Some doubt was cast upon the relationship between upper respiratory tract infections and clinically defined relapses, when MRI demonstrated new lesions with a frequency 5–10 higher than that of the clinical relapses. However, this criticism may not be justified, as studies on neurofilament light protein as a CSF marker of axonal damage revealed a temporal relationship between clinical relapses and axonal damage, with the conclusion that clinical relapses are not just the result of lesions in more eloquent CNS regions but also indicate more destructive lesions.[116]

A longer perspective was explored in a questionnaire study on past infectious events in 251 MS patients. The investigators found a more active disease, with higher symptom and attack frequencies, in the group of patients with a history of repeat respiratory infections starting in childhood.[130]

GENETIC INFLUENCE ON THE COURSE OF MULTIPLE SCLEROSIS

While genetic factors influence susceptibility to MS there are so far limited indications that genetic factors influence its natural course. An association between the severity of MS and apolipoprotein E alleles was reported but not confirmed.[131] The HLA type influenced the risk for the development of clinically definite MS after optic neuritis;[48,52] however its influence on the course of established MS seems to be marginal.[2,132] The time to disability milestones DSS 6, 8 or 10 did not differ between sporadic and familial cases, although onset was earlier in the most heavily loaded families.[133] Thus, familial disposition only marginally influenced the natural history of MS.

THE DESIGN OF NATURAL COURSE STUDIES: LIMITING VARIABILITY IN THE FLOW OF PATIENTS

Considerable variation in the prognosis exists between reports from different regions. While marked differences exist between European and some eastern Asian patients, we confine the present discussion to European- and North American-type MS with probably only moderate genetic differences between areas. In Asia, a change was reported in the disease phenotype, while we presently assume that the phenotype of Western MS is relatively constant. However, some doubt was recently cast upon

that assumption when a major change in the sex ratio was reported to have occurred over the last three decades.[134]

CASE MIX

A decisive factor for the outcome, the case mix resulting from recruitment, which may be from a hospital series, from MS rehabilitation centers, from centers performing clinical trials, from prevalence studies or from geographically defined 'spider' studies, is not easily controlled in natural history studies. There is a major difference between searching and retrieving patients from a defined onset cohort and recruiting consecutive patients at contact with a clinic. Time from onset to initial clinic contact was provided in some studies ('seen from onset' cases by Weinshenker et al,[3] 60% of remitting cases seen from onset in Runmarker and Andersen 1993[2] and average 6 years delay by Confavreux et al[1]). A particularly representative base for the follow-up study may be patients from a prevalence survey or repeat surveys already performed.[5,6,135] Incidence-based studies come closer to a random sample. An incidence cohort is defined not only by the geographical boundaries but also by time limits for onset of MS. Ideally, the recruitment effort needs to 1) overlap with the incidence period to retrieve all 'CISs' but also to 2) go on for several years afterwards, to ascertain patients who do not seek advice until their second or later bout, and then verify the onset retrospectively (Fig. 8.15).[2,72] A cohort may mature and be more representative for a local population of MS patients if it is based upon repeat surveys.[83]

FOLLOW-UP

The Kaplan–Meier survival analysis – which is the basic statistical method for this type of follow-up – has the distinct advantage of accepting nonparametric endpoints but demands information on endpoint or censoring for each unit time (year). Therefore, a transverse (prevalence) study is not enough, longitudinal follow-up is necessary. However, investigators may well contend that the quality of their clinical data is more important than the exact ratio between retrospective/prospective follow-up data.[2,3,45]

REGIONAL RESULTS – WHEN CAN THEY BE GENERALIZED?

Consequently, it is impossible to control all factors in a clinical study (as in a laboratory study). Nevertheless, local results on prognosis could be useful for the patient flow at a certain time and place. For instance, early hospital-based series with a preponderance of severe cases (extensively reviewed by Müller[136]) were conceivably representative for the patients in the hospital setting. A subgroup of 'seen from onset' patients had a moderate preponderance of cases with worse prognosis, as pointed out in a classical study[3] and may be relevant for similar subgroups. However, the risk of too limited a prognosis is not only associated with extremes of benign or malignant course but with any restriction in ascertainment, e.g. the inclusion of a tier of medium severity patients in MS clinics (Fig. 8.15). The EDSS at first contact was 4.9 or 5 for primary progressive MS,[95,102] while corresponding data for relapsing–remitting onset patients are not available. The British Columbia study, ideally based on four large MS clinics, presents a long retrospective course, which may be quite sufficient for the follow-up but raises questions on the crucial inclusion procedure. If there is no strict prevalence or incidence base, the resulting case mix may be determined by later admission policy for the activities at the MS clinics.[95] A prospective study based on prevalence surveys of the Icelandic population presented an exceptionally favorable prognosis.

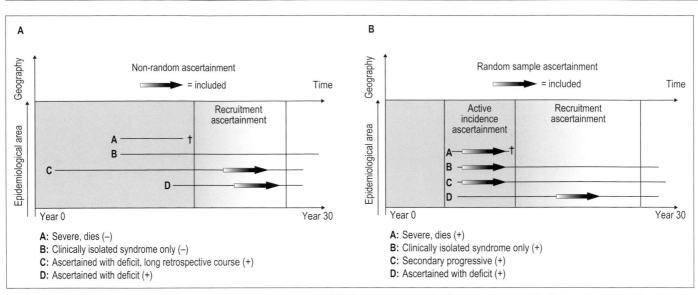

FIG. 8.15 A. Nonrandom case ascertainment. Vertical axis: geographical area. Horizontal axis: time. Geographically based study with recruitment at relatively late stage. Thin lines, disease course; broad arrows, actual recruitment to the study, with some delay. 'Ascertained with deficit' indicates that the patient already developed some neurological deficit and sought advice for treatment or rehabilitation. Retrospective reconstruction of course need not be a problem. However, benign and malignant course may be missed, skewing the ascertainment.
B. Random sample ascertainment. Vertical axis: geographical area. Horizontal axis: time. Thin lines, disease course; broad arrows, actual recruitment to the study. Incidence cohort included, and recruitment effort continued only for patients with onset during the incidence period.

However, their analysis probably did not account for the possible omission of severe (and mortal) cases from the cohort.[137]

NATURAL HISTORY STUDIES AND FUTURE TRIALS

Based on the dissociation between attack frequency and rate of secondary progression,[1] investigators contended that the current anti-inflammatory and immunomodulating drugs, which reduce relapse frequency and modify MRI parameters, would probably have no effect on long-term disability due to axonal degeneration. They proposed that the focus instead should be on neuroprotection[33] or on immediate attempts to induce remyelination.[138] However, the relationship between inflammation and neurodegeneration is complex and the relationship may be mutual throughout the course. Slow progression may be a feature of the presymptomatic stage.[20] And in addition to axonal degeneration severe immunopathology develops during the progressive phases, such as the establishment of a chronic blood–brain-barrier lesion in the plaques.[139]

At the present time, randomized placebo-controlled phase III studies of immunomodulatory drugs for therapy of MS are designed as 2- or 3-year trials (and one 2-year study with a 2-year randomized extension). These trials provided pivotal information on short-term therapeutic efficacy. However, further desired information on the capacity of these immunomodulatory drugs to prevent disease progression and the accrual of irreversible handicap cannot be gained from these studies. Moreover, ethical considerations restrain the institution of new randomized placebo-controlled trials in the relapsing–remitting phase when therapy, admittedly only moderately efficacious, is available, let alone trials of longer duration. This situation has been anticipated by designers of natural history studies, who have constructed models for dimensioning and evaluation of future trials.[73,140]

A direct comparison between data from long-term extensions of clinical trials and natural history data was reported in two studies.[141,142] An open-label extension study was performed after up to 35 months in the placebo-controlled pivotal phase III trial of glatiramer acetate. A total of 208 of the 251 patients originally randomized chose to continue in the open-label phase over 3 years. At the end of the open-label phase 40.6% showed sustained progression. This was compared with data concerning one-step EDSS progression from onset after 6 years in the tables of Weinshenker,[140] showing that only 23% of the untreated patients escaped progression at that stage.[141] However, a major incongruity exists between patients in the open-label and the natural history cohorts, as the latter contains 30% of primary progressive MS patients, thereby expanding the apparent therapeutic effect.

Another follow-up study was performed at an average of 6.1 years after the end of a 2-year pivotal placebo-controlled study of weekly intramuscular IFNβ-1a. Patients were managed by their own neurologists until an 8-year follow-up, which was achieved for 93% of eligible patients. The proportion who had reached EDSS 6 was compared with a natural history group of relapsing–remitting MS patients. The percentages reaching the endpoint were 63.3% for the original placebo group and 55.8% for the original IFNβ-1a group. The proportion expected to reach the endpoint with frequencies for transition from EDSS 1 to EDSS 2, EDSS 2 to 3, etc. was calculated in a complex manner from Weinshenker's data,[3] indicating treatment effect sizes of 75–90%. The authors conclude that the cohorts are probably not comparable, leaving the efficacy question without an answer for the present time and questioning the usefulness of historical controls.[142] Secular trends due to improved general medical care change mortality[117] and possibly disability endpoints. Probably, comparisons of treated groups with natural history cohorts need more precise comparisons, similar to case-control techniques, with stratifications of patients having the same predictors in both cohorts.

KEY FEATURES OF MULTIPLE SCLEROSIS NATURAL HISTORY

- There is a presymptomatic stage of intrathecal immunological reaction that may last for decades. This immunopathy may develop to clinically manifest MS or remain asymptomatic.
- There is a presymptomatic stage of insidious function loss, documented in the visual tracts.
- The initial dichotomy of the course of MS into relapsing–remitting or primary progressive course is the single most decisive prognostic factor. Common genetics and the continuity of clinical characteristics argue against the idea that these are two different diseases.
- There is a cluster of predictors in the early stages of relapsing–remitting course, predicting the time to secondary progression and disability milestones. Some of these predictors are constitutional, such as the capacity for restitution, and some are symptoms of the early course, such as the number and type of functional systems involved.
- The rate of secondary progression is unpredictable from the onset of the disease. The primary and secondary progression courses have a similar rate, and the medians of their development of disability show the same age-dependence. These events are under control of factors independent of factors controlling the attacks.
- The hazard function for secondary progression (of each age at onset group) has an age-related maximum.
- Pregnancy and the puerperium have a profound short-term effect on relapse frequency and are associated with a lower risk of secondary progression.
- Epidemiological methods reveal only slight effects of acute infections in manifest MS.
- While it is established that genetic factors influence susceptibility, there is so far not much evidence that single genetic factors influence the course of MS. However, results from experimental studies suggest that polygenetic effects control a number of factors of inflammation, degeneration and restitution, which determine the natural course.

BIOLOGY OF NATURAL HISTORY KEY FEATURES

Inflammation and neurodegeneration seem to be intimately and mutually related throughout the course of MS. Neurodegenera-

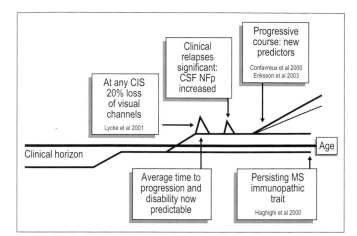

FIG. 8.16 A summary of the course, from presymptomatic course, to detectable deficit of which the individual is not aware, premonitory symptoms, relapses, progression and the possibility of remaining in an asymptomatic MS immunopathic trait stage. The limitation of prediction is outlined.

tion seems to be important for the symptoms, as inferred from cases with extensive demyelination seen at MRI or autopsy but with few symptoms. Relapses and progression dominate in early and late phases of the disease, yet they often occur in combination. The preclinical course is often described as remitting; however, evidence is lacking and the disease may well be progressive from its preclinical onset, as suggested from the insidious nature of deficit at onset (Fig. 8.16).[20] While new lesions are revealed by MRI at a frequency 5–10 higher than new relapses, the clinical relapses are associated with shedding of neurofilament protein into the CSF, indicating that they are destructive, not simply hitting more eloquent regions.[116] The existence of a large number of susceptibility genes was established in experimental studies, and some of these genes were syntenic with human genes.[143] A number of quantitative trait loci, each with possible immunological and environmental interactions, may thus be associated with any of the above key features, in particular the degree of inflammation, the capacity for restitution and the propensity for neurodegeneration, shaping the individual natural course of MS.

REFERENCES

1. Confavreux C, Vukusic S, Moreau T, Adelaine P. Relapses and progression of disability in multiple sclerosis. N Engl J Med 2000; 343: 1430–1438.
2. Runmarker B, Andersen O. Prognostic factors in a multiple sclerosis incidence cohort with twenty-five years of follow-up. Brain 1993; 116: 117–134.
3. Weinshenker B, Bass B, Rice G et al. The natural history of multiple sclerosis: a geographically based study 1. Clinical course and disability. Brain 1989; 112: 133–146.
4. Hammond S, McLeod J, Macaskill, English D. Multiple sclerosis in Australia: prognostic factors. J Clin Neurosci 2000; 7: 16–19.
5. Myhr KM, Riise T, Vedeler C et al. Disability and prognosis in multiple sclerosis: demographic and clinical variables important for the ability to walk and awarding of disability pension. Mult Scler 2001; 7: 59–65.
6. Phadke J. Clinical aspects of multiple sclerosis in north-east Scotland with particular reference to its course and prognosis. Brain 1990; 113: 1597–1628.
7. Pittock S, McClelland R, Mayr W et al. Clinical implications of benign multiple sclerosis: a 20-year population-based follow-up study. Ann Neurol 2004; 56: 303–306.
8. Massacesi L, Parigi A, Barilaro A et al. Efficacy of azathioprine on multiple sclerosis new brain lesions evaluated using magnetic resonance imaging. Arch Neurol 2005; 62: 1843–1847.
9. Fernandez O, Fernandez V, De Ramon E. Azathioprine and methotrexate in multiple sclerosis. J Neurol Sci 2004; 223: 29–34.
10. Patzold U, Pocklington P. Azathioprine in multiple sclerosis – a 3-year controlled study of its effectiveness. J Neurol 1980; 223: 97–117.
11. Weinshenker BG, Sibley WA. Natural history and treatment of multiple sclerosis. Curr Opin Neurol Neurosurg 1992; 5: 203–211.
12. Rot U, Mesec A. Clinical, MRI, CSF and electrophysiological findings in different stages of multiple sclerosis. Clin Neurol Neurosurg 2006; 108: 271–274.
13. Andersen O, Lindholm A. Tissue typing of CSF lymphocytes in MS. Acta Neurol Scand 1976; 54: 464–466.
14. Haghighi S, Andersen O, Rosengren L et al. Incidence of CSF abnormalities in siblings of multiple sclerosis patients and

unrelated controls. J Neurol 2000; 247: 616–622.

15. Lycklama à Nijeholt GJ, Uitdehag BMJ, Bergers E et al. Spinal cord magnetic resonance imaging in suspected multiple sclerosis. Eur Radiol 2000; 10: 368–376.

16. Sailer M, O'Riordan J, Thompson AJ et al. Quantitative MRI in patients with clinically isolated syndromes suggestive of demyelination. Neurology 1999; 52: 599–606.

17. Lucchinetti CF, Kiers L, O'Duffy A et al. Risk factors for developing multiple sclerosis after childhood optic neuritis. Neurology 1997; 49: 1413–1418.

18. Beck RW, Kupersmith MJ, Cleary PA, Katz B. Fellow eye abnormalities in acute unilateral optic neuritis. Experience of the optic neuritis treatment trial. Ophthalmology 1993; 100: 691–7.

19. Frisén L. High-pass resolution perimetry: central-field neuroretinal correlates. Vision Res 1995; 35: 293–301.

20. Lycke J, Tollesson PO, Frisén L. Asymptomatic visual loss in multiple sclerosis. J Neurol 2001; 248: 1079–1086.

21. Sullivan MJ, Weinshenker B, Mikail S, Edgley K. Depression before and after diagnosis of multiple sclerosis. Mult Scler 1995; 1: 104–108.

22. Joffe R, Lippert G, Gray T et al. Mood disorder and multiple sclerosis. Arch Neurol 1987; 44: 376–377.

23. Polliack ML, Barak Y, Achiron A. Late-onset multiple sclerosis. J Am Geriatr Soc 2001; 49: 168–171.

24. Whitlock FA, Siskind MM. Depression as a major symptom of multiple sclerosis. J Neurol Neurosurg Psychiatr 1980; 43: 861–865.

25. Kurtzke JF. Further notes on disability evaluation in multiple sclerosis, with scale modifications. Neurology 1965; 15: 654–661.

26. Weinshenker BG, Rice GPA, Noseworthy JH et al. The natural history of multiple sclerosis: a geographically based study 3. Multivariate analysis of predictive factors and models of outcome. Brain 1991; 114: 1045–1056.

27. Poser CM. Clinical diagnostic criteria in epidemiological studies of multiple sclerosis. Ann NY Acad Sci 1965; 122: 506–519.

28. McDonald WI, Compston A, Edan G et al. Recommended diagnostic criteria for multiple sclerosis: guidelines from the International Panel on the diagnosis of multiple sclerosis. Ann Neurol 2001; 50: 121–127.

29. Brex P, Ciccarelli O, O'Riordan J et al. A longitudinal study of abnormalities on MRI and disability from multiple sclerosis. N Engl J Med 2002; 346: 158–164.

30. Jacobs LD, Beck RW, Simon JH et al. Intramuscular interferon beta-1a therapy initiated during a first demyelinating event in multiple sclerosis. CHAMPS study group. N Engl J Med 2000; 343: 898–904.

31. Comi G, Filippi M, Barkhof F et al. Early Treatment of Multiple Sclerosis Study Group. Effect of early interferon treatment on conversion to definite multiple sclerosis: a randomised study. Lancet 2001; 357: 1576–1582.

32. Confavreux C, Vukusic S. Age at disability milestones in multiple sclerosis. Brain 2006; 129: 595–605.

33. Confavreux C, Vukusic S. Accumulation of irreversible disability in multiple sclerosis: from epidemiology to treatment. Clin Neurol Neurosurg 2006; 108: 327–332.

34. Eriksson M, Andersen O, Runmarker B. Long-term follow up of patients with clinically isolated syndromes, relapsing–remitting and secondary progressive multiple sclerosis. Mult Scler 2003; 9: 260–274.

35. Svenningsson A, Runmarker B, Lycke J, Andersen O. Incidence of MS during two fifteen-year periods in the Gothenburg region of Sweden. Acta Neurol Scand 1990; 82: 161–168.

36. Poser CM. Onset symptoms of multiple sclerosis. J Neurol Neurosurg Psychiatr 1995; 58: 253–254.

37. Andersen O. Restricted dissemination of clinically defined attacks in an MS incidence material. Acta Neurol Scand 1980; 66(suppl): 77.

38. Fukazawa T, Moriwaka F, Hamada K et al. Facial palsy in multiple sclerosis. J Neurol 1997; 244: 631–633.

39. Hanner P, Andersen O, Frisén L et al. Clinical observations of effects on central nervous system in patients with acute facial palsy. Arch Otolaryngol Head Neck Surg 1987; 113: 516–520.

40. Nilsson P, Larsson E, Maly-Sundgren P et al. Predicting the outcome of optic neuritis. J Neurol 2005; 253: 396–402.

41. Weinshenker B, Bass B, Rice G et al. The natural history of multiple sclerosis: A geographically based study 2. Predictive value of the early clinical course. Brain 1989; 112: 1419–1428.

42. Miller DH, McDonald I, Compston A. Multiple sclerosis in the individual and in groups: a conspectus. In: Compston A, ed. McAlpine's multiple sclerosis. Edinburgh: Churchill Livingstone; 2006: 442.

43. Polman CH, Wolinsky JS, Reingold SC. Multiple sclerosis diagnostic criteria: three years later. Mult Scler 2005; 11: 5–12.

44. Kappos L, Polman CH, Freedman MS et al. Treatment with interferon beta-1b delays conversion to clinically definite and McDonald MS in patients with clinically isolated syndromes. Neurology 2006; 67: 1242–1249.

45. Confavreux C, Vukusic S, Adelaine P. Early clinical predictors and progression of irreversible disability in multiple sclerosis: an amnesic process. Brain 2003; 126: 770–782.

46. Miller DH, Ormerod IEC, McDonald WI et al. The early risk of multiple sclerosis after optic neuritis. J Neurol Neurosurg Psychiatr 1988; 51: 1569–1571.

47. Paty DW, Oger JJ, Kastrukoff LF et al. MRI in the diagnosis of MS: a prospective study with comparison of clinical evaluation, evoked potentials, oligoclonal banding, and CT. Neurology 1988; 38: 180–185.

48. Söderström M, Ya-Ping J, Hillert J, Link H. Optic neuritis: prognosis for multiple sclerosis from MRI, CSF, and HLA findings. Neurology 1998; 50: 708–714.

49. Rolak LA, Beck RW, Paty DW et al. Cerebrospinal fluid in acute optic neuritis: experience of the optic neuritis treatment trial. Neurology 1996; 46: 368–372.

50. Beck RW, Smith CH, Gal RL et al. Optic Neuritis Study Group. Neurologic impairment 10 years after optic neuritis. Arch Neurol 2004; 61: 1386–1389.

51. Francis DA, Compston DA, Batchelor JR, McDonald WI. A reassessment of the risk of multiple sclerosis developing in patients with optic neuritis after extended follow-up. J Neurol Neurosurg Psychiatr 1987; 50: 758–765.

52. Sandberg-Wollheim M, Bynke H et al. A Long-term prospective study of optic neuritis: Evaluation of risk factors. Ann Neurol 1990; 27: 386–393.

53. Tintoré M, Rovira A, Martinez MJ et al. Isolated demyelinating syndromes: comparison of different MR imaging criteria to predict conversion to clinically definite multiple sclerosis. Am J Neuroradiol 2000; 21: 702–706.

54. Rodriguez M, Siva A, Cross SA et al. Optic neuritis: a population-based study in Olmsted County, Minnesota. Neurology 1995; 45: 244–250.

55. De Seze J, Stojkovic T, Breteau G et al. Acute myelopathies. Clinical, laboratory and outcome profiles in 79 cases. Brain 2001; 124: 1509–1521.

56. Miller DH, Ormerod IEC, Rudge P et al. The early risk of multiple sclerosis following isolated acute syndromes of the brainstem and spinal cord. Ann Neurol 1989; 26: 635–639.

57. Morrissey SP, MillerDH, Kendall BE et al. The significance of brain magnetic resonance imaging abnormalities at presentation with clinically isolated syndromes suggestive of multiple sclerosis. Brain 1993; 116: 135–146.

58. O'Riordan JI, Losseff NA, Phatouros C et al. Asymptomatic spinal cord lesions in clinically isolated optic nerve, brain stem, and spinal cord syndromes suggestive of demyelination. J Neurol Neurosurg Psychiatr 1998; 64: 353–357.

59. Daumer M, Griffith LM, Meister W et al. Survival, and time to an advanced disease state or progression, of untreated patients with moderately severe multiple sclerosis in a multicenter observational database: relevance for design of a clinical trial for high dose immunosuppressive therapy with autologous stem cell transplantation. Mult Scler 2006; 12: 174–179.

60. Sørensen TL, Frederiksen JL, Brønnum-Hansen H, Petersen HC. Optic neuritis as onset manifestation of multiple sclerosis. A nationwide, long-term survey. Neurology 1999; 53: 473–480.

61. Held U, Heigenhauer L, Shang C et al; the Sylvia Lawry Centre for MS Research. Predictors of relapse rate in MS clinical trials. Neurology 2005; 65: 1769–1773.

62. Liu C, Blumhardt LD. Disability outcome measures in therapeutic trials of relapsing–remitting multiple sclerosis: effects of heterogeneity of disease course in placebo cohorts. J Neurol Neurosurg Psychiatr 2000; 68: 450–457.

63. Scott T, Schramke C, Novero J, Chieffe C. Short-term prognosis in early relapsing–remitting multiple sclerosis. Neurology 2000; 55: 689–693.

64. Berger T, Rubner P, Schautzer F et al. Antimyelin antibodies as a predictor of clinically definite multiple sclerosis after a first demyelinating event. N Engl J Med 2003; 349: 139–145.

65. Kuhle J, Pohl C, Mehling M et al. Lack of association between antimyelin antibodies and progression to multiple sclerosis. N Engl J Med 2007; 356: 371–378.

66. Villar LM, Masjuan J, González-Porqué P et al. Intrathecal IgM synthesis predicts the onset of new relapses and a worse disease course in MS. Neurology 2002; 59: 555–559.

67. Martinez-Yelamos A, Saiz A, Sanchez-Valle R et al. 14-3-3- protein in the CSF as prognostic marker in early multiple sclerosis. Neurology 2001; 57: 722–724.

68. Barkhof F, Filippi M, Miller D et al. Comparison of MRI criteria at first presentation to predict conversion to clinically definite multiple sclerosis. Brain 1997; 120: 2059–2069.

69. Brettschneider J, Petzold A, Junker A, Tumani H. Axonal damage markers in the cerebrospinal fluid of patients with clinically isolated syndrome improve predicting conversion to definite multiple sclerosis. Mult Scler 2006; 12: 143–148.

70. Andersen O, Runmarker B. Natural history of multiple sclerosis. State of the art conference jointly organized by the World Health Organization, International Federation of Multiple Sclerosis Societies and Société Suisse de la Sclérose en Plaque, Geneva, 1998: 20–21.

71. McAlpine D, Compston N. Some aspects of the natural history of disseminated sclerosis. Q J Med 1951; 82: 135–167.

72. Broman T, Andersen O, Bergmann L. Clinical studies on multiple sclerosis. Acta Neurol Scand 1981; 63: 6–33.

73. Andersen O. Multiple sclerosis incidence material data used in the design of clinical trials. In: Immunological and clinical aspects of multiple sclerosis. Boston, MA: MTP Press; 1984: 110–118.

74. Sundström P, Nyström L, Svenningsson A, Forsgren L. Sick leave and professional assistance for multiple sclerosis individuals in Västerbotten County, northern Sweden. Mult Scler 2003; 9: 515–520.

75. Pittion-Vouyovitch S, Debouverie M, Guillemin F et al. Fatigue in multiple sclerosis is related to disability, depression and quality of life. J Neurol Sci 2006; 243: 39–45.

76. Jönsson A, Andresen J, Storr L et al. Cognitive impairment in newly diagnosed multiple sclerosis patients: A 4-year follow-up study. J Neurol Sci 2006; 245: 77–85.

77. Beatty WW, Goodkin ED, Hertsgaard D, Monson N. Clinical and demographic predictors of cognitive performance in multiple sclerosis. Arch Neurol 1990; 47: 305–308.

78. Kujala P, Portin R, Ruutiainen J. The progress of cognitive decline in multiple sclerosis. Brain 1997; 120: 289–297.

79. Amato MP, Ponziani G, Siracusa G, Sorbi S. Cognitive dysfunction in early-onset multiple sclerosis: a reappraisal after 10 years. Arch Neurol 2001; 58: 1602–1606.

80. Tellez N, Rio J, Tintoré M et al. Fatigue in multiple sclerosis persists over time : a longitudinal study. J Neurol 2006; 253: 1466–1470.

81. Achiron A, Polliack M, Rao SM et al. Cognitive patterns and progression in multiple sclerosis: construction and validation of percentile curves. J Neurol Neurosurg Psychiatr 2005; 76: 744–749.

82. Eriksson M, Ben-Menachem E, Andersen O. Epileptic seizures, cranial neuralgias and paroxysmal symptoms in remitting and progressive multiple sclerosis. Mult Scler 2002; 8: 495–499.

83. Kremenchutzky M, Rice G, Baskerville J et al. The natural history of multiple sclerosis: a geographically based study 9: observations on the progressive phase of the disease. Brain 2006; 129: 584–594.

84. Minderhoud JM, van der Hoeven JH, Prange AJ. Course and prognosis of chronic progressive multiple sclerosis. Results of an epidemiological study. Acta Neurol Scand 1988; 78: 10–15.

85. Weinshenker B, Issa M, Baskerville J. Long-term and short-term outcome of multiple sclerosis. Arch Neurol 1996; 53: 353–358.

86. Confavreux C, Aimard G, Devic M. Course and prognosis of multiple sclerosis assessed by the computerized data processing of 349 patients. Brain 1980; 103: 281–300.

87. Waubant E, Goodkin D. Methodological problems in evaluating efficacy of a treatment in multiple sclerosis. Pathol Biol 2000; 48: 104–113.

88. Cottrell DA, Kremenchutzky M, Rice GPA et al. The natural history of multiple sclerosis: A geographically based study 5. The clinical features and natural history of primary progressive multiple sclerosis. Brain 1999; 122: 625–639.

89. Lublin FD, Reingold SC. Defining the clinical course of multiple sclerosis: results of an international survey. Neurology 1996; 46: 907–911.

90. Andersson PB, Waubant E, Gee L, Goodkin DE. Multiple sclerosis that is progressive from the time of onset. Arch Neurol 1999; 56: 1138–1142.

91. Kremenchutzky M, Cottrell D, Rice G et al. The natural history of multiple sclerosis: a geographically based study 7. Progressive-relapsing and relapsing-progressive multiple sclerosis: a re-evaluation. Brain 1999; 122:1941–1945.

92. Wolinsky J. New insights in primary progressive multiple sclerosis (conference proceedings: 20th Congress of the European Committee for Treatment and Research in Multiple Sclerosis). Mult Scler 2004; 10(suppl 2): S110.

93. Pittock SJ, Mayr, WT, McClelland RL et al. Disability profile of MS did not change over 10 years in a population based prevalence cohort. Neurology 2004; 62: 601–606.

94. Tremlett H, Paty D, Devonshire V. The natural history of primary progressive MS in British Columbia, Canada. Neurology 2005; 65: 1919–1923.

95. Sayao A, Devonshire V, Tremlett H. Longitudinal follow-up of 'benign' multiple sclerosis at 20 years. Neurology 2007; 68: 496–500.

96. Runmarker B, Andersson, Odén A, Andersen O. Prediction of outcome in multiple sclerosis based on multivariate models. J Neurol 1994; 241: 597–604.

97. Ebers GC. Natural history of multiple sclerosis. J Neurol Neurosurg Psychiatr 2001; 71(suppl II): 16–19.

98. Wingerchuk DM, Lennon VA, Pittock SJ et al. Revised diagnostic criteria for neuromyelitis optica. Neurology 2006; 66: 1485–1489.

99. Kurtzke JF, Beebe GW, Nagler B et al. Studies on the natural history of multiple sclerosis. 8. Early prognostic features of the later course of the illness. J Chronic Dis 1977; 30: 819–830.

100. Amato MP, Ponziani G, Bartolozzi, ML, Siracusa G. A prospective study on the natural history of multiple sclerosis: clues to the conduct and interpretation of clinical trials. J Neurol Sci 1999; 168: 96–106.

101. Thompson A, Hutchinson M, Brazil J et al. A clinical and laboratory study of benign multiple sclerosis. Q J Med N Ser 1986; 58, 225: 69–80.

102. Ebers GC. The natural history of multiple sclerosis. Neurol Sci 2000; 21: S815-S817.

103. Campbell B. The factor of safety in the safety in the nervous system. Bull Los Angel Neuro Soc 1960; 25: 109–117.

104. Fog T, Linnemann F. The course of multiple sclerosis in 73 cases with computer-designed curves. Acta Neurol Scand 1970; 47: 3–175.

105. Andersen O, Runmarker B, Lycke J. Video presentation of a sensitive scoring system, the RFSS. Eur J Neurol 1996; 3(suppl 5): 115–116.

106. Rudick RA, Cutter G, Baier M et al. Use of the Multiple Sclerosis Functional Composite to predict disability in relapsing MS. Neurology 2001; 56: 1324–1330.

107. Achiron A, Barak Y, Rotstein Z. Longitudinal disability curves for predicting the course of relapsing–remitting multiple sclerosis. Mult Scler 2003; 9: 486–491.

108. Roxburgh RH, Seaman SR, Masterman T et al. Multiple Sclerosis Severity Score: using disability and disease duration to rate disease severity. Neurology 2005; 64: 1144–1151.

109. Charcot JM. Leçons sur les maladies du système nerveux faites a la Salpêtrière, 2nd edn. Paris: A Delahaye; 1875.

110. McAlpine D. The benign form of multiple sclerosis. A study based on 241 cases seen within three years of onset and followed up until the tenth year or more of the disease. Brain 1961; 84: 186–203.

111. Skoog B, Runmarker B, Andersen O. A 37–50 year follow-up of the Gothenburg multiple sclerosis cohort. Mult Scler 2004; 10(suppl 2): S156.

112. Gilbert J, Sadler M. Unsuspected multiple sclerosis. Arch Neurol 1983; 40: 533–536.

113. Engell T. A clinical patho-anatomical study of clinically silent multiple sclerosis. Acta Neurol Scand 1989; 79: 428–430.

114. Fog T, Hyllested K, Andersen SR. Acta Neurol Scand Suppl 1972; 51: 369–370.

115. Marburg O. Die sogenannte 'multiple Sklerose'. Jahrb Psychiatr Neurol 1906; 27: 211–312.

116. Lycke J, Karlsson JE, Andersen O, Rosengren LE. Neurofilament protein in cerebrospinal fluid: a potential marker of activity in multiple sclerosis. J Neurol Neurosurg Psychiatr 1998; 64: 402–404.

117. Brønnum-Hansen H, Koch-Henriksen N, Stenager E. Trends in survival and cause of death in Danish patients with multiple sclerosis. Brain 2004; 127: 840–850.

118. Sadovnick AD, Eisen K, Ebers GC, Paty DW. Cause of death in patients attending muktiple sclerosis clinics. Neurology 1991; 41: 1193–1196.

119. Vukusic S, Hutchinson M, Hours M et al, the Pregnancy In Multiple Sclerosis Group. Pregnancy and multiple sclerosis (the

PRIMS study): clinical predictors of post-partum relapse. Brain 2004; 127: 1353–1360.

120. Roullet E, Verdier-Taillefer MH, Amarenco P et al. Pregnancy and multiple sclerosis: a longitudinal study of 125 remittent patients. J Neurol Neurosurg Psychiatr 1993; 56: 1062–1065.

121. Runmarker B, Andersen O. Pregnancy is associated with a lower risk of onset and a better prognosis in multiple sclerosis. Brain 1995; 118: 253–261.

122. Sibley WA, Foley JM. Infection and immunization in multiple sclerosis. Ann NY Acad Sci 1965; 122: 457–466.

123. Sibley WA, Bamford CR, Clark K. Clinical viral infections and multiple sclerosis. Lancet 1985; 1: 1313–1315.

124. Andersen O, Lygner P, Bergström T et al. Viral infections trigger multiple sclerosis relapses: a prospective seroepidemiological study. J Neurol 1993; 240: 417–422.

125. Panitch H. Influence of infection on exacerbations of multiple sclerosis. Ann Neurol 1994; 36S: 25–28.

126. Edwards S, Zvartau M, Clarke H et al. Clinical relapses and disease activity on magnetic resonance imaging associated with viral upper respiratory tract infections in multiple sclerosis. J Neurol Neuropsychiatr 1998; 64: 736–741.

127. Buljevac D, Flach H, Hop W et al. Prospective study on the relationship between infections and multiple sclerosis exacerbations. Brain 2002; 125: 952–960.

128. Confavreux C, Suissa S, Saddier P et al, Vaccines in Multiple Sclerosis Study Group. Vaccinations and the risk of relapse in multiple sclerosis. N Engl J Med 2001; 344: 319–326.

129. Kriesel JD, White A, Hayden FG et al. Multiple sclerosis attacks are associated with picorna virus infections. Mult Scler 2004; 10: 145–148.

130. Lamoureux G, Lapierre Y, Ducharme G. Past infectious events and disease evolution in multiple sclerosis. J Neurol 1983; 230: 81–90.

131. Burwick RM, Ramsay PP, Haines JL et al. APOE epsilon variation in multiple sclerosis susceptibility and disease severity: some answers. Neurology 2006; 66: 1373–1383.

132. Masterman T, Hillert J. HLA-DR15 and age at onset in multiple sclerosis. Eur J Neurol 2002; 9: 179–180.

133. Ebers GC, Koopman WJ, Hader W et al. The natural history of multiple sclerosis; a geographically based study 8: familial multiple sclerosis. Brain 2000; 123: 641–649.

134. Orton SM, Herrera BM, Yee IM et al, Canadian Collaborative Study Group. Sex ratio of multiple sclerosis in Canada: a longitudinal study. Lancet Neurol 2006; 5: 932–936.

135. Midgard R, Albrektsen G, Riise T et al. Prognostic factors for survival in multiple sclerosis: a longitudinal, population based study in Möre and Romsdal Norway. J Neurol Neurosurg Psychiatr 1995; 58: 417–421.

136. Müller R. Studies on disseminated sclerosis with special reference to symptomatology: course and prognosis. Acta Med Scand 1949; 222(suppl): 1–214.

137. Benedikz J, Stefánsson M, Gudmundsson J et al. The natural history of untreated multiple sclerosis in Iceland. A total population-based 50 year prospective study. Clin Neurol Neurosurg 2002; 104: 208–210.

138. Rodriguez M. A function of myelin is to protect axons from subsequent injury: implications for deficits in multiple sclerosis. Brain 2003; 126: 751–752.

139. Broman T. The permeability of the cerebrospinal vessels in normal and pathological conditions. Copenhagen: Munksgaard, 1949.

140. Weinshenker BG, Rice GPA, Noseworthy JH et al. The natural history of multiple sclerosis: a geographically based study 4. Applications to planning and interpretation of clinical therapeutric trials. Brain 1991; 114: 1057–1067.

141. Johnson KP, Brooks BR, Ford CC et al. Sustained clinical benefits of glatiramer acetate in relapsing multiple sclerosis patients observed for 6 years. Mult Scler 2000; 6: 255–266.

142. Rudick RA, Cutter GR, Baier M et al. Estimating long-term effects of disease-modifying drug therapy in multiple sclerosis patients. Mult Scler 2005; 11: 626–634.

143. Ockinger J, Serrano-Fernandez P, Moller S et al. Definition of a 1.06 Mb region linked to neuroinflammation in humans, rats and mice. Genetics 2006; 173: 1539–1545.

M. Pugliatti and G. Rosati

EPIDEMIOLOGY AND MEASURES OF OCCURRENCE

Epidemiology is the study of the occurrence of disease according to time, space and person.[1] Its ultimate goal is to detect the causes underlying disease occurrence and explaining its patterns by testing hypotheses.[2]

The most commonly used measures in multiple sclerosis (MS) are the incidence rate, the mortality rate and the point prevalence ratio. The incidence rate refers to the number of new cases of disease during a defined time interval and in a specified population. An incident case of MS is usually defined as any individual who experiences symptoms or shows signs that are later related to MS.[3] The mortality rate, or death rate, is the number of deaths from disease over a specified population and time interval. For MS, annual incidence and death rates are usually expressed per 100 000 population (as are the rates cited in this chapter). The case-fatality rate represents the proportion of those with a disease who die from it. When this proportion is low, as for MS, this rate is not suitable to describe the mortality rate. Point prevalence is commonly expressed as a rate but is really a ratio, as it is the proportion of individuals with MS (prevalent cases) within a specified population at one time. If the mortality rate is stable over time, the point prevalence rate is the average annual incidence rate times the average duration of the disease. Crude rates are computed from the rate numerator and denominator referring to the same specified population, such as a community. These can be expressed as age- or sex-specific rates. Because study samples and the target population usually differ in sex and age distribution, rates should be adjusted for these variables. This is achieved by multiplying the rate specific to a particular group of people defined by one of the variables (such as age group 20–29 years) by a factor representing the proportion of that specific defined group in a standard population.

Given the low frequency of MS in the general population and the wide spectrum of age of onset, cross-sectional studies are much more frequently used in MS research than perspective cohort studies. Population surveys on MS are prevalence studies based on people receiving health care rather than based on surveying general populations. By retrospectively investigating historical cohorts, incidence studies on MS often report incidence proportions or cumulative incidence: the proportion of individuals developing the disease during a given period of time in a closed population at risk rather than true rates expressed in person–time.[2] Morbidity data for MS come from investigating the general population or a community or from health system records, whereas mortality data usually come from national official sources, such as death certificates.

THE DEFINITION OF A CASE AND DIAGNOSTIC CRITERIA

Case ascertainment relies on a definition of case. This is accomplished by using conventionally approved diagnostic criteria. In epidemiology, the degree of case ascertainment in a population may vary consistently.[4] This can lead to rate underestimation. Further, even if proper diagnosis is made shortly after clinical onset, the use of conventional diagnostic criteria implies different levels of diagnostic certainty and inter- and intraobserver biases.

Poser & Brinar[5] conducted a comprehensive historical review of the diagnostic criteria used for MS. Since Charcot defined MS as a triad of nervous system signs more than 130 years ago, several more structured and stringent classifications and subsequent revisions have been made. In 1982, Charles Poser and a panel of European and Northern American experts established new diagnostic criteria aimed at meeting epidemiological research needs.[6] Discrepancy in terms and subjective judgment were reduced, and more objective measures from laboratory and neurophysiological tests were included. The criteria of Poser et al consisted of two large categories for definite and probable MS, each applicable on a purely clinical and paraclinical basis or with laboratory support. The categories eventually identified were clinically definite MS, laboratory-supported definite MS, clinically probable MS and laboratory-supported probable MS. The routine increasing use of magnetic resonance imaging (MRI) in diagnosing people with MS and its role as outcome in many clinical trials led to a further revision of the criteria. In 2001, an international committee of neurologists headed by W. Ian McDonald published the new diagnostic guidelines by incorporating MRI (defining progressive MS), eliminating the category of probable MS and reintroducing that of possible MS.[7]

Because of the retrospective methods used in MS epidemiological studies and the lack of MRI facilities in some populations, the Poser et al criteria still comprise the most common classification in such surveys. The use of the new diagnostic criteria is associated with greater interobserver variability and with the need for more routine investigations.[8] Both sets of criteria were applied to 76 patients at the first diagnosis of MS.[9] MS was diagnosed more often according to the McDonald et al criteria than the Poser et al clinically definite MS (52% vs 38%). However, the number of diagnosed MS cases increased when the Poser et al clinically definite MS and laboratory-supported definite MS were combined (84% versus 52%). 75% of the patients who had MS with the McDonald et al criteria could be assigned to Poser's clinically definite MS and 83% of the patients with possible MS had laboratory-supported definite MS. Although interobserver agreement was moderate for the overall diagnosis of MS using both Poser et al and McDonald et al criteria,[10] agreement was moderate to substantial with the McDonald et al criteria and fair to substantial with the Poser et al criteria. Based on clinical information, the agreement on dissemination in time was substantially greater than that for dissemination in space, whereas agreement was greater for spatial dissemination when MRI was considered in the criteria.

METHODS OF ASCERTAINMENT

According to Kurtzke,[11] population-based surveys assessing MS morbidity rates have three main epidemiological approaches: the Assyrian, the in-law and the spider survey. The first is the commonest type of ascertainment and is used for both population-based prevalence surveys (such as door-to-door surveys) and community-based prevalence studies based on healthcare resources. A group of investigators is deployed briefly in the community and leaves after collecting data. The second approach differs: the researchers establish direct surveillance in the community for a longer time period and can therefore assess incidence, prevalence and survival rates and investigate risk factors. These surveys can be very informative but expensive. The spider survey design aims at catching patients in the study network, consisting of or assisted by peripheral health-care structures under one qualified community health-care resource. This approach represents the basis for registry systems, allowing researchers to assess population-specific exposure, and can thus potentially produce valid epidemiological studies.

REGISTRIES

Registries are systems or agencies that compile data on all occurrences of a disease within a defined area.[12] Population-based registries provide relevant information on the epidemiology of MS; some examples follow. Although formally established in 1956, the Danish Multiple Sclerosis Registry has collected MS cases since 1948. It has been updated by prospectively and retrospectively recording information on MS incident cases from multiple sources: departments of neurology, practicing neurologists, rehabilitation centers, the National Patient Registry, the Danish Multiple Sclerosis Society and departments of neuropathology.[13] The Registry is estimated to be 90% complete, and diagnostic validity for definite MS was an estimated 94% based on autopsy cases. Its strength lies in its links with Denmark's Centralized Civil Registry, including the National Registry of Causes of Death, and the Danish Twin Registry. Registered cases are classified according to updated standardized diagnostic criteria. More than 14 000 MS patients were registered at a follow-up in 1997, of whom nearly 11 000 had their onset from 1948 to 1996. The Danish Multiple Sclerosis Registry has proved to be a valuable tool for multiple assessments of incidence, prevalence and survival, for studying the natural history of MS and for case–control and prospective studies providing unselected patient samples.[14–17]

The Rochester Epidemiology Project is a unique health-care record-linkage system applied to the population of Rochester and Olmsted County, Minnesota, USA. It was created in 1966 as a comprehensive population-based data resource in which clinical records from the Mayo Clinic were merged with those from other community providers, such as the Olmsted Medical Group and Olmsted Community Hospital.[18] The Rochester Epidemiology Project has provided surveillance for almost all serious illnesses and supported population-based studies, especially analyzing disease occurrence and natural history. The strength of the Rochester Epidemiology Project lies in 1) the close correspondence between a geographically defined population and the health-care providers, 2) the accurate longitudinal collection of medical information, 3) the easy access to data through diagnostic indexes, 4) the linking system with other health-care providers and 5) the infrastructure developed to support studies in clinical epidemiology, biostatistics and public health. In 1987, 83% of the Olmsted County population referred to one of the health-care structures providing data to the Project.

Among the first surveys of the Rochester Epidemiology Project was an incidence study on MS.[19] Because of the high degree of assessment, a saturation effect is often reported to apply to data from the Rochester Epidemiology Project.

The Consortium of Multiple Sclerosis Centers started the North American Research Committee on Multiple Sclerosis (NARCOMS) Project in 1993 to facilitate multicenter research on MS. As part of this objective, the NARCOMS Registry, a large patient self-report registry for MS, was started.[20] The Registry includes more than 29 000 participants enrolled between 1996 and 2004 via post mailings, MS centers, support groups and the NARCOMS Registry website. Data on demographics, MS-related medical history (including performance scales), immune and symptomatic therapies and health-care services are recorded.

The European Database for Multiple Sclerosis (EDMUS) has been available since 1992. It was designed within the European Concerted Action for Multiple Sclerosis funded by the European Commission[21,22] as a fast dataset containing a minimal set of obligatory information serving MS population-based studies and multicenter collaborative research. EDMUS can automatically generate data by means of algorithms, ensuring a uniform approach and automatically updating new information. EDMUS has served international multicenter trials, such as EVALUED,[23] assessing EDMUS interrater variability; PRIMS,[24,25] examining how pregnancy and the postpartum period influence the course of MS; VACCIMUS,[26] investigating the association between vaccines and MS; and KIDMUS, focusing on MS starting in childhood.[27,28] EDMUS has been relevant in studying the natural history and physiopathology of MS.[29,30]

The Canadian Collaborative Project on Genetic Susceptibility to MS (CCPGSMS) started in the early 1980s with a study on sib pairs,[31] the first population-based study of MS in twins.[32] The CCPGSMS was converted into a more structured network crucially contributing to studies on familial recurrence.[33] The CCPGSMS involves 15 MS clinics across Canada. All MS patients referred to these clinics have their family histories recorded and annually updated as part of the overall assessment. Structured questionnaires are administered in a standardized way to index cases, spouses and relatives. These data are longitudinally collected along with clinical information and biological material. The CCPGSMS represents a uniquely valuable resource for MS studies on clinical genetics, genetic epidemiology and molecular genetics.[33]

The Norwegian National Multiple Sclerosis Registry was established in 2001 at the Norwegian Multiple Sclerosis National Competence Centre, Haukeland University Hospital, Bergen, aimed at collecting clinical and demographic information of all prevalent MS patients in Norway. In 2007, a biobank unit for collection of biological samples (DNA and serum) from all available MS patients was implemented.[34]

THE GEOGRAPHY OF MULTIPLE SCLEROSIS

The geography of MS and its variation over time have been systematically investigated for the past 70 years (Fig. 9.1).[35]

EUROPE

The most relevant epidemiological patterns of MS distribution in time and space across Europe are summarized here. Reviews[36-38] and Tables 9.1 and 9.2 provide further detail.

Systematic surveys in the UK for more than 70 years[87] show three main epidemiological trends: a north-to-south gradient: the northeast mainland and the Scottish offshore islands versus southern England and Wales; a markedly increased prevalence up to tenfold in Wales[88] partly related to repeated assessments

over time and increased awareness of MS; and the subsequent tendency for the latitudinal gradient to level off.[78] Scotland and the Scottish offshore islands (Shetland and Orkney) have the highest prevalence and incidence rates in the UK and in Europe, although based on small populations and older diagnostic criteria.[88,89] Scotland's rates are at least twice those of England and Wales and, despite methodological differences, the north-to-south latitudinal gradient of MS prevalence across the UK is unquestionable, with a discrete change in risk at the Scottish border.[78-81] The MS prevalence in Northern Ireland is comparable with that in Scotland, probably because of the close ethnic origins and genetic composition of the two populations. Differing genetic susceptibility and a greater reduction in mortality rates over time in Scotland and Northern Ireland than in England and Wales might explain higher prevalence rates and the action of exposure intrinsic to Scottish ethnicity.[80,91,92] In Ireland, the prevalence of MS is similar to that in the UK at comparable latitudes.[55]

The MS prevalence in the Nordic countries is notably high, with some heterogeneity in temporal trends and across regions. The higher prevalence rates of MS reported in some regions compared with the respective national means was referred to as the Fennoscandian focus of MS. This extended from western to southeastern Norway, Denmark, southern Sweden, southwestern Finland and back to northeastern Sweden.[93] A correlation with the distribution of environmental exposure was hypothesized.

Norway has an uneven distribution of prevalence and incidence, with peaks in central areas (Nord-Trøndelag County).[65] Mean annual incidence rates have increased significantly from 3 to 6 per 100 000 per year in the western regions in the past

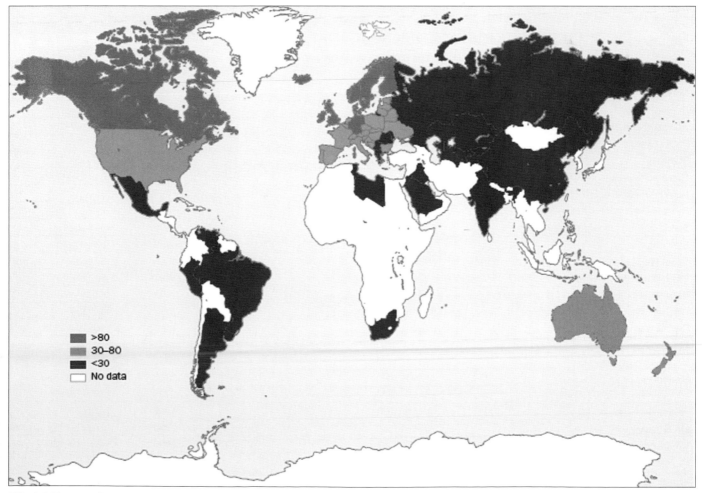

FIG. 9.1 The prevalence of multiple sclerosis worldwide (per 100 000 population). Reproduced with permission from Marrie 2004.[35]

Legend:
- >80
- 30–80
- <30
- No data

TABLE 9.1 Prevalence (per 100 000) of multiple sclerosis in Europe

Country	Study population size (% of country population)	Year	Crude rate (95% CI)
Albania[36]	3 091 400 (98.8)	1988	10 (–)*
Austria[39]	Nationwide	1999	98 (92–104)
Belarus[36]	–	1980	55 (–)
Belgium (Flanders)[40]	250 393 (2.5)	1991	88 (76–99)
Bulgaria (Svoge and Trojan)[41]	53 573 (0.7)	1995	39 (24–60)
Croatia (Osijek-Baranya)[42]	298 600 (6.8)	1998	50 (42–59)†
Cyprus[44]	108 600 (13.6)	1988	39 (28–52)
Denmark (Brønnum-Hansen, personal data)	Nationwide	1996	122 (115–120)
Estonia (south)[46]	392 009 (29.5)	1989	51 (44–59)
Finland (Seinäjoki)[47]	197 042 (3.9)	1993	188 (168–211)†
Finland (Uusimaa)[47]	1 277 932 (25.1)	1993	93 (87–99)†
Finland (Vaasa)[47]	179 079 (3.5)	1993	107 (91–125)†
Finland (central)[48]	263 886 (5.1)	2000	105 (93–118)
France[49]	Nationwide	1986	50 (–)‡
Germany[51]	Nationwide	1990s	127 (–)
Greece (Evros)[52]	143 752 (1.4)	1999	39 (29–51)
Hungary (Csongrad County)[53]	400 128 (3.9)	1999	62 (55–70)
Iceland[54]	285 000 (98.3)	1999	119 (106–133)
Ireland (County Donegal)[55]	129 994 (3.5)	2001	185 (162–210)
Ireland (County Wexford)[55]	104 372 (2.8)	2001	121 (101–144)
Italy (Ferrara, north)[56]	358 808 (0.6)	1993	69 (62–79)
Italy (Sicily, insular)[57]	337 332 (0.6)	1995	58 (51–68)§
Italy (L'Aquila, central)[58]	297 838 (0.5)	1996	53 (45–62)
Italy (Sardinia, insular)[59]	454 904 (0.8)	1997	144 (134–156)
Italy (Genoa)[60]	913 218 (1.6)	1997	94 (88–100)
Italy (Padua, north)[61]	820 318 (1.4)	1999	81 (70–91)
Latvia[36]	–	1980	55 (–)
Lithuania[36]	–	1980	35 (–)
Malta[62]	378 518 (94.6)	1999	17 (13–22)
Netherlands (Groningen)[36]	560 000 (3.5)	1992	76 (–)
Norway (Troms and Finnmark Counties)[63]	224 724 (4.9)	1993	73 (62–85)
Norway (Oslo)[64]	483 401 (10.5)	1995	120 (111–131)†
Norway (Nord-Trøndelag County)[65]	127 108 (2.7)	2000	164 (142–188)
Poland (west)[67]	50 000 (0.1)	1995	55 (–)
Portugal[68]	61 496 (0.6)	1998	47 (30–64)
Romania (Mures County)[69]	615 032 (2.7)	1986	21 (18–25)†
Russian Federation (Novosibirsk)[70]	–	1990s	60 (–)
Russian Federation (Ufa)[70]	–	1990s	31 (–)
Serbia and Montenegro (Belgrade)[71]	1 602 226 (15.2)	1996	51 (47–55)
Slovenia[36]	–	1992	83 (–)
Spain (Teruel, east)[72]	143 680 (0.4)	1996	32 (23–41)
Spain (Valladolid, north)[73]	92 632 (0.2)	1997	58 (44–76)
Spain (Mostoles, central)[74]	195 979 (0.5)	1998	43 (35–54)
Sweden (Västerbotten County)[75]	259 163 (2.9)	1997	154 (139–170)
Switzerland (Canton of Berne)[76]	920 000 (12.7)	1986	110 (103–117)‡
Former Yugoslav Republic of Macedonia	–	1991	16 (–)
Ukraine (Vinnytsya)[77]	390 500 (0.8)	2001	41 (35–48)
UK (north Cambridgeshire)[78]	378 959 (0.6)	1993	107 (98–118)‡
UK (south-eastern Scotland)[79]	864 300 (1.5)	1995	187 (178–196)
UK (eastern Scotland)[80]	395 600 (0.7)	1996	184 (171–198)
UK (Leeds Health Authority)[81]	732 061 (1.2)	1996	97 (90–105)‡
UK (Northern Ireland)[82]	151 000 (0.3)	1996	168 (148–189)

CI, confidence interval.
*Rose et al definite prevalence and probable MS.[78] †Only Poser Committee et al definite MS.[6] ‡Approximately. §Onset-adjusted prevalence rate.
Source: modified from Pugliatti et al 2006[38] with the permission of Blackwell Publishing.

TABLE 9.2 Incidence (per 100 000 population per year) of multiple sclerosis in European countries

Country	Time interval	Study population size	Rate (95% CI)
Albania[36]	1968–1987	3 091 000	0.5 (0.4–0.6)*
Croatia (northern Adriatic islands)[42]	1956–1998	50 552	1.3 (–)
Croatia (Osijek-Baranya)[42]	1991–1998	298 600	3.5 (–)†
Denmark[16]	1980–1989	nationwide	5.0 (4.8–5.2)
Finland (Seinäjoki)[84]	1979–1993	197 000	11.6 (10.1–13.1)†
Finland (Uusimaa)[84]	1979–1993	1 278 000	5.1 (4.1–6.3)†
Finland (Vaasa)[84]	1979–1993	179 000	5.2 (4.8–5.5)†
Finland (central)[48]	1994–1998	263 886	9.2 (7.4–10.9)
France[85]	1993–1997	94 000	4.3 (2.9–7.2)
Germany (Lauer, personal data)	1979–1992	100 000	4.2 (–)
Greece (Evros)[52]	1994–1999	143 000	2.4 (1.4–3.7)
Hungary[53]	1997–1998	400 128	5.5 (–)
Iceland[54]	1991–1995	255 000	0–5 (–)
Ireland (County Donegal)[55]	2001	129 994	5.1 (1.6–11.7)
Ireland (County Wexford)[55]	2001	104 372	4.5 (0.3–8.7)
Italy (Ferrara, north)[56]	1990–1993	368 000	2.4 (1.6–3.4)
Italy (Sicily, insular)[57]	1990–1994	338 000	3.9 (3.0–5.0)
Italy (Sardinia, insular)[59]	1995–1999	454 000	6.1 (5.1–7.2)
Italy (Padua, north)[61]	1995–1999	820 000	4.2 (3.7–4.7)
Malta[62]	1989–1998	400 000	0.8 (–)
Netherlands (Groningen)[36]	1985–1990	560 000	3.0 (–)
Norway (Nord-Trøndelag County)[65]	1974–1998	127 000	5.3 (3.7–7.5)
Norway (Oslo)[64]	1992–1996	484 000	8.7 (6.3–11.9)†
Norway (Troms and Finnmark Counties)[63]	1989–1992	225 000	4.3 (3.0–5.9)
Poland (west)[67]	1993–1995	50 000	2.2 (–)
Romania (Mures County)[69]	1976–1986	600 000	0.9 (–)†
Russian Federation (Iaroslavl)[70]	1996–2001	–	3.0 (–)
Slovenia[36]	1990s	2.9 (–)	
Spain (Mostoles, central)[74]	1994–1998	196 000	3.8 (2.7–5.3)
Spain (Teruel, east)[72]	1992–1996	143 000	2.2 (–)
Sweden (Västerbotten County)[75]	1988–1997	256 000	5.2 (4.4–6.2)
Switzerland (Canton of Berne)[76]	1961–1980	920 000	4.0 (3.7–4.3)
Former Yugoslav Republic of Macedonia[36]	1990s	–	0.2–1.2 (–)
Ukraine (Vinnytsya)[86]	1990–1994	390 000	0.7 (–)
UK (northern Cambridgeshire)[78]	1990–1995	379 000	4.8 (3.8–6.0)
UK (southeastern Scotland)[79]	1992–1995	864 000	12.0 (10.6–13.3)

CI, confidence interval.
*Rose et al definite and probable MS.[83] †Only Poser Committee et al definite MS.[6]
Source: modified from Pugliatti et al 2006[36] with the permission of Blackwell Publishing.

three decades,[94,95] probably because of change in the population age structure and improved ascertainment over time. However, the clinical phenotypes also appeared to have changed in Norway over time, with increased proportions of relapsing–remitting versus primary progressive MS[95] and among women versus men.[96] A fluctuating incidence pattern was reported for Vestfold, with peak rates of about 4 in 1953–7 and 1973–97,[96] and for Hordaland County with a peak of 6.9 in 1978–1982.[66]

Native Norwegians in Oslo had a prevalence rate of 136, which was higher than that in the city's general population yet underestimated because only one of the Poser et al definite criteria for MS was used.[64] In Hordaland County, prevalence was 151 in 2003.[66] Prevalence increased 3.5 times to 73 between 1973 and 1993 but the northernmost counties of Troms and Finnmark, largely populated by Sami, had a rather steady pattern of incidence.[63] The overall lower risk for MS in this ethnic group can be explained by genetically based resistance to MS and/or a small population size effect.[63]

Based on a registry system established in the early 1950s, prevalence in Göteborg in southwestern Sweden was 96 in 1988 and the mean annual incidence rate 2.6 in 1974–88.[97] Multiple assessments carried out in Västerbotten County in northern Sweden showed an increase of prevalence from 125 in 1990 to 154 in 1997[75,98] and a mean annual incidence rate of 5.2 in 1988–97.[75]

In Finland, regional differences in MS prevalence and incidence have persisted over a 30-year follow-up period, with the highest rates reported in the western district of Seinäjoki, intermediate rates in central Finland and coastal Vaasa and relatively lower rates in Uusimaa in the south.[47,48,84] Prevalence increased between 1983 and 1993 in all these districts and in Vaasa, especially among women.[47] Based on the evidence of frequent familial MS recurrence in western Finland, a genetically based susceptibility to MS due to genetic drift in isolated rural communities was hypothesized to explain the absolute persisting rate differences across regions and over time.[36] Environmental factors and improved case ascertainment are instead probably responsible for the increasing occurrence of MS in western and central Finland.[47,48]

The Danish Multiple Sclerosis Registry[14–16] provides epidemiological data on MS in Denmark that appear to be consistent with the findings in Norway and Sweden,[45] probably indicating a similar genetic and environmental background for susceptibility to MS.

Iceland provides a 50-year observational period in a well-defined and stable population.[54] The threefold increase of MS prevalence up to 119 in 1999 compared with 1950 was related to improved case ascertainment over time. The MS risk in Iceland is similar to that in the other Nordic countries. The mean annual incidence rate in Iceland fluctuated between 0 and 5 from 1900–2000, peaking in 1981–90.[54]

The MS prevalence in Germany has been rather homogeneously distributed over time and space, with prevalence rates between 83 and 127[38] and an estimated mean annual incidence rate of 4.2 (Lauer, personal data) for the past two decades. Similar prevalence rates were found in the Netherlands,[36] Belgium,[40] Slovenia,[36] Switzerland[76] and Austria,[39] in comparable time periods. The geographical distribution of MS prevalence was heterogeneous in Poland, with a peak rate of 110 in the south,[36] in the Czech Republic, with rates up to 160 in three small northern Bohemian districts,[36] and in Hungary, with rates up to 79 in Fejer County.[36,53,99] Among Roma in Hungary, the prevalence ranged from 5 in Baranya County to 98 in Fejer County.[36] Mean annual incidence rates in these areas ranged from 2–8 in the 1980s and 1990s.[36,53,67]

In the 1980s, the prevalence rate in France ranged from 37–58.[36] A nationwide survey in 1986 based on questionnaires returned by people with MS responding to a television announcement reported a mean prevalence rate of 50 and clustering patterns in the northeast.[49] Concerns about ascertainment bias were raised in relation to the differential response rate among the regions participating in the study. The hypothesis of a northeast-to-southwest gradient of MS distribution in France is supported by mortality studies[59,100] and by a survey on the whole farming population, in which prevalence varied from 100–50.[101] Further studies showed that regional differences applied to prevalence but not to incidence rates, indicating a focal distribution of MS in ethnic groups with different susceptibility.[85]

Parallel to improvement of the national health-care system, multiple large population-based assessments conducted in northern, eastern and central Spain found prevalence rates of 32–58 and mean annual incidence rates from 2–4 in the 1990s.[72–74] Prevalence data are in the same range for Portugal.[68]

Several prevalence surveys on MS have been conducted in Italy in the past two decades and some regions have been multiply assessed.[38] The overall prevalence rates and the reported increase over time in the mainland and in Sicily probably resulted from improved diagnostic accuracy, epidemiological methods, multiple assessments and increased survival. Prevalence and incidence rates in the island of Sardinia were significantly higher than the national mean rates and showed a significantly increasing temporal trend over the past 30 years.[59,102–104] The fourfold increase in Malta's prevalence rate since 1978 was explained by changing population age structure, generally increased life expectancy and previous diagnoses.[62] The genetic influence from northern Africa, an area at low risk for MS, is believed to account for the low absolute MS risk in the Maltese.

Prevalence rates between 20 and 55 have been reported for Croatia,[42] Serbia and Montenegro,[71] Romania[69] and Bulgaria[41] in the past three decades. Where they are available, mean annual incidence rates ranged from 1.0–3.4.[38] An exception was the prevalence rate of 152 in 1999 reported for Gorski Kotar, Croatia and Kocevje region[43] and the mean annual incidence rate of 4.1 in 1948–1987 for Gorski Kotar.[42] A high inbreeding rate in this isolated mountainous Germanic community and survey methods might have accounted for such a high rate. Prevalence rates ranged from 10–45 in Albania, the former Yugoslav Republic of Macedonia, Greece, Cyprus and Turkey in the past two decades.[38] Where available for these areas, mean annual incidence rates ranged from 0.2–2.4 in comparable periods.[38] Methodological issues, such as hospital-based study designs and under-reporting, may account for underestimation of rates in these areas.

Results from MS prevalence studies carried out in the Russian Federation and other countries of the former Soviet Union[36,105] are difficult to interpret because of differences in ethnic features, high migration rates and epidemiological methods used in different areas. In these countries, including Ukraine,[79] prevalence rates range from 35–60 but are likely to be underestimated to differing degrees. A recent incidence study for the Russian Federation showed a mean annual rate of 3 in Iaroslavl in 1996–2001.[70]

THE AMERICAS

Table 9.3 reports the MS prevalence rates for the Americas.

Prior to the 1990s, Canada had two relevant MS prevalence patterns: higher rates in populations of northern European ancestry and an east-to-west gradient, with the lowest rates in Newfoundland.[37] These two patterns converged in a higher proportion of northern European ancestry, e.g. British ancestry, in western Canada. In 2001, however, a rate of 94 was also reported for Newfoundland,[106] with stable mean annual incidence rates for 1994–2001. Such evidence, in accordance with that from the rest of Canada, was explained by better access to diagnostic facilities and more neurologists in Newfoundland over time. Increased prevalence rates have been reported for Alberta[107] and for Saskatoon, Saskatchewan.[108] Given the lack of relevant ethnic differences between these populations and the rest of western Canada, epidemiological surveillance was carried out to identify community-specific environmental risk factors. The reported high rates probably reflected a saturation effect from exceptionally thorough case ascertainment instead of a true association with risk factors.[126] MS risk is lower, yet increasing in native Canadians (Indians)[107] and those with MS have Caucasian ancestry.[127] The Canadian Hutterites, immigrants from southern Germany with rare social mixing and high inbreeding rates, have a low prevalence of MS.[128] This exception to the association between low MS risk and northern European ancestry in Canada may be explained by a drift of susceptibility genes and/or by lower concentrations of population-specific exposure.

TABLE 9.3 Prevalence of multiple sclerosis (per 100 000 population) in the Americas

Country	Year	Crude rate
Canada		
Newfoundland[106]	2001	94
Barrhead County, Alberta[107]	1990	196
Saskatoon, Saskatchewan[108]	1999	248
London, Ontario[109]	1984	94
USA		
Olmsted County, MN[110]	2000	177
Galion, OH[111]	1987	112
Weld-Larimer County CO[112]	1982	65
Key West island, FL[114]	1983	110
Hawaii[115]	1969	24 (Caucasians) 9 (Orientals)
NINCDS National survey[116]	1976	46 53 north of 37°N 30 south of 37°N
National Health Interview Survey[117]		85
Central and South America		
Venezuela[118]	1970	2
Peru[118]	1970	4
Brazil[118]	<1990	4
Mexico City, Mexico[119]	review	1.5
Cuba[120]	1990s	5–10
Rio de Janeiro[121]	1999	5
São Paulo, Brazil[122]	1997	15*
Colombia[123]	2000	1–5*
Buenos Aires, Argentina[124]	1996	18
Uruguay National Survey[125]	1996	30

*Only Poser Committee et al definite MS.6

Local investigations in 1948–1967 suggested a north-to-south gradient of MS prevalence for the USA,[4] as did a survey in the 1970s.[116] An overall prevalence of 46 was estimated in 1976, with a cut-off at latitude 37°N: north of this the rate was 53 and south of this 30. However, as the study had randomly sampled physicians and general hospitals across the USA, a similar method could have underestimated MS prevalence by up to 40%, and differentially across the country.[112] A study of a cohort of more than 20 million people in the USA who had been in the military in World War II or in the Korean conflict provides the major support for the north-to-south gradient theory of MS distribution in the USA.[129] Of these veterans, 5305 developed MS 'in connection with the service': during the service or within 7 years after discharge. Not only did MS distribution differ by latitude but also according to a west-to-east gradient. The differential distribution of MS by latitude was further reanalyzed for ancestry; high rates were correlated with northern European ancestry.[130] The Nurses' Health Study (NHS) and the Nurses' Health Study II (NHS II), conducted on two cohorts of women born in 1920–46 and in 1947–64, also investigated the relationship between MS and latitude.[131] Women residing in the northern tier had a higher MS incidence than women in the southern tier after adjusting for age, ancestry and longitude zone. MS did not increase among the NHS II women living in the north, and the different incidence patterns between the two cohorts over time were due to the leveling-off effect of improved case ascertainment over the MS latitudinal gradient.

Olmsted County, Minnesota had a prevalence rate of 177 in 2000 and a mean annual incidence rate of 7.5 for 1985–2000.[110] Based on a 100-year disease surveillance system, a recent survey undertaken within the Rochester Epidemiology Project demonstrated that MS occurrence in Olmsted County had not really significantly increased over the past two decades and that the apparently increasing rates from 1915 to 1978 can be ascribed to improved ascertainment[110] (Fig. 9.2). The overall pattern of geographical distribution in the USA is affected by the low level of comparability between studies, especially the effect of ascertainment saturation in some areas.

Data on the widespread distribution of MS in Latin America are still limited. Nevertheless, the interest in epidemiological studies on MS has increased in recent years, probably related to starting procedures for prescribing disease-modifying treatments. The few studies conducted before 1990 showed low prevalence rates in Venezuela, Peru and Brazil[118] and in Mexico.[119] In the 1990s, the overall prevalence rate of MS in Latin America ranged from 1–18[119,121–124] (Table 9.3). In particular, a prevalence survey based only on Poser et al criteria for definite MS and conducted on a population of more than 9 million in São Paulo, Brazil showed a rate of 15 in 1997.[122] The threefold increase observed since 1990 was attributed to improved diagnostic procedures. A prevalence rate of 30 was recorded in a national survey in Uruguay, where most of the population is of European ancestry.[125] In 1994, the Atlantic South Project was started, aimed at defining MS in Brazil through the use of registry systems. Among 509 patients classified according to the Poser et al criteria, 72% were Caucasian Brazilian and the rest were Afro-Brazilian, indicating ethnic heterogeneity as the cause for rate underestimation.[37]

ASIA

Table 9.4 reports the prevalence rates of MS in Asia.[132]

MS is rare in Korea,[133] Malaysia[140] and Thailand[133] and among Chinese.[133,134] A recent study based on records from the National Health Insurance, which covers 96% of the Chinese population and has mandatorily enrolled individuals since 1995, revealed a prevalence of 1.9 in Taiwan in 2002.[141] MS prevalence in a hospital-based study in Hong Kong was 1 in 10:1 ratio of women to men. A door-to-door survey in a county of Yunnan province in 1986 found a prevalence of 2.[136] A recent population-based survey conducted on a population of nearly 9 million in Shanghai showed a prevalence of 1.4 per 100 000 in 2004.[137]

MS in Japan was rarely reported prior to the 1950s, and the few cases registered presented with opticospinal disease (neuromyelitis optica).[132] In 1975–1983, the MS prevalence rate was 1–4, with no differences in geographical distribution.[138,139] Two decades later, the prevalence rates for Hokkaido and Asahikawa in the north were 8.6 and 10, respectively, attributed to previous underascertainment.[142] The validity of MS diagnosis in these reports is undermined by the use of the 1972 Japanese criteria, which also affected some Chinese reports.[37] The different clinical features of MS in Japan – predominant opticospinal forms, a rapid progression based on high inflammation rate and a low proportion of familial cases – indicate a different disease from that among Caucasians, with implications for comparability among studies.[132] The proportion of conventional forms is now reported to be increasing for the youngest cohorts.[151] However, relapsing–remitting neuromyelitis optica is now more often classified as MS, so the proportion of the opticospinal forms of MS in Japanese may have only apparently decreased.[132,142]

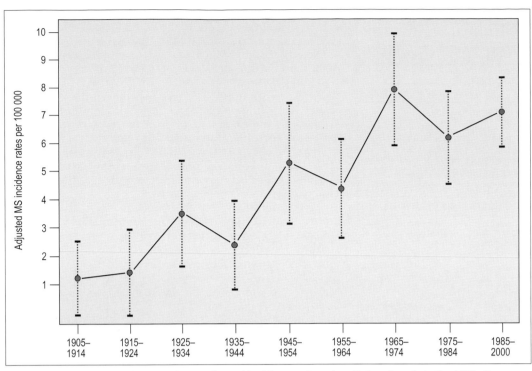

FIG. 9.2 Temporal trend of sex- and age-adjusted incidence rates of multiple sclerosis in the USA. Bars represent 95% confidence intervals. Redrawn from Mayr et al 2003[105] with permission from Lippincott Williams & Wilkins.

MS is believed to be rare in India but relatively higher rates were found in northern areas, which were settled by Indo-Europeans, than in the south, where Tamils and Dravidians predominate.[37] Studies conducted in Bombay and Poona in the late 1980s found prevalence rates from 26–58 among the Parsis.[143] The risk of MS in this population of Persian origin that migrated to the Bombay area in the 7th century is believed to be higher than that in the background population. Prevalence data on other ethnic groups are not available.

Clinical series of MS patients are reported for Pakistan, but no prevalence data.[152] Inferring MS epidemiology in the Middle East is complex because of the admixture of genetics, ethnicity and historical events. Arabs in Jordan[145] and Saudi Arabia[150] had prevalence rates between 7 and 8 as compared to the Jordanian/Palestinian prevalence of 39.[146]

In Kuwait, the prevalence in 1988 was 10 among Arabs and 13 among Kuwaitis, Palestinians and Egyptians.[147] Among non-Arabs, 95% of whom were southeastern Asians, the rate was 3. The frequencies of the ABO blood groups and the distribution of the HLA-DR and HLA-DW haplotypes differed between Kuwaitis and Palestinians, the latter retaining Caucasian features.[147] A mean rate of 15 was recently reported for Kuwait, with a significant difference between Kuwaitis (31) and non-Kuwaitis (6).[148] Because of the Arab make-up of nearly 75% of Kuwaitis, the reversal pattern compared with previous data is difficult to interpret.[148] The mean annual incidence rate increased from 1.0–2.6 from 1993–2000, especially among Kuwaiti women.

In Israel, MS prevalence has been investigated in the native born population and among immigrants of different origins. The prevalence rates among native-born Israelis of European or North American ethnic origin were as high as those among immigrants from Europe and North America, whereas the prevalence among immigrants from Africa and Asia was lowest and that among native-born Israelis of African or Asian ethnic origin was intermediate.[144,153,154] A survey was conducted in Greater Jerusalem on an admixed population of immigrant Jews from Europe and North America and from Africa and Asia, of Israel-born Jews of European and North American ethnic origin, Israel-born Jews of African and Asian ethnic origin and Arabs.[144] In 1995, the prevalence rates in the two groups of Jews of Caucasian origin were comparable at 64 versus 22 among African and Asian immigrants, 52 among native-born Israeli Jews of African and Asian ethnic origin and 19 among Arabs.

In Iran, the mean prevalence for the period 2004–2005 was 36 per 100 000.[149]

The prevalence of MS in the Asian part of the Russian Federation has gradually increased over time, probably related to the migration of Russians to the east, to a large-scale process of industrialization and to a marked demographic increase. A review of epidemiological data from the late 1980s, proceedings of local meetings and Russian publications found prevalence rates of 12–41 with no clear geographical pattern.[36,105] The higher rates were reported in the Amur, Khabarovsk and Primorski regions in populations of Russian ancestry. MS is very rare among native Siberians. The discrepancy of MS prevalence between indigenous populations and Russians was explained by the possible causative role of factors associated with ethnicity and not by restricted access of native Siberians to specialist health care.

AFRICA

In the Canary Islands, populated by individuals of European ancestry but at the same latitude as northwestern Africa, the prevalence of MS was between 6 and 15 in the 1980s, similar to that reported from Spain in the same years, based on hospital records.[37] In 2002, prevalence in the Canary Islands ranged between 74 and 78 depending on the diagnostic criteria used.[155] The same study showed a mean annual incidence rate of 4.1, with rates gradually decreasing from 6.1 in 1998 to 2.4 in 2002, possibly due to delay in diagnosis. MS prevalence rates ranged from 6–10 in Tunisia in 1975, in Libya in 1984 and in Kelibia, Tunisia in 1985.[37]

Reports on MS in the black African population are extremely scarce, because of the lack of epidemiological studies, a low proportion of recognized and diagnosed cases or population-specific resistance to MS. In these epidemiological settings, case recognition from investigators with poor neurological expertise

TABLE 9.4 Prevalence (per 100 000 population) of multiple sclerosis in Asia

Country	Ethnic group	Year	Prevalence
Areas of prevalence <1/100 000 population			
Taiwan[133]	Southern Chinese	1970–1980	0.8
Hong Kong[134]	Southern Chinese	1999	0.77
India[135]	Indian	1970s	0.22–0.6
Areas of prevalence 1–5/100 000 population			
China (Yunnan Province)[136]	Southern Chinese	1986	2
Japan[138,139]	Japanese	1957–1984	0.70–4.0
Korea[133]	Korean	1970s	1.8*
Malaysia[140]	80% southern Chinese	1980s	2*
Taiwan[141]	Southern Chinese	2002	1.9
Thailand[142]	Thai	2002	2
Areas of prevalence >5/100 000 population			
India[143]	Parsis	1988	26–58
Israel[144]	Immigrant Caucasian Jews and Israel-born Caucasian Jews	1995	64
Israel[144]	Immigrant African and Asian Jews	1995	22
Israel[144]	Israel-born African and Asian Jews	1995	52
Israel[144]	Arab	1995	19
Japan[142]	Japanese	2002	10
Jordan[145]	Arab	1977	7
Jordan[146]	Jordanian	1992–1993	20
Jordan[146]	Palestinian	1992–1993	42
Kuwait[147]	Arab	1988	10
Kuwait[147]	Kuwaiti, Palestinian and Egyptian	1988	13
Kuwait[147]	Palestinian	1988	23.8
Kuwait[148]	Kuwaitis	2000	31
Kuwait[148]	Non-Kuwaitis	2000	6
Russian Federation (Asia)[105]	Caucasian Russian and native Russian	1980s	12–41
Saudi Arabia[150]	Gulf Arab	1977	8*

*Estimation based on the ratio of MS versus amyotrophic lateral sclerosis
Source: modified from Kira 2003[132] with the permission of The Lancet Publishing Group.

and inadequate survey resources can represent a concern in determining the distribution of MS in the continent. Black Africans are believed to be resistant to MS because of low genetic susceptibility or endemic exposure to protective environmental factors (viral infections) in childhood. In South Africa, the reported prevalence in 1960 was 13 among English-speaking white South Africans and 4 among Afrikaners, but no cases were found among black Africans.[156] Later 12 cases were described among South African and Zimbabwean blacks,[157] six of whom presented with a different clinical phenotype characterized by very severe visual disturbances and progressive course from onset. A review of MS in tropical countries documented the occurrence of MS among blacks in Senegal.[158] The extremely small number of MS cases reported among black South Africans by highly trained observers supports this high resistance to MS. Ethnic groups such as Zulu and Xhosa that exclusively settled in South Africa might carry such low susceptibility.[158] Progressive improvement of diagnostic sensitivity and of the knowledge on nervous system disorders classically occurring in populations in industrialized countries has enabled greater detection of MS

cases and to increasing reports over time.[159] Seven MS cases were reported among 2831 indigenous Bantu Kenyans consecutively referred to a health structure over a 10-year period based on clinical criteria.[160] As 'the disease continues to appear', Kioy 'feels' that MS in Bantu Africans might not be as rare as previously believed and suggests that such populations might provide information on the role of exogenous factors in increasing rates over time in otherwise resistant populations.[160]

AUSTRALASIA

Epidemiological studies into MS conducted in the early 1980s in different areas of Australia and New Zealand reported rates between 11 in north Queensland, Australia to 69 in Otago-Southland, New Zealand, indicating a south-to-north gradient in the distribution of exogenous risk factors.[37] MS risk is low among Maoris, who represent 16% of the Waikato, 7% of the Wellington and 3% of the Otago-Southland populations.[37] Maori ancestry probably therefore provides low susceptibility to MS to the white Waikato population versus the southern populations with less Maori ancestry and a considerable proportion of Scottish ancestry. Prevalence increased significantly over time from 21–34 in Newcastle, Perth and Hobart from 1961–81, associated with increased incidence.[37] The rates from Newcastle were revisited for the decade 1986–96, showing a further significant increase to 59 even using less comprehensive diagnostic criteria.[161] The annual mean incidence rate doubled to 2.4 from 1950–60 followed by no further significant rise in the latest three decades, thus indicating increased survival in the MS population and improved ascertainment over the years. In the Australian Capital Territory, an area never investigated for MS, prevalence was 80 using the Rose et al criteria[78] and 71 using the Poser et al[6] criteria.[162]

In northern New Zealand, the reappraised prevalence rate in 2001 was 50 for the province of Bay of Plenty.[163] Maoris were 24% of the whole study population, with a prevalence of 7.

AGE

MORTALITY

Multiple sclerosis is associated with an increased risk of death. In Europe, mortality rates range from 0.5–3.6 per 100 000 population per year, with decreasing temporal trends in Austria, Denmark, Germany, the Netherlands, Portugal, Scotland and Switzerland and increasing trends in Bulgaria, Italy and Sweden.[38] Based on the Danish Multiple Sclerosis Registry, an analysis of all deaths with MS reported among other conditions on the certificate and of those with MS as the underlying cause of death showed a mean crude death rate of 2.6 for all ages and for total deaths and 2.0 when MS was the underlying cause, with no substantial difference in gender.[164] The highest rates were among those 55–64 years old for both distributions by cause and in both genders. The same analysis was conducted in 1955 in the USA among whites and nonwhites, mostly African-Americans.[164] Among whites and for all ages, the total death rate was 1.3 versus 0.9 with MS as the underlying cause, with no difference by gender. Among nonwhites, the respective rates were 0.5 and 0.4. The age-specific death rate with MS as the underlying cause remained stable at 3 from age 45 years. In both Denmark and the USA, the proportion of deaths with MS as the underlying cause tended to decline with increasing age. MS mortality was investigated in all Canadian provinces for 1965–1994.[165] The highest mean annual MS mortality rates of 4.4 and 3.9 were registered in Quebec and Ontario, respectively. A rate of 2.1 was reported for the western provinces and of 1.2 for eastern Canada, following a fluctuating pattern. Mortality was higher among women in each time period and for each geographical area. The highest mortality rate was for age 65

years and older among both genders, and the distribution of prevalence and mortality rates were not correlated. Standardized mortality data from the World Health Organization for affluent industrialized countries distributed by age and gender for various diseases of the nervous system and mental disorders showed that the mortality rates for MS in 1979–97 were 0.1 in Japan, 1.4 in Canada, Germany and the Netherlands and 1.7 in the UK, with most countries between 0.5 and 1.0.[166] Such rates were higher among women and no substantial change over time was reported.

MORBIDITY

In Europe, the highest prevalence estimates were reported among people 35–49 years for all countries except for Ireland, the UK (Northern Ireland and Scotland) and Norway, where the rates peaked at 50–64 years.[38] The absolute age-specific rates varied by country in relation to the disease prevalence in the population at large.

Age- and gender-specific annual incidence rates are higher among women and at age 25–29 years among Caucasians and Asians.[167,168] Based on the Danish Multiple Sclerosis Registry, the mean age at onset in Denmark was 34.7 years among men and 34.1 years among women for 1949–96 and age at onset increased by 2.3 years over time.[169]

The diagnostic criteria for MS apply to individuals aged 10–59 years.[6] Nevertheless, MS onset in childhood is common[170] (Table 9.5). The difficulty in collecting clinical information from children, the classification controversies[178] and the polysymptomatic onset of MS among children[179] all affect ascertainment and ultimately interpretation of epidemiological evidence from this subpopulation. Reports on the female:male ratio in childhood MS have been controversial, from significantly lower[175] to significantly higher[177] than for adults. Prognosis and course appear to be similar to the adult forms.[179]

Late-onset MS refers to initial clinical manifestations at age 50 years or older, which occurs in 4.0–9.4% of MS cases.[29,180] Up to 70% have monosymptomatic motor or cerebellar onset and a progressive course.[169] Because of the higher incidence of disorders mimicking MS, such as ischemic encephalopathy, late-onset cerebellar ataxia, vasculitides and cervical spondylosis, differential diagnosis can be problematic in this age group.

GENDER

Women have a higher incidence of MS, with ratios ranging from 1 to over 3.[38] The female:male sex ratio of MS has been increasing in Canada for at least 50 years and now exceeds 3.2:1.[180] This is in line with the widespread perception that incidence

TABLE 9.5 **Studies of multiple sclerosis among children**

Country	Year	Study design	Patients (n)	Mean age at onset, year (range)	Female:male ratio
Canada[171]	2002	Retrospective longitudinal (1980–1999)	116	12.7 (3–15)	2.87:1
Russian Federation[172]	2002	Retrospective	67	11.7 (4–15)	1.31:1
Italy[173]	2002	Retrospective	83	14.3 (1.3–15.9)	1.86:1
Review[174]	1999	Cross-sectional and literature review	49	3.2 (0.8–5.3)	1.4:1
Italy (multicenter)[175]	1997	Retrospective	149	12.6	2.2:1
Scotland[176]	1995	Retrospective	28	11.5 (1–15)	1.54:1
Canada (multicenter)[177]	1987	Retrospective population based	125	13 (5–15)	3.03:1

Source: modified from Banwell 2004[170] with the permission of Current Medicine.

and prevalence of MS have generally increased. The National Health Interview Survey reported a 50% increase among women in the USA from 1982–6 to 1991–4.[117] The relative risk for MS was compared among women from the old USA veterans cohort, represented by USA veterans who took part in World War II and the Korean conflict, and the new one, with entry into the military service between 1960 and 1994.[182] The relative risk for MS among all women was higher than previously reported, including 2.86 for blacks, 2.99 for whites and 3.51 for other races. A gender effect in MS was described in relation to age of disease onset and geography[171,177] and has been supported by genetic studies on MS transmission.[33]

RACE

Mortality and morbidity data show that Asians and Africans have a lower risk of MS.[132,156] Among US army veterans,[183] the risk of MS among blacks was half that among whites regardless of state of residence.[129] The risk was also notably lower among Asians and native Americans. In Hawaii, prevalence was 24 for Caucasians and 9 for Asians.[115] Foreign-born and USA–born Japanese and Chinese on the west coast of the USA have low MS rates.[133] Although the relative risk was lower than in Caucasians, the relative risk for MS in blacks from the recent cohort of USA veterans was 0.67 versus 0.44 in the previous cohort.[182] The clinical phenotype also differed between African-Americans and Caucasian-Americans with MS residing in the same area. Among African-Americans, age at onset was 2.5 years later and onset was more frequently polysymptomatic, followed by an opticospinal and more aggressive course.[184] Similarly, in the French population a more aggressive course was reported in North Africa compared to European patients.[185]

SURVIVAL

The results of several studies on mean survival after onset in the past two decades vary from 28 years among men in Denmark[17] to 43 years among white women in the USA[186] and 45 years in Finland.[187] Based on the Danish Multiple Sclerosis Registry, the secular trends of survival probabilities, excess mortality and causes of death were calculated, adjusting for the change in the general population death rate and distribution of causes of death over the past 50 years.[169] A total of 4254 people with MS (1980 men and 2274 women) had died before 1 January 2000 versus the expected 1471 deaths (746 men and 725 women) in the matched general population. The standardized mortality ratio was 2.89 for the whole group (2.66 for men and 3.14 for women). The excess death rates, a measure of the number of deaths due to MS exceeding the expected number, increased more rapidly among men than women in subsequent periods. The median survival time from onset was 28 years for men and 33 years for women versus 38 and 45 years respectively in the matched general population. Figure 9.3 shows the 10- and 25-year survival probability after onset. The survival probability has improved substantially since the 1950s (Fig. 9.4) and was not attributed to declining general population mortality but rather to improved case management.[169] MS was indicated on 82% of the death certificates as the underlying or contributing cause of death and the underlying cause of death in 56%. Excess death rates increased with the increasing number of years from onset (Table 9.6) and when cerebellar symptoms presented at onset. It was lowest for optic neuritis as a presenting symptom.[17]

Survival improved from 1953–87 in an MS population in Norway with a median survival time of 27 years.[188] A reduced mortality rate in the general population could partly explain this trend. Survival rates improved in cohorts with more recent onset.[169,188] Survival was also analyzed for nearly 2500 USA veterans of World War II whose MS was connected with military service.[186] The median survival time was 43 years for white women, 30 years for black men and 34 years for white men. Survival among white men was two-thirds that of white male controls 20 years after onset and one-third after 40 years, but improved over time. Rates did not differ significantly in the northern versus southern tiers. Female gender, lower socioeconomic status and younger age at MS onset were associated with improved survival, although confounders such as ethnicity and socioeconomic status must be considered. Conversely, the survival rate analyzed prospectively from disease onset showed no change over 80 years in Rochester, Minnesota.[189]

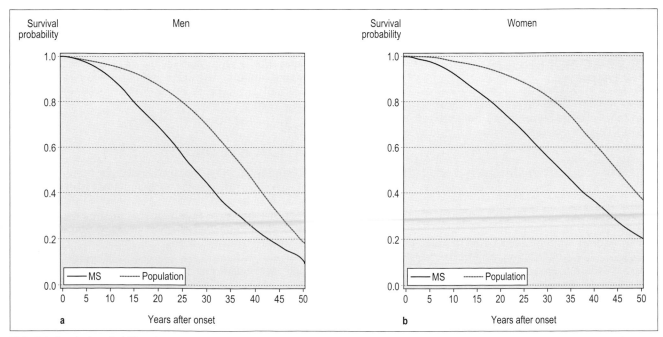

FIG. 9.3 Survival probability of people with multiple sclerosis and of the matched general population. Redrawn from Brønnum-Hansen et al 2004[169] with permission from Oxford University Press.

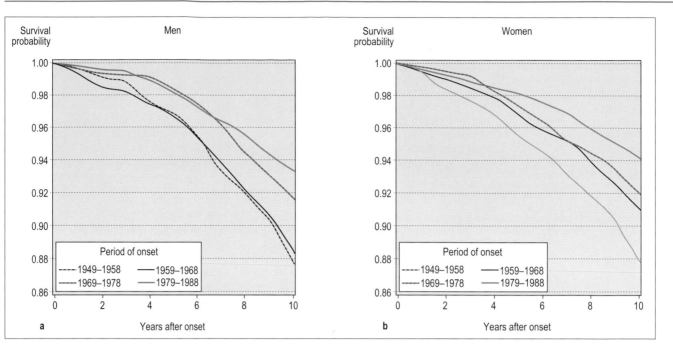

FIG. 9.4 10-year survival probability of people with multiple sclerosis aged 35 years at onset, by period of onset. Redrawn from Brønnum-Hansen et al 2004[169] with permission from Oxford University Press.

TABLE 9.6 **Excess death rates* by sex and years after onset for people with multiple sclerosis in Denmark**

Years after onset	Excess death rate (95% confidence interval)		
	Men	Women	All
0–1	1.0 (–0.6–3.4)	2.3 (0.8–4.2)	1.8 (0.7–3.2)
1–5	1.9 (0.9–3.2)	4.1 (3.2–5.2)	3.2 (2.5–4.0)
5–10	9.7 (8.0–11.5)	7.7 (6.5–9.0)	8.5 (7.5–9.5)
10–15	18.1 (15.6–20.8)	12.2 (10.5–14.0)	14.6 (13.1–16.1)
15–20	19.9 (16.8–23.3)	15.7 (13.6–18.1)	17.4 (15.6–19.3)
20–50	28.2 (25.1–31.5)	22.3 (20.3–24.5)	24.6 (22.8–26.3)
0–50	15.0 (14.0–16.1)	12.3 (11.6–13.1)	13.4 (12.8–14.0)

Observed minus expected number of deaths per 1000 person–years.
Source: modified from Brønnum-Hansen et al 2004[169] with permission from Oxford University Press.

THE MULTIPLE SCLEROSIS LATENCY PERIOD

The manifestation of the first symptom(s) or sign(s) eventually attributed to MS[3] is referred to as the clinical onset of MS. The age at onset is therefore the age at which such clinical manifestations occur. However, biological initiation of MS is believed not to coincide with the clinical initiation: the disease process starts earlier in life. Poser[190] hypothesized a 'premorbid stage of MS' or 'MS trait' to be a systemic, nonpathological condition developing in prepuberty in genetically susceptible individuals, as 'a disease waiting to happen'. The conversion of the trait into overt disease might follow subsequent triggering events, such as increased permeability of the blood–brain barrier. The time elapsing between disease initiation (induction) and clinical onset is referred to as the latency period.[191] As the cause of MS is unknown, the induction period cannot be determined, so the term 'susceptibility period' is used to refer to the time of putative disease acquisition. Because of the possible variable length of the latency period and the unknown exact temporal location of the susceptibility period within an individual's life, the study designs used to investigate risk factors, such as case–control studies, may not be informative and may instead be undermined by confounding. Migration and cluster studies represent other epidemiological approaches for investigating the MS susceptibility period.

MIGRATION STUDIES

Migration studies can help determine whether MS is related to genetic or environmental factors. Relevant studies include those conducted among immigrants from Europe to South Africa and in the population born in South Africa.[156,192] Age-adjusted prevalence and incidence rates were highest in European immigrants, lower in South African English and Afrikaners and lowest among admixed black and Caucasian Africans. Age of migration was crucial in determining the risk; adult immigrants from Europe to South Africa had a threefold higher risk of MS than those migrating at age 15 years or younger.[193] The risk of MS was higher among the children of immigrants to the UK from India, Africa and the Caribbean than among their parents, and it was similar to that among children born in the UK.[194] In France, the risk of MS was higher among people with Vietnamese mothers who had migrated from Vietnam at age 20 years or younger.[195] These individuals, however, were likely to have admixed genes from French fathers.

The prevalence of MS was 7 among Japanese living in Hawaii, 10.5 among native Hawaiians and 34 among migrant populations from North America,[115] largely reflecting the rates of Japanese and Caucasians living in California[133] and in Japan.[138]

The relevant role of age at migration was demonstrated in a study conducted on Ashkenazi (from northern Europe) and Sephardic Jews (from Asia and Africa) in Israel.[196] The risk was higher in the Ashkenazis in relation to older age at migration (after adolescence), suggesting that the age effect is probably related to the first two decades of life. The variation in the prevalence of Israel's different population groups according to ancestry or migration has already been discussed.[144,153]

A study on prevalence in a migrant population from the UK and Ireland to different regions in Australia showed that the risk among individuals who migrated before age 15 years to low-risk areas in Australia did not differ from that among individuals migrating at age 15 years or older, suggesting that environmental factors may operate over a longer period of time after childhood.[197]

The validity of migration studies is undermined by methodological issues, such as small sample sizes, the difficulty of identifying a denominator for the migrant target population,[198] the age of MS onset relative to that of migration, selection bias and confounding based on demographic features such as age, gender proportion and health status.[199] Further, too few studies have been conducted on MS incidence among migrants from low- to high-risk areas,[198] and relevant secular changes in the prevalence within the general population over time can mask prevalence in subgroups.

CLUSTER STUDIES

Clusters of disease are deviations from a random distribution of cases, most commonly in time and/or in space.[200] In contrast to post-hoc cluster analysis aimed at revealing disease clustering based on empirical evidence, space–time cluster analysis is used without any perceived excess of cases to infer on disease causation. Based on individuals' places of residence at different ages before clinical onset, it allows MS latency and susceptibility periods to be explored.[200] Riise et al[221] found clustering in Norway between 13 and 20 years, with a peak at 18 years. The degree of clustering was high among people with younger age at onset and low among those with later onset, consequently leading to latency periods of different length.[202] Among Sardinians clustering was substantial in early childhood,[203] and most marked in the most recent cases, among women, and among patients with early age at onset, and a relapsing-remitting course. MS did not cluster at a fixed time before onset, suggesting that MS is not triggered by exposure with fixed latency incubation periods (such as viral agents).[201,203] The degree of clustering was high among people with younger age at onset and low among those with later onset, consequently leading to latency periods of different length.[202] Based on diagnosed patients, space–time cluster studies cannot assess the disease status of individuals migrating from the target population before disease onset who could have potentially contributed to clustering.[198]

EPIDEMICS

Epidemics have a shorter and better defined latency period and could ideally be more successful for characterizing the susceptibility period. In this respect, epidemics are a special case of space–time clustering. The most comprehensive report on MS epidemics is Kurtzke's 30-year observational study on the pattern of MS in the Faroe Islands in the North Atlantic.[204] The adjusted MS prevalence rate was 66 in 1998. The first MS case among native residents since 1900 was reported in 1943. Based on the analysis of patterns of MS occurrence and patients' residence history, MS was hypothesized to be acquired at least 2 years after exposure to an exogenous factor and during puberty (age 11 years). After the first case, 21 new cases developed MS in a type 1 epidemic (occurrence due to initial exposure to an exogenous 'virulent' factor in a susceptible population virgin to that specific exposure). The source of such exposure was believed to be a widespread, specific, persistent infectious yet unknown agent introduced by the British troops occupying the Faroe Islands during World War II. The consequent asymptomatic infection, the 'primary MS affection', would convert into clinically detectable MS years later and only in subsets of individuals. Susceptibility to the primary MS affection would be limited to age 11–45 years at the start of exposure, whereas the primary MS affection would be transmitted at age 13–26 years and before clinical onset. The first epidemic was followed by three successive epidemics of 10, 10 and 13 cases, respectively, defined by calendar time and age of exposure, with peaks at 13-year intervals.[204] This led Kurtzke et al to conclude that MS was the result of a specific infection transmissible from person to person. After reanalyzing the data, Cooke et al[205] critiqued the 'pubertal hypothesis' with a 'protective hypothesis', hypothesizing that the pubertal exposure consisted of a childhood infection with later onset, and that early childhood would instead be the susceptibility period. Methodological issues were raised against the evidence of MS epidemics due to small sample sizes, multiple assessments over time based on registries, the use of old and more inclusive diagnostic criteria and the plausibility of the role of the British troops in determining the epidemic.[206]

In the Orkney and Shetland Islands, MS prevalence rates steadily increased by almost threefold to 110 in Orkney and from 134 to 184 in Shetland between 1954 and 1974. Over the same time period, however, general awareness of MS improved.[207] Incidence rates were stable in 1930–69, but a slight reduction at the end of the period was attributed to underascertainment and to more stringent diagnostic criteria.

In 1979, incidence in Iceland was studied based on the 168 MS cases retrospectively ascertained since 1900.[208] Until 1922, MS cases had been sporadic. The mean annual incidence rate was 1.6 in 1923–44 and 3.2 in 1945–54, followed by plateau and a decline to 1.9 in 1955–74. The age at onset also increased from 1945–9 to 1950–4. This whole incidence pattern was interpreted as a postwar epidemic of MS. This trend was reanalyzed[36,54] and explained by improved diagnostic accuracy due to the increased number of neurologists in the 1930s and in the 1970s and easier access to neurological care. It was also argued that the epidemic could be an artifact secondary to underascertainment at the end of the study period because prevalence rates were based on diagnosis rather than onset, thus not including patients who already had the first symptoms of MS but had not been diagnosed yet.[209] After adjustment for onset, prevalence rates were higher at the end of the study period.

GENETIC EPIDEMIOLOGY

Ethnic groups resistant to MS living in areas at high risk for MS demonstrate that genetics is important in shaping overall population susceptibility.[37,63] MS is a genetic complex trait. Few or multiple genes are believed to interplay independently or interactively with nonheritable exogenous agents and start MS. Although familial aggregation per se can have both genetic and exogenous causes, analyzing the pattern of occurrence can be informative in testing genetic hypotheses.[33]

TABLE 9.7 Degree of relatedness and familial risk for multiple sclerosis

Relation to subject with MS	% Sharing	Recurrence risk (%)	Lambda value
Monozygotic twins[211]	100	30.8	308
Dizygotic twins[211]	50	4.7	47
Full-siblings[212]	50	3.46	34.6
Half-siblings[212]	25	1.47	14.7
Cousins[213]	12.5	0.88	5.9

Source: modified from Dyment et al 1997[196] with the permission of Oxford University Press.

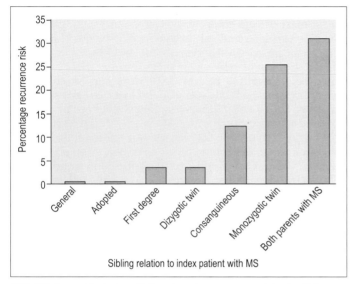

FIG. 9.5 Age-adjusted multiple sclerosis recurrence risks in siblings of index MS cases. Redrawn from Dyment et al 2004[33] with permission from The Lancet Publishing Group.

The change in the recurrence risk ratio (λ) in families of people with MS shows that first-, second- and third-degree relatives are more likely to develop MS than the general population, and this is according to the degree of biological relatedness[33,210] (Table 9.7 and Fig. 9.5). Despite the low absolute recurrence risk in the relatives, the steep drop in rates observed between monozygotic twins and first-degree relatives, and the further, yet less dramatic declines between first- and second-degree relatives and second- and third-degree relatives, favor oligogenic or polygenic inheritance with epistatic interactions among susceptibility loci.[33]

Factors contributing to an increased familial risk for MS include gender, age at onset and affected parents. For the 1567 index cases in Canada with half-siblings, the risk of MS was compared between 3436 half-siblings and 2706 full siblings.[214] The age-adjusted risk of 3.11% (95% confidence interval (CI) 2.39–3.83%) found among full siblings was higher than the 1.89% (95% CI 1.36–2.41%) among half-siblings. The risk was 2.35% (95% CI 1.57–3.13%) among maternal and 1.31% (95% CI 0.65–1.96%) among paternal half-siblings, suggesting a maternal parent-of-origin effect. Based on 1083 MS index cases, 2166 parents and 3112 sibs, the Canadian Collaborative Project on Genetic Susceptibility to MS (CCPGSMS) showed that the risk of developing MS was 2.18 times as high among the sisters of index cases as among brothers.[215] The hazard ratio for MS in siblings declined with increasing age of MS onset of index cases: 0.55-fold (95% CI 0.32–0.96) if the index case had MS onset at age 30 years or older versus that for siblings of index cases with onset at 20 years or younger.[215] Having one parent with MS doubled the risk among the siblings of MS index cases.[216] The

CCPGSMS study on conjugal MS[217] based on six MS cases among 49 offspring showed an age-adjusted risk of 30.5%, similar to that of monozygotic twins in Canada and higher than that of 2.7% among the offspring of matings with only one parent having MS.

Based on the Danish Multiple Sclerosis Registry, the lifetime familial risk for MS was analyzed for 8205 people with MS in 1968–97.[218] The relative risk of MS among first-degree relatives was 7.1 (95% CI 5.8–8.8): sevenfold that of the general population. After stratifying by kinship, similar estimates were found for parents (6.4, 95% CI 3.4–12.4), offspring (6.8, 95% CI 5.3–8.7) and nontwin siblings (8.6, 95% CI 5.2–14.2). The relative risk of MS was lower among women (5.9, 95% CI 4.5–7.9) than men (9.3, 95% CI 6.8–12.5). The relatives of men with MS (8.8, 95% CI 6.6–11.8) tended to have a higher risk than relatives of women with MS (6.0, 95% CI 4.5–8.0). Adjusted to the general population risks, familial lifetime risks were 2.9% among female first-degree relatives of MS cases and 2.8% among males.

Population-based screening of more than 16 000 people with MS revealed that the rate of MS among 1201 nonbiological first-degree relatives of people with MS adopted in early infancy was similar to that of the background population.[219] These data are in keeping with those from studies on half-siblings, in which the recurrence risk is 1.32%, much lower than the 3.46% observed for full siblings in the same population.[212] The half-siblings living with the person with MS and those living apart did not differ significantly in risk. This indicates a genetically based aggregation of MS at the familial level. A study on consanguineous matings[220] showed that the risk was nearly four-fold higher among the siblings of MS patients with third-degree-related unaffected grandparents versus that among siblings with unrelated ancestors. Although potentially biased by small numbers, these findings may suggest a low-penetrance recessive type of inheritance or low-frequency, low-penetrance dominant inheritance.

The study of conjugal MS can help determine whether MS can be transmitted in adulthood, despite concern about small sample sizes and recall bias. A population-based sample of 15 504 patients was investigated for conjugal MS within the CCPGSMS.[217] Based on 23 MS cases, the recurrence rate was 0.17%, which was intermediate between the prevalence (0.1%) and the lifetime risk (0.2%) for the general population. Similar findings were reported for Denmark.[218]

Population-based studies on twins are a classical approach for investigating the relative roles of genes and exogenous exposure in determining MS.[221] The rate of MS among monozygotic twins (30%) is about tenfold that among dizygotic twins, indicating that genes are involved in the process of susceptibility[32,33,211,222–225] (Table 9.8). Based on the CCPGSMS, the probandwise concordance rates analyzed for more than 19 938 probands were 25.3% (SE±4.4%) in monozygotic twins, 5.4% (SE±2.8%) in dizygotic twins and 2.9% (SE±0.6) in their nontwin siblings.[230] The excess concordance in monozygotic twins was primarily ascribed to like-sexed female pairs with a

TABLE 9.8 Selected multiple sclerosis twin studies since 1980	
Pairwise monozygotic twin concordance	Pairwise dizygotic twin concordance
6/12 (50%)[226]	2/12 (16.7%)[226]
8/22 (36.4%)[227]	3/29 (10.3%)[227]
4/19 (21.1%)[223]	1/28 (3.57%)[223]
1/11 (9.1%)[224]	0/10[224]
2/7 (28.6%)[228]	0/6[228]
1/17 (5.9%)[229]	1/37 (2.7%)[229]
11/44 (25%)[225]	2/61 (3.3%)[225]
24/133 (18.0%)[230]	9/221 (4.1%)[230]
Total 57/265 (21.5%)	Total 18/404(4.5%)

Source: modified from Dyment et al 2004[33] with the permission of The Lancet Publishing Group.

probandwise concordance rate of 34% (SE±5.7%) versus 3.8% (SE±2.8%) for female dizygotic twin pairs.

ENVIRONMENTAL RISK FACTORS

Reviews of the role of environmental factors[35,231,232] in causing MS highlight the complexity in identifying proper design approaches and interpreting the findings obtained. Potentially any environmental agent can have a role in determining MS in susceptible populations and yet be neither a necessary nor a sufficient cause. Potential risk factors investigated have been infectious disorders, vaccines, stress, occupation, climate and nutrition. Chapter 13 discusses infectious agents and MS, and Lauer,[233] Martinelli,[234] Marrie,[35] Coo & Aronson[235] and Schwartz & Leweling[236] review this topic.

OCCUPATIONAL EXPOSURE AND TOXINS

Among all types of occupational exposures, organic solvents have raised most concern in studies of MS causation.[35] The prevalence of MS was five times higher in a group of employees in a leather factory in Italy than in the background and the employed population. Odd ratios varying from 0.8–4.0 are reported from case–control studies using a sufficiently large number of cases, but statistical significance is almost never reached. The cumulative incidence rate ratio of MS was found to be increased in female nurse anesthetists compared to teachers.[237] Several methodological issues have been raised, such as the cross-sectional nature of most studies based on prevalence, self-reported exposure assessment reflecting recall bias, the lack of adjustment to confounders and the small sample sizes. Few studies have focused on the putative period elapsing between exposure and onset as well as defining 'exposed' by the necessary duration of exposure. The results from cohort studies are also controversial.

GEOCLIMATIC FACTORS

Sun exposure, ultraviolet (UV) radiation and latitude are inversely correlated with MS.[35,232,235,238] As MS has long been reported to vary with latitude, an association with UV radiation has been hypothesized, also based on the suppressive effects of UV radiation on T-cell functioning.[238] Ecological studies showed strong inverse correlations between UV radiation and MS and between residential and occupational exposure to sunlight and MS mortality and showed that the incidence of skin cancer in

the MS population was significantly lower than expected. In a study conducted on monozygotic twins, sun exposure-related activities during childhood seemed to convey a strong protection against MS.[239] Higher vitamin D intake was associated with a lower risk of MS.[232,240] Vitamin D receptor polymorphisms were associated with MS in the population of Japan but not Canada. Because of confounding related to dietary factors and inconsistent measurements of sunlight exposure, the evidence is too weak to even partly explain the geographical variation in MS risk as an effect of sunlight.

STRESS

Several authors have supported the causative role of traumatic brain injuries such as cervical whiplash injury, closed head trauma and cervical compression by spondylosis in the incidence of MS due to disruption of the blood–brain barrier, impaired blood supply to the spinal cord or compression.[35,234] Physical trauma (especially head trauma) is not associated with MS onset, exacerbation or progression, and only weakly with emotional stress. Compared with controls, people with MS had more frequently undergone intense mental stress or severely threatening life events, such as the death of a child, a few years before onset. The limitations of studies on the role of physical and emotional stress in causing MS derive from inconsistent measurements of exposure, recall bias, small sample sizes and confounding.

SEX HORMONES

As MS is predominant in women, sex hormones have been hypothesized to play a causative role, the biological plausibility lying in the effect of such hormones on the immune system.[235] Epidemiological studies on sex hormones and MS have focused on four major risk factors: age at menarche, pregnancy, parity and use of oral contraceptives. None has provided sufficient evidence on the role of these hormones in causing MS. Whether pregnancy is associated with fewer relapses and postpartum with more is still debated.

DIET

Diet as a risk factor has been of interest in MS studies for over 50 years because it implies potentially toxic agents and because it varies with ethnicity and geographical areas in which MS occurrence also differs.[23,235,236] Because most studies are cross-sectional, the role of nutrition in causing MS is inferred from observations on individuals' current nutritional status. Several population-based ecological studies conducted in different areas reported that MS is correlated with the consumption of milk, dairy products, meat and especially animal fat but few case–control studies have confirmed this. Dietary fat has been reported to correlate with MS and mortality and fatty acids are reported to have a role in the MS course. Lower levels of linoleic acid, an omega-6 fatty acid, have been found in the blood, blood cells, cerebrospinal fluid and brain of MS patients, but the interpretation of such findings is controversial. Other dietary factors such as the consumption of brain, sweets and confectionery, new potatoes, alcohol, smoked meat products, pasta, bread, horsemeat, minestrone, coffee, tea and breastmilk have been investigated as potential risk factors in MS. Vitamin B_{12} deficiency is not unusual in MS patients but no evidence indicates its causative role. No consistent data from analytical studies and clinical trials confirm any relationship between MS and nutrition. Methodological problems have mostly consisted of selection bias, differential recall on diet between patients and controls and within patients before and after diagnosis, the lack of objective measurements of dietary factors and the scarce control for confounders.

OTHER FACTORS

Results from case–control and cohort studies indicate that cigarette smoking is a risk factor for MS.[232,241] The risk of developing MS was 1.81 times as high (rate ratio, 95% CI 1.1–2.9) among smokers as among never-smokers in a population in Norway in 1997–9.[242] Smoking was found to be a significant independent factor for MS in a case-control study conducted in Serbia (OR=2.4).[243] In the Nurses' Health Study and Nurses' Health Study II, the incidence relative rate was 1.6 (95% CI 1.2–2.1) among smokers and 1.2 (95% CI 0.9–1.6) among ex-smokers versus women who never smoked.[244] The relative risk increased significantly with cumulative exposure to smoking from 1.1 for 1–9 pack-years to 1.7 for 25 or more pack-years. All rates were adjusted for potential confounders. A nested case–control study of 201 people with MS found an odds ratio of 1.3 (95% CI 1.0–1.7) for ever-smokers versus never-smokers.[245]

Individuals with MS have an excess of spring births.[246–248] A population-based study of 17 874 people with MS in Canada and 11 502 in Great Britain showed that significantly fewer were born in November versus controls from the population census and unaffected siblings.[246] Pooled analysis of datasets from Canada, Great Britain, Denmark and Sweden (n = 42 045) showed that fewer (8.5%) people with MS were born in November and more (9.1%) were born in May. The association between seasonal variation and risk of MS onset, or disease activity,[249] has been interpreted as a climate-related interaction between genes and environment during gestation or shortly after birth, at least for northern Caucasian populations. Methodological issues such as random variation, misclassification and statistical methods applied, however, may partly explain such results.

CONCLUSIONS

The prevalence of MS has increased substantially worldwide. Environmental changes have been hypothesized to account for such change, as genetics requires longer to shape prevalence. However, the geographical distribution of absolute rates might depend on the distribution of genetic susceptibility alleles and their interaction with specific environmental factors. Environmental and genetic determinants of such rate gradients are not mutually exclusive, so the nature-versus-nurture controversy is a sterile debate. Ethnicity and ancestry are often used to refer to populations' genetic origin but can also refer to cultural habits and lifestyle factors, which can confound results.

However, whether the reported increases in disease rates partly reflect a true change in MS risk or merely improved case ascertainment, demographic factors, such as increased survival, or better study methods over time is still debated. The outlining of geographical patterns is undermined by the variation in the size, age structure and ethnicity of the populations surveyed;[250] case ascertainment;[126] the level of health care and expertise, degree of public awareness of MS and access to diagnostic procedures;[126] and the methods applied to study designs and statistical analysis. Prevalence rates almost invariably increase with multiple-source repeated assessments over time and when small populations are used.[251]

Finally, the most relevant and to some extent hopeless concern in MS epidemiology is that its clinical heterogeneity probably reflects diverse causes. Histopathological evidence[252] suggests that at least four distinct types of demyelinating disorder of the central nervous system might be contained under the diagnosis of MS. Such definition would rather serve a syndromic nosological entity, comprising undistinguished diseases and consequently biasing the effect size, if any, of the action of any exposure detected. Efforts in future epidemiological research on MS need to be directed towards such clinical and epidemiological distinction by reliable variables, hence the need for large comprehensive multicenter networks.

REFERENCES

1. Cole P. The evolving case–control study. J Chronic Dis 1979; 32: 15–27.
2. Rothman KJ, Greenland S. Measures of disease frequency. In: Rothman KJ, Greenland S, eds. Modern epidemiology, 2nd edn. Baltimore, MD: Lippincott Williams & Wilkins; 1998: 29–46.
3. Poser CM. Onset symptoms of multiple sclerosis. J Neurol Neurosurg Psychiatry 1995; 58: 253–264.
4. Kurtzke JF, Kurland LT, Goldberg ID et al. Multiple sclerosis. In: Kurland LT, Kurtzke JF, Goldberg ID, eds. Epidemiology of neurologic and sense organ disorders. Cambridge, MA: Harvard University Press; 1973: 604–607.
5. Poser CM, Brinar VV. Diagnostic criteria for multiple sclerosis: an historical review. Clin Neurol Neurosurg 2004; 106: 147–158.
6. Poser CM, Paty DW, Scheinberg L, et al. New diagnostic criteria for multiple sclerosis: guidelines for research protocols. Ann Neurol 1983; 13: 227–231.
7. McDonald WI, Compston A, Edan G et al. Recommended diagnostic criteria for multiple sclerosis: guidelines from the International Panel on the Diagnosis of Multiple Sclerosis. Ann Neurol 2001; 50: 121–127.
8. Fox CM, Bensa S, Bray I, Zajicek JP. The epidemiology of multiple sclerosis in Devon: a comparison of the new and old classification criteria. J Neurol Neurosurg Psychiatry 2004; 75: 56–60.

9. Fangerau T, Schimrigk S, Haupts M et al. Diagnosis of multiple sclerosis: comparison of the Poser criteria and the new McDonald criteria. Acta Neurol Scand 2004; 109: 385–389.
10. Zipoli V, Portaccio E, Siracusa G et al. Interobserver agreement on Poser's and the new McDonald's diagnostic criteria for multiple sclerosis. Mult Scler 2003; 9: 481–485.
11. Kurztke JF. Multiple sclerosis from an epidemiological viewpoint. In: Field EJ, ed. Multiple sclerosis. A critical conspectus. Lancaster: MTP Press; 1977: 83–142.
12. Buehler JW. Surveillance. In: Rothman KJ, Greenland S, eds. Modern epidemiology, 2nd edn. Baltimore, MD: Lippincott Williams & Wilkins; 1998: 435–457.
13. Koch-Henriksen N, Rasmussen S, Stenager E et al. The Danish Multiple Sclerosis Registry. History, data collection and validity. Dan Med Bull 2001; 48: 91–94.
14. Koch-Henriksen N, Hyllested K. Epidemiology of multiple sclerosis: incidence and prevalence rates in Denmark 1948–64 based on the Danish Multiple Sclerosis Registry. Acta Neurol Scand 1988; 78: 369–380.
15. Koch-Henriksen N, Brønnum-Hansen H, Hyllested K. Incidence of multiple sclerosis in Denmark 1948–1982: a descriptive nationwide study. Neuroepidemiology 1992; 11: 1–10.

16. Koch-Henriksen N. The Danish Multiple Sclerosis Registry: a 50-year follow-up. Mult Scler 1999; 5: 293–296.
17. Brønnum-Hansen H, Koch-Henriksen N, Hyllested K. Survival of patients with multiple sclerosis in Denmark: a nationwide, long-term epidemiologic survey. Neurology 1994; 44: 1901–1907.
18. Melton LJ III. History of the Rochester Epidemiology Project. Mayo Clin Proc 1996; 71: 266–274.
19. MacLean AR, Berkson J, Woltman HW et al. Multiple sclerosis in a rural community. In: Woltman HW, Merritt HH, Wortis SB et al, eds. Association for research in nervous and mental disease. Multiple sclerosis and the demyelinating diseases. Baltimore, MD: Williams & Wilkins; 1950: 25–27.
20. Consortium of Multiple Sclerosis Centers (CMSC). NARCOMS Multiple Sclerosis Registry (www.mscare.org/patient. cfm?doc_id=65, accessed 23 Oct 2005).
21. Confavreux C, Compston DA, Hommes OR et al. EDMUS, a European database for multiple sclerosis. J Neurol Neurosurg Psychiatr 1992; 55: 671–676.
22. Confavreux C. Establishment and use of multiple sclerosis registers – EDMUS. Ann Neurol 1994; 36(suppl): S136–S139.
23. Amato MP, Grimaud J, Achiti I et al for the Evaluation of the EDMUS system (EVALUED) Study Group. European validation of a standardized clinical

description of multiple sclerosis. J Neurol 2004; 251: 1472–1480.

24. Confavreux C, Hutchisnon M, Hours MM et al. Rate of pregnancy-related relapse in multiple sclerosis. Pregnancy in Multiple Sclerosis Group. N Engl J Med 1998; 339: 285–291.

25. Vukusic S, Hutchinson M, Hours M et al. and the Pregnancy in Multiple Sclerosis Group. Pregnancy and multiple sclerosis (the PRIMS study): clinical predictors of post-partum relapse. Brain 2004; 127: 1353–1360.

26. Confavreux C, Suissa S, Saddier P et al. Vaccination and the risk of relapse in multiple sclerosis. N Engl J Med 2001; 344: 319–326.

27. Mikaeloff Y, Adamsbaum C, Husson B et al and the KIDMUS study group on Radiology. MRI prognostic factors for relapse after a first episode of acute CNS inflammatory demyelination in childhood. Brain 2004; 124: 1942–1947.

28. Mikaeloff Y, Suissa S, Vallée L et al and the KIDMUS Study Group. First episode of acute CNS inflammatory demyelination in childhood: prognostic factors for multiple sclerosis and disability. J Pediatrics 2004; 144: 246–252.

29. Confavreux C, Vukusic S, Moreau T et al. Relapses and progression of disability in multiple sclerosis. N Engl J Med 2000; 343: 1430–1438.

30. Confavreux C, Vukusic S, Adeleine P. Early clinical predictors and progression of irreversible disability in multiple sclerosis: an amnesic process. Brain 2003; 126: 770–782.

31. Ebers GC, Paty DW, Stiller CR et al. HI A-typing in multiple sclerosis sibling pairs. Lancet 1982; 2: 88–90.

32. Ebers GC, Bulman DE, Sadovnick AD et al. A population-based study of multiple sclerosis in twins. N Engl J Med 1986; 15: 1638–1642.

33. Dyment DA, Ebers GC, Sadovnick AD. Genetics of multiple sclerosis. Lancet Neurol 2004; 3: 104–110.

34. Myhr KM, Grytten N, Aarseth JH, Nyland H. The Norwegian Multiple Sclerosis National Competence Centre and National Multiple Sclerosis registry – a resource for clinical practice and research. Acta Neurol Scand 2006; 183(Suppl): 37–40.

35. Marrie RA. Environmental risk factors in multiple sclerosis aetiology. Lancet Neurol 2004; 3: 709–718.

36. Firnhaber W, Lauer K eds. Multiple sclerosis in Europe: an epidemiological update. Darmstadt: Leuchtturm-Verlag/LTV Press; 1994.

37. Rosati G. The prevalence of multiple sclerosis in the world: an update. Neurol Sci 2001; 22: 117–139.

38. Pugliatti M, Rosati G, Carton H et al. The epidemiology of multiple sclerosis in Europe. 2006; 13: 700–722.

39. Baumhackl U, Eibl G, Ganzinger U et al. Prevalence of multiple sclerosis in Austria. Results of a nationwide survey. Neuroepidemiology 2002; 21: 226–234.

40. Van Ooteghem P, De Hooghe MB, Vlietnick R et al. Prevalence of multiple sclerosis in Flanders, Belgium. Neuroepidemiology 1994; 13: 220–225.

41. Milanov I, Georgiev D, Kmetska K et al. Prevalence of multiple sclerosis in Bulgaria. Neuroepidemiology 1997; 16: 304–307.

42. Materljan E, Sepcic J. Epidemiology of multiple sclerosis in Croatia. Clin Neurol Neurosurg 2002; 104: 192–198.

43. Peterlin B, Ristic S, Sepcic J et al. Region with persistent high frequency of multiple sclerosis in Croatia and Slovenia. J Neurol Sci 2006; 247: 169–172.

44. Middleton LT, Dean G. Multiple sclerosis in Cyprus. J Neurol Sci 1991; 103: 29–36.

45. Brønnum-Hansen H, Stenager E, Hansen T, Koch-Henriksen H. Survival and mortality rates among Danes with MS. Int MS J 2006; 13: 66–71.

46. Gross K, Kokk A, Kaasik AE. Prevalence of MS in south Estonia. Evidence of a new border of the Fennoscandian focus. Acta Neurol Scand 1993; 88: 241–246.

47. Sumelahti ML, Tienari PJ, Wikström J et al. Increasing prevalence of multiple sclerosis in Finland. Acta Neurol Scand 2001; 103: 153–158.

48. Sarasoja T, Wikstrom J, Paltamaa J et al. Occurrence of multiple sclerosis in central Finland: a regional and temporal comparison during 30 years. Acta Neurol Scand 2004; 110: 331–336.

49. Kurtzke JF, Delasnerie-Lauprêtre N. Reflection on the geographic distribution of multiple sclerosis in France. Acta Neurol Scand 1996; 93: 110–117.

50. Vukusic S, Van Bockstael V, Gosselin S, Confavreux C. Regional variations in the prevalence of multiple sclerosis in French farmers. J Neurol Neurosurg Psychiatry 2007; 78: 707–709.

51. Hein T, Hopfenmüller W [Projection of the number of multiple sclerosis patients in Germany]. Nervenartz 2000; 71: 288–294.

52. Piperidou HN, Holiopoulos IN, Maltezos ES et al. Epidemiological data of multiple sclerosis in the province of Evros, Greece. Eur Neurol 2003; 49: 8–12.

53. Bencsik K, Rajda C, Füvesi J et al. The prevalence of multiple sclerosis, distribution of clinical forms of the disease and functional status of patients in Csongrád County, Hungary. Eur Neurol 2001; 46: 206–209.

54. Benedikz J, Magnus S, Gudmundsson J et al. The natural history of untreated multiple sclerosis in Iceland. A total population-based 50 year prospective study. Clin Neurol Neurosurg 2002; 104: 208–210.

55. McGuigan C, McCarthy A, Quigley C et al. Latitudinal variation in the prevalence of multiple sclerosis in Ireland, an effect of genetic diversity. J Neurol Neurosurg Psychiatr 2004; 75: 572–576.

56. Granieri E, Malagú S, Casetta I et al. Multiple sclerosis in Italy. A reappraisal of incidence and prevalence in Ferrara. Arch Neurol 1996; 53: 793–798.

57. Nicoletti A, Lo Bartolo ML, Lo Fermo S et al. Prevalence and incidence of multiple sclerosis in Catania, Sicily. Neurology 2001; 56: 62–66.

58. Totaro R, Marini C, Cialfi A et al. Prevalence of multiple sclerosis in the L'Aquila district, central Italy. J Neurol Neurosurg Psychiatr 2000; 68: 349–352.

59. Pugliatti M, Sotgiu S, Solinas G et al. Multiple sclerosis epidemiology in Sardinia: evidence for a true increasing risk. Acta Neurol Scand 2001; 103: 20–26.

60. Solaro C, Allemani C, Messmer Uccelli M et al. The prevalence of multiple sclerosis in the north-west Italian province of Genoa. J Neurol 2005; 252: 436–440.

61. Ranzato F, Perini P, Tzintzeva E et al. Increasing frequency of multiple sclerosis in Padova, Italy: a 30-year epidemiological survey. Mult Scler 2003; 9: 387–392.

62. Dean G, Elian M, Galea de Bono A et al. Multiple sclerosis in Malta in 1999: an update. J Neurol Neurosurg Psychiatr 2002; 73: 256–260.

63. Grønlie SA, Myrvoll E, Hansen G et al. Multiple sclerosis in north Norway, and first appearance in an indigenous population. J Neurol 2000; 247: 129–133.

64. Celius EG, Vandvik B. Multiple sclerosis in Oslo, Norway: prevalence on 1 January 1995 and incidence over a 25-year period. Eur J Neurol 2001; 8: 463–469.

65. Dahl OP, Aarseth JH, Myhr KM et al. Multiple sclerosis in Nord-Trøndelag County, Norway: a prevalence and incidence study. Acta Neurol Scand 2004; 109: 378–384.

66. Grytten N, Glad SB, Aarseth JH et al. A 50-year follow-up of the incidence of multiple sclerosis in Hordaland County, Norway. Neurology 2006; 66: 182–186.

67. Potemkowski A. Epidemiology of multiple sclerosis in the region of Szczecin: prevalence and incidence 1993–1995. Neurol Neurochir Pol 1999; 33: 575–585.

68. De Sã J, Paulos A, Mendes H et al. The prevalence of multiple sclerosis in the District of Santarem, Portugal. J Neurol 2006; 253: 914–918.

69. Becus T, Popoviciu L. Epidemiologic survey of multiple sclerosis in Mures County, Romania. Rom J Neurol Psychiatr 1994; 32: 115–122.

70. Boiko A, Zavalishin IA, Spirin NN et al. Epidemiology of MS in Russia: first data of United Study of Multiple Sclerosis epidemiology in Russia. Mult Scler 2004; 10(suppl 2): 157.

71. Pekmezovic T, Jarebinski M, Drulovic J et al. Prevalence of multiple sclerosis in Belgrade, Yugoslavia. Acta Neurol Scand 2001; 104: 353–357.

72. Modrego Pardo PJ, Pina Latorre MA, López A et al. Prevalence of multiple sclerosis in the province of Teruel, Spain. J Neurol 1997; 244: 182–185.

73. Tola MA, Yugueros MI, Fernández-Buey N et al. Prevalence of multiple sclerosis in Valladolid, northern Spain. J Neurol 1999; 246: 170–174.

74. Benito-Léon J, Martín E, Vela L et al. Multiple sclerosis in Móstoles, central Spain. Acta Neurol Scand 1998; 98: 238–242.

75. Sundström P, Nyström L, Forsgren L. Incidence (1988–97) and prevalence (1997) of multiple sclerosis in Västerbotten County in northern Sweden. J Neurol Neurosurg Psychiatr 2003; 74: 29–32.

76. Beer S, Kesserling J. High prevalence of multiple sclerosis in Switzerland. Neuroepidemiology 1994; 19: 14–18.

77. Korbut AL, Konryichuk AG. MS in the population of Vinnytsya City, central Ukraine. In: Abstracts of the 33rd International Danube Symposium, Lublin, August 29–September 1, 2001. Neurol Neurochir Pol 2000; suppl. 2: 1–60.

78. Robertson N, Compston A. Surveying multiple sclerosis in the United Kingdom. J Neurol Neurosurg Psychiatr 1995; 58: 2–6.

79. Rothwell PM, Charlton D. High incidence and prevalence of multiple sclerosis in

south east Scotland: evidence of a genetic predisposition. J Neurol Neurosurg Psychiatr 1998; 64: 733–735.

80. Forbes RB, Wilson SV, Swingler RJ. The prevalence of multiple sclerosis in Tayside, Scotland: do latitudinal gradients really exist? J Neurol 1999; 246: 1033–1040.

81. Ford HL, Gerry E, Airey CM et al. The prevalence of multiple sclerosis in the Leeds Health Authority. J Neurol Neurosurg Psychiatr 1998; 64: 605–610.

82. McDonnell GV, Hawkins SA. An epidemiologic study of multiple sclerosis in Northern Ireland. Neurology 1998; 50: 423–428.

83. Rose AS, Ellison GW, Myers LW et al. New diagnostic criteria for the clinical diagnosis of multiple sclerosis. Neurology 1976; 26(suppl): 20–22.

84. Sumelahti ML, Tienari P, Wikström J et al. Regional and temporal variation in the incidence of multiple sclerosis in Finland in 1979–1993. Neuroepidemiology 2000; 19: 67–75.

85. Moreau T, Manceau E, Lucas B et al. Incidence of multiple sclerosis in Dijon, France: a population-based ascertainment. Neurol Res 2000; 22: 156–159.

86. Konryichuk AG, Zheliba OV. Epidemiology of MS in Vinnytsia Oblast, south-west Ukraine. In: The 11th European Congress on Multiple Sclerosis. Abstracts. J Neuroimmunol 1995; suppl 1: 1–86.

87. Allison R. Disseminated sclerosis in north Wales: an inquiry into its incidence, frequency, distribution and other aetiological factors. Brain 1931; 53: 391–430.

88. Swingler RJ, Compston D. The distribution of multiple sclerosis in the United Kingdom. J Neurol Neurosurg Psychiatr 1986; 49: 1115–1124.

89. Cook SD, Cromarty MB, Tapp W et al. Declining incidence of multiple sclerosis in the Orkney Islands. Neurology 1985; 35: 545–551.

90. Cook SD, MacDonald J, Tapp W, Poskanzer D, Dowling PC. Multiple sclerosis in the Shetland Islands: an update. Acta Neurol Scand 1988; 77: 148–151.

91. McDonnell GV, Hawkins SA. Multiple sclerosis in Northern Ireland: a historical and global perspective. Ulster Med J 2000; 69: 97–105.

92. Williams ES, Jones DR, McKeran RO. Mortality rates from multiple sclerosis: geographical and temporal variations revisited. J Neurol Neurosurg Psychiatr 1991; 54: 104–109.

93. Kurtzke JF. A Fennoscandian focus of multiple sclerosis. Neurology 1968; 18: 16–20.

94. Larsen JP, Kvaale G, Riise T et al. An increase in the incidence of multiple sclerosis in western Norway. Acta Neurol Scand 1984; 70: 96–103.

95. Midgard R, Riise T, Kvale G et al. Disability and mortality in multiple sclerosis in western Norway. Acta Neurol Scand 1996; 93: 307–314.

96. Edland A, Nyland H, Riise T et al. Epidemiology of multiple sclerosis in the county of Vestfold, eastern Norway: incidence and prevalence calculations. Acta Neurol Scand 1996; 93: 104–109.

97. Svenningsson A, Runmarker B, Lycke J et al. Incidence of multiple sclerosis during two fifteen-year periods in the Gothenburg region of Sweden. Acta Neurol Scand 1990; 82: 161–168.

98. Sundström P, Nyström L, Forsgren L. Prevalence of multiple sclerosis in Västerbotten County in northern Sweden. Acta Neurol Scand 2001; 103: 214–218.

99. Bencsik K, Rajda C, Klivényi P et al. The prevalence of multiple sclerosis in the Hungarian city of Szeged. Acta Neurol Scand 1998; 97: 315–319.

100. Alperovitch A, Bouvier MH. Geographical pattern of death rates from multiple sclerosis in France. An analysis of 4912 deaths. Acta Neurol Scand 1982; 66: 454–461.

101. Van Bockstael V, Gosselin S, Vukusic S et al. Prevalence of multiple sclerosis in French farmers: a national survey. Mult Scler 2004; 10(suppl 2): S156.

102. Granieri E, Casetta I, Govoni V et al. The increasing incidence and prevalence of MS in a Sardinian province. Neurology 2000; 55: 842–847.

103. Pugliatti M, Riise T, Sotgiu MA et al. Increasing incidence of multiple sclerosis in the province of Sassari, northern Sardinia. Neuroepidemiology 2005; 25: 129–134.

104. Sotgiu S, Pugliatti M, Sanna A et al. Multiple sclerosis complexity in selected populations: the challenge of Sardinia, insular Italy. Eur J Neurol 2002; 9: 329–341.

105. Boiko A, Deomina T, Favorova O et al. Epidemiology of multiple sclerosis in Russia and other of the former Soviet Union: investigations of environmental and genetic factors. Acta Neurol Scand 1995; 91(suppl 161): 71–76.

106. Sloka JS, Pryse-Phillips WE et al. Incidence and prevalence of multiple sclerosis in Newfoundland and Labrador. Can J Neurol Sci 2005; 32: 37–42.

107. Svenson LW, Warren S, Warren KG et al. Prevalence of multiple sclerosis in First Nations people of Alberta. Can J Neurol Sci 2007; 34: 175–180.

108. Hader WJ. The incidence and prevalence of multiple sclerosis in Saskatoon, Saskatchewan: a reappraisal. Neuroepidemiology 1999; 18: 331.

109. Hader WJ, Elliot M, Ebers GC. Epidemiology of multiple sclerosis in London and Middlesex County, Ontario, Canada. Neurology 1988; 38: 617–621.

110. Mayr WT, Pittock SJ, McClelland RL et al. Incidence and prevalence of multiple sclerosis in Olmsted County, Minnesota, 1985–2000. Neurology 2003; 61: 1373–1377.

111. Hopkins RS, Indian RW, Pinnow E et al. Multiple sclerosis in Galion, Ohio: prevalence and results of a case–control study. Neuroepidemiology 1991; 10: 192–199.

112. Nelson LM, Hamman RF, Thomson DS et al. Higher than expected prevalence of multiple sclerosis in northern Colorado: dependence on methodologic issues. Neuroepidemiology 1986; 5: 17–28.

113. Williamson DM, Henry JP, Schiffer R, Wagner L. Prevalence of multiple sclerosis in 19 Texas counties, 1998–2000. J Environ Health 2007; 69: 41–45.

114. Sheremata WA, Poskanzer DC, Withum DG et al. Unusual occurrence on a tropical island of multiple sclerosis. Lancet 1985; 2: 618.

115. Alter M, Okihiro M, Rowley W et al. Multiple sclerosis among Orientals and Caucasians in Hawaii. Neurology 1971; 21: 122–130.

116. Baum HM, Rothschild BB. The incidence and prevalence of reported multiple sclerosis. Ann Neurol 1981; 10: 420–428.

117. Noonan CW, Kathman SJ, White MC. Prevalence estimates for MS in the United States and evidence of an increasing trend for women. Neurology 2002; 58: 136–138.

118. Christensen JC. Multiple sclerosis: some epidemiological clues to its etiology. Acta Neurol Latinoam 1975; 21: 66–85.

119. De la Maza M, Garcia J, Bernal J et al. [A review of the epidemiology of multiple sclerosis in Mexico]. Rev Neurol 2000; 31: 494–495.

120. Cabrera-Gomez JA, Rivera-Olmos V. Multiple sclerosis in Cuba and Central America countries: a review. Rev Neurol 2000; 156(suppl 3): 162–163.

121. Alvarenga RMM, Santos CMM, Vasconcelos CCF et al. Multiple sclerosis in Rio de Janeiro. Rev Neurol 2000; 156(suppl 3): 159–160.

122. Callegaro D, Goldbaum M, Morais L et al. The prevalence of multiple sclerosis in the city of São Paulo, Brazil, 1997. Acta Neurol Scand 2001; 104: 208–213.

123. Toro J, Sarmiento OL, Díaz del Castillo A et al. Prevalence of multiple sclerosis in Bogotá, Colombia. Neuroepidemiology 2007; 28: 33–38.

124. Cristiano E, Patrucco L, Garcea O et al. Prevalence of multiple sclerosis in Argentina estimated by the capture–recapture method. Mult Scler 1997; 3: 282.

125. Oehninger C, Ketzoian C, Buzó R et al. Multiple sclerosis in Uruguay: epidemiologic study. Mult Scler 1998; 4: 371.

126. Sadovnick AD, Ebers GC. Epidemiology of multiple sclerosis: a critical overview. Can J Neurol Sci 1993; 20: 17–29.

127. Ebers GC, Sadovnick AD. The role of genetic factors in multiple sclerosis susceptibility. J Neuroimmunol 1994; 54: 1–17.

128. Hader WJ, Seland TP, Hader MB et al. The occurrence of multiple sclerosis in the Hutterites of North America. Can J Neurol Sci 1996; 23: 291–295.

129. Kurtzke JF, Beebe GW, Norman JE Jr. Epidemiology of multiple sclerosis in US veterans. 1. Race, sex, and geographic distribution. Neurology 1979; 29: 1228–1235.

130. Page WF, Kurtzke JF, Murphy FM et al. Epidemiology of multiple sclerosis in US veterans. V. Ancestry and the risk of multiple sclerosis. Ann Neurol 1993; 33: 632–639.

131. Hernán MA, Olek MJ, Ascherio A. Geographic variations of multiple sclerosis incidence in two prospective studies of US women. Neurology 1999; 53: 1711–1718.

132. Kira J. Multiple sclerosis in the Japanese population. Lancet Neurology 2003; 2: 117–127.

133. Kuroiwa Y, Kurland LT, eds. Multiple sclerosis: east and west. Fukuoka: Kyuhu University; 1982: 83–96.

134. Lau KK, Wong LK, Li LS et al. Epidemiological study of multiple sclerosis in Hong Kong Chinese: questionnaire survey. Hong Kong Med J 2002; 8: 77–80.

135. Singhal BS. Clinical profile and HLA-studies in Indian multiple sclerosis patients

from the Bombay region. In: Kuroiwa Y, Kurland LT, eds. Multiple sclerosis east and west. Fukuoka: Kyushu University Press; 1982: 123–134.

136. Hou JB, Zang ZX. Prevalence of multiple sclerosis: a door to door survey in Lan Cang La Hu Zu autonomous county, Yunnan Province of China. Neuroepidemiology 1992; 11: 52.

137. Cheng Q, Miao L, Zhang J et al. A population-based survey of multiple sclerosis in Shanghai, China. Neurology 2007; 68: 1495–1500.

138. Kuroiwa Y, Shibasaki H, Ikeda M. Prevalence of multiple sclerosis and its north-to-south gradient in Japan. Neuroepidemiology 1983; 2: 62–69.

139. Araki S, Uchino M, Kumamoto T. Prevalence studies of multiple sclerosis, myasthenia gravis, and myopathies in Kumamoto District, Japan. Neuroepidemiology 1987; 6: 120–129.

140. Tan CT. Multiple sclerosis in Malaysia. Arch Neurol 1988; 45: 624–627.

141. Tsai CP, Yuan CL, Yu HY et al. Multiple sclerosis in Taiwan. J Chin Med Assoc 2004; 67: 500–505.

142. Itoh T, Aizawa H, Hashimoto K et al. Prevalence of multiple sclerosis in Asahikawa, a city in northern Japan. J Neurol Sci 2003; 214: 7–9.

143. Wadia NH, Bhatia K. Multiple sclerosis is prevalent in the Zoroastrians (Parsis) of India. Ann Neurol 1990; 28: 177–179.

144. Alter M, Kahana E, Zilber N, Miller A. Multiple sclerosis frequency in Israel's diverse populations. Neurology 2006; 66: 1061–1066.

145. Kurdi A, Abdallat A, Ayesh I et al. Different B lymphocyte alloantigens associated with multiple sclerosis in Arabs and northern Europeans. Lancet 1977; 1123–1125.

146. El-Salem K, Al-Shimmery E, Horany K et al. Multiple sclerosis in Jordan: a clinical and epidemiological study. J Neurol 2006; 253: 1210–1216.

147. Al-Din AS, Khogali M, Poser CM et al. Epidemiology of multiple sclerosis in Arabs in Kuwait: a comparative study between Kuwaitis and Palestinians. J Neurol Sci 1990; 100: 137–141.

148. Alshubaili AF, Alramzy K, Ayyad YM et al. Epidemiology of multiple sclerosis in Kuwait: new trends in incidence and prevalence. Eur Neurol 2005; 53: 125–131.

149. Etemadifar M, Janghorbani M, Shaygannejad V, Ashtari F. Prevalence of multiple sclerosis in Isfahan, Iran. Neuroepidemiology 2006; 27: 39–44.

150. Yaqub BA, Daif AK. Multiple sclerosis in Saudi Arabia. Neurology 1988; 38: 621–623.

151. Kira J, Yamasaki K, Horiuchi I et al. Changes in the clinical phenotypes of multiple sclerosis during the past 50 years in Japan. J Neurol Sci 1999; 166: 53–57.

152. Wasay M, Ali S, Khatri IA et al. Multiple sclerosis in Pakistan. Mult Scler 2007; 13: 668–669.

153. Kahana E, Zilber N, Abramson JH et al. Multiple sclerosis: genetic versus environmental etiology: epidemiology in Israel updated. J Neurol 1994; 241: 341–346.

154. Karni A, Kahana E, Zilber N et al. The frequency of multiple sclerosis in Jewish and Arab populations in greater Jerusalem. Neuroepidemiology 2003; 22: 82–86.

155. Aladro Y, Alemany MJ, Perez-Vieitez MC et al. Prevalence and incidence of multiple sclerosis in Las Palmas, Canary Islands, Spain. Neuroepidemiology 2005; 24: 70–75.

156. Dean G. Annual incidence, prevalence and mortality of multiple sclerosis in white South African-born and in white immigrants to South Africa. Br Med J 1967; 2: 724–730.

157. Dean G, Bhigjee A, Bill PLA. Multiple sclerosis in black South Africans and Zimbabweans. J Neurol Neurosurg Psychiatry 1994; 57: 1064–1069.

158. Poser CM. Multiple sclerosis. In: Shakir RA, Newman PK, Poser CM, eds. Tropical neurology. London: WB Saunders; 1996: 437–455.

159. Casanova-Sotolongo P, Casanova-Carrillo P, Rodriguez-Costa J. [A neuroepidemiological study in Beira, Mozambique]. Rev Neurol 2000; 30: 1135–1140.

160. Kioy PG. Emerging picture of multiple sclerosis in Kenya. East Afr Med J 2001; 78: 93–96.

161. Barnett MH, Williams DB, Day S et al. Progressive increase in incidence and prevalence of multiple sclerosis in Newcastle, Australia: a 35-year study. J Neurol Sci 2003; 213: 1–6.

162. Simmons RD, Hall CA, Gleeson P et al. Prevalence survey of multiple sclerosis in the Australian Capital Territory. Intern Med J 2001; 31: 161–167.

163. Chancellor AM, Addidle M, Dawson K. Multiple sclerosis is more prevalent in northern New Zealand than previously reported. Intern Med J 2003; 33: 79–83.

164. Kurtzke JF. Multiple sclerosis death rates from underlying cause and total deaths. Acta Neurol Scand 1972; 48: 148–162.

165. Warren S, Warren KG, Svenson LW et al. Geographic and temporal distribution of mortality rates for multiple sclerosis in Canada, 1965–1994. Neuroepidemiology 2003; 22: 75–81.

166. Pritchard C, Baldwin D, Mayers A. Changing patterns of adult (45–74 years) neurological deaths in the major Western world countries 1979–1997. Public Health 2004; 118: 268–283.

167. Kurtzke JF, Hamtoft H. Multiple sclerosis and Hodgkin's disease in Denmark. Acta Neurol Scand 1976; 53: 358–375.

168. Shibasaki H, Okihiro MM, Kuroiwa Y. Multiple sclerosis among Orientals and Caucasians in Hawaii: a reappraisal. Neurology 1978; 28: 113–118.

169. Brønnum-Hansen H, Koch-Henriksen N, Stenager E. Trends in survival and cause of death in Danish patients with multiple sclerosis. Brain 2004; 127: 844–850.

170. Banwell BL. Pediatric multiple sclerosis. Curr Neurol Neurosci Rep 2004; 4: 245–252.

171. Boiko A, Vorobeychik G, Paty D et al. Early onset multiple sclerosis. A longitudinal study. Neurology 2002; 59: 1006–1010.

172. Gusev E, Boiko A, Bikova O et al. The natural history of early onset multiple sclerosis: comparison of data from Moscow and Vancouver. Clin Neurol Neurosurg 2002; 104: 203–207.

173. Simone IL, Carrara D, Tortorella C et al. Course and prognosis in early-onset MS: comparison with adult-onset forms. Neurology 2002; 59: 1922–1928.

174. Ruggieri M, Polizzi A, Pavone L et al. Multiple sclerosis in children under 6 years of age. Neurology 1999; 53: 478–484.

175. Ghezzi A, Deplano V, Faroni J et al. Multiple sclerosis in childhood: clinical features of 149 cases. Mult Scler 1997; 3: 43–46.

176. Cole GF, Stuart CA. A long perspective on childhood multiple sclerosis. Dev Med Child Neurol 1995; 37: 661–666.

177. Duquette P, Murray TJ, Pleines J et al. Multiple sclerosis in childhood: clinical profile in 125 patients. J Pediatrics 1987; 111: 359–363.

178. Belman AL, Chitnis T, Renoux C, Waubant E; International Pediatric MS Study Group. Challenges in the classification of pediatric multiple sclerosis and future directions. Neurology 2007; 68: S70–74.

179. Gadoth N. Multiple sclerosis in children. Brain Dev 2003; 25: 229–232.

180. Paty DW, Boiko AN, Vorobeychi GK. Multiple sclerosis with early and late disease onset. In: McDonald WI, Noseworthy JM, eds. Multiple sclerosis 2. Oxford: Butterworth-Heinemann; 2003: 285–302.

181. Orton SM, Herrera BM, Yee IM et al. Sex ratio of multiple sclerosis in Canada: a longitudinal study. Lancet Neurol 2006; 5: 932–936.

182. Wallin MT, Page WF, Kurtzke JF. Multiple sclerosis in US veterans of the Vietnam era and later military service: race, sex, and geography. Ann Neurol 2004; 55: 65–71.

183. Beebe GW, Kurtzke JF, Kurland LT et al. Studies on the natural history of multiple sclerosis. 3. Epidemiologic analysis of the Army experience in World War II. Neurology 1967; 17: 1–17.

184. Cree BA, Khan O, Bourdette D et al. Clinical characteristics of African Americans vs Caucasian Americans with multiple sclerosis. Neurology 2004; 63: 2039–2045.

185. Debouverie M, Lebrun C, Jeannin S et al. More severe disability of North Africans vs Europeans with multiple sclerosis in France. Neurology 2007; 68: 29–32.

186. Wallin MT, Page WF, Kurtzke JF. Epidemiology of multiple sclerosis in US veterans. VIII. Long-term survival after onset of multiple sclerosis. Brain 2000; 123: 1677–1687.

187. Sumelahti ML, Tienari PJ, Wikström J et al. Survival of multiple sclerosis in Finland between 1964 and 1993. Mult Scler 2002; 8: 350–355.

188. Riise T, Grønning M, Aarli JA et al. Prognostic factors for life expectancy in multiple sclerosis analysed by Cox-models. J Clin Epidemiol 1988; 41: 1031–1036.

189. Wynn DR, Rodriguez M, O'Fallon WM et al. A reappraisal of the epidemiology of multiple sclerosis in Olmsted County, Minnesota. Neurology 1990; 40: 780–786.

190. Poser CM. Multiple sclerosis trait: the premorbid stage of multiple sclerosis. A hypothesis. Acta Neurol Scand 2004; 109: 239–243.

191. Rothman KJ. Induction and latent periods. Am J Epidemiol 1981; 114: 253–259.

192. Kurtzke JF, Dean G, Botha DP. A method for estimating the age at immigration of white immigrants to South Africa, with an example of its importance. S Afr Med J 1970; 44: 663–669.

193. Dean G, Kurtzke JF. On the risk of multiple sclerosis according to age at immigration to South Africa. Br Med J 1971; 3: 725–729.

194. Elian M, Nightingale S, Dean G. Multiple sclerosis among United Kingdom-born children of immigrants from the Indian

subcontinent, Africa and the West Indies. J Neurol Neurosurg Psychiatry 1990; 53: 906–911.

195. Kurtzke JF, Bui-Quoc H. Multiple sclerosis in a migrant population. 2. Half-orientals immigrating in childhood. Ann Neurol 1980; 8: 256–260.

196. Alter M, Kahana E, Lowenson R. Migration and risk of multiple sclerosis. Neurology 1978; 28: 1089–1093.

197. Hammond SR, English DR, McLeod JG. The age range of risk of developing multiple sclerosis. Evidence from a migrant population in Australia. Brain 2000; 123: 968–974.

198. Wolfson C, Wolfson DB. The latent period of multiple sclerosis: a critical review. Epidemiology 1993; 4: 464–470.

199. Gale CR, Martyn CN. Migrant studies in multiple sclerosis. Prog Neurobiol 1995; 47: 425–448.

200. Riise T. Cluster studies in multiple sclerosis. Neurology 1997; 49(suppl 2): S27–S32.

201. Riise T, Grønning M, Klauber R et al. Clustering of residence of multiple sclerosis patients at age 13 to 20 years in Hordaland, Norway. Am J Epidemiol 1991; 133: 932–939.

202. Riise T, Klauber MR. Relationship between the degree of individual space-time clustering and age at onset of disease among multiple sclerosis patients. Int J Epidemiol 1992; 21: 528–532.

203. Pugliatti M, Riise T, Sotgiu MA et al. Evidence of early childhood as the susceptibility period in multiple sclerosis: space-time cluster analysis in a Sardinian population. Am J Epidemiol 2006; 164: 326–333.

204. Kurtzke JF, Heltberg A. Multiple sclerosis in the Faroe Islands: an epitome. J Clin Epidemiol 2001; 54: 1–22.

205. Cooke RG. MS in the Faroe Islands and the possible protective effect of early childhood exposure to the 'MS agent'. Acta Neurol Scand 1990; 82: 230–233.

206. Poser CM, Hibberd PL. Analysis of the 'epidemic' of multiple sclerosis in the Faroe Islands. II. Biostatistical aspects. Neuroepidemiology 1988; 7: 181–189.

207. Poskanzer DC, Prenney LB, Sheridan JL et al. Multiple sclerosis in the Orkney and Shetland Islands. I. Epidemiology, clinical factors and methodology. J Epidemiol Community Health 1980; 34: 229–239.

208. Kurtzke JF, Gudmundsson KR, Bergmann S. Multiple sclerosis in Iceland. I. Evidence of a postwar epidemic. Neurology 1982; 32: 143–150.

209. Poser CM, Benedikz J, Hibberd PL. The epidemiology of multiple sclerosis: the Iceland model. Onset-adjusted prevalence rate and other methodological considerations. J Neurol Sci 1992; 111: 143–152.

210. Dyment DA, Sadovnick AD, Ebers GC. Genetics of multiple sclerosis. Hum Mol Genet 1997; 6: 1693–1698.

211. Sadovnick AD, Armstrong H, Rice GP et al. A population-based study of twins: update. Ann Neurol 1993; 33: 281–285.

212. Sadovnick AD, Ebers GC, Dyment DA et al, and the Canadian Collaborative Group. A population-based half-sib study of multiple sclerosis. Lancet 1996; 347: 1728–1730.

213. Robertson N, Fraser Deans J, Clayton D et al. Age-adjusted recurrence risks for relatives of patients with multiple sclerosis. Brain 1996; 119: 449–455.

214. Ebers GC, Sadovnick AD, Dyment DA et al. Parent-of-origin effect in multiple sclerosis: observations in half-siblings. Lancet 2004; 363: 1773–1774.

215. Sadovnick AD, Yee IML, Ebers GC and the Canadian Collaborative Study Group. Factors influencing sib risks for MS. Clin Genet 2000; 58: 431–435.

216. Sadovnick AD, Yee IML, Ebers GC et al. The effect of age onset and parental disease status on sib risks for multiple sclerosis. Neurology 1998; 50: 719–723.

217. Ebers GC, Yee IML, Sadovnick AD et al. and the Canadian Collaborative Study Group. Conjugal multiple sclerosis: population-based prevalence and recurrence risks in offspring. Ann Neurol 2000; 48: 927–931.

218. Nielsen NM, Westergaard T, Rostgaard K et al. Familial risk of multiple sclerosis: a nationwide cohort study. Am J Epidemiol 2005; 162: 774–778.

219. Ebers GC, Sadovnick AD, Risch NJ and the Canadian Collaborative Study Group. A genetic basis for familial aggregation in multiple sclerosis. Nature 1995; 377: 150–151.

220. Sadovnick AD, Yee IML, Ebers GC and the Canadian Collaborative Study Group. Recurrence risks to sibs of MS index cases: impact of consanguineous mating. Neurology 2001; 56: 784–785.

221. Ristori G, Cannoni S, Stazi MA et al. Multiple sclerosis in twins from continental Italy and Sardinia: a nationwide study. Ann Neurol 2006; 59: 27–34.

222. Heltberg A, Holm N. Concordance in twins and recurrence in sibships in multiple sclerosis. Lancet 1982; 1: 1068.

223. Kinnunen E, Koskenvuo M, Kaprio J et al. Multiple sclerosis in a nationwide series of twins. Neurology 1987; 37: 1627–1629.

224. Mumford CJ, Wood NW, Kellar-Wood H et al. The British Isles survey of multiple sclerosis in twins. Neurology 1994; 44: 11–15.

225. Hansen T, Skytthe A, Stenager E et al. Concordance for multiple sclerosis in Danish twins: an update of a nationwide study. Mult Scler 2005; 11: 504–510.

226. Williams A, Eldridge R, McFarland H et al. Multiple sclerosis in twins. Neurol 1980; 30: 1139–1147.

227. Currier RD, Eldridge R. Possible risk factors in multiple sclerosis as found in a national twin study. Arch Neurol 1982; 39: 140–144.

228. Kinnunen E, Juntunen J, Ketonen L et al. Genetic susceptibility to multiple sclerosis: a co-twin study of a nationwide series. Arch Neurol 1988; 45: 1108–1011.

229. French Research Group on Multiple Sclerosis. Multiple sclerosis in 54 twinships: concordance rate is independent of zygosity. Ann Neurol 1992; 32: 724–727.

230. Willer CJ, Dyment DA, Sadovnick AD et al. Twin concordance and sibling recurrence rates in multiple sclerosis: the Canadian Collaborative Study. Proc Natl Acad Sci USA 2003; 100: 12877–12882.

231. Giovannoni G, Ebers G. Multiple sclerosis: the environment and causation. Curr Opin Neurol 2007; 20: 261–268.

232. Ascherio A, Munger KL. Environmental risk factors for multiple sclerosis. Part II: Noninfectious factors. Ann Neurol 2007; 61: 504–513.

233. Lauer K. Diet and multiple sclerosis. Neurology 1997; 49(suppl 2): S55–S61.

234. Martinelli V. Trauma, stress and multiple sclerosis. Neurol Sci 2000; 21: S849–S852.

235. Coo H, Aronson KJ. A systematic review of several potential non-genetic risk factors for multiple sclerosis. Neuroepidemiology 2004; 23: 1–12.

236. Schwarz S, Leweling H. Multiple sclerosis and nutrition. Mult Scler 2005; 11: 24–32.

237. Landtblom AM, Tondel M, Hjalmarsson P et al. The risk for multiple sclerosis in female nurse anaesthetists: a register based study. Occup Environ Med 2006; 63: 387–389.

238. Dumas M, Jaubertau-Marchan MO. The protective role of Langerhans' cells and sunlight in multiple sclerosis. Med Hypotheses 2000; 55; 517–520.

239. Islam T, Gauderman WJ, Cozen W, Mack TM. Childhood sun exposure influences risk of multiple sclerosis in monozygotic twins. Neurology 2007; 69: 381–388.

240. Munger KL, Levin LI, Hollis BW et al. Serum 25-hydroxyvitamin D levels and risk of multiple sclerosis. JAMA 2006; 296: 2832–2838.

241. Hawkes CH. Smoking is a risk factor for multiple sclerosis: a metanalysis. Mult Scler 2007; 13: 610–615.

242. Pekmezovic T, Drulovic J, Milenkovic M et al. Lifestyle factors and multiple sclerosis: A case-control study in Belgrade. Neuroepidemiology 2006; 27: 212–216.

243. Riise T, Nortvedt MW, Ascherio A. Smoking is a risk factor for multiple sclerosis. Neurology 2003; 61: 1122–1124.

244. Hernan MA, Olek MJ, Ascherio A. Cigarette smoking and incidence of multiple sclerosis. Am J Epidemiol 2001; 154: 69–74.

245. Hernan MA, Jick SS, Logroscino G et al. Cigarette smoking and the progression of multiple sclerosis. Brain 2005; 128: 1461–1465.

246. Willer CJ, Dyment DA, Sadovnick AD et al. for the Canadian Collaborative Study Group. Timing of birth and risk of multiple sclerosis: population based study. Br Med J 2005; 330: 120–124.

247. Torrey EF, Miller J, Rawlings R et al. Seasonal birth patterns of neurological disorders. Neuroepidemiology 2000; 19: 177–185.

248. Sotgiu S, Pugliatti M, Sotgiu MA et al. Seasonal fluctuation of multiple sclerosis births in Sardinia. J Neurol 2006; 253: 38–44.

249. Jin Y, de Pedro-Cuesta J, Soderstrom M et al. Seasonal patterns in optic neuritis and multiple sclerosis: a meta-analysis. J Neurol Sci 2000; 181: 56–64.

250. Rosati G. Descriptive epidemiology of multiple sclerosis in Europe in the 1980s: a critical overview. Ann Neurol 1994; 36(suppl 2): S164–S174.

251. Martyn C. The epidemiology of multiple sclerosis. In: Matthews WB, ed. McApine's multiple sclerosis, 2nd edn. Edinburgh: Churchill Livingstone; 1991: 5–6.

252. Lassmann H, Bruck W, Lucchinetti C. Heterogeneity of multiple sclerosis pathogenesis: implications for diagnosis and therapy. Trends Molec Med 2001; 7: 115–121.

F. K. Cantor and T. J. Lehky

INTRODUCTION

Sensory evoked potentials (EPs) – visual evoked potentials (VEP), short latency somatosensory evoked potentials (SSEP) and brainstem auditory evoked potentials (BAEP) – and motor evoked potentials (MEP) can provide objective evidence of central nervous system (CNS) abnormalities that complement the clinical and radiological findings in establishing the diagnosis of multiple sclerosis (MS).[1-5] While the early diagnostic criteria were based on a purely clinical definition of MS,[6] Poser et al[1] recognized the diagnostic advantage of paraclinical studies to improve the sensitivity of MS diagnosis. Abnormal EPs can provide evidence for pathology to satisfy the diagnostic criteria of lesions disseminated in space in the absence of clinical findings and for a relapse in patients with new symptoms but no changes on clinical examination.[7] However, EP abnormalities can be caused by a number of disorders and are not specific for MS.

Since magnetic resonance imaging (MRI) plays a critical role in the current diagnostic criteria of MS,[5] it is important to consider the relationship between EPs and MRI. Evoked potentials provide neurophysiological information about CNS functional abnormalities, while MRI provides anatomical localization of CNS lesions. MRI is a more sensitive diagnostic test than EPs in establishing the diagnosis of MS because MRI shows more lesions than are detected by EPs.[8-11] Some patients show corresponding abnormalities on both MRI and EPs, but other patients have abnormalities detected by only one or the other mode of testing.[9,12-16] VEP is more sensitive than MRI in detecting acute and old prechiasmatic optic nerve lesions.[8,17,18] The revised diagnostic criteria for MS[5] include a provision for an abnormal VEP to serve as a diagnostic factor in patients who have at least four but fewer than nine lesions demonstrated by MRI. Rarely, patients with spinal cord pathology may have an abnormal SEP or MEP without an observed lesion on MRI.[8,19] Combining multimodality evoked potentials and MRI results in the greatest diagnostic yield.[8,19-21]

There are other neurophysiological studies that can be used to assess cranial nerve and brainstem lesions in MS patients, although none of these are part of the established diagnostic criteria for MS diagnosis.[5] These include electronystagmography (ENG),[22-24] electroretinography (ERG)[25] and the blink reflex.[26] Optical coherence tomography (OCT) is a new imaging technique that correlates with ERG and clinical visual deficits.[27] These tests are also used in the diagnosis of other diseases than MS.

SENSORY EVOKED POTENTIALS: TECHNICAL AND STATISTICAL ASPECTS OF TESTING AND INTERPRETATION

Sensory evoked potentials are brain or spinal cord responses to sensory stimuli that are 'time-locked' to the stimulus. The amplitudes of these potentials range from $0.1\,\mu V$ for some BAEP and SEP components to $20\,\mu V$ for the major VEP component. Because most of these waveforms have amplitudes that are less than the background electroencephalographic (EEG) and electrocardiographic activity, computer averaging is employed to improve the signal-to-noise ratio and to extract the desired evoked potential signal from other unwanted electrical activity. Latencies of the peaks are the most consistent measurements used in clinical evaluation.[28,29] Peak latencies are considered to be abnormal if they are longer than the upper limit of the normal values of the laboratory (usually 2.5 or 3 standard deviations (SD) above the mean).[7,28,29] Latencies in an individual are reproducible over time, provided that the test situations are identical.[28,30,31] An increase in response latency from baseline in a patient with a suspected new MS lesion can be considered as abnormal even if both results are within the normal range. Amplitude variability limits the usefulness of measures of absolute amplitudes for clinical evaluation.[28,29] Amplitude differences between the two sides or between two components of a response can yield useful clinical information. Absence of a response is also an important diagnostic finding.

For the diagnostic evaluation of an individual patient, the determination that an EP measurement is abnormal is based on comparison with values in a population of normal subjects.

This differs from research studies that evaluate differences between groups. For those comparisons, which usually involve a research or a treatment protocol, a statistical analysis for the significance of the difference between the means of the groups is appropriate regardless of overlap between the two groups.

VISUAL EVOKED POTENTIALS

The pattern shift VEP (sometimes designated PVEP) is the standard paradigm used in clinical testing. The stimulus consists of an alternating checkerboard pattern of black and white squares displayed on a video screen. Each eye is tested separately with two sets of stimuli – a small checkerboard pattern and a large checkerboard pattern. The smaller checkerboard pattern primarily stimulates the central retina and larger checkerboard pattern includes more peripheral portions of the retina. The VEP response is usually averaged from at least 100 stimuli. The response is recorded with standard EEG electrodes in the midline and bilateral occipital regions. This VEP technique[28,32] has great reliability in identifying MS patients with optic nerve impairment compared to other techniques such as flash VEPs evoked by a strobe light.[31,33] Multifocal VEP is a newer technique that allows simultaneous stimulation of multiple retinal areas while recording the responses from each of these areas. The result is a greater ability to find a smaller, more peripheral optic nerve lesion.[34,35] This technique may also be useful in delineating retinal abnormalities from optic neuritis.

The VEP response consists of a complex waveform produced primarily from the striate cortex.[36] For clinical purposes, the most reliable measurement is the latency of a large positive component (P100) that occurs at approximately 100 ms after the stimulus (Fig. 10.1A).[28,32] Normal latency will depend upon the check sizes of the stimuli and should be standardized for each laboratory. Both an increased absolute latency beyond 3 SD and an interocular difference greater than 11 ms or 3 SD above the mean interocular difference are considered abnormal (Fig.10.1B). Prolongation of a unilateral P100 latency or increased interocular differences are suggestive of demyelination in the prechiasmatic portion of the optic nerve.[28,29] Bilateral optic nerve, chiasmatic or postchiasmatic lesions can produce abnormal responses in each eye, which makes anatomical localization of the abnormality more difficult. Unilateral postchiasmatic lesions are not reliably diagnosed with VEPs even when using a hemifield checkerboard in patients with homonymous hemianopsia[28] because of the bilateral and diffuse distribution of the postchiasmatic visual pathways. VEP amplitude is not ordinarily useful because of the variability found in normal subjects but a marked decrease in amplitude or dispersion of the P100 waveform would suggest a destructive lesion with axonal loss rather than simple demyelination.[28] Marked amplitude asymmetry between the two eyes also suggests a possible postchiasmatic abnormality. Interocular amplitude asymmetries may also be caused by refractive differences, cataracts and other ocular pathologies that affect visual acuity, particularly if smaller checkerboard patterns are used.[28,37] Other causes of abnormal VEPs include diabetes,[38] leukoencephalopathies,[39,40] sarcoidosis,[41] vitamin B_{12} deficiency,[42] thyroid disease[43] and other disorders.[44]

The VEP is important in establishing the diagnosis of isolated optic neuritis either as an isolated demyelinating event or as an abnormality in a patient with MS.[45,46] It was initially included in the diagnostic criteria in 1983[1] and is still an important component of the revised diagnostic criteria for MS.[5] Because of technical difficulties in MRI imaging of the optic nerve and chiasm, VEP has shown to have greater sensitivity than the MRI in identifying prechiasmatic optic lesions.[8,17,47] In patients with

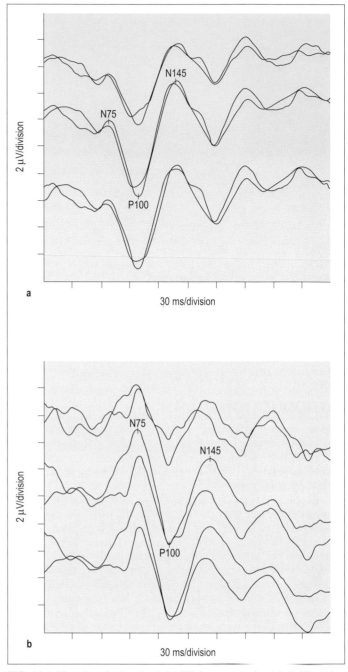

FIG. 10.1 Visual evoked potential. VEP from normal subject (**A**) and patient with demyelinating disease (**B**) using full-field, size 16, checkerboard pattern at 1.9 and 1 Hz frequency respectively, with 200 averages. Sensitivity 2 μV/div. The normal subject (**A**) has a normal configuration of the P100 with a latency of 98.7 ms. The patient (**B**) has marked delay in the P100 with a latency of 130.8 ms, suggesting a prechiasmal lesion. Courtesy of Dr Susumu Sato, EEG Section, NINDS.

a history of optic neuritis, an abnormal VEP has been found in 89–100%.[28,37] In a large group of MS patients classified primarily on clinical criteria, VEP was abnormal in 81% with definite MS, 52% with probable MS and 26% with possible MS.[28] Abnormal VEPs can be found in MS patients in the absence of visual symptoms or abnormal eye examinations – including evaluation of visual field tests, visual acuity, color vision and pupillary responses,[28,48–50] thereby uncovering 'silent' MS lesions. Because the VEP remains abnormal[28,51] after recovery from optic neuritis, VEP can verify the earlier occurrence of optic neuritis in a patient with unclear prior history of demyelinating disease. Therefore, VEP abnormalities are useful for initial diagnosis as well as to document disease progression by the presence of a new optic nerve lesion.

OTHER NEUROPHYSIOLOGICAL MEASUREMENTS OF VISUAL PATHWAY: ELECTRORETINOGRAPHY AND OPTICAL COHERENCE TOMOGRAPHY

Electroretinography (ERG) records the response of the retina to visual stimuli. Amplitude and latency measurements of different components of the ERG waveform correlate with the response of different retinal elements. The diagnostic value of ERG is its ability to distinguish retinal pathology from optic nerve pathology in patients with unilateral visual symptoms.[25,52,53] The pattern-evoked ERG records the response of the ganglion cells of the optic nerve with relative exclusion of responses from other retinal structures[25] and correlates with ganglion cell and optic nerve pathology. An abnormal pattern-evoked ERG can be found with demyelinating optic neuritis[54,55] though it may also be found in other pathologies including glaucoma, ischemic optic neuritis and Alzheimer's disease.[56]

Optical coherence tomography (OCT) is an imaging (rather than a physiological) test that provides information concerning atrophy or edema in specific retinal layers.[27] OCT demonstration of thinning of the retinal fiber layer can correlate with abnormalities found in optic neuritis[54,57,58] and may correlate with ganglion cell pathology demonstrated by pattern-evoked ERG,[54] MRI and VEP[57,58] abnormalities. In acute optic neuritis, there may be swelling of the nerve fiber layer caused by edema. In patients with prior optic neuritis, residual thinning of the nerve fiber layer may be present.[59,60]

BRAINSTEM AUDITORY EVOKED POTENTIALS

The BAEP is generated by eighth cranial nerve and brainstem structures in response to a click stimulus.[28,61] Clicks are delivered through headphones, averaging a minimum of 1000 responses.[28,61] Recording is done from EEG electrodes placed over the vertex (Cz) linked to each ear or to each mastoid.[28,61] The resultant waveform consists of five components identified as waves I–V (Fig. 10.2A). Clinical testing is generally based upon the absolute latency of waves I, III and V and the interpeak latencies. The absence of waves I, III or V is also considered a significant clinical finding but waves II and IV can be absent in normals. Amplitudes are variable in normals.[28,61]

Wave I, generated by the eighth nerve, usually has a normal latency in MS patients whose cochleae are normal except in rare instances of a plaque located at the VIIIth nerve root entry zone. The origins of the other waves are thought to be as follows: wave II from the cochlear nucleus in the caudal pons, wave III from the midpons in the area of the superior olive, waves IV and V from the upper pons and low midbrain in the areas of the lateral lemniscus and inferior colliculus respectively.[28,51] Brainstem lesions may produce an absence of waves generated rostral to the pathology or a prolongation of latency based on the location of the pathology. Accordingly, a large lower pontine lesion may cause absence of all components beyond wave I. A smaller lesion may cause an increased I–V interpeak latency. A large lesion in the mid- to upper pons may cause loss of waves IV and V. A smaller lesion in the same location may show a normal I–III latency but a prolonged I–V and III–V latency (Fig. 10.2B). A delay of all latencies with normal interpeak latencies

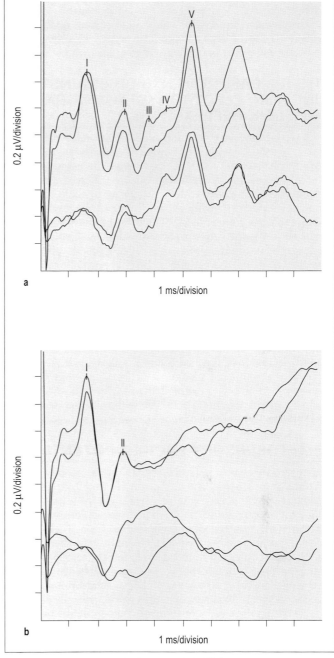

FIG. 10.2 Brainstem evoked potential. BAEP from normal subject (**A**) and patient with demyelinating disease (**B**) using click stimulus at 80 and 85 dB respectively, delivered at 11 Hz frequency with 2000 averages. Sensitivity 0.2 μV/div. The upper two traces are ipsilateral responses. In the normal subject (**A**), the peaks are marked as I (1.68 ms), II (3.03 ms), III (3.91 ms), IV (4.52 ms), V (5.46 ms). The I–V interpeak latency is 3.78 ms with I–III interpeak latency of 2.23 ms and III–V interpeak latency of 1.55 ms. In a person with demyelinating disease (**B**), the peak I is 1.67 and peak II is 2.96 with absence of all subsequent waveforms suggesting pathology in the lower to midpontine region. Courtesy of Dr Susumu Sato, EEG Section NINDS.

is consistent with cochlear or VIIIth nerve pathology. Lateralization of the pathology is uncertain above the upper brainstem because of the bilateral course of the acoustic pathway.[28]

BAEPs have been shown to be abnormal in 46% of all MS patients.[28] The BAEP was originally part of the supportive paraclinical evidence used in the diagnosis of MS.[1] This was because early data showed BAEPs to be superior to MRI in detecting brainstem lesions.[15,62] Higher-resolution MRI imaging has supplanted BAEPs for the demonstration of brainstem and posterior fossa pathology.[5,10,63,64] Infrequently, a patient with brainstem symptoms will have an abnormal BAEP with a normal MRI.[9] BAEP abnormalities also occur with other pathologies that disrupt the brainstem auditory pathways.[65,28]

OTHER MEASUREMENTS OF BRAINSTEM FUNCTION: ELECTRONYSTAGMOGRAPHY AND BLINK REFLEX

Electronystagmography records and quantifies nystagmus induced by caloric testing, positioning maneuvers and the ability to track visual stimuli.[22,23] ENG may help to distinguish imbalance or vertigo due to brainstem pathology from peripheral causes. An asymmetric caloric response usually indicates peripheral pathology, while downbeating nystagmus or the inability to track a target or optokinetic stimulus smoothly and symmetrically is indicative of central pathology. The pattern of responses to positioning maneuvers also helps to distinguish central from peripheral pathology. ENG abnormalities indicating CNS pathology do not differentiate MS lesions from other brainstem pathologies.

The blink reflex is elicited by unilateral electrical stimulation of the supraorbital branch of the trigeminal nerve while recording from the ipsilateral and contralateral orbicularis oculi. This is analogous to the direct and consensual corneal responses. Abnormal latency or absence of blink reflexes can be used to distinguish a peripheral trigeminal or facial nerve lesion from brainstem pathology.[26] This modality may be abnormal in MS in some cases of trigeminal neuralgia with minimal or negative MRI findings.[66]

SOMATOSENSORY EVOKED POTENTIALS

Somatosensory evoked potentials[28,67] are produced by stimulation of a mixed nerve, activating muscle and large-diameter cutaneous afferent fibers[68] with propagation of the sensory signal though the dorsal column to the somatosensory cortex. Cerebral waveforms are recorded from contralateral C3'/C4' electrodes, which are located midway between C3 and P3 and between C4 and P4 respectively, and from electrodes on the extremities and spine. The upper extremity SSEP, typically produced by stimulating the median nerve, also has recording sites at Erb's point and the cervical spine. The lower extremity SSEP, typically produced by stimulating the tibial nerve (but in some circumstances by peroneal nerve stimulation) also has recording sites in the popliteal fossa and lumbar spine. The responses are averaged from 1000–2000 stimuli. The peaks are named as N or P to indicate polarity, followed by an integer to indicate the typical latency.[67]

In the upper extremity SSEP (Fig. 10.3A) the first potential, N9, is generated at Erb's point, followed by P11 at the dorsal root entry zone. The N13/P13 peaks are generated in the sensory interneurons in the cervical cord. The P14 peak is thought to be generated in the medial lemniscus and the N18 peak is generated by upper brainstem nuclei. The most prominent cortical peak, N20, is generated within the somatosensory cortex, as is the P22 peak.[67] Some small cord or brain stem components may not be visible in all normals.

In the lower extremity SSEP (Fig. 10.4A) a response recorded at the popliteal fossa after stimulation of the tibial nerve at the ankle serves to determine if there is peripheral pathology in the tibial nerve. The absolute latencies of the lower extremity SSEP correlate to some extent with the subject's height. The first spinal peak is a postsynaptic potential generated at the lumbar spine or 'lumbar point' area (LP) with an 18–24 ms latency. This is followed by the N28 and P31 peaks, generated within the cervical cord and caudal portion of the medial lemniscus, and

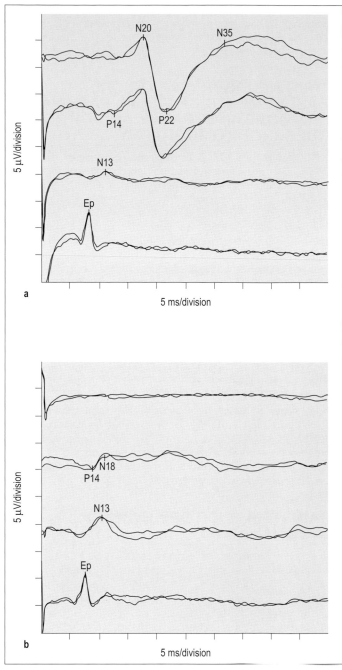

FIG. 10.3 Upper extremity somatosensory evoked potential. USSEP from normal subject (**A**) and patient with demyelinating disease (**B**) stimulating from the median nerve with an intensity of 9 mA and at a rate of 5 Hz for 1000 averages. Sensitivity 5 μV/div. In the normal subject (**A**), the waveform latencies are Erb's point (Ep) (8.25 ms), N13 (11.10 ms), P14 (12.70 ms), N20 (17.75 ms), P22 (21.75 ms) and N35 (31.75 ms). In the subject with central demyelination (**B**), the waveform latencies are Ep (7.70 ms), N13 (10.50 ms), P14 (9.05 ms) and N18 (11.00 ms) with absent cortical waveforms. The absence of the N20 and subsequent cortical potentials suggest that there is a lesion between the upper pontine region and the cortex. Courtesy of Dr Susumu Sato, EEG Section, NINDS.

the N34 peak, which is generated by more rostral brainstem nuclei. The P37 peak is the most prominent cortical peak and is generated in the ipsilateral primary somatosensory cortex.[67]

The parameters measured are the latencies of peaks, interpeak latency and, to a lesser extent, amplitude. The interpeak latency between the N13 and N18 or N20 peaks in the upper extremity SSEP and the N22–N34 or P37 peaks in the lower extremity SSEP are measures of conduction through the spinal cord. Prolonged interpeak latencies suggests spinal cord pathology such as demyelination[28,69] (Figs 10.3B and 10.4B). Absence of or markedly decreased amplitude of individual peaks (Fig. 10.4B) can indicate axonal loss or conduction block through

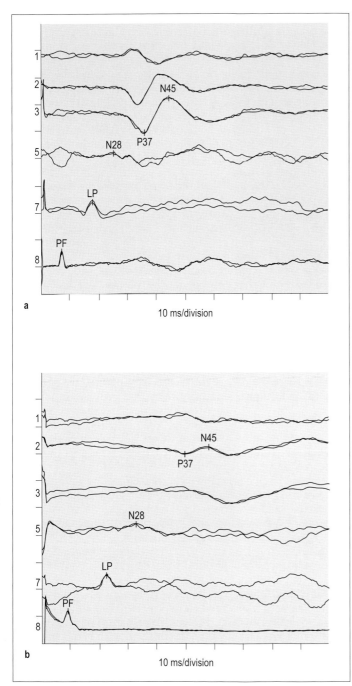

FIG. 10.4 Lower extremity somatosensory evoked potential. LSSEP from a normal subject (**A**) and patient with demyelinating disease (**B**) stimulating from the tibial nerve with an intensity of 15 mA and at a rate of 4 Hz for 1000 averages. Sensitivity 5 µV/div (A/B 1, 2, 3 and 8) and 2 µV/div (A/B 5 and 7). In the normal subject (**A**), the waveform latencies are popliteal fossa (PF) (7.0 ms), lumbar potential (LP) (17.8 ms), N28 (25.0 ms), P37 (35.7 ms) and N45 (44.1 ms). In the subject with central demyelination (**B**), the waveform latencies are PF (8.9 ms) and LP (22.3 ms), N28 (32.5), P37 (49.4 ms) and N45 (57.7 ms). The interpeak latency between the LP and P37 peaks for the normal subject and patient are 17.9 ms and 27.1 ms respectively, suggesting central demyelination. Courtesy of Dr Susumu Sato, EEG Section, NINDS.

that region. Care must be taken to rule out peripheral nerve or nerve root pathology because both can slow conduction and increase the absolute peak latency. Since not all small components may be visible, a normal USSEP with a prolonged LSSEP is indicative of cord pathology.

The SSEP is abnormal in 82–89% of patients with clinically definite MS but only in 58% of those with a suspected but not clinically definite diagnosis.[70–72] Prolongation of SSEP latency occurs with some but not all cervical cord lesions demonstrable on MRI and occasionally SSEP will be abnormal in a myelopathy when the MRI does not show a cord lesion.[16,64,73–75] There is little correlation between white matter lesions in the brain and SSEP cortical potentials.[73] There are a variety of neurological diseases that may affect conduction through the multisynaptic somatosensory pathway,[76] including neuropathies, spinal cord disease of multiple etiologies, and strokes. The use of SSEP as an outcome measure in clinical trials has shown correlation with other outcome measures in some studies[77,78] but not in others.[2,79,80]

As diagnostic MRI modalities have become more refined the SSEP has been relegated to a more adjunctive role and is no longer part of the MS diagnostic criteria.[5] SSEPs can be useful in the evaluation of MS, particularly when the presentation is atypical and MRI lesions are nonspecific in their appearance.[81] They may also have some prognostic value in early MS.[82] As an isolated study, the SSEP has less significance than the MRI and VEP both in diagnosis and for clinical correlation.

MOTOR EVOKED POTENTIALS

Motor evoked potentials (MEP) are produced by stimulating the motor cortex using transcranial electrical stimulation (TES)[83,84] or, more commonly, transcranial magnetic stimulation (TMS).[85,86] This technique allows assessment of the length and function of the corticospinal tract. TMS is a well tolerated, noninvasive technique that has shown promise as an electrophysiological parameter to monitor MS patients since its introduction in 1985.[87–91] TMS uses the principle of induction to produce a magnetic field a few centimeters below the skull from a coil placed on the scalp over the motor cortex.[92,93] Corticospinal neurons are activated by the electrical field induced by the magnetic field. The corticospinal volleys activate motor neurons and the responses are recorded from the muscle as the MEP (Fig. 10.5A). The number of synchronously firing motor units determines the amplitude of the MEP.[94] The latency of MEP reflects the time from initial activation of cortical motor neurons, conduction through descending corticospinal tracts, synaptic transmission in the motor neurons within the anterior horn of the spinal cord, and conduction through the motor nerve to the target muscle. The central motor conduction time (CMCT) is the time for the cortically generated impulse to reach the motor neuron in the spinal cord. CMCT is calculated by subtracting the peripheral contribution from the MEP latency using F-wave latency measurements or MEPs generated from the spine to estimate the peripheral latency.[95,96] The CMCT is a reproducible measurement. MEP amplitude is more variable because it is affected by the degree of muscle contraction and desynchronization of the corticospinal volleys. Approaches for improving the reproducibility of the MEP amplitude include standardizing the optimal voluntary muscle contraction for each muscle[85] or optimizing the synchronization of the motor volleys using the triple stimulation technique, a combination of TMS with peripheral collision techniques.[97] Following the MEP is a period with no electrical activity referred to as the silent period. The initial portion of the silent period is generated by a refractory state and reflexes within spinal circuits, whereas the much longer later portion of the silent period is produced by inhibitory

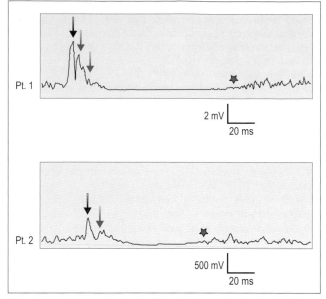

FIG. 10.5 Motor evoked potentials. Motor evoked potentials from a normal subject (**A**) and a patient with demyelinating disease (**B**), recorded from the arm (abductor pollicis brevis). The motor evoked potential is composed of an initial direct wave (left arrow) followed by one or more indirect waves (grey arrow). After the MEP, there is a cortical silent period (★), related to spinal and cortical inhibition, ending with the resumption of low voltage cortical activity. In the normal subject (**A**), the MEP latency recorded from the arm was 16.0 ms. The CMCT, using the F-latency method, was 3.7 ms. In the patient with demyelinating disease (**B**), the MEP latency recorded from the arm was 33.9. The CMCT was 15.8 ms, suggesting delayed conduction through the corticospinal tracts.

circuits within the motor cortex that are also activated by the TMS pulse.[98,99]

In MS patients, slowed conduction occurs through demyelinated portions of the corticospinal tracts. Conduction may be blocked with axonal loss or severe demyelination.[100–102] This results in prolongation of CMCT (Fig. 10.5B) or dispersion of impulse, leading to a decrease in MEP amplitude.[87,103] The CMCT has a diagnostic sensitivity of 0.68 and specificity of 0.77, comparable to the MRI sensitivity of 0.84–0.62 and specificity of 0.87–0.82.[21] In a comparison study, MEPs were abnormal in 83% of MS patients compared to VEPS (67%), BAEP (42%) and SSEPs (67%).[104] The silent period can be prolonged in MS, reflecting alterations in the intracortical connections or, possibly, cerebellar dysfunction.[105,106]

In comparison with MRI, prolongation of the MEP in the lower extremity has been chronologically associated with the appearance of new MRI lesions in the spinal cord, suggesting that the two modalities can be used as corroborative evidence of disease progression, but some patients progress without changes in spinal cord lesion load or increased CMCT.[107] In some other studies, the two modalities provide divergent information. Spinal motor conduction time was more prolonged in secondary progressive MS than in relapsing–remitting patients and showed better correlation with EDSS than brain MRI lesion load, suggesting that secondary progressive MS has more perturbations in conduction through the motor pathways than is radiologically discernible.[108]

MEP has been followed in several clinical trials. Treatment of acute exacerbations with methylprednisolone resulted in an 80–87% decrease in the CMCT by day 6 that persisted for 2 months following treatment.[109] CMCT detected a greater improvement from 2 g of daily intravenous methylprednisolone compared to a 1 g dose.[110] CMCT changes correlated with improved fatigue in treatment studies with β-interferon.[111] Future clinical trials may be able to combine the MEPs with radiological and functional parameters to more completely capture subtle changes as a result of treatment.

PRACTICAL CONSIDERATIONS

Evaluating the utility of a paraclinical test raises several questions. How sensitive and specific is this test in establishing the diagnosis of definite MS? Does it have prognostic implications, particularly in clinically isolated syndromes? Can it be used to differentiate the subtypes of MS? Does it have the reproducibility and sensitivity to be used serially in clinical trials?

Numerous studies have examined the sensitivity and specificity of evoked potentials and compared EPs to MRI.[19,21,104,112,113] All the evoked potential studies offer some insight into the functioning of parts of the CNS – the VEP and the optic nerve; the BAEP and the auditory pathway through the brainstem; the SSEP and the spinal and brainstem somatosensory pathways; and the MEP and the corticospinal pathways. Individually, the sensitivity of each EP does not exceed the sensitivity of MRI in establishing the diagnosis of MS. It is likely that some demyelinating lesions do not cause sufficient conduction dysfunction to cause an abnormal EP. In addition, the white matter lesion observed on MRI may not always be within the pathway being evaluated by the specific EP. However, the combined use of multimodality EPs enhances the ability to identify lesions separated by space so critical for the diagnosis of MS.[10] The combination of MRI and multimodality sensory and motor EPs results in a greater diagnostic yield than MRI alone.[15,19–21,64,114]

In clinically isolated syndromes such as optic neuritis, only the VEP has been consistently used to support the early diagnosis of MS for inclusion in clinical trials.[115] An abnormal VEP, when combined with abnormal cerebrospinal fluid (CSF) and MRI findings, is highly specific for MS.[46,116] This same relationship with MRI and CSF findings does not hold for other EPs. Longitudinal studies of EPs in MS have suggested that they may have a predictive value in prognosis and disability,[16,48,117–123] but this approach has not been widely used clinically. Thus far, EPs have not been useful for classification of subtypes of MS.[119] In clinical trials, EPs were used for several decades as secondary endpoints.[51,78,124–127] Since the 1990s, the MRI has largely supplanted EPs as the critical outcome measurement.[115,128,129] There is still importance in being able to use the neurophysiological parameters measured by EPs, particularly VEP and MEP, to complement clinical and MRI outcome measures. Since serial EPs show little latency variability in normals, changes occurring during a clinical trial would be indicative of functional changes caused by demyelination. More widespread use of multimodality EPs in combination with MRI might lead to better outcome measurement in clinical trials, where one compares the difference between group means, as opposed to the clinical situation, where an individual's response is either within or outside of the normal range.

For the clinical evaluation of an individual patient with signs and symptoms suspicious of MS, it is reasonable to perform a VEP even when the MRI is strongly suggestive of the diagnosis of MS. An abnormal VEP, which is noninvasive and simple to perform, markedly increases the probability that the abnormal white matter lesions observed in the MRI are due to MS. Of course, the addition of abnormal CSF findings of oligoclonal bands or increased IgG Index would further strengthen the diagnosis of MS. Testing with additional EP modalities can be considered when the clinical examination, MRI and VEP do not definitively establish the diagnosis of MS. In the established MS patient, multimodality EPs may help to determine whether a new episode of demyelination has occurred, especially if there are no definite examination or MRI changes. In particular, an abnormal VEP can establish an MS exacerbation with the onset of optic neuritis even in the absence of new clinical findings or MRI changes. Though EPs have some limitations, they remain an important adjunct in the diagnosis and clinical management of MS patients.

REFERENCES

1. Poser CM, Paty DW, Scheinberg L et al. New diagnostic criteria for multiple sclerosis: guidelines for research protocols. Ann Neurol 1983; 13: 227–231.

2. Anderson DC, Slater GE, Sherman R, Ettinger MG. Evoked potentials to test a treatment of chronic multiple sclerosis. Arch Neurol 1987; 44: 1232–1236.

3. Filippini G, Comi GC, Cosi V et al. Sensitivities and predictive values of paraclinical tests for diagnosing multiple sclerosis. J Neurol 1994; 241: 132–137.

4. Andersson T, Siden A. Multimodality evoked potentials and neurological phenomenology in patients with multiple sclerosis and potentially related conditions. Electromyogr Clin Neurophysiol 1991; 31: 109–117.

5. Polman CH, Reingold SC, Edan G et al. Diagnostic criteria for multiple sclerosis: 2005 revisions to the 'McDonald Criteria'. Ann Neurol 2005; 58: 840–846.

6. Schumacher GA. Multiple sclerosis. Med Clin North Am 1963; 47: 1603–1617.

7. Gronseth GS, Ashman EJ. Practice parameter: the usefulness of evoked potentials in identifying clinically silent lesions in patients with suspected multiple sclerosis (an evidence-based review): Report of the Quality Standards Subcommittee of the American Academy of Neurology. Neurology 2000; 54: 1720–1725.

8. Farlow MR, Markand ON, Edwards MK et al. Multiple sclerosis: magnetic resonance imaging, evoked responses, and spinal fluid electrophoresis. Neurology 1986; 36: 828–831.

9. Comi G, Filippi M, Martinelli V et al. Brain stem magnetic resonance imaging and evoked potential studies of symptomatic multiple sclerosis patients. Eur Neurol 1993; 33: 232–237.

10. Paty DW, Oger JJ, Kastrukoff LF et al. MRI in the diagnosis of MS: a prospective study with comparison of clinical evaluation, evoked potentials, oligoclonal banding, and CT. Neurology 1988; 38: 180–185.

11. Uhlenbrock D, Seidel D, Gehlen W et al. MR imaging in multiple sclerosis: comparison with clinical, CSF, and visual evoked potential findings. Am J Neuroradiol 1988; 9: 59–67.

12. Comi G, Leocani L, Medaglini S et al. Evoked potentials in diagnosis and monitoring of multiple sclerosis. Electroencephalogr Clin Neurophysiol Suppl 1999; 49: 13–18.

13. Comi G, Locatelli T, Leocani L et al. Can evoked potentials be useful in monitoring multiple sclerosis evolution? Electroencephalogr Clin Neurophysiol Suppl 1999; 50: 349–357.

14. Comi G, Filippi M, Rovaris M et al. Clinical, neurophysiological, and magnetic resonance imaging correlations in multiple sclerosis. J Neurol Neurosurg Psychiatr 1998; 64(suppl 1): S21–S25.

15. Comi G, Martinelli V, Medaglini S et al. Correlation between multimodal evoked potentials and magnetic resonance imaging in multiple sclerosis. J Neurol 1989; 236: 4–8.

16. Comi G, Canal N, Martinelli V et al. Comparison between magnetic resonance imaging and other techniques in 39 multiple sclerosis patients. Riv Neurol 1987; 57: 44–47.

17. Acar G, Ozakbas S, Cakmakci H et al. Visual evoked potential is superior to triple dose magnetic resonance imaging in the diagnosis of optic nerve involvement. Int J Neurosci 2004; 114: 1025–1033.

18. Davies MB, Williams R, Haq N et al. MRI of optic nerve and postchiasmal visual pathways and visual evoked potentials in secondary progressive multiple sclerosis. Neuroradiology 1998; 40: 765–770.

19. Rossini PM, Zarola F, Floris R et al. Sensory (VEP, BAEP, SEP) and motor-evoked potentials, liquoral and magnetic resonance findings in multiple sclerosis. Eur Neurol 1989; 29: 41–47.

20. Giang DW, Grow VM, Mooney C et al. Clinical diagnosis of multiple sclerosis. The impact of magnetic resonance imaging and ancillary testing. Rochester-Toronto Magnetic Resonance Study Group. Arch Neurol 1994; 51: 61–66.

21. Beer S, Rosler KM, Hess CW. Diagnostic value of paraclinical tests in multiple sclerosis: relative sensitivities and specificities for reclassification according to the Poser committee criteria. J Neurol Neurosurg Psychiatr 1995; 59: 152–159.

22. Shepard N. Electronystagmography (ENG) testing. In: Goebel JA, ed. Practical management of the dizzy patient. Philadelphia, PA: Lippincott Williams & Wilkins, 2001.

23. Bhansali SA, Honrubia V. Current status of electronystagmography testing. Otolaryngol Head Neck Surg 1999; 120: 419–426.

24. NT S. Electronystagmography (ENG) testing. In: Goebel JA, ed. Practical management of the dizzy patient. Philadelphia, PA: Lippincott Williams & Wilkins, 2001.

25. Lam B. Electrophysiology of vision: clinical testing and applications. Boca Raton, FL: Taylor & Francis, 2005.

26. Kimura J. Conduction abnormalities of the facial and trigeminal nerves in polyneuropathy. Muscle Nerve 1982; 5: S139–144.

27. Schuman J PC, Fujimoto J. Optical coherence tomography of ocular diseases, 2nd ed. Thorofare, NJ: Slack, 2004.

28. Chiappa K. Evoked potentials in clinical medicine, 3rd ed. Philadelphia, PA: Lippincott-Raven, 1997.

29. Epstein C, Bej D et al. American Clinical Neurophysiology Society: Guideline 9A: Guidelines on evoked potentials. J Clin Neurophysiol 2006; 23: 125–137.

30. Emerson RG. Evoked potentials in clinical trials for multiple sclerosis. J Clin Neurophysiol 1998; 15: 109–116.

31. Aunon JI, Cantor FK. VEP and AEP variability: interlaboratory vs. intralaboratory and intersession vs. intrasession variability. Electroencephalogr Clin Neurophysiol 1977; 42: 705–708.

32. American Clinical Neurophysiology Society. Guideline 9B: guidelines on visual evoked potentials. J Clin Neurophysiol 2006; 23: 138–156.

33. Kooi KA, Guevener AM, Bagchi BK. Visual evoked responses in lesions of the higher optic pathways. Neurology 1965; 15: 841–854.

34. Hedges TR III, Quireza ML. Multifocal visual evoked potential, multifocal electroretinography, and optical coherence tomography in the diagnosis of subclinical loss of vision. Ophthalmol Clin North Am 2004; 17: 89–105.

35. Hood DC, Odel JG, Winn BJ. The multifocal visual evoked potential. J Neuroophthalmol 2003; 23: 279–289.

36. Di Russo F, Martinez A, Sereno MI et al. Cortical sources of the early components of the visual evoked potential. Hum Brain Mapp 2002; 15: 95–111.

37. Halliday AM, McDonald WI, Mushin J. Visual evoked response in diagnosis of multiple sclerosis. Br Med J 1973; 4: 661–664.

38. Puvanendran K, Devathasan G, Wong PK. Visual evoked responses in diabetes. J Neurol Neurosurg Psychiatr 1983; 46: 643–647.

39. Neubauer BA, Stefanova I, Hubner CA et al. A new type of leukoencephalopathy with metaphyseal chondrodysplasia maps to Xq25–q27. Neurology 2006; 67: 587–591.

40. Husain AM, Altuwaijri M, Aldosari M. Krabbe disease: Neurophysiologic studies and MRI correlations. Neurology 2004; 63: 617–620.

41. Streletz LJ, Chambers RA, Bae SH, Israel HL. Visual evoked potentials in sarcoidosis. Neurology 1981; 31: 1545–1549.

42. Fine EJ, Hallett M. Neurophysiological study of subacute combined degeneration. J Neurol Sci 1980; 45: 331–336.

43. Salvi M, Spaggiari E, Neri F et al. The study of visual evoked potentials in patients with thyroid-associated ophthalmopathy identifies asymptomatic optic nerve involvement. J Clin Endocrinol Metab 1997; 82: 1027–1030.

44. Nguyen KV, Ostergaard E, Ravn SH et al. POLG mutations in Alpers syndrome. Neurology 2005; 65: 1493–1495.

45. Beck RW. The Optic Neuritis Treatment Trial. Arch Ophthalmol 1988; 106: 1051–1053.

46. Beck RW, Trobe JD, Moke PS et al. High- and low-risk profiles for the development of multiple sclerosis within 10 years after optic neuritis: experience of the optic neuritis treatment trial. Arch Ophthalmol 2003; 121: 944–949.

47. Miller DH, Newton MR, van der Poel JC et al. Magnetic resonance imaging of the optic nerve in optic neuritis. Neurology 1988; 38: 175–179.

48. Weinstock-Guttman B, Baier M, Stockton R et al. Pattern reversal visual evoked potentials as a measure of visual pathway pathology in multiple sclerosis. Mult Scler 2003; 9: 529–534.

49. Corallo G, Cicinelli S, Papadia M et al. Conventional perimetry, short-wavelength automated perimetry, frequency-doubling technology, and visual evoked potentials in the assessment of patients with multiple sclerosis. Eur J Ophthalmol 2005; 15: 730–738.

50. Kupersmith MJ, Nelson JI, Seiple WH et al. The 20/20 eye in multiple sclerosis. Neurology 1983; 33: 1015–1020.

51. Nuwer M. Evoked potentials in multiple sclerosis. In: Raine C, McFarland H, Tourtellotte W, eds. Multiple sclerosis: clinical and pathogenetic basis. London: Chapman & Hall, 1997: 43–55.

52. Celesia GG, Kaufman D, Cone SB. Simultaneous recording of pattern electroretinography and visual evoked potentials in multiple sclerosis. A method to separate demyelination from axonal damage to the optic nerve. Arch Neurol 1986; 43: 1247–1252.

53. Kaufman D, Celesia GG. Simultaneous recording of pattern electroretinogram and visual evoked responses in neuro-ophthalmologic disorders. Neurology 1985; 35: 644–651.

54. Parisi V, Manni G, Spadaro M et al. Correlation between morphological and functional retinal impairment in multiple sclerosis patients. Invest Ophthalmol Vis Sci 1999; 40: 2520–2527.

55. Stefano E, Cupini LM, Rizzo P et al. Simultaneous recording of pattern electroretinogram (PERG) and visual evoked potential (VEP) in multiple sclerosis. Acta Neurol Belg 1991; 91: 20–28.

56. Parisi V. Correlation between morphological and functional retinal impairment in patients affected by ocular hypertension, glaucoma, demyelinating optic neuritis and Alzheimer's disease. Semin Ophthalmol 2003; 18: 50–57.

57. Trip SA, Schlottmann PG, Jones SJ et al. Retinal nerve fiber layer axonal loss and visual dysfunction in optic neuritis. Ann Neurol 2005; 58: 383–391.

58. Trip SA, Schlottmann PG, Jones SJ et al. Optic nerve atrophy and retinal nerve fibre layer thinning following optic neuritis: evidence that axonal loss is a substrate of MRI-detected atrophy. Neuroimage 2006; 31: 286–293.

59. Noval S, Contreras I, Rebolleda G, Munoz-Negrete FJ. Optical coherence tomography versus automated perimetry for follow-up of optic neuritis. Acta Ophthalmol Scand 2006; 84: 790–794.

60. Pro MJ, Pons ME, Liebmann JM et al. Imaging of the optic disc and retinal nerve fiber layer in acute optic neuritis. J Neurol Sci 2006; 250: 114–119.

61. American Neurophysiology Society. Guideline 9C: guidelines on short-latency auditory evoked potentials. J Clin Neurophysiol 2006; 23: 157–167.

62. Chiappa KH. Use of evoked potentials for diagnosis of multiple sclerosis. Neurol Clin 1988; 6: 861–880.

63. Mani J, Chaudhary N, Ravat S, Shah PU. Multiple sclerosis: experience in neuroimaging era from western India. Neurol India 1999; 47: 8–11.

64. Cutler JR, Aminoff MJ, Brant-Zawadzki M. Evaluation of patients with multiple sclerosis by evoked potentials and magnetic resonance imaging: a comparative study. Ann Neurol 1986; 20: 645–648.

65. Chiappa KH, Parker SW. Diagnosis of acoustic tumors. Neurology 1984; 34: 131–132.

66. Jaaskelainen SK, Forssell H, Tenovuo O. Electrophysiological testing of the trigeminofacial system: aid in the diagnosis of atypical facial pain. Pain 1999; 80: 191–200.

67. American Clinical Neurophysiology Society. Guideline 9D: guidelines on short-latency somatosensory evoked potentials. J Clin Neurophysiol 2006; 23: 168–179.

68. Halonen JP, Jones S, Shawkat F. Contribution of cutaneous and muscle afferent fibres to cortical SEPs following median and radial nerve stimulation in man. Electroencephalogr Clin Neurophysiol 1988; 71: 331–335.

69. Strenge H, Tackmann W, Barth R, Sojka-Raytscheff A. Central somatosensory conduction time in diagnosis of multiple sclerosis. Eur Neurol 1980; 19: 402–408.

70. Khoshbin S, Hallett M. Multimodality evoked potentials and blink reflex in multiple sclerosis. Neurology 1981; 31: 138–144.

71. Eisen A, Odusote K, Li D et al. Comparison of magnetic resonance imaging with somatosensory testing in MS suspects. Muscle Nerve 1987; 10: 385–390.

72. Baumhefner RW, Tourtellotte WW, Syndulko K et al. Quantitative multiple sclerosis plaque assessment with magnetic resonance imaging. Its correlation with clinical parameters, evoked potentials, and intra-blood-brain barrier IgG synthesis. Arch Neurol 1990; 47: 19–26.

73. Turano G, Jones SJ, Miller DH et al. Correlation of SEP abnormalities with brain and cervical cord MRI in multiple sclerosis. Brain 1991; 114: 663–681.

74. Misra UK, Kalita J, Das A. Vitamin B_{12} deficiency neurological syndromes: a clinical, MRI and electrodiagnostic study. Electromyogr Clin Neurophysiol 2003; 43: 57–64.

75. Fushimi S, Nagano I, Deguchi K et al. [A case of subacute myelitis associated with primary Sjogren syndrome showing no MRI abnormality and diagnosed by somatosensory evoked potentials]. No To Shinkei 2004; 56: 1029–1034.

76. Aminoff MJ, Eisen AA. AAEM minimonograph 19: somatosensory evoked potentials. Muscle Nerve 1998; 21: 277–290.

77. Hellwig K, Stein FJ, Przuntek H, Muller T. Efficacy of repeated intrathecal triamcinolone acetonide application in progressive multiple sclerosis patients with spinal symptoms. BMC Neurol 2004; 4: 18.

78. Dau PC, Petajan JH, Johnson KP et al. Plasmapheresis in multiple sclerosis: preliminary findings. Neurology 1980; 30: 1023–1028.

79. Smith T, Zeeberg I, Sjo O. Evoked potentials in multiple sclerosis before and after high-dose methylprednisolone infusion. Eur Neurol 1986; 25: 67–73.

80. De Weerd AW. Variability of central conduction in the course of multiple sclerosis. Serial recordings of evoked potentials in the evaluation of therapy. Clin Neurol Neurosurg 1987; 89: 9–15.

81. Bashir K, Whitaker JN. Importance of paraclinical and CSF studies in the diagnosis of MS in patients presenting with partial cervical transverse myelopathy and negative cranial MRI. Mult Scler 2000; 6: 312–316.

82. Kallmann BA, Fackelmann S, Toyka KV et al. Early abnormalities of evoked potentials and future disability in patients with multiple sclerosis. Mult Scler 2006; 12: 58–65.

83. Berardelli A, Inghilleri M, Cruccu G et al. Stimulation of motor tracts in multiple sclerosis. J Neurol Neurosurg Psychiatr 1988; 51: 677–683.

84. Mills KR, Murray NM. Corticospinal tract conduction time in multiple sclerosis. Ann Neurol 1985; 18: 601–605.

85. Ravnborg M, Dahl K. Examination of central and peripheral motor pathways by standardized magnetic stimulation. Acta Neurol Scand 1991; 84: 491–497.

86. Wassermann EM, McShane LM, Hallett M, Cohen LG. Noninvasive mapping of muscle representations in human motor cortex. Electroencephalogr Clin Neurophysiol 1992; 85: 1–8.

87. Eisen AA, Shtybel W. AAEM minimonograph #35: Clinical experience with transcranial magnetic stimulation. Muscle Nerve 1990; 13: 995–1011.

88. Hess CW, Mills KR, Murray NM, Schriefer TN. Magnetic brain stimulation: central motor conduction studies in multiple sclerosis. Ann Neurol 1987; 22: 744–752.

89. Ravnborg M. The role of transcranial magnetic stimulation and motor evoked potentials in the investigation of central motor pathways in multiple sclerosis. Dan Med Bull 1996; 43: 448–462.

90. Jones SM, Streletz LJ, Raab VE et al. Lower extremity motor evoked potentials in multiple sclerosis. Arch Neurol 1991; 48: 944–948.

91. Mills KR, Murray NM, Hess CW. Magnetic and electrical transcranial brain stimulation: physiological mechanisms and clinical applications. Neurosurgery 1987; 20: 164–168.

92. Hallett M, Chokroverty S. Magnetic stimulation in clinical neurophysiology, 2nd ed. Philadelphia, PA: Butterworth-Heinemann, 2005.

93. Maccabee PJ, Zeimann U, Wassermann E, Deletis V. Emerging applications in neuromagnetic stimulation. In: Kerry H. Levin HOL, ed. Comprehensive clinical neurophysiology. Philadelphia, PA: WB Saunders, 2000: 325–347.

94. Rosler KM, Petrow E, Mathis J et al. Effect of discharge desynchronization on the size of motor evoked potentials: an analysis. Clin Neurophysiol 2002; 113: 1680–1687.

95. Rossini PM, Rossi S. Clinical applications of motor evoked potentials. Electroencephalogr Clin Neurophysiol 1998; 106: 180–194.

96. Di Lazzaro V, Oliviero A, Profice P et al. The diagnostic value of motor evoked potentials. Clin Neurophysiol 1999; 110: 1297–1307.

97. Humm AM, Z'Graggen WJ, von Hornstein NE et al. Assessment of central motor conduction to intrinsic hand muscles using the triple stimulation technique: normal values and repeatability. Clin Neurophysiol 2004; 115: 2558–2566.

98. Brasil-Neto JP, Cammarota A, Valls-Sole J et al. Role of intracortical mechanisms in the late part of the silent period to transcranial stimulation of the human motor cortex. Acta Neurol Scand 1995; 92: 383–386.

99. Wilson SA, Thickbroom GW, Mastaglia FL. Topography of excitatory and inhibitory muscle responses evoked by transcranial magnetic stimulation in the human motor cortex. Neurosci Lett 1993; 154: 52–56.

100. Bjartmar C, Yin X, Trapp BD. Axonal pathology in myelin disorders. J Neurocytol 1999; 28: 383–395.

101. Peterson JW, Trapp BD. Neuropathobiology of multiple sclerosis. Neurol Clin 2005; 23: 107–129, vi-vii.

102. Thickbroom GW, Byrnes ML, Archer SA et al. Corticomotor organisation and motor function in multiple sclerosis. J Neurol 2005; 252: 765–771.

103. Hess W MK, Marray NMF. Magnetic brain stimulation: central motor conduction in multiple sclerosis. Ann Neurol 1988; 22: 744–752.

104. Ravnborg M, Liguori R, Christiansen P et al. The diagnostic reliability of magnetically evoked motor potentials in multiple sclerosis. Neurology 1992; 42: 1296–1301.

105. Tataroglu C, Genc A, Idiman E et al. Cortical silent period and motor evoked potentials in patients with multiple sclerosis. Clin Neurol Neurosurg 2003, 105. 105–110.

106. Caramia MD, Palmieri MG, Desiato MT et al. Brain excitability changes in the relapsing and remitting phases of multiple sclerosis: a study with transcranial magnetic stimulation. Clin Neurophysiol 2004; 115: 956–965.

107. Kidd D, Thompson PD, Day BL et al. Central motor conduction time in progressive multiple sclerosis. Correlations with MRI and disease activity. Brain 1998; 121: 1109–1116.

108. Facchetti D, Mai R, Micheli A et al. Motor evoked potentials and disability in secondary progressive multiple sclerosis. Can J Neurol Sci 1997; 24: 332–337.

109. Salle JY, Hugon J, Tabaraud F et al. Improvement in motor evoked potentials and clinical course post-steroid therapy in multiple sclerosis. J Neurol Sci 1992; 108: 184–188.

110. Fierro B, Salemi G, Brighina F et al. A transcranial magnetic stimulation study evaluating methylprednisolone treatment in multiple sclerosis. Acta Neurol Scand 2002; 105: 152–157.

111. White AT, Petajan JH. Physiological measures of therapeutic response to interferon beta-1a treatment in remitting-relapsing MS. Clin Neurophysiol 2004; 115: 2364–2371.

112. Kandler RH, Jarratt JA, Gumpert EJ et al. The role of magnetic stimulation in the diagnosis of multiple sclerosis. J Neurol Sci 1991; 106: 25–30.

113. Mayr N, Baumgartner C, Zeitlhofer J, Deecke L. The sensitivity of transcranial cortical magnetic stimulation in detecting pyramidal tract lesions in clinically definite multiple sclerosis. Neurology 1991; 41: 566–569.

114. David P, Ristori GP, Elia M et al. Multiple sclerosis. Magnetic resonance imaging, evoked potentials and cerebrospinal fluid analysis. Acta Neurol (Napoli) 1990; 12: 200–206.

115. Jacobs LD, Beck RW, Simon JH et al. Intramuscular interferon beta-1a therapy initiated during a first demyelinating event in multiple sclerosis. CHAMPS Study Group. N Engl J Med 2000; 343: 898–904.

116. Jin YP, de Pedro-Cuesta J, Huang YH, Soderstrom M. Predicting multiple sclerosis at optic neuritis onset. Mult Scler 2003; 9: 135–141.

117. Bednarik J, Kadanka Z. Multimodal sensory and motor evoked potentials in a two-year follow-up study of MS patients with relapsing course. Acta Neurol Scand 1992; 86: 15–18.

118. Leocani L, Rovaris M, Boneschi FM et al. Multimodal evoked potentials to assess the evolution of multiple sclerosis: a longitudinal study. J Neurol Neurosurg Psychiatr 2006; 77: 1030–1035.

119. Rot U, Mesec A. Clinical, MRI, CSF and electrophysiological findings in different stages of multiple sclerosis. Clin Neurol Neurosurg 2006; 108: 271–274.

120. O'Connor PW, Tansay CM, Detsky AS et al. The effect of spectrum bias on the utility of magnetic resonance imaging and evoked potentials in the diagnosis of suspected multiple sclerosis. Neurology 1996; 47: 140–144.

121. O'Connor P, Marchetti P, Lee L, Perera M. Evoked potential abnormality scores are a useful measure of disease burden in relapsing-remitting multiple sclerosis. Ann Neurol 1998; 44: 404–407.

122. Sand T, Sulg IA. Evoked potentials and CSF-immunoglobulins in MS: relationship to disease duration, disability, and functional status. Acta Neurol Scand 1990; 82: 217–221.

123. Sater RA, Rostami AM, Galetta S et al. Serial evoked potential studies and MRI imaging in chronic progressive multiple sclerosis. J Neurol Sci 1999; 171: 79–83.

124. Nuwer MR, Packwood JW, Myers LW, Ellison GW. Evoked potentials predict the clinical changes in a multiple sclerosis drug study. Neurology 1987; 37: 1754–1761.

125. Neiman J, Nilsson BY, Barr PO, Perrins DJ. Hyperbaric oxygen in chronic progressive multiple sclerosis: visual evoked potentials and clinical effects. J Neurol Neurosurg Psychiatr 1985; 48: 497–500.

126. Rostami AM, Sater RA, Bird SJ et al. A double-blind, placebo-controlled trial of extracorporeal photopheresis in chronic progressive multiple sclerosis. Mult Scler 1999; 5: 198–203.

127. Van Diemen HA, Polman CH, van Dongen MM et al. 4-aminopyridine induces functional improvement in multiple sclerosis patients: a neurophysiological study. J Neurol Sci 1993; 116: 220–226.

128. Johnson KP. A review of the clinical efficacy profile of copolymer 1: new US phase III trial data. J Neurol 1996; 243: S3–S7.

129. Interferon beta-1b in the treatment of multiple sclerosis: final outcome of the randomized controlled trial. The IFNB Multiple Sclerosis Study Group and the University of British Columbia MS/MRI Analysis Group. Neurology 1995; 45: 1277–1285.

CHAPTER

11   The neuropathology of multiple sclerosis

S. K. Ludwin and C. S. Raine

INTRODUCTION

Multiple sclerosis (MS) remains a complex and mysterious disease, despite extensive work that has delineated advances in its biology. MS researchers have been greatly aided by the explosion of new knowledge in immunology, genetics and cell biology. However, continued study of the pathology of the lesions in MS remains crucial in understanding the etiopathology, clinical course, diagnosis and basis for treatment.[1,2] It is of great interest to note that the pathological features described by Charcot[3] among others in the mid-19th century remain relevant today. However, what has changed throughout these intervening years is not the description of the actual pathology but rather the way this has been reinterpreted in the light of advances in both clinical medicine and basic science. The search for surrogate markers has meant that a pathological gold-standard must be established by which these putative markers may be measured. This is relevant for neuroimaging, which has become advanced to the stage of not only providing sophisticated diagnosis but also assisting in the staging, response to therapy and individual make-up of each patient.

Many aspects of the pathology of MS, even though well described, remain laden with controversy. The role played by damaged axons in the course of the disease, observed for decades, is of uncertain cause; this has major practical ramifications in management and treatment. This is well seen with current therapies, which have played a major role in the modification of disease and amelioration of symptoms. Enough knowledge exists to begin these therapies, and the results of the therapy have in turn helped the understanding of the basic science involved.[4,5]

There has been much discussion as to the validity of animal models in understanding the pathology of MS. Over the years, the use of animal models has contributed significantly to understanding the components of, if not the entire disease. It has also become clear that many of the features of these models demonstrate what could be happening in MS rather than always what necessarily is. As will be discussed below, extrapolations need to be made with caution.

Understanding MS requires solving the complex genetics underlying the disease, as demonstrated by population and family studies[6,7] and genome and protein screening to identify genes associated with either disease etiology or course.[8,9] Clinical and epidemiological observation, as well as animal models, have also facilitated elucidation of the environmental component of the etiology, with agents being studied ranging from viruses to vitamin D levels in sun exposure.[10] There is still much controversy over what constitute the earliest early stages and the inciting factors of the MS lesion. It is widely held that MS occurs in genetically predisposed individuals and is triggered by an unknown process(es). Most workers in the field concur that early events in the evolution of MS, usually related to relapses and remissions, are part of an inflammatory, probably immune, process. It is also widely recognized, however, that the disease, both in its primary and secondary form, usually develops a chronic progressive course. Whether this is related to inflammation or to some other factor leading to axonal degeneration is still open to question.

The emerging interest in cortical pathology and in events occurring in the apparently normal white matter away from the lesions have assumed considerable importance in understanding and correlating the clinical aspects of the disease. The answers to these questions have practical ramifications. Does the progressive phase of the disease need to be treated with anti-inflammatory or neurotrophic agents, or both? How great is the ability of the brain to repair itself with regard to both axonal regeneration and remyelination? Finally, of emerging interest and importance, is MS all one disease with different manifestations?

Therefore, the pathology of the MS lesion requires an analysis not only of the whole lesion but also of its components and the relationship of these components to similar components in other conditions. Such an analysis remains one of the central pillars in understanding and managing this devastating disease.

HISTORY OF MULTIPLE SCLEROSIS PATHOLOGY

Over the last 150 years, theories and concepts on the etiology and pathogenesis of MS have reflected those of the emerging fields of infectious disease, developmental disease, environmental medicine, immunology and genetics. Full accounts of the history of the disease can be found in the work of Murray[11] and Chapter 1.

With the emergence of one of the golden ages of clinical neurology in the mid 1800s, the first proper descriptions of the disease appeared both from Cruveilhier and also from Carswell.[12] In his Atlas in 1829–1832, Cruveilhier also depicted some fine illustrations of the lesions of MS. In 1863, Rindfleisch published seminal works on the pathology and the clinical picture, as well as postulating as to the cause of the disease. Perhaps the most important of the early workers in MS was Charcot,[3] who described both the clinical and the pathologic findings extensively in 1886 and did much to publicize the nature of the disease. Dawson in Edinburgh in 1916[13] left wonderful observations on the pathology that remain accurate to this day. The advent of microscopic examination allowed for the recognition that myelin sheaths were being lost and that the debris was taken up by macrophages. However, in the early works of Charcot and later of Marburg in 1906, changes in the axon were already observed.[14] In addition, although many authors had noted the presence of thin sheaths, it was Charcot who hinted at the possibility of regeneration, while most of his contemporaries felt that they represented demyelination.

From even the earliest days, investigators were debating the etiology of MS. For some, such as Strumpfel, MS was a developmental disease, and Charcot felt that the underlying cause lay with the glia. Rindfleisch very astutely noted the collection of cells around blood vessels and first postulated the vascular theory of the disease, emphasizing its inflammatory nature. The debates between those postulating inflammation and those postulating degeneration of glia are slightly reminiscent of today's debate as to the relative roles of inflammation and neurodegeneration in the course of MS. Dawson also agreed with the vascular theory and extended it to suggest that factors emanating from the blood vessels were responsible for the tissue damage. In concert with the clinical observations, investigators turned to the laboratory in an attempt to understand the disease using animal models. The emerging sciences of neurochemistry and immunology in the 1930s, together with the discovery of experimental immune disease in the brain, ushered in an era of studies on the autoimmune basis for MS that continues to this day. Years of investigation to find an infectious agent have yielded little success, although this hypothesis is continually revisited. Modern studies on molecular biology and genetics, as well as genetic epidemiology, continue to put together the pieces of the puzzle.

In all these studies, as in those over the last century, we keep returning to pathology for clues and for checks. In this respect, the pathologist of today truly stands on the shoulders of the giants of the last 150 years, and sometimes even falls short of the standards they set.

DEMYELINATING DISEASE

The classical definition of a demyelinating disease is one in which the myelin is preferentially destroyed with relative sparing of the axon, in contrast to wallerian degeneration where myelin loss is secondary to axon destruction. This classical distinction has attracted some questioning recently, with the demonstration that many diseases thought to be demyelinating do in fact have significant axonal damage either as part of the primary disease or secondary to it. This will be dealt with below when considering axonal pathology, but some of the inherited leukodystrophies, and indeed MS, are examples of this.

There are four main groups of diseases in which myelin is selectively destroyed:

- Group 1 comprises acquired inflammatory demyelinating diseases with no established infectious etiology, including MS and its variants, neuromyelitis optica (NMO), Balo's concentric sclerosis, acute disseminated encephalomyelitis and acute hemorrhagic leukoencephalomyelitis.
- Group 2 progressive multifocal leukoencephalopathy, subacute sclerosing panencephalitis and human immunodeficiency virus (HIV) vacuolar myelopathy represent examples of inflammatory demyelinating diseases with a known infectious background or proven infectious etiology.
- Group 3 covers the acquired noninflammatory diseases of myelin, which include toxic diseases such as vitamin B^{12} deficiency and central pontine myelinolysis as well as other environmental agents such as trauma, radiation, drugs and chemotherapy, etc.
- Group 4 consists of the hereditary metabolic diseases of myelin, including adrenoleukodystrophy, metachromatic leukodystrophy and globoid leukodystrophy (Krabbe's disease), for which defective genes have been isolated. Diseases in this group may either become manifest during development, leading to hypomyelination, or following the establishment of myelin, in which they lead to loss of myelin. These diseases are usually referred to as dysmyelinating diseases and invariably display extensive involvement of axons. They may also at times have a secondary autoimmune response to myelin breakdown.

ANIMAL MODELS AND/OR OTHER HUMAN CONDITIONS IN UNDERSTANDING THE DEVELOPMENT OF MULTIPLE SCLEROSIS

In any discussion on the etiopathogenesis of MS, reference will be made to numerous animal models as well as to other human diseases of known etiology. In using animal models, one has to establish whether the model replicates exactly the disease under consideration and whether it occurs spontaneously or secondary to an appropriate insult. Such models include spontaneous cancer or hypertension in rodents, or the development of stroke after arterial ligation. In MS there is no spontaneous model, nor even a convincing induced model. What animal models have shown extensively are similarities to elements of the MS lesion (such as immune-mediated inflammation, demyelination, axonal damage and remyelination), which has allowed us to infer that their known mechanisms may explain events in MS. Undoubtedly, the most important model is experimental autoimmune encephalomyelitis (EAE), an immune-mediated neurological disease induced by the injection of myelin, myelin peptides or myelin-sensitized cells into genetically-susceptible animals, with or without adjuvant. This disease is described in full in Chapter 16. It has many features in common with MS.

In its original form, EAE is monophasic, resembling acute MS or acute disseminated encephalomyelitis (ADEM). By manipulating the induction protocol and by using different species and/or strains, other forms of EAE may be produced, including chronic relapsing or progressive variants, with greater similarities to MS. Indeed, many of the same chronic pathological features of MS may be recapitulated in the experimental disease.

Similarly, in the absence of a perfect fit, other models are used to demonstrate features of individual components of the disease. Exogenous toxins such as Cuprizone, lysolecithin and ethidium bromide are used as demyelinating agents in animals and are also the basis for studies in remyelination. Viruses such as MHV, canine distemper, herpes and Theiler's virus all produce varying degrees of demyelination and subsequent remyelination, while many may also lead to axonal degeneration. Inflammatory and immune diseases may also cause abnormalities of the blood–brain barrier, while all these conditions may lead to gliosis of varying degrees. The use of gene deletions, transgenic models or spontaneously dysmyelinating mutants in understanding the genesis of myelin and axon pathology has increased dramatically in recent years.

Because of the lack of a true-matched model, some authors have rejected the extrapolation of animal work to the clinical disease. However, as long as the caveats are recognized, the judicious use of animal models can be of enormous value in trying to understand and dissect mechanisms of causation and progression in MS.

STAGING AND DEFINITION OF LESION PATHOLOGY

In discussing, comparing and defining any lesion, accurate or at least consistent staging becomes very important.[15,16] Indeed, the subject was considered of enough importance to warrant a consensus document, which has, however, failed to become widely accepted,[17] probably because of its complexity and lack of true applicability to a broad spectrum of researchers. The acuity of the lesion, as described in different pathological staging schemes, is often discordant with the assessment of the acuity of the clinical presentation. The usual categories in common usage include terms such as active/acute, chronic–active and chronic–inactive/classical to describe MS lesions. Active/acute lesions have traditionally been defined as showing demyelination with inflammatory infiltrates, whereas chronic lesions show demyelination with little or no inflammation or myelin breakdown. Most authors will accept that the subacute or chronic–active lesion is one with a chronic core and active edge, or a plaque with a low level of inflammatory activity. The active edge of plaque may represent continual expansion of a lesion with an inactive core, or it could represent new activity around the edge of a pre-existing plaque.

Because cellularity may often be a misleading sign of acuity, as lymphocytes and macrophages and debris may remain in the tissue for prolonged periods, some investigators have attempted to use the contents of macrophages to assess the stage of myelin breakdown more accurately.[18-21] Early activated macrophages may stain positively for MRP14 and 27E10; these cells will also show reactivity for the minor myelin proteins, myelin/oligodendrocyte glycoprotein (MOG) and myelin-associated glycoprotein (MAG), which disappears within a week or two. The major myelin proteins, myelin basic protein (MBP) and proteolipid protein (PLP), are retained in macrophages for up 3–4 weeks, seen also with Luxol fast blue (LFB) staining. Most staging and classifications, however, either lack or do not consider other important elements, including axonal and cortical damage, the gliotic reaction and remyelination. These probably play as much

of a role in the development of symptoms and prognosis than the degree of myelin breakdown, as do changes in the so-called normal-appearing white matter (NAWM). It is hoped that future staging or classification systems will also take these features into account.

THE MORPHOLOGY OF THE MULTIPLE SCLEROSIS LESION

There have been numerous descriptions of the classical pathology of MS lesions.[22-28] For descriptive purposes, it will be of value to describe the common lesions before continuing to a more detailed discussion of the pathology and pathogenesis of some of the component features that make up these various lesions.

THE CHRONIC OR INACTIVE (CLASSICAL) PLAQUE

The most common type of MS lesion is the chronic plaque, seen at autopsy in patients who die after a protracted course. Grossly, this type of plaque is seen as a firm grayish-brown, well circumscribed lesion in the brain or spinal cord. Although this may occasionally be single, sometimes found incidentally, in most cases the plaques are multiple. Most affected sites include the centrum semiovale and the corpus callosum in the cerebral hemispheres (Figs 11.1–11.3), as well as the white matter of the cerebellum, and may range in size from less than a centimeter to a diffuse lesion (Fig. 11.4) extending to adjacent gray matter structures of the cortex and the deep nuclei. They are classically found in a periventricular distribution (Figs 11.1 and 11.2), in particular in the region adjacent to the caudate nucleus and the corpus callosum. Plaques are also found at the corticomedullary junction, and small plaques may be found in the cortex and other gray matter structures (see below). The latter have proved to be more common than previously thought, may be isolated or continuous with underlying white matter plaques and may play a role in cognitive defects.[29] MRI studies have also related memory dysfunction to juxtacortical lesions.[30] Other sites of predilection include optic nerves and chiasm (Fig. 11.5), and brainstem (Fig. 11.6), where involvement of the medial longitudinal fasciculus causes internuclear ophthalmoplegia. The spinal cord is often shrunken and gray-white following involvement with primary demyelinated lesions as well as secondary

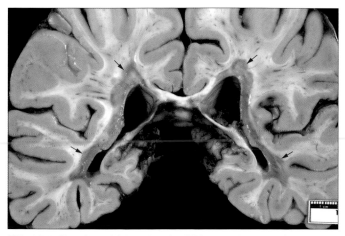

FIG. 11.1 Chronic multiple sclerosis. Widespread gray periventricular plaques with well defined edges (arrows) surround the ventricles and extend into the centrum semiovale and the corpus callosum. The ventricles are enlarged.

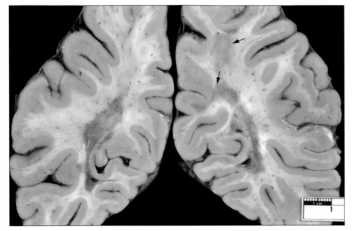

FIG. 11.2 Multiple plaques from a case of chronic multiple sclerosis demonstrate a predominantly periventricular position in the occipital lobes but extend widely into the white matter up to the cortex (arrows). Some plaques are less clearly defined and blend into the surrounding white matter.

(Wallerian) degeneration (Fig. 11.7). The upper cervical and thoracic cord is usually affected. Spinal cord atrophy is seen, particularly in the progressive stages of the disease, either primary or secondary, and contributes significantly to clinical debility. In both brainstem and spinal cord, lesions may be subpial, often around cranial and spinal nerve roots. MRI studies of these areas are difficult but have confirmed the atrophy and have shown good clinical correlation with the progressive forms of the disease.[31,32]

Besides obvious plaques, the pathologist is often struck by more diffuse alterations in neighboring white matter, including granularity and discoloration (Fig. 11.8), which have been the basis of further pathology. In addition, in recent years, it has been well demonstrated that MRI changes at post-mortem (Fig. 11.9) have guided the pathologist to grossly normal regions that histologically show significant pathology. It is apparent that many lesions have been under-represented in the past, emphasizing a need for the use of imaging in the pathological examination of MS cases.

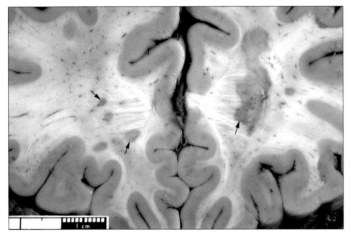

FIG. 11.3 In this case of chronic multiple sclerosis, plaques are seen extending along the very anterior fibres of the genu of the corpus callosum in the frontal lobe (arrows) as well as being around the ventricle in a very anterior frontal position. This pattern of radiation through the corpus callosum can frequently be seen on MRI.

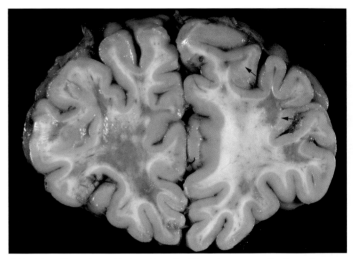

FIG. 11.4 Chronic multiple sclerosis. The plaques are both well circumscribed and diffuse. They often abut the corticomedullary junction and at times involve the cortex (arrows). The distribution of the plaques is far more diffuse and ill defined than in the previous figures.

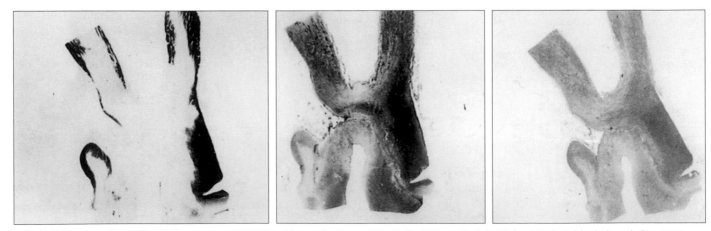

FIG. 11.5 A series of paraffin sections across the optic chiasm shows severe myelin loss on the left, stained with Heidenhain, relative axon sparing in the middle, stained with Bodian, and the general rarefaction of tissue in the hematoxylin and eosin (H&E) section on the right. Reproduced with permission from Raine 1997.[27]

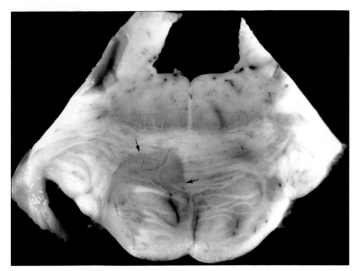

FIG. 11.6 A chronic plaque is seen in the basis pontis (arrows) in this case of chronic multiple sclerosis.

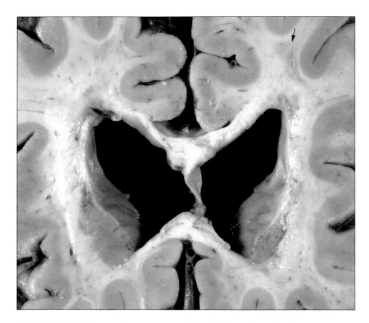

FIG. 11.8 This image from a case of multiple sclerosis demonstrates diffuse granularity of the white matter in the presence of only subtle images of plaques at the left angle of the ventricle. The involvement of the white matter is extensive extending up into the superior frontal lobe (arrow) and the surrounding so-called normal appearing white matter in this case showed histological changes.

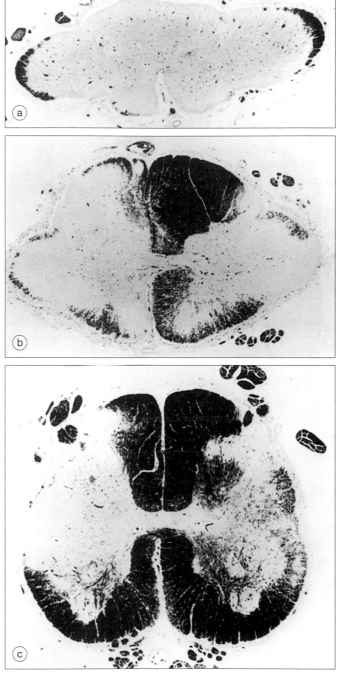

FIG. 11.7 Three different levels of spinal cord from a case of chronic multiple sclerosis demonstrate variation in degree of involvement. Note the almost total loss of myelin in **A** (cervical), the large, asymmetrical lesions in **B** (midthoracic) and the disseminated involvement in **C** (lumbar). Heidenhain stain. Reproduced with permission from Raine 1997.[27]

Generalized atrophy is often striking in the brains of MS patients, either focally or diffusely, as manifested by enlargement of the ventricles and shrinkage of structures such as the corpus callosum and deep white matter (Figs 11.1 and 11.8), as well as cortex and, in severe cases, deep gray matter. This mirrors changes seen on MRI.[33] Atrophy of optic nerves and spinal cord has already been noted. In rare instances, cavity formation may be seen grossly.

Histologically, the hallmark of the disease is loss of myelin (Figs 11.10 and 11.11). In most chronic plaques, the border between demyelinated areas and normal tissue is sharp, although within the plaque there may be varying degrees of myelin preservation (Figs 11.12–11.14). Demyelination may be detected either with conventional stains such as LFB or with immunochemical stains against myelin components, such as myelin basic protein (MBP) and proteolipid protein (PLP), as well as minor proteins (MOG and MAG). Often, axons appear to lose their sheaths as they enter the plaque. There may be almost no myelinated fibers present, or axons with either thin or normal myelin sheaths may be present, representing remyelination and myelin preservation respectively. At times, there is an extension of demyelination following the walls of blood vessels into the surrounding tissue, a feature known as a Dawson's finger. Oli-

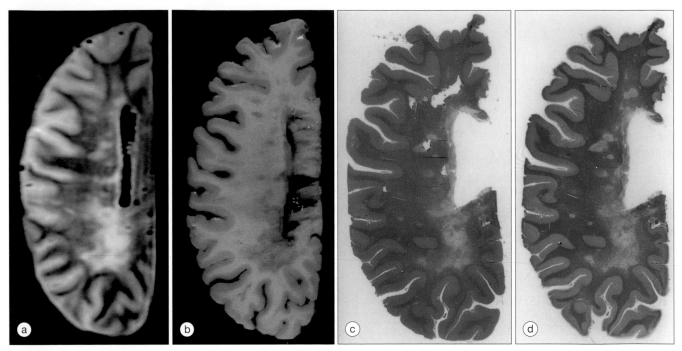

FIG. 11.9 A series of images depicting a single horizontal slice from a patient with chronic multiple sclerosis. Multiple areas of plaque involvement of the white matter, especially prominent in the occipital lobes, are seen in the post-mortem MRI (**a**), and confirmed grossly (**b**) and with H&E (**c**) and myelin stains (**d**). Although the figures are complementary, the extent of involvement shown on the MRI is more widespread than that seen either grossly or histologically. Courtesy of Dr G. R. W. Moore, University of British Columbia, Vancouver, Canada.

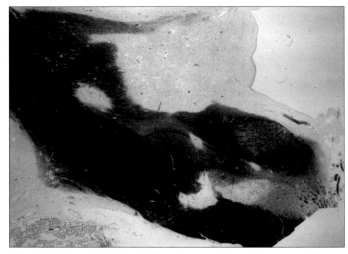

FIG. 11.10 Luxol fast blue (LFB)-stained section of the area of the thalamus and internal capsule. The third ventricle is to the right and the temporal horn of the lateral ventricle to the left inferiorly. There is extensive demyelination in the thalamus and patches of myelin loss within the internal capsule and the area of the subthalamus.

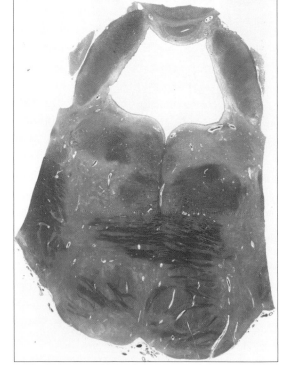

FIG. 11.11 LFB/H&E-stained section of the pons showing large areas of demyelination, leaving patches of myelinated tracts stained blue. The myelin loss in this case is less well circumscribed and more diffuse and inferiorly extends to and is based on the pia. The superior cerebellar peduncle shows some pallor bilaterally, due either to wallerian degeneration or to partial demyelination.

godendrocyte loss, which may be extensive and near total at times, is usually most severe in the center of the lesion and may accompany loss of myelin (Figs 11.11–11.13). In chronic plaques, there is almost invariably no evidence of ongoing oligodendrocyte necrosis or apoptosis. Around the periphery of the lesion, there is often a rim in which there is a greater density of oligodendrocytes, which may be associated with an increase in the number of thin sheaths representing remyelination (Fig. 11.12).

The chronic inactive (silent) lesion contains extensive areas of gliosis, with elongated astrocytic processes forming a fibrillary

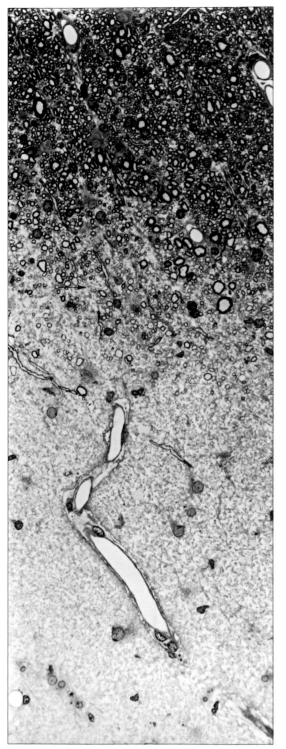

FIG. 11.12 Toluidine-blue-stained section of a chronic MS plaque showing normally myelinated white matter (top) and a relatively acellular demyelinated area, with extensive oligodendrocyte loss (below). At the interface (arrow) there are numerous thinly myelinated fibres suggestive of remyelination, as well as an increase in rounded dark nuclei consistent with oligodendrocytes. Reproduced with permission from Prineas et al 2002.[26]

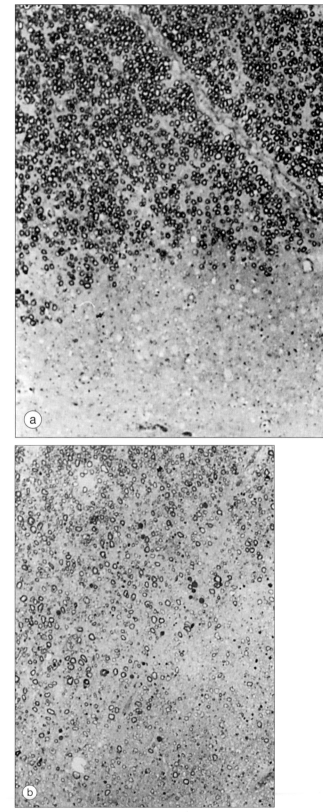

FIG. 11.13 Toluidine blue semi-thin sections of the edge (**A**) and centre (**B**) of two MS plaques. In **A** the plaque shows little remyelination except at the edge, whereas in **B** there are numerous fibres with inappropriately thinned myelin sheaths.

meshwork. Astrocytes within a chronic plaque may appear to be hypertrophic (gemistocytes), particularly towards the margin, where recent activity (demyelination) may be found, but most tend to have scant cytoplasm and are characterized by their fibrillary processes, an appearance typical for established silent lesions (Fig. 11.15). The latter cells are no longer gemistocytic,

unless there is concomitant demyelination, and have small nuclei with imperceptible processes. Some gemistocytes may remain, suggestive of ongoing activity, and may be multinucleated. Ultrastructurally, naked axons are surrounded by astro-

157

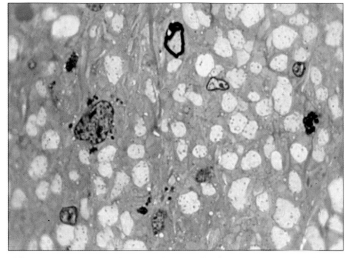

FIG. 11.14 High magnification of a toluidine-blue-stained semi-thin section of a chronic multiple sclerosis plaque showing extensive demyelination on a background of dense gliosis. Although relatively spared, the number of axons is decreased. There is still residual myelin debris in macrophages, and a fibre with a thin sheath.

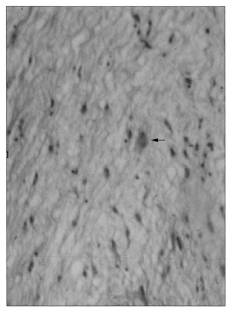

FIG. 11.15 H&E section of a chronic multiple sclerosis plaque showing dense gliosis on a fibrillary background and an increased number of astrocytes. Although some of these are rounded with pink cytoplasm (arrow), the rest are relatively inert with spindly nuclei.

cytic processes and junctional structures may be found between astrocytes, and also between axons and glia in these chronic plaques[34,35] (Fig. 11.16). While inflammation (see below) is not a striking feature of the chronic plaque (indeed this is often used to define the chronic lesion), scant collections of mononuclear cells, including lymphocytes and sometimes plasma cells and mast cells, may frequently be seen, usually in a perivascular position. In the silent lesion, B cells may be more common than T cells. Similarly, specific markers show many more monocytes and macrophages than might otherwise have been seen, and lipid-laden macrophages may be found scattered throughout the tissue. These macrophages contain periodic acid–Schiff (PAS)-positive material but, within the lesion itself, rarely contain significant amounts of myelin-specific proteins. There is usually prominent loss of axons within the plaque, ranging from mild to severe (Figs 11.14 and 11.16), even though at first sight this is often less apparent than the more obvious loss of myelin. If axonal loss is severe, the remaining neuropil may be rarified, even extending to cavity formation. Blood vessels within the plaque may show some alterations in the form of sclerosis or perivascular fibrosis (hyalinization) and blood–brain barrier abnormalities[36] but may often appear to be histologically normal. In many plaques, both at the center and at the edge, there is an increase in vessel number.[37]

New evidence is emerging that the extent of lesions is far greater than was originally believed. Involvement of deep gray matter is quite common and, as will be discussed below, there is often widespread involvement of white matter that had appeared normal on gross examination, the so-called NAWM. In addition, evidence suggests that cortical pathology and demyelination is widespread and common.

The periplaque, or the rim of tissue around the classical inactive or burnt-out plaque, frequently shows changes in composition and disease activity. Myelin in this area may be less well stained than normal (Figs 11.10 and 11.12), forming a penumbra of myelin pallor. This may be the result both of thinner sheaths, representing remyelination, and fewer axons, due to Wallerian degeneration emanating from damaged axons in the plaque center. Accompanying this myelin alteration is an increase in gliosis, seen to best advantage with the astrocytic marker glial fibrillary acidic protein (GFAP) (see below). Macro-

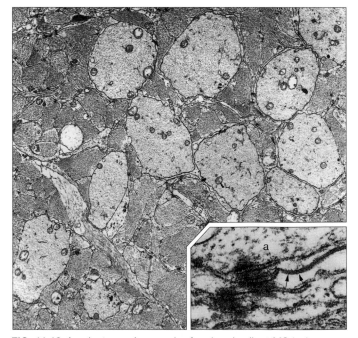

FIG. 11.16 An electron micrograph of a chronic silent MS lesion showing the demyelinated axons and the background astroglial scar tissue. (Inset) An axoglial junction exists between a demyelinated axon (a) and an astroglial process. Desmosomes and a gap junction (arrows) exist between other astroglial cell processes. With permission from reference 29.

phage markers will show an increase in these cells in this area. At times, myelin changes can be most extreme, with alternating areas of myelin loss and preservation, resembling the pattern seen in Balo's disease (see below). In these areas, the number of oligodendrocytes may be normal or even increased in areas where the myelin is present, or decreased in areas of myelin loss.

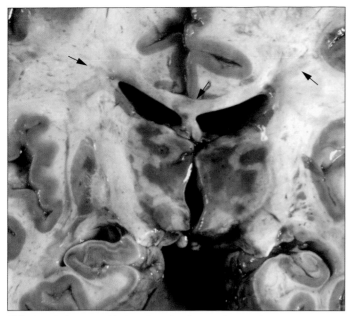

FIG. 11.17 Acute multiple sclerosis plaques from a freshly cut brain demonstrating well circumscribed but reddish plaques, in this case seen extensively in the thalamus and putamen. Although subtle, there are abnormalities seen in the white matter around the ventricle, as well as in the corpus callosum (arrows).

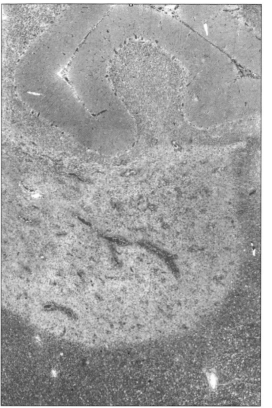

FIG. 11.18 Toluidine-blue-stained semi-thin section of a late acute multiple sclerosis plaque in the cerebellum. There is a well defined border of demyelination but the plaque itself is extremely cellular and there is extensive cellular infiltrate around the blood vessels.

Ultrastructural examination of plaques has typically shown loss of myelin and variable loss of axons, separated by numerous processes of filament-filled astrocytes (Fig. 11.16). Despite years of searching, and the occasional descriptions of virus-like inclusions in MS tissue, a virus has not been identified. The loss of oligodendrocytes from the lesion center and their preservation at the periphery has been confirmed by electron microscopy studies.[38]

THE ACTIVE OR ACUTE LESION

For some, the term 'acute' should be reserved for the clinical situation. However, one can use the term, recognizing that an acute plaque can be found in a chronic clinical case and vice versa. The definition and dating of acute plaques pathologically has been described above.

Grossly, the acute plaque may sometimes appear to differ from the chronic plaque in that the color tends to be slightly pinker and it may sometimes appear to be softer and swollen rather than shrunken and retracted as in the chronic situation (Fig. 11.17). A characteristic of some of these lesions, noted recently with the extensive use of imaging techniques, is their alarming size and confluent nature; these cases of tumefactive MS invoke the differential diagnosis of a rapidly developing neoplasm. It will be of interest to see, with prospective imaging studies, whether these lesions will be shown to develop into the more diffuse forms of MS described below.

Histologically, the acute plaque is characterized by an extensive loss of myelin (Figs 11.18 and 11.19). This may be in the form of a well demarcated area of demyelination although, in the acute situation, the edges of the plaque are usually less well defined and demyelination and attendant cellular processes extend into the surrounding rim. Demyelinated fibers may be recognized by an axon devoid of a sheath as seen histochemically or immunohistochemically (Fig. 11.20) or, on electron microscopy, by the presence of naked axons. In addition, thinly myelinated fibers may be seen within the lesion, suggesting

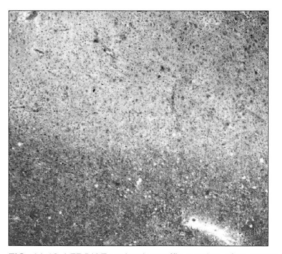

FIG. 11.19 LFB/H&E-stained paraffin section of an acute plaque showing the border between demyelination and normal tissue. Although reasonably well demarcated, to the right of the figure the border appears fuzzy. The plaque itself is very cellular.

either partially demyelinated or remyelinated fibers. The presence of oligodendrocytes showing the re-expression of developmental proteins, seen during myelination, suggests that the latter event is occurring in a significant number of these fibers. Edema may be severe and is seen as an expansion of the extracellular space, spreading apart both fibers and cells. Striking changes are seen in and around blood vessels corresponding to the breakdown of the blood–brain barrier, seen as gadolinium

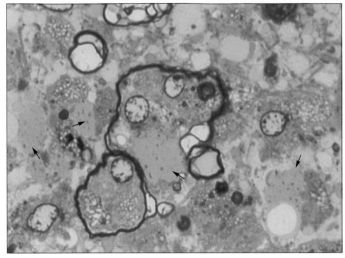

FIG. 11.20 Toluidine-blue-stained semi-thin section of an acute plaque showing demyelinated axons (arrows) as well as lipid-laden macrophages, some in the process of removing myelin from an axon (centre). There is edema and some myelin vacuolation seen in the upper left.

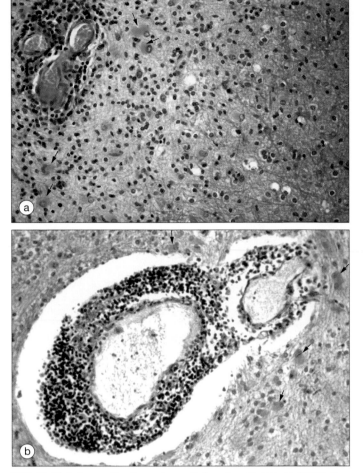

FIG. 11.21 Inflammation in acute multiple sclerosis lesions (H&E). **A.** A perivascular cuff of small mononuclear cells (left) abuts a lesion area infiltrated by inflammatory cells. Note the edematous nature of the tissue, the many hypertrophic astrocytes (arrows) and the adjacent less affected white matter (right). **B.** Perivascular mononuclear cells and reactive astrocytes (arrows) are seen in another case.

enhancement on the MRI. These include lymphocytic infiltrates (Figs 11.21 and 11.22), deposition of serum proteins such as albumin in the vessels and the surrounding tissue and, in very severe cases, mural necrosis. Accompanying myelin loss is a large infiltrate of foamy or debris-filled macrophages (Fig. 11.23) lying in sheets that appear to have replaced the normal neuropil, or may be around the blood vessels or percolating through more preserved areas of tissue as single cells. They may be associated with denuded axons or axons surrounded by thin sheaths suggestive of remyelination (Fig. 11.23a).

Depending on the age of the lesion, macrophages may demonstrate the myelin proteins mentioned above. Many macrophages and microglia are MHC-II positive (Fig. 11.23c), as are some astrocytes and even endothelial cells. Normal CNS tissue does not express MHC-II and its presence in diseased tissue suggests an ability to interact with lymphocytes.[39] The inflammatory infiltrate varies but in most acute cases it is extensive. Lymphocytes staining with the leukocyte common antigen (CD45) comprise the majority of cells, although plasma cells and even mast cells have been found, together with less well characterized monocytes. Although present throughout the tissue, lymphocytes are particularly prominent around blood vessels and at times may be so severe as to mimic a vasculitis (Fig. 11.2). Both CD4+ helper T cells (Fig. 11.22a) and CD8+ suppressor, cytotoxic T cells (Fig. 11.22b) may be found in acute lesions. CD4+ cells are usually felt to predominate in early lesions, with CD8+ cells taking over at later stages, but this is variable and a fixed pattern has not been defined. The importance of the latter cells in the pathogenesis of the disease is growing and these appear to be clonally expanded.[40] The occurrence of γδ T cells has been described in these lesions and their association with acute phase reactant or stress proteins such as heat shock protein on oligodendrocytes has been well recognized[41–43] (Fig. 11.24).

The pattern of damage and loss of oligodendrocytes is variable.[44] In some acute lesions, they are clearly decreased, as recognized with cell specific markers, while in others the cell number may be normal. In general, cell loss is more profound in the lesion center than at the periphery, where the numbers may even be increased. Lucchinetti and colleagues[45] found that oligodendrocyte loss was often striking in very acute cases, challenging previously held views that this was a function of chronicity. They found that for each patient there was a uniform type of oligodendrocyte loss and the numbers correlated with the extent of remyelination. The pattern of cell death in oligodendrocytes is somewhat controversial, with apoptosis being rare in some studies[46] and common in others,[47] and Bcl-2, a marker of cell survival, has been shown to be expressed by oligodendrocytes in MS tissue.[46,48] More recently, TRAIL death receptors have been described on oligodendrocytes in MS and normal brain but were not associated with apoptosis which was exceedingly rare on these cells.[49] Of great importance has been the finding that in some oligodendrocytes, even in the acute plaque, molecules expressed early in development during myelination are re-expressed, suggesting that remyelination recapitulates development and is an early phenomenon within the plaque[50] (see below under Remyelination). Changes in oligodendrocytes extend into the surrounding rim or penumbra.

Axonal damage is regularly seen, especially in the earliest lesions. Using silver stains and neurofilament proteins as markers, Trapp and colleagues[51] demonstrated truncated and swollen axons indicative of acute axonal injury (Fig. 11.25). Axonal numbers are often decreased, although the difficulty of

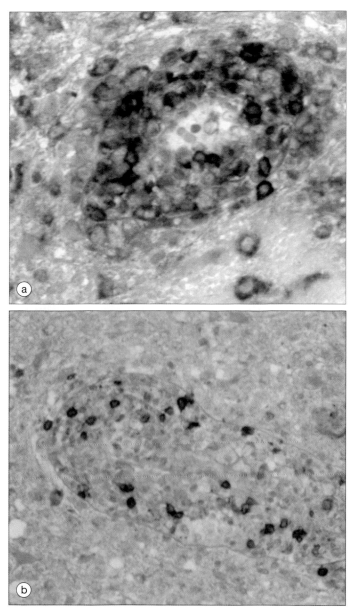

FIG. 11.22 Lymphocytes in acute multiple sclerosis lesions. The vessel walls, perivascular space and surrounding tissue are infiltrated by CD4+ (**A**) and CD8+ (**B**) T cells. Immunoperoxidase stain.

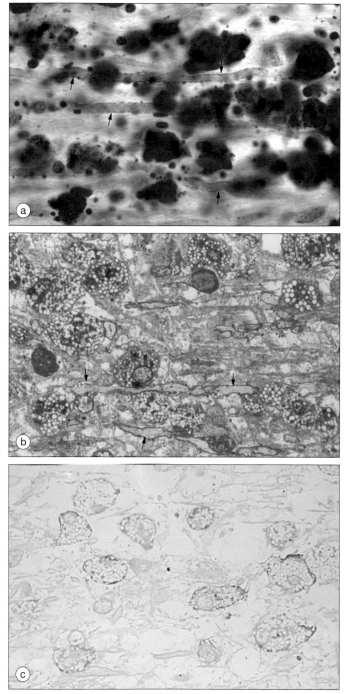

FIG. 11.23 Macrophages from acute plaques. **A**. Stained with oil red O, multiple lipid-filled macrophages are seen lying adjacent to axons, which show thin sheaths suggestive of remyelination (arrows). **B**. A semi-thin section stained with toluidine blue; there are multiple sheaths of lipid-laden macrophages surrounding axons, some of which are demyelinated while others show thin remyelinated sheaths (arrows) adjacent to macrophages. An axonal spheroid (ax) is also apparent. **C**. Stained immunochemically for MHC-II; macrophages among remyelinated fibres contain foamy debris and demonstrate membrane staining. **A** courtesy of Dr John W. Prineas, University of Sydney, Sydney, Australia.

assessing this in tissue infiltrated by cells and edema fluid is recognized. Other indicators of axonal damage, such as expression of the precursor protein for β amyloid, have also been demonstrated in these axons.[52] Similar changes have been noted in the surrounding periplaque rim (discussed in detail below).

The astrocytic response in the acute plaque, recognized by astrocytes or gemistocytes showing evidence of hypertrophy with swollen eosinophilic cytoplasm, is early and vigorous (Fig. 11.26). These cells may be so numerous in biopsies as to raise the possibility of neoplasia in biopsies of the tissue. Although some very atypical nuclei may be found, the generally benign nature of gemistocytes, as well as the accompanying inflammatory infiltrate, helps rule out this diagnosis. These cells have short, blunt processes and are heavily reactive with antibodies against GFAP (see below). Occasionally, nuclear structures suggestive of mitoses can be seen (Creutzberg cells). Some of these

cells contain oligodendrocytes within their cytoplasm, a process known as emperipolesis; this is possibly a nonspecific indicator of oligodendrocyte injury or protection[53,54] (Fig. 11.27). At this stage, the plaque lacks the heavy fibrillary astrocytic meshwork of the chronic plaque. This astrocytosis can be seen in the

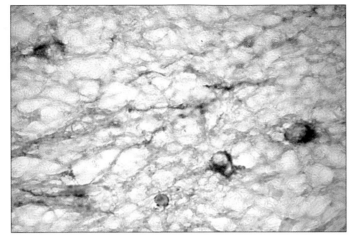

FIG. 11.24 An acute MS plaque edge is double-stained with antibodies against heat-shock protein 60 (blue), a molecule believed to be protective, and HNK-1 (brown), a marker for immature oligodendrocytes. Oligodendrocytes demonstrate double staining. Some thinly (re)myelinated fibers are also shown. Reproduced with permission from Jurewicz 2006.[96]

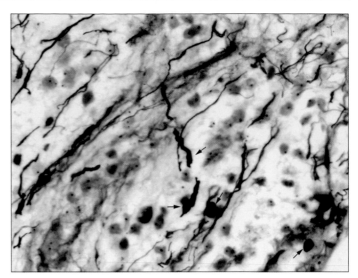

FIG. 11.25 Acute multiple sclerosis plaque stained with a Bodian silver stain. The number of fibers is decreased and, in addition, separated by edema. Many of the fibers show spheroids, shortening and irregularities indicative of axonal damage (arrows).

periplaque rim and surrounding tissue, where it usually accompanies infiltration of macrophages and inflammatory cells. As the acuteness of the plaque diminishes, the intensity of this cytoplasmic reaction abates and a correspondingly greater degree of fibrillary astrogliosis develops.

As in many inflammatory reactions, neovascularization has been described in MS lesions;[37] this may extend outside the lesion to the periplaque and even the NAWM and may have consequences both for diagnosis and for the generation of future lesions. Although several cDNA microarray studies in MS have attempted to detect gene regulation abnormalities,[55–58] they have so far demonstrated only upregulation of inflammation-related molecules and have failed to show any definitive etiological agents.

The prototypical acute form of MS, although relatively rare, is Marburg's disease, in which the severe clinical course generally lasts less than 1 year. Some of the more florid cases now being seen on MRI and on biopsy may be examples of this variant. The pathology is generally highly destructive[59] and affects the entire nervous system. A wide range of plaque size is seen, from small to confluent, even resembling the diffuse sclerosis of Schilder's disease. However, there are almost always signs of lesional activity in cases of Marburg's disease, even if macrophages no longer contain recognizable myelin products.

Ultrastructural studies have shown vesicular transformation of the myelin sheath (Fig. 11.28) and stripping of myelin by macrophages, similar to patterns seen in EAE.[27] Phagocytosis of myelin by macrophages through clathrin-coated pits and IgG-Fc receptors has been well demonstrated[27] and was early on thought to denote an immune etiology, and the interaction between lymphocytes and damaged oligodendrocytes has been confirmed. A dying-back gliopathy shown in experimental demyelination[60] has been proposed in acute MS lesions.[61] Ultrastructural studies have also played a large role in the designation of axons with thinned myelin sheaths as remyelinated fibers.[22,27,38]

THE CHRONIC ACTIVE OR SUBACUTE PLAQUE

This is a loosely defined entity, and both terms are used almost interchangeably in the literature. These plaques contain an inactive hypocellular gliotic core with the features of a chronic silent plaque described above, surrounded by an active periphery with the features of active or acute plaques (Fig. 11.29A,B). The periphery may display demyelination, edema, increased astrocytes and oligodendrocytes, mononuclear cell infiltration, demyelination and even some remyelination. Frequently, however, the degree of activity is less than that seen in acute plaques.

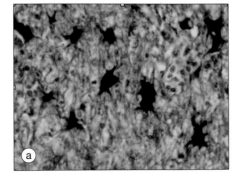

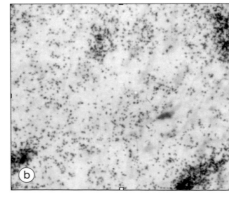

FIG. 11.26 Acute multiple sclerosis demonstrating reactive astrocytes. Large gemistocytes stained with immunoperoxidase show increased GFAP (**A**) and upregulation of mRNA for GFAP (**B**). With permission from Raine 1997.[25]

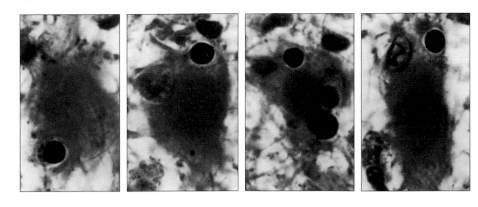

FIG. 11.27 An acute MS lesion showing hypertrophic astrocytes investing small rounded oligodendrocytes. H&E stain.

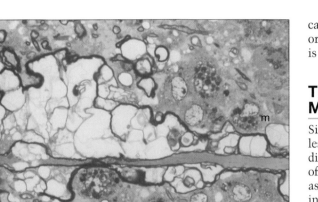

FIG. 11.28 Toluidine-blue-stained semi-thin section from an acute multiple sclerosis plaque demonstrating vesiculation of the myelin sheath during the course of demyelination. Flanked by macrophages (m) containing recognizable myelin debris typical of very recent activity, at the left of the figure, the axon is demyelinated (arrow).

The consensus document[17] refers to the chronically active plaque as one containing inflammatory cells and late markers of macrophage activity, as defined earlier. Some people have accepted the presence of significant numbers of lymphocytes and macrophages as indicators of lesions with some residual activity, even in the absence of the macrophage-defined markers of activity. Precise dating of the lesions is of great value in these

cases. Whether this pattern represents ongoing activity from the original process or a new extension superimposed on old lesion is not clear, and will be discussed further below.

THE INFLAMMATORY RESPONSE IN MEDIATING DISEASE AND REGENERATION

Since the time of Rindfleisch, the inflammatory infiltrate in MS lesions has defined the thinking of investigators about this disease. Cellular infiltrates have been recognized as the source of tissue injury mediators and studied for clues they may reveal as to the immune basis of the disease.[4,62] The inflammatory infiltrate is most developed and florid in the acute lesion and may also be scattered in chronic lesions, where it is predominantly lymphocytic. In some cases, clusters of plasma cells may be seen, suggesting a basis for the local production of intra-CNS immunoglobulins (Ig). Infiltrates may also form the active rim of expanding acute-on-chronic or subacute lesions. Both CD4+ and CD8+ T cells are seen in MS (Fig. 11.22) and EAE. Two subtypes of CD4+ T cells, based on the array of cytokines they produce are known as T helper (Th)-1 and Th-2 with pro- and anti-inflammatory characteristics respectively (see Ch. 13). Molecules known to facilitate cell trafficking are present on infiltrating cells within the MS lesion, either macrophages or lymphocytes, some of which may be activated by antigen-presenting dendritic cells within the normal and MS brain.[63] Proinflammatory cytokines can be demonstrated, including tumor necrosis factor (TNF)α, interferon (IFN)γ, and interleukin (IL)-2.[64]

In recent times, the role of CD8+ cytotoxic cells has assumed much greater importance;[65] in the MS lesion, they may

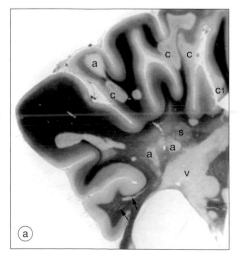

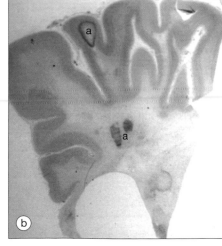

FIG. 11.29 Chronic active multiple sclerosis showing a combination of acute and chronic plaques. In **A**, stained with Luxol fast blue, there are numerous chronic plaques both around the ventricles (v) as well as within the gyri extending to the cortex. Within the centrum semiovale, there are also paler areas (s) suggestive of shadow plaques with remyelination. Some of the plaques appear to follow the path of the radiating blood vessels suggestive of Dawson's fingers (arrows). **C.** Cortical involvement with demyelination, at times extending from white matter plaques, is prominent. Some of these appear to be entirely within the cortex (C1). The plaques labeled (a), when stained with the Nissl stain as depicted in **B**, show a very active cellular rim indicating ongoing activity.

predominate.[40] They interact with MHC I molecules supposedly present on oligodendrocytes, neurons and axons, as well as other tissue elements. The pathogenetic role of blood and CSF Ig in MS patients has always puzzled researchers; in recent years the importance of B cells has become evident.[66,67] The interplay between B and T cells in the MS lesion mirrors that seen in the genesis of many forms of EAE. Ig and complement are deposited on myelin and on the axon and, in addition, antibodies against MOG and MBP have been demonstrated in CSF and sera of MS patients[68] as well as in tissue.[69] These may be related to the CSF oligoclonal bands.

Some authors have suggested that MS is neurodegenerative, despite the features of immune activation.[70] They have pointed out that the presence of inflammation and of oligoclonal banding is nonspecific and can be seen in many infectious and degenerative diseases; in these cases, immune phenomena could also be secondary events. Inflammatory infiltrates may be seen in adrenoleukodystrophy, poliomyelitis and ALS, and the complement deposition seen in MS is also found in numerous other conditions, including ischemia. The search for an infectious trigger has proved elusive (see Ch. 15). Cells autoreactive to myelin proteins, as well as antimyelin antibodies, may well be seen in healthy controls and indeed may be part of the normal repertoire of the immune system. In contrast to rheumatoid arthritis and Crohn's disease, no association with disease-specific immune markers or genes exist in patients with MS. Some authors have also suggested that, in many cases, the autoimmune response may follow a primary CNS event (infection, ischemia), with the target antigens subsequently presented within lymph nodes. These in turn produce activated lymphocytes, which re-enter the CNS and cause damage.[70]

Other authors have pointed out similarities between the pathology of MS and the Th-1 type bias in EAE[71] in defending the concept of MS as an inflammatory T-cell mediated autoimmune disease. These include activated T cells in the blood and CSF, T-cell reactivity to myelin antigens, Th1-type inflammation in the brain, chemokine expression and deposition of Ig. T cells reactive against myelin antigens have been found in normal patients and previously it has not been proven that the myelin-reactive T cells circulating in MS patients were capable of inducing tissue damage. Recently, however,[72,73] using transgenic mice humanized for the human T-cell receptor, it has been shown that MS-patient-derived T cells, when passively-transferred to these mice, are capable of inducing inflammation, demyelination and axonal damage. Other features supporting involvement of the immune system in pathogenesis include the response to therapy with interferons, glatiramer acetate, natalizumab (Tysabri) and immunosuppression, which, although not conclusive, have been used to bolster the argument. Relationships to other autoimmune diseases in family members, as well as reduction of disease during pregnancy, are further indicators of an autoimmune component. However, it should be pointed out that, although disease-modifying therapies reduce the incidence of relapses and new gadolinium-enhancing lesions indicative of breakdown of the blood–brain barrier, they do not alter the long-term inexorable progression of the disease. Some investigators suggest that there may be two pathways to immunity,[70] one originating with activated immune cells in the periphery and the other secondary to CNS tissue destruction and the development of subsequent autoimmunity.

THE PATHOGENESIS OF DEMYELINATION IN MULTIPLE SCLEROSIS

Demyelination defines the disease and is the dominant feature of the plaque. The outward extension of demyelination from the main lesion in a perivascular sleeve (Dawson's finger) (Fig. 11.29) hints at the role of vascular-mediated inflammation in the pathogenesis. Demyelination is also seen early in the acute plaque together with its disseminated distribution and this usually distinguishes it from acute disseminated encephalomyelitis, in which, as in EAE, demyelination is often less prominent than inflammation and tends to be subpial. Myelin preservation may cause some confusion with remyelination (see below). Immunochemical stains for myelin proteins (MBP, PLP, MOG) often reveal more subtle degrees of myelin loss than classical staining methods.

Demyelination may occur in a variety of different ways. In toxin-induced and antibody-mediated EAE models, demyelination can occur following damage to oligodendrocytes; demyelination may also be caused by a direct attack on the myelin sheath, as in lysolethicin-induced membrane damage and in EAE. MS may show many features of these demyelination models. In acute cases of MS, where there is infiltration by T cells and deposition of Ig, myelin breakdown can occur with a significant degree of preservation of oligodendrocytes, suggesting a direct attack on the myelin sheath (Fig. 11.28). In other plaques, there is significant decrease in the number of oligodendrocytes, especially in the lesion center, indicating direct damage to the oligodendrocyte.[45,74] Oligodendrocytes and their precursors may be killed by necrosis, and a variety of experiments have demonstrated their susceptibility in vitro to numerous toxic inflammatory mediators.[75] Such dying oligodendrocytes have been claimed to be seen in MS lesions. Most authors suggest that oligodendrocytes undergoing apoptosis are present in MS,[48] although the extent varies.[76,77] The so-called dying-back gliopathy demonstrated experimentally in chronic Cuprizone poisoning,[60] where the inner cell tongue of the oligodendrocyte is seen to degenerate before the perikaryon of the oligodendrocyte, may also occur in MS tissue.[36,61] The tempo and pace of demyelination varies according to how myelin is primarily damaged. In early EAE, macrophage stripping of myelin occurs rapidly during the first few days.[27] Traditionally, it has been held that, in models where oligodendrocytes are damaged, demyelination may be much slower, but recent observations in MS[76] have suggested that this may occur much more rapidly.

Inflammation induces individual mediators of tissue injury to damage oligodendrocytes, myelin and axons.[78] These include direct and indirect attack by CD8+ T cells with the discharge of cytotoxic granules and Fas ligation, excitotoxicity through glutamate,[79,80] antibody and terminal complement component attack on the membranes,[81–84] and pro-inflammatory molecules (TNFα,[85] IFNγ, IL-12, lymphotoxin, etc.). Although most authors have considered macrophages to be important mediators of this damage, others have postulated that they act only as scavengers.[86,87] It should be noted that human oligodendrocytes, unlike rodent cells, have a lower level of ionotropic AMPA and kainate receptors[88,89] and may be more resistant to AMPA-mediated excitotoxic damage. The role of heat shock proteins such as αβ crystalline and γδ T cells in causing oligodendrocyte damage has been well described,[41,42,90–93] although recent evidence suggests that αβ crystalline may have protective and therapeutic effects.[94] Oligodendrocytes in MS tissue can also upregulate TRAIL receptors in response to injury, rendering them more vulnerable when a second injury occurs.[95,96] Nitrous oxide and other reactive oxygen species are also important mediators of damage. Finally, the release of components of tissue damage such as the matrix metalloproteinases (MMPs), which facilitate the entry of circulating cells into the CNS, as well as perforin, granzyme, caspases and calpain, have all been implicated in oligodendrocyte and axonal damage.[62] The development of ongoing demyelination in chronic plaques devoid of florid inflammation has been linked to the development of secondary progressive MS.[97]

The distribution of plaques in the brain, optic nerves and spinal cord has always aroused interest and many investigators have sought to understand the etiology of the disease through a differential localization. The periventricular location of many plaques has raised the possibility of circulating CSF agents. Plaques, however, may be found anywhere in the CNS. However, experimental studies have shown that myelin in different parts of the nervous system has differing susceptibilities to damage. In the Cuprizone model, the superior cerebellar peduncle, the corpus callosum and the centrum semiovale are routinely affected whereas optic nerve and spinal cord are unaffected. Interestingly, demyelination and remyelination in a transgenic mouse model[98] in which there is over-expression of DM-20 shows a distribution similar to Cuprizone. Therefore, it is apparent that certain epigenetic modifying factors and perhaps the local anatomical environment may render certain oligodendrocytes more susceptible to damage. This may be operating in MS as well. It is possible that different genetic backgrounds may render certain areas more susceptible, as in NMO (discussed below). In addition, CNS myelin in different areas may vary; different charge isomers of MBP and highly citrullinated forms, generally seen in development, may be found in MS brains, and may be more susceptible to attack.[99]

In a recent series of publications on active MS lesions, Lucchinetti and colleagues described a large, unique collection of cases with acute/active MS, diagnosed mainly on biopsy but also with autopsy material, and suggested new ways of interpreting the pathology and pathogenesis of the demyelination leading to MS lesions.[47,100] Morphologically, they described four lesion patterns. The patterns varied from patient to patient but all the lesions in any one given patient were claimed to be of the same type. Cases in Type 1 (15%) showed inflammatory demyelination marked by T-cell and macrophage infiltration. Type 2, the most common (58%), consisted of lesions with well demarcated zones of demyelination and striking T-cell inflammation. When lesions were studied with antibodies against myelin proteins, all these were lost simultaneously. This pattern was marked by the striking deposition of complement around blood vessels and on the myelin. Oligodendrocytes were relatively well preserved and remyelination was frequently found. In all, the morphological features resembled those seen in T-cell, antibody-mediated, MOG-induced EAE. In Type 3, the next most common type at 26%, the plaque was less sharply delineated but demyelination and inflammation still occurred. The prominent feature in these cases was loss of oligodendrocytes and no remyelination. Another prominent finding was loss of MAG, greater than that of MBP or PLP. This feature suggested pathology in the inner cell tongue of the oligodendrocyte, perhaps suggestive of a dying-back or distal gliopathy of the type seen in Cuprizone demyelination.[60] In these cases, Balo-like rings were often found. Significantly, the changes also resembled damage seen with anoxic and toxic damage to the oligodendrocyte.[101] Type 4, a very rare form (1%), showed oligodendrocyte degeneration in the periplaque white matter. The demographic and clinical features of patients with these four types have been found to be comparable to a cohort of typical MS patients.[102] The authors have now studied a total of 286 acute cases (mostly as biopsies) and in their hands the distinction between patterns remains valid. Chemokine receptor expression differs between types 2 and 3, which could potentially indicate differing inflammatory microenvironments. In addition, patients with type 2 lesions are said to show a greater response to plasmapheresis than those with type 3, supporting the proposed antibody/complement-mediated nature of the former.[103]

These observations suggest an heterogeneous etiopathogenesis in MS patients. If true, this would also suggest different therapies depending on the etiological background. This analy-

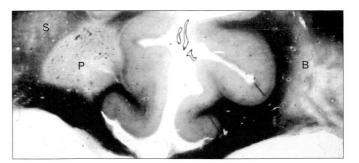

FIG. 11.30 Chronic multiple sclerosis plaques show a variety of features in the same case. At (P) is a classical well demarcated inactive plaque extending to the base of the cingulate gyrus. In addition, there is a plaque with the features of a shadow plaque (S), as well as a plaque on the right with the tigroid alternating bands of myelin and myelin loss typical of Balo's concentric sclerosis (B). With permission from reference 23.

sis, if valid, could represent an opportunity to evaluate clinical outcomes and MRI findings in light of the etiology, as well as the possibility of defining a group of surrogate markers. Unfortunately, few other groups have access to a similar population of acute cases and the findings have been difficult to confirm. It is also possible that the pathological variability represents not differences in etiology but a difference in severity from one case to another. In addition, an overlap of features from one type to another can sometimes be seen (Fig. 11.30). Finally, there has been no convincing segregation of clinical features between different patterns.[1]

Barnett and Prineas[76] described the case of a young girl with known MS who developed acute neurological and respiratory symptoms and died 17 hours later. Besides typical chronic MS plaques, an unusual acute lesion was seen in the brainstem that showed a region of myelin pallor, claimed to contain oligodendrocytes undergoing cell death and some macrophage activity, but in which there was no or sparse inflammatory activity. The authors felt that this represented the very earliest form of the disease and postulated that this was the way all MS lesions started. They called this the early apoptotic lesion, although the usual criteria for apoptosis were not demonstrated. They attributed an anoxic or toxic etiology to this lesion, primarily affecting the oligodendrocyte, with myelin breakdown and secondary macrophage and/or lymphocytic involvement. They argued against heterogeneity of MS types, pointed out some overlap between types and indirectly questioned the primary immunological basis for the development of the disease as well as the role of antibody and complement. They also questioned the extrapolation from EAE. While the findings and the etiological implications closely resemble the etiology and pathology of the type 3 lesion described by Lucchinetti and colleagues, these authors differ in that they believe that this is the way all MS starts and that differences in pathology represent differences in timing rather than etiology.

Whether the lesion represents acute MS, an artifact of autopsy interval or an episode secondary to MS, such as terminal brainstem ischemia, remains a question. In addition, it should be noted that secondary immune phenomena do not usually occur after strokes or other anoxic/toxic episodes in non-MS patients, even though many strokes probably occur in patients with an immunogenetic make-up similar to that of MS patients. Prineas has attempted to reconcile these two views by suggesting that, since complement and IgG may be found in ischemic infarcts, perhaps the type 2 lesions start that way; with time these may evolve into different types.[104] More recently, a study on active

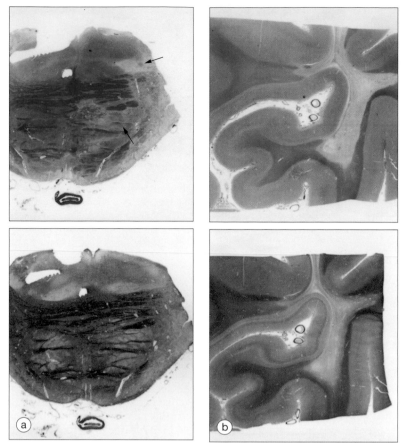

FIG. 11.31 Variable axon loss in chronic plaques in the same case. **A**. The plaque in the pons, the top figure stained for Luxol fast blue, shows areas of myelin loss (arrows), whereas the lower figure stained with Bodian shows almost no corresponding loss of axons. **B**. A hemispheral plaque, the upper figure stained with Luxol-fast blue, shows extensive white matter loss and there is a corresponding severe loss of axons as denoted in the lower figure stained with Bodian.

lesions from cases of established MS, lesions which display many features in common with early active MS, Breij et al,[105] found them to be homogeneous, consistently positive for complement activation and negative for oligodendrocyte apoptosis, questioning the criteria of Lucchinetti et al.[47] Lack of oligodendrocyte apoptosis has also been the conclusion of previous communications[46,49] and indeed protective mechanisms for the cells have been proposed.[93] These controversies need to be resolved, as they may have profound implications for management of patients.[106]

AXONAL DAMAGE IN MULTIPLE SCLEROSIS

In the past, damage to the myelin sheath dominated our thinking about MS; only passing reference was made to loss of axons. However, pathologists need to be reminded that descriptions of axonal damage in MS are almost as old as descriptions of the disease itself.[107]

Trapp and colleagues[51] described axonal loss in very early cases and emphasized the pivotal role of axonal pathology in the progression and refractoriness of the disease. Most investigators now correlate axonal degeneration both with increasing disability and with the transition from relapsing–remitting disease to progressive forms. It is also one of the striking features of primary progressive MS. It is at the basis of brain and especially spinal cord atrophy and is the reason for extensive areas of rarefaction and necrosis.[28] Axonal loss is also one of the substrates for the presence of the 'black holes' seen on MRI[108–109] and the reduction in the neuronal marker N-acetyl

aspartic acid (NAA) found on MR-spectroscopy and the reduced magnetization transfer ratio.

Axonal loss varies from 20–90% as seen with silver stains and antibodies to neurofilaments (Fig. 11.31). Wallerian degeneration emanating from damaged axons within lesions may also lead to axonal degeneration and loss in tracts distal to lesions. Early damage to axons corresponds to an accumulation of β-amyloid precursor protein, nonphosphorylated neurofilament proteins and axonal swellings or spheroids (Fig. 11.25). Peterson and Trapp demonstrated that, while normal white matter contains fewer than 1 transected axon per mm^3, active lesions contained more than 11 000 terminal ovoids and the core of chronic active lesions contained about 10^5; chronic (inactive) lesions show ongoing loss.[110,111]

These observations suggest that there is probably as much need for neuroprotection in MS as in some of the more traditionally denoted axonal conditions,[112] and this requires an understanding of its etiology.[113] It would seem intuitive that inflammatory[114] and immune factors either target axons directly in the first instance or else damage them as a bystander reaction secondary to an attack on myelin. Although antineurofilament antibodies can be demonstrated in MS patients, antimyelin antibodies are far more prevalent, which suggests that the axon may not be a primary immune target. However, others have questioned this.[115,116] Axons can be damaged by agents causing oligodendroglial damage, including cytotoxic T cells, complement, proinflammatory molecules, free-radicals including nitric oxide, cytokines, granzyme, matrix-metalloproteases and glutamate.[117] Voltage-gated calcium channels also accumulate at sites of axonal damage and allow for calcium influx, leading to damage.[112] Observations on sodium channel distribution suggest that different mechanisms underlie axonal damage in acute and chronic lesions.[118]

The cause of ongoing axonal degeneration in chronic progressive cases is not at all certain. It is possible that a slow subclinical inflammatory process continues throughout the disease course that is not manifest through the usual indicators of acute inflammation such as clinical relapses or gadolinium enhancement. In most plaques, even chronic ones, occasional inflammatory cells can be found and, in culture, it has been found that it takes only one cell releasing proteolytic enzymes to destroy an axon. However, the paucity of these cells, the lack of gadolinium enhancement even during clinical progression, and the progression of disease even when anti-inflammatory therapies control the relapse rate, have suggested that other factors are operating in the chronic situation. There is often an associated loss of axons in noninflammatory conditions of primary myelin damage,[119] exemplified in animal models of chronic demyelination such as mice with MAG and PLP mutations. Either loss of trophic factors from oligodendrocytes and myelin[120] or loss of a physical barrier protecting the axon from exposure to destructive factors could be the cause. Remyelination may be the best neuroprotective strategy possible.[121] In addition, the rearrangement of Na and K channels on demyelinated axons may place undue metabolic stress on axons by increasing the need for ATP.[122] There is therefore an opportunity for therapeutic intervention.

PATHOLOGY OF CORTEX AND GRAY MATTER

The exclusive characterization of MS as a disease of white matter ignored the symptoms and signs of cortical disease, despite frequent evidence of plaques and demyelination in gray matter (Fig. 11.17) and descriptions of involvement of the gray matter in MS.[123] The importance of cortical lesions has been stimulated by an increasing recognition of cognitive changes in patients; it may be more frequent in progressive MS.[124] Cortical lesions have been reported frequently,[123] in some series in up to 93% of cases, and probably correlate with atrophy and cognitive changes in patients; they may be more frequent in progressive MS.[124] In the spinal cord, it appears that most of the atrophy is caused by white matter rather than gray matter loss.[125]

Using antibodies to myelin basic protein, a more sensitive indicator than LFB, Bo et al[29] described three different types of cortical lesion in 50 cases (Figs 11.29 and 11.32). Type 1 lesions occurred at the corticomedullary junction, often in continuity with a lesion in the white matter, whereas type 2 lesions were found completely within the cortex. Type 3 lesions abut on the pia, most commonly in the depths of the sulci, and may result directly from oligodendrocytolytic or other demyelinative factors in the CSF. Microscopic changes seen in these areas included demyelination, macrophage activation and axonal and neuritic changes, including transection, spheroids, apoptosis and neuronal drop-out. Significantly in all types, inflammation was much less than than seen in white matter lesions, even when the two were adjacent,[126] perhaps explained by the differences in the expression of cell-adhesion molecules in the cortex and the white matter. This commonly involves the hippocampus[127] and cerebellum.[128] Cortical involvement, together with the paucity of inflammation in chronic MS with axonal disease and with changes in the NAWM, highlights the so-called degenerative stage described above. Recently, Kutzellnig et al have reported[129] that, in contrast to the usual inflammatory demyelinated white matter lesions where cells are clearly derived from the circulation, in the cortex and NAWM, inflammation may derive from

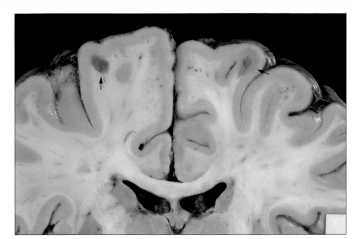

FIG. 11.32 Cortical involvement in multiple sclerosis plaques (see also Fig. 11.29). On the left side (arrow) a white matter plaque extends into the base of the superior frontal gyrus. On the right (arrow), there is a corresponding white matter plaque but it is surrounded by a diffuse area of extension into the cortex extending almost to the surface.

cells that have become sequestered behind the blood–brain barrier. Significantly, MTR imaging studies in primary progressive cases show significant changes in the normal appearing gray matter.[130] Cortical demyelination may not correlate with white matter changes.[131]

PATHOLOGY OF NORMAL APPEARING WHITE MATTER

The long-standing ignorance of changes in the extraplaque white matter continued despite early studies that showed numerous abnormalities, albeit subtle, in this location.[132] These include loss of myelin and axons as well as a variety of biochemical and histological changes indicating active pathology, such as the demonstration of lysosomal enzymes, and changes in myelin proteins.[133] The term 'normal-appearing white matter' is thus a misnomer. Of interest is the suggestion that the myelin in MS patients is inherently abnormal, demonstrated by an immature form of MBP charge isomer.[99] Two factors have highlighted the importance of the NAWM. First, in many patients, the volume and location of plaques is not sufficient to explain the severity or nature of many of the clinical signs and symptoms. Progressive brain atrophy (Fig. 11.8), even in patients with a relatively moderate plaque load, suggests more widespread loss in the NAWM. Secondly, sophisticated forms of MR examination of grossly normal regions of white matter previously ignored by pathologists[134] (Fig. 11.9) have highlighted changes, including reduced magnetization transfer ratios,[135,136] thought to represent a marker of myelin loss, changes in diffusion coefficient and decreases in NAA, a neuronal marker, on MR spectroscopy.[137,138] Examination of these image guided areas has shown active demyelination, with macrophages filled with myelin in varying stages of degradation, scattered inflammatory cells, axonal spheroids and even some remyelination.[109] The finding of reactive astrocytes is always a reasonable indicator of ongoing or recent activity. These changes have been well-summarized by Moore.[139]

Wallerian degeneration of damaged axons in the plaque undoubtedly accounts for some of these changes, demonstrated in studies on the corpus callosum in MS patients[140] that showed

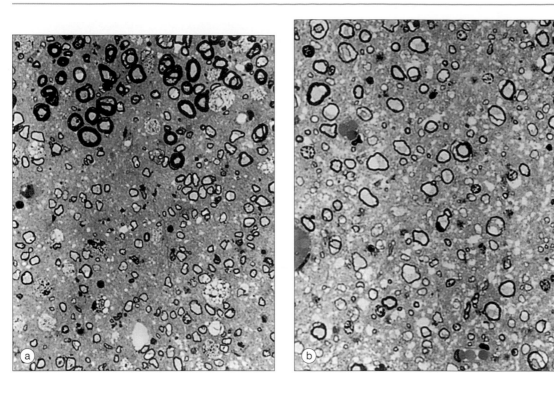

FIG. 11.33 Remyelination in multiple sclerosis plaques. In these toluidine-stained semi-thin sections, the edge of the plaque is seen at the top of **A** and the center of the lesion is seen at higher magnification in **B**. Extensive remyelination recognized by inappropriately thin sheaths is seen both at the edge of the lesion and in the center. In a myelin-stained preparation (LFB), this lesion would give the appearance of a shadow plaque.

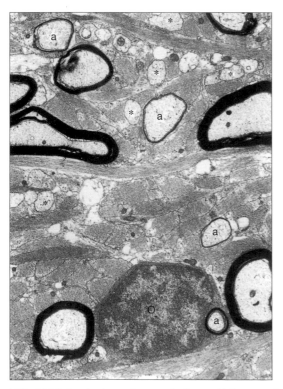

FIG. 11.34 An electron micrograph shows thinly remyelinated nerve fibers (a) intermixed with normally myelinated fibers at the periphery of a chronic silent multiple sclerosis plaque. Densely packed astroglial processes separate the nerve fibers. One remyelinated fiber is intimately associated with an oligodendrocyte (O). Demyelinated axons (*) are numerous. Reproduced with permission from Prineas et al 2002.[26]

that regions containing plaques in the centrum semiovale corresponded anatomically to areas of atrophy in the corpus callosum. Another, perhaps more intriguing suggestion is that they represent the first stages of lesions, or what has been termed 'preactive lesions',[16] or even that the white matter of such patients is inherently more susceptible to disease. Serial imaging has demonstrated subtle changes in the white matter that subsequently develop into typical plaques. These areas have possibly been the site of prior plaque formation, now undergoing further demyelination. As noted earlier, lesion formation is accompanied by vascular changes, seen also in the NAWM, that alter the background vascular architecture, potentially rendering the tissue more susceptible to subsequent attack.[37]

REMYELINATION AND SHADOW PLAQUES

Remyelination by oligodendrocytes occurs with surprising regularity in MS[24–26,50,141–146] (Figs 11.33 and 11.34). The use of animal models, such as EAE and Theiler's virus, have shown specifically how remyelination in MS may be affected by autoimmune disease[27] and have revealed striking similarities. Experimental remyelination, either because of age or species adaptability, is generally more robust and complete than is usually seen in the human. Restitution of the myelin sheath is still probably the best way of protecting the axon from progressive ongoing damage by exogenous factors and loss of trophic substances. Morphologically, remyelination recapitulates the process seen in developmental myelination but the thickness of the myelin sheath (Fig. 11.34) and the length of the internode never achieve the same degree as in the normal; the usual ratio of thickness to the axon diameter appears to be laid down in development and, once destroyed, does not return.

Under unusual chronic situations, aberrant Schwann cells in the CNS have been shown to myelinate CNS axons[147] (Fig. 11.35) but the vast majority of remyelinating cells are oligoden-

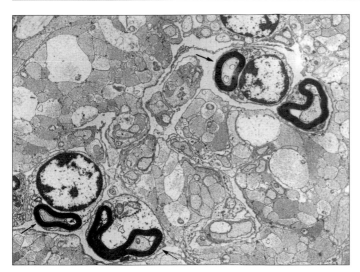

FIG. 11.35 An area of chronically demyelinated plaque in a spinal cord contains Schwann cells, which have elaborated PNS-type myelin around CNS axons (arrows). Elsewhere, gliotic cell processes and demyelinated axons can be seen.

drocyte precursors, which proliferate and mature, displaying the markers of differentiation (Fig. 11.36) (described in detail below). The role of mature surviving oligodendrocytes[38] in helping remyelination is unclear, although experimentally these cells may be capable of cell division.[148]

The extent of remyelination is surprising. Up to 28% of plaques were remyelinated and another 27% were partially remyelinated in one study,[102] whereas in another,[149] up to 47% of the lesion area was remyelinated. Despite such extensive remyelination, it is not known how continuous it is; an axon that is myelinated in one plane may very well be demyelinated at another level, leading to residual disability. This may also involve the cortex.[150]

Efficient remyelination requires undamaged axons and a sufficient number of residual oligodendrocytes.[151] These can be recognized by typical precursor markers such as NG2[152] and, when remyelinating, by differential expression of certain exons of myelination molecules, e.g. of the MBP–Golli complex.[98] These precursors may be susceptible to further damage[75] either by T cells or by antibodies. Progenitors are more common in acute than in chronic lesions.

There are a number of myelination-associated and myelin-inhibitory molecules found in MS lesions, correlating with the occurrence of remyelination or its absence. Olig-1 and -2 are basic helix–loop–helix transcription factors found on oligodendrocytes and are differentially expressed either in repair in MS (olig1)[153] or in normal development (olig2). Other molecular factors present in lesions include the inhibitory Jagged/Notch/Hes5 pathway, the activation of which is believed to lead to the inhibition of oligodendrocyte maturation, recruitment and remyelination,[154] the migration guidance molecule netrin, and NoGoA, a myelin-associated neurite outgrowth inhibitor on oligodendrocytes in MS.[155,156] Neurotrophins, ILGF, BDNF and PDGF[157] and the extracellular matrix[158] may all lead to increased myelin repair through the promotion of proliferation, differentiation, survival and regeneration of oligodendrocytes and their precursors, and chemokines produced by reactive astrocytes may play a role in oligodendrocyte migration and myelin repair.[159]

Finally, it should be pointed out that inflammation, while at the root of tissue damage, may also play a large role in repair. Oligodendrocytes may be damaged by some molecules, such as TNF and NO, as can their precursors[75] but, in addition, under

certain circumstances, B cells, T cells[160] and macrophages and their products may also be required for remyelination.[75] Interestingly, oligodendrocytes in situ have been shown to express a number of cytokine receptors,[161] which may render them capable of interacting with T cells. IgG has been found to promote remyelination in the Theiler's virus demyelination model.[162,163] Transplantation of oligodendrocyte, glial, neural or stem cell precursors, which can migrate and mature, can lead to extensive remyelination.[164–166] Following experimental intraventricular injection, precursors have been shown to be able to migrate throughout the brain. The finding that human precursor cells can have many similar properties leads to exciting prospects for therapy.

Early descriptions of the histological appearance of MS noted plaques and parts of plaques appearing less completely demyelinated than the usual chronic lesion (Fig. 11.37). These *Markschattenherde*, or shadow plaques, can be found with regularity anywhere in the CNS in typical cases of MS. Similar areas of 'shadow' demyelination can be frequently found forming a rim around the periphery of more typical chronic plaques. Long thought to represent zones of incomplete demyelination, in the chronic lesion they consist of sheaths thinner than normal, typical of remyelinated fibres. In addition, in the shadow rims, they are frequently accompanied by an increased density of small cells suggestive of oligodendrocytes, a phenomenon consistent with remyelination. These rims may be the site of new lesions causing recurrent demyelination[167] similar to that seen in recurrent experimental demyelination and remyelination with Cuprizone.[147]

BALO'S CONCENTRIC SCLEROSIS

This is a most striking condition, which has proved to be of major interest in understanding the etiopathogenesis and progression of MS. For a long time considered to be a distinct entity, it presents clinically as an acute condition similar to Marburg's disease.[168] It is more common in Chinese people, suggesting that phenotypic heterogeneity may relate to different immunogenetic backgrounds. It may also present as an acute episode in a known case of more typical MS.

Balo lesions consist of multiple ring-shaped areas (Fig. 11.38) composed of alternating bands of demyelination and normally preserved myelin (Fig. 11.39). In many cases, the pathology of all the lesions may appear uniform. The presence of similar tigroid lesions in typical MS cases associated with classical lesions (Fig. 11.30), and the not infrequent concomitant presence of typical plaques in more typical Balo's cases, suggest that this condition belongs within the spectrum of MS. The demyelinating bands show inflammation, axonal loss and astrocytic hyperplasia. The age of the demyelination bands varies, as judged by the tissue reaction, and the acuity usually increases centrifugally through the lesions.

Despite the clinical acuity of the presentation, the pathology does not always reflect this severe inflammation, and on imaging, the lesions do not always enhance as much as might be expected. Earlier ultrastructural studies[169] reported that the bands represented remyelination, but subsequent studies suggested that these may represent zones of preserved myelin. A recent study of 14 cases[170] has cast light on the pathogenesis of this condition. The demyelinated bands contain high levels of iNOS, a typical mediator of inflammatory damage, whereas the preserved myelin contains high levels of hypoxia inducing factor (HIF) and D-110, an epitope associated with hypoxic stress. These authors hypothesize that the inflammatory process induces a preconditioning hypoxic response in the periphery of the lesion, the preserved band, which renders this area more resistant to subsequent ischemic assaults and is in keeping with

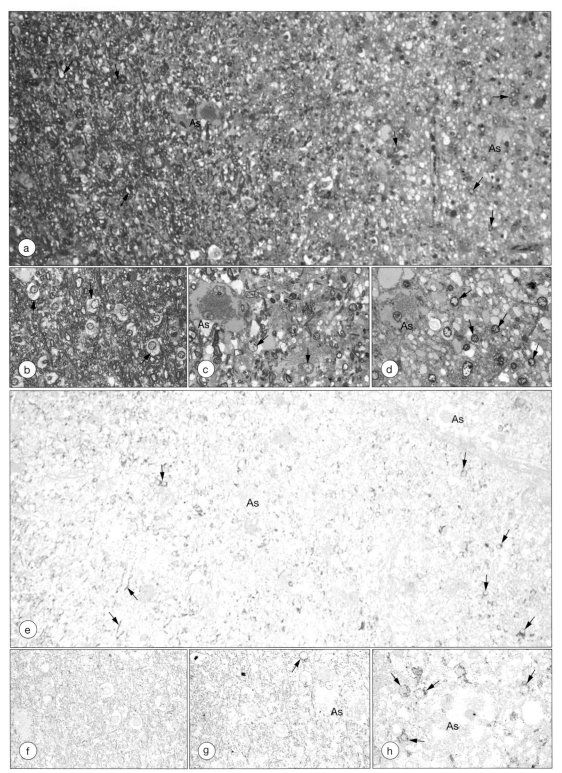

FIG. 11.36 Oligodendrocyte precursors in an active multiple sclerosis plaque. **A**. Taken from a 1 μm epoxy section stained with toluidine blue. Periplaque white matter lies to the left (note myelinated nerve fibers at arrows), plaque edge is in the center (note myelin droplets and hypertrophic astrocyte at As) and the cellular plaque center is to the right (note hypertrophic astrocyte at As and the population of small rounded cells at arrowheads). **B–D**. Higher magnification of the same lesion. **B**. Rounded mature oligodendrocytes (arrows) in the periplaque white matter. **C**. A hypertrophic astrocyte (As), also seen in **A**, oligodendrocytes (arrows) and scattered droplets of myelin debris. **D**. A hypertrophic astrocyte (As) and numerous small, rounded cells (arrows), which represent immature, precursor oligodendrocytes. **E**. The same plaque is shown in an epoxy section immunoreacted for HNK-1, a marker for immature, precursor oligodendrocytes. Note the staining of myelin and myelin droplets in the periplaque area (arrows) and increasing number of small rounded cells towards the center of the plaque (arrowheads) to the right. Hypertrophic astrocytes are seen at As. Details of **E** are seen in **F–H**. **F**. Several HNK-1-negative oligodendrocytes are seen in the periplaque white matter. **G**. HNK-1-negative and one HNK-1-positive (arrow) oligodendrocytes are present at the lesion edge. **H**. Numerous HNK-1 positive immature precursor oligodendrocytes (arrows) are seen in the plaque center. As, hypertrophic astrocytes.

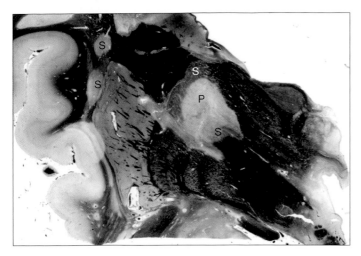

FIG. 11.37 Shadow plaques (S) in the basal ganglia of a chronic MS patient. The central plaque (P) in the internal capsule is surrounded by a rim of poorly staining myelin consistent with a shadow plaque (S). Similarly, other zones of partially stained plaque areas are seen in the area of the external capsule.

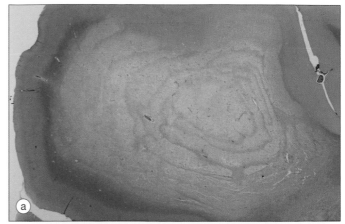

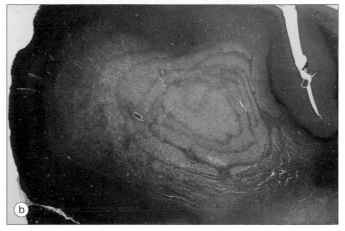

FIG. 11.39 The concentric rings are seen to be made up of alternating bands of demyelination and preserved myelin in **A**, stained with LFB, and in **B** with the Bodian stain. There is also a severe drop-out of axons in the zones of myelin loss.

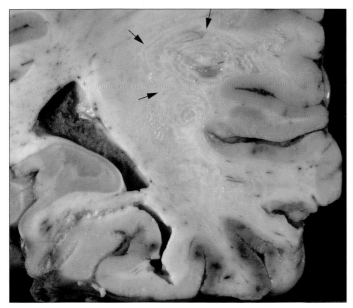

FIG. 11.38 Balo's concentric sclerosis. A tigroid lesion consisting of concentric rings of alternating bands is seen in the inferior parietal and superior temporal lobes (arrows).

the demonstration of Balo-like changes in the type 3 lesions of Lucchinetti and colleagues, in which a possible hypoxic etiology has been postulated.[101]

NEUROMYELITIS OPTICA

Neuromyelitis optica (NMO; Devic's disease) is a very severe form of inflammatory demyelination located in the optic chiasm and nerves, the spinal cord and occasionally, the brain.[171] Epidemiological observation, as well as more recent biological studies, has suggested that it might be a process different from MS. It is particularly common in Japanese patients and is found more frequently in females. Interestingly, Japanese patients with established and typical MS also have a high incidence of

optic nerve and spinal cord involvement; as the genetic background of these patients differs from Western patients, it furthers the theory that this factor may be responsible for phenotypic variability in MS. NMO can be either monophasic or relapsing. Spinal cord lesions are characterized by extensive necrosis, demyelination and axonal damage as well as inflammation and deposition of complement, especially C9neo, mainly around vessels. B cells are prominent and T cells less common. Neutrophils and eosinophils (absent in MS) are common. Remyelination is, however, not a frequent finding. Recent observations have demonstrated that patients with NMO have a high incidence of a specific IgG marker, related to aquaporin-4,[172] which binds to laminin and other elements of the blood–brain barrier.[24,173] To date, this marker distinguishes NMO patients from those with MS, again suggesting that they may be different diseases.[174–176]

DIFFUSE MULTIPLE SCLEROSIS OR SCHILDER'S DISEASE

Schilder's disease occupies a murky position in the pantheon of MS variants. Two of the three cases described originally by Schilder in 1912 have been shown to be different conditions (adrenoleukodystrophy and subacute sclerosing panencephalitis), while the third was probably a case of diffuse MS. However, true diffuse MS is rare (Fig. 11.40). It is sometimes seen in younger patients and sometimes in very acute conditions such

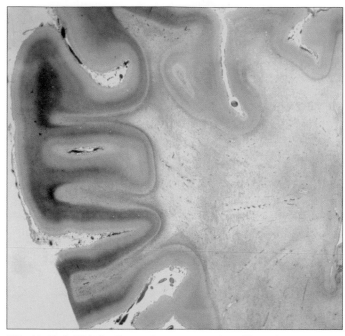

FIG. 11.40 Schilder's disease in a young patient. There is extensive loss of myelin, at times sparing the U fibers but in other places extending all the way to the cortex. Differentiation from other causes of leukodystrophy may be difficult, and such multiple sclerosis cases are probably rare.

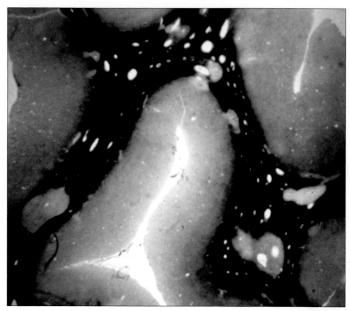

FIG. 11.41 Acute disseminated encephalomyelitis. This Loyez-stained section demonstrates the multiple zones of myelin loss, many of them centered on blood vessels, ranging from tiny foci to larger areas consistent with the appearance of plaques. These latter lesions may be the result of coalescence of such small zones.

as Marburg's disease. Usually, there will be more typical MS plaques but, in their absence, the designation as MS is questionable. Pathologically, there is diffuse loss of myelin throughout the brain, usually more than the spinal cord, with resultant gliosis. There may be also a diffuse loss of axons. It remains a puzzling and controversial entity.

ACUTE DISSEMINATED ENCEPHALOMYELITIS

Acute disseminated encephalomyelitis is the purest form of an immune-mediated inflammatory disease in humans and usually presents following viral infection or vaccination. It is relatively common, especially among children. It typically presents as an encephalopathy and can be distinguished from encephalitis on MRI by its multifocality and its location in white matter. Only rarely is it severe enough to lead to biopsy or death. It is probably the human counterpart of EAE and, in many instances, it resembles the first attack of acute MS. Whether it is not part of the MS spectrum,[177] or whether it leads to MS at a later stage, is still controversial. Some authors have been adamant that differences in the pathology, the lack of oligoclonal banding and the monophasic nature of the disease imply a different condition, whereas others[168] have reported the same findings but have not taken a definitive stand. In ADEM, in contrast to acute MS, the lesions are generally more dispersed (Fig. 11.41) and more inflammatory in a perivenous and subpial distribution than demyelinative, although the latter feature can be prominent (Fig. 11.41). They often lack the sharply delineated demyelinated profile of the MS plaque. There is also a very severe form, acute hemorrhagic leukoencephalopathy (Weston–Hurst disease), which is almost invariably postviral and characterized by fibrinoid necrosis, vasculitis and hemorrhage. It is felt to be the human immune equivalent of hyperacute EAE induced by the administration of pertussis vaccine. To complicate matters, some cases of ADEM may recur (multiphasic or recurrent ADEM) and some go on to develop typical MS. On the other hand, some cases of acute clinically isolated MS may be ADEM.

GLIOSIS

The reaction of astrocytes to injury is one of the most sensitive markers of CNS damage, in MS lesions as well as in NAWM, where it draws attention to subtle myelin and axonal damage. In the cortex of MS cases, reactive astrocytes, although present, are less obvious. Gliosis in MS shows dense scarring of the chronic plaque, with glial processes containing filament bundles lying between demyelinated axons and replacing lost axons (Figs 11.15 and 11.16). GFAP, the astrocytic filament protein, was first isolated from MS plaques. Although the gliotic astrocytic scar has long been thought to be a barrier to successful remyelination and axonal regeneration, gliosis should not be considered to be a unidimensional process. The acute lesion shows a completely different picture. Reactive swollen gemistocytes or hypertrophic astrocytes (Fig. 11.21), often showing a proliferative response with mitoses and the so-called Creutzfeldt cells, characterize the inflammatory lesion. These changes may also be seen in EAE.[178] In contrast to inactive chronic plaques, where astrocytes show diminished mRNA for GFAP, gemistocytes in acute lesions have a major upregulation of this gene and its protein (Fig. 11.26) Astrocytes in acute lesions show a marked production of other trophic factors, including BDNF and TrK receptors,[179,180] as well as VEGF,[37] suggesting a major role in remyelination, neuroregeneration and neuroprotection. Astrocytes have been suggested to play a role in antigen presentation in the immune reaction,[181] although this is far from proven. Gliosis is a complex biphasic reaction,[2] with astrocytes in the acute phase providing both structural and neurotrophic support and demonstrating plasticity. As the lesion advances, gliosis becomes chronic, rigid and non-plastic, inhibiting regeneration.[182] Studies on Wallerian degeneration in the optic nerve show that the scar becomes impervious to axonal ingrowth,[183] confirmed in clinical studies on spinal cord trauma. The course and type of gliosis is therefore determined by the degree and nature of tissue damage and loss. Future therapies will involve maximizing the period of facilitation while minimizing the development of inhibition.

PATHOLOGY–IMAGING CORRELATES

The explosion of information and techniques for imaging the brain and spinal cord has allowed investigators to begin to relate these results to the pathology of MS[184,185] to diagnose, manage and monitor progression or remission. Some findings are quite clear. Gadolinium enhancement is a well-accepted marker of breakdown of the blood–brain barrier and usually denotes an acute lesion with inflammation and edema.. However, lesions with low levels of activity may not enhance, even if they are still active. Experimentally, traffic of cells across blood vessels in demyelination can occur in the absence of blood–brain barrier markers.[186] T2 lesions, commonly accepted as the marker of the presence of established acute or chronic lesion, are not specific pathologically; their cause is heterogeneous and includes inflammation, edema, demyelination, gliosis and axonal loss. The T2 lesion load is a marker of severity of involvement, as is brain volume, which can be a marker for atrophy.[187] Loss of axons can be inferred by MR spectroscopy, which may show a reduction in NAA,[1,188,189] both in early and the late phases, as well as in the development of nonresolving 'black holes'. In addition, changes in choline peaks can also indicate myelin damage. Imaging studies showing significant cord atrophy,[109] often confirmed at later stages on histology, usually indicates a progressive form. Reduction in the MTR and the diffusion coefficient, thought to represent demyelination and tissue loss, may also be the predictor of early white matter changes, preceding plaque development. Similarly, imaging of cortex[190] and spinal cord[191] is improving steadily. Imaging remyelination has proved difficult. Although smaller, more subtle changes in MTR may indicate recovery of myelin,[192] a more promising avenue may turn out to be the development of myelin mapping as a tool to specifically show both loss and recovery of myelin.[193–195]

The evolution of these lesions toward normality often signals reparative processes, including abatement of edema, remyelination[196] or diminution of gliosis, with restoration of normal architecture.

CONCLUSIONS

The study of the pathology of the patterns and the components of MS and its experimental models continues to play a pivotal role in understanding the genesis, evolution, progression and clinical presentation of the MS lesion. However, considerably more studies must be done to achieve this fully. The problem of what constitutes the earliest lesion still needs to be resolved and will necessitate a combination of modalities, with ever-increasingly sophisticated diagnostic techniques correlated in vivo with the pathology. Pathological studies will be crucial in testing the validity of the use of these techniques as surrogate markers for the in vivo diagnosis and management of the disease in vivo. This will apply to imaging as well as biochemical and cellular markers. Similarly, further studies on MS and experimental tissue will be important in solving the problem of what is primary in the disease and what is secondary. The current investigation of the role of axon damage in MS is a good example of this. However, many other pathways still remain to be explored. The role of infectious agents has never been truly proved or disproved, and pathological manifestation of infectious damage or localization in the brain by increasingly sophisticated methodology will continue to be sought. Experimentally, the pathological study of how myelin breaks down in animals with myelin mutations or genetic defects is proving to be valuable and instructive. Will we be able to garner similar clues from the study of MS tissue, which will expand our understanding of how the genetic predisposition affects myelin damage in patients? Finally, insights gained from continued pathological study will prove invaluable in devising appropriate therapies for the disease, whether these involve alterations of cellular trafficking and function, axon and neuron protection or myelin stabilization and remyelination.

ACKNOWLEDGMENTS

We thank Linda Oster and Patricia Cobban-Bond for administrative assistance, Drs Barbara Cannella, Stefanie Gaupp and Kakuri Omari for helpful discussion and photographic help, and Miriam Pakingan and Mirta Chiong for expert technical assistance.

SKL supported in the past by the Canadian Institute for Health Research (MRC) and the Multiple Sclerosis Society of Canada; CSR by USPHS grants NS 08952, NS 11920 and NS 07098, NMSS grant RG-1001-K-11 and the Wollowick Family Foundation for Multiple Sclerosis Research.

REFERENCES

1. Frohman EM, Racke MK, Raine CS. Multiple sclerosis – the plaque and its pathogenesis. N Engl J Med 2006; 354: 942–955.

2. Ludwin SK. The pathogenesis of multiple sclerosis: relating human pathology to experimental studies. J Neuropathol Exp Neurol 2006; 65: 305–318.

3. Charcot JM. Histologie de la sclérose en plaque. Gaz Hop (Paris) 1868; 41: 554–566.

4. Prat A, Antel J. Pathogenesis of multiple sclerosis. Curr Opin Neurol 2005; 18: 225–230.

5. Hafler D, Slavic JM, Anderson DE et al. Multiple sclerosis. Immunol Rev 2005; 204: 208–231.

6. Willer CJ, Dyment DA, Sadovnick AD et al. Twin concordance and sibling recurrence rates in multiple sclerosis. Proc Natl Acad Sci USA 2003; 100: 12877–12882.

7. Ebers GC, Sadovnick AD, Dyment DA et al. A parent of origin effect in multiple sclerosis: observations in half siblings. Lancet 2004; 363: 857–860.

8. Lincoln MB, Montpetit A, Cader MZ et al. A predominant role for the HLA class 11 region in the association of the MHC region with multiple sclerosis. Nat Genet 2005; 37: 1108–1112.

9. Dyment DA, Sadovnick AD, Willer CJ et al. Canadian Collaborative Study Group. An extended genome scan in 442 Canadian multiple sclerosis-affected sibships a report form the Canadian Collaborative Study Group. Hum Mol Genet 2004; 13: 1005–1115.

10. Ponsonby AL, Lucas RM, Van der Mei IA. UVR, vitamin D and three autoimmune diseases – MS, type 1 diabetes, rheumatoid arthritis. Photochem Photobiol 2005; 81: 1267–1275.

11. Murray TJ. Multiple sclerosis: the history of a disease.New York: Demos Medical; 2005.

12. Carswell R. Pathological anatomy: illustrations of the elementary forms of the disease. London: Longman, Orme, Brown, Green and Longman; 1838.

13. Dawson JD. The histology of disseminated sclerosis. Trans R Soc Edin 1916; 50: 517–740.

14. Vos JP, Giudici ML, Vangolde LMG et al. Cultured oligodendrocytes metabolize a fluorescent analogue of sulphatide – inhibition by monensin. Biochim Biophys Acta 1992; 1126: 269–276.

15. Ludwin SK. Pathogenic classification systems in MS: what is their significance? Mult Scler 2005; 11: 106–107.

16. Van der Valk P, De Groot CJ. Staging of multiple sclerosis (MS) lesions: pathology

of the time frame of MS. Neuropathol Appl Neurobiol 2000; 26: 2–10.

17. Lassmann H, Raine CS, Antel J, Prineas JW. Immunopathology of multiple sclerosis: report on an international meeting held at the Institute of Neurology of the University of Vienna. J Neuroimmunol 1998; 86: 213–217.

18. Friede RL, Bruck W. Macrophage functional properties during myelin degradation. In: Seil FJ, ed. Advances in neurology, vol 59. New York: Raven Press; 1993: 327.

19. Bruck W, Sommermeier N, Bergmann M et al. Macrophages in multiple sclerosis. Immunobiology 1996; 195: 588–600.

20. Bruck W, Porada P, Poser S et al. Monocyte/macrophage differentiation in early multiple sclerosis lesions. Ann Neurol 1995; 38: 788–796.

21. Lucchinetti CF, Bruck W, Rodriguez M, Lassmann H. Distinct patterns of multiple sclerosis pathology indicates heterogeneity in pathogenesis. Brain Pathol 1996; 6: 259–274.

22. Prineas JW. The neuropathology of multiple sclerosis. In: Koetsier JC, Vinken PJ, Bruyn GW, Klawans HL, eds. Handbook of clinical neurology, vol 3(47): Demyelinating diseases. Amsterdam: Elsevier; 1985: 213.

23. Ludwin SK. Neuropathology of multiple sclerosis. Neuroimag Clin North Am 2000; 10: 625–648.

24. Lucchinetti CF, Parisi J, Bruck W. The pathology of multiple sclerosis. Neurol Clin 2005; 23: 77–105.

25. Raine CS. The neuropathology of multiple sclerosis. In: Raine CS, McFarland HF, Tourtellotte W W, eds. Multiple sclerosis: clinical and pathogenetic basis. London: Chapman & Hall; 1997: 151.

26. Prineas JW, McDonald WI, Franklin RJM. Demyelinating diseases. In: Graham DI, Lantos P L, eds. Greenfield's neuropathology. London: Arnold; 2002: 471.

27. Raine CS. The lesion in multiple sclerosis and chronic relapsing experimental allergic encephalomyelitis: a structural comparison. In: Raine CS, McFarland H F, Tourtellotte W W, eds. Multiple sclerosis: clinical and pathogenetic basis, London: Chapman & Hall; 1997: 243.

28. Bruck W, Lucchinetti C, Lassmann H. The pathology of primary progressive multiple sclerosis. Mult Scler 2002; 8: 93–97.

29. Bo L, Nyland H, Trapp BD, Mork S. Cortical demyelination in multiple sclerosis. J Neuropathol Exp Neurol 2000; 59: 431.

30. Moriarty DM, Blackshaw AJ, Talbot PR et al. Memory dysfunction in multiple sclerosis corresponds to juxtacortical lesion load on fast fluid-attenuated inversion-recovery MR images. Am J Neuroradiol 1999; 20: 1956–1962.

31. Losseff NA, Webb SL, O'Riordan JI et al. Spinal cord atrophy and disability in multiple sclerosis. A new reproducible and sensitive MRI method with potential to monitor disease progression. Brain 1996; 119: 701–708.

32. Silver NC, Barker GJ, Losseff NA et al. Magnetisation transfer ratio measurement in the cervical spinal cord: a preliminary study in multiple sclerosis. Neuroradiology 1997; 39: 441–445.

33. Fox NC, Jenkins R, Leary SM et al. Progressive cerebral atrophy in MS: a serial study using registered, volumetric MRI. Neurology 2000; 54: 807–812.

34. Raine CS. Membrane specialisations between demyelinated axons and astroglia in chronic EAE lesions and multiple sclerosis plaques. Nature 1978; 275: 326–327.

35. Soffer D, Raine CS. Morphologic analysis of axo-glial membrane specializations in the demyelinated central nervous system. Brain Res 1980; 186: 301–313.

36. Kwon EE, Prineas JW. Blood brain barrier abnormalities in longstanding multiple sclerosis lesions. An immunohistochemical study. J Neuropathol Exp Neurol 1994; 53: 625–636.

37. Ludwin SK, Henry JM, McFarland H. Vascular proliferation and angiogenesis in multiple sclerosis: clinical and pathogenetic implications. J Neuropathol Exp Neurol 2001; 60: 505.

38. Raine CS, Scheinberg L, Waltz JM. Multiple sclerosis. Oligodendrocyte survival and proliferation in an active established lesion. Lab Invest 1981; 45: 534–546.

39. Cannella B, Aquino DA, Raine CS. MHC II expression in the CNS after long-term demyelination. J Neuropathol Exp Neurol 1995; 54: 521–530.

40. Babbe H, Roers A, Waisman A et al. Clonal expansion of CD8+ T cells dominate the T cell infiltrate in multiple sclerosis lesions as shown by micromanipulation and single cell polymerase chain reaction. J Exp Med 2000; 192: 393–404.

41. Selmaj K, Brosnan CF, Raine CS. Colocalization of lymphocytes bearing gamma delta T-cell receptor and heat shock protein hsp65+ oligodendrocytes in multiple sclerosis. Proc Natl Acad Sci USA 1991; 88: 6452–6456.

42. Battistini L, Salvetti M, Ristori G et al. Gamma delta T cell receptor analysis supports a role for HSP 70 selection of lymphocytes in multiple sclerosis lesions. Mol Med 1995; 1: 554–562.

43. Brosnan CF, Battistini L, Gao YL et al. Heat shock proteins and multiple sclerosis: a review. J Neuropathol Exp Neurol 1996; 55: 389–402.

44. Raine CS. The Norton Lecture: a review of the oligodendrocyte in the multiple sclerosis lesion. J Neuroimmunol 1997; 77: 135–152.

45. Lucchinetti C, Bruck W, Parisi J et al. A quantitative analysis of oligodendrocytes in multiple sclerosis lesions. A study of 113 cases. Brain 1999; 122: 2279–2295.

46. Bonetti B, Raine CS. Multiple sclerosis: oligodendrocytes display cell death-related molecules in situ but do not undergo apoptosis. Ann Neurol 1997; 42: 74–84.

47. Lucchinetti C, Bruck W, Parisi J et al. Heterogeneity of multiple sclerosis lesions: implications for the pathogenesis of demyelination. Ann Neurol 2000; 47: 707–717.

48. Kuhlmann T, Lucchinetti C, Zettl UK et al. Bcl-2-expressing oligodendrocytes in multiple sclerosis lesions. Glia 1999; 28: 34–39.

49. Cannella B, Gaupp S, Omari K, Raine CS. Multiple sclerosis: death receptor expression and oligodendrocyte apoptosis in established lesions. J Neurosci 2007; 188: 128–137.

50. Capello E, Voskuhl RR, McFarland HF, Raine CS. Multiple sclerosis: re-expression of a developmental gene in chronic lesions correlates with remyelination. Ann Neurol 1997; 41: 797–805.

51. Trapp BD, Peterson J, Ransohoff RM et al. Axonal transections in the lesions of multiple sclerosis. N Engl J Med 1998; 338: 278–285.

52. Ferguson B, Matyszak MK, Esiri MM, Perry VH. Axonal damage in acute multiple sclerosis lesions. Brain 1997; 120: 393–399.

53. Wu E, Raine CS. Multiple sclerosis. Interactions between oligodendrocytes and hypertrophic astrocytes and their occurrence in other, nondemyelinating conditions. Lab Invest 1992; 67: 88–99.

54. Ghatak NR. Occurrence of oligodendrocytes within astrocytes in demyelinating lesions. J Neuropathol Exp Neurol 1992; 51: 40–46.

55. Mycko MP, Papoian R, Boschert U et al. cDNA microarray analysis in multiple sclerosis lesions: detection of genes associated with disease activity. Brain 2003; 126: 1048–1057.

56. Whitney LW, Ludwin SK, McFarland HF, Biddison WE. Microarray analysis of gene expression in multiple sclerosis and EAE identifies 5-lipoxygenase as a component of inflammatory lesions. J Immunol 2001; 121: 40–48.

57. Mycko MP, Papoian R, Boschert U et al. Microarray gene expression profiling of chronic active and inactive lesions in multiple sclerosis. Clin Neurol Neurosurg 2004; 106: 223–229.

58. Lock C, Hermans G, Pedotti R et al. Gene-microarray analysis of multiple sclerosis lesons yields new targets validated in autoimmune encephalomyelitis. Nat Med 2002; 8: 451–453.

59. Bitsch A, Wegener C, da Costa C et al. Lesion development in Marburg's type of acute multiple sclerosis: from inflammation to demyelination. Mult Scler 1999; 5: 138–146.

60. Ludwin SK, Johnson ES. Evidence for a 'dying-back' gliopathy in demyelinating disease. Ann Neurol 1981; 9: 301–305.

61. Rodriguez M, Scheithauer B. Ultrastructure of multiple sclerosis. Ultrastruct Pathol 1994; 18: 3–13.

62. Bar-Or A. Immunology of multiple sclerosis. Neurol Clin 2005; 23 : 149–175.

63. Wu GF, Laufer TM. The role of dendritic cells in multiple sclerosis. Curr Neurol Neursci Rep 2007; 7: 245–252.

64. Cannella B, Raine CS. The adhesion molecule and cytokine profile of multiple sclerosis lesions. Ann Neurol 1995; 37: 424–435.

65. Kalkers NF, Ameziane N, Bot JCJ et al. Longitudinal brain volume measurement in multiple sclerosis: rate of brain atrophy is independent of the disease subtype. Arch Neurol 2002; 59: 1572–1576.

66. Raine CS, Cannella B, Hauser SL, Genain CP. Demyelination in primate autoimmune encephalomyelitis and acute multiple sclerosis lesions: a case for antigen-specific antibody mediation. Ann Neurol 1999; 46: 144–160.

67. Klawiter EC, Cross AH. B cells: no longer the nondominant arm of multiple sclerosis. Curr Neurol Neurosci Rep 2007; 7: 231–238.

68. Markovic-Plese S, Pinilla C, Martin R. The initiation of the autoimmune response in multiple sclerosis. Clin Neurol Neurosurg 2004; 106: 218–222.

69. Genain CP, Cannella B, Hauser SL, Raine CS. Identification of autoantibodies associated with myelin damage in multiple sclerosis. Nat Med 1999; 5: 170–175.

70. Hemmer B, Archelos JJ, Hartung HP. New concepts in the immunopathogenesis of multiple sclerosis. Nat Rev Neurosci 2002; 3: 291–301.

71. Weiner HL. Multiple sclerosis is an inflammatory T-cell-mediated autoimmune disease. Arch Neurol 2004; 61: 1613–1616.

72. Kleine TO, Zwerenz P, Graser C, Zofel P. Approach to discriminate subgroups in multiple sclerosis with cerebrospinal fluid (CSF) basic inflammation indices and TNF-α, IL-1β, IL-6, IL-8. Brain Res Bull 2003; 61: 327–346.

73. Quandt JA, Baig M, Yao K et al. Unique clinical and pathological findings in HLA-DRB1*0401-restricted MBP 111–129-specific humanized TCR transgenic mice. J Exp Med 2004; 200: 223–234.

74. Bruck W, Stadelmann C. The spectrum of multiple sclerosis: new lessons from pathology. Curr Opin Neurol 2005; 18: 221–224.

75. Ruffini F, Kennedy TE, Antel J. Inflammation and remyelination in the central nervous system: a tale of two systems. Am J Pathol 2004; 164: 1519–1522.

76. Barnett MH, Prineas JW. Relapsing and remitting multiple sclerosis: pathology of the newly forming lesion. Ann Neurol 2004; 55: 458–468.

77. Lucchinetti C, Bruck W, Parisi J et al. A quantitative analysis of oligodendrocytes in multiple sclerosis lesions. A study of 113 cases. Brain 1999; 122: 2279–2295.

78. Wosik K, Antel J, Kuhlmann T et al. Oligodendrocyte injury in multiple sclerosis. J Neurochem 2003; 85: 635–644.

79. Werner P, Pitt D, Raine CS. Multiple sclerosis: altered glutamate homeostasis in lesions correlates with oligodendrocyte and axonal damage. Ann Neurol 2001; 50: 169–180.

80. Werner P, Pitt D, Raine CS. Glutamate excitotoxicity – a mechanism for axonal damage and oligodendrocyte death in multiple sclerosis? J Neural Transm Suppl 2000; 375–385.

81. Compston DAS, Morgan BP, Oleesky D et al. Cerebrospinal fluid C9 in demyelinating disease. Neurology 1986; 36: 1503–1506.

82. Piddlesden SJ, Lassmann H, Zimprich F et al. The demyelinating potential of antibodies to myelin oligodendrocyte glycoprotein is related to their ability to fix complement. Am J Pathol 1993; 143: 555–564.

83. Wood A, Wing MG, Benham CD, Compston DA. Specific induction of intracellular calcium oscillations by complement membrane attack on oligodendroglia. J Neurosci 1993; 13: 3319–3332.

84. Shirazi Y, Rus HG, Macklin WB, Shin ML. Enhanced degradation of messenger RNA encoding myelin proteins by terminal complement complexes in oligodendrocytes. J Immunol 1993; 150: 4581–4590.

85. Selmaj K, Raine CS. Tumor necrosis factor mediates myelin and oligodendrocyte damage in vitro. Ann Neurol 1988; 23: 339–346.

86. Epstein LG, Prineas JW, Raine CS. Attachment of myelin to coated pits on macrophages in experimental allergic encephalomyelitis. J Neurol Sci 1983; 61: 341–348.

87. Barnett MH, Henderson E, Prineas JW. The macrophage in MS: just a scavenger after all? Pathology and pathogenesis of the acute MS lesion. Mult Scler 2006; 12: 121–132.

88. Wosik K, Ruffini F, Almazan G, et al. Resistance of human adult oligodendrocytes to AMPA/kainate receptor-mediated glutamate injury. Brain 2004; 127: 2636–2648.

89. Spassky N, Olivier C, Perez Villegas EM et al. Single or multiple oligodendroglial lineages: a controversy. Glia 2000; 29: 143–148.

90. Selmaj K, Brosnan CF, Raine CS. Expression of heat shock protein-65 by oligodendrocytes in vivo and in vitro: implications for multiple sclerosis. Neurology 1992; 42: 795–800.

91. Van Noort JM, van Sechel AC, Bajramovic JJ et al. The small heat-shock protein alpha B-crystallin as candidate autoantigen in multiple sclerosis. Nature 1995; 375: 798–801.

92. Cwiklinska H, Mycko MP, Luvsannorov O et al. Heat shock protein 70 associations with myelin basic protein and proteolipid protein in multiple sclerosis brains. Int Immunol 2003; 15: 241–249.

93. Raine CS, Wu E, Ivanyi J et al. Multiple sclerosis: a protective or a pathogenic role for heat shock protein 60 in the central nervous system? Lab Invest 1996; 75: 109–123.

94. Ousmann SS, Tomooka BH, van Noort JM et al. Protective and therapeutic role for alphaB-crystallin in autoimmune demyelination. Nature 2007; 448: 474–479.

95. Matysiak M, Jurewicz A, Jaskolski D, Selmaj K. TRAIL induces death of human oligodendrocytes isolated from adult brain. Brain 2002; 125: 2469–2480.

96. Jurewicz A, Matysiak M, Andrzejak S, Selmaj K. TRAIL-induced death of human adult oligodendrocytes is mediated by JNK pathway. Glia 2006; 53: 158–166.

97. Prineas JW, Kwon EE, Cho ES et al. Immunopathology of secondary-progressive multiple sclerosis. Ann Neurol 2001; 5: 646–657.

98. Moscarello MA, Mak B, Nguyen TA et al. Paclitaxel (Taxol) attenuates clinical disease in a spontaneously demyelinating transgenic mouse and induces remyelination. Mult Scler 2002; 8: 130–138.

99. Wood DD, Bilbao JM, O'Connors P, Moscarello MA. Acute multiple sclerosis (Marburg's type) is associated with developmentally immature myelin basic protein. Ann Neurol 1996; 40: 18–24.

100. Kornek B, Lassmann H. Neuropathology of multiple sclerosis-new concepts. Brain Res Bull 2003; 61: 321–326.

101. Aboul-Enein F, Rauschka H, Kornek B et al. Preferential loss of myelin-associated glycoprotein reflects hypoxia-like white matter damage in stroke and inflammatory brain diseases. J Neuropathol Exp Neurol 2003; 62: 25–33.

102. Lucchinetti C. Update on the International Project on Pathological Correlates in MS. Mult Scler 2004; 11: 99–100.

103. Keegan M, Konig F, McClelland R et al. Relation between humoral pathological changes in multiple sclerosis and response to therapeutic plasma exchange. Lancet 2005; 366: 579–582.

104. Barnett MH, Henderson APD, Prineas JW. The macrophage in MS: just a scavenger after all? Pathology and pathogenesis of the acute MS lesion. Mult Scler 2006; 12: 121–132.

105. Breij ECW, Brink BP, Veerhuis R et al. Homogeneity of active demyelinating lesions in established multiple sclerosis. Ann Neurol 2008; 63: 16–25.

106. Lassmann H. Multiple sclerosis pathology: evolution of pathogenetic concepts. Brain Pathol 2005; 15: 217–222.

107. Kornek B, Lassmann H. Axonal pathology in multiple sclerosis. A historical note. Brain Pathol 1999; 9: 651–656.

108. Van Walderveen MA, Kamphorst W, Scheltens P et al. Histopathologic correlate of hypointense lesions on T1-weighted spin-echo MRI in multiple sclerosis. Neurology 1998; 50: 1282–1288.

109. Van Waesberghe JH, Kamphorst W, De Groot CJ et al. Axonal loss in multiple sclerosis lesions: magnetic resonance imaging insights into substrates of disability. Ann Neurol 1999; 46: 747–754.

110. Peterson JW, Trapp BD. Neuropathobiology of multiple sclerosis. Neurol Clin 2005; 23: 107–129.

111. Kuhlmann T, Lingfeld G, Bitsch A et al. Acute axonal damage in multiple sclerosis is most extensive in early disease stages and decreases over time. Brain 2002; 125: 2202–2212.

112. Stys PK. Axonal degeneration in multiple sclerosis: is it time for neuroprotective strategies? Ann Neurol 2004; 55: 601–603.

113. Dutta R, Trapp BD. Pathogenesis of axonal and neuronal damage in multiple sclerosis. Neurol 2007; 68(Suppl 3): S22–31.

114. Bitsch A, Schuchardt J, Bunkowski S et al. Acute axonal injury in multiple sclerosis. Correlatation with demyelination and inflammation. Brain 2000; 123: 1174–1183.

115. DeLuca GC, Williams K, Evangelou N et al. The contribution of demyelination to axonal loss in multiple sclerosis. Brain 2006; 129: 1507–1516.

116. Evangelou N, DeLuca GC, Owens T, Esiri MM. Pathological study of spinal cord atrophy in multiple sclerosis suggests limited role of local lesions. Brain 2005; 128: 29–34.

117. Diaz-Sanchez M, Williams K, DeLuca GC, Esiri MM. Protein co-expression with axonal injury in multiple sclerosis plaques. Acta Neuropathol (Berl) 2006; 111: 289–299.

118. Black JA, Newcombe J, Trapp BD, Waxman SG. Sodium channel expression within chronic multiple sclerosis plaques. J Neuropathol Exp Neurol 2007; 66: 828–837.

119. Raine CS, Cross AH. Axonal dystrophy as a consequence of long-term demyelination. Lab Invest 1989; 60: 714–725.

120. Bjartmar C, Wujek JR, Trapp BD. Axonal loss in the pathology of MS: consequences for understanding the progressive phase of the disease. J Neurol Sci 2003; 206: 165–171.

121. Grigoriadis N, Ben-Hur T, Karussis D, Milonas I. Axonal damage in multiple sclerosis: a complex issue in a complex disease. Clin Neurol Neurosurg 2004; 106: 211–217.

122. Smith KJ, Hall SM. Factors directly affecting impulse transmission in inflammatory demyelinating disease: recent advances in our understanding. Curr Opin Neurol 2001; 14: 289–298.

123. Kidd D, Barkhof F, McConnell R et al. Cortical lesions in multiple sclerosis. Brain 1999; 122: 17–26.

124. Kutzelnigg A, Lassmann H. Cortical demyelination in multiple sclerosis: a substrate for cognitive deficits? J Neurol Sci 2006; 245: 123–126.

125. Gilmore CP, DeLuca GC, Bo L et al. Spinal cord atrophy in multiple sclerosis caused by white matter volume loss. Arch Neurol 2006; 62: 1859–1862.

126. Bo L, Vedeler CA, Nyland H et al. Intracortical multiple sclerosis lesions are not associated with increased lymphocyte infiltration. Mult Scler 2003; 9: 323–331.

127. Geurts JJ, Bö L, Roosendaal SD et al. Extensive hippocampal demyelination in multiple sclerosis. J Neuropathol Exp Neurol 2007; 66: 819–827.

128. Kutzelnigg A, Faber-Rod JC, Bauer J et al. Widespread demyelination in the cerebellar cortex in multiple sclerosis. Brain Pathol 2007; 17: 38–44.

129. Kutzelnigg A, Lucchinetti CF, Stadelmann C et al. Cortical demyelination and diffuse white matter injury in multiple sclerosis. Brain 2005; 128: 2705–2712.

130. Dehmeshki J, Chard DT, Leary SM et al. The normal appearing grey matter in primary progressive multiple sclerosis: a magnetisation transfer imaging study. J Neurol 2003; 250: 67–74.

131. Bö L, Geurts JJ, van der Valk P et al. Lack of correlation between cortical demyelination and white matter pathologic changes in multiple sclerosis. Arch Neurol 2007; 64: 76–80.

132. Allen IV. Pathology of multiple sclerosis. In: Matthews WB, ed. McAlpine's multiple sclerosis. Edinburgh: Churchill Livingstone; 1991: 341.

133. Allen IV, McQuaid S, Mirakhur M, Nevin G. Pathological abnormalities in the normal-apppearing white matter in multiple sclerosis. Neurol Sci 2001; 22: 141–144.

134. De Stefano N, Narayanan S, Francis SJ et al. Diffuse axonal and tissue injury in patients with multiple sclerosis with low cerebral lesion load and no disability. Arch Neurol 2002; 59: 1565–1571.

135. Werring DJ, Clark CA, Barker GJ et al. Diffusion tensor imaging of lesions and normal-appearing white matter in multiple sclerosis. Neurology 1999; 52: 1626–1632.

136. Leary SM, Silver NC, Stevenson VL et al. Magnetisation transfer of normal appearing white matter in primary progressive multiple sclerosis. Mult Scler 1999; 5: 313–316.

137. Leary SM, Davie CA, Parker GJ et al. [1]H magnetic resonance spectroscopy of normal appearing white matter in primary progressive multiple sclerosis. J Neurol 1999; 246: 1023–1026.

138. De Stefano N, Narayanan S, Matthews PM et al. In vivo evidence for axonal dysfunction remote from focal cerebral demyelination of the type seen in multiple sclerosis. Brain 1999; 122: 1933–1939.

139. Moore GRW. Neuropathology and pathophysiology of the multiple sclerosis lesion. In: Paty DW, Ebers G C, eds. Multiple sclerosis. Philadelphia, PA: FA Davis; 2000: 257.

140. Evangelou N, Konz D, Esiri MM et al. Size-selective neuronal changes in the anterior optic pathways suggest a differential susceptibility to injury in multiple sclerosis. Brain 2001; 124: 1813–1820.

141. Suzuki K, Andrews JM, Waltz JM, Terry RD. Ultrastructural studies of multiple sclerosis. Lab Invest 1969; 20: 444–454.

142. Prineas JW, Connell F. Remyelination in multiple sclerosis. Ann Neurol 1979; 5: 22–31.

143. Prineas JW, Barnard RO, Kwon EE et al. Multiple sclerosis – remyelination of nascent lesions. Ann Neurol 1993; 33: 137–151.

144. Raine CS. Multiple sclerosis: prospects for remyelination. Mult Scler 1996; 2: 195–197.

145. Bruck W, Kuhlmann T, Stadelmann C. Remyelination in multiple sclerosis. J Neurol Sci 2003; 206: 181–185.

146. Raine CS, Wu E. Multiple sclerosis: remyelination in acute lesions. J Neuropathol Exp Neurol 1993; 52: 199–204.

147. Johnson ES, Ludwin SK. The demonstration of recurrent demyelination and remyelination of axons in the central nervous system. Acta Neuropathol (Berl) 1981; 53: 93–98.

148. Ludwin SK, Bakker DA. Can oligodendrocytes attached to myelin proliferate? J Neurosci 1988; 8: 1239–1244.

149. Patani R, Balaratnam M, Vora A et al. Remyelination can be extensive in multiple sclerosis despite a long disease course. Neuropathol Appl Neurobiol 2007; 33: 277–287.

150. Albert M, Antel J, Brück W et al. Extensive cortical remyelination in patients with chronic multiple sclerosis. Brain Pathol 2007; 17: 129–138.

151. Wolswijk G. Oligodendrocyte survival, loss and birth in lesions of chronic-stage multiple sclerosis. Brain 2000; 123: 105–115.

152. Chang A, Nishiyama A, Peterson J et al. NG2-positive oligodendrocyte progenitor cells in adult human brain and multiple sclerosis lesions. J Neurosci 2000; 20: 6404–6412.

153. Arnett HA, Fancy SP, Alberta JA et al. bHLH transcripton factor oligo1 is required to repairr demyelinated lesions in the CNS. Science 2004; 306: 2111–2115.

154. John GR, Shankar SL, Shafit-Zagardo B et al. Multiple sclerosis: Re-expression of a developmental pathway that restricts oligodendrocyte maturation. Nat Med 2002; 8: 1115–1121.

155. Satoh J, Onoue H, Arima K, Yamamura T. Nogo-A and nogo receptor expression in demyelinating lesions of multiple sclerosis. J Neuropathol Exp Neurol 2005; 64: 129–138.

156. Kuhlmann T, Remington L, Maruschak B et al. Nogo-A is a reliable oligodendroglial marker in adult human and mouse CNS and in demyelinated lesions. J Neuropathol Exp Neurol 2007; 66: 238–246.

157. Althaus H-H. Remyelination in multiple sclerosis: a new role for neurtrophins? Prog Brain Res 2004; 146: 415–432.

158. van Horssen J, Dijkstra CD, de Vries HE. The extracellular matrix in multiple sclerosis pathology. J Neurochem 2007; 103: 1293–1301.

159. Omari KM, John G, Lango R, Raine CS. Role for CXCR2 and CXCL1 on glia in multiple sclerosis. Glia 2006; 53: 24–31.

160. Bieber AJ, Rodriguez M. Efficient central nervous system remyelination requires T cells. Ann Neurol 2003; 53: 680–684.

161. Cannella B, Raine CS. Multiple sclerosis: cytokine receptors on oligodendrocytes predict innate regulation. Ann Neurol 2004; 55 : 46–57.

162. Das GD. Gliogenesis and ependymogenesis during embryonic development of the rat. J Neurol Sci 1979; 43: 193–204.

163. Asakura K, Miller DJ, Murray K et al. Monoclonal autoantibody SCH94.03, which promotes central nervous system remyelination, recognizes an antigen on the surface of oligodendrocytes. J Neurosci Res 1996; 43: 273–281.

164. Duncan ID. Glial cell transplantation and remyelination of the central nervous system. Neuropathol Appl Neurobiol 1996; 22: 87–100.

165. Vitry S, Avellana-Adalid V, Hardy R et al. Mouse oligospheres: from pre-progenitors to functional oligodendrocytes. J Neurosci Res 2000; 58: 735–751.

166. Dunning MD, Lakatos A, Loizou L et al. Superparamagnetic iron oxide-labeled Schwann cells and olfactory ensheathing cells can be traced in vivo by magnetic resonance imaging and retain functional properties after transplantaion into the CNS. J Neurosci 2004; 24: 9799–9810.

167. Prineas JW, Barnard RO, Revesz T et al. Multiple sclerosis: Pathology of recurrent lesions. Brain 1993; 116: 681–693.

168. Stadelmann C, Bruck W. Lessons from the neuropathology of atypical forms of multiple sclerosis. Neurol Sci 2004; 25: 319–322.

169. Moore GRW, Neumann PE, Suzuki K et al. Balo's concentric sclerosis: new observations on lesion development. Ann Neurol 1985; 17: 604–611.

170. Stadelmann C, Ludwin SK, Tabira T et al. Tissue conditioning may explain concentric lesions in Balo's type of multiple sclerosis. Brain 2005; 128: 979–987.

171. Hengstman GJ, Wesseling P, Frenken CW et al. Neuromyelitis optica with clinical and histopathological involvement of the brain. Mult Scler 2007; 13: 679–682.

172. Lennon VA, Kryzer TJ, Pittock SJ et al. IgG marker of optic-spinal multiple sclerosis binds to the aquaporin-4 water channel. J Exp Med 2005; 202: 473–477.

173. Lennon VA, Wingerchuk DM, Kryzer TJ et al. A serum autoantibody marker of neuromyelitis optica: distinction from multiple sclerosis. Lancet 2006; 364: 2106–2112.

174. Wingerchuk DM, Lennon VA, Pittock SJ et al. Revised diagnostic criteria for neuromyelitis optica. Neurology 2006; 66: 1485–1489.

175. Pittock SJ, Lennon VA, Krecke K et al. Brain abnormalities in neuromyelitis optica. Arch Neurol 2006; 63: 390–396.

176. Weinshenker BG, Wingerchuk DM, Vukovic S et al. Neuromyelitis optica IgG predicts relapse after longitudinally extensive

transverse myelitis. Ann Neurol 2006; 59: 566–569.

177. Poser CM, Brinar VV. The nature of multiple sclerosis. Clin Neurol Neurosurg 2004; 106: 159–171.

178. Bannerman P, Hahn A, Soulika A et al. Astrogliosis in EAE spinal cord: derivation from radial glia and relationships to oligodendroglia. Glia 2007; 55: 57–64.

179. Valdo P, Stegagno C, Mazzucco S et al. Enhanced expression of NGF receptors in multiple sclerosis lesions. J Neuropathol Exp Neurol 2002; 61: 91–98.

180. Stadelmann C, Kerschensteiner M, Misgeld T et al. BDNF and gp145trkB in multiple sclerosis brain lesions: neuroprotective interactions between immune and neuronal cells? Brain 2002; 125: 75–85.

181. De Keyser J, Zeinstra E, Frohman E. Are astrocytes central players in the pathophysiology of multiple sclerosis? Arch Neurol 2003; 60: 132–136.

182. Williams A, Piaton G, Lubetzki C. Astrocytes – friends or foes in multiple sclerosis? Glia 2007; 55: 1300–1312.

183. Ludwin SK. Oligodendrocytes from optic nerves subjected to long term Wallerian degeneration retain the capacity to myelinate. Acta Neuropathol (Berl) 1992; 84: 530–537.

184. Katz D, Taubenberger JK, Cannella B et al. Correlation between magnetic resonance imaging findings and lesion development in chronic, active multiple sclerosis. Ann Neurol 1993; 34: 661–669.

185. Bruck W, Bitsch A, Kolenda H et al. Inflammatory central nervous system demyelination: correlation of magnetic resonance imaging findings with lesion pathology. Ann Neurol 1997; 42: 783–793.

186. Bakker DA, Ludwin SK. Blood- brain barrier permeability during Cuprizone-induced demyelination. Implications for the pathogenesis of immune-mediated demyelinating diseases. J Neurol Sci 1987; 78: 125–137.

187. Lazeron RH, Boringa JB, Schouten M et al. Brain atrophy and lesion load as explaining parameters for cognitive impairment in multiple sclerosis. Mult Scler 2005; 11: 524–531.

188. Bitsch A, Bruhn H, Vougioukas V et al. Inflammatory CNS demyelination: histopathologic correlation with in vivo quantitative proton MR spectroscopy. Am J Neuroradiol 1999; 20: 1619–1627.

189. Lycklama à Nijeholt G, Barkhof F. Differences between subgroups of MS: MRI findings and correlation with histopathology. J Neurol Sci 2003; 206: 173–174.

190. Geurts JJ, Bo L, Pouwels PJ, Castelijns JA et al. Cortical lesions in multiple sclerosis: combined postmortem MR imaging and histopathology. Am J Neuroradiol 2005; 26: 572–577.

191. Barkhof F, McKinstry RC. Quantifying spinal cord demyelination with magnetic transfer imaging. Neurology 2005; 64: 1677–1678.

192. Chen JT, Kuhlmann T, Jansen GH Collins DL et al. Voxel-based analysis of the evolution of magnetization transfer ratio to quantify remyelination and demyelination with histopathological validation in a multiple sclerosis lesion. Neuroimage 2007; 36: 1151–1158.

193. Vavasour IM, Clark CM, Li DK, Mackay AL. Reproducibility and reliability of MR measurements in white matter: clinical implications. NeuroImage 2006; 32: 637–642.

194. Laule C, Vavasour IM, Moore GR et al. Water content and myelin water Fraction in multiple sclerosis. A T2 relaxation study. J Neurol 2004; 251: 284–293.

195. Moore GR, Leung E, Mackay AL et al. A pathology-MRI study of the short-T2 component in formalin-fixed multiple sclerosis brain. Neurology 2000; 55: 1506–1510.

196. Barkhof F, Bruck W, De Groot CJ et al. Remyelinated lesions in multiple sclerosis: magnetic resonance image appearance. Arch Neurol 2003; 60: 1073–1081.

Neurophysiology of demyelination

J. D. Kocsis and S. G. Waxman

INTRODUCTION

Demyelinating diseases, including multiple sclerosis (MS) and Guillain–Barré disease and hereditary neurodegenerative diseases, such as the leukodystrophies, affect millions of people worldwide. Demyelination is also associated with contusive spinal cord injury. A common thread in these disorders is the occurrence of conduction abnormalities such as conduction block and slowing which are associated with loss of or damage to myelin. MS is associated with variable degrees of axonal transection and demyelination,[1] both of which will contribute to conduction abnormalities and functional deficits. The array of neurological symptoms associated with these disorders, including motor abnormalities, visual and somatosensory disturbances, bladder and bowel dysfunction, reflect, at least in part, abnormal impulse conduction associated with axonal demyelination.

This chapter addresses the electrophysiological and molecular substrates for abnormal impulse conduction in demyelinated axons. Abnormal impulse conduction following demyelination is the result of both passive and active electrical changes in the axon. Molecular changes of the axon membrane, including reorganization of ion channels, may account not only for changes in axonal conduction but also for remission of clinical deficits. It is possible that pharmacological and/or cell transplantation strategies may permit development of novel therapeutic interventions that can improve conduction in demyelinated axons.

THE MYELINATED AXON

Vertebrate axons are surrounded by a myelin sheath. In the central nervous system (CNS) of mammals the sheath is formed by oligodendrocytes and in the peripheral nervous system by Schwann cells. The action potential of myelinated axons is generated at the relatively narrow node of Ranvier where the myelin is absent and 'skips' in a saltatory manner from node to node. An internode of a large myelinated axon can be as long as a millimeter but the node of Ranvier is typically only several microns in length. A single teased regenerating peripheral nerve fiber where internode lengths are shorter than in normal fibers is shown in Figure 12.1, and gives a sense of the relative sizes of the node of Ranvier and the internodal axon region. Early experimental evidence for saltatory conduction in nerve by Huxley and Stampfli[2] is illustrated in Figure 12.2. Longitudinal currents were recorded at small increments along the course of a single nerve fiber. The recordings obtained at three points along an internode are very similar. However, as each node is sequentially excited, there is a discontinuity in the current and an incremental jump in latency. This is evident in Figure 12.2b, where the latency of the responses from the shock artifact 'jumps', i.e. increases incrementally, when a node is reached.

Because conduction velocity in myelinated axons is proportional to diameter while conduction velocity in nonmyelinated axons is proportional to the square root of the diameter[3] (Fig. 12.3), saltatory conduction can greatly increase the speed of an action potential and preserve space by allowing for smaller-diameter axons with rapid conduction. For example, the conduction velocity of a 500 μm giant squid axon is about the same as a 10 μm myelinated axon. It has been suggested that oligodendrocytes in the CNS developed from selection pressure to further economize space and maintain conduction velocity. A given oligodendrocyte can form as many as 100 myelinated segments as opposed to only one for a peripheral Schwann cell.[4] Thus, axons myelinated by oligodendrocytes in the brain and spinal cord have the advantage of rapid conduction where space constraints are critical to keep the size of the brain and head manageable. However, disruption of a single oligodendrocyte will have a greater adverse effect on conduction than will disruption of a single Schwann cell because more myelin segments are affected. A number of important anatomical and biophysical specializations occur at and near the node of Ranvier and its myelin-forming partner. In this chapter, key features of these specializations will be discussed, as will experimental strategies to repair myelin and improve conduction following demyelination.

IONIC CHANNEL ORGANIZATION OF NORMAL MYELINATED AXONS: HETEROGENEOUS DISTRIBUTION OF SODIUM AND POTASSIUM CHANNELS

Much work indicates that sodium channels are present at the node in relatively high concentration. Early experiments suggest that nodal sodium channel density is about 1000 sodium channels per μm^2 of nodal membrane while internodal membrane has a density of about 25 sodium channels per μm^2.[5] While the density of sodium channels is very high at the node, the absolute number of channels at the internodal axonal membrane is of the same order of magnitude because of its extensive area. A number of other early studies using immunohistochemical techniques,[6] freeze-fracture[7] and electrophysiological techniques[8] also indicate a high density of nodal sodium current. The very high density of voltage-gated sodium channels at the node is important because synchronous activation of these channels provides substantial current to assure the efficacy of activation of the next set of nodes and high fidelity saltatory conduction.

Of the multiple voltage-gated sodium channel (Na_v) isoforms expressed in nervous tissue,[10] $Na_v 1.6$ is the predominant Na_v

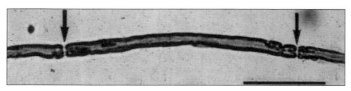

FIG. 12.1 Teased osmium-stained regenerating myelinated peripheral nerve fiber showing relative lengths of internodal (under the myelin) and nodal regions.

channel at mature nodes of Ranvier in both the peripheral nervous system (PNS) and CNS.[11,12] $Na_v 1.6$ is a kinetically fast channel and is sensitive to tetrodotoxin (TTX). It has been reported that a transition from $Na_v 1.2$ to $Na_v 1.6$ occurs during development of myelinated axons.[12–15] The clustering of Na_v channels[16,17] and the transition from $Na_v 1.2$ to $Na_v 1.6$[12,15] at nodes have been reported to be critically dependent upon interaction of the axon with ensheathing or myelinating glial cells.[18–20] Immunostaining for $Na_v 1.6$ at a peripheral node of Ranvier flanked by paranodal Caspr staining is shown in Figure 12.4.

Myelinated axons also express multiple potassium channels. Intra-axonal recording and pharmacological studies indicated that three pharmacologically distinct types of potassium channels could be identified on mammalian axons: 'fast' K^+ channels, 'slow' K^+ channels and an inward rectifier current that was permeable to both Na^+ and K^+. The fast and slow K^+ channels probably reflect transient and sustained currents that are sensitive to 4-aminopyridine (4-AP) and tetraethylammonium (TEA) respectively.[21] The axonal K^+ currents are expressed in relatively low density at the node but are present in higher density under the myelin.[8,9,22–25] It has been suggested that the density of fast (4-AP-sensitive) K current is highest in the paranodal region and falls to about one-sixth at the node.[26] Molecular studies indicate that Kv 1.1 and Kv1.2 are present in the juxtaparanodal region.[27–29] While the functional reasons for this segregation on Na and K channels on the myelinated axon are not fully understood, it has been suggested that the juxtaparanodal K channels may prevent hyperexcitability or reentry phenomena.[30]

The clustering at high density of sodium channels at the node and the paucity of these channels at the internodal axon membrane under the myelin, together with the expression of K channels under the myelin, has important pathophysiological consequences. Upon demyelination, loss of the myelin capacitative shield together with the low density of sodium channels at

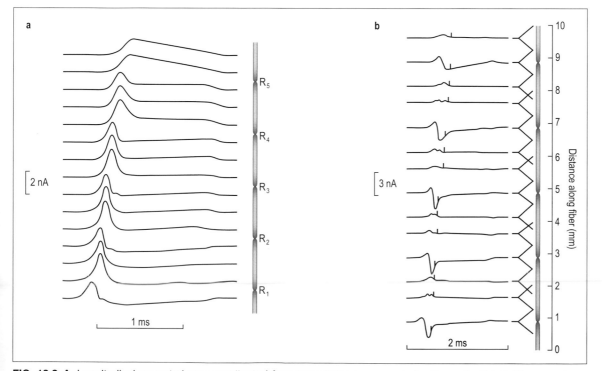

FIG. 12.2 A. Longitudinal current along a myelinated frog axon during a propagated action potential. **B.** Transmembrane current at different points along a single myelinated fiber (inward current is downward). Note the high inward current at nodes of Ranvier, indicating saltatory conduction. A schematic of a myelinated axon is shown between **A** and **B**. Nodes are labeled R1–R5. Modified from Huxley and Stampfli 1949.[2]

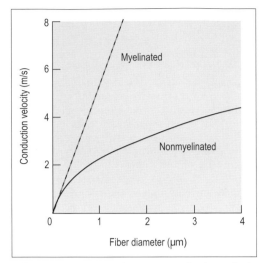

FIG. 12.3 Relationship between conduction velocity and diameter for myelinated and nonmyelinated axons. Modified from Waxman and Bennett 1972.[3]

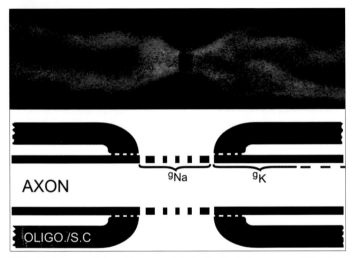

FIG. 12.4 A. Na channel immunostaining (red) at the node of Ranvier flanked by paranodal Caspr staining (blue). Green is GFP in the cytoplasm of the myelin forming cell. **B**. Schematic showing nodal and paranodal distribution of Na$^+$ and K$^+$ channels.

the axon membrane under the myelin places a capacitive load on the axon region that is nonelectrogenic. Thus, current density is reduced at the next node of Ranvier and the probability of conduction block or slowing is increased. Moreover, the exposure of K channels at the demyelinated region will tend to 'clamp' the axon near the equilibrium potential for K and thus impede action potential conduction.[9]

ELECTRICAL BASIS FOR CONDUCTION SLOWING AND BLOCK IN DEMYELINATED AXONS

Acute demyelination is associated with conduction block and conduction slowing.

In healthy myelinated axons, the inward current generated at a given node can depolarize the axon membrane at the next node without wasting charge or time by depolarizing the internodal membrane that is covered by myelin (Fig. 12.5A). The majority of the current generated by a node passes across the

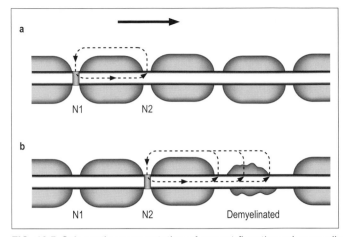

FIG. 12.5 Schematic representation of current flow through normally myelinated (**A**) and demyelinated regions of axons. Action potential conduction is from left to right. Dashed arrows indicate direction of current flow. Notice that current generated from a node is targeted toward the next node with little current loss across the myelin (**A**). At a focal site of demyelination (**B**), current is longitudinally distributed across the demyelinated segment, leading to capacitive and resistive shunting.

axon membrane at the next node by local current flow, thereby allowing for a high current density to be generated at a site distal to the previous node. Activation of sodium channels at this previously quiescent node will now generate an action potential. However, if the myelin is disrupted, as illustrated in Figure 12.5B, current generated by a given node will now be distributed longitudinally and 'leak' across the former internodal membrane, which has a low sodium channel density. The current density at the next node will be reduced and the time to charge the membrane capacitance will be increased. The consequence of this longitudinal redistribution of current subsequent to myelin disruption will be either impulse failure, because insufficient potential develops across the node to activation sodium channels, or a delay in action potential activation from the increased membrane charging time.[31] These two changes, impulse failure and conduction slowing, are hallmark signs of conduction impairment in demyelinating disorders.

Impedance mismatch reflects the passive properties of the nerve fiber and is due largely to electrical loading (capacitive) that occurs at sites of axon inhomogeneity, such as transition sites between myelinated and demyelinated regions. Impedance mismatch can prevent or delay action potential invasion into a demyelinated axon region. Figure 12.6 shows computer-simulated action potentials[32] in an axon with one segment in which the myelin has been lost (between nodes D1 and D4). Conduction failure occurs at the junction between the normal and demyelinated axon regions (D1), despite a high density of sodium channels built into the demyelinated segment, because impedance mismatch prevents threshold from being reached. Mechanisms for overcoming impedance mismatch include development of relatively short myelinated segments proximal to the demyelination site,[32] decrease in axon diameter of the demyelinated site[33] and development of an increased sodium channel density at the node upstream to the demyelinated segment.[34] An example of overcoming impedance mismatch by inserting short myelin segments proximal to the demyelination site is shown in Figure 12.6B. Thus, both passive and active electrical properties are responsible for conduction slowing and block in demyelinated axons.

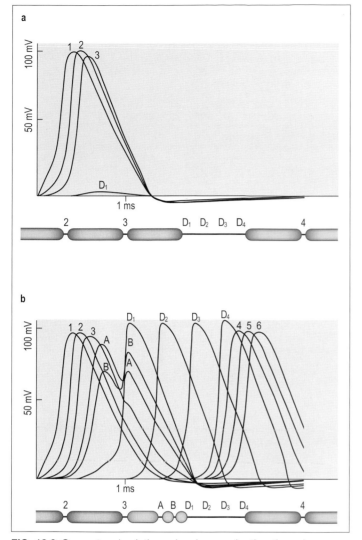

FIG. 12.6 Computer simulations showing conduction through a focally demyelinated axon. Action potentials are numbered and correspond to numbered nodes. Demyelinated regions are labeled D_1–D_4. **A.** Action potential failure occurs following removal of one myelin internode. **B.** Insertion of two short internodes in the proximal demyelinated segment restores conduction through the lesion. Modified from Waxman and Brill 1978.[32]

In some chronically demyelinated axons, demyelinated regions display a slow but continuous mode of conduction.[35] This suggests that sodium channels can increase in density with time in the internodal region after demyelination. In most experimental models of chronic demyelination, conduction can occur, but is slowed. For example, conduction is slowed but secure in the myelin-deficient rat[36] and following chemically induced demyelination.[37] The conduction velocity of a demyelinated axon can be reduced from tens of m/s to less than 1 m/s, much slower than would be predicted for a normally myelinated axon with the same diameter.[36,37] While such radical reductions in conduction velocity could lead to functional impairments by altering temporal coding of information, it is notable that some information can be extracted from the delayed impulses so that, for instance, clinical recovery from optic neuritis can occur even though visual evoked responses are delayed for tens of milliseconds.[38] However, non-uniformity of slow conduction of demyelinated axons with different diameters and functional properties

would reduce the fidelity and integrative properties of the information conveyed by these fibers.

CONDUCTION ABNORMALITIES IN DEMYELINATED AXONS

Conduction abnormalities in demyelinated axons include decreased conduction velocity, reduced ability to transmit high-frequency trains of action potentials and conduction block.[39,40] Internodal conduction time can increase to nearly half a second in demyelinated ventral root fibers as compared to 20 µs in a normal fiber.[41] If several regions of an axon are demyelinated, this could result in considerable conduction slowing even if the demyelination is focal. Moreover, if a number of axons are demyelinated within a given tract, loss of synchrony occurs with temporal dispersion of the impulses (Fig. 12.7C). This can be functionally significant within neural circuits where timing of impulse activity is important. For example, temporally dispersed and slowed afferent inputs in demyelinating polyneuropathies can result in loss of deep tendon reflexes.

Demyelinated axons can display various forms of conduction block. Conduction block can be frequency-dependent, a form of conduction block in which high-frequency impulse trains fail to conduct but low-frequency trains can conduct, albeit with a time delay (Fig. 12.6D). Conduction block can be complete for even single impulses (Fig 12.7E). High-frequency conduction block may result from hyperpolarization due to electrogenic pump (Na^+,K^+ ATPase) activity.[42] It has also been suggested that increased intracellular Na^+ concentration at the ' driving node'[41] and accumulation of extracellular K^+ in the demyelinated areas could lead to Na^+ channel inactivation and conduction block.[43]

Positive (hyperexcitable) events also occur in demyelinated axons. Ectopic action potential generation was reported for demyelinated cat dorsal column axons.[44] There are differences in the accommodative properties of demyelinated sensory vs motor fibers; this is consistent with the more frequent appearance of paresthesia than increased motor activity in MS patients. Demyelinated fibers also display increased mechanosensitivity (Fig. 12.7G), which probably accounts for clinical phenomena such as Lhermitte's sign.[44] Abnormal electrical interactions between fibers (electrical cross-talk; Fig. 12.6H), may occur between demyelinated axons and contribute to hyperexcitability.[45,46] Impulse reflection (Fig. 12.7I) may occur in some demyelinated axons[47] and may result in paresthesia, pain or tonic spasms. These reflected ectopic (antidromic) impulses could collide with normal orthodromic impulse flow and further reduce the fidelity of impulse signaling.

As outlined above, the macrostructural organization of demyelinated axons, which dictates its passive membrane properties, and the organization of ion channels on the demyelinated axons both contribute to the pathophysiology of conduction in demyelinated axons; both are potential therapeutic targets.

EXPERIMENTAL STRATEGIES TO IMPROVE CONDUCTION IN DEMYELINATED AXONS

PHARMACOLOGICAL STRATEGIES TO IMPROVE CONDUCTION IN DEMYELINATED AXONS

Pharmacological strategies designed to improve safety factor have been studied in an effort to overcome conduction block in demyelinated axons. Knowledge of the spatially heterogeneous distribution of fast K^+ channels and of their location under the

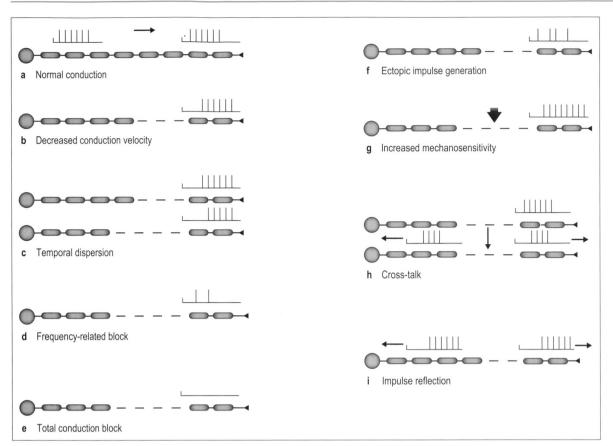

FIG. 12.7 Classes of conduction abnormality in demyelinated axons. Demyelinated regions are schematically shown as dashed lines. Cell bodies are represented as circles on the left and axon terminals are on the right. Arrows indicate the direction of conduction.

myelin led to studies using the fast K+ channel blocking agent 4-AP in an attempt to overcome conduction block. The rationale is that blockade of these channels should prolong the action potential duration by slowing repolarization and thus provide greater depolarizing current density at sites of demyelination and increase the probability of reaching threshold. 4-AP has in fact been shown to overcome conduction block in demyelinated spinal roots,[48] sciatic nerve[49] and dorsal column axons of the spinal cord.[50] Focal application of 4-AP to overcome conduction block in experimentally demyelinated axons is shown in Figure 12.8. Single axon recordings were obtained from one site of a focal demyelinating lesion and the nerve was stimulated on both sites to permit conduction through a normal region and through the zone of demyelination to be assessed (Fig. 12.8A). Stimulation on the side proximal to the lesion (S₁) resulted in an action potential that propagated through the normally myelinated part of the fiber, but stimulation on the side opposite of the demyelinating lesion (S₂) resulted in conduction block at the site of demyelination (Fig. 12.8B). After focal administration of 4-AP, which blocks fast K+ currents, the action potential was widened and impulse conduction occurred through the demyelinated lesion, albeit with an increased latency (Fig. 12.8C).

Transient improvement in motor function, reduction in scotoma and improved flicker fusion in MS patients following treatment with 4-AP and a related drug, 3,4 diaminopyridine, were reported in early studies.[51,52] Since then, a number of larger studies[53–56] have been carried out. However, more work is needed to fully assess the efficacy of this approach in the clinical domain.

Pharmacological inhibition of Na+, K+ ATPase has also been demonstrated to improve conduction in rats with demyelinated spinal cord lesions.[57] The rationale is that partial blockade of the electrogenic pump will depolarize axons and bring them closer to threshold. While depolarization will bring the membrane potential closer to threshold, it may increase resting inactivation of sodium channels, an action that would counteract any beneficial effect on threshold.

While additional clinical studies are necessary to more fully determine the therapeutic potential of these agents, the results demonstrate at a minimum the rationale for use of pharmacological approaches to improve conduction in demyelinating disorders.

REMYELINATION AS A CELL THERAPY APPROACH TO IMPROVE CONDUCTION IN MULTIPLE SCLEROSIS

Cellular transplantation approaches are being considered in an attempt to remyelinate demyelinated axons in MS and to improve impulse conduction and functional outcome. One concern surrounding such an approach is that MS is an immunological disease with central myelin presenting antigens that elicit white matter inflammation, so that introduction of exogenous oligodendrocytes or their precursors could exacerbate the disease. However, with recent advances in immunological therapies for MS, it is conceivable that, in the future, the basic immune process in MS could be controlled. Many patients would have residual demyelinated plaques that could be associated with neurological symptoms. Under these conditions, an

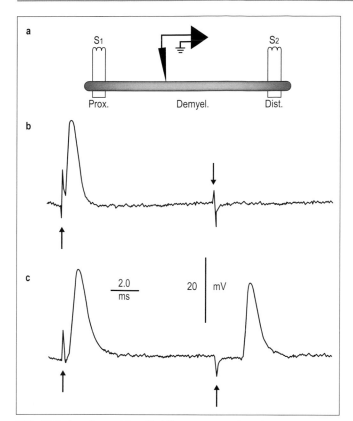

FIG. 12.8 4-aminopyridine (4-AP) can restore impulse conduction in demyelinated axons. **A**. Stimulation (S₁ and S₂) at both ends of a peripheral nerve and single axon recordings obtained on one site of a focal demyelination site. **B**. S₁ stimulation results in an action potential but S₂ stimulation, where conduction must travel through the demyelination site, does not. **C**. After focal application of 4-AP, the action potential widens and impulses can now propagate through the demyelination site. Modified from Targ and Kocsis 1985.[49]

effective cell therapy that targets sites of demyelination could produce remyelination, thereby improving axonal function and reducing neurological symptoms.

There are several experimental questions that must be resolved in the consideration of such an approach. These include determination of an appropriate and safe donor cell type, demonstration of whether there is stable anatomical myelination by the transplants and appropriate functional reorganization of Na⁺ and K⁺ channels on the myelinated axons, and finally whether there is improvement in axonal conduction properties. As discussed above, Na⁺ and K⁺ channels are heterogeneously distributed on myelinated axons and specific channel isoforms are expressed. If there is failure to achieve this organization in remyelinated axons, this could result in abnormal impulse conduction or even in the generation of ectopic or spontaneous action potential generation, which could lead to pain or paresthesia. These events would severely limit the use of transplantation of myelin-forming cells as a therapeutic approach. However, much experimental work, as reviewed below, indicates that axons remyelinated by transplanted cells generally show improvement in impulse conduction without these adverse effects.

Remyelination by endogenous cells and conduction improvement

While some endogenous remyelination can occur in MS patients it is rare.[58,59] However, a recent study indicates extensive remyelination in a subset of MS patients[60] following experimental chemically induced demyelination in spinal cord of rodents,

robust remyelination is observed, even after a few weeks.[61–63] After remyelination in the CNS, the new internodes are both thinner and shorter, implying that new nodes of Ranvier have regenerated on these axons.[61,64] Smith et al[62] demonstrated that endogenous remyelination in rat spinal cord is accompanied by restoration of rapid and secure conduction. The remyelinated axons, while structurally different from normal axons (thinner myelin and shorter internodal lengths), were able to follow high-frequency stimuli. Moreover, functional improvement occurs after endogenous remyelination of dorsal column axons.[65] Recent work indicates that nodal sodium channels (Nav1.6) and paranodal potassium channels (Kv1.2) are restored on the remyelinated axons.[66] The short length of the internode along the remyelinated axons indicates that new nodes of Ranvier are formed and that these nodes incorporate appropriate sodium channels compatible with stable and secure impulse conduction. Unfortunately, demyelinated primate CNS does not demonstrate robust endogenous myelin repair as does the CNS of rodents.[67] Thus, strategies such as stimulating endogenous precursors or introducing myelin-forming cells need to be developed.

Remyelination of axons by cellular transplants

Remyelination has been demonstrated by transplantation of oligodendrocyte lineage cells,[36,68–70] Schwann cells,[71] olfactory ensheathing cells[72,73] and a number of stem cell types.[74–77] The first demonstration of improved conduction in axons remyelinated by cell transplantation was carried out using neonatal optic-nerve-derived glial cells transplanted into the spinal cord of the myelin-deficient (md) rat.[36] The md rat has a point mutation in proteolipid protein and does not form central myelin. Conduction velocity of all axons in the amyelinated md rat is about 1 m/s or less compared to conduction velocities of over 10 m/s in normal controls.

At about 3 weeks post-transplantation into the dorsal funiculus of the md rat spinal cord, extensive remyelination is observed. Conduction velocity and the ability to follow high-frequency stimulation are significantly improved in the remyelinated axons. Figure 12.9C is a plot of conduction velocity through the dorsal columns versus conduction velocity in normal dorsal root from single fibers recorded from intracellular recordings in dorsal root ganglion neurons. The amyelinated dorsal column axons have conduction velocities of 1 m/s or less, regardless of the conduction velocity of their corresponding normal dorsal root trajectory. This implies that, as fiber diameter increases in the amyelinated axons, conduction velocity remains relatively fixed at about 1 m/s. Thus, information conveyed by different sensory modalities with different conduction velocities is compromised. In contrast, in axons that have been remyelinated after transplantation, the linear relation with conduction velocity in central and peripheral trajectories of primary afferent axons are restored (Fig. 12.9C). Thus, remyelination by transplanted glial cells restores conduction velocity and possibly the integrative properties of axons. As encouraging as these results are, the md rat is not a true demyelinating disorder but is an amyelinated developmental disorder. Therefore, it was important to determine whether demyelinated adult CNS axons could be remyelinated by cell transplantation and whether adult axons could reconstruct appropriate myelin and nodal organization to support normal impulse conduction.

Transplantation of peripheral myelin-forming cells for remyelination of central nervous system axons

Indeed, transplantation of Schwann cells into the demyelinated adult rodent spinal cord results in remyelination with a characteristic peripheral pattern.[37,78,79] Moreover, when anatomical

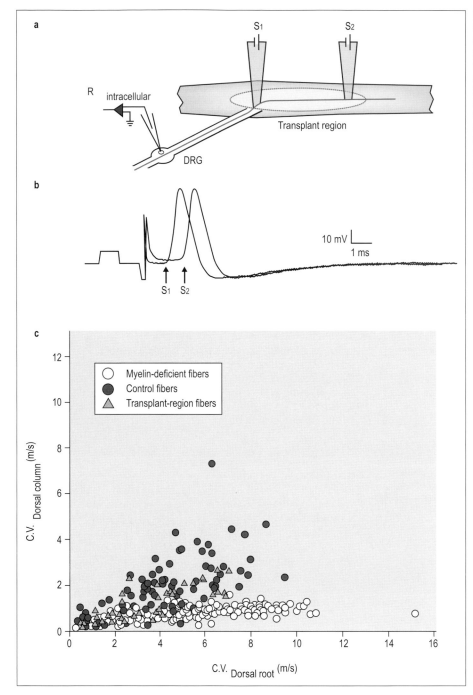

FIG. 12.9 Conduction velocities in dorsal columns for myelin-deficient, normal and remyelinated dorsal columns after optic nerve glial transplantation. **A**. Schematic of stimulating and recording arrangement. Two points were stimulated that straddled the lesion zone and intracellular recordings were obtained in the dorsal root ganglia. **B**. Intracellular recordings after S_1 and S_2 stimulation. Calculated conduction velocities for trajectory within lesion and transplant zone as a function of conduction velocity of the corresponding dorsal root trajectory. Note that conduction velocities in the transplant region approach normal conduction values. Modified from Utzschneider et al 1994.[36]

repair is achieved subsequent to Schwann cell transplantation, near-normal conduction velocity of the remyelinated axons is achieved.[37] Transplantation of human Schwann cells derived from human sural nerve can remyelinate spinal cord axons in the immunosuppressed rat.[71] In these experiments, a focal demyelinated lesion was created in the dorsal column of the spinal cord of 12-week-old rats by X-irradiation and ethidium bromide injection (X-EB) (see Kohama et al[71] for technical details). This lesion presents as a persistent area of demyelination that lacks astrocytes. An example of a remyelinated region of the spinal cord 3 weeks after focal injection of reconstituted cryopreserved human Schwann cells is shown in Figure 12.10. Note the relatively large number of myelinated axons and typical Schwann cell morphology, i.e. large cytoplasmic and nuclear regions. Electron micrographs (not shown) reveal the presence of a basement membrane and extracellular collagen deposition. The conduction velocity of axons remyelinated by the human Schwann cells was improved (Fig. 12.11), indicating that electrophysiological function of the remyelinated axons was enhanced.

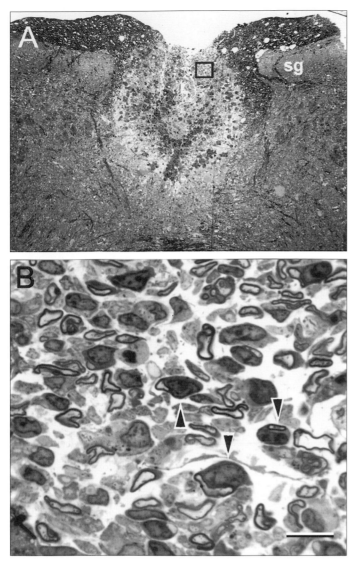

FIG. 12.10 Remyelination of rat dorsal columns by transplantation of human Schwann cells. **A.** Low-power micrograph showing area of cell transplantation into the demyelinated dorsal columns. **B.** Higher-power micrograph showing remyelinated axons from the boxed area in **A.** Scale bar in **B**=5 μm. Modified from Kohama et al. 2001.[71]

Autologous tissue represents one possible source of Schwann cells for transplantation into patients with demyelinating disease. Presumably, Schwann cells are not antigenically predisposed to the immunological attack seen in MS as are oligodendrocytes. The demonstration of anatomical and electrophysiological repair of demyelinated axons by adult human Schwann cells is an important prerequisite for future consideration of these cells as candidates for autologous transplantation studies in humans. One potential problem with the use of Schwann cells to remyelinate lesions in MS patients is the presence of a glial scar in MS lesion sites, which could limit cell migration and remyelination potential. In the X-EB lesion in the rat where relatively extensive remyelination is observed, it is important to note that the lesion is agliotic and thus the potential impediment of gliosis is not an issue. But, Schwann cells transplanted into a contusion injury model in the spinal cord, where gliosis does occur, produce increased myelination, axon sparing/regeneration and improved functional outcome in rodents.[80]

Another cell type that has attracted much attention over the past decade as a cell candidate to both encourage axonal remyelination and regeneration is the olfactory ensheathing cell (OEC). OECs are located in olfactory nerves and the outer nerve layer of the olfactory bulb. Adult olfactory receptor neurons continually undergo turnover from an endogenous progenitor pool and their nascent axons, which are ensheathed by OECs, grow through the olfactory nerves and cross the PNS–CNS interface, where they form new synaptic connections in the olfactory bulb.[81] This apparent support role of OECs in axonal growth in the adult CNS has spawned extensive research aimed at studying the potential of OEC transplants to encourage axonal regeneration and to potentially remyelinate axons in the CNS.[82–86] OECs normally do not form myelin but can do so when transplanted into the CNS.[72,73] OECs are an unusual population of glial cells in that they share characteristics with both astrocytes in the CNS and Schwann cells in the PNS[87] and are the only glial cells known to cross the PNS–CNS transitional zone, accompanying the axons that they ensheath.[88] An interesting observation with both Schwann cells and OECs is that, in addition to remyelinating CNS axons, they can enhance axonal regeneration in the spinal cord when transplanted into axonal transection lesion sites.[66,82,83–85,89]

A large body of work supports the proposal that transplantation of OECs into various spinal cord injury and demyelination models can promote axonal regeneration, remyelination and functional recovery.[72,82,83–86,90–92] Yet there is an important controversy as to whether the transplanted OECs associate with axons and form peripheral myelin, as opposed to recruiting endogenous Schwann cells that form myelin.[80,93] OECs can express a number of trophic factors, transcription factors and extracellular matrix molecules,[83,94–96] which could facilitate endogenous Schwann cell invasion, angiogenesis and activation of progenitor cells to facilitate repair.

A recent study failed to observe myelination in vitro in a coculture experiment with dorsal root ganglion neurons and immunoselected (p75) OECs under culture conditions permissive for myelination by Schwann cells.[97] This study raises the important question as to whether transplanted OECs might induce or enhance the migration of endogenous Schwann cells into the transplantation site.[98] Moreover, while numerous reports suggest that OECs can form myelin when transplanted into the demyelinated[63,67,72,73,99,100] or injured spinal cord,[82,84,85] a recent study was unable to find evidence of OEC myelination in the compressed spinal cord and suggests that OEC (derived from embryos) transplantation may facilitate endogenous SC invasion into the lesion site.[93] To address this issue, Akiyama et al[63] prepared cell suspensions of OECs from the olfactory bulb of alkaline-phosphatase-expressing adult transgenic rats.[101] The marker gene human placental alkaline phosphatase (hPAP) is linked to the ubiquitous active R26 gene promoter, and its stable expression has been demonstrated by neural precursor cells in culture and after transplantation into the CNS.[102,103] Transplantation of cell suspensions enriched in adult OECs (>95% p75+ and S100+) derived from hPAP[63] or eGFP transgenic rats[66,89,104] can be readily identified in vivo and are associated with myelin formation (Fig. 12.12). Moreover, conduction properties are improved following OEC remyelination.[73] The extensive degree of remyelination by identified Schwann cells and OECs indicates that both cell types, under appropriate in vivo conditions, are capable of forming myelin in the spinal cord.

Most of the experimental work showing axonal repair using OECs was done in a rodent system and the OEC preparations

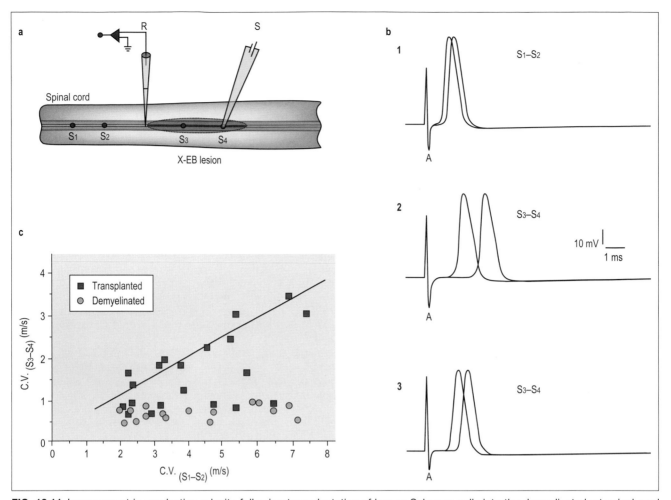

FIG. 12.11 Improvement in conduction velocity following transplantation of human Schwann cells into the demyelinated rat spinal cord. **A**. Schematic showing arrangement of intra-axonal recording and stimulation sites. Intra-axonal recordings were obtained from dorsal column axons outside of the lesion where the axons were normally myelinated. Stimulating electrodes were positioned outside (S_1–S_2) and within (S_3–S_4) the X-EB lesion zone, to assess single axon conduction velocity over both the demyelinated or remyelinated axon segment and the normally myelinated axon segment of the same axon. **B**. Pairs of action potentials recorded from (1) S_1–S_2 stimulation, (2) S_3–S_4 in the demyelinated dorsal columns and (3) S_3–S_4 following cell transplantation. Recordings were obtained at comparable conduction distances. **C**. Plot of the conduction velocity of axon segments within the lesion (S_3–S_4) versus conduction velocity of the axon segment outside the lesion (S_1–S_2) for X-EB lesioned spinal cord without (circles) and with (squares) transplantation. Modified from Kohama et al 2001.[71]

were of varying purity and cellular composition. The robust capability of rodents for endogenous myelin repair may differ from that in primates. Nonetheless, initial studies in the non-human primate are promising. Unlike the rodent, very little endogenous repair was observed after EB lesions in the nonhuman primate spinal cord at 4 weeks post-injection.[67] However, after grafting of OECs derived from a transgenic pig model expressing H-transferase to alter carbohydrate structure of the cells to mimic that of the human Type O blood group, considerable peripheral-like myelin was observed in the primate spinal cord (Fig. 12.13). These results suggest that, while endogenous repair of myelin may be less robust in primates than in rodents, transplanted peripheral myelin forming cells are capable of remyelinating primate spinal cord axons, a preclinical observation that will be important for potential future cell therapy studies in humans.

MOLECULAR REORGANIZATION OF ION CHANNELS ON SPINAL AXONS REMYELINATED BY TRANSPLANTED CELLS

As noted above, remyelinated axons display inappropriately short internodal lengths,[61,105–107] indicating that new nodes are formed. Despite their location at formerly internodal sites, remyelinated PNS axons have been shown to display high densities of Na_v channels at nodes[105,108,109] and K_v1 aggregations within juxtaparanodal domains.[27] Our recent results demonstrate that, following remyelination by OECs derived from GFP-expressing rats, nodes of Ranvier achieve a Na_v and K_v1 channel organization similar to that exhibited at mature control central nodes, with clustering of $Na_v1.6$ at remyelinated nodes and $K_v1.2$ within juxtaparanodal regions (Fig. 12.14).[66] Moreover, in

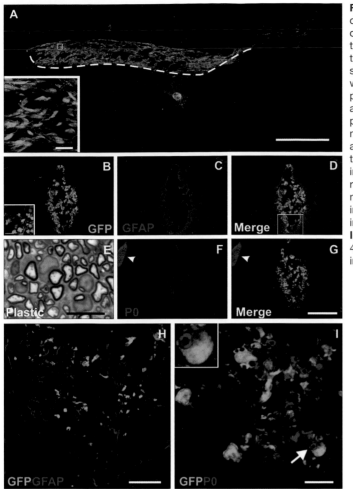

FIG. 12.12 A. Sagittal frozen section through demyelinated spinal cord demonstrates the distribution of transplanted GFP-OEC. Transplanted cells are primarily confined to the lesion site. Some cells migrated into the deep white matter. **B.** Coronal frozen sections in the lesion show the presence of GFP-OEC within a lesion site. Transplanted cells survived primarily in the dorsal funiculus. There was little GFAP staining within the lesion zone. GFAP-positive cells were present at the peripheral margin of the lesion (**C, D, H**). These results indicate that few astrocytes are present in the transplant region and that there is a preponderance of GFP-OEC in the lesion zone. **E.** High-magnification micrographs of semi-thin plastic sections stained with methylene blue/ azure II through the OEC transplanted lesion, demonstrating that the transplanted dorsal funiculus was extensively myelinated. **F.** P0-immunostaining of the frozen coronal section reveals that most axons remyelinated by transplanted OECs are surrounded by peripheral-type myelin. Peripheral roots are strongly immunostained by P0 (arrowheads in **F** and **G**). **I.** Red P0 rings are associated with green cellular elements, indicating that transplanted OECs remyelinate the demyelinated axons. **Inset in I.** Enlargement of cell indicated by arrow. Scale bars: 1 mm (**a**), 400 μm (**B, C, D, F, G**), 10 μm (**E**), 30 μm (**H**), 10 μm (**I**); inset in **A**, 20 μm; inset in **B**, 10 μm. Modified from Sasaki et al 2006.[104]

vivo recordings of GFP-OEC remyelinated spinal cord axons demonstrate conduction velocities approaching normal levels at 3 weeks post-transplantation. Proper nodal construction has also been observed on congenitally dysmyelinated axons following remyelination by adult neural precursor cells.[110] These observations demonstrate that exogenous myelin-forming cells are able to support the establishment and maintenance of mature ion channel distributions at nodal regions and to support functional recovery of demyelinated axons. Using intra-axonal recordings, we have not observed ectopic or spontaneous impulse generation following transplantation of CNS glia, Schwann cells and OECs. It is important to note that Hofstetter et al[111] report allodynia following intraspinal injections of neural stem cell grafts, but not from grafts with directed differentiation which were reported to improve functional outcome. It will be important to determine that cells being used for clinical studies do not result in aberrant action potential activity which could lead to neurological side effects.

CONCLUSIONS

Impulse conduction is compromised to various degrees in MS, resulting in conduction slowing and failure, as well as hyperexcitability, which can produce positive neurological signs such as pain or paresthesias. These conduction abnormalities can result from changes in the passive electrical properties of the axon secondary to the loss of myelin or from reorganization of ion channels on the axon membrane. The normal node of Ranvier has a high density of sodium channel Nav1.6 and a paucity of potassium channels; potassium channels (Kv1) cluster in the paranodal and juxtaparanodal region. In acutely demyelinated axons sodium channel density at the internodal axon membrane is insufficient to support secure action potential conduction but with time sodium channel density can increase in the demyelinated internode to support slow continuous conduction. Potential therapeutic strategies to improve conduction in demyelinated axons include pharmacological approaches to increase sodium currents such as by blocking repolarizing potassium currents, or to reduce threshold for action potential initiation. Transplantation of myelin forming cells into experimental demyelinated spinal cord can lead to remyelination, which significantly increases conduction velocity. It is encouraging that these remyelinated fibers can reconstruct the axon membrane so that it contains appropriate sodium and potassium channels at the nodal and adjacent regions of the axon, and that hyperexcitability-related phenomena have not been observed. Challenges for cell-based therapies for MS in the future include the development of appropriate cell types that are safe, the establishment of delivery systems that can be used clinically, and the development of clinically applicable functional assays including in vivo electrophysiological analysis that can be used to assess efficacy.

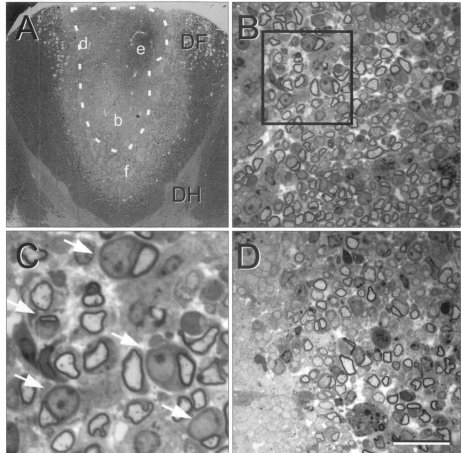

FIG. 12.13 Transplantation of transgenic pig OECs into the demyelinated monkey spinal cord. **A**. Low-power micrograph of lesion following cell transplantation into the dorsal funiculus (DF). Remyelination was observed within the white dashed lines and most of the dorsal funicular region outside of the dashed lines remained demyelinated. **B**. The central core of the lesion was densely remyelinated. **C**. The boxed area in **B**, showing myelinated axon profiles, exhibits a peripheral pattern of remyelination. **D**. The edge of the densely remyelinated zone to a transition from demyelinated (left) to remyelinated axons, can be seen. Arrows in **C** point to large cytoplasmic and nuclear regions of the myelin-forming cells. Scale bar: **A**, 1.25 mm; **B, D**, 50 μm; **C**, 10 μm. Modified from Radtke et al 2004.[67]

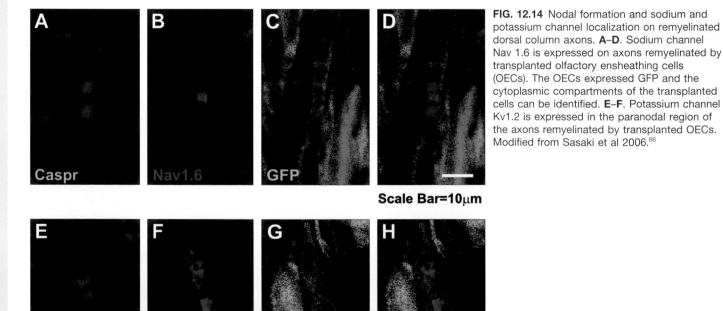

FIG. 12.14 Nodal formation and sodium and potassium channel localization on remyelinated dorsal column axons. **A–D**. Sodium channel Nav 1.6 is expressed on axons remyelinated by transplanted olfactory ensheathing cells (OECs). The OECs expressed GFP and the cytoplasmic compartments of the transplanted cells can be identified. **E–F**. Potassium channel Kv1.2 is expressed in the paranodal region of the axons remyelinated by transplanted OECs. Modified from Sasaki et al 2006.[66]

REFERENCES

1. Trapp BD, Peterson J, Ransohoff RM et al. Axonal transection in the lesions of multiple sclerosis. N Engl J Med 1998; 338: 278–285.

2. Huxley AF, Stampfli R. Evidence for saltatory conduction in peripheral myelinated nerve fibres. J Physiol 1949; 108: 315–339.

3. Waxman SG, Bennett WVL. Relative conduction velocities of small myelinated and non-myelinated fibers in the central nervous system. Nat N Biol 1972; 238: 217–219.

4. Bjartmar C, Hildebrand C, Loinder K. Morphological heterogeneity of rat oligodendrocytes: Electron microscopic studies on serial sections. Glia 1994; 11: 235–244.

5. Howe JR, Ritchie JM. Sodium currents in Schwann cells from myelinated and nonmyelinated nerves of neonatal and adult rabbits. J Physiol (Lond) 1990; 425: 169–210.

6. Waxman S G. Conduction in myelinated, unmyelinated, and demyelinated fibers. Arch Neurol 1977; 34: 585–590.

7. Black JA, Foster RE, Waxman SG. Rat optic nerve: freeze-fracture studies during development of myelinated axons. Brain Res 1982; 250: 1–10.

8. Chiu SY, Ritchie JM. Evidence for the presence of potassium channels in the paranodal region of acutely demyelinated mammalian nerve fibres. J Physiol (Lond) 1981; 313: 415–437.

9. Chiu SY, Ritchie JM. Potassium channels in nods and internodal axonal membrane in mammalian myelinated fibers. Nature 1980; 284: 170–171.

10. Goldin AL, Barchi RL, Caldwell JH et al. Nomenclature of voltage-gated sodium channels. Neurons 2000; 28: 365–368.

11. Caldwell JH, Schaller KL, Lasher RS et al. Sodium channel Nav1.6 is localized at nodes of Ranvier, dendrites, and synapses. Proc Natl Acad Sci USA 2000; 97: 5616–5620.

12. Boiko T, Rasband MN, Levinson SR et al. Compact myelin dictates the differential targeting of two sodium channel isoforms in the same axon. Neuron 2001; 30: 91–104.

13. Kaplan MR, Cho MH, Ullian EM et al. Differential control of clustering of the sodium channels Nav1.2 and Nav1.6 at developing CNS nodes of Ranvier. Neuron 2001; 30: 105–1119.

14. Jenkins SM, Bennett V. Developing nodes of Ranvier are defined by ankyrin-G clustering and are independent of paranodal axoglial adhesion. Proc Natl Acad Sci USA 2002; 99: 2303–2308.

15. Rios JC, Rubin M, St Martin M et al. Paranodal interactions regulate expression of sodium channel subtypes and provide a diffusion barrier for the node of Ranvier. J Neurosci 2003; 23: 7001–7011.

16. Vabnick I, Messing A, Chiu SY et al. Sodium channel distribution in axons of hypomyelinated and MAG null mutant mice. J Neurosci Res 1997; 50: 321–336.

17. Rasband MN, Peles E, Trimmer JS et al. Dependence of nodal sodium channel clustering on paranodal axoglial contact in the developing CNS. J Neurosci 1999; 19: 7516–7528.

18. Waxman SG, Foster RE. Development of the axon membrane during differentiation of myelinated fibres in spinal nerve roots. Proc R Soc Lond B 1980: 209: 441–446.

19. Kaplan MR, Meyer-Franke A, Lambert S et al. Induction of sodium channel clustering by oligodendrocytes. Nature 1997; 386: 724–728.

20. Eshed Y, Feinberg K, Poliak S et al. Gliomedin mediates Schwann cell-axon interaction and the molecular assembly of the nodes of Ranvier. Neuron 2005; 47: 215–229.

21. Everill B, Kocsis JD. Reduction in potassium currents in identified cutaneous afferent dorsal root ganglion neurons after axotomy. J Neurophysiol 1999; 82: 700–708.

22. Eng DL, Gordon TR, Kocsis JD et al. Development of 4-AP and TEA sensitivities in mammalian myelinated nerve fibers. J Neurophysiol 1988; 60: 2168–2179.

23. Foster RE, Connors BW, Waxman SG. Rat optic nerve: Electrophysiological, pharmacological and anatomical studies during development. Dev Brain 1982; 3: 361–376.

24. Kocsis JD, Waxman SG, Hildebrand C. Regenerating mammalian nerve fibres: changes in action potential waveform and firing characteristics following blockage of potassium conductance. Proc R Soc Lond B 1982; 217: 277–278.

25. Ritchie JM, Rang HP, Pellegrino R. Sodium and potassium channels in demyelinated and remyelinated mammalian nerve. Nature 1981; 294: 257–259.

26. Roper J. Schwarz JR. Heterogeneous distribution of fast and slow potassium channels in myelinated rat nerve fibers. J Physiol (Lond) 1989; 416: 93–110.

27. Rasband M, Trimmer JS, Schwarz TL et al. Potassium channel distribution, clustering, and function in remyelinating rat axons. J Neurosci 1998; 18: 36–47.

28. Vabnick I, Shrager P. Ion channel redistribution and function during development of the myelinated axon. J Neurobiol 1998; 37: 80–96.

29. Wang H, Kunkel DD, Martin TM et al. Heteromultimeric K$^+$ channels in terminal and juxtaparanodal regions of neurons. Nature 1993; 365: 75–79.

30. Zhou L, Zhang CL, Messing A et al. Temperature-sensitive neuromuscular transmission in Kv1.1 null mice: role of potassium channels under the myelin sheath in your nerves. J Neurosci 1998; 18: 7200–7215.

31. Brill MH, Waxman SG, Moore JW et al. Conduction velocity and spike configuration in myelinated fibers: computed dependence on internode distance. J Neurol Neurosurg Psychiatr 1977; 40: 769–774.

32. Waxman SG, Brill MH. Conduction through demyelinated plaques in multiple sclerosis: computer simulations of facilitation by short internodes. J Neurol Neurosurg Psychiatr 1978; 41: 408–417.

33. Sears TA, Bostock H. Conduction failure in demyelination: is it inevitable? Adv Neurol 1981; 31: 357–375.

34. Waxman SG, Wood SL. Impulse conduction in inhomogeneous axons: Effects of variation in voltage-sensitive ionic conductances on invasion of demyelinated axon segments and preterminal fibers. Brain Res 1984; 294: 111–122.

35. Bostock H, Sears TA. Continuous conduction in demyelinated mammalian nerve fibres. Nature 1976; 263: 786–787.

36. Utzschneider DA, Archer DR, Kocsis JD et al. Transplantation of glial cells enhances action potential conduction of a myelinated spinal cord axons in the myelin-deficient rat. Proc Natl Acad Sci USA 1994; 91: 53–57.

37. Honmou O, Felts PA, Waxman SG et al. Restoration of normal conduction properties in demyelinated spinal cord axons in the adult rat by transplantation of exogenous Schwann cells. J Neurosci 1996; 16: 3199–3208.

38. McDonald I. Pathophysiology of multiple sclerosis. In: Compston A et al, eds. McAlpine's multiple sclerosis, 3rd ed. Edinburgh: Churchill Livingstone; 1998: 359–378.

39. McDonald WI. The effects of experimental demyelination on conduction in peripheral nerve: a histological and electrophysiological study. Electrophysiological observations. Brain 1963; 86: 501–524.

40. McDonald WI, Sears TA. The effects of experimental demyelination on conduction in the central nervous system. Brain 1970; 93: 583–598.

41. Rasminsky M, Sears TA. Internodal conduction in undissected demyelinated nerve fibers. J Physiol (Lond) 1972; 227: 323–350.

42. Bostock H, Grafe P. Activity-dependent excitability changes in normal and demyelinated rat spinal root axons. J Physiol (Lond) 1985; 365: 239–257.

43. Brismar T. Specific permeability properties of demyelinated rat nerve fibers. Acta Physiol Scand 1981; 113: 167–176.

44. Smith KJ, McDonald WI. Spontaneous and mechanically evoked activity due to central demyelinating lesions. Nature 1980; 286: 154–155.

45. Rasminsky M. Hyperexcitability of pathologically myelinated axons and positive symptoms in multiple sclerosis In: Waxman SG, Ritchie JM, eds. Demyelinating disease: basic and clinical electrophysiology. New York: Raven Press; 1981: 289–297.

46. Devor M, Seltzer Z. Pathophysiology of damaged nerves in relation to chronic pain. In: Wall PD, Melzack R. Textbook of pain, 4th ed. Edinburgh: Churchill Livingstone; 1999: 129–164.

47. Burchiel K. Abnormal impulse generation in focally demyelinated trigeminal roots. J Neurosurg 1980; 53: 674–683.

48. Bostock H, Sears TA, Sherratt RM. The effects of 4-aminopyridine and tetraethylammonium ions on normal and demyelinated mammalian nerve fibers. J Physiol (Lond) 1981; 313: 301–315.

49. Targ EF, Kocsis JD. 4-aminopyridine leads to restoration of conduction in demyelinated rat sciatic nerve. Brain Res 1985; 328: 358–361.

50. Blight AR. Effect of 4-AP on axonal conduction block in chronic spinal cord injury. Brain Res Bull 1989; 22: 47–52.

51. Stefoski D, Davis FA. Faut M et al. 4-aminopyridine improves clinical signs in multiple sclerosis. Ann Neurol 1987; 21: 71–77.

52. Davis FA, Stefoski D, Rush J. Orally administered 4-aminopyridine improves clinical signs in multiple sclerosis. Ann Neurol 1990; 27: 186–192.

53. Van Diemen HAM, Polman CH, vanDongen MMM et al. The effect of 4-aminopyridine on clinical signs in multiple sclerosis: a randomized placebo-controlled, double-blind crossover study. Ann Neurol 1992; 32: 123–130.

54. Bever, CT Jr, Anderson PA, Leslie J et al. Treatment with oral 3,4 diaminopyridine improves leg strength in multiple sclerosis patients: results of a randomized double-blind placebo-controlled, crossover trail. Neurology 1996; 47: 1457–1462.

55. Polman CH, Bertelsmann FW, vanLoenen AC et al. 4-aminopyridine in the treatment of patients with multiple sclerosis: long term efficacy and safety. Arch Neurol 1994; 51: 292–296.

56. Polman CH, Bertelsmann FW, deWaal R et al. 4-aminopyridine is superior to 3,4 diaminopyridine in the treatment of multiple sclerosis. Arch Neurol 1994; 51: 1136–1139.

57. Kaji R, Sumner A. Effects of digitalis on CNS demyelinative conductive block. Ann Neurol 1989; 25: 159–166.

58. Prineas JW, Connell F. Remyelination in multiple sclerosis. Ann Neurol 1979; 5: 22–31.

59. Prineas JW, Barnard RO, Kwon EE et al. Multiple sclerosis: remyelination of nascent lesions. Ann Neurol 1993; 33: 137–151.

60. Patrikios P, Stadelmann C, Kutzelnigg A et al. Remyelination is extensive in a subset of multiple sclerosis patients. Brain 2006; 129: 3165–3172.

61. Gledhill RF, McDonald WI. Morphological characteristics of central demyelination and remyelination: a single-fiber study. Ann Neurol 1977; 1: 552–560.

62. Smith KJ, Blakemore WF, McDonald WI. Central remyelination restores secure conduction. Nature 1979; 280: 395–396.

63. Akiyama Y, Lankford KL, Radtke C et al. Remyelination of spinal cord axons by olfactory ensheathing cells and Schwann cells derived from a transgenic rat expressing alkaline phosphatase marker gene. Neuron Glia Biol 2004; 1: 1–9.

64. Harrison BM, McDonald WI, Ochoa J. Remyelination in the central diphtheria toxin lesion. J Neurol Sci 1972; 17: 293–302.

65. Jeffery ND, Blakemore WF. Locomotor deficits induced by experimental spinal cord demyelination are abolished by spontaneous remyelination. Brain 1997; 120: 27–37.

66. Sasaki M, Black JA, Lankford KL et al. Molecular reconstruction of nodes of Ranvier after remyelination by transplanted olfactory ensheathing cells in the demyelinated spinal cord. J Neurosci 2006; 26: 1803–1812.

67. Radtke C, Akiyama Y, Brokaw J et al. Remyelination of the nonhuman primate spinal cord by transplantation of H-transferase transgenic adult pig olfactory ensheathing cells. FASEB J 2004; 18: 335–337.

68. Duncan ID, Hammang, JP, Gilmore SA. Schwann cell myelination of the myelin deficient rat spinal cord following X-irradiation. Glia 1988; 1: 233–239.

69. Kierstead HS, Nistor G, Bernal G et al. Human embryonic stem cell-derived oligodendrocyte progenitor cell transplants remyelinate and restore locomotion after spinal cord injury. J Neurosci 2005; 25: 4694–4705.

70. Lachapelle F, Lapie P, Gumpel M. Oligodendrocytes from jimpy and normal mature tissue can be 'activated' when transplanted in a newborn environment. Dev Neurosci 1992; 14: 105–113.

71. Kohama I, Lankford KL, Preiningerova J et al. Transplantation of cryopreserved adult human Schwann cells enhances axonal conduction in demyelinated spinal cord. J Neurosci 2001; 21: 944–950.

72. Franklin RJ, Gilson JM, Franceschini IA et al. Schwann cell-like myelination following transplantation of an olfactory bulb-ensheathing cell line into areas of demyelination in the adult CNS. Glia 1996; 17: 217–224.

73. Imaizumi T, Lankford KL, Waxman SG et al. Transplanted olfactory ensheathing cells remyelinate and enhance axonal conduction in demyelinated dorsal column of the rat spinal cord. J Neurosci 1998; 18: 6176–6185.

74. Brustle O, Jones KN, Learish RD et al. Embryonic stem cell-derived glial precursors: a source of myelinating transplants. Science 1999; 285: 754–756.

75. Kierstead HS, Ben-Hur T, Rogister B et al. Polysialylated neural cell adhesion molecule-positive CNS precursors generate both oligodendrocytes and Schwann cells to remyelinate the CNS after transplantation. J Neurosci 1999; 19: 7529–7536.

76. Akiyama Y, Honmou O, Kato T et al. Transplantation of clonal neural precursor cells derived from adult human brain establishes functional peripheral myelin in the rat spinal cord. Exp Neurol 2001; 167: 27–39.

77. Akiyama Y, Radtke C, Kocsis JD. Remyelination of the rat spinal cord by transplantation of identified bone marrow stromal cells. J Neurosci 2002; 15: 6623–6630.

78. Blakemore WF, Crang AJ. The use of cultured autologous Schwann cells to remyelinate areas of persistent demyelination in the central nervous system. J Neurol Sci 1985; 70: 207–223.

79. Baron-Van Evercooren A, Gansmuller A, Duhamel E et al. Repair of a myelin lesion by Schwann cells transplanted in the adult mouse spinal cord. J Neuroimmunol 1992; 40: 235–242.

80. Takami T, Oudega M, Bater ML. Schwann cell but not olfactory ensheathing glia transplants improve hindlimb locomotor performance in the moderately confused adult rat thoracic spinal cord. J Neurosci 2002; 22: 6670–6681.

81. Graziadei PP, Levine RR, Graziadei GA. Regeneration of olfactory axons and synapse formation in the forebrain after bulbectomy in neonatal mice. Proc Natl Acad Sci USA 1978; 75: 5230–5234.

82. Li Y, Field PM, Raisman G. Regeneration of adult rat corticospinal axons induced

83. Ramon-Cueto A, Plant GW, Avila J et al. Long-distance axonal regeneration in the transected adult rat spinal cord is promoted by olfactory ensheathing glia transplants. J Neurosci 1998; 18: 3803–3815.

84. Imaizumi T, Lankford KL, Kocsis JD. Transplantation of olfactory ensheathing cells or Schwann cells restores rapid and secure conduction across the transected spinal cord. Brain Res 2000; 854: 70–78.

85. Imaizumi T, Lankford KL, Burton WV et al. Xenotransplantation of transgenic pig olfactory ensheathing cells promotes axonal regeneration in rat spinal cord. Nat Biotechnol 2000; 18: 949–953.

86. Ramon-Cueto A, Cordero MI, Santos-Benito FF et al. Functional recovery of paraplegic rats and motor axon regeneration in their spinal cords by olfactory ensheathing glia. Neuron 2000; 25: 425–435.

87. Ramon-Cueto A, Valverde F. Olfactory bulb ensheathing glia: a unique cell type with axonal growth-promoting properties. Glia 1995; 14: 163–173.

88. Doucette R. PNS-CNS transitional zone of the first cranial nerve. J Comp Neurol 1991; 312: 451–466.

89. Sasaki M, Lankford KL, Zemedkun M et al. Identified olfactory ensheathing cells transplanted into the transected dorsal funiculus bridge the lesion and form myelin. J Neurosci 2004; 24: 8485–8493.

90. Lu J, Feron F, Mackay-Sim A et al. Olfactory ensheathing cells promote locomotor recovery after delayed transplantation into transected spinal cord. Brain 2002; 125: 14–21.

91. Keyvan-Fouladi N, Raisman G, Li Y. Functional repair of the corticospinal tract by delayed transplantation of olfactory ensheathing cells in adult rats. J Neurosci 2003; 28: 9428–9434.

92. Plant GW, Christensen CL, Oudega M et al. Delayed transplantation of olfactory ensheathing glia promotes sparing/regeneration of supraspinal axons in the contused adult rat spinal cord. J Neurotrauma 2003; 20: 1–16.

93. Boyd JG, Lee J, Skihar V et al. LacZ-expressing olfactory ensheathing cells do not associate with myelinated axons after implantation into the compressed spinal cord. Proc Natl Acad Sci USA 2004; 17: 2162–2166.

94. Chuah MI, West AK. Cellular and molecular biology of ensheathing cells. Microsc Res Tech 2002; 58: 216–227.

95. Au E, Roskams AJ. Olfactory ensheathing cells of the lamina propria in vivo and in vitro. Glia 2003; 41: 224–236.

96. Ramer LM, Au E, Richter MW et al. Peripheral olfactory ensheathing cells reduce scar and cavity formation and promote regeneration after spinal cord injury. J Comp Neurol 2004; 473: 1–15.

97. Plant GW, Currier PF, Cuervo EP et al. Purified adult ensheathing glia fail to myelinate axons under culture conditions that enable Schwann cells to form myelin. J Neurosci 2002; 22: 6083–6091.

98. Brook GA, Plate D, Franzen R et al. Spontaneous longitudinally orientated

SECTION 2

axonal regeneration is associated with the Schwann cell framework within the lesion site following spinal cord compression injury of the rat. J Neurosci Res 1998; 53: 51–65.

99. Barnett SC, Alexander CL, Iwashita Y et al. Identification of a human olfactory ensheathing cell that can effect transplant-mediated remyelination of demyelinated CNS axons. Brain 2000; 123: 1581–1588.

100. Kato T, Honmou O, Uede T et al. Transplantation of human olfactory ensheathing cells elicits remyelination of demyelinated rat spinal cord. Glia 2000; 30: 209–218.

101. Kisseberth WC, Brettingen NT, Lohse JK et al. Ubiquitous expression of marker transgenes in mice and rats. Devel Biology 1999; 214: 128–138.

102. Mujtaba T, Han SS, Fischer I et al. Stale expression of the alkaline phosphatase marker gene by neural cells in culture and after transplantation into the CNS using cells derived from a transgenic rat. Exper Neurol 2002; 174: 48–57.

103. Han SS, Kang DY, Mujtaba T et al. Grafted lineage-restricted precursors differentiate exclusively into neurons in the adult spinal cord. Exper Neurol 2002; 177: 360–375.

104. Sasaki M, Hains BC, Lankford KL et al. Protection of corticospinal tract neurons following dorsal spinal cord transection and engraftment of olfactory ensheathing cells. Glia 2006; 53: 352–359.

105. Weiner LP, Waxman SG, Stohlman SA et al. Remyelination following viral-inducted demyelination: ferric ion-ferrocyanide staining of nodes of Ranvier within the CNS. Ann Neurol 1980; 8: 580–583.

106. Blakemore WF, Murray JA. Quantitative examination of internodal length of remyelinated nerve fibres in the central nervous system. J Neurol 1981; 49: 273–284.

107. Hildebrand C, Kocsis JD, Berglund S et al. Myelin sheath remodeling in regenerated rat sciatic nerve. Brain Res 1985; 358: 163–170.

108. Novakovic SD, Deerinck TJ, Levinson SR et al. Cluster of axonal Na$^+$ channels adjacent to remyelinating Schwann cells. J Neurocytol 1996; 25: 403–412.

109. Novakovic SD, Levinson SR, Schachner M et al. Disruption and reorganization of sodium channels in experimental allergic neuritis. Muscle Nerve 1998; 21: 1019–1032.

110. Eftekharpour E, Karimi-Abdolrezaee S, Wang J et al. Myelination of congenitally dysmyelinated spinal cord axons by adult neural precursor cells results in formation of nodes of Ranvier and improved axonal conduction. J Neurosci 2007; 27: 3416–3428.

111. Hofstetter CP, Holmstrom NA, Lilja JA et al. Allodynia limits the usefulness of intraspinal neural stem cell grafts: directed differentiation improves outcome. Nat Neurosci 2005; 8: 346–353.

CHAPTER 13

Immunology of multiple sclerosis

M. Sospedra and R. Martin

INTRODUCTION

Multiple sclerosis (MS) is considered a CD4+ T-cell-mediated autoimmune disease of the central nervous system (CNS).[1,2] Pathologically, it is characterized by inflammatory foci in the CNS with various degrees of demyelination, axonal damage/loss and glial proliferation.[3,4] Both the pathology and the clinical characteristics are covered elsewhere in this book. MS affects mainly young adults between 20 and 40 years of age and is approximately twice as frequent in women as in men.[2] Prevalence rates in northern European countries and the USA vary from 60–200/100 000. While the exact etiology of the disease is not known, it is clear that a complex genetic susceptibility trait represents the most important etiologic component and that environmental triggers such as infectious agents and others also contribute to disease manifestation and expression. The presence of a large number of quantitative trait loci translates into immune abnormalities but it is becoming clear that genetic susceptibility also includes factors that are relevant for CNS vulnerability to inflammatory insult and/or reduced ability to repair damage that occurs during the disease process. Immunological events in the CNS and the response of the target tissue to them are intricately connected and, while research in the last decades focused on the immunological factors of MS, it has to be kept in mind that these should not be viewed in isolation. In this chapter, we will focus, however, on the immunological components.

The above notion that MS is mediated by autoreactive, proinflammatory CD4+ T cells stems from data in the animal model experimental allergic encephalomyelitis (EAE), which can be induced by injecting susceptible rodent strains such as, e.g. SJL mice with myelin proteins or peptides.[5] These animals subsequently develop either a monophasic inflammatory CNS disease or various forms of chronic or relapsing–remitting EAE and, in their CNS lesions, CD4+ T cells, monocytes/activated microglia and other cell populations and humoral factors are found.[5] The demonstration that EAE can be transferred from sick to naive/healthy animals merely by transferring myelin-specific CD4+ T cells firmly established the pathogenic role of these cells.[5] The transfer of antibodies alone or of activated monocytes does not result in disease, and myelin-specific CD8+

T cells induce EAE only under special circumstances. Parallel work in MS patients showed that myelin-specific CD4+ T cells are also relevant for the human disease; however, there is no doubt that the immunological processes during MS involve many different cell types and humoral factors. Another reason for suggesting a central role for CD4+ T cells is the fact that MS, like many other autoimmune diseases, is associated with distinct human leukocyte antigen (HLA)-class II molecules, in particular those of the HLA-DR15 haplotype. This haplotype, which contains the molecules DRB1*1501, DRB5*0101, DQA1*0102 and DQB1*0602, confers by far the largest part, between 10–50%, of the genetic susceptibility to MS.[6] While it is currently not known how the presence of a certain HLA-class II molecule translates into risk for an autoimmune disease, the main biological role of HLA-class II molecules is the presentation of antigenic peptides to CD4+ T cells. It is therefore reasonable to assume that the interaction of disease-associated HLA-class II molecules, the sets of peptides that they present and the activation of antigen-specific CD4+ T cells upon recognition of these HLA-class II/peptide complexes is important for the pathogenesis of MS.

We and others have recently reviewed the immunology of MS in great detail[1,7–11] and the reader is referred to these reviews, which will be mentioned throughout the article. Here, we will follow a different structure and discuss the most important immunological events in the sequence that is expected to occur during the disease: 1) activation of autoreactive CD4+ T cells in the periphery, 2) migration through the blood–brain barrier and formation of the inflammatory lesion and finally 3) events involved in CNS tissue damage. Mechanisms of lesion resolution and those controlling pathogenic immune activation in the periphery in MS are covered as part of these sequential steps.

STEP 1: ACTIVATION OF AUTOREACTIVE CD4+ T CELLS IN THE PERIPHERY

The first important event in MS is the activation of peripheral autoreactive CD4+ T helper (Th)1 cells in the periphery (Fig. 13.1). Therefore, we will first describe the evidence for their involvement, their specificity, function and HLA restriction.

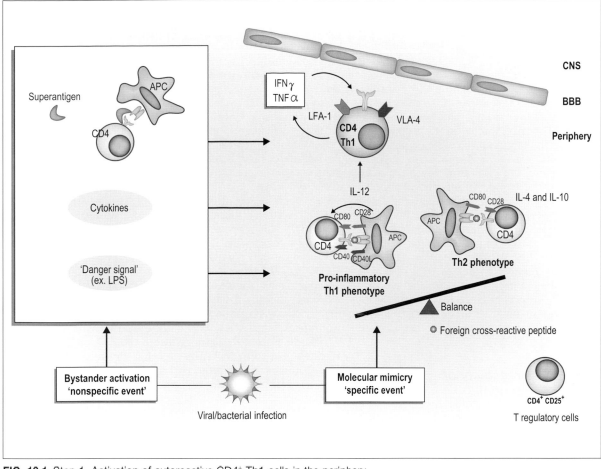

FIG. 13.1 Step 1. Activation of autoreactive CD4[+] Th1 cells in the periphery.

EVIDENCE FOR INVOLVEMENT OF CD4[+] CELLS IN MULTIPLE SCLEROSIS

More than two decades ago several investigators[5] showed that the injection of defined protein components of the myelin sheath, e.g. myelin basic protein (MBP) or proteolipid protein (PLP), together with an adjuvant into naive susceptible recipient animals caused either an acute, chronic or relapsing–remitting EAE. EAE could be induced not only by active immunization with myelin protein in adjuvant (active EAE) but also by adoptive transfer of in vitro reactivated myelin-specific CD4[+] T cells (passive or adoptive transfer EAE).[5,12] The latter observation documented convincingly that an autoimmune disease could be directly induced with an isolated autoreactive cell population in naive animals, leading to the conclusion that MS is probably a T-cell-mediated autoimmune disease. This view is probably too simplistic today and certainly does not apply to every form and stage of the MS pathogenesis. However, current evidence on the induction and perpetuation of MS still favors CD4[+] autoreactive T cells as the single most important component of the autoimmune pathogenesis of MS.

Important arguments supporting this statement are the following:

- CD4[+] T cells among others contribute to the CNS- and cerebrospinal fluid (CSF)-infiltrating inflammatory cells in MS
- Genetic risk is to a substantial degree conferred by HLA-DR and HLA-DQ molecules, and these serve primarily as recognition receptors for CD4[+] T cells

- EAE can be transferred into naive animals by autoreactive CD4[+] T cells but not by antibodies, and so far only in two models by CD8[+] T cells.[13,14] Humanized transgenic mice expressing either HLA-DR or HLA-DQ molecules are susceptible to EAE[15,16] and mice expressing both MS-associated HLA-DR molecules and MS patient-derived MBP-specific T cell receptor (TCR) develop spontaneous disease[17,18]
- A therapeutic trial with an altered peptide ligand of MBP (83–99) induced cross-reactive CD4[+] T cells with Th1 phenotype that led to disease exacerbations of MS patients in vivo[19]
- Antibody production, CD8[+] maturation and many other steps of adaptive and innate immune function are at least in part controlled by CD4[+] helper T cells.

CHARACTERIZATION OF AUTOREACTIVE CD4[+] T CELLS IN MULTIPLE SCLEROSIS

Frequency of CD4[+] myelin-specific T cells

Although the specificity of autoreactive CD4[+] T cells in MS is still incompletely understood, several pieces of evidence suggest that myelin-specific T cells are relevant. Frequencies of myelin autoreactive T cells in MS patients and healthy controls vary greatly depending on the methodology.[20–23] While tissue-culture-based techniques have shown precursor frequencies in the range of, for instance, 1 MBP-specific cell per 10^6–10^7 peripheral blood mononuclear cells (PBMCs),[20,22] approximately 1–2 orders of magnitude higher numbers were observed with enzyme-linked immunospot (ELISPOT) assays that detect, for example, interferon (IFN)γ secreting cells.[21] More recently, frequencies of 1 T cell per 10^4 or even higher have been observed using quantitative polymerase chain reaction (PCR) to follow individual T cell clones via their specific TCR CDR3 regions[23,24] or using flow-cytometry-based techniques that follow the fraction of PBMCs that proliferate upon stimulation with a myelin antigen.[25] Therefore, only studies that used similar methodologies can be compared. While some studies have found comparable frequencies of myelin-specific T cells in MS patients and healthy controls, the majority have reported elevated precursor frequencies in MS patients, e.g. of IFNγ-producing myelin-specific T cells.[21] Furthermore, the number of myelin-specific T cells with mutations of the hypoxanthine phosphoribosyl transferase (HPRT) gene, which occur in the proliferating T cell pool, is elevated in MS.[26] We could show up to 2000-fold expansions of T cells specific for the immunodominant MBP peptide (83–99) during exacerbation of patients in a treatment trial with an altered peptide ligand (APL) based on the MBP (83–99) peptide.[19] The exacerbations coincided with increased inflammatory activity in the brain. At that point, the majority of the cells induced by APL treatment cross-reacted with MBP (83–99), were also observed in the CSF and exhibited a Th1 phenotype, all supporting their involvement in the disease exacerbation.[19]

Antigen avidity and cross-reactivity of autoreactive CD4+ T cell recognition

It is now accepted that the ability of T cells to cross-react is a normal phenomenon required for thymic positive selection and for efficient host protection against potential antigens that outnumber the available T cells/TCRs by several orders of magnitude. For self-antigens that are expressed in the thymus, e.g. MBP, it is expected that only T cells recognizing these with low functional avidity will be positively selected. In agreement with this hypothesis, most MBP-specific T cell lines respond to antigen only at relatively high concentrations in the micromolar range.[20,27,28] Using combinatorial peptide libraries to search for the entire range of antigens that activate such T cell lines, we identified pathogen-derived peptides that activate MBP-specific T cell clones at concentrations several orders of magnitude lower.[29] However, high-avidity myelin-reactive T cell clones also exist in the periphery, and they are elevated in MS patients compared to controls.[30] Furthermore, during the trial with an APL peptide derived from MBP (83–99), some of the T cell clones responding to both the APL peptide and MBP (83–99) recognized these peptides at subnanomolar concentrations.[19] With respect to self-antigens that are not or barely expressed in the thymus, such as myelin oligodendrocyte glycoprotein (MOG) or the full length PLP isoform, it is expected that autoreactive T cells are deleted less efficiently in the thymus. This has been confirmed for PLP (139–154)-specific T cells in SJL mice.[31] Their frequency in the peripheral blood is clearly elevated. Furthermore, our studies documented that high-avidity T cells recognize six myelin peptides (three MBP peptides, one PLP peptide and two MOG peptides) that are immunodominant, are all derived from proteins that are not expressed in the thymus (PLP (139–154) and the two MOG peptides) or reside in areas that poorly bind to the MS-associated HLA-DR alleles, and thus also are less efficient in thymic negative selection.[30]

Phenotype of autoreactive CD4+ T cells

Auto-reactive CD4+ T cells are relatively skewed toward a pro-inflammatory Th1 phenotype.[21,30] Interleukin (IL)-12 is an important factor for the differentiation of naive T cells into IFNγ-producing Th1 cells. Conflicting results have been reported

with respect to the role of IL-12 in MS. In EAE, IL-12 has been established as a proinflammatory cytokine that is relevant for disease pathogenesis.[32] In MS patients, some studies have reported higher numbers of blood mononuclear cells expressing IL-12 p40 mRNA[33] compared with controls, while others found no differences. Interestingly, it has been reported that the percentages of PHA-activated CD4+ T cells expressing IL-12 receptors were elevated in MS patients, indicating that CD4+ T cells in MS are skewed toward Th1.[34] The proinflammatory cytokine IL-17 has also been found to be increased in the blood from MS patients.[35] Despite all these pieces of evidence supporting a critical role of IFNγ-producing Th1 cells in autoimmune pathogenesis, some questions emerged after the observation that IFNγ−/−,[36] IFNγR−/−,[37] IL-12Rβ2−/−,[38] and IL-12p35−/− mice,[39,40] which all lack critical components of the Th1–IFNγ pathway, are highly susceptible to inflammatory autoimmune diseases. Recently,[41] it has been demonstrated that IL-23, which shares the p40 subunit with IL-12, promotes the expansion of a new pathogenic T cell population characterized by the production of IL-17, IL-17F, tumor necrosis factor (TNF), IL-6 and other additional novel factors. Upon adoptive transfer to naive recipient mice, this IL-23-dependent T cell subset invades the target organ and can promote the development of organ-specific autoimmune inflammation. The pathogenic role of IL-17-secreting Th17 cells is now well established in the EAE model,[42,43,44] and research is ongoing to clarify their role in multiple sclerosis as well.[45] In contrast, a protective role has been ascribed to Th2 cells, because these cells can antagonize Th1 cell functions in several ways. However, under certain circumstances Th2 cells can induce EAE[46] and cell populations that are under Th2 control, e.g. mast cells, contribute to tissue damage at least in some MS patients. Fluctuations of cytokine secretion have, for example, been linked to the MRI-documented inflammatory activity, and elevated expression of IFNγ and TNFα have been observed before or during inflammatory disease activity, while IL-10 showed relatively higher levels during remissions.[47] Even though the inflammatory bouts decrease in number during secondary progressive disease, the secretion of proinflammatory cytokines including IL-12, IL-18 and IFNγ appears clearly elevated during the later stage,[48] the activation of Th1 cells is less strictly controlled and Th1-associated surface markers such as CCR5 and TIM-3 are upregulated.[49] When the specificity and cytokine expression of high-avidity T cells has been linked to MRI characteristics in MS patients, correlations between MOG-specific Th0/2 cells and less inflammation and between MBP-specific Th1 cells and a more destructive disease process have been observed.[30]

Costimulation of autoreactive CD4+ T cells

The requirement for costimulation, i.e. the interaction of CD80/86 on antigen presenting cells (APCs) with CD28 on T cells, as well as the control of T cell activation via the negative costimulatory molecule CTLA-4, is perturbed in CD4+ T cells in MS. CD4+ myelin-specific T cells, but also T cells with specificity for other antigens, are less dependent on or independent of the costimulatory signal 2[50–52] and do not respond or respond less to the negative signal via CTLA-4 engagement.[52,53] The latter is in part due to the absence of CTLA-4 expression upon activation on CD4+ CD28− T cells, and in addition this cell population is characterized by a clear Th1 skew, seemingly increased proliferative capacity and relative enrichment for autoreactive T cells.[52] The susceptibility to activation-induced cell death via Fas/Fas-L interactions is not generally impaired. However, data including the increased expression of the anti-apoptotic molecules survivin, Bcl-2 and inhibitor of apoptosis (IAP) family members IAP, IAP-2 and X-IAP in MS T cells, their heightened expression during disease exacerbations and down-regulation by IFN-β all suggest that the regulation of apoptosis is perturbed in MS,[54,55] although some aspects are not different from controls.

T cell receptor repertoire

Early observations of a highly restricted TCR variable chain repertoire in MBP-induced EAE in the Lewis rat and in B10.PL and PL mice[5] led to the formulation of the V-region hypothesis,[56] i.e. that susceptibility to certain autoimmune diseases is closely related to the expression of certain TCRs, most notably Vβ8.2. Research along similar lines in MS patients initially appeared to confirm these data, and a restricted expression of Vβ17 was for example described for MBP-specific T cell lines in MS;[57] however, this particular report was heavily influenced by the large number of T cell lines from one individual. Subsequent research went back and forth between describing a restricted TCR repertoire either within single MS patients (but not inter-individually[58]) or across the entire MS population,[59] while other studies in different MS populations failed to confirm an over-representation of certain TCR V chains.[60] Among the Vβ chains that were most often found were Vβ5.2, Vβ5.3 and Vβ6.2,[59,61,62] or in PLP-specific T cells Vβ2.[63] Subsequent studies examined not only the Vβ chain repertoire but also the CD3 spectratype patterns or oligoclonality by single strand conformational polymorphism typing and TCR sequencing.[1] They described:

- An association of oligoclonal TCR CDR3 spectratypes particularly in the Vβ5.2 expressing population and MS development[64]
- A correlation between TCR Vβ13-associated junctional sequences at disease onset[65]
- Increased MBP reactivity and IFNγ and IL-2 secretion in CD4+ and CD8+ T cells with altered CD3 length distributions[66]
- An oligoclonal expansion of T cells with distinct TCRs in the CSF[67,68]
- The observation of Vβ5.2-associated junctional sequences from MS brain-derived TCRs that shared similarities with MBP T cell clones,[1] and CDR3 motifs in PLP (105–124)- and PLP(95–116)-specific T cells that showed homologies with TCRs from MS brains.[63]

Tracking individual MBP-specific T cell clones by a quantitative PCR-based technique showed that such clones exist in the peripheral blood for a long time and may be reactivated during disease exacerbation.[24] Finally the comparison of the TCR Vα chain usage in monozygous concordant and discordant twins showed that the overall TCR Vα chain repertoire in discordant twins is different; however, not only in MBP-specific but also in tetanus-specific T cells.[69] A recent study focusing on the CDR3 spectratypes in naive T cells of discordant monozygous twins found similar distortions in both healthy and diseased twins.[70] Such repertoire shifts in naive T cells may predispose to MS development but are probably not sufficient.

MECHANISMS OF ACTIVATION OF AUTOREACTIVE CD4+ T CELL

According to current data MS develops in genetically susceptible individuals and may require additional environmental triggers. The relatively low concordance rate of identical twins (25–30%) indicates a role of nongenetic factors in MS etiology.[71] Environmental and behavioral influences have been proposed as putative exogenous factors that could induce or contribute to disease expression. Among environmental influences, numerous reports indicate a contribution of infectious agents to the etiology of MS.[1] The proposed mechanisms for how infections could induce MS have been grouped under two independent concepts. The first is referred to as molecular mimicry and considers that autoreactive cells are activated as a consequence of a specific recognition event of the humoral or cellular immune system; i.e. autoreactive T cells cross-react with an infectious agent. The second concept, called bystander activation, assumes that auto-reactive cells are activated as a result of nonspecific inflammatory events that occur during infection. Recently, it has been suggested that autoimmunity in some instances may be the consequence of the interaction of molecular mimicry and bystander activation.[72]

Molecular mimicry

The recognition of self-antigens at intermediate levels of affinity by T cells during thymic maturation leads to positive selection and export of these T cells to the periphery. Cross-reactivity of these potentially self-reactive T cells with foreign antigens can lead to activation during infection. MBP is one candidate auto-antigen in MS, based on numerous pieces of evidence. Although MBP-specific T cells can be isolated from both MS patients and healthy individuals,[1] the activation state of these T cells in MS patients, their proinflammatory phenotype, higher antigen avidity and preferential memory origin suggest that they had been activated in vivo, e.g. by cross-reactive infectious antigens during infections. Following the hypothesis that molecular mimicry may play a role in the activation of MBP-specific T cells, many studies have searched for cross-reactive antigens between MBP and foreign agents. Initially this search was guided by the concept that immune reactivity (humoral and cellular) is exquisitely specific and that complete homology between foreign-proteins and MBP was required for molecular mimicry. Although examples of such stringent homology have been reported for MBP and infectious agents,[73,74] complete matching of sequence stretches between different proteins is a rare event. Subsequent research into the molecular requirements for T cell recognition found that certain amino acid positions in the peptide sequence are more critical than others for the interactions within the tri-molecular complex, and most residues except for the primary TCR contact allowed for some degree of variation.[75] Based on these observations, Wucherpfennig and Strominger formulated a search algorithm that assumed that molecular mimicry can occur as long as a MHC and TCR contact motif is preserved.[76] The activation of MBP-specific T cell clones derived from MS patients by viral and bacterial peptides sharing this motif with MBP confirmed the prediction that sequence homology was not required for cross-recognition.[76]

Subsequently, the recognition by a T cell clone specific of the immunodominant peptide MBP (83–99) was systematically dissected using single amino acid substitutions in each position of the peptide sequence.[77] These data demonstrated that cross-reactivity can occur with peptides that share no amino acids in their sequence and, rather than preservation of a contact motif, the authors demonstrated that each amino acid in the peptide contributes independently and additively to recognition by the TCR.[77] Recently, the molecular concept has evolved even further. Lang and colleagues showed that different peptides bound to different class II molecules can lead to cross-reactivity by the same TCR as long as the complexes share similarity in charge distribution and overall shape.[78]

Together these observations offer new perspectives on the concept of molecular mimicry and suggest that cross-reactivity occurs probably much more frequently than originally thought. Additional evidence for molecular mimicry stems from animal experiments showing that mice expressing viral proteins as tissue-specific transgenes develop autoimmune diseases after viral infection.[79,80] Subsequently, a study using mimic peptides in complete Freund's adjuvant[17] has demonstrated that mimic sequences can initiate cross-reactive immune responses; however, these experiments failed to provide definitive evidence for infection-induced autoimmune disease. Recently, a model for virus infection that leads to molecular mimicry has been developed, in which an encephalitogenic virus (TEMV) encodes a mimic peptide for an encephalitogenic myelin proteolipid protein (PLP) that is naturally expressed by *Haemophilus influenzae*. The infection with this recombinant virus induces early onset of disease, indicating that CNS infection with a pathogen containing a mimic epitope for a self-myelin antigen can induce a cross-reactive T cell response resulting in autoimmune demyelinating disease.[81] Although all these findings demonstrate that molecular mimicry is a viable hypothesis that can explain the link between infection and MS, evidence for this phenomenon in human autoimmune diseases is still scarce.

Bystander activation

Bystander activation refers to a mechanism by which autoreactive T cells are activated as a consequence of nonspecific inflammatory events during infections. Among these inflammatory events is the production of several proinflammatory cytokines and chemokines. For a long time these molecules have been considered the main activators of responding virus-specific CD8[+] T cells. Subsequent data showed, however, that most of the activated CD8[+] T cells are specific for viral antigens[82] and that cytokines alone are unlikely to cause the activation and functional changes of T cells in the absence of a specific antigen.[82]

The exposure to superantigens has also been proposed as a bystander activation mechanism. Superantigens are microbial toxins capable of stimulating T cells via engagement of the TCR Vβ chain. These toxins can induce relapses in the EAE model[83] and stimulate MBP-specific T cell clones.

In addition to cytokines and superantigens, the infectious context ('danger signal') can also be capable of activating autoreactive T cells. One of these infection-derived and proinflammatory agents responsible for the 'danger signal' is lipopolysaccharide.[84] Lipopolysaccharide is recognized by toll-like receptor (TLR)-4, a transmembrane receptor that initiates the innate immune response to common Gram-negative bacteria such as *Chlamydophila* (formerly *Chlamydia*) *pneumoniae*. The recognition of lipopolysaccharide by TLR4 increases the expression of cytokines as well as reactive oxygen species. The adjuvant effect on APCs could activate autoreactive T cells in the periphery. The observations that the activation of autoreactive T cells in the periphery requires the presence of both specific autoantigen and immunostimulatory agents and that bacteria injected into the brain parenchyma are able to induce inflammatory responses only after peripheral sensitization support the idea that lipopolysaccharide might directly activate peripheral autoreactive T cells.

PERTURBATIONS IN THE REGULATORY NETWORK THAT FACILITATES THE ACTIVATION OF AUTOREACTIVE CD4[+] T CELLS

CD4[+] regulatory T cells

Besides proinflammatory function and potentially damaging roles, it has recently been described that CD4[+] T cells contain an important immunoregulatory population that is currently characterized by the expression of CD4[+]CD25[+] and to various degrees also the transcription factor Fox-P3[85] and other molecules. CD4[+]CD25[+] T regulatory (Treg) cells suppress T cell proliferation, and both cell–cell contact- and cytokine-mediated mechanisms are involved in their function. The number and function of CD4[+]CD25[+] Treg are reduced in MS patients,[86,87] which could facilitate the activation of autoreactive CD4[+] T cells in the periphery. CD4[+] Th2/3 cells and their cytokines

IL-4, IL-10 and transforming growth factor (TGF)β are probably largely beneficial in MS, according to most of the available data.[88]

Immunoregulation by natural killer cells

Immunoregulation may also be mediated by natural killer (NK) cells, which show reduced activity in MS.[89,90] NK cell lytic activity is decreased in patients with acute exacerbations compared with chronic diseases[90] and it is relatively normal in patients during stable phases. Furthermore, it has been demonstrated in EAE models that the depletion of NK cells exacerbates disease, while the transfer of in vitro generated NK cells decreases autoimmunity.[91,92] The mechanisms by which NK cells could suppress autoimmunity are presently not clear. The major NK effector activities that have been identified are cytokine production and the induction of target lysis via perforin and/or TRAIL-dependent mechanisms. It has been suggested that some Th2-associated cytokines, such as IL-5 and IL-13, that are produced by NK cells may indirectly suppress Th1 autoimmunity responses, although there is no direct evidence for this notion. TGFβ, another cytokine produced by NK cells, could synergize with cytokines produced by CD4[+] cells and result in immunoregulatory/suppressive activity[93] or alternatively regulate the expansion of Th cells. As another possibility NK cells could moderate autoimmune responses by regulating B and T cell survival and expansion by killing these cells via perforin and/or TRAIL-dependent mechanisms. Support for this possibility stems from data indicating that perforin-deficient lpr mice develop severe autoimmunity,[94] and that blockage of TRAIL exacerbated EAE in a mouse model.[95] In a recent phase II clinical trial with a humanized monoclonal antibody against the IL-2 receptor α chain, daclizumab, in MS we observed marginal effects on CD4[+] T cells but an expansion of CD56[bright] immunoregulatory NK cells.[96] The relative and absolute expansion of the latter CD56[bright] NK cell population and their increased perforin expression correlate strongly with the reduction of the inflammatory activity in the brains of treated patients, and in vitro experiments demonstrated that they can directly lyse activated CD4[+] T cells via perforin-mediated lysis.[96] These novel observations not only indicate that NK cells may exert important immunoregulatory functions in MS but furthermore, that certain NK subpopulations may be generally relevant for the maintenance of tolerance and, for instance, transplant acceptance. Interestingly, the same NK cell populations appear to be involved in establishing tolerance of the fetus in the maternal placenta.

HLA-RESTRICTION AND FUNCTIONAL CHARACTERISTICS OF AUTOREACTIVE CD4[+] T CELLS – THE ROLE OF THE HLA GENE COMPLEX

The overwhelming majority of myelin-specific CD4[+] T cells are restricted by HLA-DR molecules.[1] It is important to note that the genes that confer higher risk for MS are HLA-DR and HLA-DQ genes, particularly in Caucasians the HLA-DR15 haplotype (DRB1*1501, DRB5*0101, DQA1*0102, DQB1*0602).[97] Most of the risk appears to be associated with the two DR alleles,[6] which are in very tight linkage disequilibrium, i.e. almost never inherited separately, and it was recently demonstrated that there is also a dose effect, since individuals homozygotic for DR15 carry a higher risk than heterozygotes.[98] Immunologically, higher CSF immunoglobulins,[98] oligoclonal bands and matrix metalloproteinase (MMP)-9 levels[98] have been reported. Patients expressing HLA-DR4 alleles on the other hand often have a worse clinical outcome and/or progressive course.[100] Individual HLA-class II alleles have also been associated with other genes, such as TGFβ family, CTLA-4, alleles in the TNF cluster, an IL-1 receptor antagonist allele and IL-1, a CD45 isoform, the MHC-class II transactivator (*MHC2TA*), the IL-7 receptor, the programmed-cel-death-related molecule PD1, an estrogen receptor polymorphism, and others (for details see reference 1).

While the involvement of HLA loci in MS has been demonstrated consistently for more than 20 years, our knowledge as to how the presence of certain HLA-class II genes translates into increased risk and by which molecular mechanisms is still sketchy, and this statement also holds for any MHC-class II association in other autoimmune diseases such as type 1 diabetes or rheumatoid arthritis. Several potential mechanisms have been considered:

- Disease-associated HLA-DR and –DQ molecules have binding characteristics that lead to preferential presentation of specific sets of self peptides, e.g. peptides derived from myelin proteins in the case of MS. There is currently little data to support this hypothesis and comparisons of polymorphic residues in the HLA-DR- and DQ binding pockets have not been conclusive.[101]

- As a variation of the above, it was speculated that disease-associated MHC molecules could have binding characteristics that allow only limited sets of peptides to bind, accounting for less 'complete' thymic negative selection of self-reactive T cells. Diabetes-prone NOD mice and their MHC-class II (I-A^{NOD}) have been viewed as an example of this situation.[102] Given the high frequency of most autoimmune-disease-associated HLA-DR and HLA-DQ alleles in the human population and the normal cellular immune function in the vast majority of individuals, it is unlikely that this mechanism alone accounts for the HLA-class II association in MS.

- Either polymorphic residues of the TCR-exposed surfaces of the α-helical regions of DR/DQ-α and -β chain such as the 'shared motif' in rheumatoid-arthritis-associated class II molecules[103] or TCR-contacting amino acids of the antigenic peptide or both could select a T cell repertoire with overall higher propensity to respond to self peptides. Gross abnormalities in T cell repertoires do not exist in MS patients according to current data (see below). We recently observed that clonally expanded T cells from the CSF of MS patients are capable of utilizing multiple HLA-class II molecules, i.e. all MS-associated HLA-DR/DQ molecules in the DR15 haplotype, for recognition of large sets of peptides.[104]

- The gene and protein expression of one/several disease-associated DR and DQ alleles could be altered, i.e. generally be elevated in MS patients or enhanced in the target tissue, the CNS, and thus lead to more potent antigen presentation and T cell activation.[105,106] Our comparative studies of the expression of the two MS-associated DR molecules in the DR15 haplotype, DR2a (DRA1*0101 and DRB5*0101) and DR2b (DRA1*0101 and DRB1*1501), in MS patients and controls did not reveal general or tissue-specific upregulation of one DR allele[107] but differential expression on B cells and monocytes.

- Antigen presentation in the context of certain DR molecules could be shaped by proteases involved in antigen processing or by nonpolymorphic class II molecules such as HLA-DO and HLA-DM that are tightly linked on chromosome 6p21.3 and fulfill peptide sorting and loading functions. An involvement of DM has been examined but so far no association has been found.[108]

- Engagement of HLA-class II molecules leads to intracellular signaling events, for example, anergy[109] and

this mechanism could be perturbed in patients with autoimmune diseases as well, but there is currently no information on this aspect in MS.

STEP 2: MIGRATION THROUGH THE BLOOD–BRAIN BARRIER AND FORMATION OF THE INFLAMMATORY LESION

Trafficking of activated proinflammatory and autoreactive CD4$^+$ T cells into the CNS is a crucial event in the pathogenesis of MS (Fig. 13.2).[7] The proinflammatory cytokines (IFNγ and TNFα) produced by these cells activate the adhesion molecules (ICAM-1 and VCAM-1) on the endothelium of the blood–brain barrier. Activated autoreactive CD4$^+$ T cells express the respective counterreceptors (LFA-1 and VLA-4) and adhere to the endothelium of the blood–brain barrier via these adhesion molecules;[110] following rolling and firm adhesion they transmigrate into the brain parenchyma through cerebrovascular endothelial cells. Furthermore, activated autoreactive CD4$^+$ T cells and activated monocytes also produce proteolytic enzymes (MMP-2 and MMP9) that are involved in opening the blood–brain barrier.[111] The proinflammatory cytokines produced by autoreactive CD4$^+$ T cells further activate other cell populations in the peripheral blood, including CD8$^+$ T cells, B cells, γδ T cells, granulocytes, monocytes and mast cells.

Elevated serum TNFα concentrations and higher numbers of blood cells secreting TNFα[112] have been reported in MS patients compared with controls. Nevertheless, the use of a recombinant soluble TNFα receptor immunoglobulin fusion protein as treatment in MS as well as an antibody against TNFα were found to increase and prolong MS exacerbations for as yet unclear reasons.[113,114]

Results about the prototypic proinflammatory cytokine IFNγ in the blood of MS patients are conflicting. While some studies have reported higher numbers of blood mononuclear cells expressing IFNγ mRNA and serum levels in MS patients compared with controls, others found no differences. Attempts of the direct application of IFNγ in MS resulted in disease exacerbation.[115] As already mentioned above, the role of IFNγ in EAE is also conflicting. While the prevailing perception is that proinflammatory, IFNγ-secreting T cells are encephalitogenic, IFNγ knockout animals develop much worse or even lethal EAE compared with wild-type littermates.[37]

Upon entry into the CNS, autoreactive T cells are locally reactivated (Fig. 13.2), as shown by downmodulation of their TCR,[116] presumably following recognition of local autoantigen. The autoantigens responsible for this reactivation are still unknown, although several have emerged as good candidates.

Myelin basic protein

Myelin basic protein is by far the best studied myelin component in MS. It is the second most abundant myelin protein (approximately 30–40%) after PLP. There are five MBP isoforms with 14–21.5 kDa molecular weights in mammals that result from differential splicing of 11 axons within the Golli–MBP locus.[117] The highly basic MBP is positioned at the intracellular surface of myelin membranes and via interactions with acidic lipid moieties is involved in maintaining the structure of compact myelin. The most abundant 18.5 kDa isoform (170 amino acid length) has been used in most immunological studies. Different from MOG and PLP, MBP is found in both central and peripheral myelin, and MBP transcripts have also been demonstrated in peripheral lymphoid organs such as lymph nodes and thymus.[118] Without listing all the rodent strains in which MBP induces EAE, these include several mouse and rat strains, guinea pigs and nonhuman primates.[119] The

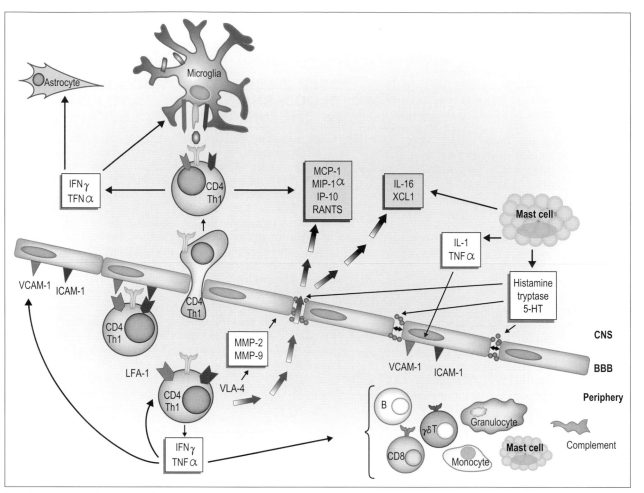

FIG. 13.2 Step 2. Trafficking of activated autoreactive CD4⁺ T cells, monocytes and other white blood cells through the blood–brain barrier (BBB) into the central nervous system (CNS) and local formation of the inflammatory lesion.

most important encephalitogenic MBP peptides in the various mouse and rat strains are summarized in references 5 and 112. While EAE in PL/J mice and Lewis rats runs an acute and monophasic course, it is relapsing–remitting in SJL/J mice.

An important parallel between mouse, rat, guinea pig and primate EAE models and MBP-specific immune responses in MS patients and healthy controls is the striking overlap between epitopes that are encephalitogenic in the context of MHC-class II alleles that confer susceptibility to EAE and the regions of MBP that are immunodominant for human MBP-specific T cells and recognized on MS-associated HLA-DR alleles, i.e. HLA-DR2a (DRB5*0101), -DRb (DRB1*1501), DRB1*0401/04 04/0405.[20,28,62] This applies to the immunodominant MBP (83–99) or (84–102) epitope, a promiscuous binder to all of the above MS-associated HLA-DR molecules,[120,121] but also to the immunodominant MBP (111–129) epitope in the context of DRB1*0401[122] and the region of MBP (140–168) that is immunodominant with DR2a[20,123] but also other DR alleles. Our recent study on high-avidity myelin-specific T cells in MS documented that, among these T cells MBP (83–99) is not immunodominant but MBP epitopes (13–32), (111–129) and (146–170) are.[30] Each of these MBP peptides has a very low predicted binding affinity to DR2a, DR2b, DR4 and other DR alleles, indicating that central tolerance mechanisms, i.e. the deletion of T cells with high functional avidity in the thymus, are incomplete. This situation is reminiscent of MBP Ac1–11 epitope in PL/J mice.[117]

The poor binding affinity of the latter MBP epitope to IAᵘ argues that complexes of MBP Ac1–11 with IAᵘ are unstable

and therefore inefficient in negative selection.[124] Transgenic expression of MBP Ac1–11-specific in different laboratories demonstrated that EAE is readily inducible with either MBP Ac1–11 or pertussis toxin only, and the MBP Ac1–11 TCR tg mice also exhibited spontaneous disease with varying frequencies depending on the level of microbial exposure.[125,126] A few years later Fugger and colleagues expressed a MBP (84–102)-specific and DR2b-restricted TCR from an MS patient in a humanized transgenic mouse model together with the DRA1*0101/DRB1*1501 heterodimer (DR2b).[17] EAE could readily be induced and about 4% of these animals developed spontaneous disease, clearly arguing that MS-patient-derived MBP-specific T cells have encephalitogenic potential. The complex of HLA-DR2b and MBP (84–102) was also detected in the brains of MS patients via staining with a monoclonal antibody that recognizes this peptide/HLA-DR complex, supporting the notion that the relevant complex of MS-associated HLA-DR molecule and immunodominant autoantigenic peptide is available in the CNS of MS patients.[127]

Finally, as already mentioned above, data from a therapeutic trial with an APL based on MBP (83–99) support the relevance of APL-specific Th1 cells that cross-reacted with the native MBP (83–99) peptide.[19] While the MBP (83–99) or (84–102) epitope has received by far the most attention, we could recently demonstrate encephalitogenicity in another humanized transgenic mouse model in which an MBP (111–129)-specific MS-patient-derived TCR was expressed as transgene together with the restriction element DRB1*0401.[18] Interestingly, only adoptive transfer EAE was inducible, there was no spontaneous disease development and a considerable percentage of animals not only developed signs of conventional EAE, i.e. limp tail, flaccid hind limb paresis or paralysis, but also involvement of caudal cranial nerves with swallowing difficulties and ataxia, indicating that clinical/phenotypic heterogeneity is related to the inducing myelin peptide.[128]

Additional evidence supporting the relevance of MBP as a target for the cellular immune response in MS include the following. Cross-reactivity between a large fraction of MBP (84–102)-specific Th1 cells and an identical sequence in the U24 antigen of HHV-6, a candidate infectious agent for MS, have been reported.[74] Mazza et al showed that MS patients had generally broader responses to MBP, i.e. recognized more epitopes,[129] and, like Vergelli et al, observed substantial intra- and interindividual fluctuations of the specificities of MBP-reactive T cells over time without clear relation to inflammatory MRI activity.[130]

Proteolipid protein

Proteolipid protein is the most abundant protein in CNS compact myelin (about 50%), highly hydrophobic and evolutionarily conserved across species. There are two main transcripts, the full-length 276 amino acid isoform and DM-20, an isoform that lacks 35 amino acids and is mainly expressed in brain and spinal cord prior to myelination, but also in peripheral lymphoid organs such as the thymus, where full-length PLP is barely found.[117,118,131] Interestingly, the major encephalitogenic and immunodominant PLP peptide (139–154) is contained in full-length PLP but not in DM-20.[118,131] This observation is thought to account for the encephalitogenicity and immunodominance of the PLP (139–154) peptide, since it is essentially not available for thymic negative selection and consequently a high precursor frequency of PLP (139–154)-specific T cells has been observed even in naive unprimed animals.[131,132]

When comparing PLP and MBP, the former is a stronger and dominant encephalitogen, at least in some EAE models, particularly in SJL/J mice, where PLP (139–151) is the dominant PLP peptide.[133] PLP TCR transgenic mice on the SJL/J background develop spontaneous EAE with very high frequency.[132] Further, upon EAE induction with whole spinal cord homogenate, the dominant T cell response is directed against PLP (139–151) and during subsequent disease relapses predictable epitope spreading has been observed to PLP (178–191) and later to MBP (89–101).[133] If EAE in SJL/J mice is induced with either the secondary PLP (178–191) epitope or with MBP (89–101), further waves of the disease always involve reactivity to the PLP (139–151) peptide.[133] Numerous other PLP peptides besides PLP (139–151) are encephalitogenic in different EAE models, e.g. PLP (178–191, 43–64, 56–70, 104–117; all subdominant in SJL mice,[134] PLP (217–233) in Lewis rats[117] and PLP (56–70) in Biozzi mice,[135] and this list is far from complete.

Although not examined quite as extensively as MBP in both EAE and in MS patients, the above parallels between encephalitogenic epitopes in EAE and immunodominant peptides in humans are also observed for PLP. PLP peptides (104–117), (142–153), (184–199) and (190–209) are immunodominant in MS patients and healthy controls, particularly in the context of the MS-associated DR2 alleles, but these peptides also bind to other HLA-DR alleles.[136] Further epitopes have been localized in the areas of PLP amino acid (30–49), (40–60), (89–106) and (95–116).[1] Our recent work on high-avidity myelin-specific T cells in MS documented that both the PLP (139–151) and the PLP (178–191) epitope are main targets of high avidity T cells and clearly elevated in MS versus healthy controls.[30]

Myelin oligodendrocyte glycoprotein

Myelin oligodendrocyte glycoprotein, a 218 amino acid transmembrane glycoprotein of the Ig superfamily, is much less abundant (0.01–0.05%) than MBP and PLP, and also different from the two major myelin proteins in being located not in compact myelin but exposed on the outermost surface of the oligodendrocyte membrane. Because of this 'strategic' location, it is directly accessible to antibodies and believed to be particularly relevant as a target for both cellular and humoral immune responses in MS. MOG is expressed relatively late during myelination and is only found in the brain/spinal cord and the retina but not in peripheral nerve. Furthermore, MOG expression is either completely or almost completely lacking in peripheral lymphoid tissues, although MOG transcripts have been seen in nonhuman primate peripheral nerve and a few samples of human tonsils and thymus.[117,118]

MOG-induced EAE is best examined in C57/BL6 mice, in which the MOG (35–55) peptide induces a chronic, nonrelapsing EAE.[137] Several other encephalitogenic MOG epitopes have been found in at least five mouse strains, four rat strains and nonhuman primates, and these data support the idea that central tolerance mechanisms for MOG are incomplete. A recently published MOG-TCR transgenic mouse model on the B6 background shows that spontaneous EAE with inflammation, demyelination and axonal damage in brain and spinal cord develops only in a small fraction of animals (about 4%), while 35% of these mice develop spontaneous optic neuritis.[138] Optic neuritis is also seen in MOG-induced EAE in DA rats,[128] and the relatively higher expression of MOG in the optic nerve has been proposed as one explanation for the involvement of the optic nerve.[138] The finding of the involvement of specific areas of the brain as well other clinical and immunological differences, i.e. involvement of antibodies versus cellular immune responses, between the various EAE models support the concept that the inducing antigens and the immunogenetic background contribute to the phenotypic expression of the disease.[128,139]

Examination of the human T cell response against MOG initially focused on the extracellular immunoglobulin domain (amino acid 1–122)[140] but later the responses to the transmembrane and intracellular components were tested as well.[141] Overall, much less information is available on the fine specificity of MOG-reactive T cells when compared to MBP and PLP, but immunodominant epitopes have been located in the Ig-like domain (amino acids 1–22, 11–30, -21–40, 31–50, 34–56), in the area of amino acids (63–87, 64–96, 71–90),[140,142] which interestingly also harbors several of the encephalitogenic regions in various EAE models,[143] and also in the intracellular parts of MOG, where amino acids (146–154) have been identified as an immunodominant epitope in the context of both DR15 (DRB1*1501; intermediate binding affinity) and DR4 (DRB1*0401; weak binding affinity).[141] The latter study found stronger responses toward intracellular as compared to extracellular portions of MOG and an overall broader reactivity to different MOG peptides in healthy controls versus controls, and the reverse was observed by Lindert.[144] When high avidity myelin-specific T cells were examined by Bielekova et al in 55 MS patients and 15 healthy controls,[30] MOG peptides (1–20) and (35–55) were among the six out of 15 immunodominant myelin peptides from MBP, PLP, MOG and CNPase that accounted for the clearly higher frequency of these cells in MS patients, supporting an important role of MOG as a target antigen of the cellular and humoral (see below) immune response in MS.

Myelin-associated glycoprotein

Myelin-associated glycoprotein (MAG) is a large (approximately 100 kDa) myelin glycoprotein that is located at the inner surface of the myelin sheath opposing the axon surface. It accounts for less than 1% of total myelin protein in the CNS and is even less abundant in the peripheral nervous system. The pathogenetic relevance of MAG has been documented for poly-neuropathies that are mediated by IgM antibodies against MAG. MAG (97–112) is encephalitogenic in ABH (H-2A[g7]) mice[145] and elevated MAG-specific T and B cell responses have been observed preferentially in the CSF of MS patients mainly by ELISPOT assays.[146] Among the few MAG peptides that have been examined, C-terminal areas, i.e. MAG (596–612) and (609–626), appeared relatively immunodominant, although the differences to the other peptides were not significant.[146] The preferential location of CNS lesions in cerebellum, centrum semiovale and forebrain in MAG-induced EAE in Lewis rats supports the notion that the antigen specificity is related to lesion location.[128]

2',3'-cyclic nucleotide 3' phosphodiesterase

2',3'-cyclic nucleotide 3' phosphodiesterase (CNPase) exists in two splice variants (CNPase I and II, 46 kDa and 48 kDa) and with about 3–4% of total myelin protein is the fourth most abundant one. It is located in oligodendrocytes mainly around the nucleus and in the paranodal loops, but also expressed in peripheral Schwann cells and much less in lymphoid tissues. Its exact role for myelin function is not clear. It has not been possible so far to demonstrate encephalitogenicity;[145] however, immunization of Lewis rats with a CNPase peptide with homology with a HSP65 peptide from mycobacteria resulted in protection from EAE.[147] CNPase is immunogenic both in rodents and in humans, and studies of the reactivity to either recombinant or native CNPase and to overlapping CNPase peptides have located a number of areas with promiscuous binding to several HLA-DR alleles, including the MS-associated DR15 molecules.[148,149] A C-terminal area (CNPase (343–373)) is among these and also one of the immunodominant epitopes that is recognized preferentially by high-avidity myelin-specific T cells of MS patients.[30]

Myelin-associated oligodendrocytic basic protein

Myelin-associated oligodendrocytic basic protein (MOBP) was discovered only recently. Several splice variants exist and the 81 amino acid isoform appears to be the most abundant in rodent and human myelin. According to current knowledge MOBP is exclusively expressed in oligodendrocytes, appears late in myelination and is located in the major dense line of compact myelin. MOBP is encephalitogenic in SJL/J mice and the encephalitogenic epitope was located within amino acid (37–60).[150,151] Preliminary studies of cellular anti-MOBP responses in MS patients and controls identified one immunodominant region (MOBP (21–39)).[150] The reactivity of MOBP-specific T cells cofluctuated with inflammatory MRI activity in some MS patients.[152]

Oligodendrocyte-specific glycoprotein

Oligodendrocyte-specific glycoprotein (OSP) is the third most abundant myelin protein (7%), expressed in the CNS and testis and located in the tight junctions, which led to it being grouped in the family of tight junction proteins and renaming it OSP/claudin-11. Several OSP peptides induce EAE in SJL/J mice[153,154] and OSP-specific antibodies are found in the CSF of relapsing–remitting MS patients.[155] Testing of PBMC from relapsing–remitting MS and secondary progressive MS patients and healthy controls with overlapping OSP peptides identified a number of immunogenic areas and overall strong responses in both healthy controls and relapsing–remitting MS patients, but decreased reactivity in secondary progressive MS.[156]

Alpha-B crystallin (αB-C)

Different from all the above listed myelin proteins αB crystallin (αB-C) was identified as an interesting candidate target first in MS patients and not in EAE models. Van Noort and colleagues fractionated MS brain-derived proteins and then systematically tested the proliferation of PBMC from MS patients and healthy controls against the brain protein fractions.[157] They observed prominent reactivity in one of the fractions and identified the small heat shock protein αB-C as the protein responsible for the strong immunogenicity.[157] αB-C is a major constituent of the eye lens but is also expressed in astrocytes and oligodendrocytes in active MS lesions.[158] A cryptic epitope of αB-C (amino acid 1–6) is weakly encephalitogenic in Biozzi ABH mice.[159] In addition to the above demonstration of strong responses to αB-C-containing MS brain-derived protein fractions, Chou and colleagues found DRB1*1501-restricted CD4[+] Th1 T cells in MS patients that responded to peptides (21–40), (41–60) and less to (131–150).[160] Other investigators documented comparable T cell responses to αB-C in MS patients and healthy controls.[161]

S100β protein

Linington and colleagues examined the encephalitogenicity of the astrocyte-derived calcium-binding protein S100 in Lewis rats and observed a strong immune response against the S100β epitope (amino acid 76–91) restricted by the RT1B1 Lewis MHC-class II molecule.[162] Unlike myelin antigens, S100 immunization or adoptive transfer of S100-specific T cells led to a panencephalitis and uveoretinitis but little if any clinical deficit.[162] The lack of clinical disease was related to the decreased recruitment of macrophages despite massive T cell infiltrates.[162] Further, unlike MBP-specific T cell lines, S100-specific T cells did not show cytotoxic activity. These observations were paralleled by data from MS patients and controls. Both CD4[+] and CD8[+] T cells specific for S100β could be isolated, with no differences between the groups.[161,163] S100-specific CD4[+] T cells less often exhibited cytotoxic activity compared with MBP-specific T cells from the same donors, and their HLA restriction could be established in about 50% of the T cell lines.[163]

In summary, myelin-reactive CD4[+] T cells are relevant in MS based on the following observations. They are increased in number and have relatively higher antigen avidity. Multiple different myelin proteins and peptides are recognized, and for therapeutic purposes one needs to know the specificity profile of the individual patient if one wants to achieve antigen-specific tolerization or immunomodulation. Myelin-specific CD4[+] T cells are skewed towards Th1 phenotypes and most often restricted by those HLA-DR molecules that are associated with MS. Finally, data from the APL trial and from humanized transgenic mice clearly demonstrate that myelin-specific CD4[+] T cells can be pathogenic.

Local reactivation of myelin-specific T cells

Local reactivation of invading T cells probably involves bystander activation and unveiling of host antigens. Destruction of CNS tissue during autoimmune inflammation leads to release of self-antigens, which can then be processed and presented by APCs resulting in the de novo activation of autoreactive T cells. This cascade of events can also lead to epitope spreading. It has been observed in the TMEV mouse model for MS, where an initial virus-specific T cell response broadens/spreads to myelin proteins during persistent infection of the CNS.[164] In addition, epitope spreading can include the presentation of cryptic epitopes that usually are not processed and presented as efficiently as immunodominant epitopes but that can be presented during specific conditions associated with viral infection.[165] During viral infection the expression of self-proteins in the infected tissue is often upregulated,[166] tissue-specific APCs are activated and the expression pattern of proteases in these APCs can be altered, leading to processing of cryptic epitopes that are not generated during 'normal' processing.[167] The recognition of such cryptic epitopes probably plays a more important role in the progression and perpetuation of the autoimmune response compared with the initial activation of autoreactive T cells.

AMPLIFICATION OF LOCAL INFLAMMATION

After reactivation in the CNS, autoreactive CD4+ T cells release both proinflammatory cytokines (IFNγ, TNFα, LT) and a number of chemokines (RANTES, IP-10, IL-8 and others) that orchestrate formation of the initial inflammatory lesion (Fig. 13.2) that resembles in many aspects a secondary lymphoid organ.[168] The proinflammatory cytokine release can activate resident cells such as microglia and astrocytes, which can then phagocytose myelin, increasing the reactivation of CD4+ T cells. The chemokine release by autoreactive CD4+ T cells in the CNS is crucial for the recruitment from the peripheral blood of other immune cells, including monocytes, CD8+ T cells, B cells.

Mast cells

Mast cells have also an important role in the recruitment of cells to the CNS. They can be attracted to the CNS via chemokines as RANTES, a potent chemoattractant for mast cells that is elevated in MS lesions.[169] Interestingly, not only the number of mast cells but also the concentration of mast-cell-released mediators such as tryptase[170] and histamine[171] have been found to be increased in the CSF of MS patients, suggesting increased mast cell degranulation in MS. The mast-cell-derived mediators could facilitate the development of MS participating in blood–brain barrier opening, as has been demonstrated by intramuscular injection of a mast cell degranulator that caused brain mast cell degranulation and blood–brain barrier alterations.[172] Mast cell mediators such as the chemokines lymphotactin and IL-16 have been shown to recruit leukocytes to the site of inflammation.[173] Other products such as TNFα and IL-1 can induce ICAM-1 and VCAM-1 expression and facilitate the adhesion of leukocytes to the endothelium. Histamine and tryptase can play a critical role in leukocyte-rolling.[174] Finally, mast cell proteases such as tryptase and chymase are capable of activating precursors of matrix metalloproteinases (MMPs) that are essential for leukocyte extravasation[175] and even the direct synthesis of MMP-2 and MMP-9 by mast cells has been reported.[176]

Role of chemokines

Numerous observations about the roles of chemokines and their receptors in MS have been reported.[177] The expression of CCR5 on circulating T cells has been found to be increased in MS patients compared with control populations.[178,179] Elevated CCR5 expression during disease relapse suggests a pathogenic role of CCR5+ T cells.[180] Increased CXCR3 expression on circulating T cells has also been shown in MS patients.[179] T cells expressing CCR5 and CXCR3 in MS patients were reported to produce high quantities of IFNγ and TNFα,[179] and MBP-specific Th1 cells express high levels of CXCR3 and CXCR6 chemokine receptors.[181]

The chemokines CCL5 (RANTES) and CXCL10 (IP-10) are elevated in the CSF of MS patients compared with controls, while CCL2 (MCP-1) was significantly decreased.[178] The increase of CXCL10 (IP-10) and decrease of CCL2 (MCP-1) in MS has been confirmed by other groups and appears to characterize the CSF of patients only during attacks and not during periods of disease inactivity.[182] In addition, the CCL2 (MCP-1) decrease correlated with active MRI, i.e. presence of inflammation and gadolinium-enhancing lesions in the brain,[182] suggesting that decreased CSF CCL2 (MCP-1) in active MS might

reflect a polarization of the immune response toward Th1 cytokine profile. CCL3 (MIP-1α↓Σ) has been found in the CSF of MS patients; however, it has also been found in patients with other neuroinflammatory diseases. Since comparable production of CCL2 and CCL5 by mononuclear cells in the CSF of MS patients and controls has been shown,[183] the source of these chemokines in the CSF remains to be elucidated.

Regarding the expression of chemokine receptors in the CSF of MS patients, initial studies documented a higher proportion of CSF-infiltrating T cells expressing CXCR3 and CCR5[178] compared with peripheral T cells. Since CSF T cells are enriched for the CD4+/CD45RO+ subset, corrections were introduced to ensure that comparable cell populations were analyzed in blood and CSF. This new analysis indicated that only CXCR3, not other receptors (CCR1–3, CCR5 and CCR6), was present at higher levels on CSF cells than on the corresponding blood population.[184] Interestingly, the same was observed in controls and interpreted as indicating that the presence of CXCR3+ cells in the CSF is independent of CNS inflammation.[178] CXCR3 expression probably facilitates the entry of T cells into the CSF and, through interactions with its intrathecal ligand, CXCL10 (IP-10), mediates the retention of T-cells in the inflamed CNS. Recently, an enrichment of CCR7+ memory Th1 lymphocytes coexpressing CCR5 and CXCR3 within the CSF in MS patients has been also reported.[185] Furthermore CSF infiltrating monocytes expressed comparably higher CCR1 and CCR5 levels than peripheral blood mononuclear cells,[186] but similar results were again obtained in controls, suggesting that the presence of CCR1+/CCR5+ monocytes in the CSF was independent of CNS inflammation.

A significant number of chemokines and the corresponding receptors have been detected in MS brain lesions, supporting a pathogenic role for these elements in MS and indicating that they might evolve into interesting therapeutic targets. CCL3 (MIP-1α), CCL4 (MIP-1β) and CCL5 (RANTES) are expressed within MS lesions, CCL4 (MIP-1β) in parenchymal inflammatory cells (macrophages and microglia), CCL3 (MIP-1α) also in parenchymal inflammatory cells and in activated neuroglial cells,[187] and CCL5 (RANTES) in perivascular inflammatory cells and to a lesser extent in astrocytes.[169,188] Other chemokines that have been found in active MS lesions, particularly in the center of the lesion expressed by astrocytes and inflammatory cells, include CCL2 (MCP-1),[178,182] CCL7 (MCP-3), CCL8 (MCP-2)[187] and CXCL10 (IP-10), which is expressed by astrocytes in MS lesions.[178,179]

From the standpoint of chemokine receptors, CXCR3 is expressed on the majority of perivascular T cells in MS brain lesions and CCR5 on a subset of these cells,[178,179] while CCR1 has been found on newly infiltrating monocytes, CCR2 and CCR3 on macrophages and CCR5 on infiltrating monocytes and also activated microglia cells.[178,179] More recently,[189] CXCR1, -2 and -3 have been shown to be expressed by oligodendrocytes in MS (and non-MS conditions, although at lower levels), and these cells colocalized with reactive astrocytes expressing the respective ligands (CXCL8, CXCL1 and CSCL10). The latter chemokines were not expressed by normal astrocytes in MS or in control CNS.

Further data supporting a role of chemokines and their receptors in MS comes from EAE models. Increased expression of chemokines such as CCL2 (MCP-1), CCL3 (MIP-1α), CCL5 (RANTES) and CXCL10 (IP-10) in EAE animals is closely associated with disease progression, while in vivo depletion results in decreased severity of EAE.[190] Data on the chemokine receptor CCR2 are controversial in that, in one study, mice deficient in CCR2[191] have been claimed to be resistant to EAE, while another on three different strains showed CCR2 mice to be susceptible to EAE, albeit to a lesser degree than wild-type. In contrast,

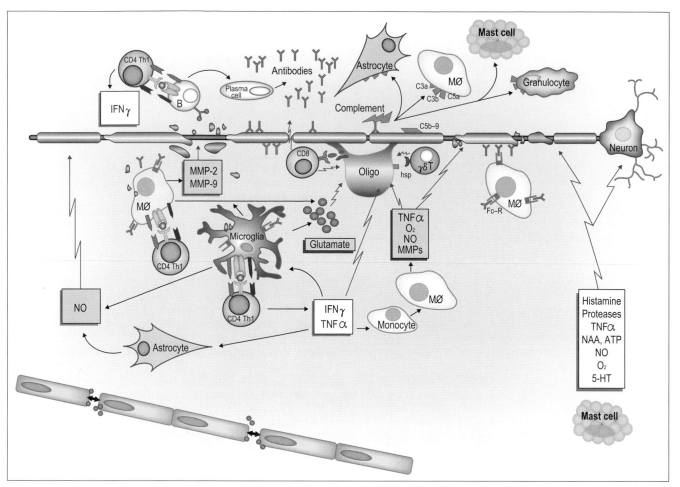

FIG. 13.3 Step 3. Effector mechanisms leading to damage of central nervous system tissue and factors involved in lesion resolution.

CCR5-deficient mice showed the same level of disease severity as control animals,[192] suggesting that T cell accumulation in the CNS during EAE does not function through CCR5.

STEP 3: DAMAGE WITHIN THE CENTRAL NERVOUS SYSTEM

The last step is the damage of CNS tissue, i.e. of the myelin sheath and oligodendrocytes but also of axons, and the activation of the astroglial scarring response (Fig. 13.3). In contrast to the above events, during which CD4+ autoreactive T cells are most probably driving the process, their role in the effector phase is probably secondary, and many other cells and processes mediate tissue damage.[193] In this section we will describe the main components of the immune system that participate in myelin/oligodendrocyte and axonal damage and also refer to events in the CNS involved in lesion resolution.

B cells and antibodies

Despite the mostly accepted view that MS is a T-cell-mediated autoimmune disease, antibodies are probably very important during other steps such as the development of demyelinating plaques. The observation of elevated Igs in the CSF of MS patients[194] has been the most important and earliest evidence suggesting a role of B cells and antibodies in the pathology of MS. The correlations between increased concentrations of antibodies in the CSF of MS patients with episodes of worsening and the absence of oligoclonal bands (OCB) in patients with more benign course[195] also suggest the involvement of humoral responses in MS.

B cells do not cross the intact blood–brain barrier; however, once inflammation has started and led to blood–brain barrier disruption, B cells, antibodies and complement factors can enter the CNS parenchyma.[196] B cells can be activated outside or within the CNS. The observation of increased Igs in MS patients in the CSF, i.e. intrathecally,[194] but not in the serum, indicates that they are produced locally within the CNS. Different mechanisms may be involved in B cell activation and the corresponding antibody production, e.g. as a result of stimulation with antigen from either self or foreign proteins, through a random bystander effect of the inflammatory response observed in MS lesions or by superantigen stimulation. Sequence analysis of the antigen binding Ig variable regions revealed a high frequency of clonally expanded memory B cells and a predominance of the variable heavy chain-4 (VH4) type in CSF B cells of MS patients[197,198] and also in lesions,[199,200] suggesting selection by a specific antigen and not by unspecific bystander activation. In addition CSF Igs of MS patients show an oligoclonal distribution, i.e. only a limited number of B cell clones contribute to the increased CSF Igs.[198,201]

B cells and antibodies can contribute to MS disease pathogenesis in various ways.

- B cells can act as antigen presenting cells that take up and present antigen to autoreactive T cells. The observation that the epitope specificity of the Abs generated during EAE and the encephalitogenic T cell epitopes as well as the immunodominant T- and B-cell epitopes in humans can be overlapping or identical[202,203] supports this mechanism.

- B cells can also act by providing co-stimulation to autoreactive T cells. This is indicated by data that the number of circulating B cells expressing B7–1 is higher during MS exacerbations,[204] although this observation has not been confirmed by others.[205]
- It has been reported that B cells and autoantibodies bound to tissues can recruit autoreactive T cells to the site of inflammation resulting in infiltration of T cells, monocytes and eosinophils.[206]
- Recently a new mechanism has been proposed by which idiotope-specific T cells are activated by CSF Igs, and subsequently these activated T cells activate and sustain B cells producing such idiotopes.[207]
- Finally, the production of myelin-specific antibodies and the destruction of myelin within plaques appears to be the most important way how B cells contribute to disease pathogenesis and also the one for which the most convincing data has been reported.[208]

The first evidence for an important contribution of humoral factors to inflammatory demyelination in EAE was already provided in 1959,[209] when it was demonstrated that a serum factor from animals affected with EAE, which was later identified as myelin-specific Igs, displayed demyelinating activity in vitro.[210] Similar activity was also demonstrated in vitro with serum from MS patients.[211] Further support came from histopathological studies of CNS tissue and the analysis of CSF. B cells, plasma cells and myelin-specific antibodies are detected in MS plaques and in areas of active demyelination in MS patients.[208,212,213]

Antibodies can cause demyelination by several effector mechanisms. One of these is the opsonization of myelin for subsequent phagocytosis by macrophages, which has been observed in MS and EAE.[214] Serum antimyelin antibodies raise macrophage phagocytosis, and the uptake by macrophages of CNS myelin increases after opsonization with complement.[215] Another mechanism of demyelination that involves autoantibodies is through activation of the entire complement cascade leading to membrane attack complex (MAC) deposition and complement-mediated cytolysis.[216] Studies of acute MS lesions found complement localized to areas of active demyelination.[217,218] A correlation of neurological disability and CSF concentrations of the terminal complement complex has been demonstrated in MS patients.[219] The presence of MAC-enriched vesicles in the CSF of MS further suggests a contribution of complement-mediated injury to myelin damage in vivo,[220] and EAE data support this mechanism. The demyelinating potential of an Ab in EAE has been correlated with its ability to fix complement and the soluble complement receptor (sCR1), which blocks complement activation, inhibited EAE severity.[221]

Although these data collectively argue for an involvement of B cells and antibodies in demyelinaton in MS, it is important to note that there is considerable heterogeneity in lesion composition in different patients. Antibody deposition and/or complement activation appear relevant for lesion pathogenesis in some MS patients, while different immunologic mechanisms or oligodendrocyte apoptosis dominate in others[217] (and see below).

It was hoped that the identfication of the specificity of intrathecal Igs in MS patients would provide clues as to which targets are recognized and how they might participate in disease pathogenesis. Despite intensive research, the antigenic specificity/ies for CSF antibodies in MS have yet to be established. It is important to point out that CSF oligoclonal bands do not usually contain autoantibodies against the major myelin components[222] but are sometimes directed against infectious agents.[223]

Despite the fact that MBP is an immunodominant T cell antigen, a pathogenic contribution of MBP-specific antibodies in EAE has not been established and the presence of anti-MBP antibodies in the serum and CSF of MS patients is controversial. While some studies emphasized the relevance of MBP-specific antibodies.[224,225] others failed to confirm these data.[226–228] Furthermore, unbiased screenings of antigen libraries with CSF-derived antibodies did not identify MBP epitopes as antibody targets.[229,230] Technical considerations as well as the low-affinity interactions that characterized these antibodies[231] may contribute to the controversial results. Increased numbers of anti-PLP secreting B cells have been detected in the CSF of MS patients.[232] It has been proposed that MS patients with a prominent antibody response against PLP are distinct from those showing antibody responses against MBP.[233]

Antibodies with specificity against minor myelin components have also been detected in MS patients. MOG is the most interesting candidate B-cell autoantigen in MS. Because of its location it is an ideal target for antibody-mediated demyelination. Anti-MOG antibodies are indeed able to cause myelin destruction in EAE models,[234–236] while other antibodies against major myelin proteins such as MBP or PLP, which are both not located on the myelin surface, do not cause myelin destruction on their own. Anti-MOG Abs mediate a characteristic vesicular transformation of compact myelin in acutely demyelinated lesions that also has been documented in human MS lesions[208] strongly suggesting a role of anti-MOG Abs in MS. The B-cell response to MOG is enhanced in MS[144,237] also supporting the pathogenic importance of anti-MOG Abs. Interestingly, the presence of serum anti-MOG antibodies, with or without anti-MBP antibodies, in patients presenting with an initial clinical event suggestive of central nervous system demyelination and evidence of multifocal lesions on MRI studies, is predictive of subsequent clinical events that establish the diagnosis of clinically definitive MS.[238] However, the presence of anti-MOG antibodies in patients with nondemyelinating diseases of the CNS, as well as in a substantial number of healthy individuals, has raised important questions about the role of these antibodies in MS, and these need to be addressed in future studies.

Another minor component of myelin is MAG, and antibodies specific for this protein have also been observed in MS patients.[239] The low level of anti-MAG antibodies suggest that the immune response to MAG might be secondary to the demyelinating process but that it could play a role in the progression of the disease.[240] Antibodies against two other minor myelin components, OSP[149] and CNPase,[241] as well as against the enzyme transaldolase H have been detected in MS patients.[242]

Interestingly, humoral responses against nonprotein components of myelin or axons such as various glycolipids including glycosphingolipids,[243] sulfatide[244] or GD1a[245] and GM-3[246] have also been described, and a pathological role in demyelination has been suggested, particularly for antibodies against galactocerebroside (GalC), a major galactosphingolipid of myelin. The evidence includes similarities between the patterns of anti-GalC-induced demyelination in CNS cultures of mouse cerebellum and whole-spinal-cord-induced EAE, the elevated antibody titers to GalC found in sera from rabbits with whole-spinal-cord-induced EAE,[247] absorption studies on antimyelin serum tested in vitro[248] and the pathogenic effect of anti-GalC mAb exacerbating inflammation in the CNS in EAE mice,[249] although there is at present no hint as to these antibodies in MS.

αB-crystallin is another interesting candidate autoantigen in MS, since stress induces its expression in the CNS. Anticrystallin antibodies have been detected in sera from MS patients in two different studies.[250,251] However, the data about the isotype of these antibodies is controversial. While IgM and IgG responses have been detected in the sera of MS patients in one study,[250] the other found only IgM antibodies.[251] The lack of anti-αB-C antibodies in the CSF of MS patients indicates that their role in MS pathogenesis is limited.

The light neurofilament subunit (NF-L), a major component of the axonal cytoskeleton, represents another interesting candidate autoantigen. Elevated CSF levels of NF-L have suggested that it as an indicator of axonal damage in several neurological diseases, including MS.[252] The intrathecal production of IgG antibodies to NF-L appears to be raised in progressive MS and may serve as a marker of axonal loss and disease progression.[253] The CSF from MS patients also contains antibodies against a cell surface glycoprotein called AN2, which is expressed by oligodendrocyte precursor cells. In vitro, these antibodies are able to suppress the synthesis of myelin proteins and lyse oligodendrocyte precursor cells.[254] Nogo-A is a protein associated with CNS myelin that is thought to impair regenerative responses and the sprouting and plastic changes of synaptic terminals. Interestingly, autoantibodies to Nogo-A are frequent in the CSF of MS patients as well as in the serum in MS, inflammatory and noninflammatory neurological diseases but not in neurodegenerative diseases.[255]

Finally, antibodies with specificity against ubiquitous proteins have also been related with MS; for example, antibodies against the proteasome, a family of proteases, have been found in the serum and CSF in more than 60% of MS patients, suggesting that proteasome members serve as autoantigens in MS. Interestingly, 40% of these MS patients also showed T cell responses against some subunits of the proteasome complex.[256] High affinity anti-DNA antibodies have been mentioned as a major component of the intrathecal B cell response in MS. Anti-DNA antibodies from some patients suffering from systemic lupus erythematosus bound efficiently to the surface of neuronal cells and oligodendrocytes supporting a role for these antibodies in the demyelinating process.[233] Using completely unbiased approaches additional antibodies have been identified. In a recent study, antibodies binding to intact cultured human oligodendrocyte cell lines have been identified in sera from MS patients and other inflammatory CNS diseases.[257] Although the antigens targeted by these antibodies still have to be elucidated, this represents a promising approach to identify cell surface autoantigens that are accessible to antibodies and could initiate demyelination at least in some MS patients.

Another unbiased approach employs proteomics technologies. Proteomics is the large-scale study of expression, function and interaction of proteins that can be applied to identify the specificity of autoantibodies utilizing cDNA expression libraries, peptide libraries or arrayed fractions of autoimmune target tissues. Once candidate autoantigens are identified, proteomics technologies can characterize the sensitivity and specificity of autoantibodies directed against candidate antigens in cohorts of autoimmune and control patients as well as in experimental autoimmune conditions.[258]

Complement

Complement serves as an auxiliary effector system in immunity and the antimicrobial defense. Its activation occurs via a cascade of proteolytic steps. Three different pathways of activation are distinguished, the classical pathway triggered by target-bound antibody, the lectin pathway triggered by microbial repetitive polysaccharide structures and the alternative pathway triggered by recognition of other foreign surface structures. All three merge in the pivotal activation of C3 and subsequently of C5 by highly specific enzymatic complexes. In the common terminal pathway, additional complement components are activated and assembled into the MAC. The entire activation machinery is controlled by numerous inhibitors, which are expressed on the surface of most cells, protecting them against autologous complement attack.

The human brain is considered an immunologically privileged tissue, and as part of this privilege separated from the peripheral immune system via the blood–brain barrier. Nevertheless, all major cell types in the brain, including oligodendrocytes, were shown to produce most of the complement proteins.[259] Astrocytes, the most abundant glial cells, are the major source of complement in the brain, thereby providing immune defense against invading pathogens but also contributing to brain damage in some diseases. The process of demyelination characteristic of MS not only results from an autoimmune response against myelin components with production of antibodies and subsequent activation of the classical pathway but also from direct activation of the complement cascade by binding of some complement factors to myelin. Purified CNS myelin, but not peripheral nervous system myelin, can activate the classical pathway of complement.[260] Furthermore, mature rat oligodendrocytes cultured in vitro are lysed by complement in the absence of antimyelin antibodies.[261] MOG may represent the myelin component that is capable of binding and activating the C1q component of complement.[262] MOG harbors a protein domain similar to the C1q-binding sequence previously identified in antibodies. Complement activation results in oligodendrocyte lysis and chemoattraction of macrophages. It has been suggested that the high susceptibility of oligodendrocytes to injury by complement could be facilitated by the lack of the protective, and otherwise ubiquitously distributed complement inhibitors. CR1 (CD35), membrane cofactor protein (MCP, CD46) and homologous restriction factor (HRF) were not expressed on oligodendrocytes while CD59 showed substantial heterogeneity.[262,263]

CD8+ T cells

In contrast to the extensive data on CD4+ T cells and their role in both EAE and MS, much less is known about CD8+ T cells, not only in MS but in general in human autoimmune diseases. However, several lines of evidence suggest a contribution of CD8+ T cells in MS pathogenesis and particularly in the effector phases that lead to tissue damage.[8,10] These data are:

- Except for microglia, none of the resident CNS cells express MHC-class II constitutively. It can be induced on astrocytes by IFNγ;[264] however, oligodendrocytes and neurons do not express class II molecules at all, and can thus not serve as APCs to CD4+ T cells, but nevertheless be recognized by CD8+ T cells[265]
- Strong oligoclonal expansions of CD8+ memory T cells have been found in the CSF[266] and in MS brain tissue,[267] and a persistence of certain CD8+ T cell clones in CSF and blood[267]
- CD8+ T cells are more prevalent in MS brain tissue than CD4+ T cells[268]
- MHC-class I can be induced on neurons that are functionally compromised[269] and CD8+ virus-specific T cells can directly lyse neurons via Fas/Fas-L-mediated cytolysis[270]
- A number of HLA-class I-restricted myelin epitopes have been described for MBP, PLP, MAG and others[25,271–273] and the CD8+ cytotoxic T cell response to MBP is increased in MS patients[273]
- CD8+ myelin-specific T cells secrete chemoattractants (IL-16 and IP-10) for CD4+ myelin-specific T cells[274]
- The MBP (79–87)-specific CD8+ T cell clones from wild-type C3H mice are encephalitogenic and induce a disease phenotype that resembles MS more closely with respect to the presence of ataxia and spasticity than some of the CD4+ T cell-mediated EAE models.[13]

MOG-specific CD8+ T cells can also mediate EAE.[14] Further data supporting a role of CD8+ T cells is the increased production of lymphotoxin in SP-MS patients,[275] their selectively increased adhesion to brain venules,[276] an increased frequency of CD8+ T cells against EBV epitopes in MS patients[277] and a correlation between cytokine production by CD8+ T cells and MRI-documented tissue destruction.[278] As a caveat, the studies on the specificity of CD8+ T cells and their restriction largely employed HLA-A2-transfected cells. HLA-A2 is found in MS patients at lower frequency than in the general populations and the MS-associated class I alleles HLA-A3 and –B7 have so far received little attention. Furthermore, unlike the extensive studies on CD4+ autoreactive T cells in EAE and MS, which have been repeated and confirmed by several groups, the observations on CD8+ autoreactive T cells in most instances await confirmation.

Nitric oxide synthase

Phagocytes (granulocytes and macrophages) are equipped with the enzymatic machinery that generates highly toxic reactive oxygen and nitrogen intermediates, which exert potent antimicrobial activities. The enzyme inducible nitric oxide synthase (iNOS) generates large amounts of nitric oxide (NO), a short-lived and bioactive free radical that is toxic to bacteria, and other reactive nitrogen species such as peroxynitrite. NOS has been found in MS lesions, suggesting that NO may play a role in MS pathology.[279] Although initial studies have shown that NO can mediate microglia-induced cytotoxicity[280] and also necrosis of rodent oligodendrocytes,[281] suggesting that NO could mediate CNS injury, the actual role of NOS in MS is not clear. The results from blocking NOS in EAE are not conclusive[282] and additional data suggest that NO may even have an anti-apoptotic effect under certain conditions[283] or modulate immune response in a beneficial way.[284]

γδ T cells

In MS patients, a significantly increased number of γδ T cells was detected in the CSF[285] and in some brain lesions.[286,287] These γδ T cells can lyse oligodendrocytes, mainly via the perforin pathway,[288] suggesting a role in MS. Two main fractions of γδ T cells have been described: one expressing Vγ1 resides within epithelial tissues, where it may provide a first line of defense against infections and cancer. The second fraction expressing Vγ2 represents the majority of peripheral blood γδ T cells, infiltrates chronic lesions and is detected in the CSF of MS patients.[289,290] Interestingly, it has been observed that oligodendrocytes selectively stimulate the expansion of the Vγ2 subtype of γδ T cells.[291] The limited TCR heterogeneity that has been shown for CSF-infiltrating γδ T cells in MS suggests a common antigen reactivity for these cells.[292,293] Pointing in the same direction, it has been observed that human γδ T cells can lyse oligodendrocytes without the need for intermediary APCs, possibly involving the recognition of heat shock proteins (hsp),[290,291,294] αB-C, a member of the hsp family present in the oligodendrocyte/myelin complex and candidate autoantigen in MS,[157] or even nonpeptide antigens.[295,296] Interestingly, the Vγ2 subtype of γδ T cells, when selectively stimulated by oligodendrocytes, is particularly reactive to hsps.[291] These findings, together with EAE studies, in which γδ T cells appear to be important early mediators of damage,[297] support a role of γδ T cells in MS pathogenesis.

Cytotoxic CD4+ T cells

With respect to biological function, the cytotoxic activity of CD4+ T cells is relatively poorly understood compared to CD8+ T cells. MBP-specific CD4+ T cells mediate both perforin- and Fas/Fas-L-mediated cytotoxicity of MBP- or MBP-peptide-pulsed targets.[298] When we compared MBP-specific T cells that were restricted by either DR2a or DR2b, we observed that the former only employ the more efficient perforin-mediated killing or are noncytotoxic, whereas DR2b-restricted MBP-specific CD4+ T cells exclusively exhibit Fas/Fas-L-mediated cytolysis.[298] Currently, it is not known how this relates to the pathogenesis of MS, i.e. whether the differences in cytolysis indicate special roles of autoreactive CD4+ T cells that use different restriction elements. It is unlikely that direct lysis of oligodendrocytes and even less neurons involves CD4+ T cells since both types of CNS cells do not express HLA-class II. A subtype of MBP-specific CD4+ TCRα/β+ T cells expresses the neural cell adhesion molecule (NCAM) family member CD56 (also a marker for NK cells) and is capable of lysing CD56+ target cells via homotypic CD56–CD56 interactions without requirement of HLA restriction.[299] A number of CNS cells including oligodendrocytes express CD56, and it has been shown that CD4+ CD56+ T cells can lyse oligodendrocytes in an HLA-unrestricted fashion.[300]

Cytokines

Although the administration of cytokines can induce disease relapses in an animal model of EAE,[301] there are very few examples where the local overexpression of inflammatory cytokines or chemokines alone can break tolerance to autoantigens in healthy animals. The local expression of IL-2, IL-12 and IP-10 in diabetes has been shown to lead to inflammation but not clinical disease,[302] and only the overexpression of IFNγ in pancreatic β cells disrupted tolerance to autoantigens,[303] probably because IFNγ strongly enhances the presentation of self-antigens.

In EAE and MS, a number of proinflammatory cytokines have been shown to contribute to both neuroinflammation and neurodegeneration, and these include IFNγ, TNFα, LT-α, IL-1, IL-6, IL-8, IL-12, IL-17, IL-18 and IL-23.[301–305] Proinflammatory cytokines are produced either by activated infiltrating CD4+ T cells (IFNγ, TNFα, LT-α)[168] or by microglia (IL-1, IL-6)[306] and contribute to blood–brain barrier opening, recruitment and local activation of cells, formation of the inflammatory focus and its maintenance. Recent studies indicated that cytokines such as IL-17 and IL-23 may be particularly relevant for the proinflammatory processes,[305–307] although these data await further confirmation and are so far mainly derived from animal studies. Furthermore, it needs to be noted that not only may inflammation in the target tissue, i.e. the CNS, have detrimental effects but that at least parts of the inflammatory response are required for removing debris of damaged cells and membranes and for restoring the local cytoarchitecture. Besides local macrophage/microglia activation, even proinflammatory T cells themselves can be involved in such beneficial effects.[308,309] Furthermore, the growth factor milieu that is created during inflammatory responses is not relevant only for the maturation and migration of precursor cells[310] but also for preventing the deposition of sclerotic tissue by astroglia, which would further impair reconstitution of damage.[311,312]

Glutamate-mediated damage

Increased production and decreased degradation or reuptake of the excitatory neurotransmitter glutamate by astrocytes leads to glutamate-mediated excitotoxicity of oligodendrocytes via AMPA receptor-mediated calcium influx.[313] Calcium accumulation in the myelin sheath, however, appears to be mediated by NMDA receptors.[314] While glutamate-mediated excitotoxicity as a mechanism of tissue damage is well established in neurodegenerative disorders and stroke, this topic clearly merits further study in MS and EAE.[315]

Apoptosis and its role in central nervous system tissue damage in multiple sclerosis

Cell damage via apoptosis plays different roles in the CNS. Initial observations documented that CD95/CD95L-mediated apoptosis is an important process for eliminating invading activated T cells.[316] Together with the upregulation of the inhibitory costimulatory ligand CTLA-4 on astrocytes[317] and the downregulation of adhesion molecule and MHC class II expression on microglia by astrocyte-derived factors such as TGFβ[317] and the tryptophan-metabolizing enzyme indoleamine 2,3 dioxygenase,[316–318] apoptosis induction in T cells is one of the mechanisms that constitutes the immune privilege of the CNS. In distinction to other immunoprivileged sites, the TNF-related apoptosis inducing ligand (TRAIL) is not expressed in the brain; however, both apoptosis-mediating and -blocking TRAIL receptors are found on neurons, microglia and astrocytes[319,320] and encephalitogenic T cells can injure neurons[321] and oligodendrocytes via TRAIL and induction of the c-Jun terminal kinase pathway.[322,323] Consistent with these observations, one of the pathological lesion patterns described by Lucchinetti et al shows prominent oligodendrocyte apoptosis[208] and another study of very early lesions in relapsing–remitting MS also emphasizes its role.[324]

CONCLUSIONS

With the better understanding of basic immunological mechanisms and the steady addition of new factors, receptors and effector molecules, our concepts of the immunology of MS have continuously evolved. It may still be accurate to describe MS as a CD4+ Th1-mediated autoimmune disease, but this is only a rough approximation and does not account for many other factors that play important roles during the various stages of the disease. Not only does MS have a highly complex genetic background that affects numerous aspects of the immune system, but in addition the different contributing factors vary from patient to patient. The latter fact complicates research of the human disease considerably and has led to some investigators even stratifying the MS lesion patterns into different subtypes,[217] a pattern yet to be confirmed. Dissecting MS disease heterogeneity further and addressing which immunological mechanisms or CNS factors influence its phenotypic expression will be central aims of clinical and basic MS research in the future.

REFERENCES

1. Sospedra M, Martin R. Immunology of multiple sclerosis. Annu Rev Immunol 2005; 23: 683–747.
2. Frohman EM, Racke MK, Raine CS. Multiple sclerosis: the plaque and its pathogenesis. N Engl J Med 2006; 354: 942–955.
3. Raine CS, Scheinberg LC. On the immunopathology of plaque development and repair in multiple sclerosis. J Neuroimmunol 1988; 20: 189–201.
4. Bruck W, Stadelmann C. Inflammation and degeneration in multiple sclerosis. Neurol Sc 2003; 24(suppl 5): S265–S267.
5. Martin R, McFarland HF, McFarlin DE. Immunological aspects of demyelinating diseases. Annu Rev Immunol 1992; 10: 153–187.
6. Oksenberg JR, Barcellos LF, Cree BA et al. Mapping multiple sclerosis susceptibility to the HLA-DR locus in African Americans. Am J Hum Genet 2004; 74: 160–167.
7. Engelhardt B, Ransohoff RM. The ins and outs of T-lymphocyte traficking to the CNS: anatomical sites and molecular mechanisms. Trends Immunol 2005; 26: 485–495.
8. Friese MA, Fugger L. Autoreactive CD8+ T cells in multiple sclerosis: a new target for therapy? Brain 2005; 128: 1747–1763.
9. Kieseier BC, Hemmer B, Hartung HP. Multiple sclerosis – novel insights and new therapeutic strategies. Curr Opin Neurol 2005; 18: 211–220.
10. Goverman J, Perchellet A, Huseby ES. The role of CD8+ T cells in multiple sclerosis and its animal models. Curr Drug Targets Inflamm Allergy 2005; 4: 239–245.
11. Owens T. Animal models for multiple sclerosis. Adv Neurol 2006; 98: 77–89.
12. Zamvil S, Nelson P, Trotter J et al. T-cell clones specific for myelin basic protein induce chronic relapsing paralysis and demyelination. Nature 1985; 317: 355–358.
13. Huseby ES, Liggitt D, Brabb T et al. A pathogenic role for myelin-specific CD8+ T cells in a model for multiple sclerosis. J Exp Med 2001; 194: 669–676.
14. Sun D, Whitaker JN, Huang Z et al. Myelin antigen-specific CD8+ T cells are encephalitogenic and produce severe disease in C57BL/6 mice. J Immunol 2001; 166: 7579–7587.
15. Das P, Drescher KM, Geluk A et al. Complementation between specific HLA-DR and HLA-DQ genes in transgenic mice determines susceptibility to experimental autoimmune encephalomyelitis. Hum Immunol 2000; 61: 279–289.
16. Kawamura K, Yamamura T, Yokoyama K et al. Hla-DR2-restricted responses to proteolipid protein 95–116 peptide cause autoimmune encephalitis in transgenic mice. J Clin Invest 2000; 105: 977–984.
17. Madsen LS, Andersson EC, Jansson L et al. A humanized model for multiple sclerosis using HLA-DR2 and a human T-cell receptor. Nat Genet 1999; 23: 343–347.
18. Shukaliak Quandt J, Baig M et al. Unique clinical and pathological features in HLA-DRB1*0401-restricted MBP 111–129-specific humanized transgenic mice. J Exp Med 2004; 200: 223–234.
19. Bielekova B, Goodwin B, Richert N et al. Encephalitogenic potential of the myelin basic protein peptide (amino acids 83–99) in multiple sclerosis: results of a phase II clinical trial with an altered peptide ligand. Nat Med 2000; 6: 1167–1175.
20. Ota K, Matsui M, Milford EL et al. T-cell recognition of an immunodominant myelin basic protein epitope in multiple sclerosis. Nature 1990; 346: 183–187.
21. Olsson T, Sun J, Hillert J et al. Increased numbers of T cells recognizing multiple myelin basic protein epitopes in multiple sclerosis. Eur J Immunol 1992; 22: 1083–1087.
22. Martin R, Voskuhl R, Flerlage M et al. Myelin basic protein-specific T-cell responses in identical twins discordant or concordant for multiple sclerosis. Ann Neurol 1993; 34: 524–535.
23. Bieganowska KD, Ausubel LJ, Modabber Y et al. Direct ex vivo analysis of activated, Fas-sensitive autoreactive T cells in human autoimmune disease. J Exp Med 1997; 185: 1585–1594.
24. Muraro PA, Wandinger KP, Bielekova B et al. Molecular tracking of antigen-specific T cell clones in neurological immune-mediated disorders. Brain 2003; 126: 20–31.
25. Crawford MP, Yan SX, Ortega SB et al. High prevalence of autoreactive, neuroantigen-specific CD8+ T cells in multiple sclerosis revealed by novel flow cytometric assay. Blood 2004; 103: 4222–4231.
26. Allegretta M, Nicklas JA, Sriram S, Albertini RJ. T cells responsive to myelin basic protein in patients with multiple sclerosis. Science 1990; 247: 718–721.
27. Martin R, Jaraquemada D, Flerlage M et al. Fine specificity and HLA restriction of myelin basic protein-specific cytotoxic T cell lines from multiple sclerosis patients and healthy individuals. J Immunol 1990; 145: 540–548.
28. Pette M, Fujita K, Kitze B et al. Myelin basic protein-specific T lymphocyte lines from MS patients and healthy individuals. Neurology 1990; 40: 1770–1776.
29. Hemmer B, Fleckenstein BT, Vergelli M et al. Identification of high potency microbial and self ligands for a human autoreactive class II-restricted T cell clone. J Exp Med 1997; 185: 1651–1659.
30. Bielekova B, Sung MH, Kadom N et al. Expansion and functional relevance of high-avidity myelin-specific CD4+ T cells in multiple sclerosis. J Immunol 2004; 172: 3893–3904.
31. Anderson AC, Nicholson LB, Legge KL et al. High frequency of autoreactive myelin proteolipid protein-specific T cells in the periphery of naive mice: mechanisms of selection of the self-reactive repertoire. J Exp Med 2000; 191: 757–760.
32. Segal BM, Dwyer BK, Shevach EM. An interleukin (IL) 10/IL 12 immunoregulatory circuit controls susceptibility to autoimmune disease. J Exp Med 1998; 187: 537–546.
33. Matusevicius D, Kivisakk P, Navikas V et al. Interleukin-12 and perforin mRNA expression is augmented in blood mononuclear cells in multiple sclerosis. Scand J Immunol 1998; 47: 582–590.
34. Ozenci V, Pashenkov M, Kouwenhoven M et al. IL-12/IL-12R system in multiple

sclerosis. J Neuroimmunol 2001; 114: 242–252.

35. Matusevicius D, Kivisakk P, He B et al. Interleukin-17 mRNA expression in blood and CSF mononuclear cells is augmented in multiple sclerosis. Mult Scler 1999; 5: 101–104.

36. Ferber IA, Brocke S, Taylor-Edwards C et al. Mice with a disrupted IFN-gamma gene are susceptible to the induction of experimental autoimmune encephalomyelitis (EAE). J Immunol 1996; 156: 5–7.

37. Willenborg DO, Fordham S, Bernard CC et al. IFN-gamma plays a critical down-regulatory role in the induction and effector phase of myelin oligodendrocyte glycoprotein-induced autoimmune encephalomyelitis. J Immunol 1996; 157: 3223–3227.

38. Zhang GX, Yu S, Gran B et al. Role of IL-12 receptor beta 1 in regulation of T cell response by APC in experimental autoimmune encephalomyelitis. J Immunol 2003; 171: 4485–4492.

39. Becher B, Durell BG, Noelle RJ. Experimental autoimmune encephalitis and inflammation in the absence of interleukin-12. J Clin Invest 2002; 110: 493–497.

40. Gran B, Zhang GX, Yu S et al. IL-12p35-deficient mice are susceptible to experimental autoimmune encephalomyelitis: evidence for redundancy in the IL-12 system in the induction of central nervous system autoimmune demyelination. J Immunol 2002; 169: 7104–7110.

41. Langrish CL, Chen Y, Blumenschein WM et al. IL-23 drives a pathogenic T cell population that induces autoimmune inflammation. J Exp Med 2005; 201: 233–240.

42. Korn T, Bettelli E, Gao W et al. IL-21 initiates an alternative pathway to induce proinflammatory T(H)17 cells. Nature 2007; 448: 484–487.

43. Bettelli E, Carrier Y, Gao W et al. Reciprocal developmental pathways for the generation of pathogenetic effector TH17 and regulatory T cells. Nature 2006; 441: 235–238.

44. Langrish CL, Chen Y, Blumenschein WM et al. IL-23 drives a pathogenic T cell population that induces autoimmune inflammation. J Exp Med 2005; 201: 233–240.

45. Lock C, Hermans G, Pedotti R et al. Harvest of gene microarray analysis of multiple sclerosis lesions yields new targets validated in the experimental autoimmune encephalomyelitis model. Nature Med 2002; 8: 500–508.

46. Lafaille JJ, Keere FV, Hsu AL et al. Myelin basic protein-specific T helper 2 (Th2) cells cause experimental autoimmune encephalomyelitis in immunodeficient hosts rather than protect them from the disease. J Exp Med 1997; 186: 307–312.

47. Correale J, Gilmore W, McMillan M et al. Patterns of cytokine secretion by autoreactive proteolipid protein-specific T cell clones during the course of multiple sclerosis. J Immunol 1995; 154: 2959–2968.

48. Balashov KE, Smith DR, Khoury SJ et al. Increased interleukin 12 production in progressive multiple sclerosis: induction by activated CD4+ T cells via CD40 ligand.

Proc Natl Acad Sci USA 1997; 94: 599–603.

49. Khademi M, Illes Z, Gielen AW et al. T Cell Ig- and mucin-domain-containing molecule-3 (TIM-3) and TIM-1 molecules are differentially expressed on human Th1 and Th2 cells and in cerebrospinal fluid-derived mononuclear cells in multiple sclerosis. J Immunol 2004; 172: 7169–7176.

50. Scholz C, Patton KT, Anderson DE et al. Expansion of autoreactive T cells in multiple sclerosis is independent of exogenous B7 costimulation. J Immunol 1998; 160: 1532–1538.

51. Lovett-Racke AE, Trotter JL, Lauber J et al. Decreased dependence of myelin basic protein-reactive T cells on CD28-mediated costimulation in multiple sclerosis patients. A marker of activated/memory T cells. J Clin Invest 1998; 101: 725–730.

52. Markovic-Plese S, Cortese I, Wandinger KP et al. CD4+CD28- costimulation-independent T cells in multiple sclerosis. J Clin Invest 2001; 108: 1185–1194.

53. Oliveira EM, Bar-Or A, Waliszewska AI et al. CTLA-4 dysregulation in the activation of myelin basic protein reactive T cells may distinguish patients with multiple sclerosis from healthy controls. J Autoimmun 2003; 20: 71–81.

54. Zipp F, Otzelberger K, Dichgans J et al. Serum CD95 of relapsing remitting multiple sclerosis patients protects from CD95-mediated apoptosis. J Neuroimmunol 1998; 86: 151–154.

55. Sharief MK, Matthews H, Noori MA. Expression ratios of the Bcl-2 family proteins and disease activity in multiple sclerosis. J Neuroimmunol 2003; 134: 158–165.

56. Heber-Katz E, Acha-Orbea H. The V-region disease hypothesis: evidence from autoimmune encephalomyelitis. Immunol Today 1989; 10: 164–169.

57. Wucherpfennig KW, Ota K, Endo N et al. Shared human T cell receptor V beta usage to immunodominant regions of myelin basic protein. Science 1990; 248: 1016–1019.

58. Ben Nun A, Liblau RS, Cohen L et al. Restricted T-cell receptor Vβ gene usage by myelin basic protein-specific T-cell clones in multiple sclerosis: predominant genes vary in individuals. Proc Natl Acad Sci USA 1991; 88: 2466–2470.

59. Kotzin BL, Karuturi S, Chou YK et al. Preferential T-cell receptor Vβ-chain variable gene use in myelin basic protein-reactive T-cell clones from patients with multiple sclerosis. Proc Natl Acad Sci USA 1991; 88: 9161–9165.

60. Afshar G, Muraro PA, McFarland HF, Martin R. Lack of over-expression of T cell receptor Vbeta5.2 in myelin basic protein-specific T cell lines derived from HLA-DR2 positive multiple sclerosis patients and controls. J Neuroimmunol 1998; 84: 7–13.

61. Oksenberg JR, Stuart S, Begovich AB et al. Limited heterogeneity of rearranged T-cell receptor V alpha transcripts in brains of multiple sclerosis patients. Nature 1990; 345: 344–346.

62. Martin R, Howell MD, Jaraquemada D et al. A myelin basic protein peptide is recognized by cytotoxic T cells in the context of four HLA-DR types associated with multiple sclerosis. J Exp Med 1991; 173: 19–24.

63. Kondo T, Yamamura T, Inobe J et al. TCR repertoire to proteolipid protein (PLP) in multiple sclerosis (MS): homologies between PLP-specific T cells and MS-associated T cells in TCR junctional sequences. Int Immunol 1996; 8: 123–130.

64. Matsumoto Y, Yoon WK, Jee Y et al. Complementarity-determining region 3 spectratyping analysis of the TCR repertoire in multiple sclerosis. J Immunol 2003; 170: 4846–4853.

65. Demoulins T, Mouthon F, Clayette P et al. The same TCR (N)Dbeta(N)Jbeta junctional region is associated with several different vbeta13 subtypes in a multiple sclerosis patient at the onset of the disease. Neurobiol Dis 2003; 14: 470–482.

66. Laplaud DA, Ruiz C, Wiertlewski S et al. Blood T-cell receptor beta chain transcriptome in multiple sclerosis. Characterization of the T cells with altered CDR3 length distribution. Brain 2004; 127: 981–995.

67. Gestri D, Baldacci L, Taiuti R et al. Oligoclonal T cell repertoire in cerebrospinal fluid of patients with inflammatory diseases of the nervous system. J Neurol Neurosurg Psychiatr 2001; 70: 767–772.

68. Sospedra M, Zhao Y, Zur Hausen H et al. Recognition of conserved amino acid motifs of common viruses and its role in autoimmunity. PLoS Pathog 2005; 1: 335–348.

69. Utz U, Biddison WE, McFarland HF et al. Skewed T-cell receptor repertoire in genetically identical twins correlates with multiple sclerosis. Nature 1993; 364: 243–247.

70. Haegert DG, Galutira D, Murray TJ et al. Identical twins discordant for multiple sclerosis have a shift in their T-cell receptor repertoires. Clin Exp Immunol 2003; 134: 532–537.

71. Dyment DA, Ebers GC, Sadovnick AD. Genetics of multiple sclerosis. Lancet Neurol 2004; 3: 104–110.

72. Von Herrath MG, Fujinami RS, Whitton JL. Microorganisms and autoimmunity: making the barren field fertile? Nat Rev Microbiol 2003; 1: 151–157.

73. Fujinami RS, Oldstone MB. Amino acid homology between the encephalitogenic site of myelin basic protein and virus: mechanism for autoimmunity. Science 1985; 230: 1043–1045.

74. Tejada-Simon MV, Zang YC, Hong J et al. Cross-reactivity with myelin basic protein and human herpesvirus-6 in multiple sclerosis. Ann Neurol 2003; 53: 189–197.

75. Evavold BD, Sloan-Lancaster J, Hsu BL, Allen PM. Separation of T helper 1 clone cytolysis from proliferation and lymphokine production using analog peptides. J Immunol 1993; 150: 3131–3140.

76. Wucherpfennig KW, Strominger JL. Molecular mimicry in T cell-mediated autoimmunity: viral peptides activate human T cell clones specific for myelin basic protein. Cell 1995; 80: 695–705.

77. Hemmer B, Vergelli M, Gran B et al. Predictable TCR antigen recognition based on peptide scans leads to the identification of agonist ligands with no sequence homology. J Immunol 1998; 160: 3631–3636.

78. Lang HL, Jacobsen H, Ikemizu S et al. A functional and structural basis for TCR

cross-reactivity in multiple sclerosis. Nat Immunol 2002; 3: 940–943.

79. Ohashi PS, Oehen S, Buerki K et al. Ablation of 'tolerance' and induction of diabetes by virus infection in viral antigen transgenic mice. Cell 1991; 65: 305–317.

80. Oldstone MB, Nerenberg M, Southern P et al. Virus infection triggers insulin-dependent diabetes mellitus in a transgenic model: role of anti-self (virus) immune response. Cell 1991; 65: 319–331.

81. Olson JK, Ludovic Croxford J, Miller SD. Innate and adaptive immune requirements for induction of autoimmune demyelinating disease by molecular mimicry. Mol Immunol 2004; 40: 1103–1108.

82. Murali-Krishna K, Altman JD, Suresh M et al. Counting antigen-specific CD8 T cells: a reevaluation of bystander activation during viral infection. Immunity 1998; 8: 177–187.

83. Brocke S, Gaur A, Piercy C et al. Induction of relapsing paralysis in experimental autoimmune encephalomyelitis by bacterial superantigen. Nature 1993; 365: 642–644.

84. Rocken M, Urban JF, Shevach EM. Infection breaks T-cell tolerance. Nature 1992; 359: 79–82.

85. Hori S, Nomura T, Sakaguchi S. Control of regulatory T cell development by the transcription factor Foxp3. Science 2003; 299: 1057–1061.

86. Viglietta V, Baecher-Allan C, Weiner HL, Hafler DA. Loss of functional suppression by CD4+CD25+ regulatory T cells in patients with multiple sclerosis. J Exp Med 2004; 199: 971–979.

87. Haas J, Hug A, Viehover A et al. Reduced suppressive effect of CD4+CD25high regulatory T cells on the T cell immune response against myelin oligodendrocyte glycoprotein in patients with multiple sclerosis. Eur J Immunol 2005; 35: 3343–3352.

88. Weiner HL, Friedman A, Miller A et al. Oral tolerance: immunologic mechanisms and treatment of animal and human organ-specific autoimmune diseases by oral administration of autoantigens. Annu Rev Immunol 1994; 12: 809–837.

89. Benczur M, Petranyi GG, Palffy G et al. Dysfunction of natural killer cells in multiple sclerosis: a possible pathogenetic factor. Clin Exp Immunol 1980; 39: 657–662.

90. Kastrukoff LF, Morgan NG, Zecchini D et al. A role for natural killer cells in the immunopathogenesis of multiple sclerosis. J Neuroimmunol 1998; 86: 123–133.

91. Zhang B, Yamamura T, Kondo T et al. Regulation of experimental autoimmune encephalomyelitis by natural killer (NK) cells. J Exp Med 1997; 186: 1677–1687.

92. Smeltz RB, Wolf NA, Swanborg RH. Inhibition of autoimmune T cell responses in the DA rat by bone marrow-derived NK cells in vitro: implications for autoimmunity. J Immunol 1999; 163: 1390–1397.

93. Gray JD, Hirokawa M, Horwitz DA. The role of transforming growth factor beta in the generation of suppression: an interaction between CD8+ T and NK cells. J Exp Med 1994; 180: 1937–1942.

94. Peng SL, Moslehi J, Robert ME, Craft J. Perforin protects against autoimmunity in lupus-prone mice. J Immunol 1998; 160: 652–660.

95. Hilliard B, Wilmen A, Seidel C et al. Roles of TNF-related apoptosis-inducing ligand in experimental autoimmune encephalomyelitis. J Immunol 2001; 166: 1314–1319.

96. Bielekova B, Catalfamo M, Reichert-Scrivner S et al. Regulatory CD56(bright) natural killer cells mediate immunomodulatory effects of IL-2Ralpha-targeted therapy (daclizumab) in multiple sclerosis. Proc Natl Acad Sci USA 2006; 103: 5941–5946.

97. Hillert J, Olerup O. HLA and MS. Neurology 1993; 43: 2426–2427.

98. Barcellos LF, Oksenberg JR, Begovich AB et al. HLA-DR2 dose effect on susceptibility to multiple sclerosis and influence on disease course. Am J Hum Genet 2003; 72: 710–716.

99. Sellebjerg F, Jensen J, Madsen HO, Svejgaard A. HLA DRB1*1501 and intrathecal inflammation in multiple sclerosis. Tissue Antigens 2000; 55: 312–318.

100. Olerup O, Hillert J, Fredrikson S et al. Primarily chronic progressive and relapsing/remitting multiple sclerosis: two immunogenetically distinct disease entities. Proc Natl Acad Sci USA 1989; 86: 7113–7137.

101. Vartdal F, Sollid LM, Vandvik B et al. Patients with multiple sclerosis carry DQB1 genes which encode shared polymorphic amino acid sequences. Hum Immunol 1989; 25: 103–110.

102. Ridgway WM, Ito H, Fasso M et al. Analysis of the role of variation of major histocompatibility complex class II expression on nonobese diabetic (NOD) peripheral T cell response. J Exp Med 1998; 188: 2267–2275.

103. Merryman PF, Crapper RM, Lee S et al. Class II major histocompatibility complex gene sequences in rheumatoid arthritis. The third diversity regions of both DR beta 1 genes in two DR1, DRw10-positive individuals specify the same inferred amino acid sequence as the DR beta 1 and DR beta 2 genes of a DR4 (Dw14) haplotype. Arthritis Rheum 1989; 32: 251–258.

104. Sospedra M, Muraro PA, Stefanova I et al. Redundancy in antigen-presenting function of the HLA-DR and -DQ molecules in the multiple sclerosis-associated HLA-DR haplotype. J Immunol 2006; 176: 1951–1961.

105. Andersen LC, Beaty JS, Nettles JW et al. Allelic polymorphism in transcriptional regulatory regions of HLA-DQB genes. J Exp Med 1991; 173: 181–192.

106. Sospedra M, Obiols G, Babi LF et al. Hyperinducibility of HLA class II expression of thyroid follicular cells from Graves' disease. A primary defect? J Immunol 1995; 154: 4213–4222.

107. Prat E, Tomaru U, Sabater L et al. HLA-DRB5*0101 and -DRB1*1501 expression in the multiple sclerosis-associated HLA-DR15 haplotype. J Neuroimmunol 2005; 167: 108–119.

108. Ristori G, Carcassi C, Lai S et al. HLA-DM polymorphisms do not associate with multiple sclerosis: an association study with analysis of myelin basic protein T cell specificity. J Neuroimmunol 1997; 77: 181–184.

109. Matsuoka T, Tabata H, Matsushita S. Monocytes are differentially activated through HLA-DR, -DQ, and -DP molecules via mitogen-activated protein kinases. J Immunol 2001; 166: 2202–2208.

110. Baron J, Madri J, Ruddle N et al. Surface expression of α4 integrin by CD4+ cells is required for their entry into brain parenchyma. J Exp Med 1993; 177: 57–68.

111. Sindern E. Role of chemokines and their receptors in the pathogenesis of multiple sclerosis. Front Biosci 2004; 9: 457–463.

112. Ozenci V, Kouwenhoven M, Huang YM et al. Multiple sclerosis is associated with an imbalance between tumour necrosis factor-alpha (TNF-alpha)- and IL-10-secreting blood cells that is corrected by interferon-beta (IFN-beta) treatment. Clin Exp Immunol 2000; 120: 147–153.

113. The Lenercept Multiple Sclerosis Study Group and The University of British Columbia MS/MRI Analysis Group. TNF neutralization in MS: results of a randomized, placebo-controlled multicenter study. Neurology 1999; 53: 457–465.

114. Van Oosten BW, Barkhof F, Truyen L et al. Increased MRI activity and immune activation in two multiple sclerosis patients treated with the monoclonal anti-tumor necrosis factor antibody cA2. Neurology 1996; 47: 1531–1534.

115. Panitch HS, Hirsch RL, Schindler J, Johnson KP. Treatment of multiple sclerosis with gamma interferon: exacerbations associated with activation of the immune system. Neurology 1987; 37: 1097–1102.

116. Flugel A, Berkowicz T, Ritter T et al. Migratory activity and functional changes of green fluorescent effector cells before and during experimental autoimmune encephalomyelitis. Immunity 2001; 14: 547–560.

117. Seamons A, Perchellet A, Goverman J. Immune tolerance to myelin proteins. Immunol Res 2003; 28: 201–221.

118. Bruno R, Sabater L, Sospedra M et al. Multiple sclerosis candidate autoantigens except myelin oligodendrocyte glycoprotein are transcribed in human thymus. Eur J Immunol 2002; 32: 2737–2747.

119. Wekerle H, Kojima K, Lannes-Vieira J et al. Animal models. Ann Neurol 1994; 36: S47–S53.

120. Wucherpfennig KW, Sette A, Southwood S et al. Structural requirements for binding of an immunodominant myelin basic protein peptide to DR2 isotypes and for its recognition by human T cell clones. J Exp Med 1994; 179: 279–290.

121. Vogt AB, Kropshofer H, Kalbacher H et al. Ligand motifs of HLA-DRB5*0101 and DRB1*1501 molecules delineated from self-peptides. J Immunol 1994; 153: 1665–1673.

122. Muraro PA, Vergelli M, Kalbus M et al. Immunodominance of a low-affinity major histocompatibility complex-binding myelin basic protein epitope (residues 111–129) in HLA-DR4 (B1*0401) subjects is associated with a restricted T cell receptor repertoire. J Clin Invest 1997; 100: 339–349.

123. Vergelli M, Kalbus M, Rojo SC et al. T cell response to myelin basic protein in the context of the multiple sclerosis-associated HLA-DR15 haplotype: peptide binding, immunodominance and effector functions of T cells. J Neuroimmunol 1997; 77: 195–203.

124. Fairchild PJ, Wraith DC. Peptide-MHC interaction in autoimmunity. Curr Opin Immunol 1992; 4: 748–753.

125. Goverman J, Woods A, Larson L et al. Transgenic mice that express a myelin basic protein-specific T cell receptor develop spontaneous autoimmunity. Cell 1993; 72: 551–560.

126. Lafaille JJ, Nagashima K, Katsuki M, Tonegawa S. High incidence of spontaneous autoimmune encephalomyelitis in immunodeficient anti-myelin basic protein T cell receptor transgenic mice. Cell 1994; 78: 399–408.

127. Krogsgaard M, Wucherpfennig KW, Cannella B et al. Visualization of myelin basic protein (MBP) T cell epitopes in multiple sclerosis lesions using a monoclonal antibody specific for the human histocompatibility leukocyte antigen (HLA)-DR2-MBP 85–99 complex. J Exp Med 2000; 191: 1395–1412.

128. Berger T, Weerth S, Kojima K et al. Experimental autoimmune encephalomyelitis: the antigen specificity of T lymphocytes determines the topography of lesions in the central and peripheral nervous system. Lab Invest 1997; 76: 355–364.

129. Mazza G, Ponsford M, Lowrey P et al. Diversity and dynamics of the T-cell response to MBP in DR2+ve individuals. Clin Exp Immunol 2002; 128: 538–547.

130. Vergelli M, Mazzanti B, Traggiai E et al. Short-term evolution of autoreactive T cell repertoire in multiple sclerosis. J Neurosci Res 2001; 66: 517–524.

131. Klein L, Klugmann M, Nave K-A et al. Shaping of the autoreactive T-cell repertoire by a splice variant of self protein expressed in thymic epithelial cells. Nat Med 2000; 6: 56–62.

132. Waldner H, Whitters MJ, Sobel RA et al. Fulminant spontaneous autoimmunity of the central nervous system in mice transgenic for the myelin proteolipid protein-specific T cell receptor. Proc Natl Acad Sci USA 2000; 97: 3412–3417.

133. Kennedy MK, Tan LJ, Dal Canto MC et al. Inhibition of murine relapsing experimental autoimmune encephalomyelitis by immune tolerance to proteolipid protein and its encephalitogenic peptides. J Immunol 1990; 144: 909–915.

134. Whitham RH, Jones RF, Hashim GA et al. Location of a new encephalitogenic epitope (residues 43–64) in proteolipid protein that induces relapsing experimental autoimmune encephalomyelitis in PL/J and (SJLxPL)F1 mice. J Immunol 1991; 147: 3803–3808.

135. Amor S, Baker D, Groome N, Turk JL. Identification of a major encephalitogenic epitope of proteolipid protein (residues 56–70) for the induction of experimental allergic encephalomyelitis in Biozzi AB/H and nonobese diabetic mice. J Immunol 1993; 150: 5666–5672.

136. Greer JM, Csurhes PA, Cameron KD et al. Increased immunoreactivity to two overlapping peptides of myelin proteolipid protein in multiple sclerosis. Brain 1997; 120: 1447–1460.

137. Mendel I, Kerlero de Rosbo N, Ben Nun A. A myelin oligodendrocyte glycoprotein peptide induces typical chronic experimental autoimmune encephalomyelitis in H-2b mice: fine specificity and T cell receptor V beta expression of encephalitogenic T cells. Eur J Immunol 1995; 25: 1951–1959.

138. Bettelli E, Pagany M, Weiner HL et al. Myelin oligodendrocyte glycoprotein-specific T cell receptor transgenic mice develop spontaneous autoimmune optic neuritis. J Exp Med 2003; 197: 1073–1081.

139. Tsunoda I, Kuang LQ, Theil DJ, Fujinami RS. Antibody association with a novel model for primary progressive multiple sclerosis: induction of relapsing–remitting and progressive forms of EAE in H2s mouse strains. Brain Pathol 2000; 10: 402–418.

140. Wallstrom E, Khademi M, Andersson M et al. Increased reactivity to myelin oligodendrocyte glycoprotein peptides and epitope mapping in HLA DR2(15)+ multiple sclerosis. Eur J Immunol 1998; 28: 3329–3335.

141. Weissert R, Kuhle J, de Graaf KL et al. High immunogenicity of intracellular myelin oligodendrocyte glycoprotein epitopes. J Immunol 2002; 169: 548–556.

142. Kerlero de Rosbo N, Hoffman M, Mendel I et al. Predominance of the autoimmune response to myelin oligodendrocyte glycoprotein (MOG) in multiple sclerosis: reactivity to the extracellular domain of MOG is directed against three main regions. Eur J Immunol 1997; 27: 3059–3069.

143. Iglesias A, Bauer J, Litzenburger T et al. T- and B-cell responses to myelin oligodendrocyte glycoprotein in experimental autoimmune encephalomyelitis and multiple sclerosis. Glia 2001; 36: 220–234.

144. Lindert RB, Haase CG, Brehm U et al. Multiple sclerosis: B- and T-cell responses to the extracellular domain of the myelin oligodendrocyte glycoprotein. Brain 1999; 122: 2089–2100.

145. Morris-Downes MM, McCormack K, Baker D et al. Encephalitogenic and immunogenic potential of myelin-associated glycoprotein (MAG), oligodendrocyte-specific glycoprotein (OSP) and 2′,3′-cyclic nucleotide 3′-phosphodiesterase (CNPase) in ABH and SJL mice. J Neuroimmunol 2002; 122: 20–33.

146. Andersson M, Yu M, Soderstrom M et al. Multiple MAG peptides are recognized by circulating T and B lymphocytes in polyneuropathy and multiple sclerosis. Eur J Neurol 2002; 9: 243–251.

147. Birnbaum G, Kotilinek L, Schlievert P et al. Heat shock proteins and experimental autoimmune encephalomyelitis (EAE): I. immunization with a peptide of the myelin protein 2′,3′ cyclic nucleotide 3′ phosphodiesterase that is cross-reactive with a heat shock protein alters the course of EAE. J Neurosci Res 1996; 44: 381–396.

148. Rosener M, Muraro PA, Riethmuller A et al. 2′,3′-cyclic nucleotide 3′-phosphodiesterase: a novel candidate autoantigen in demyelinating diseases. J Neuroimmunol 1997; 75: 28–34.

149. Muraro PA, Kalbus M, Afshar G et al. T cell response to 2′,3′-cyclic nucleotide 3′-phosphodiesterase (CNPase) in multiple sclerosis patients. J Neuroimmunol 2002; 130: 233–242.

150. Holz A, Bielekova B, Martin R, Oldstone MB. Myelin-associated oligodendrocytic basic protein: identification of an encephalitogenic epitope and association with multiple sclerosis. J Immunol 2000; 164: 1103–1109.

151. Kaye JF, Kerlero de Rosbo N, Mendel I et al. The central nervous sytem-specific myelin oligodendrocytic basic protein (MOBP) is encephalitogenic and a potential target antigen in multiple sclerosis (MS). J Neuroimmunol 2000; 102: 189–198.

152. Arbour N, Holz A, Sipe JC et al. A new approach for evaluating antigen-specific T cell responses to myelin antigens during the course of multiple sclerosis. J Neuroimmunol 2003; 137: 197–209.

153. Stevens DB, Chen K, Seitz RS et al. Oligodendrocyte-specific protein peptides induce experimental autoimmune encephalomyelitis in SJL/J mice. J Immunol 1999; 162: 7501–7509.

154. Zhong MC, Cohen L, Meshorer A et al. T-cells specific for soluble recombinant oligodendrocyte-specific protein induce severe clinical experimental autoimmune encephalomyelitis in H-2(b) and H-2(s) mice. J Neuroimmunol 2000; 105: 39–45.

155. Bronstein JM, Lallone RL, Seitz RS et al. A humoral response to oligodendrocyte-specific protein in MS: a potential molecular mimic. Neurology 1999; 53: 154–161.

156. Vu T, Myers LW, Ellison GW et al. T-cell responses to oligodendrocyte-specific protein in multiple sclerosis. J Neurosci Res 2001; 66: 506–509.

157. Van Noort JM, van Sechel AC, Bajramovic JJ et al. The small heat-shock protein alpha B-crystallin as candidate autoantigen in multiple sclerosis. Nature 1995; 375: 798–801.

158. Bajramovic JJ, Lassmann H, van Noort JM. Expression of alphaB-crystallin in glia cells during lesional development in multiple sclerosis. J Neuroimmunol 1997; 78: 143–151.

159. Thoua NM, van Noort JM, Baker D et al. Encephalitogenic and immunogenic potential of the stress protein alphaB-crystallin in Biozzi ABH (H-2A(g7)) mice. J Neuroimmunol 2000; 104: 47–57.

160. Chou YK, Burrows GG, LaTocha D et al. CD4 T-cell epitopes of human alpha B-crystallin. J Neurosci Res 2004; 75: 516–523.

161. Saez-Torres I, Brieva L, Espejo C et al. Specific proliferation towards myelin antigens in patients with multiple sclerosis during a relapse. Autoimmunity 2002; 35: 45–50.

162. Kojima K, Berger T, Lassmann H et al. Experimental autoimmune panencephalitis and uveoretinitis transferred to the Lewis rat by T lymphocytes specific for the S100 beta molecule, a calcium binding protein of astroglia. J Exp Med 1994; 180: 817–829.

163. Schmidt S, Linington C, Zipp F et al. Multiple sclerosis: comparison of the human T-cell response to S100 beta and myelin basic protein reveals parallels to rat experimental autoimmune panencephalitis. Brain 1997; 120: 1437–1445.

164. Miller SD, Vanderlugt CL, Begolka WS et al. Persistent infection with Theiler's virus leads to CNS autoimmunity via epitope spreading. Nat Med 1997; 3: 1133–1136.

165. Horwitz MS, Bradley LM, Harbertson J et al. Diabetes induced by Coxsackie virus: initiation by bystander damage and not molecular mimicry. Nat Med 1998; 4: 781–785.

166. Barnaba V. Viruses, hidden self-epitopes and autoimmunity. Immunol Rev 1996; 152: 47–66.

167. Opdenakker G, Van Damme J. Cytokine-regulated proteases in autoimmune diseases. Immunol Today 1994; 15: 103–107.

168. Suen WE, Bergman CM, Hjelmstrom P, Ruddle NH. A critical role for lymphotoxin in experimental allergic encephalomyelitis. J Exp Med 1997; 186: 1233–1240.

169. Baranzini SE, Elfstrom C, Chang SY et al. Transcriptional analysis of multiple sclerosis brain lesions reveals a complex pattern of cytokine expression. J Immunol 2000; 165: 6576–6582.

170. Rozniecki JJ, Hauser SL, Stein M et al. Elevated mast cell tryptase in cerebrospinal fluid of multiple sclerosis patients. Ann Neurol 1995; 37: 63–66.

171. Tuomisto L, Kilpelainen H, Riekkinen P. Histamine and histamine-N-methyltransferase in the CSF of patients with multiple sclerosis. Agents Actions 1983; 13: 255–257.

172. Zhuang X, Silverman AJ, Silver R. Brain mast cell degranulation regulates blood-brain barrier. J Neurobiol 1996; 31: 393–403.

173. Rumsaeng V, Cruikshank WW, Foster B et al. Human mast cells produce the CD4+ T lymphocyte chemoattractant factor, IL-16. J Immunol 1997; 159: 2904–2910.

174. Ley K. Histamine can induce leukocyte rolling in rat mesenteric venules. Am J Physiol 1994; 267: H1017–H1023.

175. Lees M, Taylor DJ, Woolley DE. Mast cell proteinases activate precursor forms of collagenase and stromelysin, but not of gelatinases A and B. Eur J Biochem 1994; 223: 171–177.

176. Kanbe N, Tanaka A, Kanbe M et al. Human mast cells produce matrix metalloproteinase 9. Eur J Immunol 1999; 29: 2645–2649.

177. Trebst C, Ransohoff RM. Investigating chemokines and chemokine receptors in patients with multiple sclerosis: opportunities and challenges. Arch Neurol 2001; 58: 1975–1980.

178. Sorensen TL, Tani M, Jensen J et al. Expression of specific chemokines and chemokine receptors in the central nervous system of multiple sclerosis patients. J Clin Invest 1999; 103: 807–815.

179. Balashov KE, Rottman JB, Weiner HL, Hancock WW. CCR5(+) and CXCR3(+) T cells are increased in multiple sclerosis and their ligands MIP-1α and IP-10 are expressed in demyelinating brain lesions. Proc Natl Acad Sci USA 1999; 96: 6873–6878.

180. Misu T, Onodera H, Fujihara K et al. Chemokine receptor expression on T cells in blood and cerebrospinal fluid at relapse and remission of multiple sclerosis: imbalance of Th1/Th2-associated chemokine signaling. J Neuroimmunol 2001; 114: 207–212.

181. Calabresi PA, Yun SH, Allie R, Whartenby KA. Chemokine receptor expression on MBP-reactive T cells: CXCR6 is a marker of IFNgamma-producing effector cells. J Neuroimmunol 2002; 127: 96–105.

182. Sindern E, Niederkinkhaus Y, Henschel M et al. Differential release of beta-chemokines in serum and CSF of patients with relapsing–remitting multiple

sclerosis. Acta Neurol Scand 2001; 104: 88–91.

183. Kivisakk P, Teleshova N, Ozenci V et al. No evidence for elevated numbers of mononuclear cells expressing MCP-1 and RANTES mRNA in blood and CSF in multiple sclerosis. J Neuroimmunol 1998; 91: 108–112.

184. Kivisakk P, Trebst C, Liu Z et al. T-cells in the cerebrospinal fluid express a similar repertoire of inflammatory chemokine receptors in the absence or presence of CNS inflammation: implications for CNS trafficking. Clin Exp Immunol 2002; 129: 510–518.

185. Giunti D, Borsellino G, Benelli R et al. Phenotypic and functional analysis of T cells homing into the CSF of subjects with inflammatory diseases of the CNS. J Leukoc Biol 2003; 73: 584–590.

186. Sellebjerg F, Madsen HO, Jensen CV et al. CCR5 delta32, matrix metalloproteinase-9 and disease activity in multiple sclerosis. J Neuroimmunol 2000; 102: 98–106.

187. Simpson JE, Newcombe J, Cuzner ML, Woodroofe MN. Expression of monocyte chemoattractant protein-1 and other beta-chemokines by resident glia and inflammatory cells in multiple sclerosis lesions. J Neuroimmunol 1998; 84: 238–249.

188. Woodroofe N, Cross AK, Harkness K, Simpson JE. The role of chemokines in the pathogenesis of multiple sclerosis. Adv Exp Med Biol 1999; 468: 135–150.

189. Omari KM, John G, Sealfon S, Raine CS. CXC chemokine receptors on human oligodendrocytes: Implications for multiple sclerosis. Brain 2005; 128: 1003–1015.

190. Fife BT, Huffnagle GB, Kuziel WA, Karpus WJ. CC chemokine receptor 2 is critical for induction of experimental autoimmune encephalomyelitis. J Exp Med 2000; 192: 899–905.

191. Gaupp S, Pitt D, Kuziel WA et al. Experimental autoimmune encephalomyelitis (EAE) in CCR2−/− mice: susceptibility in multiple strains. Am J Pathol 2003; 162: 139–150.

192. Tran EH, Kuziel WA, Owens T. Induction of experimental autoimmune encephalomyelitis in C57BL/6 mice deficient in either the chemokine macrophage inflammatory protein-1alpha or its CCR5 receptor. Eur J Immunol 2000; 30: 1410–1415.

193. Lassmann H. Mechanisms of demyelination and tissue destruction in multiple sclerosis. Clin Neurol Neurosurg 2002; 104: 168–171.

194. Kabat EA, Freedman DA, Murray JP, Knaub V. A study of the cristalline albumin, gamma globulin and total protein in the cerebrospinal fluid of one hundred cases of multiple sclerosis and in other diseases. Am J Med Sci 1950; 219: 55–64.

195. Zeman AZ, Kidd D, McLean BN et al. A study of oligoclonal band negative multiple sclerosis. J Neurol Neurosurg Psychiatr 1996; 60: 27–30.

196. Corcione A, Aloisi F, Serafini B et al. B-cell differentiation in the CNS of patients with multiple sclerosis. Autoimmun Rev 2005; 4: 549–554.

197. Qin Y, Duquette P, Zhang Y et al. Clonal expansion and somatic hypermutation of V(H) genes of B cells from cerebrospinal fluid in multiple sclerosis. J Clin Invest 1998; 102: 1045–1050.

198. Haubold K, Owens GP, Kaur P et al. B-lymphocyte and plasma cell clonal expansion in monosymptomatic optic neuritis cerebrospinal fluid. Ann Neurol 2004; 56: 97–107.

199. Owens GP, Kraus H, Burgoon MP et al. Restricted use of VH4 germline segments in an acute multiple sclerosis brain. Ann Neurol 1998; 43: 236–243.

200. Baranzini SE, Jeong MC, Butunoi C et al. B cell repertoire diversity and clonal expansion in multiple sclerosis brain lesions. J Immunol 1999; 163: 5133–5144.

201. Walsh MJ, Tourtellotte WW, Roman J, Dreyer W. Immunoglobulin G, A, and M–clonal restriction in multiple sclerosis cerebrospinal fluid and serum–analysis by two-dimensional electrophoresis. Clin Immunol Immunopathol 1985; 35: 313–327.

202. Wang LY, Fujinami RS. Enhancement of EAE and induction of autoantibodies to T-cell epitopes in mice infected with a recombinant vaccinia virus encoding myelin proteolipid protein. J Neuroimmunol 1997; 75: 75–83.

203. Wucherpfennig KW, Catz I, Hausmann S et al. Recognition of the immunodominant myelin basic protein peptide by autoantibodies and HLA-DR2-restricted T cell clones from multiple sclerosis patients. Identity of key contact residues in the B-cell and T-cell epitopes. J Clin Invest 1997; 100: 1114–1122.

204. Genc K, Dona DL, Reder AT. Increased CD80(+) B cells in active multiple sclerosis and reversal by interferon beta-1b therapy. J Clin Invest 1997; 99: 2664–2671.

205. Boylan MT, Crockard AD, McDonnell GV et al. CD80 (B7–1) and CD86 (B7–2) expression in multiple sclerosis patients: clinical subtype specific variation in peripheral monocytes and B cells and lack of modulation by high dose methylprednisolone. J Neurol Sci 1999; 167: 79–89.

206. Lou YH, Park KK, Agersborg S et al. Retargeting T cell-mediated inflammation: a new perspective on autoantibody action. J Immunol 2000; 164: 5251–5257.

207. Holmoy T, Vandvik B, Vartdal F. T cells from multiple sclerosis patients recognize immunoglobulin G from cerebrospinal fluid. Mult Scler 2003; 9: 228–234.

208. Genain CP, Cannella B, Hauser SL, Raine CS. Identification of autoantibodies associated with myelin damage in multiple sclerosis. Nat Med 1999; 5: 170–175.

209. Bornstein MB, Appel SH. Demyelination in cultures of rat cerebellum produced by experimental allergic encephalomyelitic serum. Trans Am Neurol Assoc 1959; 84: 165–166.

210. Raine CS, Bornstein MB. Experimental allergic encephalomyelitis: An ultrastructural study of demyelination in vitro. J Neuropathol Exp Neurol 1970; 29: 177–191.

211. Raine CS, Hummelgard A, Swanson E, Bornstein MB. Multiple sclerosis: serum-induced demyelination in vitro. A light and electron microscope study. J Neurol Sci 1973; 20: 127–148.

212. Esiri MM. Immunoglobulin-containing cells in multiple-sclerosis plaques. Lancet 1977; 2: 478.

213. Mattson DH, Roos RP, Arnason BG. Isoelectric focusing of IgG eluted from

multiple sclerosis and subacute sclerosing panencephalitis brains. Nature 1980; 287: 335–337.

214. Trotter J, DeJong LJ, Smith ME. Opsonization with antimyelin antibody increases the uptake and intracellular metabolism of myelin in inflammatory macrophages. J Neurochem 1986; 47: 779–789.

215. Van der Laan LJ, Ruuls SR, Weber KS et al. Macrophage phagocytosis of myelin in vitro determined by flow cytometry: phagocytosis is mediated by CR3 and induces production of tumor necrosis factor-alpha and nitric oxide. J Neuroimmunol 1996; 70: 145–152.

216. Mead RJ, Singhrao SK, Neal JW et al. The membrane attack complex of complement causes severe demyelination associated with acute axonal injury. J Immunol 2002; 168: 458–465.

217. Lucchinetti C, Bruck W, Parisi J et al. Heterogeneity of multiple sclerosis lesions: implications for the pathogenesis of demyelination. Ann Neurol 2000; 47: 707–717.

218. Storch MK, Piddlesden S, Haltia M et al. Multiple sclerosis: in situ evidence for antibody- and complement-mediated demyelination. Ann Neurol 1998; 43: 465–471.

219. Sellebjerg F, Jaliashvili I, Christiansen M, Garred P. Intrathecal activation of the complement system and disability in multiple sclerosis. J Neurol Sci 1998; 157: 168–174.

220. Scolding NJ, Morgan BP, Houston WA et al. Vesicular removal by oligodendrocytes of membrane attack complexes formed by activated complement. Nature 1989; 339: 620–622.

221. Piddlesden SJ, Storch MK, Hibbs M et al. Soluble recombinant complement receptor 1 inhibits inflammation and demyelination in antibody-mediated demyelinating experimental allergic encephalomyelitis. J Immunol 1994; 152: 5477–5484.

222. Trotter JL, Rust RS. Human cerebrospinal fluid immunology. Amsterdam: Martinus Nyhoff, 1989: 179–226.

223. Sindic CJ, Monteyne P, Laterre EC. The intrathecal synthesis of virus-specific oligoclonal IgG in multiple sclerosis. J Neuroimmunol 1994; 54: 75–80.

224. Warren KG, Catz I. Increased synthetic peptide specificity of tissue-CSF bound anti-MBP in multiple sclerosis. J Neuroimmunol 1993; 43: 87–96.

225. Reindl M, Linington C, Brehm U et al. Antibodies against the myelin oligodendrocyte glycoprotein and the myelin basic protein in multiple sclerosis and other neurological diseases: a comparative study. Brain 1999; 122: 2047–2056.

226. Chou CH, Tourtellotte WW, Kibler RF. Failure to detect antibodies to myelin basic protein or peptic fragments of myelin basic protein in CSF of patients with MS. Neurology 1983; 33: 24–28.

227. Olsson T, Baig S, Hojeberg B, Link H. Antimyelin basic protein and antimyelin antibody-producing cells in multiple sclerosis. Ann Neurol 1990; 27: 132–136.

228. Brokstad KA, Page M, Nyland H, Haaheim LR. Autoantibodies to myelin basic protein are not present in the serum and CSF of

MS patients. Acta Neurol Scand 1994; 89: 407–411.

229. Cortese I, Tafi R, Grimaldi LM et al. Identification of peptides specific for cerebrospinal fluid antibodies in multiple sclerosis by using phage libraries. Proc Natl Acad Sci USA 1996; 93: 11063–11067.

230. Williamson RA, Burgoon MP, Owens GP et al. Anti-DNA antibodies are a major component of the intrathecal B cell response in multiple sclerosis. Proc Natl Acad Sci USA 2001; 98: 1793–1798.

231. O'Connor KC, Chitnis T, Griffin DE et al. Myelin basic protein-reactive autoantibodies in the serum and cerebrospinal fluid of multiple sclerosis patients are characterized by low-affinity interactions. J Neuroimmunol 2003; 136: 140–148.

232. Sun JB, Olsson T, Wang WZ et al. Autoreactive T and B cells responding to myelin proteolipid protein in multiple sclerosis and controls. Eur J Immunol 1991; 21: 1461–1468.

233. Warren KG, Catz I, Johnson E, Mielke B. Anti-myelin basic protein and anti-proteolipid protein specific forms of multiple sclerosis. Ann Neurol 1994; 35: 280–289.

234. Linington C, Bradl M, Lassmann H et al. Augmentation of demyelination in rat acute allergic encephalomyelitis by circulating mouse monoclonal antibodies directed against a myelin/oligodendrocyte glycoprotein. Am J Pathol 1988; 130: 443–454.

235. Storch MK, Stefferl A, Brehm U et al. Autoimmunity to myelin oligodendrocyte glycoprotein in rats mimics the spectrum of multiple sclerosis pathology. Brain Pathol 1998; 8: 681–694.

236. Litzenburger T, Fassler R, Bauer J et al. B lymphocytes producing demyelinating autoantibodies: development and function in gene-targeted transgenic mice. J Exp Med 1998; 188: 169–180.

237. Sun J, Link H, Olsson T et al. T and B cell responses to myelin-oligodendrocyte glycoprotein in multiple sclerosis. J Immunol 1991; 146: 1490–1495.

238. Berger T, Rubner P, Schautzer F et al. Antimyelin antibodies as a predictor of clinically definite multiple sclerosis after a first demyelinating event. N Engl J Med 2003; 349: 139–145.

239. Wajgt A, Gorny M. CSF antibodies to myelin basic protein and to myelin-associated glycoprotein in multiple sclerosis. Evidence of the intrathecal production of antibodies. Acta Neurol Scand 1983; 68: 337–343.

240. Moller JR, Johnson D, Brady RO et al. Antibodies to myelin-associated glycoprotein (MAG) in the cerebrospinal fluid of multiple sclerosis patients. J Neuroimmunol 1989; 22: 55–61.

241. Walsh MJ, Murray JM. Dual implication of 2′,3′-cyclic nucleotide 3′ phosphodiesterase as major autoantigen and C3 complement-binding protein in the pathogenesis of multiple sclerosis. J Clin Invest 1998; 101: 1923–1931.

242. Banki K, Colombo E, Sia F et al. Oligodendrocyte-specific expression and autoantigenicity of transaldolase in multiple sclerosis. J Exp Med 1994; 180: 1649–1663.

243. Endo T, Scott DD, Stewart SS et al. Antibodies to glycosphingolipids in patients with multiple sclerosis and SLE. J Immunol 1984; 132: 1793–1797.

244. Ilyas AA, Chen ZW, Cook SD. Antibodies to sulfatide in cerebrospinal fluid of patients with multiple sclerosis. J Neuroimmunol 2003; 139: 76–80.

245. Mata S, Lolli F, Soderstrom M et al. Multiple sclerosis is associated with enhanced B cell responses to the ganglioside GD1a. Mult Scler 1999; 5: 379–388.

246. Sadatipour BT, Greer JM, Pender MP. Increased circulating antiganglioside antibodies in primary and secondary progressive multiple sclerosis. Ann Neurol 1998; 44: 980–983.

247. Saida T, Saida K, Silberberg DH. Demyelination produced by experimental allergic neuritis serum and anti-galactocerebroside antiserum in CNS cultures. An ultrastructural study. Acta Neuropathol (Berl) 1979; 48: 19–25.

248. Raine CS, Johnson AB, Marcus DM et al. Demyelination in vitro: absorption studies demonstrate that galactocerebroside is a major target. J Neurol Sci 1981; 52: 117–131.

249. Morris-Downes MM, Smith PA, Rundle JL et al. Pathological and regulatory effects of anti-myelin antibodies in experimental allergic encephalomyelitis in mice. J Neuroimmunol 2002; 125: 114–124.

250. Agius MA, Kirvan CA, Schafer AL et al. High prevalence of anti-alpha-crystallin antibodies in multiple sclerosis: correlation with severity and activity of disease. Acta Neurol Scand 1999; 100: 139–147.

251. Celet B, Akman-Demir G, Serdaroglu P et al. Anti-alpha B-crystallin immunoreactivity in inflammatory nervous system diseases. J Neurol 2000; 247: 935–939.

252. Lycke JN, Karlsson JE, Andersen O, Rosengren LE. Neurofilament protein in cerebrospinal fluid: a potential marker of activity in multiple sclerosis. J Neurol Neurosurg Psychiatr 1998; 64: 402–404.

253. Silber E, Semra YK, Gregson NA, Sharief MK. Patients with progressive multiple sclerosis have elevated antibodies to neurofilament subunit. Neurology 2002; 58: 1372–1381.

254. Niehaus A, Shi J, Grzenkowski M et al. Patients with active relapsing–remitting multiple sclerosis synthesize antibodies recognizing oligodendrocyte progenitor cell surface protein: implications for remyelination. Ann Neurol 2000; 48: 362–371.

255. Reindl M, Khantane S, Ehling R et al. Serum and cerebrospinal fluid antibodies to Nogo-A in patients with multiple sclerosis and acute neurological disorders. J Neuroimmunol 2003; 145: 139–147.

256. Mayo I, Arribas J, Villoslada P et al. The proteasome is a major autoantigen in multiple sclerosis. Brain 2002; 125: 2658–2667.

257. Lily O, Palace J, Vincent A. Serum autoantibodies to cell surface determinants in multiple sclerosis: a flow cytometric study. Brain 2004; 127: 269–279.

258. Robinson WH, Fontoura P, Lee BJ et al. Protein microarrays guide tolerizing DNA vaccine treatment of autoimmune encephalomyelitis. Nat Biotechnol 2003; 21: 1033–1039.

259. Gasque P, Dean YD, McGreal EP et al. Complement components of the innate immune system in health and disease in the CNS. Immunopharmacology 2000; 49: 171–186.

260. Vanguri P, Shin ML. Activation of complement by myelin: identification of C1-binding proteins of human myelin from central nervous tissue. J Neurochem 1986; 46: 1535–1541.

261. Scolding NJ, Morgan BP, Houston A et al. Normal rat serum cytotoxicity against syngeneic oligodendrocytes. Complement activation and attack in the absence of anti-myelin antibodies. J Neurol Sci 1989; 89: 289–300.

262. Johns TG, Bernard CC. Binding of complement component C1q to myelin oligodendrocyte glycoprotein: a novel mechanism for regulating CNS inflammation. Mol Immunol 1997l 34: 33–38.

263. Scolding NJ, Morgan BP, Compston DA. The expression of complement regulatory proteins by adult human oligodendrocytes. J Neuroimmunol 1998; 84: 69–75.

264. Head JR, Griffin WST. Functional capacity of solid tissue transplants in brain: evidence for immonological privilege. Proc R Soc Lond Ser B 1985; 224: 375–387.

265. Jurewicz A, Biddison WE, Antel JP. MHC class I-restricted lysis of human oligodendrocytes by myelin basic protein peptide-specific CD8 T lymphocytes. J Immunol 1998; 160: 3056–3059.

266. Jacobsen M, Cepok S, Quak E et al. Oligoclonal expansion of memory CD8[+] T cells in cerebrospinal fluid from multiple sclerosis patients. Brain 2002; 125: 538–550.

267. Skulina C, Schmidt S, Dornmair K et al. Multiple sclerosis: brain-infiltrating CD8[+] T cells persist as clonal expansions in the cerebrospinal fluid and blood. Proc Natl Acad Sci USA 2004; 101: 2428–2433.

268. Cabarrocas J, Bauer J, Piaggio E et al. Effective and selective immune surveillance of the brain by MHC class I-restricted cytotoxic T lymphocytes. Eur J Immunol 2003; 33: 1174–1182.

269. Neumann H. Molecular mechanisms of axonal damage in inflammatory central nervous system diseases. Curr Opin Neurol 2003; 16: 267–273.

270. Medana IM, Gallimore A, Oxenius A et al. MHC class I-restricted killing of neurons by virus-specific CD8[+] T lymphocytes is effected through the Fas/FasL, but not the perforin pathway. Eur J Immunol 2000; 30: 3623–3633.

271. Tsuchida T, Parker KC, Turner RV et al. Autoreactive CD8[+] T-cell responses to human myelin protein-derived peptides. Proc Natl Acad Sci USA 1994; 91: 10859–10863.

272. Honma K, Parker KC, Becker KG et al. Identification of an epitope derived from human proteolipid protein that can induce autoreactive CD8[+] cytotoxic T lymphocytes restricted by HLA-A3: evidence for cross-reactivity with an environmental microorganism. J Neuroimmunol 1997; 73: 7–14.

273. Zang YC, Li S, Rivera VM et al. Increased CD8[+] cytotoxic T cell responses to myelin basic protein in multiple sclerosis. J Immunol 2004; 172: 5120–5127.

274. Biddison WE, Cruikshank WW, Center DM et al. CD8[+] myelin peptide-specific T cells can chemoattract CD4[+] myelin peptide-specific T cells: importance of IFN-inducible protein 10. J Immunol 1998; 160: 444–448.

275. Buckle GJ, Hollsberg P, Hafler DA. Activated CD8[+] T cells in secondary progressive MS secrete lymphotoxin. Neurology 2003; 60: 702–705.

276. Battistini L, Piccio L, Rossi B et al. CD8[+] T cells from patients with acute multiple sclerosis display selective increase of adhesiveness in brain venules: a critical role for P-selectin glycoprotein ligand-1. Blood 2003; 101: 4775–4782.

277. Hollsberg P, Hansen HJ, Haahr S. Altered CD8[+] T cell responses to selected Epstein-Barr virus immunodominant epitopes in patients with multiple sclerosis. Clin Exp Immunol 2003; 132: 137–143.

278. Killestein J, Eikelenboom MJ, Izeboud I et al. Cytokine producing CD8[+] T cells are correlated to MRI features of tissue destruction in MS. J Neuroimmunol 2003; 142: 141–148.

279. Bo L, Dawson TM, Wesselingh S et al. Induction of nitric oxide synthase in demyelinating regions of multiple sclerosis brains. Ann Neurol 1994; 36: 778–786.

280. Merrill JE, Ignarro LJ, Sherman MP et al. Microglial cell cytotoxicity of oligodendrocytes is mediated through nitric oxide. J Immunol 1993; 151: 2132–2141.

281. Mitrovic B, Ignarro LJ, Vinters HV et al. Nitric oxide induces necrotic but not apoptotic cell death in oligodendrocytes. Neuroscience 1995; 65: 531–539.

282. Parkinson JF, Mitrovic B, Merrill JE. The role of nitric oxide in multiple sclerosis. J Mol Med 1997; 75: 174–186.

283. Dimmeler S, Haendeler J, Nehls M, Zeiher AM. Suppression of apoptosis by nitric oxide via inhibition of interleukin-1β-converting enzyme (ICE)-like and cysteine protease protein (CPP)-32-like proteases. J Exp Med 1997; 185: 601–607.

284. Kolb H, Kolb-Bachofen V. Nitric oxide in autoimmune disease: cytotoxic or regulatory mediator? Immunol Today 1998; 19: 556–561.

285. Shimonkevitz R, Colburn C, Burnham JA et al. Clonal expansions of activated gamma/delta T cells in recent-onset multiple sclerosis. Proc Natl Acad Sci USA 1993; 90: 923–927.

286. Selmaj K, Brosnan CF, Raine CS. Colocalization of lymphocytes bearing gamma delta T-cell receptor and heat shock protein hsp65[+] oligodendrocytes in multiple sclerosis. Proc Natl Acad Sci USA 1991; 88: 6452–6456.

287. Wucherpfennig KW, Newcombe J, Li H et al. Gamma delta T-cell receptor repertoire in acute multiple sclerosis lesions. Proc Natl Acad Sci USA 1992; 89: 4588–4592.

288. Zeine R, Pon R, Ladiwala U et al. Mechanism of gammadelta T cell-induced human oligodendrocyte cytotoxicity: relevance to multiple sclerosis. J Neuroimmunol 1998; 87: 49–61.

289. Triebel F, Hercend T. Subpopulations of human peripheral T gamma delta lymphocytes. Immunol Today 1989; 10: 186–188.

290. Battistini L, Salvetti M, Ristori G et al. Gamma delta T cell receptor analysis supports a role for HSP 70 selection of lymphocytes in multiple sclerosis lesions. Mol Med 1995; 1: 554–562.

291. Freedman MS, Bitar R, Antel JP. γδ T-cell-human glial cell interactions. II. Relationship between heat shock protein expression and susceptibility to cytolysis. J Neuroimmunol 1997; 74: 143–148.

292. Battistini L, Selmaj K, Kowal C et al. Multiple sclerosis: limited diversity of the V δ 2-J δ 3 T-cell receptor in chronic active lesions. Ann Neurol 1995; 37: 198–203.

293. Nick S, Pileri P, Tongiani S et al. T cell receptor gamma delta repertoire is skewed in cerebrospinal fluid of multiple sclerosis patients: molecular and functional analyses of antigen-reactive gamma delta clones. Eur J Immunol 1995; 25: 355–363.

294. Birnbaum G, Kotilinek L, Albrecht L. Spinal fluid lymphocytes from a subgroup of multiple sclerosis patients respond to mycobacterial antigens. Ann Neurol 1993; 34: 18–24.

295. Constant P, Davodeau F, Peyrat MA et al. Stimulation of human gamma delta T cells by nonpeptidic mycobacterial ligands. Science 1994; 264: 267–270.

296. Bukowski JF, Morita CT, Tanaka Y et al. V γ 2V δ 2 TCR-dependent recognition of non-peptide antigens and Daudi cells analyzed by TCR gene transfer. J Immunol 1995; 154: 998–1006.

297. Rajan AJ, Gao YL, Raine CS, Brosnan CF. A pathogenic role for gamma delta T cells in relapsing–remitting experimental allergic encephalomyelitis in the SJL mouse. J Immunol 1996; 157: 941–949.

298. Vergelli M, Hemmer B, Muraro PA et al. Human autoreactive CD4[+] T cell clones use perforin- or Fas/Fas ligand-mediated pathways for target cell lysis. J Immunol 1997; 158: 2756–2761.

299. Vergelli M, Le H, van Noort JM et al. A novel population of CD4[+]CD56[+] myelin-reactive T cells lyses target cells expressing CD56/neural cell adhesion molecule. J Immunol 1996; 157: 679–688.

300. Antel JP, McCrea E, Ladiwala U et al. Non-MHC-restricted cell-mediated lysis of human oligodendrocytes in vitro: relation with CD56 expression. J Immunol 1998; 160: 1606–1611.

301. Ahmed Z, Gveric D, Pryce G et al. Myelin/axonal pathology in interleukin-12 induced serial relapses of experimental allergic encephalomyelitis in the Lewis rat. Am J Pathol 2001; 158: 2127–2138.

302. Von Herrath MG, Allison J, Miller JF, Oldstone MB. Focal expression of interleukin-2 does not break unresponsiveness to 'self' (viral) antigen expressed in beta cells but enhances development of autoimmune disease (diabetes) after initiation of an anti-self immune response. J Clin Invest 1995; 95: 477–485.

303. Lee MS, von Herrath M, Reiser H et al. Sensitization to self (virus) antigen by in situ expression of murine interferon-gamma. J Clin Invest 1995; 95: 486–492.

304. Allan SM, Rothwell NJ. Cytokines and acute neurodegeneration. Nat Rev Neurosci 2001; 2: 734–744.

305. Becher B, Durell BG, Noelle RJ. IL-23 produced by CNS-resident cells controls T cell encephalitogenicity during the effector phase of experimental autoimmune encephalomyelitis. J Clin Invest 2003; 112: 1186–1191.

306. Cua DJ, Sherlock J, Chen Y et al. Interleukin-23 rather than interleukin-12 is the critical cytokine for autoimmune inflammation of the brain. Nature 2003; 421: 744–748.

307. Wheeler RD, Owens T. The changing face of cytokines in the brain: perspectives from EAE. Curr Pharm Des 2005; 11: 1031–1037.

308. Moalem G, Gdalyahu A, Shani Y et al. Production of neurotrophins by activated T cells: implications for neuroprotective autoimmunity. J Autoimmun 2000; 15: 331–345.

309. Kerschensteiner M, Stadelmann C, Dechant G et al. Neurotrophic cross-talk between the nervous and immune systems: implications for neurological diseases. Ann Neurol 2003; 53: 292–304.

310. Legos JJ, Whitmore RG, Erhardt JA et al. Quantitative changes in interleukin proteins following focal stroke in the rat. Neurosci Lett 2000; 282: 189–192.

311. Albrecht PJ, Murtie JC, Ness JK et al. Astrocytes produce CNTF during the remyelination phase of viral-induced spinal cord demyelination to stimulate FGF-2 production. Neurobiol Dis 2003; 13: 89–101.

312. Pluchino S, Zanotti L, Rossi B et al. Neurosphere-derived multipotent precursors promote neuroprotection by an immunomodulatory mechanism. Nature 2005; 436: 266–271.

313. Pitt D, Werner P, Raine CS. Glutamate excitotoxicity in a model of multiple sclerosis. Nat Med 2000; 6: 67–70.

314. Micu I, Jiang Q, Coderre E et al. NMDA receptors mediate calcium accumulation in myelin during chemical ischemia. Nature 2006; 439: 988–992.

315. Matute C, Domercq M, Sanchez-Gomez MV. Glutamate-mediated glial injury: mechanisms and clinical importance. Glia 2006; 53: 212–224.

316. Pender MP, McCombe PA, Yoong G, Nguyen KB. Apoptosis of alpha beta T lymphocytes in the nervous system in experimental autoimmune encephalomyelitis: its possible implications for recovery and acquired tolerance. J Autoimmun 1992; 5: 401–410.

317. Gimsa U, ORen A, Pandiyan P et al. Astrocytes protect the CNS: antigen-specific T helper cell responses are inhibited by astrocyte-induced upregulation of CTLA-4 (CD152). J Mol Med 2004; 82: 364–372.

318. Hailer NP, Heppner FL, Haas D, Nitsch R. Astrocytic factors deactivate antigen presenting cells that invade the central nervous system. Brain Pathol 1998; 8: 459–474.

319. Dorr J, Bechmann I, Waiczies S et al. Lack of tumor necrosis factor-related apoptosis-inducing ligand but presence of its receptors in the human brain. J Neurosci 2002; 22: RC209.

320. Dorr J, Roth K, Zurbuchen U et al. Tumor-necrosis-factor-related apoptosis-inducing-ligand (TRAIL)-mediated death of neurons in living human brain tissue is inhibited by flupirtine-maleate. J Neuroimmunol 2005; 167: 204–209.

321. Aktas O, Smorodchenko A, Brocke S et al. Neuronal damage in autoimmune neuroinflammation mediated by the death ligand TRAIL. Neuron 2005; 46: 421–432.

322. Jurewicz A, Matysiak M, Andrzejak S, Selmaj K. TRAIL-induced death of human adult oligodendrocytes is mediated by JNK pathway. Glia 2006; 53: 158–166.

323. Jurewicz A, Matysiak M, Tybor K et al. Tumour necrosis factor-induced death of adult human oligodendrocytes is mediated by apoptosis inducing factor. Brain 2005; 128: 2675–2688.

324. Barnett MH, Prineas JW. Relapsing and remitting multiple sclerosis: pathology of the newly forming lesion. Ann Neurol 2004; 55: 458–468.

Genetics of multiple sclerosis

J. R. Oksenberg and S. L. Hauser

MULTIPLE SCLEROSIS AS A GENETIC DISEASE

Multiple sclerosis (MS) clusters with the so-called complex genetic diseases, a group of common disorders characterized by modest disease risk heritability and multifaceted gene-environment interactions. The genetic component in MS is suggested by familial aggregation of cases and the high incidence in some ethnic populations (particularly those of northern European origin) compared with others (African and Asian groups), irrespective of geographical location. High frequency rates are found in Scandinavia, Iceland, the British Isles and North America (about 1–2/1000). Lower frequencies are found among southern Europeans. The disease is uncommon among Samis, Turkmen, Uzbeks, Kazakhs, Kyrgyzis, native Siberians, North and South Amerindians, Chinese, Japanese, African blacks and New Zealand Maori.[1] According to some observers, this characteristic geographical distribution implicates a pathogen that is not ubiquitously distributed. However, this prevalence pattern can also be explained, at least in part, by the geographical clustering of northern Europeans and their descendants. Further, the overall distribution of MS in Europe, showing many exceptions to the previously described north–south gradient, requires more explanation than simply an environmental relationship.[2] The relative high risk among Sardinians, Parsis and Palestinians, and the observation of resistant ethnic groups residing in high-risk regions, as for example gypsies in Bulgaria[3] or Japanese in the USA,[4,5] support the hypothesis that the differential risk observed in different population groups results primarily from genetic susceptibility or resistance.

Evidence of risk heritability in the form of familial recurrence has long been known.[6–8] The degree of familial aggregation can be determined by estimating the ratio of the prevalence in siblings versus the population prevalence of the disease (λ_s).[9] For MS, λ_s is between 20 (0.02/0.001) and 40 (0.04/0.001). Half-sibling,[7] adoptee[10] and spouse[11] risk assessment studies performed in Canada appear to confirm that genetic and not environmental factors are primarily responsible for the familial clustering of cases. However, an intriguing association with month of birth was observed in the Canadian familial cases, reflecting perhaps an interaction between genes and an environmental factor operating during gestation or shortly after birth.[12] Concordant sibs tend to share age of symptom onset rather than year of onset, and second- and third-degree relatives of MS patients are also at an increased risk.

Twin studies from different populations consistently indicate pairwise concordance (20–40% in identical twin pairs compared to 2–5% in like-sex fraternal twin pairs) providing additional evidence for a genetic etiology in MS.[13,14] Surprisingly, twin concordance appears to exhibit, at least in the Canadian series, gender dimorphism (i.e. affectation concordance was only detectable in female twins).[15] On the other hand, the disease concordance ratio was reported to be similar in males and females in a recently published MS twin study.[16] Among the monozygotic twin pairs included in this study, disease concordance was 1.9 times greater in the northern twin pairs residing in Canada and adjacent US states, at or above 41–42°N, 1.9 times greater among twins with high-risk ancestry and 2.1 times greater if diagnosis was early. Ancestry and early diagnosis made independent contributions to the differential concordance by latitude. Altogether, this study indicates that MS is similarly heritable by gender, and the apparent variation in monozygotic concordance by latitude is influenced by both environmental and genetic factors. Exposure to sunlight has received considerable attention as one possible environmental factor that might explain the effect of latitude on MS risk.

Finally, parent-of-origin effects may also influence both disease susceptibility and outcome,[17–19] and concordance in families for early and late clinical features has been observed as well, suggesting that, in addition to susceptibility, genes may influence disease severity or other aspects of the clinical phenotype.[20–22] Overall, neither the recurrence familial rate nor the twin concordance supports the presence of a mendelian trait. Modeling of the available data predicts that the MS-prone genotype results from multiple interacting polymorphic genes, each exerting a small or at most a moderate effect on the overall risk (Fig. 4.1 and Table 14.1).

MULTIPLE SCLEROSIS GENOMICS

In an attempt to map the full array of susceptibility loci and identify the genes that predispose to MS, whole-genome screens

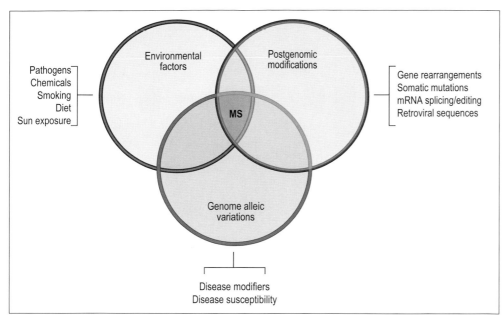

Pathogens
Chemicals
Smoking
Diet
Sun exposure

Environmental factors

Postgenomic modifications

Gene rearrangements
Somatic mutations
mRNA splicing/editing
Retroviral sequences

MS

Genome alleic variations

Disease modifiers
Disease susceptibility

FIG. 14.1 Multiple sclerosis is a complex disease. Compelling epidemiological and molecular data indicate that genes play a role in determining who is at risk for developing MS. However, a simple mendelian model of inheritance for all MS is unlikely because it cannot account for the nonlinear decrease in disease risk in families with increasing genetic distance from the proband. Recurrence risk estimates in families, combined with twin data, predict that the MS-prone genotype results from multiple independent or interacting polymorphic genes, each exerting a small or at most a moderate effect to the overall risk. Hence, although a mendelian-like genetic etiology cannot be ruled out for a small subset of pedigrees, overall the data supports the long-held view that MS is a polygenic and multifactorial disorder.

TABLE 14.1 **Model of genetic contributions in complex genetic disorders**
Multiple genes of moderate and cumulative effect dictate susceptibility and influence disease course
Postgenomic (transcriptional) mechanisms
Difficult-to-identify nonheritable (environmental) factors
Unknown genetic parameters and mode of inheritance
Complex gene–gene and gene–environment interactions
Gender effect in susceptibility
Etiological heterogeneity – identical genes, different phenotype
Genetic heterogeneity – different genes, identical phenotype
Allelic heterogeneity – identical genes, different alleles, identical phenotype

for linkage and/or associations have now been completed in over 30 datasets.[23] Altogether these studies detected a number of genomic regions with potential involvement in disease susceptibility, consistent with the long-held view that MS is a polygenic disorder. However, comparative analysis reveals only partial replication of results across the various screens. This is in part due to the limited power of the datasets, incomplete genomic maps available at the time the (early) studies were performed resulting in poor average information extraction, unknown genotyping error rates, and low statistical thresholds. It is also possible that the study design in each case underestimated the confounding influence of disease heterogeneity and the limitations of parametric methods of statistical analysis. A notable exception is the *MHC* region mapping to the short arm of chromosome 6 (Fig. 14.2), where strong linkage and association signals consistently indicate the presence of a major susceptibility gene or genes. This signal segregates primarily with

the *HLA-DR15* haplotype *DQB1*0602, DQA1*0102, DRB1*1501, DRB5*0101*.[21,24] The association of MS with the HLA-class II locus has been a reproducible finding across nearly all populations studied. Interestingly, a dose effect of *HLA* on disease risk has also been detected;[25–27] this observation was to a certain degree unexpected because if HLA molecules confer susceptibility in MS by presenting an encephalitogenic peptide, then a dominant effect might be anticipated. In the animal model of MS, experimental autoimmune encephalomyelitis or EAE, a single copy of a disease-associated *MHC* haplotype, when expressed in the context of an appropriate genetic background, is generally sufficient for the induction of susceptibility.

Attempts to identify the primary susceptibility gene in the *HLA* region have not provided consensus. The identification of the true predisposing gene or genes within the class II haplotype has been held back by the extensive linkage disequilibrium (LD) across the region and by the presence of many other potential candidate genes with roles in the immune response within this region. LD refers to the presence of alleles at neighboring loci segregating together at the population level more frequently than would be expected according to the genetic distance that separates them. When the effect of *DRB1*1501* is removed from the DR15 haplotype, inconclusive evidence against[28,29] or in favor[30,31] of a primary role for *DQB1*0602* in MS susceptibility has been reported. There is also debate as to the role of non-HLA genes mapping to this region.[32] Results suggesting that genes of interest exist within the *class III*[33,34] and/or telomeric to the *class I*[35–39] regions have been reported as well. The recent availability of genetic LD maps defining haplotype bins in the *HLA* extended region[40,41] will provide a useful reference and tools to identify the true disease gene or genes for MS operating within this superlocus.

Because LD patterns differ between populations, the most direct and practical approach to resolve this complex genetic obstacle will be to scrutinize and compare a large number of MS haplotypes in well characterized datasets from distinct

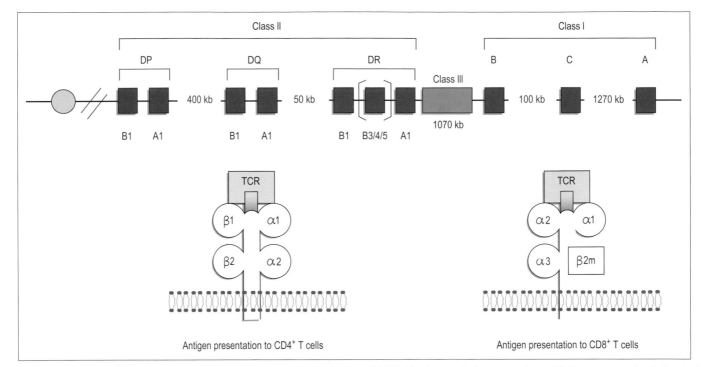

FIG. 14.2 Genomic organization of the major histocompatibility complex (MHC). The human leukocyte antigen (*HLA*) gene complex is located on the short arm of chromosome 6 at p21.3, spanning almost 4000 kb of DNA. The full sequence of this superlocus was completed and reported by the MHC Sequencing Consortium in 1999. Gene density in this region is greater than expected. From 224 identified loci, 128 are predicted to be expressed and about 40% to have immune recognition and response functions. There are two major classes of HLA-encoding genes. The telomeric stretch contains the class I genes, whereas the centromere proximal region encodes HLA-class II genes.

populations. For example, some combinations in *cis* of *DRB1* and *DQB1* alleles are unique in African-Americans. Specifically the *DRB1*1501*, *DQB1*0602* haplotype does not display the rigidity and high degree of LD that is characteristic of northern Europeans. In a recent study of *DRB1* and *DQB1* alleles and haplotypes in a well characterized African-American MS cohort, a selective association with *HLA-DRB1*15* was revealed, indicating a primary role for the *DRB1* locus in MS independent of *DQB1*0602*.[42] It is then likely that *HLA-DRB1* constitutes the centromeric boundary of the class II *DR-DQ* association in MS. African-American patients also exhibited a high degree of allelic heterogeneity as disease association at the *DRB1* locus was found for *DRB1*1501*, *DRB1*1503* and *DRB1*0301* alleles. The haplotypic features of the *DRB1*1501-DQB1*X* (non 0602) and *DRB1*1503*-positive chromosomes indicated an older African origin for the HLA-associated MS susceptibility gene(s), predating the divergence of human ethnic groups, rather than being solely due to genetic admixture with people of European descent. *HLA-DRB1*1501* has a relative low frequency in Africa. Positive selection for this allele appears to have occurred in Europeans but not in Africans and, although the factors that drove this selection, presumably some infectious pathogen, are unknown, one possible consequence was a heightened susceptibility in Europe to MS, a disorder almost nonexistent in Africa.

Compared to European-Americans, African-Americans are at low-risk for MS,[5,43] supporting the presence of genetic risk factors that occur at higher frequency in Europeans. Because the sections of the genome in African-Americans inherited from their European or African ancestors have only had an average of six generations of recombination, extended LD is present in these segments and non-MHC disease genes are potentially amenable to identification through admixture mapping using reasonable numbers of ancestry-informative genetic markers (Fig. 14.3).[44,45] Admixture mapping is based on the observation

that on average 80% of the ancestry of African-Americans is west African and about 20% is European, and works by searching through the genome for sections in which the proportion of European or African ancestry differs from the genome-wide average. In regions of susceptibility, it is expected that African-Americans affected with MS will inherit a higher than average proportion of African or European ancestry, depending on which population has a higher risk for disease at the genetic level. We have already had success with admixture mapping and have just recently identified a locus on chromosome 1 where there is a significant higher proportion of European ancestry in MS chromosomes compared to the genome-wide average; follow-up studies should identify the responsible gene.[46]

A primary role for *HLA-DRB1* in susceptibility to MS is consistent with a pathogenesis model that involves a T-cell-mediated autoimmune response against the 85–99 peptide of myelin basic protein (MBP).[47–50] The crystal structure of DRβ1501 differs from other non *DR2*-related DRβ molecules in that aromatic residues in the ligand are preferred in the large hydrophobic P4 pocket of the peptide binding domain.[51] For MBP, this pocket is primarily occupied by the aromatic side chain Phe92, acting as an important primary anchor and accounting for its high-affinity binding to the HLA-DRα0101/DRβ1501 heterodimer. The polymorphic residue at DRβ71 is also critically important in creating the necessary space for Phe92 of MBP, and Ala at this position has only been observed for *DR15* alleles (*DRB1*1501-DRB1*1506*) and *DRB1*1309*.

*HLA-DRB1*1501*, *DRB1*1503* and *DRB1*0301* alleles all share a critical Val residue at position 86, where the HLA-DRβ chain is also polymorphic, and can encode either Val or Gly. DRβVal86 at the base of the P1 pocket results in a smaller pocket than that observed for *DR1* and *DR4* (Gly) for example, influencing not only binding and presentation of a number of self antigens including MBP, but also DRαβ dimer stability.[50–53] The Val86/Val86 genotype has been implicated in association

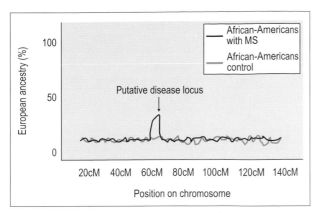

FIG. 14.3 How a disease locus will appear in an admixture scan. Admixture mapping is designed to study populations descended, at least in part, from the recent mixing of ethnic groups from multiple parts of the world (such as African- and Hispanic Americans). In chromosomal regions containing variants contributing to disease risk, there will be an overrepresentation of ancestry from whichever population has a higher proportion of risk alleles at the locus. The peak can be identified not only in a case-control comparison but also in a comparison of the estimate of ancestry in cases at that point in their genome to the rest of their genomes. The width of the peak of association is determined by the number of generations since mixture.

TABLE 14.2 Top results from the nonparametric analysis of linkage data

Chromosome	MLS	Sib allele sharing (%)	λ_s
6p21	11.66	58.5	1.51
17q23	2.45	53.8	1.18
5q33	2.18	54.0	1.19
20p12	1.83	54.0	1.09
3p26	1.74	53.4	1.16

The most recent and comprehensive linkage study in MS was recently completed by the International MS Genetics Consortium.[24] Data from 4506 markers in 2692 individuals were included in the analysis. This set of markers achieved a mean information extraction across the genome of 79.3%. Multipoint nonparametric linkage analysis reveals highly significant linkage in the MHC on chromosome 6p21 together with suggestive linkage on chromosome 17q23 and 5q33. Stratification based on carriage of the MS associated DRB1*1501 allele failed to identify any other region of linkage with genome wide significance. However, ordered-subset analysis suggests that there may be an additional locus on chromosome 19p13 acting independently of the main MHC locus. These data illustrate the substantial increase in power that can be achieved using the latest tools emerging from the Human Genome Project and indicate that future attempts to identify susceptibility genes in multiple sclerosis will have to involve large sample sizes and an association-based methodology.

studies in Swedish and Australian MS populations.[28,54] Glatiramer acetate binds to purified HLA-DR1, -DR2, and -DR4 molecules with high affinity. Interestingly, none of the amino acid residues in glatiramer acetate (Tyr, Glu, Ala, Lys) is able to bind with high affinity to the P1 pocket of HLA-DR2. Tyr is, however, appropriate for the P4 pocket and thus can serve to anchor binding of glatiramer acetate to DR2. Altered peptide ligands (APL) were developed to bind DR2 but not trigger T-cell responses against MBP86–99; despite the apparent failure of APL to modulate clinical disease activity in MS, a new generation of therapeutic synthetic peptides developed based upon a better understanding of the molecular structure of HLA molecules may be available for clinical trials in the near future.[55]

Using family data, the proportion of total genetic susceptibility explained by the *HLA* locus in MS can be estimated; at the lower end, under an additive model it could explain as little as 15% and at the upper end under a multiplicative genetic model the *HLA* association can explain as much as 60% of the genetic etiology.[56] In either case, much of the genetic effect in MS remains to be explained but there is no consensus on which are the best supported non-MHC regions in the genome.[57–59] The most powerful linkage study performed so far in MS (4506 markers in 2692 individuals from 730 multiplex families of northern European descent) was recently published. Analysis reveals highly significant linkage in the MHC, together with suggestive linkage on chromosome 17q23 and 5q33 (Table 14.2).[24]

Unfortunately, the direct testing by association of possibly relevant candidate genes, identified by speculation based upon concepts of pathogenesis, has been also unproductive for gene identification in this disease. Recently reported associated genes such as *NOS2a*,[60] *IL4R*,[61] *CD24*,[62] *TAC1*,[63] *CCLs*,[64] *MHC2TA*[65] and *PRKCA*[66] constitute promising leads but remain to be replicated (Table 14.3). Variations in the interleukin 7 receptor alpha chain have recently been identified as having a consistent, albeit small effect in MS.[67] Surprisingly, genes found to be associated with multiple autoimmune diseases such as *CTLA4* and *PTN22* do not appear to play a major role in MS, indicating a fundamentally different disease pathogenesis.[68,69] Progress in developing affordable high-throughput genotyping technology and a

better understanding of the complex structure encoded within the human genome[70–72] suggest that the tools may finally be at hand to achieve the elusive goal of whole-genome association studies.[73] Although most SNPs are likely to be neutral with no phenotypic consequences, some may mark the 'causative' sequence difference contributing to disease susceptibility and/or resistance. Association studies of this type harbor great potential for complex disorders but a number of very important challenges, including how to interpret results obtained from large numbers of statistical tests and how to detect biologically meaningful interactions between polymorphisms that confer disease risk, will need to be overcome. A screen of such type in 931 MS trio families was recently completed by an international consortium.[74] The study yielded a large number of promising leads, which were pursued in a confirmatory data set. A combined analysis from more than 12,000 samples identified a number of genes involved in disease susceptibility, including the interleukin 2 receptor (also known as CD25), on chromosome 10p15 and the interleukin 7 receptor (CD127) on chromosome 5p13.

GENETIC HETEROGENEITY IN MULTIPLE SCLEROSIS

A noteworthy conceptual development in the understanding of MS genetics has been the recognition of locus heterogeneity, meaning that different genes or alleles can cause identical or similar forms of the disease in different individuals (Fig. 14.4). In a study of 184 multicase US MS families, linkage and association to the *HLA-DRB1* locus and a strong association with the specific DR2 haplotype (*DRB1*1501, DQB1*0602*) was confirmed.[21] Remarkably, all the linkage information and evidence for association derived from the families in which *DRB1*1501* was present in at least one nuclear member. No genetic effect of the *HLA* locus could be discerned in the clinically indistinguishable *DRB1*1501*-negative family set. In fact, the results excluded linkage for at least 20 cM around *HLA-DRB1* in the *DRB1*1501*-negative families, providing strong evidence that heterogeneity at the *HLA* locus exists in MS.

Another example of *HLA* locus heterogeneity in MS is provided by studies in Japanese patients. In this group, one form of MS is characterized by disseminated CNS involvement and is associated with the *HLA-DRB1*1501* haplotype, whereas

TABLE 14.3 **Examples of non-MHC candidate gene variants that have recently been associated with multiple sclerosis**

Gene	Chromosomal location	Population(s)	Biological function(s)	Reference
CD24 molecule (CD24)	6q21	Central Ohio case-control	Apoptosis Immune response	62
Neuropeptide preprotachykinin-1 (TAC1)	7q21–22	Northern Irish case-control	Neurotransmission Vasodilatation Behavior	63
Interleukin 4 receptor (IL4R)	16p11–12	Single case US MS families	Immune response	61
MHC class II transactivator (MHC2TA)	16p13	Nordic case-control	Regulation of MHC class II expression	65
Nitric acid synthase (NOS2a)	17q11	Multicase US families and African-American case-control	Neurotransmission Antimicrobial Immune response	60
β-chemokines or CC chemokine ligands (CCLs)	17q11	Multicase US and Canadian families	Immune response	64
Protein kinase C α (PRKCA)	17q24	Multi-case Finnish and Canadian MS families	Cell adhesion Cell transformation Cell cycle checkpoint	66
Interleukin-7 receptor α	5p13	Single and multi-case US and UK families	Immune response Immune maturation	67

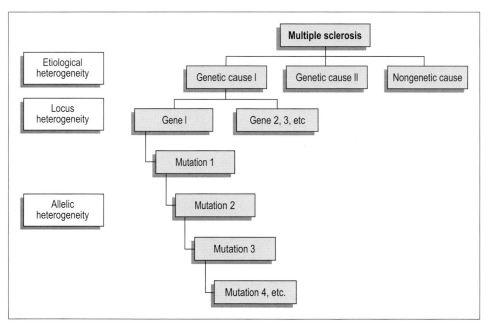

FIG. 14.4 Possible levels of heterogeneity in MS. The clinical thinking that MS is a single disorder with varied clinical manifestations and courses may be at odds with data derived from a variety of disciplines – clinical, pathological, imaging, immunological and genetic – all suggesting that biological diversity is an important feature of the MS syndrome. The implications of this heterogeneity are considerable because fundamentally distinct immunopathogenic mechanisms may be acting in different affected individuals. Progress in deciphering the MS genome is necessarily linked to a full description of heterogeneity at all etiological levels.

more restricted forms of disease in which optic nerve and/or spinal cord involvement predominate and lesions are more severe and necrotizing, are not associated with *HLA-DRB1*1501*.[75] The strength of the association between primary progressive MS (PPMS) and *HLA-DRB1*1501* is also uncertain. A number of small studies failed to show any association between PPMS and *DRB1*1501*, although a larger study from Northern Ireland appeared to show the association.[76] Our recent data also clearly reveal an association between PPMS and *DRB1*1501*.[77]

We recently studied *HLA* class II alleles in an MS dataset carefully ascertained in Sicily, an island 3 km apart from continental Italy, with a population of just over 5 100 000 but a unique demo-graphic history and high prevalence and incidence of MS.[78] Evidence for excess transmission to affected individuals was observed for *HLA-DRB1*1501, DRB1*04, DQB1*02* and *DQB1*0302* alleles but not for *DQB1*0602*. When *HLA* alleles were analyzed as haplotypes, we observed an excess transmission for the *DRB1*04, DQB1*0302* haplotype. Overall, Sicilian patients share the *HLA-DRB1*1501* susceptibility allele with patients living in continental Italy, but also display allelic heterogeneity, specifically a strong association with the *HLA-DR4* haplotype. The *HLA-DR3* haplotype observed in association with MS in neighboring Sardinia[37] was negative in Sicilians. However, *HLA-DR3* may confer a low relative risk compared to *HLA-DRB1*1501*, and large datasets may be necessary to detect its effect. Interestingly, a dose effect for *HLA-DR3* has also been proposed in MS cases and controls[27] and confirmed in family studies.[77] However, in contrast to *HLA-DRB1*1501*, the risk conferred by *DR3* appears to be minor and recessive, with two copies (*DR3/DR3*) modestly increasing risk, compared to no risk for *DR3/DRX* individuals. The preferential transmission of the *DRB1*08* allele in *trans* with *DRB1*1* haplotypes and the undertransmission of *DRB1*14* was detected in MS families,[77,79] underscoring the complex genetic nature of this disease. Together these data are helping to upgrade the conceptual model of MS pathogenesis and suggest that complex *trans DRB1* allelic interactions may determine the balance between susceptibility and resistance.

SUSCEPTIBILITY GENES VERSUS MODIFIERS

Clinical symptoms in MS are extremely variable. The course may be relapsing–remitting or progressive, severe or mild, and involve the neuraxis in a widespread fashion or predominantly affect the spinal cord and optic nerve. Very little is known about the underlying cause of disease variability in MS but it is important to recognize that the aggregate contribution of germline genetic variants to the disease course may be quite modest. This is highlighted by observations that the clinical expression of MS may be different even between monozygotic twin siblings. Nevertheless, the demonstration of even a modest genetic effect of a known gene on the course of MS could represent a major therapeutic opportunity. A large number of studies have focused, with inconclusive findings, on the relevance of *HLA* variation to the clinical features of MS. To date, *HLA-DRB1*1501* has been reported to be associated with an earlier age of disease onset, female gender, severe, relapsing–remitting, and mild MS courses[26,80–84] or to have no influence on disease course.[85–90]

To assess the state of genotype-phenotype research in MS we have identified from the literature a set of gene polymorphisms that have been reported to be significantly associated with phenotypic endpoints (Table 14.4). The list omits many reports and probably includes type I errors due to small sample sizes. In addition, the clinical assessments were determined retrospectively in most series, some phenotypic endpoints are questionable or not validated, and the confounding effects of drug treatment and/or stratification have not been generally considered. Finally, the assessment of modifier effects has often been piggybacked upon candidate-gene susceptibility studies, further limiting their informativeness. Parenthetically, it may also be difficult to discriminate whether phenotypic diversity reflects etiological heterogeneity, as suggested above, a modifying role of a specific gene or some combination of the two. These caveats aside, the studies summarized in Table 14.4 highlight the range and scope of published reports suggesting genetic influences on the natural history of MS.

GENES AND ENVIRONMENTAL FACTORS

Epidemiological, twin concordance, clusters or outbreaks, and migration studies have been widely used to search for potential environmental influences on MS. Although the interpretation of most of these studies has been difficult, in part because of the small number of study participants in the individual reports, the results have been influential and do suggest a role for environmental factors in MS and, in some cases, the existence of critical time periods for exposure to putative environmental disease agents. A large number of environmental exposures have been investigated. Those include viral and bacterial infections, nutritional and dietary factors, well water consumption, exposure to animals, minerals, trauma due to accident or surgery, pollution, solar radiation, temperature, rainfall, humidity, chemical agents, metals, organic solvents and various occupational hazards. Viruses are among the most frequently studied and biologically plausible putative infectious agents related to MS pathogenesis, and many have been proposed to be the causative MS agent. Prominent candidates have included measles, rubella, mumps and the herpes viruses including Epstein–Barr virus (EBV), herpes simplex virus 1 and 2 and varicella zoster virus. Higher antibody titers against each of these have been detected in the serum and CSF samples of MS patients when compared to control individuals. Strong evidence for a role of EBV in particular has been indicated by epidemiological[91,92] and laboratory studies.[93,94] Similar to other autoimmune diseases, exposure to cigarette smoke has also emerged as a potential environmental risk factor for MS. In a recent prospective study, researchers defined a 60% greater incidence rate of MS in current smokers than in never-smokers.[95] Interestingly, the relative rate also increased significantly with cumulative exposure to smoking.

However, most attempts to isolate the causative environmental trigger(s) in MS have been largely unproductive and have failed to provide major insights into mechanisms of disease susceptibility and pathogenesis. This may be because of heterogeneity operating also at the level of causative factors. Whether the genotype dictates different forms of the same disease in response to a common causative agent or other trigger, or whether the genotype reflects different diseases with completely separate environmental causes is not known. The expectation that any single agent would have enough specificity and universality to account for all cases of a single disorder may be unrealistic. On the other hand, the identification and confirmation of true environmental factors might lead to the discovery of important variation in relevant susceptibility genes such as cell membrane molecules serving as pathogen receptors, base excision repair or detoxification enzymes.

GENETICS IN ANIMAL MODELS OF MULTIPLE SCLEROSIS

Experimental allergic (or autoimmune) encephalomyelitis (EAE) can be induced in a variety of animal species, including nonhuman primates, by immunization with myelin proteins or their peptide derivatives, as well as by adoptive transfer of CD4+ activated cells specific for myelin components.[96,97] A second, virally induced animal model for MS uses the Theiler's murine virus from the picorna family to induce brain inflammation and injury of the myelin sheath. When studied in genetically susceptible animals, immunization induces brain inflammation accompanied by varied signs of neurological disease, ataxia and paralysis, first in the tail and hind limbs then progressing to forelimb paralysis and eventual death. EAE and MS share common clinical, histological, immunological and genetic features; hence EAE is widely considered to be a relevant model for the human disease.[98] The concept of susceptibility versus resistance in EAE is relative rather than absolute, as evidence demonstrates that modifications of the experimental protocol will induce detectable disease in strains previously considered resistant. Genetic studies in EAE have been informative in defining the complex interplay of multiple genes that can result in brain inflammation and demyelination. Furthermore, like MS, EAE is sensitive to environmental factors, including age and season at immunization.[99,100] The best characterized EAE susceptibility gene resides within the *MHC* on murine chromosome 17.[101] Induction and full clinical manifestations of EAE

TABLE 14.4 Examples of gene variants that have been associated with the MS phenotype

Gene/locus	Chromosomal location	Allele	Associate phenotype	Reference
GSTM1	1p13.3	Ile105	Severe disability	110
IL-1ra/IL-1β	2q14.2	IL-1β exon 5 C/T	High protein expression and favorable prognosis	111, 112
		IL-1ra intron 4 VNTR	High protein expression and favorable prognosis	113, 114
PD-1	2237	G/A 7146, enhancer in intron 4	An allele associated with impaired secretion of interferon-γ progressive disease course	115
CCR5	3p21–24	Δ32 bp deletion	Age of onset was approximately 3 years later in patients carrying the deletion	116
			Progression to disability was delayed in homozygotes and heterozygotes for the deletion	117
			Lower risk of recurrent disease activity	118
			Trend to reduced frequency in PPMS	119
			Trend to smaller lesion burden	120
			Early death	121
OPN	4q21-q25	1284A/C	Patients with the wild type 1284A genotype are less likely to have mild disease course and are at increased risk for a secondary progressive clinical type	122
		9583 G/A	Patients with the 9583 G/G genotype showed later disease onset	123
		Rs# 4754, Rs# 1126616, Rs# 4660, Rs# 1126772, Rs# 1126859, Rs# 9138, Rs# 1126880, Rs# 1126893	No association with disease severity	124
Il-4	5q31.1	VNTR B1	Late onset / Late onset in homozygotes	125, 126
HLA	6p21.3	DRB1*1501	HLA haplotypes have been reported to be associated with an earlier age of disease onset, gender dimorphism, severe, relapsing–remitting, and mild MS courses	26,80–84
			HLA haplotypes have been reported to have no influence on disease course	85–90
			No DRB1 association in some Asian populations who have a restricted disease, termed neuromyelitis optica in which optic nerve and/or spinal cord involvement predominates.	75
			A high prevalence of DR2 was observed in patients with acute unilateral optic neuritis. Its presence was associated with increased odds for developing definite MS. The association was most apparent among patients with signal abnormalities on the baseline brain MRI	127
			A number of small studies failed to show any association between PPMS and DR2, although a larger study from Northern Ireland appeared to show the association. Others suggested an association between PPMS and the HLA-DR4 haplotype although a post-hoc analysis is consistent with an effect decreasing the risk for RRMS in HLA-DR4+ individuals, rather than increasing the risk for PPMS	22, 76, 87, 128, 129
			Glutamic acid at position 71 or 74 in pocket 4 of DRβ1 is associated with PPMS	130
CD24	6q21	ORF A/V	50% of CD24 V/V patients with expanded disability status scale 6.0 reached the milestone in 5 years, whereas the CD24 A/V and CD24 A/A patients did so in 16 and 13 years, respectively	64
ESR1	6q21.5	PvuII and XbaI RFLP	P-allele-positive patients had a significantly higher progression of disability and a worse ranked MS severity score. The study also suggests an interaction between the ESR1 genotype and DR2 in women with MS. Esr1 and -2 appear to regulate the severity of clinical EAE	131, 132
		PvuII RFLP	The study suggests an interaction between the ESR1 genotype and DR2 in women with MS	133
CD59	10q24.1	−670A or exon 7 74C	Gender dimorphism	134

TABLE 14.4 Examples of gene variants that have been associated with the MS phenotype—cont'd

Gene/locus	Chromosomal location	Allele	Associate phenotype	Reference
CNTF	11q12	Exon 2/–6, G→A null mutation	Patients with the CNTF –/– genotype had significantly earlier onset (17 vs 27 years) with predominant motor symptoms	135
			No correlation with age of onset, course or severity	136
CRYAB	11q22.3–q23.1	Promoter region C650G	Carriers of the rare allele CRYAB-650*C have an increased likelihood of a noninflammatory, neurodegenerative phenotype characterized by a relatively rapid, primary progressive clinical disease course	137
IFNG	12q14	3'(325)*G/A	Gender dimorphism	138
MEFV	16p13.3	M694V	Rapid progression to disability in non-Ashkenazi Jewish patients	139
APOE	19q13.2	APOE-4	Increased severity, rate of progression, or disease brain activity	140–146
			Disease course (PPMS) in women not carrying HLA susceptibility haplotypes	147
			No effect	120, 148–151
		APOE-2	Decreased severity and progression to chronic progressive disease	152–154
TGFB1	19q13	–509/C and codon 10/+869	Decreased severity defined as an EDSS score <3 after 10 years of symptoms	155
		codon 10/+869	C allele associated with higher annual increase of central brain atrophy and matrix destruction	156

EAE, experimental autoimmune encephalomyelitis; PPMS, primary progressive multiple sclerosis; RRMS, relapsing–remitting multiple sclerosis.

are strongly influenced by inherited polymorphisms of *MHC* class II region genes; certain *MHC* haplotypes are more permissive for EAE whereas others are more resistant. In addition, the various EAE models underscore the importance of locus heterogeneity, with different *MHC*-encoded genes and alleles mediating highly specific autoimmune responses induced by different triggering encephalitogenic peptides.

The use of classic genetics and whole-genome screening in different strains has identified several additional genetic regions that contain QTLs conferring EAE susceptibility, including loci on chromosomes 2, 3, 7, 8, 15, 16, 17 (*MHC* in the mouse), 17 (distal to *MHC*) and 18.[102] Other regions in the genome, including the Y chromosome,[103] have been implicated as containing disease-modifying genes affecting severity, course, duration and CNS pathology. All together 27 non-MHC have been identified. Interestingly, the linkage peaks are, in part, gender-specific. More recently, genetic control of CNS repair-related traits in virally induced EAE (less axonal damage, progressive remyelination and stabilization of motor function) was demonstrated, highlighting the significant extent to which genetic factors can influence disease course.[104] These studies provide compelling evidence for the hypothesis that susceptibility to autoimmune demyelination is genetically determined. Similar to human diseases, a multiple-locus model is applicable: each locus may contribute to a specific stage of EAE pathology, although some loci are probably involved in several steps of the autoimmune process.[105] However, no locus seems to be an absolute requirement for the susceptible phenotype; i.e. a susceptible EAE phenotype can be achieved in different crosses by different combinations of genotypes. As the roster of genes that contribute to EAE is fully identified, such genes will represent strong candidates for testing in human disease.

GENETIC VARIATION AND THE CLINICAL RESPONSE TO THERAPY IN MULTIPLE SCLEROSIS

Perhaps the most significant advance in MS therapeutics has been the approval of interferons.[106] Interferons are small inducible proteins secreted by nucleated cells in response to viral infection or other stimuli, which act in a paracrine fashion on other cells in their immediate vicinity. Overall, interferon (IFN)β has been shown to decrease clinical relapses, reduce brain MRI activity and possibly slow progression of disability. However, the effect of this treatment is partial and a substantial proportion of patients are not responders. Therapy has been associated with a number of adverse reactions, including flu-like symptoms, transient laboratory abnormalities, menstrual disorders, increased spasticity and skin reactions. Furthermore, the significance of long-term effects and especially the impact of treatment on disease progression has not been determined. Lacking predictive clinical, neuroradiological and/or immunological markers of response, and given that some patients have a relatively benign form of the disease, what should be the appropriate indications for treatment of an MS therapy with substantial side effects, inconvenience and cost?

The pharmacogenomic MS literature is relatively sparse but a substantial effort is currently under way in different laboratories to directly address the question of genetic heterogeneity and the response to immunotherapy by analysis of the correlation between different genotypes and clinical response to therapeutic modalities. In recently published studies, for example, an effect of the *HLA-DRB1*1501* haplotype was observed in MS patients treated with glatiramer acetate but not with IFNβ.[90,107] The analysis of eight SNPs in the interferon receptor genes failed to show significant evidence of pharmacogenomic influences.[108] More recently, we applied advanced data-mining and predictive modeling tools to a longitudinal gene expression dataset generated from MS patients treated with IFNβ in order to discover higher-order predictive patterns associated with treatment outcome.[109] We identified nine sets of gene triplets whose expression, when tested before the initiation of therapy, can predict favorable response with up to 87% accuracy. Notably, the genes in the top-scoring triplet were Caspase-2, Caspase-10 and *FLIP*, three apoptosis-related molecules. The second highest scoring triplet was that of Caspase 2, Caspase 3 and *IRF4* (86.8%). Other high scoring triplets included *IL4Ra* and *MAP3K1*, in addition to other apoptotic molecules. Despite the relatively high predictive accuracy of these models, the functional link between genes and therapeutic effects of this drug is still unclear.

CONCLUSIONS

Compelling epidemiological and molecular data indicate that genes play a primary role in determining who is at risk for developing MS. The genetic component of MS etiology is believed to result from the action of common allelic variants in several genes. Some loci may be involved in the initial pathogenic events while others could influence the development and progression of the disease. Their incomplete penetrance and moderate individual effect probably reflects interactions with other genes, post-transcriptional regulatory mechanisms, and significant environmental and epigenetic influences. Equally significantly, it is also likely that genetic heterogeneity exists, meaning that specific genes influence susceptibility and pathogenesis in some individuals with MS but not others.

The past few years have seen real progress in the development of laboratory and analytical approaches to study non-mendelian complex genetic disorders and in defining the pathological basis of demyelination, setting the stage for the final characterization of the genes involved in MS susceptibility and pathogenesis. Large-scale molecular explorations in human genetics are now virtually routine. With the aid of high-capacity technologies, the combined and integrative analysis of genomic, transcriptional, proteomic and extensive phenotypic information, including environmental exposure data, is expected, in the near future, to revolutionize concepts of MS pathogenesis, provide a framework for understanding the mechanisms of action of existing therapies and lead to the conception of novel curative strategies. To paraphrase Einstein, we can anticipate discoveries that will simplify the problem of MS.

ACKNOWLEDGMENTS

The authors are supported by the National Multiple Sclerosis Society, the National Institute of Health and the Nancy Davis and Montel Williams Foundations.

REFERENCES

1. Rosati G. The prevalence of multiple sclerosis in the world: an update. Neurol Sci 2001; 22: 117–139.

2. Sotgiu S, Pugliatti M, Sotgiu A et al. Does the 'hygiene hypothesis' provide an explanation for the high prevalence of multiple sclerosis in Sardinia? Autoimmunity 2003; 36: 257–260.

3. Milanov I, Topalov N, Kmetski T. Prevalence of multiple sclerosis in Gypsies and Bulgarians. Epidemiol 1999; 18: 218–222.

4. Detels R, Visscher BR, Malmgren RM et al. Evidence for lower susceptibility to multiple sclerosis in Japanese-Americans. Am J Epidemiol 1977; 105: 303–310.

5. Kurtzke JF, Beebe GW, Norman JE Jr. Epidemiology of multiple sclerosis in U.S. veterans: 1. Race, sex, and geographic distribution. Neurology 1979; 29: 1228–1235.

6. Robertson NP, Fraser M, Deans J et al. Age-adjusted recurrence risks for relatives of patients with multiple sclerosis. Brain 1996; 119: 449–455.

7. Sadovnick AD, Ebers GC, Dyment DA, Risch NJ. Evidence for genetic basis of multiple sclerosis. Lancet 1996; 347: 1728–1730.

8. Sadovnick AD, Yee IM, Ebers GC. Factors influencing sib risks for multiple sclerosis. Clin Genet 2000; 58: 431–435.

9. Risch N. Corrections to linkage strategies for genetically complex traits. III. The effect of marker polymorphism on anlaysis of affected relative pairs. Am J Hum Genet 1992; 51: 673–675.

10. Ebers GC, Sadovnick AD, Risch NJ. A genetic basis for familial aggregation in multiple sclerosis. Nature 1995; 377: 150–151.

11. Ebers GC, Yee IM, Sadovnick AD, Duquette P. Conjugal multiple sclerosis: population-based prevalence and recurrence risks in offspring. Ann Neurol 2000; 48: 927–931.

12. Willer CJ, Dyment DA, Sadovnick AD et al. Timing of birth and risk of multiple sclerosis: population based study. Br Med J 2005; 330: 120.

13. Sadovnick AD, Armstrong H, Rice GP et al. A population-based study of multiple sclerosis in twins: update. Ann Neurol 1993; 33: 281–285.

14. Mumford CJ, Wood NW, Kellar-Wood H et al. The British Isles survey of multiple sclerosis in twins. Neurology 1994; 44: 11–15.

15. Willer CJ, Dyment DA, Risch NJ et al. Twin concordance and sibling recurrence rates in multiple sclerosis. Proc Natl Acad Sci USA 2003; 100: 12877–12882.

16. Islam T, Gauderman J, Cozen W et al. Differential twin concordance for multiple sclerosis by latitude of birthplace. Ann Neurol 2006; 60: 56–64.

17. Hupperts R, Broadley S, Mander A et al. Patterns of disease in concordant parent-child pairs with multiple sclerosis. Neurology 2001; 57: 290–295.

18. Ebers GC, Sadovnick AD, Dyment DA et al. Parent-of-origin effect in multiple sclerosis: observations in half-siblings. Lancet 2004; 363: 1773–1774.

19. Kantarci OH, Barcellos LF, Atkinson EJ et al. Men transmit MS more often to their children vs. women: the Carter effect. Neurology 2006; 67: 305–310.

20. Brassat D, Azais-Vuillemin C, Yaouanq J et al. Familial factors influence disability in MS multiplex families. Neurology 1999; 52: 1632–1636.

21. Barcellos LF, Oksenberg JR, Green AJ et al. Genetic basis for clinical expression in multiple sclerosis. Brain 2002; 125: 150–158.

22. Hensiek AE, Seaman SR, Barcellos LF et al. Familial effects on the clinical course of multiple sclerosis. Neurology 2007; 68: 373–383.

23. Fernald GH, Yeh RF, Hauser SL et al. Mapping gene activity in complex disorders: Integration of expression and genomic scans for multiple sclerosis. J Neuroimmunol 2005; 167: 157–169.

24. Sawcer S, Ban M, Maranian M et al. A high-density screen for linkage in multiple sclerosis. Am J Hum Genet 2005; 77: 454–467.

25. Rasmussen HB, Kelly MA, Clausen J. Addictive effect of the HLA-DR15 haplotype in susceptibility to multiple sclerosis. Mult Scler 2001; 7: 91–93.

26. Barcellos LF, Oksenberg JR, Begovich AB et al. HLA-DR2 dose effect on susceptibility to multiple sclerosis and influence on disease course. Am J Hum Genet 2003; 72: 710–716.

27. Modin H, Olsson W, Hillert J, Masterman T. Modes of action of HLA-DR

susceptibility specificities in multiple sclerosis. Am J Hum Genet 2004; 74: 1321–1322.

28. Allen M, Sandberg-Wollheim M, Sjogren K et al. Association of susceptibility to multiple sclerosis in Sweden with HLA class II DRB1 and DQB1 alleles. Hum Immunol 1994; 39: 41–48.

29. Lincoln MR, Montpetit A, Cader MZ et al. A predominant role for the HLA class II region in the association of the MHC region with multiple sclerosis. Nat Genet 2005; 37: 1108–1112.

30. Spurkland A, Ronningen K, Vandvik B et al. HLA-DQA1 and HLA-DQB1 genes may jointly determine susceptibility to develop multiple sclerosis. Hum Immunol 1991; 30: 69–75.

31. Boon M, Nolte IM, Bruinenberg M et al. Mapping of a susceptibility gene for multiple sclerosis to the 51kb interval between G511525 and D6S1666 using a new method of haplotype sharing analysis. Neurogenetics 2001; 3: 221–230.

32. Ligers A, Dyment DA, Willer CJ et al. Evidence of linkage with HLA-DR in DRB1*15-negative families with multiple sclerosis. Am J Hum Genet 2001; 69: 900–903.

33. De Jong BA, Huizinga TW, Zanelli E et al. Evidence for additional genetic risk indicators of relapse-onset MS within the HLA region. Neurology 2002; 59: 549–555.

34. Palacio LG, Rivera D, Builes JJ et al. Multiple sclerosis in the tropics: genetic association to STR's loci spanning the HLA and TNF. Mult Scler 2002; 8: 249–255.

35. Shinar Y, Pras E, Siev-Ner I et al. Analysis of allelic association between D6S461 marker and multiple sclerosis in Ashkenazi and Iraqi Jewish patients. J Mol Neurosci 1998; 11: 265–269.

36. Fogdell-Hahn A, Ligers A, Gronning M et al. Multiple sclerosis: a modifying influence of HLA class I genes in an HLA class II associated autoimmune disease. Tissue Antigens 2000; 55: 140–148.

37. Marrosu MG, Murru R, Murru MR et al. Dissection of the HLA association with multiple sclerosis in the founder isolated population of Sardinia. Hum Mol Genet 2001; 10: 2907–2916.

38. Lie BA, Akselsen HE, Bowlus CL et al. Polymorphisms in the gene encoding thymus-specific serine protease in the extended HLA complex: a potential candidate gene for autoimmune and HLA-associated diseases. Genes Immun 2002; 3: 306–312.

39. Rubio JP, Bahlo M, Butzkueven H et al. Genetic dissection of the human leukocyte antigen region by use of haplotypes of Tasmanians with multiple sclerosis. Am J Hum Genet 2002; 70: 1125–1137.

40. Walsh EC, Mather KA, Schaffner SF et al. An integrated haplotype map of the human major histocompatibility complex. Am J Hum Genet 2003; 73: 580–590.

41. Miretti MM, Walsh EC, Ke X et al. A high-resolution linkage-disequilibrium map of the human major histocompatibility complex and first generation of tag single-nucleotide polymorphisms. Am J Hum Genet 2005; 76: 634–646.

42. Oksenberg JR, Barcellos LF, Cree BA et al. Mapping multiple sclerosis

susceptibility to the HLA-DR locus in African Americans. Am J Hum Genet 2004; 74: 160–167.

43. Wallin MT, Page WF, Kurtzke JF. Multiple sclerosis in US veterans of the Vietnam era and later military service: race, sex, and geography. Ann Neurol 2004; 55: 65–71.

44. Patterson N, Hattangadi N, Lane B et al. Methods for high-density admixture mapping of disease genes. Am J Hum Genet 2004; 74: 979–1000.

45. Seldin MF, Morii T, Collins-Schramm HE et al. Putative ancestral origins of chromosomal segments in individual African Americans: implications for admixture mapping. Genome Res 2004; 14: 1076–1084.

46. Reich DE, Patterson N, De Jager PL et al. A whole-genome admixture scan localizes a candidate gene for multiple sclerosis susceptibility. Nat Genet 2005; 37: 1113–1118.

47. Allegretta M, Nicklas JA, Sriram S, Albertini RJ. T cells responsive to myelin basic protein in patients with multiple sclerosis. Science 1990; 247: 718–721.

48. Pette M, Fujita K, Kitze B et al. Myelin basic protein specific T cell lines from MS patients and healthy individuals. Neurology 1990; 40: 1770–1776.

49. Oksenberg JR, Panzara MA, Begovich AB et al. Selection for T-cell receptor Vb-Db-Jb gene rearrangements with specificity for a myelin basic protein peptide in brain lesions of multiple sclerosis. Nature 1993; 362: 68–70.

50. Krogsgaard M, Wucherpfennig KW, Canella B et al. Visualization of myelin basic protein (MBP) T cell epitopes in multiple sclerosis lesions using a monoclonal antibody specific for the human histocompatibility leukocyte antigen (HLA)-DR2-MBP 85–99 complex. J Exp Med 2000; 191: 1395–1412.

51. Smith KJ, Pyrdol J, Gauthier L et al. Crystal structure of HLA-DR2 (DRA*0101, DRB1*1501) complexed with a peptide from human myelin basic protein. J Exp Med 1998; 188: 1511–1520.

52. Verreck FA, Termijtelen A, Koning F. HLA-DR beta chain residue 86 controls DR alpha beta dimer stability. Eur J Immunol 1993; 23: 1346–1350.

53. Wucherpfennig KW, Sette A, Southwood S et al. Structural requirements for binding of an immunodominant myelin basic protein peptide to DR 2 isotypes and for its recognition by human T cell clones. J Exp Med 1994; 179: 279–290.

54. Teutsch SM, Bennetts BH, Buhler MM et al. The DRB1 Val86/Val86 genotype associates with multiple sclerosis in Australian patients. Hum Immunol 1999; 60: 715–722.

55. Stern JN, Illes Z, Reddy J et al. Peptide 15-mers of defined sequence that substitute for random amino acid copolymers in amelioration of experimental autoimmune encephalomyelitis. Proc Natl Acad Sci USA 2005; 102: 1620–1625.

56. Haines JL, Terwedow HA, Burgess K et al. Linkage of the MHC to familial multiple sclerosis suggests genetic heterogeneity. Hum Mol Genet 1998; 7: 1229–1234.

57. Pericak-Vance MA, Rimmler JB, Martin ER et al. Linkage and association analysis of chromosome 19q13 in multiple sclerosis. Neurogenetics 2001; 3: 195–201.

58. Transatlantic Genetics Cooperative. A meta-analysis of whole genome linkage screens in multiple sclerosis. J Neuroimmunol 2003; 143: 39–46.

59. Kenealy SJ, Babron MC, Bradford Y et al. A second-generation genomic screen for multiple sclerosis. Am J Hum Genet 2004; 75: 1070–1078.

60. Barcellos LF, Begovich AB, Reynolds RL et al. Linkage and association with the NOS2A locus on chromosome 17q11 in multiple sclerosis. Ann Neurol 2004; 55: 793–800.

61. Mirel DB, Barcellos LF, Wang J et al. Analysis of IL4R haplotypes in predisposition to multiple sclerosis. Genes Immun 2004; 5: 138–141.

62. Zhou Q, Rammohan K, Lin S et al. CD24 is a genetic modifier for risk and progression of multiple sclerosis. Proc Natl Acad Sci USA 2003; 100: 15041–15046.

63. Cunningham S, Patterson CC, McDonnell G et al. Haplotype analysis of the preprotachykinin-1 (TAC1) gene in multiple sclerosis. Genes Immun 2005; 6: 265–270.

64. Vyshkina T, Shugart YY, Birnbaum G et al. Association of haplotypes in the beta-chemokine locus with multiple sclerosis. Eur J Hum Genet 2005; 13: 240–247.

65. Swanberg M, Lidman O, Padyukov L et al. MHC2TA is associated with differential MHC molecule expression and susceptibility to rheumatoid arthritis, multiple sclerosis and myocardial infarction. Nat Genet 2005; 37: 486–494.

66. Saarela J, Kallio SP, Chen D et al. PRKCA and multiple sclerosis: association in two independent populations. PLoS Genet 2006; 2: e42.

67. Gregory SG, Schmidt S, Seth P et al. Interleukin 7 receptor alpha chain shows allelic and functional association with multiple sclerosis. Nat Genet 2007; 39: 1083–1091.

68. Dyment DA, Steckley JL, Willer CJ et al. No evidence to support CTLA-4 as a susceptibility gene in MS families: the Canadian Collaborative Study. J Neuroimmunol 2002; 123: 193–198.

69. Begovich AB, Caillier SJ, Alexander HC et al. The R620W polymorphism of the protein tyrosine phosphatase PTPN22 is not associated with multiple sclerosis. Am J Hum Genet 2005; 76: 184–187.

70. Daly MJ, Rioux JD, Schaffner SF et al. High-resolution haplotype structure in the human genome. Nat Genet 2001; 29: 229–232.

71. Rioux JD, Daly MJ, Silverberg MS et al. Genetic variation in the 5q31 cytokine gene cluster confers susceptibility to Crohn disease. Nat Genet 2001; 29: 223–228.

72. Gabriel SB, Schaffner SF, Nguyen H et al. The structure of haplotype blocks in the human genome. Science 2002; 296: 2225–2229.

73. Carlson CS, Eberle MA, Kruglyak L, Nickerson DA. Mapping complex disease loci in whole-genome association studies. Nature 2004; 429: 446–452.

74. The International Multiple Sclerosis Genetics Consortium. Risk alleles for

multiple sclerosis identified by a genome wide study. N Engl J Med 2007; 357: 851–862.

75. Kira J, Kanai T, Nishimura Y et al. Western versus Asian types of multiple sclerosis: immunogenetically and clinically distinct disorders. Ann Neurol 1996; 40: 569–574.

76. McDonnell GV, Hawkins SA. Clinical study of primary progressive multiple sclerosis in Northern Ireland, UK. J Neurol Neurosurg Psychiatr 1998; 64: 451–454.

77. Barcellos LFS, Sawcer S, Ramsay PP et al. Heterogeneity at the HLA-DRB1 locus and the risk for multiple sclerosis. Hum Mol Genet 2006; 15: 2813–2824.

78. Brassat D, Salemi G, Barcellos L et al. The HLA locus and multiple sclerosis in Sicily. Neurology 2005; 64: 361–363.

79. Dyment DA, Herrera BM, Cader MZ et al. Complex interactions among MHC haplotypes in multiple sclerosis: susceptibility and resistance. Hum Mol Genet 2005; 14: 2019–2026.

80. Engell T, Raun NE, Thomsen M, Platz P. HLA and heterogeneity of multiple sclerosis. Neurology 1982; 32: 1043–1046.

81. Madigand M, Oger JJ, Fauchet R et al. HLA profiles in multiple sclerosis suggest two forms of disease and the existence of protective haplotypes. J Neurol Sci 1982; 53: 519–529.

82. Duquette P, Decary F, Pleines J et al. Clinical sub-groups of multiple sclerosis in relation to HLA: DR alleles as possible markers of disease progression. Can J Neurol Sci 1985; 12: 106–110.

83. Masterman T, Ligers A, Olsson T et al. HLA-DR15 is associated with lower age at onset in multiple sclerosis. Ann Neurol 2000; 48: 211–219.

84. Hensiek AE, Sawcer SJ, Feakes R et al. HLA-DR 15 is associated with female sex and younger age at diagnosis in multiple sclerosis. J Neurol Neurosurg Psychiatr 2002; 72: 184–187.

85. Poser S, Ritter G, Bauer HJ et al. HLA-antigens and the prognosis of multiple sclerosis. J Neurol 1981; 225: 219–221.

86. Runmarker B, Martinsson T, Wahlstrom J, Andersen O. HLA and prognosis in multiple sclerosis. J Neurol 1994; 241: 385–390.

87. Weinshenker BG, Santrach P, Bissonet AS et al. Major histocompatibility complex class II alleles and the course and outcome of MS: a population-based study. Neurology 1998; 51: 742–747.

88. McDonnell GV, Mawhinney H, Graham CA et al. A study of the HLA-DR region in clinical subgroups of multiple sclerosis and its influence on prognosis. J Neurol Sci 1999; 165: 77–83.

89. Celius EG, Harbo HF, Egeland T et al. Sex and age at diagnosis are correlated with the HLA-DR2, DQ6 haplotype in multiple sclerosis. J Neurol Sci 2000; 178: 132–135.

90. Villoslada P, Barcellos L, Rio J et al. The HLA locus and multiple sclerosis in Spain. Role in disease susceptibility, clinical course and response to interferon-beta. J Neuroimmunol 2002; 130: 194–201.

91. Ascherio A, Munger KL, Lennette ET et al. Epstein–Barr virus antibodies and risk of multiple sclerosis: a prospective study. JAMA 2001; 286: 3083–3088.

92. Ponsonby AL, van der Mei I, Dwyer T et al. Exposure to infant siblings during early life and risk of multiple sclerosis. JAMA 2005; 293: 463–469.

93. Cepok S, Zhou D, Srivastava R et al. Identification of Epstein–Barr virus proteins as putative targets of the immune response in multiple sclerosis. J Clin Invest 2005; 115: 1352–1360.

94. Ascherio A, Munger KL. Environmental risk factors for multiple sclerosis. Part I: the role of infection. Ann Neurol 2007; 61: 288–299.

95. Hernan MA, Olek MJ, Ascherio A. Cigarette smoking and incidence of multiple sclerosis. Am J Epidemiol 2001; 154: 69–74.

96. Steinman L. Assessment of animal models for MS and demyelinating disease in the design of rational therapy. Neuron 1999; 24: 511–514.

97. Sobel RA. Genetic and epigenetic influence on EAE phenotypes induced with different encephalitogenic peptides. J Neuroimmunol 2000; 108: 45–52.

98. Steinman L and Zamvil SS. How to successfully apply studies in experimental allergic encephalomyelitis to research on multiple sclerosis Ann Neurol 2006; 60: 12–21.

99. Blankenhorn EP, Butterfield RJ, Rigby R et al. Genetic analysis of the influence of pertussis toxin on experimental allergic encephalomyelitis susceptibility: an environmental agent can override genetic checkpoints. J Immunol 2000; 164: 3420–3425.

100. Teuscher C, Bunn JY, Fillmore PD et al. Gender, age, and season at immunization uniquely influence the genetic control of susceptibility to histopathological lesions and clinical signs of experimental allergic encephalomyelitis: implications for the genetics of multiple sclerosis. Am J Pathol 2004; 165: 1593–1602.

101. Encinas JA, Weiner HL, Kuchroo VK. Inheritance of susceptibility to experimental autoimmune encephalomyelitis. J Neurosci Res 1996; 45: 655–669.

102. Andersson A, Karlsson J. Genetics of experimental autoimmune encephalomyelitis in the mouse. Arch Immunol Ther Exp (Warsz) 2004; 52: 316–325.

103. Teuscher C Noubade R, Spach KV. Evidence that the Y chromosome influences autoimmune disease in male and female mice. Proc Natl Acad Sci USA 2007; 103: 8024–8029.

104. Bieber AJ, Ure DR, Rodriguez M. Genetically dominant spinal cord repair in a murine model of chronic progressive multiple sclerosis. J Neuropathol Exp Neurol 2005; 64: 46–57.

105. Butterfield RJ, Blankenhorn EP, Roper RJ et al. Identification of genetic loci controlling the characteristics and severity of brain and spinal cord lesions in experimental allergic encephalomyelitis. Am J Pathol 2000; 157: 637–645.

106. Polman CH, Herndon RM, Pozzilli C. Interferons. In: Rudick RA, Goodkin DE, eds. Multiple sclerosis therapeutics. London: Martin Dunitz; 1999: 243–276.

107. Fusco C, Andreone V, Coppola G et al. HLA-DRB1*1501 and response to copolymer-1 therapy in relapsing-remitting multiple sclerosis. Neurology 2001; 57: 1976–1979.

108. Sriram U, Barcellos LF, Villoslada P et al. Pharmacogenomic analysis of interferon receptor polymorphisms in multiple sclerosis. Genes Immun 2002; 4: 147–152.

109. Baranzini SE, Mousavi P, Rio J et al. Transcription-based prediction of response to IFN beta using supervised computational methods. PLoS Biol 2005; 3: e2.

110. Mann CL, Davies MB, Boggild MD et al. Glutathione S-transferase polymorphisms in MS: their relationship to disability. Neurology 2000; 54: 552–557.

111. Schrijver HM, Crusius JB, Uitdehaag BM et al. Association of interleukin-1beta and interleukin-1 receptor antagonist gene with disease severity in MS. Neurology 1999; 52: 595–599.

112. Kantarci OH, Atkinson EJ, Hebrink DD et al. Association of two variants in IL-1beta and IL-1 receptor antagonist genes with multiple sclerosis. J Neuroimmunol 2000; 106: 220–227.

113. Sciacca FL, Ferri C, Vandenbroeck K et al. Relevance of interleukin 1 receptor antagonist intron 2 polymorphism in Italian MS patients. Neurology 1999; 52: 1896–1898.

114. Feakes R, Sawcer S, Broadley S et al. Interleukin 1 receptor antagonist (IL-1ra) in multiple sclerosis. J Neuroimmunol 2000; 105: 96–101.

115. Kroner A, Mehling M, Hemmer B et al. A PD-1 polymorphism is associated with disease progression in multiple sclerosis. Ann Neurol 2005; 58: 50–57.

116. Barcellos LF, Schito AM, Rimmler JB et al. CC-chemokine receptor 5 polymorphism and age of onset in familial multiple sclerosis. Immunogenetics 2000; 51: 281–288.

117. Kantor R, Bakhanashvili M, Achiron A. A mutated CCR5 gene may have favorable prognostic implications in MS. Neurology 2003; 61: 238–240.

118. Sellebjerg F, Madsen HO, Jensen CV et al. CCR5 delta32, matrix metalloproteinase-9 and disease activity in multiple sclerosis. J Neuroimmunol 2000; 102: 98–106.

119. Haase CG, Schmidt S, Faustmann PM. Frequencies of the G-protein beta3 subunit C825T polymorphism and the delta 32 mutation of the chemokine receptor-5 in patients with multiple sclerosis. Neurosci Lett 2002; 330: 293–295.

120. Schreiber K, Otura AB, Ryder LP et al. Disease severity in Danish multiple sclerosis patients evaluated by MRI and three genetic markers (HLA-DRB1*1501, CCR5 deletion mutation, apolipoprotein E). Mult Scler 2002; 8: 295–298.

121. Gade-Andavolu R, Comings DE, MacMurray J et al. Association of CCR5 delta32 deletion with early death in multiple sclerosis. Genet Med 2004; 6: 126–131.

122. Caillier S, Barcellos LF, Baranzini SE et al. Osteopontin polymorphisms and disease course in multiple sclerosis. Genes Immun 2003; 4: 312–315.

123. Niino M, Kikuchi S, Fukazawa T et al. Genetic polymorphisms of osteopontin in association with multiple sclerosis in Japanese patients. J Neuroimmunol 2003; 136: 125–129.

124. Hensiek AE, Roxburgh R, Meranian M et al. Osteopontin gene and clinical severity

of multiple sclerosis. J Neurol 2003; 250: 943–947.

125. Vandenbroeck k, Martino G, Marrosu A et al. Occurrence and clinical relevance of an interleukin-4 gene polymorphism in patients with multiple sclerosis. J Neuroimmunol 1997; 76: 189–192.

126. Kantarci OH, Schaefer-Klein JL, Hebrink DD et al. A population-based study of IL4 polymorphisms in multiple sclerosis. J Neuroimmunol 2003; 137: 134–139.

127. Hauser SL, Oksenberg JR, Lincoln R et al. Interaction between HLA-DR2 and abnormal brain MRI in optic neuritis and early MS. Neurology 2000; 54: 1859–1861.

128. Olerup O, Hillert J, Fredrikson S et al. Primarily chronic progressive and relapsing/remitting multiple sclerosis: two immunogenetically distinct disease entities. Proc Natl Acad Sci USA 1989; 86: 7113–7117.

129. De la Concha EG, Arroyo R, Crusius JBA et al. Combined effect of HLA-DRB1*1501 and interleukin-1 receptor antagonist gene allele 2 in susceptibility to relapsing/remitting multiple sclerosis. J Neuroimmunol 1997; 80: 172–178.

130. Greer JM, Pender MP. The presence of glutamic acid at positions 71 or 74 in pocket 4 of the HLA-DRβ1 chain is associated with the clinical course of multiple sclerosis. J Neurol Neurosurg Psychiatr 2005; 76: 656–662.

131. Kikuchi S, Fukazawa T, Niino M et al. Estrogen receptor gene polymorphism and multiple sclerosis in Japanese patients: interaction with HLA-DRB1*1501 and disease modulation. J Neuroimmunol 2002; 128: 77–81.

132. Polanczyk M, Yellayi S, Zamora A et al. Estrogen receptor-1 (Esr1) and -2 (Esr2) regulate the severity of clinical experimental allergic encephalomyelitis in male mice. Am J Pathol 2004; 164: 1915–1924.

133. Mattila KM, Luomala M, Lehtimaki T et al. Interaction between ESR1 and HLA-DR2 may contribute to the development of MS in women. Neurology 2001; 56: 1246–1247.

134. Kantarci OH, Hebrink DD, Achenbach SJ et al. CD95 polymorphisms are associated with susceptibility to MS in women. A population-based study of CD95 and CD95L in MS. J Neuroimmunol 2004; 146: 162–170.

135. Giess R, Maurer M, Linker R et al. Association of a null mutation in the CNTF gene with early onset of multiple sclerosis. Arch Neurol 2002; 59: 407–409.

136. Hoffmann V, Hardt C. A null mutation in the CNTF gene is not associated with early onset of multiple sclerosis. Arch Neurol 2002; 59: 1974.

137. Van Veen T, van Winsen L, Crusius JB et al. αB-crystallin genotype has impact on the multiple sclerosis phenotype. Neurology 2003; 61: 1245–1249.

138. Kantarci OH, Goris A, Hebrink DD et al. IFNG polymorphisms are associated with gender differences in susceptibility to multiple sclerosis. Genes Immun 2005; 6: 153–161.

139. Shinar Y, Livneh A, Villa Y et al. Common mutations in the familial Mediterranean fever gene associate with rapid progression to disability in non-Ashkenazi Jewish multiple sclerosis patients. Genes Immun 2003; 4: 197–203.

140. Evangelou N, Jackson M, Beeson D, Palace J. Association of the APOE epsilon4 allele with disease activity in multiple sclerosis. J Neurol Neurosurg Psychiatr 1999; 67: 203–205.

141. Fazekas F, Strasser-Fuchs S, Schmidt H et al. Apolipoprotein E genotype related differences in brain lesions of multiple sclerosis. J Neurol Neurosurg Psychiatr 2000; 69: 25–28.

142. Hogh P, Oturai A, Schreiber K et al. Apolipoprotein E and multiple sclerosis: impact of the epsilon-4 allele on susceptibility, clinical type and progression rate. Mult Scler 2000; 6: 226–230.

143. Chapman J, Vinokurov S, Achiron A et al. APOE genotype is a major predictor of long-term progression of disability in MS. Neurology 2001; 56: 312–316.

144. Fazekas F, Strasser-Fuchs S, Kollegger H et al. Apolipoprotein E epsilon 4 is associated with rapid progression of multiple sclerosis. Neurology 2001; 57: 853–857.

145. Enzinger C, Ropele S, Strasser-Fuchs S et al. Lower levels of N-acetylaspartate in multiple sclerosis patients with the apolipoprotein E ε4 allele. Arch Neurol 2003; 60: 65–70.

146. Enzinger C, Ropele S, Smith S et al. Accelerated evolution of brain atrophy and 'black holes' in MS patients with APOE-ε4. Ann Neuro 2004; I 55: 563–569.

147. Cocco E, Sotgiu A, Costa G et al. HLA-DR,DQ and APOE genotypes and gender influence in Sardinian primary progressive MS. Neurology 2005; 64: 564–566.

148. Ferri C, Sciacca FL, Veglia F et al. APOE ε2–4 and −491 polymorphisms are not associated with MS. Neurology 1999; 53: 888–889.

149. Weatherby SJ, Mann CL, Davies MB et al. Polymorphisms of apolipoprotein E; outcome and susceptibility in multiple sclerosis. Mult Scler 2000; 6: 32–36.

150. Masterman T, Zhang Z, Hellgren D et al. APOE genotypes and disease severity in multiple sclerosis. Mult Scler 2002; 8: 98–103.

151. Savettieri G, Andreoli V, Bonavita S et al. Apolipoprotein E genotype does not influence the progression of multiple sclerosis. J Neurol 2003; 250: 1094–1098.

152. Ballerini C, Campani D, Rombola G et al. Association of apolipoprotein E polymorphism to clinical heterogeneity of multiple sclerosis. Neurosci Lett 2000; 296: 174–176.

153. Schmidt S, Barcellos LF, DeSombre K et al. Association of polymorphisms in the apolipoprotein E region with susceptibility to and progression of multiple sclerosis. Am J Hum Genet 2002; 70: 708–717.

154. Kantarci OH, Hebrink DD, Achenbach SJ et al. Association of APOE polymorphisms with disease severity in MS is limited to women. Neurology 2004; 62: 811–814.

155. Green AJ, Barcellos LF, Rimmler JB et al. Sequence variation in the transforming growth factor-beta1 (TGFB1) gene and multiple sclerosis susceptibility. J Neuroimmunol 2001; 116: 116–124.

156. Schrijver HM, Crusius JB, Garcia-Gonzalez MA et al. Gender-related association between the TGFB1+869 polymorphism and multiple sclerosis. J Interferon Cytokine Res 2004; 24: 536–542.

CHAPTER 15

Infectious agents and multiple sclerosis

J. L. Bennett, X. Yu, D. H. Gilden, M. P. Burgoon and G. P. Owens

INTRODUCTION

Multiple sclerosis (MS) is the most common demyelinating disease of humans in the developed world. The disease affects about 400 000 people in the USA (National MS Society, http://www.nationalmssociety.org) and is a major cause of nervous system disability in young adults.[1] Disease usually takes a relapsing–remitting course that begins between ages 15–50, although a substantial proportion of patients eventually develop chronic progressive disease. Although the cause of MS is unknown, clinicopathological and immunological data support the notion that an infectious organism triggers disease. This chapter critically reviews data supporting an infectious etiology in MS and examines novel approaches to antigen identification in demyelinating disease.

PATHOLOGY OF MULTIPLE SCLEROSIS

The pathological hallmark of disease is the plaque, an area of white matter demyelination characterized by early inflammation and later astrogliosis.[2] Although it is generally believed that inflammation is an obligatory and possibly primary feature of demyelination in MS, myelin destruction has recently been reported to occur before inflammation.[3] Thus, endogenous glia, such as microglia or astrocytes, or infectious agents might serve as a source of injury mediators.[4] The inflammatory cell profile of active lesions is characterized by the perivascular infiltration of oligoclonal T cells,[5] consisting of CD4+ and CD8+ α/β[6–8] and γ/δ[5] T cells. Macrophages containing myelin debris are most prominent in the center of plaques, where the number of oligodendrocytes is reduced, and IgG and complement are found at the periphery of plaques.[9,10] Lymphocytes are also found in normal-appearing white matter beyond the margin of active demyelination.[11] B lymphocytes and plasma cells are present in both chronic plaques and areas of active myelin breakdown[12–14] and the prevalence of mature plasma cells increases with longer disease duration.[15] In some MS lesions, inflammation is less prominent and restricted mostly to the rim of the plaque, suggesting the presence of chronic activity along the lesion edge.[9,16]

THE CAUSE OF MULTIPLE SCLEROSIS IS UNKNOWN

Leading theories contend that MS is infectious or a virus-triggered immunopathology, perhaps directed against an autoantigen. These two theories are not mutually exclusive. The causative agent may be a virus that reactivates after years of latency and lyses oligodendrocytes, as occurs in progressive multifocal leukoencephalopathy (PML). Alternatively, a virus might initiate an immunopathology leading to demyelination, as seen in animals infected with certain strains of Theiler's murine encephalomyelitis virus (TMEV), coronaviruses or lentiviruses.[17] Note that β-interferon, a cytokine effective in treating relapsing–remitting MS, has potent antiviral activity.

INFECTION AS A CAUSE OF CHRONIC NEUROLOGICAL DISEASE

Several major studies in the 1960s revealed that persistent virus infections cause chronic neurological disease. First, paramyxovirus nucleocapsids were found in brains of patients with subacute sclerosing panencephalitis (SSPE), a chronic inflammatory disease of both gray and white matter.[18] This was rapidly followed by the detection of unusually high levels of antibody to measles virus in serum and cerebrospinal fluid (CSF) of SSPE patients.[19] Soon thereafter, measles virus was isolated in tissue culture from SSPE brain explants.[20]

Another seminal discovery was that a virus causes PML, a fatal human demyelinating disease characterized by rapidly progressive dementia and motor deficit. The newly discovered human papovavirus (named JC virus, after the initials of the PML patient from whom the papovavirus was isolated), was found in oligodendrocytes, the myelin-producing cell in brain. JC virus (JCV) was isolated from PML brain by cocultivation of explanted brain cells with normal human fetal brain.[21] The excitement generated by the isolation of JCV from PML brain diminished when experimental infection of JCV in rodents was found to produce tumors instead of demyelination. Nevertheless, PML is still the only demyelinating disease of humans that has been proved to have a viral etiology.

RATIONALE FOR AN INFECTIOUS ETIOLOGY OF MULTIPLE SCLEROSIS

The best evidence that MS is infectious comes from a combination of genetic and immunologic studies.

GENETIC STUDIES

While familial aggregation is a well recognized phenomenon in MS[22] and genetic studies show an association between MS and the major histocompatibility locus,[23] no tight linkage for any gene region and MS has been demonstrated. More importantly, studies of identical twins in which one has MS have shown that only 30% of second twins develop disease, suggest that more than a putative susceptible genotype determines disease.[24,25] The discordance of MS among monozygotic twins is best explained by an environmental factor.

Adoption and half-sibling studies in a large population in Canada (reviewed in reference 26) noted the increased incidence of MS in biological compared to adopted relatives, leading the investigators to dispute a viral cause of disease. The authors' conclusions, however, are flawed. Almost all viral infections with CNS involvement are associated with a low case-to-infection ratio. For example, both poliomyelitis and postinfectious encephalomyelitis (PIE) after measles occur in the order of 1 case in 500–2000 infections. Thus, the risk of acquiring MS in a shared environment of adopted, nonbiological relatives would be expected to be the same as in the general population (1 in 1000), since the case-to-infection ratio of MS is likely to be low (as in poliomyelitis and PIE) and the period over which MS is acquired is probably decades.[27] Accordingly, Dyment et al[26] found that the incidence of MS in adopted relatives does not exceed that in the general population. Overall, the increased risk of MS in siblings and twins is most probably due to a combina-

tion of an environmental factor (perhaps viral infection) and a predisposing genetic background. Even in mouse models of TMEV-induced demyelination, there is a critical genetic component. For example, SJL/J but not C57 black mice exhibit demyelination after intracerebral inoculation of TMEV. Thus, while a genetic predisposition to MS appears to exist, an environmental agent is likely to be critical for development of disease.

IMMUNOLOGICAL STUDIES

Immunological evidence that MS might be infectious is provided by the presence of high concentrations of IgG in the brain and CSF of more than 90% of MS patients manifesting as bands of oligoclonal IgG (OGBs). The human CNS diseases associated with OGBs are highly inflammatory and usually infectious (reviewed in reference 28).

Oligoclonal IgG in humans and in animal models of virus-induced demyelination is antigen-specific

Analyses addressing the specificity of oligoclonal IgG have shown that the antibody is directed against the disease-causing agent (Table 15.1). For example, the oligoclonal IgG found in SSPE brain and CSF is directed against measles virus[29] while in cryptococcal meningitis the oligoclonal IgG is directed against cryptococcus.[30] In PML, the intrathecal oligoclonal IgG is directed against the viral coat protein VP1 of JCV and the numbers of plasma cells in affected brain correlate with the oligoclonal response.[39]

In experimental models of demyelination produced by persistent virus infection, oligoclonal IgG is also directed against the agent that causes disease. For example, in the TMEV-induced model of demyelination, oligoclonal IgG is directed primarily against the causative virus.[37] Brown Norway rats infected with the wild-type JHM coronavirus exhibit subacute demyelination and the virus persists in the brain tissue for several weeks in association with large numbers of plasma cells and the synthesis of JHM-specific antibodies. All the oligoclonal IgG produced is directed against JHM virus.[38] Together, these findings provide a rationale for the hypothesis that oligoclonal IgG in MS brain and CSF is antibody directed against the foreign agent/antigen that causes MS.

TABLE 15.1 Oligoclonal IgG in human CNS infectious diseases and murine virus-induced demyelination is directed against the agent that causes disease

Disease	Oligoclonal IgG directed against	Reference
Subacute sclerosing panencephalitis	Measles virus	29
Cryptococcal meningitis	Cryptococcus	30
Mumps meningitis	Mumps virus	31
Chronic rubella panencephalitis	Rubella virus	32
Herpes simplex virus (HSV) encephalitis	HSV glycoprotein B	33
Progressive multifocal leukoencephalopathy	JC virus	34
Neurosyphilis	*Treponema pallidum*	35
Varicella zoster virus (VZV) vasculopathy	VZV	36
Theiler's virus-induced demyelination	Theiler's virus	37
Coronavirus-induced demyelination	JHM coronavirus	38

Oligoclonal IgG persists

Once OGBs appear in MS, they may increase in number but do not disappear with time.[40] Furthermore, serial magnetic resonance imaging (MRI) of MS brains reveals continuous plaque production, even in the absence of clinical disease,[41] with new MRI abnormalities occurring about seven times more frequently than clinical events.[42] The progressive development of both silent and clinically evident brain lesions in MS, together with the intrathecal synthesis and persistence of OGBs in MS, points to the continued production and presentation of a specific antigen in MS brain.

Features of oligoclonal IgG in multiple sclerosis

Although originally described as oligoclonal to emphasize their derivation from more than a single clone of an antibody-synthesizing cell, each OGB is monoclonal and has a single light-chain type[43] that is predominantly kappa and of a single idiotype.[44] Compared with the IgG repertoire in measles virus-induced SSPE, more background polyclonal IgG occurs in MS CSF, perhaps due to contamination from a damaged blood–brain barrier or to polyclonal immune stimulation. Recently, CD138[+]/CD19[+] plasmablasts were shown to be the main source of intrathecal IgG synthesis in MS CSF.[45]

Oligoclonal IgG in MS is probably synthesized locally in plaques. Plasma cells are readily detected in active and chronic lesions[12,46] and antibody deposition is readily seen in MS plaques, primarily at plaque borders and occasionally in single cells (Fig. 15.1). When analyzed by isoelectric focusing, IgG eluted from MS plaques is oligoclonal.[47] Experiments in which antigen was injected intracerebrally into the brain of animals with an intact blood–brain barrier revealed antigen-specific B and plasma cells at the site of antigen deposition, indicating that the CNS can support a localized humoral response.[48] Lymphoid-like structures resembling secondary lymphoid organs and containing proliferating B cells, T cells and a network of cells expressing dendritic cell markers can sometimes be found in the cerebral meninges of MS patients with secondary progressive disease.[49] Plasma cells are found adjacent to these structures and within the demyelinated brain parenchyma, suggesting that ectopic follicles can sustain B cell differentiation within the CNS.[50] Strongly supporting this view, a significant increase in B cell subsets constituting all stages of the B cell germinal center reaction has been found in MS CSF relative to paired peripheral blood.[51]

Oligoclonal IgG in most MS patients is primarily subclass IgG1.[52,53] OGB patterns differ among patients but remain fairly constant in an individual patient during the course of disease.[54]

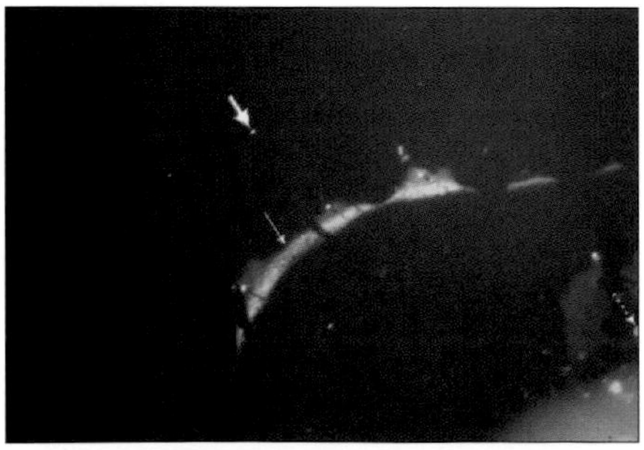

FIG. 15.1 Multiple sclerosis brain plaque–periplaque white matter. Direct immunofluorescence with a 1:20 dilution of fluorescein-conjugated antihuman IgG reveals IgG deposition (green fluorescence) at the junction of plaque–periplaque white matter (middle thin arrow), in mononuclear cells in the plaque (dotted arrow) and in a mononuclear cell in normal periplaque white matter (top thick arrow). The antigen targeted by the IgG in MS brain and cerebrospinal fluid is unknown.

When followed for years, MS patients remain positive for oligoclonal IgG in CSF,[55] confirming the earlier demonstration of clonally stable IgG production in CSF over long periods.[56] CSF IgG levels are reportedly elevated more frequently in MS patients with the most aggressive course of disease than in patients with a benign course.[57] Disease severity has also been correlated with B cell numbers in MS CSF.[58] Nevertheless, the antigenic targets of the oligoclonal IgG have remained elusive. Note that no known genetic disorder of humans is associated with the presence of oligoclonal IgG in the brain and CSF.

EPIDEMIOLOGY

The notion that MS might be infectious is further supported by epidemiological studies. A characteristic geographical pattern of increasing MS prevalence with increasing latitude north and south from the equator has been found, raising the question of whether MS prevalence would be influenced by migration between high- and low-risk regions. Earlier migration studies suggested that the risk of acquiring MS is largely determined before age 15 but more recent studies suggest that the risk may operate over many years and is not restricted to childhood and early adult life.[26,59] Analysis of data on MS from the Faeroe Islands suggests a point-source epidemic acquired over a wide age range,[60] although these data have recently been challenged (reviewed in reference 61). Most recently, the emergence of MS in the French West Indies has pointed to an environmental rather than genetic origin of disease.[62]

Two contrasting hypotheses have been offered to explain the collective epidemiological data: the 'prevalence' hypothesis posits that MS disease is most common where the causative agent is most widespread, whereas the 'polio' hypothesis proposes that antibody is acquired early in life (e.g. maternal antibody or antibody produced after infection in infancy) and reduces the likelihood that the agent will ever reach the CNS, with primary infection after puberty or in adult life resulting in a small incidence of symptomatic CNS infection.[63]

ASSOCIATION OF DEMYELINATING DISEASE IN HUMANS AND ANIMALS WITH VIRUS INFECTION

Indirect evidence consistent with a viral cause for MS comes from the association of viruses with PIE, a multifocal and diffuse inflammatory demyelinating disorder that usually begins days to weeks after virus infection, usually measles, Epstein–Barr virus (EBV), cytomegalovirus (CMV) or varicella zoster virus (VZV), or after *Mycoplasma* infection. The syndrome has also been described after vaccination with hepatitis B virus,[64] *Bordetella pertussis* and possibly influenza virus (reviewed in reference 65). An older rabies vaccine that contains brain tissue may also trigger demyelination.[66] However, both postvaccinal encephalomyelitis and PIE are now rarer, because of the omission of brain tissue in the current rabies vaccine, discontinuation of smallpox vaccination and the immunization of most people against measles virus. Nevertheless, the clear temporal association of encephalomyelitis with smallpox vaccination or naturally occurring viral infections indicates that multiple viruses can produce demyelination. The mechanism by which PIE develops is unknown. Analysis of PIE after natural measles virus infection suggested that perivascular demyelination is immune-mediated,[67] consistent with a study of autopsy tissue from seven patients with measles-associated PIE, which revealed no measles virus RNA or antigen in brain.[68]

Several viruses can produce demyelination in experimentally infected animals. The best studied is TMEV infection in

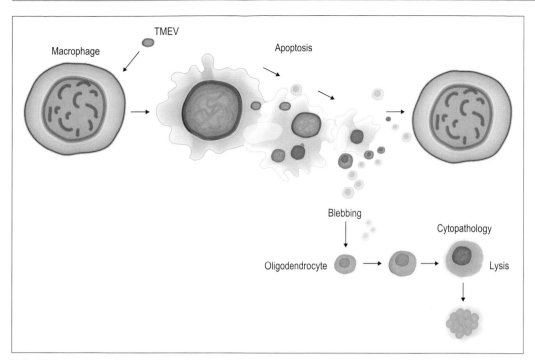

FIG. 15.2 A proposed mechanism of demyelination in mice persistently infected with Theiler's murine encephalomyelitis virus (TMEV), a highly cytolytic picornavirus. TMEV infection of oligodendrocytes is productive, resulting in cell lysis and liberation of virions (bottom), whereas TMEV infection of macrophages is restricted, resulting in apoptosis of these cells.[70] TMEV antigen is abundant in the cytoplasm of apoptotic macrophages (top center). Small amounts of TMEV are released from persistently infected macrophages, leading to infection of more macrophages and oligodendrocytes. A persistent CNS infection is established as virus spreads among macrophages, and the virus released from macrophages can infect and lyse additional oligodendrocytes, resulting in further myelin destruction.

mice,[69] although coronavirus (JHM or MHV-4) infection in mice, canine distemper virus infection in dogs, Visna virus and caprine arthritis–encephalitis virus infection in sheep and goats have all been shown to cause CNS demyelination in their natural hosts. Each of these viruses can establish a persistent infection in the respective host, continuously replicating over a long period without killing the host. Such viruses may be attenuated or restricted in their replicative capacity in the cells they infect and can avoid elimination by the immune system. Multiple laboratories are working intensely to determine the relationship of such virus persistence to demyelination.

Figure 15.2 illustrates a possible mechanism for demyelination by TMEV. While TMEV lytically infects oligodendrocytes, resulting in myelin destruction, TMEV persists in macrophages, ultimately resulting in apoptosis.[70] Sporadic liberation of TMEV from persistently infected macrophages in the CNS might result in viral propagation and secondary infection of oligodendrocytes. The spread of virus from macrophage to macrophage might result in a persistent CNS infection, and virus released from macrophages would also produce oligodendrocyte lysis and demyelination.

Based on the varying degrees of inflammation and demyelination manifested pathologically in the MS plaque, some investigators have argued that more than one infectious agent might cause MS. However, such an assumption seems unwarranted, since differing pathologies are observed in other chronic infectious disorders of the CNS caused by a single agent. For example, patients with neurosyphilis (CNS infection with *Treponema pallidum*) may have diffuse parenchymal disease (general paresis), infection and inflammation restricted to cerebral arteries (meningovascular syphilis), isolated involvement of the optic nerves (syphilitic optic atrophy), lesions restricted to the posterior roots and dorsal columns (tabes dorsalis), or a solitary mass lesion (syphilitic gumma). Similarly, MS patients may exhibit prominent perivascular inflammation, little more than optic atrophy, or develop a solitary demyelinating lesion that mimics a tumor. Besides *Treponema pallidum*, other organisms such as *Mycobacterium tuberculosis* or fungi produce chronic CNS disease with multiple pathologies.

If MS is infectious, disease might ultimately result from a virus-induced immunopathology or autoimmunity. Yet repeated attempts by our laboratory to demonstrate specific binding of IgG extracted from MS brain and CSF to MS plaque and normal human brain have not succeeded, arguing against the notion of an autoantigen involved in disease pathogenesis. While lack of specific binding can also serve as an argument against an infectious hypothesis, the putative MS virus might be latent with limited viral gene expression and low abundance in brain tissue, analogous to other well-studied examples of virus latency in the nervous system. For example, herpes simplex virus (HSV) and VZV are both latent in human ganglia, and antiviral antibody directed against either virus does not stain human ganglia. However, latent virus can produce clinical disease upon reactivation after as yet unknown stimuli. Even in the face of low-grade persistent infections with continuous virus replication, as seen in experimental models of virus-induced demyelination (e.g. TMEV infection of mice), it is virtually impossible to detect the footprint of a virus without first knowing its identity. Finally, if MS turns out to be a virus-induced immunopathology, as shown for acute lymphocytic choriomeningitis virus infection or TMEV-induced demyelination in mice, identification of the causative agent will be critical to preventing disease.

IMMUNIZATION AND MULTIPLE SCLEROSIS

If MS results from a nonbeneficial immune response to an infectious agent, then exacerbations might be expected to increase around the time of infectious episodes or vaccination. While some studies have indicated an increase in attacks around the time of infectious episodes,[71,72] a summary of published evidence by Rutschmann et al[73] revealed no increased risk of MS exacerbations during such times. Furthermore, hepatitis B, VZV, tetanus, bacille Calmette–Guérin and influenza vaccines do not increase MS exacerbations. Influenza vaccination was found not to exacerbate symptoms of MS, and a study of 180 patients with relapsing MS indicated that influenza virus infection caused neurological symptoms more often than did the virus vaccine.[74] Finally, a multicenter, randomized, double-blind, placebo-controlled trial of influenza vaccination in MS revealed no difference in attack rate for the two groups with respect to disease progression over 6 months, leading the investigators to conclude that influenza immunization in MS patients is associated with neither an increased exacerbation rate in the postvaccination period nor a change in disease course over the subsequent 6 months.[75] No association between hepatitis B vaccination and development of MS has been found.[76,77]

Overall, patients with MS have been advised to follow the recommendations of the Centers for Disease Control (http://www.cdc.gov/nip/recs/adult-schedule.pdf) for immunizations against influenza, hepatitis B, VZV and tetanus. There is no strong evidence to warrant a delay in vaccination during clinically significant relapses or until patients have stabilized or begun to improve from relapse, typically 4–6 weeks after initial symptoms. Although pneumococcal vaccine might be considered for MS patients with compromised pulmonary function, such as wheelchair-dependent or bed-bound patients, there have been no studies to assess the benefit/detriment of such vaccination.

THE SEARCH FOR AN INFECTIOUS AGENT IN MULTIPLE SCLEROSIS BRAIN CELLS

Based on the successful isolation of both measles and papovavirus from SSPE and PML brain respectively, and the demonstrated transmissibility of two presumed degenerative neurological diseases (kuru and Jakob–Creutzfeldt disease), multiple attempts have been made to demonstrate that MS is transmissible and to isolate an infectious agent from MS brain. MS brain cells were propagated in tissue culture by the same techniques used to grow ganglia and to successfully rescue HSV from human trigeminal, nodose and vagus ganglia.[78,79] Although only glial cells and brain fibroblasts from MS brain survived subcultivation,[80,81] sufficient quantities of MS brain cells were generated. Nevertheless, cocultivation of MS brain cells in tissue culture with indicator cells did not lead to a cytopathic effect characteristic of any infectious agent.

Cell fusion provides even more intimate contact between MS brain cells and indicator cells, with a fusing agent used to bring the membrane of two cells together to produce a heterokaryon (a cell containing different nuclei inside a common cytoplasm). Use of inactivated Sendai virus (a parainfluenza virus) as the fusing agent, as well as conditions at pH 7.0, which had been shown to be optimal for heterokaryon production, led to the isolation of a parainfluenza virus (6/94 virus) from MS brain.[82] However, 6/94 virus did not prove to be the cause of MS. The possibility that the Sendai parainfluenza virus had not been completely inactivated led to its replacement as a fusing agent

by lysolecithin and eventually polyethylene glycol. Explanted cells from multiple MS brains were assessed before and after fusion with indicator cells, not only for a spontaneous cytopathic effect but also for binding to antisera against measles virus, HSV, VZV, CMV, Coxsackie and echo viruses, rubella, influenza A and B and coronaviruses by indirect immunofluorescence. Explanted and fused MS brain cells were also inoculated into embryonated hen eggs, in which influenza and parainfluenza viruses are readily propagated, and into rodent species and chimpanzees in an attempt to produce neurological disease. While no agent specific for MS was found, this effort led to the isolation of an endogenous mouse picornavirus (the WW strain of TMEV) that produces demyelination.[81] In addition, one chimpanzee inoculated intracerebrally with MS brain cells developed demyelinating disease, and CMV was subsequently isolated from the brain of this animal;[83] the virus was identified as a chimpanzee strain of CMV.[84] Interestingly, inoculation of brain xenografts (MS cells) in both chimpanzee and mouse-induced reactivation of an endogenous virus capable of producing demyelination; however, none of 24 MS brains analyzed revealed virus.[85]

Another approach to rescuing a virus that might be latent in MS brain involved the search for pseudotype virus. In the early 1970s, Weiss et al[86] showed that cells in tissue culture containing an enveloped virus and superinfected with vesicular stomatitis virus (VSV) produced a pseudotype or 'transvestite' virus containing the genome of one virus and the protein coat of the second. The pseudotype virus was demonstrated by the presence of a small VSV antibody-resistant virus fraction that was completely neutralized by antiserum to the second virus. To search for a latent enveloped virus in MS brain, MS brain cells in culture were infected with VSV. When a cytopathic effect appeared, cells were harvested and assayed for a VSV non-neutralizable fraction; no enveloped virus latent in MS brain cells was found.

ASSOCIATION OF VARIOUS MICROORGANISMS WITH MULTIPLE SCLEROSIS

CHLAMYDOPHILA PNEUMONIAE

One of the most recent organisms to be implicated in MS is *Chlamydophila* (formerly *Chlamydia*) *pneumoniae*, a Gram-negative bacterium. Since the original detection of *C. pneumoniae* DNA and antibody in the CSF of some MS patients,[87] laboratories around the world have attempted to confirm this potentially important finding. An analysis of the humoral immune responses to *C. pneumoniae* in paired sera and CSF of patients with definite MS versus other inflammatory and non-inflammatory neurological diseases revealed no difference in seropositivity between the groups, although *C. pneumoniae*-specific IgG titers were significantly higher in the CSF of MS patients than in controls. Interestingly, 16/52 (30.8%) seropositive MS patients showed intrathecal synthesis of *C. pneumoniae*-specific IgG compared to only 1/43 (2.3%) seropositive controls. However, these elevated *C. pneumoniae* antibody titers in CSF did not correlate significantly with disease duration, disease course, clinical or MRI disease activity, disability or the presence of oligoclonal IgG.[88] Overall, multiple studies have not revealed a significant association between *C. pneumoniae* and MS (reviewed in reference 89). Further, if an organism larger than a virus (e.g. a rickettsial agent or a bacterium) causes MS, it would probably have been detected during the many electron microscopic analyses of MS plaque ultrastructure.

HERPESVIRUSES

In the past decade, two human herpesviruses have also been associated with MS. One is human herpesvirus-6 (HHV-6), the cause of roseola, and the other is Epstein–Barr virus (EBV), the cause of infectious mononucleosis. The detection of these two ubiquitous viruses known to be latent in blood B (EBV) or T- (HHV-6) cells is intriguing, since seroconversion to both viruses typically occurs during the same time that epidemiological evidence indicates exposure to the disease-causing agent of MS.

HHV-6

Blood HHV-6 DNA and antibody can be detected in MS patients but do not correlate with clinical disease.[90] In MS patients examined over time, HHV-6 DNA was only rarely present in serum[91] but was found more frequently during exacerbations.[92] However, these findings were not reproduced in other investigations.[93] Increased levels of anti-HHV-6 IgG can be found in blood of relapsing–remitting MS compared to patients with chronic progressive MS, other neurological diseases (ONDs) and normal controls.[94] In addition, anti-HHV-6 IgM is elevated in 80% of MS patients compared to 60% of non-MS controls.[95] Active HHV-6A infection can be detected in 14.6% of MS patients.[96]

Cerebrospinal fluid and brain A nucleotide fragment that was more than 99% identical to the major DNA-binding protein gene of HHV-6B was found in 25/32 (78%) brain specimens from MS patients and in 40/54 (74%) specimens from control subjects. In addition, HHV-6 antigen was found in oligodendrocytes in 12/15 (80%) brain specimens from MS patients and in none of 45 brain specimens from controls. Viral antigen was observed predominantly in cells associated with plaques rather than normal white matter, suggesting that virus was actively replicating and not merely latent. However, prominent antigen staining was also observed in brains with other CNS inflammatory disease. Many cell types (neurons, astrocytes, macrophages, ependymal cells, choroid plexus and endothelial cells), were positive for viral antigen, particularly macrophages.[97] Importantly, HHV-6 DNA is found not only in the brain and CSF of MS patients but also in neoplastic and normal brain.[98]

The use of sensitive polymerase chain reaction (PCR) techniques has not revealed the preferential presence of HHV-6 DNA in MS CSF or brain tissue. PCR studies did not detect HHV-6 DNA in the CSF from any of 32[99] or 23 MS patients,[100] and HHV-6 was found only in 11% of MS patients compared to 7% of HIV-infected patients and not in any control subjects with ONDs. Interestingly, when cellular instead of cell-free CSF was analyzed, the frequency of positive PCR isolates increased substantially to 29% in OND control subjects, 41% in HIV-infected patients and 39% in patients with MS,[90] suggesting that any association between HHV-6 and MS might simply reflect the presence of virus-infected cells within an inflammatory infiltrate. Such an interpretation is supported by analyses of 36 MS patients, 27 acquired immunodeficiency syndrome (AIDS) patients with neurological disease and 24 noninflammatory control patients, which revealed HHV-6 DNA in 30–40% of CSFs in all groups in which a pleocytosis was present. Moreover, another study found no difference in HHV-6 antibody titers between MS patients and controls or MS patients in different disease stages.[101]

Additional studies of HHV-6 in MS have applied in situ hybridization combined with PCR to formalin-fixed tissue sections. HHV-6 DNA, but not antigen-positive cells, was found in 11/13 sections from eight MS brain specimens, predominantly in oligodendrocytes.[102] More recently, laser microdissection was used to isolate tissue from plaques and normal-appearing white matter from 13 MS patients followed by nested PCR to amplify the HHV-6 major capsid protein gene; the percentage of samples in which HHV genome was detected (16–27%) did not differ significantly among healthy brain, normal-appearing white matter in brain from MS patients, and brain from patients with ONDs, whereas the HHV-6 genome was detected in 57% samples from MS plaques, a highly significant difference compared to controls. There were no statistically significant differences among the groups when only HHV-6-positive patients were considered.[103]

Overall, HHV-6 DNA and increased levels of antibody to HHV-6 in blood and CSF appear to be detectable only in a minority of MS patients. Furthermore, HHV-6 DNA and increased levels of HHV-6 antibody are detected in patients with ONDs. The presence of HHV-6 DNA and antigen in brain is likely to reflect reactivation of this virus from latently infected T cells that traffic through the brain of patients with chronic inflammatory CNS disease.

Epstein–Barr virus

The neurotropism of EBV and its ability to produce serious neurological disease at all levels of the human neuraxis have been extensively documented.[104] While all patients with MS have antibody against EBV compared to 86–95% of controls, it is still unknown whether EBV infection is a prerequisite for the development of MS or whether 100% EBV seropositivity is a consequence of MS.[105] A meta-analysis of EBV infection in MS, representing eight studies and a total of 1005 MS cases and 1060 controls, found an odds-ratio of 13.5 (95% confidence interval) for MS infection between EBV-seropositive and -seronegative individuals, a finding taken as supportive of a role for EBV in the etiology of MS.[106] Bray et al[107] detected antibodies to the Epstein–Barr nuclear antigen (EBNA) in 85% of MS patients compared to 13% of EBV-seropositive controls. Further, a prospective serological study of 62 439 women[108] found significant elevations in serum EBV antibody titers, particularly antibody to the EBNA-2 antigen, before the onset of MS. An unexpected finding in that study was the late onset of disease in most of the women who developed MS (median age 52 years). Unfortunately, no CSF data were available, information that would have been important, since the IgG in MS brain and CSF is synthesized intrathecally and may more accurately reflect the immune response at the site of disease. The strongest predictors of MS were found to be serum levels of IgG antibodies to the EBV capsid antigen or the EBNA complex.[109] Finally, strong associations between EBV antibodies and the risk of MS determined in samples collected from MS patients 5 or more years before onset of disease raises the possibility that late EBV infection plays a role in MS.[110] Nevertheless, in situ hybridization has not revealed EBV-specific RNA in 10 MS brains.[111]

The most recent evidence for a link between EBV and MS has come from the demonstration that EBV-specific proteins are putative targets of the immune response in MS.[112] In that study, CSF samples from MS patients and controls were applied to protein arrays generated from cDNA expression libraries of human brain. Expression clones that showed strong reactivity to MS, but not to control CSF, were further mapped to identify high-affinity epitopes. Immunoreactivity to the EBV-specific proteins BRRF2 and EBNA-1 was significantly higher in serum and CSF of MS patients than in controls, and a minority of oligoclonal IgG in MS was removed by incubation of MS CSF with purified BRRF2 and EBNA-1, suggesting that EBV may play a role in the pathogenesis of disease.

Retroviruses

Multiple investigators have searched for various retrovirus sequences in MS brain. Jocher et al[113] found no HTLV-1 sequences in peripheral blood mononuclear cells (MNCs) or in brain of MS patients and a large blinded, multipopulation, PCR-based study provided no support for an association between HTLV-1 or HTLV-II and MS.[114] Although levels of antibody to reverse transcriptase differ significantly between MS and controls,[115] analysis using three sets of oligonucleotides that detect all known human oncoretroviruses or lentiviruses revealed no evidence of retrovirus infection in the brain of MS or control patients.[116] A similar study detected no evidence of retrovirus in serum, CSF or blood MNCs of MS patients.[117] On the other hand, Rasmussen et al[118] reported the transcription of several endogenous retrovirus sequences in peripheral blood MNCs and brain from MS patients and controls. Perron et al[119] repeatedly isolated a novel retrovirus (LM7) from the leptomeninges, choroid plexus and EBV-immortalized B cells of MS patients. The same sequences were also detected in noncellular RNA from MS patient plasma and in CSF from untreated MS patients. The significance of these findings is unknown. Further epidemiological studies might help to determine the possible association of retroviruses with MS.

Coronaviruses

The ability of coronaviruses to produce demyelination in experimentally infected mice has led to a few searches for human coronaviruses in MS brain. Using in situ hybridization, Murray et al[120] detected coronavirus RNA in 12/22 MS brains, including coronavirus antigen in two patients with rapidly progressive disease; control brain was negative. Stewart et al[121] detected human coronavirus 229E RNA in four of 11 MS patients, but not in brains of six OND patients or in five normal brains. In contrast, PCR conducted with primers specific for human coronaviruses 229E and OC43, revealed no evidence of coronavirus infection in MS brain.[122]

JC virus

Polyoma JCV is the cause of PML, the only human demyelinating disease with a proven viral cause. JCV is latent in kidney and hematopoietic progenitor cells. To date, there is no strong evidence to support an association between JCV and MS. JCV was not found in the urine of 53 patients with clinically definite MS or in 53 age- and sex-matched controls.[123] PCR revealed JCV DNA in urine of 30/37 MS patients taking cyclosporin,[124] which is not unexpected since JCV is intermittently excreted in urine by 40% of the population.[125] Finally, JCV DNA was detected in the CSF of 9% of MS patients but not in any OND patients or in other controls.[126]

The possibility that MS is infectious has been extended to the consideration that the disease might even be sexually transmitted. This is based in part on a proposed correlation between sexual permissiveness and MS prevalence, and the fact that HTLV-1 myelopathy, an infectious disorder with some features in common with MS, can be transmitted sexually. Such a hypothesis might be further tested by a case-control study of MS patients and their partners, and by studies of MS in social groups adhering to a strict moral code, such as Mormons or nuns.[127]

ANTIGEN IDENTIFICATION IN MULTIPLE SCLEROSIS

A major and crucial challenge to the identification of an infectious pathogen in MS is the development of novel approaches to identify low-abundance antigen in the CNS of MS patients. As discussed above, there is significant evidence to suggest that antibodies in MS might be directed against the causative infectious agent. Therefore, the humoral response in MS patients may offer a powerful tool for the identification of a potential MS pathogen.

ANTIGEN-DRIVEN RESPONSE IN MULTIPLE SCLEROSIS

To determine the significance of the humoral response in MS, several laboratories, including ours, have used PCR methodologies to analyze the variable (V)-region sequences of immunoglobulins produced by plasma cells and B cells in MS lesions and CSF. Clonally expanded B cell populations were found in the brain and CSF of MS patients and in SSPE brain but not in noninflammatory neurological control CSFs such as migraine, amyotrophic lateral sclerosis, spinocerebellar degeneration and epilepsy[128-131] or in CSF B cells obtained from a patient on the first day of viral meningitis, before an antibody response would be expected.[129] Studies of the MS CSF cells revealed a continuum of clonally related antibody secreting cells that are predominantly plasma blasts.[132] Analysis of heavy chain V-region (VH) sequences expressed in plaque regions of several MS brains revealed a restricted Ig repertoire indicative of a targeted humoral response.[133-137] Oligoclonal VH populations were readily detected in each of the MS repertoires and displayed features indicative of affinity maturation, including extensive somatic mutation and the preferential accumulation of replacement mutations in complementarity-determining regions. In one MS brain, ≈33% of the IgG transcripts comprised a single clonal population and many of the dominant VH sequences from this brain were found in multiple plaque sites.[134] Intraclonal diversification indicative of clonally expanded B cell populations and the preferential usage of specific family germline segments were also observed in many MS repertoires. Most recently, V_H4 gene segments were shown to dominate the intrathecal humoral immune response in MS.[135] Furthermore, the antibodies expressed in MS plaques and CSF are preferentially targeted to the CNS. Colombo et al[128] found that two of the three most overrepresented VH sequences in MS CSF were not amplified from blood lymphocytes, and a comparison of the IgG repertoire of an MS plaque to that in peripheral blood lymphocytes of the same MS patient revealed no overlap between the two VH repertoires.[136]

A similar feature of the clonal expansion in MS brain and SSPE brain suggests that the CNS IgG in MS is antigen-specific. Comparison of VH sequences from MS plaques and SSPE brain revealed no significant differences in the degree or character of somatic mutations.[137] Since the humoral response in SSPE brain is antigen-driven and directed against measles virus (the cause of disease), and several prominent IgG populations and overrepresented IgGs from plasma cells in SSPE brains react specifically with measles virus proteins,[138,139,140,141] it is likely that that the oligoclonal IgG in MS is also antibody directed against disease-relevant antigen.

SINGLE-CELL ANALYSIS OF B LYMPHOCYTES AND PLASMA CELLS AND GENERATION OF RECOMBINANT ANTIBODIES IN MULTIPLE SCLEROSIS

A major advance in the analysis of the antibody response in MS has been the use of single-cell PCR to identify an exact pairing of VH and VL sequences, thus allowing an accurate comparison of clonal populations. Using fluorescence-activated cell sorting (FACS) reverse-transcriptase (RT)-PCR, several investigators have identified clonally expanded B lymphocytes and plasma cells in MS CSF and showed that the limited IgG repertoire is consistent with a targeted immune response.[129,131,142,143] The most important implication of identifying rearranged H and light (L) chain V-region sequences at the single-cell level is the ability to accurately recreate antibodies from clonal IgG populations, which can then be used to identify disease-relevant antigens in MS. Furthermore, monoclonal recombinant antibodies generated from paired VH and VL sequences of clonal IgG populations provide a virtually unlimited supply of MS antibody.

Importantly, clonal populations of IgG have also been found early in demyelinating disease in the CSF of some individuals a few months after their first clinical attack.[131,144] Subsequent follow-up of these patients has indicated a high conversion rate to definite MS. Thus, recombinant antibodies derived from these patients are likely to be directed against the inciting disease-relevant antigen.

Laser-capture microdissection has added an extra dimension to the characterization of clonal IgG populations in inflammatory CNS diseases. Using this technique, Burgoon et al[145] recently isolated individual CD138+ plasma cells from the brain of a patient with SSPE. Subsequent single-cell RT-PCR to analyze individual IgG H and L chains expressed by each cell identified overrepresented populations of CD138+ plasma cells containing somatic mutations consistent with a targeted antibody response. Functional recombinant antibodies were constructed from the overexpressed sequences and their specificities were determined; five of eight such antibodies recognized the nucleocapsid protein of measles virus. Furthermore, recombinant antibodies generated from less abundant plasma cell IgG sequences in SSPE brain are also directed against measles virus.[146] Identical strategies and techniques can be readily applied in efforts to identify the causative antigen of MS, particularly since multiple analyses of IgGs in MS brain plaques and CSF have revealed features of a targeted antibody response. Indeed, sensitive and unbiased molecular techniques such as phage-displayed random peptide libraries, cDNA expression libraries and protein and lipid arrays can be used to identify low-abundance, foreign candidate antigens in MS and to screen them for disease specificity.

PHAGE-DISPLAYED RANDOM PEPTIDE LIBRARIES

Phage-displayed random peptide libraries, in which high-affinity phage clones can be enriched by affinity selection on a monoclonal antibody,[147] represent a novel approach to identifying antigen specificity. Such libraries contain a large number of random peptides (2.7×10^9) that allows the identification of rare epitopes undetectable by conventional methods. This technology can be used to determine the target sequences for monoclonal antibodies that recognize both linear and conformational epitopes (mimotopes). Combinatorial approaches allow the selection of ligands in an unbiased functional assay without preconceptions about the nature of targets in disease.[148] Phage-displayed random peptide libraries have been used successfully to identify a rheumatoid-factor-specific mimotope[149] and allergen mimotopes,[150] and to map neutralizing antibodies to infectious agents such as the Puumala hantavirus[151] and HIV antigens.[152] Using these techniques, Zhong et al[153] identified continuous coronavirus-specific epitopes in patients with severe acute respiratory syndrome. We have recently shown that panning a phage-displayed random peptide library with recombinant antibodies generated from over-represented IgG sequences expressed by single plasma cells in MS CSF revealed several specific peptide sequences.[154] Application of phage-mediated real-time immuno-PCR (RT-IPCR) to study the reactivity of phage peptides specific for the recombinant antibodies further revealed that RT-IPCR detected binding with as few as 100 phage particles compared to standard ELISA, which required greater that 10^4 or 10^5 phage particles to detect binding to recombinant antibodies.[155] Thus, screening of random peptide libraries with MS-specific monoclonal recombinant antibodies might also identify disease-specific epitopes/mimotopes.

CONCLUSION

Multiple sclerosis is a common demyelinating disorder of the CNS that affects people worldwide. The pathological hallmark of disease is the plaque, an area of white matter demyelination often accompanied by inflammation. The CSF of many MS patients also contains inflammatory cells and nearly every MS CSF contains increased amounts of oligoclonal IgG. The cause of MS is unknown but epidemiological evidence suggests that MS is acquired. The most compelling evidence for an infectious etiology of MS derives from studies of CSF from patients with chronic infectious diseases of the CNS, where oligoclonal IgG is directed against the agent that causes disease. Indirect evidence for the infectious nature of MS is that viruses are associated with human demyelinating disease and that demyelination can be produced experimentally with viruses. However, to date, the goal of establishing a tight link between a virus and MS remains elusive. Many investigators hold that MS is an immune-mediated disease, perhaps initially triggered by an infectious agent. Molecular biological and immunological strategies and techniques available today allow studies of virus latency not previously possible. In particular, molecular analysis of the specificity of IgG in MS brain and CSF has the potential to identify an infectious antigen in MS. Application of these techniques to single B lymphocytes and plasma cells in CSF of patients with clinically isolated syndromes such as optic neuritis have already revealed features of an antigen-driven response. More importantly, recombinant antibodies prepared from over-expressed sequences in single plasma cells from the brain of a patient with SSPE were shown to be specific for measles virus, the cause of SSPE. This finding points to the promise of applying identical strategies and techniques to identify the causative antigen of MS.

ACKNOWLEDGMENTS

This study was supported by grant NS32623 from the National Institutes of Health. The authors thank Marina Hoffman for editorial review, and Cathy Allen for preparing the manuscript.

REFERENCES

1. Weinshenker BG. Epidemiology of multiple sclerosis. Neurol Clin 1996; 14: 291–308.

2. Frohman EM, Racke MK, Raine CS. Multiple sclerosis: the plaque and its pathogenesis. N Engl J Med 2006; 354: 942–955.

3. Barnett MH, Prineas JW. Relapsing and remitting multiple sclerosis: pathology of the newly formed lesion. Ann Neurol 2004; 55: 458–468.

4. Lassmann H, Raine CS, Antel J et al. Immunopathology of multiple sclerosis: report on an international meeting held at the Institute of Neurology of the University of Vienna. J Neuroimmunol 1998; 86: 213–217.

5. Wucherpfennig KW, Catz I, Hausmann S et al. Recognition of the immunodominant myelin basic protein peptide by autoantibodies and HLA-DR2-restricted T cell clones from multiple sclerosis patients.

Identity of key contact residues in the B-cell and T-cell epitopes. J Clin Invest 1997; 100: 1114–1122.

6. Babbe H, Roers A, Waisman A et al. Clonal expansions of CD8+ T cells dominate the T cell infiltrate in active multiple sclerosis lesions as shown by micromanipulation and single cell polymerase chain reaction. J Exp Med 2000; 192: 393–404.

7. Hauser SL, Bhan AK, Gilles F et al. Immunohistochemical analysis of the

cellular infiltrate in multiple sclerosis lesions. Ann Neurol 1986; 19: 578–587.

8. Traugott U, Reinherz E, Raine CS. Multiple sclerosis: distribution of T cell subsets within acute chronic lesions. Science 1983; 219: 308–310.

9. Lumsden CE. The immunogenesis of the multiple sclerosis plaque. Brain Res 1971; 28: 365–390.

10. Lucchinetti C, Bruck W, Parisi J et al. Heterogeneity of multiple sclerosis lesions: implications for the pathogenesis of demyelination. Ann Neurol 2000; 47: 707–717.

11. Prineas JW, Connell F. The fine structure of chronically active multiple sclerosis plaques. Neurology 1978; 28: 68–75.

12. Esiri MM. Immunoglobulin-containing cells in multiple sclerosis plaques. Lancet 1977; 2: 478–480.

13. Genain CP, Cannella B, Hauser SL et al. Identification of autoantibodies associated with myelin damage in multiple sclerosis. Nat Med 1999; 5: 170–175.

14. Gerritse K, Deen C, Fasbender M et al. The involvement of specific anti myelin basic protein antibody-forming cells in multiple sclerosis immunopathology. J Neuroimmunol 1994; 49: 153–159.

15. Zeman D, Adam P, Kalistova H et al. Cerebrospinal fluid cytologic findings in multiple sclerosis. A comparison between patient subgroups. Acta Cytol 2001; 45: 51–59.

16. Hafler DA. 2004. Multiple sclerosis. J Clin Invest 2004; 113: 788–794.

17. Buchmeier MJ, Lane TE. Viral-induced neurodegenerative disease. Curr Opin Microbiol 1999; 2: 398–402.

18. Bouteille M, Fontaine C, Vedrenne C et al. Sur un cas d'encéphalite subaiguë à inclusions. Étude anatomo-clinique et ultrastructurale. Rev Neurol (Paris) 1965; 113: 454–458.

19. Connolly JH, Allen IV, Hurwitz LJ et al. Measles-virus antibody and antigen in subacute sclerosing panencephalitis. Lancet 1967; 1: 542–544.

20. Payne FE, Baublis JV, Itabashi HH. Isolation of measles virus from cell cultures of brain from a patient with subacute sclerosing panencephalitis. N Engl J Med 1969; 281: 585–616.

21. Padgett BL, Walker DL, ZuRhein GM et al. Cultivation of papova-like virus from human brain with progressive multifocal leukoencephalopathy. Lancet 1971; 1: 1257–1260.

22. Mackay RP. The familial occurrence of multiple sclerosis and its implications. Res Publ Assoc Res Nerv Ment Dis 1950; 28: 149–177.

23. Sotgiu S, Rosati G, Saana A et al. Multiple sclerosis complexity in selected populations: the challenge of Sardinia, insular Italy. Eur J Neurol 2002; 9: 1–13.

24. Spielman RS, Nathanson N. The genetics of susceptibility to multiple sclerosis. Epidemiol Rev 1982; 4: 45–65.

25. Willer CJ, Dyment DA, Risch NJ et al. Twin concordance and sibling recurrence rates in multiple sclerosis. Proc Natl Acad Sci USA 2003; 100: 12877–12882.

26. Dyment DA, Ebers GC, Sadovnick AD. Genetics of multiple sclerosis. Lancet Neurol 2004; 3: 104–110.

27. Hammond SR, English DR, McLeod JG. The age-range of risk of developing multiple sclerosis. Evidence from a migrant population in Australia. Brain 2000; 123: 968–974.

28. Gilden DH, Devlin ME, Burgoon MP et al. The search for virus in multiple sclerosis brain. Mult Scler 1996; 2: 179–183.

29. Vandvik B, Norrby E, Nordal HJ et al. Oligoclonal measles virus-specific IgG antibodies isolated from cerebrospinal fluids, brain extracts, and sera from patients with subacute sclerosing panencephalitis and multiple sclerosis. Scand J Immunol 1976; 5: 979–992.

30. Porter KG, Sinnamon DG, Gillies RR. Cryptococcus neoformans-specific oligoclonal immunoglobulins in cerebrospinal fluid in cryptococcal meningitis. Lancet 1977; 1: 1262.

31. Vandvik B, Norrby E, Steen-Johnson J et al. Mumps meningitis: prolonged pleocytosis and occurrence of mumps virus-specific oligoclonal IgG in the cerebrospinal fluid. Eur Neurol 1978; 17: 13–22.

32. Coyle PK, Wolinsky JS. Characterization of immune complexes in progressive rubella panencephalitis. Ann Neurol 1981; 9: 557–562.

33. Grimaldi LM, Roos RP, Manservigi R et al. An isolelectric focusing study in herpes simplex virus encephalitis. Ann Neurol 1988; 24: 227–232.

34. Sindic CJ, Trebst C, van Antwerpen MP et al. Detection of CSF-specific oligoclonal antibodies to recombinant JC virus VP1 in patients with progressive multifocal leukoencephalopathy. J Neuroimmunol 1997; 76: 100–104.

35. Vartdal F, Vandvik B, Michaelsen TE et al. Neurosyphilis: intrathecal synthesis of oligoclonal antibodies to Treponema pallidum. Ann Neurol 1981; 11: 35–40.

36. Burgoon MP, Hammack BN, Owens GP et al. Oligoclonal immunoglobulins in cerebrospinal fluid during varicella zoster virus (VZV) vasculopathy are directed against VZV. Ann Neurol 2003; 54: 459–463.

37. Roos RP, Nalefski EA, Nitayaphan S et al. An isoelectric focusing overlay study of the humoral immune response in Theiler's virus demyelinating disease. J Neuroimmunol 1987; 13: 305–314.

38. Dorries R, Watanabe R, Wege H et al. Analysis of the intrathecal humoral immune response in Brown Norway (BN) rats, infected with the murine coronavirus JHM. J Neuroimmunol 1987; 14: 305–316.

39. Weber T, Trebst C, Frye S et al. Analysis of the systemic and intrathecal humoral immune response in progressive multifocal leukoencephalopathy. J Infect Dis 1997; 176: 250–254.

40. Whitaker JN, Benveniste EN, Zhou S-R. Cerebrospinal fluid. In: Cook SD, ed. Handbook of multiple sclerosis. New York: Marcel Dekker; 1990: 251–270.

41. Miller DH, Rudge P, Johnson G et al. Serial gadolinium enhanced magnetic resonance imaging in multiple sclerosis. Brain 1988; 111: 927–939.

42. Thompson AJ, Miller D, Youl B et al. Serial gadolinium-enhanced MRI in relapsing/remitting multiple sclerosis of varying disease duration. Neurology 1992; 42: 60–63.

43. Link H, Laurenzi MA. Immunoglobulin class and light chain type of oligoclonal bands in CSF in multiple sclerosis determined by agarose gel electrophoresis and immunofixation. Ann Neurol 1979; 6: 107–110.

44. Gerhard W, Taylor A, Wroblewska Z et al. Analysis of a predominant immunoglobulin population in the cerebrospinal fluid of a multiple sclerosis patient by means of an anti-idiotypic hybridoma antibody. Proc Natl Acad Sci USA 1981; 78: 3225–3229.

45. Cepok S, Rosche B, Grummel V et al. Short-lived plasma blasts are the main B cell effector subset during the course of multiple sclerosis. Brain 2005; 128: 1667–1676.

46. Prineas JW. The neuropathology of multiple sclerosis. In: Koetsier JC, ed. Handbook of clinical neurology, vol. 3(47): Demyelinating diseases. Amsterdam: Elsevier; 1985: 213–257.

47. Mehta PD, Frisch S, Thormar H et al. Bound antibody in multiple sclerosis brains. J Neurol Sci 1981; 49: 91–98.

48. Knopf PM, Harling-Berg CJ, Cserr HF et al. Antigen-dependent intrathecal antibody synthesis in the normal rat brain: tissue entry and local retention of antigen-specific B cells. J Immunol 1998; 161: 692–701.

49. Serafini B, Rosicarelli B, Magliozzi R et al. Detection of ectopic B-cell follicles with germinal centers in the meninges of patients with secondary progressive multiple sclerosis. Brain Pathol 2004; 14: 164–174.

50. Uccelli A, Aloisi F, Pistoia V. Unveiling the enigma of the CNS as a B-cell fostering environment. Trends Immunol 2005; 26: 254–259.

51. Corcione A, Casazza S, Ferretti E et al. Recapitulation of B cell differentiation in the central nervous system of patients with multiple sclerosis. Proc Natl Acad Sci USA 2004; 101: 11064–11069.

52. Vartdal F, Vandvik B. Characterization of classes of intrathecally synthesized antibodies by imprint immunofixation of electrophoretically separated sera and cerebrospinal fluids. Acta Pathol Microbiol Immunol Scand 1983; 91: 69–75.

53. Losy J, Mehta PD, Wisniewski HM. Identification of IgG subclasses' oligoclonal bands in multiple sclerosis CSF. Acta Neurol Scand 1990; 82: 4–8.

54. DeCastro P, Baumhefner RW, Syndulko K et al. Longitudinal intra-BBB IgG synthesis lasting up to eighteen years in patients with multiple sclerosis. Ann Neurol 1990; 28: 253.

55. Hela-Felicitas P, Reske D. Expansion of antibody reactivity in the cerebrospinal fluid of multiple sclerosis patients – follow-up and clinical implications. Cerebrospinal Fluid Res 2005; 2: 3.

56. Walsh MJ, Tourtellotte WW. Temporal invariance and clonal uniformity of brain and cerebrospinal IgG, IgA, and IgM in multiple sclerosis. J Exp Med 1986; 163: 41–53.

57. Stendahl-Brodin L, Link H. Relation between benign course of multiple sclerosis and low-grade humoral immune response in cerebrospinal fluid. J Neurol Neurosurg Psychiatr 1980; 43: 102–105.

58. Cepok S, Jacobsen M, Schock S et al. Patterns of cerebrospinal fluid pathology correlate with disease progression in multiple sclerosis. Brain 2001; 124: 2169–2176.

59. Kurtzke JF, Delasnerie-Laupretre N, Wallin MT. Multiple sclerosis in North African migrants to France. Acta Neurol Scand 1998; 98: 302–309.

60. Kurtzke JF, Hyllested K. Multiple sclerosis in the Faroe Islands: I. Clinical and epidemiological features. Ann Neurol 1979; 5: 6–21.

61. Marrie RA. Environmental risk factors in multiple sclerosis aetiology. Lancet Neurol 2004; 3: 709–718.

62. Cabre P, Signate A, Olindo S et al. Role of return migration in the emergence of multiple sclerosis in the French West Indies. Brain 2005; 128: 2899–2910.

63. Nathanson N, Miller A. Epidemiology of multiple sclerosis: critique of the evidence for a viral etiology. Am J Epidemiol 1978; 107: 451–461.

64. Tourbah A, Gout O, Liblau R et al. Encephalitis after hepatitis B vaccination: recurrent disseminated encephalitis or MS? Neurology 1999; 53: 396–401.

65. Fenichel GM. Neurological complications of immunization. Ann Neurol 1982; 12: 119–128.

66. Gupta V, Bandyopadhyay S, Bapuraj JR et al. Bilateral optic neuritis complicating rabies vaccination. Retina 2004; 24: 179–181.

67. Johnson RT, Griffin DE, Hirsch JS et al. Measles encephalomyelitis clinical and immunological studies. N Engl J Med 1984; 310: 137–141.

68. Moench TR, Griffin DE, Obriecht CR et al. Acute measles in patients with and without neurological involvement: distribution of measles virus antigen and RNA. J Infect Dis 1988; 158: 433–442.

69. Lipton HL, Dal Canto MC. Theiler's virus-induced demyelination: prevention by immunosuppression. Science 1976; 192: 62–64.

70. Schlitt BP, Felrice M, Jelachich ML et al. Apoptotic cells, including macrophages, are prominent in Theiler's virus-induced inflammatory, demyelinating lesions. J Virol 2003; 77: 4383–4388.

71. Panitch HS, Bever CT, Katz E et al. Upper respiratory tract infections trigger attacks of multiple sclerosis in patients treated with interferon. J Neuroimmunol 1991; 36: 125.

72. Andersen O, Lygner PE, Bergstrom T et al. Viral infections trigger multiple sclerosis relapses: a prospective seroepidemiological study. J Neurol 1993; 240: 417–422.

73. Rutschmann OT, McCrory DC, Matchar DB et al. Immunization and MS: a summary of published evidence and recommendations. Neurology 2002; 59: 1837–1843.

74. De Keyser J, Zwanikken C, Boon M. Effects of influenza vaccination and influenza illness on exacerbations in multiple sclerosis. J Neurol Sci 1998; 159: 51–53.

75. Miller AE, Morgante LA, Buchwald LY et al. A multicenter, randomized, double-blind, placebo-controlled trial of influenza immunization in multiple sclerosis. Neurology 1997; 48: 312–314.

76. Ascherio A, Zhang SM, Hernán MA et al. Hepatitis B vaccination and the risk of multiple sclerosis. N Engl J Med 2001; 344: 327–332.

77. Naismith RT, Cross AH. Does the hepatitis B vaccine cause multiple sclerosis? Neurology 2004; 63: 772–773.

78. Warren KG, Devlin M, Gilden DH et al. Isolation of herpes simplex virus from human trigeminal ganglia, including ganglia from one patient with multiple sclerosis. Lancet 1977; 2: 637–639.

79. Warren KG, Brown SM, Wroblewska Z et al. Isolation of latent herpes simplex virus from the superior cervical and vagus ganglions of humans. N Engl J Med 1978; 298: 1068–1069.

80. Gilden DH, Wroblewska Z, Chesler M et al. Experimental panencephalitis induced in suckling mice by parainfluenza type I (6/94) virus. II. Virologic studies. J Neuropath Exp Neurol 1976; 35: 259–270.

81. Wroblewska Z, Gilden DH, Wellish M et al. Virus-specific intracytoplasmic inclusions in mouse brain produced by a newly isolated strain of Theiler virus: I. Virologic and morphologic studies. Lab Invest 1977; 37: 595–602.

82. Ter Meulen V, Koprowski H, Iwasaki Y et al. Fusion of cultured multiple-sclerosis brain cells with indicator cells: presence of nucleocapsids and virions and isolation of parainfluenza-type virus. Lancet 1972; 2: 1–5.

83. Rorke LB, Iwasaki Y, Koprowski H et al. Acute demyelinating disease in a chimpanzee three years after inoculation of brain cells from a patient with MS. Ann Neurol 1979; 5: 89–94.

84. Wroblewska Z, Gilden DH, Devlin M et al. Cytomegalovirus isolation from a chimpanzee with acute demyelinating disease after inoculation of MS brain cells. Infect Immun 1979; 25: 1008–1015.

85. Gilden DH. A search for virus in multiple sclerosis. Hybrid Hybridomics 2002; 21: 93–97.

86. Weiss RA, Boettiger D, Love DN. Phenotypic mixing between vesicular stomatitis virus and avian RNA tumor viruses. Cold Spring Harbor Symp 1975; 39: 913–918.

87. Sriram S, Stratton CW, Yao S et al. Chlamydia pneumoniae infection of the central nervous system in multiple sclerosis. Ann Neurol 1999; 46: 6–14.

88. Krametter D, Niederwieser G, Berghold A et al. Chlamydia pneumoniae in multiple sclerosis: humoral immune responses in serum and cerebrospinal fluid and correlation with disease activity marker. Mult Scler 2001; 7: 13–18.

89. Tsai JC, Gilden DH. Chlamydia pneumoniae and multiple sclerosis: no significant association. Trends Microbiol 2001; 9: 152–154.

90. Liedtke W, Malessa R, Faustmann PM et al. Human herpesvirus 6 polymerase chain reaction findings in human immunodeficiency virus associated neurological disease and multiple sclerosis. J Neurovirol 1995; 1: 253–258.

91. Goldberg CH, Albright AV, Lisak RP et al. Polymerase chain reaction analysis of human herpesvirus-6 sequences in the sera and cerebrospinal fluid of patients with multiple sclerosis. J Neurovirol 1999; 5: 134–139.

92. Berti R, Brennan MB, Soldan SS et al. Increased detection of serum HHV-6 DNA sequences during multiple sclerosis (MS) exacerbations and correlation with parameters of MS disease progression. J Neurovirol 2002; 8: 250–256.

93. Gutierrez J, Vergara MJ, Guerrero M et al. Multiple sclerosis and human herpesvirus 6. Infection 2002; 30: 145–149.

94. Soldan SS, Berti R, Salem N et al. Association of human herpes virus 6 (HHV-6) with multiple sclerosis: increased IgM response to HHV-6 early antigen and detection of serum HHV-6 DNA. Nat Med 1997; 3: 1394–1397.

95. Friedman JE, Lyons MJ, Ablashi DV et al. The association of the human herpesvirus-6 and MS. Mult Scler 1999; 5: 355–362.

96. Alvarez-Lafuente R, Martin-Estefania C, de Las Heras V et al. Active human herpesvirus 6 infection in patients with multiple sclerosis. Arch Neurol 2002; 59: 929–393.

97. Challoner PB, Smith KT, Parker JD et al. Plaque-associated expression of human herpesvirus 6 in multiple sclerosis. Proc Natl Acad Sci USA 1995; 92: 7740–7744.

98. Cuomo L, Trivedi P, Cardillo MR et al. Human herpesvirus 6 infection in neoplastic and normal brain tissue. J Med Virol 2001; 63: 45–51.

99. Mirandola P, Stefan A, Brambilla E et al. Absence of human herpes virus 6 and 7 from spinal fluid and serum of multiple sclerosis patients. Neurology 1999; 53: 1367–1368.

100. Rodriguez Carnero S, Martinez-Vazquez C, Potel Alvarellos C et al. Lack of human herpesvirus type 6 DNA in CSF by nested PCR among patients with multiple sclerosis. Rev Clin Esp 2002; 202: 588–591.

101. Nielsen L, Larsen AM, Munk M et al. Human herpesvirus-6 immunoglobulin G antibodies in patients with multiple sclerosis. Acta Neurol Scand Suppl 1997; 169: 76–78.

102. Blumberg BM, Mock DJ, Powers JM et al. The HHV6 paradox: ubiquitous commensal or insidious pathogen? A two-step in situ PCR approach. J Clin Virol 2000; 16: 159–178.

103. Cermelli C, Bert R, Soldan SS et al. High frequency of human herpesvirus 6 DNA in multiple sclerosis plaques isolated by laser microdissection. J Infect Dis 2003; 187: 1377–1387.

104. Majid A, Galetta SL, Sweeney CJ et al. Epstein–Barr virus myeloradiculitis and encephalomyeloradiculitis. Brain 2002; 125: 1–7.

105. Wandinger K, Jabs W, Siekhaus A et al. Association between clinical disease activity and Epstein–Barr virus reactivation in MS. Neurology 2000; 55: 178–184.

106. Ascherio A, Munch M. Epstein–Barr virus and multiple sclerosis. Epidemiology 2000; 11: 220–224.

107. Bray PF, Luka J, Bray PF et al. Antibodies against Epstein–Barr nuclear antigen (EBNA) in multiple sclerosis CSF, and two pentapeptide sequence identities between EBNA and myelin basic protein. Neurology 1992; 42: 1798–1804.

108. Ascherio A, Gorham KL, Lennette ET et al. Epstein–Barr virus antibodies and risk of multiple sclerosis: a prospective study. JAMA 2002; 286: 3083–3088.

109. Lewin LI, Munger KL, Rubertone MV et al. Multiple sclerosis and Epstein–Barr virus. JAMA 2003; 289: 1533–1536.

110. Haahr S, Plesner AM, Vestergaard BF et al. A role of late Epstein–Barr virus infection in multiple sclerosis. Acta Neurol Scand 2004; 109: 270–275.

111. Hilton DA, Love S, Fletcher A et al. Absence of Epstein–Barr virus in multiple sclerosis as assessed by in situ hybridisation. J Neurol Neurosurg Psychiatry 1994; 57: 975–976.

112. Cepok S, Zhou D, Srivastava R et al. Identification of Epstein–Barr virus proteins as putative targets of the immune response in multiple sclerosis. J Clin Invest 2005; 115: 1352–1360.

113. Jocher R, Rethwilm A, Kappos L et al. Search for retroviral sequences in peripheral blood mononuclear cells and brain tissue of multiple sclerosis patients. J Neurol 1990; 237: 352–355.

114. Ehrlich GD, Glaser JB, Bryz-Gornia V et al. Multiple sclerosis, retroviruses, and PCR. The HTLV-MS Working Group. Neurology 1991; 41: 335–343.

115. Perron H, Geny C, Genoulaz O et al. Antibody to reverse transcriptase of human retroviruses in multiple sclerosis. Acta Neurol Scand 1991; 84: 507–513.

116. Rozenberg F, Lefebvre S, Lubetzki C et al. Analysis of retroviral sequences in the spinal form of multiple sclerosis. Ann Neurol 1991; 29: 333–336.

117. Hackett J Jr, Swanson P, Leahy D et al. Search for retrovirus in patients with multiple sclerosis. Ann Neurol 1996; 40: 805–809.

118. Rasmussen HB, Geny C, Deforges L et al. Expression of endogenous retroviruses in blood mononuclear cells and brain tissue from multiple sclerosis patients. Acta Neurol Scand Suppl 1997; 169: 38–44.

119. Perron H, Garson JA, Bedin F et al. Molecular identification of a novel retrovirus repeatedly isolated from patients with multiple sclerosis. The Collaborative Research Group on Multiple Sclerosis. Proc Natl Acad Sci USA 1997; 94: 7583–7588.

120. Murray RS, Brown B, Brain D et al. Detection of coronavirus RNA and antigen in multiple sclerosis brain. Ann Neurol 1992; 31: 525–533.

121. Stewart JN, Mounir S, Talbot PJ. Human coronavirus gene expression in the brains of multiple sclerosis patients. Virology 1992; 191: 502–505.

122. Dessau RB, Lisby G, Frederiksen JL. Coronaviruses in brain tissue from patients with multiple sclerosis. Acta Neuropathol (Berl) 2001;101: 601–604.

123. Boerman RH, Bax JJ, Beekhuis-Brussee JA et al. JC virus and multiple sclerosis: a refutation? Acta Neurol Scand 1993; 87: 353–355.

124. Stoner GL, Agostini HT, Ryschkewitsch CF et al. Characterization of JC virus DNA amplified from urine of chronic progressive multiple sclerosis patients. Mult Scler 1996; 1: 193–199.

125. Agostini HT, Ryschkewitsch CF, Baumhefner RW et al. Influence of JC virus coding region genotype on risk of multiple sclerosis and progressive multifocal leukoencephalopathy. J Neurovirol 2000; 6: S101–S108.

126. Ferrante P, Omodeo-Zorini E, Caldarelli-Stefano R et al. Detection of JC virus DNA in cerebrospinal fluid from multiple sclerosis patients. Mult Scler 1998; 4: 49–54.

127. Hawkes CH. Is multiple sclerosis a sexually transmitted infection? J Neurol Neurosurg Psychiatr 2002; 73: 439–443.

128. Colombo M, Dono M, Gazzola P et al. Accumulation of clonally related B lymphocytes in the cerebrospinal fluid of multiple sclerosis patients. J Immunol 2000; 164: 2782–2789.

129. Owens GP, Ritchie A, Burgoon MP et al. Single-cell repertoire analysis demonstrates that clonal expansion is a prominent feature of the B cell response in multiple sclerosis cerebrospinal fluid. J Immunol 2003; 171: 2725–2733.

130. Qin Y, Duquette P, Poole R et al. Clonal expansion and somatic hypermutation of V_H genes of B cells from cerebrospinal fluid in multiple sclerosis. J Clin Invest 1998; 102: 1046–1050.

131. Qin Y, Duquette P, Zhang Y et al. Intrathecal B-cell clonal expansion, an early sign of humoral immunity, in the cerebrospinal fluid of patients with clinically isolated syndrome suggestive of multiple sclerosis. Lab Invest 2003; 83: 1081–1088.

132. Winges KM, Gilden DH, Bernett JL et al. Analysis of multiple sclerosis cerebrospinal fluid reveals a continuum of clonally related antibody-secreting cells that are predominantly plasma blasts. J Neuroimmunol 2007; 192: 226–234.

133. Baranzini SE, Jeong MC, Butoni C et al. B cell repertoire diversity and clonal expansion in multiple sclerosis brain lesions. J Immunol 1999; 163: 5133–5144.

134. Owens GP, Kraus H, Burgoon MP et al. Restricted use of V_H4 germline segments in an acute multiple sclerosis brain. Ann Neurol 1998; 43: 236–243.

135. Owens GP, Winges KM, Ritchie AM et al. V_H4 gene segments dominate the intrathecal humoral immune esponse in multiple sclerosis. J Immunol 2007; 179: 6343–6351.

136. Owens GP, Burgoon MP, Anthony J et al. The immunoglobulin G heavy chain repertoire in multiple sclerosis plaques is distinct from the heavy chain repertoire in peripheral blood lymphocytes. Clin Immunol 2001; 98: 258–263.

137. Smith-Jensen T, Burgoon MP, Anthony J et al. Comparison of IgG heavy chain sequences in MS and SSPE brains reveals an antigen-driven response. Neurology 2000; 54: 1227–1232.

138. Burgoon MP, Williamson RA, Owens GP et al. Cloning the antibody response in humans with inflammatory CNS disease: isolation of measles virus-specific antibodies from phage display libraries of a subacute sclerosing panencephalitis brain. J Neuroimmunol 1999; 94: 204–211.

139. Burgoon MP, Owens GP, Smith-Jensen T et al. Cloning the antibody response in humans with inflammatory CNS disease: analysis of the expressed IgG repertoire in subacute sclerosing panencephalitis brain reveals disease-relevant antibodies that recognize specific measles virus antigens. J Immunol 1999; 163: 3496–3502.

140. Owens GP, Ritchie AM, Gilden DH et al. Measles virus-specific plasma cells are prominent in subacute sclerosing panencephalitis CSF. Neurology 2007; 68: 1815–1819.

141. Owens GP, Shearer AJ, Yu K et al. Screening random peptide libraries with subacute sclerosing panencephalitis brain-derived recombinant antibodies identifies multiple epitopes in the C-terminal region of the measles virus nucleocapsid protein. J Virol 2006; 80: 12121–12130.

142. Monson NL, Brezinschek H-P, Brezinschek RI et al. Receptor revision and atypical mutational characteristics in clonally expanded B cells from the cerebrospinal fluid of recently diagnosed multiple sclerosis patients. J Neuroimmunol 2005; 158: 170–181.

143. Ritchie AM, Gilden DH, Williamson RA et al. Comparative analysis of the CD19+ and CD138+ cell antibody repertoires in the cerebrospinal fluid of patients with multiple sclerosis. J Immunol 2004; 173: 649–656.

144. Haubold K, Owens GP, Kaur P et al. B-lymphocyte and plasma cell clonal expansion in monosymptomatic optic neuritis cerebrospinal fluid. Ann Neurol 2004; 56: 97–107.

145. Burgoon MP, Keays KM, Owens GP et al. Laser-capture microdissection of plasma cells from subacute sclerosing panencephalitis brain reveals intrathecal disease-relevant antibodies. Proc Natl Acad Sci USA 2005; 102: 7245–7250.

146. Burgoon MP, Caldas YA, Keays KM et al. Recombinant antibodies generated from both clonal and less abundant plasma cell IgG sequences in subacute sclerosing panencephalitis brain are directed against measles virus. J NeuroVirol 2006; 12: 389–402.

147. Scott JK, Smith GP. Searching for peptide ligands with an epitope library. Science 1990; 249: 386–390.

148. Mintz PJ, Kim J, Do KA et al. Fingerprinting the circulating repertoire of antibodies from cancer patients. Nat Biotechnol 2003; 21: 57–63.

149. Zhang M, Davidson A. A rheumatoid factor specific mimotope identified by a peptide display library. Autoimmunity 1999: 30, 131–142.

150. Rudolf MP, Vogel M, Kricek F et al. Epitope-specific antibody response to IgE by mimotope immunization. J Immunol 1998; 160: 3315–3321.

151. Heiskanen T, Lundkvist A, Soliymani R et al. Phage-displayed peptides mimicking the discontinuous neutralization sites of puumala Hantavirus envelope glycoproteins. Virology 1999; 262: 321–332.

152. Ferrer M, Sullivan BJ, Godbout KL et al. Structural and functional characterization of an epitope in the conserved C-terminal region of HIV-1 gp120. J Pept Res 1999; 54: 32–42.

153. Zhong X, Yang H, Guo ZF et al. B-cell responses in patients who have recovered from severe acute respiratory syndrome target a dominant site in the S2 domain of the surface spike glycoprotein. J Virol 2005; 79: 3401–3408.

154. Yu X, Gilden DH, Ritchie AM et al. Specificity of recombinant antibodies generated from multiple sclerosis cerebrospinal fluid probed with a random peptide library. J Neuroimmunol 2006; 172: 121–131.

155. Yu X, Burgoon MP, Shearer AJ et al. Characterization of phage peptide interaction with antibody using phage mediated immuno-PCR. J Immunol Methods 2007; 325: 33–40.

CHAPTER 16

Models of chronic relapsing experimental autoimmune encephalomyelitis

C. S. Raine and C. P. Genain

INTRODUCTION

Experimental autoimmune encephalomyelitis (EAE) has for many years been the model of choice for the validation of pathogenetic mechanisms implicated in multiple sclerosis (MS) and for the testing of therapeutic avenues.[1–3] Since its introduction as a model in the 1930s[4] to study iatrogenic acute disseminated encephalomyelitis (ADEM) resulting from antirabies vaccination (described by Pasteur at the end of the 19th century and known to be due to central nervous system (CNS) tissue in the vaccine), EAE has evolved from an acute (often fatal) form in monkeys induced by active sensitization with whole CNS tissue to a veritable catalogue of acute and chronic forms inducible in most animal species and strains using a wide spectrum of procedures and antigens. With time, however, the links to ADEM were de-emphasized and on the basis of similarities to the acute form of MS, EAE was adopted as a model for that disease. Since typical MS has a chronic relapsing–remitting or progressive course, a need for more chronic forms of EAE was perceived and throughout the 1960s and 1970s, there developed a concerted effort to produce models of chronic EAE in a number of species.[1,5] Since that time, a time when neuropathology was cutting-edge and morphology the principal tool, quantum leaps have been made in the field projecting it from a mainly descriptive discipline to neuroimmunology as we know it today, with its molecular bent, employing analytical and immunological technologies to define mechanisms. Concomitant with this trend has been a massive overhaul of our everyday vocabulary and a new heightened awareness of the broad scope of the field. Nevertheless,

although our repertoire of skills in the nervous system now freely embraces terms barely in existence 20 years ago, viz. molecules of the immunological synapse, cytokine and chemokine modulation of gene expression, polymerase chain reaction and gene chip analysis, to name but a few, a structural framework on which to attach these terms and technologies still remains a key part of our understanding of disease processes.

THE NEED FOR AN IMMUNOLOGICAL MODEL FOR MULTIPLE SCLEROSIS

Lacking a natural, nonhuman counterpart for MS, investigators investigating pathogenetic mechanisms were compelled to turn towards the development of different forms of EAE, an autoimmune demyelinating disease of laboratory animals induced by T-cell sensitization to myelin antigens (see Ch. 13). With regard to chronic relapsing EAE, the pre-eminent laboratory tool for MS today, the first reproducible model[6] was applied in the 1970s as an innovative approach to MS research and utilized active sensitization of juvenile strain 13 guinea pigs with syngeneic spinal cord tissue.[7] While providing a reliable tool with both clinical and pathological similarities to MS, the guinea pig paradigm was eventually found to have immunogenetic limitations and fell short of standards to which cellular immunologists were accustomed. In the early 1980s there occurred a redirecting of energies towards the selection of species and protocols in which the immunological terrain was less hazardous. Consequently, for studies on immune-mediated demyelination, the mouse and the rat became the species of choice. After an initial period of experimentation with active sensitization,[8-11] murine models of chronic demyelination moved for a while towards adoptive-transfer technologies whereby CNS antigen-specific bulk-isolated lymphocytes,[12] T-cell lines or T-cell clones[13] were administered intravenously into naive recipients. More recently, there has been a move back to chronic relapsing models involving active sensitization with well-defined myelin antigens, especially myelin/oligodendrocyte glycoprotein (MOG) and proteolipid protein (PLP), and their peptides or species-specific epitopes.[14-17] Facilitated by a growing battery of species- and strain-specific molecular and immunological probes, chronic relapsing EAE in the mouse, while sacrificing some of the structural hallmarks of the MS lesion seen with the strain 13 guinea pig model, has become the most widely applied tool for studies on MS. In addition to the mouse and rat,[18] actively-induced and adoptively-transferred models have been developed in the New World monkey, the marmoset,[19] which affords opportunities for evaluation of demyelination in primates and the testing of therapeutic protocols perhaps more relevant to human MS.

Historically, EAE has probably contributed as much to the understanding of delayed hypersensitivity as it has to immune-mediated demyelination.[20-23] In acute EAE, T-cell mediation is well proven and roles for antibodies to myelin components have been demonstrated.[1] More recent data suggest some of the encephalitogenicity in EAE to be related to the sharing of common T-cell receptor (TCR) variable regions in some species (see Chapter 13). Moreover, transgenic mice expressing genes encoding a rearranged TCR specific for myelin basic protein (MBP) or MOG[24-26] have been shown to develop spontaneous, late-onset EAE in the absence of active or adoptive sensitization, further supporting a key role for the T cell in this condition. Despite the multitude of contributions of acute EAE to immune-mediated myelin pathology, its direct application to MS was limited by its clinical and pathological dissimilarities to the human disease. Indeed, as stated above, it was originally developed as a model for ADEM related to postrabies encephalomyelitis and its adoption as a model for MS was a later event.[1,5] In spite of many dissimilarities to MS (enough for some authors to refute its applicability as a model[27]), acute EAE continues to provide seminal data on fundamental questions in CNS autoimmunity and on a number of therapeutic approaches to MS,[2,3,28] some involving myelin-related TCR sequences, anti-inflammatory compounds, immunosuppressive modalities and antibodies to CNS and immune system molecules (see Ch. 23). In light of the now extensively expanded forms of EAE, the overall goal of the following narrative is to present, within the same canvas, the respective values of the models to the analysis of the lesions and therapeutic approaches to multiple sclerosis.

EARLY CHRONIC MODELS

Although it has long been realized that a chronic form of EAE might have greater relevance to MS, prior to 1980 chronic EAE had been reported only sporadically.[29] The model of Stone and Lerner,[6] a model which, like MS, demonstrated a relapsing course and lesions separated in time and space,[7] was the first to be applied extensively to MS-related questions. A modified version of this model was subsequently developed and investigated in outbred guinea pigs with considerable success.[30,31] However, it was the strain 13 guinea pig model that firmly established clinical and pathological similarities between chronic relapsing EAE and human MS. The likenesses were not only morphological but also encompassed immunological, genetic and therapeutic parameters.[29] Pathogenetically, it was found that a combination of myelin antigens was required to induce

an inflammatory demyelinated lesion.[32,33] This information was then applied therapeutically, whereby it was found that chronic relapsing EAE in the guinea pig could be suppressed with MBP given before disease onset[34] but not treated with MBP (given after onset). However, MBP combined with a major glycolipid of myelin, galactocerebroside (GalC), proved to be an effective treatment protocol,[29,35] discussed later under Therapeutic approaches.

Chronic relapsing EAE in strain 13 guinea pigs involved a single subcutaneous sensitization of juveniles in the nuchal region with syngeneic spinal cord tissue and the ensuing disease had a latent period of 1–2 months after this single sensitization, during which subclinical CNS lesions could be seen before overt signs were manifest.[36] Clinical signs sometimes progressed to quadriparesis, events that were rarely fatal and remitted to varying degrees, after which relapses occurred at irregular intervals over periods of more than 3 years. Attempts to induce chronic relapsing EAE with MBP were unsuccessful and resulted in an acute syndrome that healed and did not relapse. Equally unsuccessful were attempts to induce chronic disease in strain 13 guinea pigs using adoptive transfer technology and, regardless of whether donor lymphocytes were derived from CNS antigen-sensitized juveniles or adults, the outcome was invariably acute EAE.[37]

MOUSE MODELS

The first detailed studies on mouse EAE were conducted on 10 mouse strains with different H-2 backgrounds which were tested for acute EAE, among them, EAE-susceptible and non-susceptible strains. As in most other species, this began with an examination of the acute disease induced by active sensitization with an emulsion of whole CNS tissue in adjuvant in combination with booster injections of pertussis vaccine.[8] While demyelination was a feature of the acute EAE lesion, nerve fiber damage (Wallerian degeneration) was a prominent and extensive component and the inflammatory component was severe, consisting of polymorphonuclear leukocytes (PMNs), fibrin and some hemorrhage. The axonal loss was criticized at the time as an aberration, undermining the relevance of the model to MS. However, with a resurgence of interest in axonal pathology in MS,[2,38] (see Ch. 11), in retrospect, such changes actually rendered the model quite relevant. Work on EAE in the mouse soon turned towards the development of more chronic forms and in 1981 a new model was reported in the EAE-susceptible SJL/J mouse (H-2[s]), with a protocol involving multiple (usually two or three) subcutaneous sensitizations with whole CNS tissue administered at weekly intervals, after which animals developed a chronic relapsing disease.[10] The neuropathology of this model also showed loss of axons, a severe inflammatory response, primary demyelination and remyelination and some sparing of oligodendrocytes.[11] Immunocytochemistry of both the acute and chronic relapsing forms of actively induced EAE in the mouse implicated early expression of class II MHC prior to lesion formation and a predominance of CD4+ T helper (Th)-1 type T-cells in lesion pathogenesis, in agreement with current pathogenetic thinking (see Chapter 13).

In 1984, chronic relapsing EAE in the female SJL mouse using adoptive (passive) transfer technology was reported,[12] a modification of an earlier protocol.[39] Females were selected because of their increased susceptibility to EAE[40] and the protocol involved injection, into the tail vein of a naive animal, of lymph node cells from syngeneic MBP-injected donors. Recipient mice developed acute signs 7–10 days post-transfer, a disease from which they recovered, and over the following several months multiple relapses were observed. The neuropathology of this model[41] revealed primary demyelination, heavy PMN involvement and some vascular damage during acute stages and remyelination during remissions. A subsequent study examined the age-dependence of this adoptively transferred model.[42]

As mouse EAE became more refined, so did methods of inducing the disease. With long-term cultured T-cell lines activated with MBP in vitro, it was shown not only that chronic relapsing EAE could be produced in SJL mice but also that there occurred prolonged upregulation of class II MHC (Ia) expression on endothelial and infiltrating cells within lesions and that this increased during relapses.[43] T-cell line-induced chronic relapsing EAE was later extended to work on MBP+ T-cell clones and elegantly elaborated upon at the ultrastructural level.[13] It was found that, although there was severe decrease in axons in lesions, demyelination remained prominent and was especially marked when recipient mice were 1) given whole-body X-irradiation, 2) MHC-II-compatible strains or 3) congenitally athymic. Although most early models of murine chronic EAE involved SJL/J (H-2^s) mice, other EAE-susceptible haplotypes have provided important immunogenetic pointers in the search for the morphologic basis of genetic susceptibility. Among these, the PL/J strain (H-2^u), a strain developing EAE in response to an epitope of the MBP molecule different from that responsible for the disease in the SJL/J strain (H-2^s), has been helpful.[44] The many studies on transgenic mice overexpressing specific developmental CNS or immune system genes, and on mice in which specific genes have mostly been deleted (knockout or null mice), have been carried out in mice displaying H-2^k (BalbC) or H-2^b (C57/BL6) backgrounds.

LATER CHRONIC MODELS IN MOUSE

Most of the above examples of chronic relapsing EAE were predicated upon MBP being the major encephalitogen. It has been held, as far back as the early 1950s,[45] that other protein components of the myelin sheath, most notably PLP (the major protein of myelin), might also be encephalitogenic. This was eventually confirmed and PLP-induced chronic relapsing EAE has been produced in the guinea pig[46] and Lewis rat.[47] With the need for mouse models, PLP-induced EAE was developed in the BalbC mouse (H-2^k), a strain normally resistant to EAE induced by MBP.[48,49] The encephalitogenicity of the 20 kDa protein component of PLP, DM20, was also demonstrated.[48] The ultrastructural features of the condition in euthymic and athymic mice reconstituted with T cells were similar to models reported above after MBP sensitization. The strategy was then repeated using T-cell lines to PLP in SJL mice.[50] The majority of animals developed acute EAE but a small percentage went on to display relapses. This model was not entirely compatible with MBP-induced T-cell models since priming injections of pertussis vaccine and low-dose irradiation were needed to optimize the effects of the T-cell lines. Nevertheless, a typical inflammatory demyelinating condition did ensue. Other studies have shown that MBP-epitope-specific T-cell lines can be used to induce chronic relapsing EAE,[51] this work highlighting the need for T-cell recognition of haplotype-specific antigenic epitopes for successful disease induction. The phenomenon of epitope spreading in chronic EAE,[52] further developed by others,[53-54] provides an important possible mechanism for the attenuation of pathogenetic events in this condition.

Among the remaining models of chronic relapsing EAE are several in the Lewis rat, one involving active sensitization with CNS tissue and a disease duration of 4–5 months.[9] A second rat model[18] combined active sensitization with low-dose cyclosporin A administration and has been applied in pathophysiological studies. An increasing number of models induced in rats and mice by sensitization with MOG (probably the most-used

encephalitogen for EAE today), have been reported.[55-57] MOG is also an encephalitogen favored and highly effective in transgenic and knockout mice (see below). It is noteworthy that whereas different strains of mice will mostly respond to one immunodominant epitope of MBP or PLP (e.g. H2^u to MBP$_{1-11Ac}$, or H2^s to PLP$_{139-151}$), animals are generally more susceptible to MOG and its common immunodominant epitope in rodents, MOG$_{35-5}$.[5]

With the advent of gene technology, we began to see EAE being induced in transgenic models in which, for example, the effects of different class II MHC gene products on the expression of disease were examined[58] and where mice genetically constructed to overexpress T-cell receptors specific for MBP[24,25] or MOG[26] developed EAE either spontaneously or after challenge with pertussis alone. Interestingly, transgenic mice overexpressing immune system molecules such as MHC class I display CNS hypomyelination[59] while others inducibly overexpressing the chemokine MCP-1 (CCL1) develop spontaneous inflammatory CNS pathology with similarities to EAE, due perhaps to autosensitization.[60] Chronic EAE investigations using transgenic systems (too many to give appropriate coverage here) continue to proliferate and raise fascinating questions. Also, with regard to genetic manipulations and EAE, there have been an impressive number of studies on knockout models with mice lacking, for example, CNS myelin or immune system genes, in which EAE has been induced, often with a chronic course.[61] Such models have proved extremely useful in the dissection of disease mechanisms. Many of these myelin-related null mice lack a clinical phenotype, appearing normal in all regards, and only after careful structural analysis were axonal atrophy and degeneration discerned.[62] Another common finding is that deletion of one gene with an important role (e.g. expression of a key proinflammatory cytokine) can lead to compensatory upregulation of another gene with a similar function, resulting in no change in outcome.

The above (still expanding) compendium of models of chronic relapsing EAE serves to document at least six separate trends in the field that have occurred over the years:

- a move from guinea pig to murine models, a move necessitated by the demand for precise immunological analysis
- the application of adoptive-transfer technology and antigen-specific T-cells to dissect pathogenetic mechanisms
- the demonstration that myelin proteins are complex antigens with different epitopes recognized by different TCRs depending upon the genetic make-up (strain) of the recipient and, when administered alone, may not induce a demyelinating pathology (e.g. requiring a B-cell response to myelin)
- the discovery that most myelin antigens, such as MBP, PLP and MOG, are encephalitogenic (with species-specific epitopes) and equally capable of inducing chronic disease
- the fact that, with transgenic and gene depletion (knockout) technologies, we are now able to dissect selectively the roles of different immune system molecules and relate them to therapeutic relevance.
- the adoption of MOG as the major encephalitogen for EAE in gene-manipulated strains which are normally EAE-resistant.

LESION TOPOGRAPHY IN COMPARISON TO MULTIPLE SCLEROSIS

The following paragraphs will delineate where possible the morphologic similarities between these various chronic relapsing models and will compare the picture with that of MS (see

Ch. 11). Chronic relapsing EAE in the guinea pig resembles MS in many respects, more so than other model. CNS disease is most evident in spinal cord white matter and can be detected in gross specimens as areas of discoloration (Fig. 16.1A). With myelin stains, large foci of demyelination are seen histologically, sometimes deep in the parenchyma but more usually extending as a subpial rim (Fig. 16.1D,E). Lesions in the cerebral hemispheres are equally disseminated and are pronounced in periventricular areas (Fig. 16.1B,C). Brain lesions are most common in severely affected animals 2–4 months postinoculation. The brains of less afflicted or more chronic animals display smaller areas of demyelination or shadow (remyelinated) plaques. Invariably, optic nerves are affected in chronic relapsing EAE[63] but, unlike the spinal cord (see below), optic nerve lesions rarely reflect relapsing activity and tend to be monophasic. Lesions occur in the PNS in chronic relapsing EAE in guinea pigs, more so than in MS, with involvement heaviest in the proximal (intradural) regions of the spinal nerve roots. As has been noted previously in chronic EAE in the rabbit,[64,65] PNS fibers in radicular zones are affected and can remyelinate rapidly and completely, unlike CNS fibers, which remyelinate slowly or remain demyelinated. Chronically demyelinated axons, although physiologically silent, can persist intact for months to years (also in MS – see Ch. 11).

Topography of lesions in the actively and passively induced mouse models is similar but lesions are less extensive than in the guinea pig model (Fig. 16.2A,B). Optic nerves are always affected, cerebral white matter lesions are small and involve thin paraventricular zones only, yet inflammatory activity may be extensive supependymally. Spinal cord lesions are more common caudally and are subpial and narrow (Fig. 16.2A,B), with some predilection for root entry zones. There is little or no involvement of the PNS. In the mouse, chronic relapsing EAE is typically a spinal cord disease, particularly evident at lumbosacral levels, although with time, as relapsing disease evolves, lesion activity moves rostrally. This holds true irrespective of the mode of induction and a single sensitization with a crude CNS antigenic emulsion or an intravenous injection of an MBP-specific T-cell line will both cause a severe disease, mainly of the lower spinal cord initially. In size and topography, murine EAE lesions compare poorly with typical MS plaques because of their limited extent and subpial distribution but, like MS, they reveal an abundance of axonal pathology or depletion (Fig. 16.2C). However, they do retain demyelination and remyelination as major features, particularly adoptively-transferred forms (Fig. 16.2D,E).

THE AXON IN THE ESTABLISHED LESION OF CHRONIC EXPERIMENTAL AUTOIMMUNE ENCEPHALOMYELITIS

As is the case in MS, the typical chronic EAE lesion in the strain 13 guinea pig model is well demarcated from adjacent less affected myelinated white matter and not infrequently displays a moderate amount of ongoing inflammation about its margins (Fig. 16.1E,F). The lesion center is usually a mosaic of well preserved, naked axons among an abundance of blood vessels with enlarged Virchow–Robin spaces, suggestive of neovascularization (increased angiogenesis has also been noted in MS – see Ch. 11). Sometimes, these blood vessels reveal a fenestrated endothelium.[66] The perivascular compartments contain fibroblasts, collagen deposits and macrophages (Figs 16.1G and 16.3A). The overlying meninges are usually severely fibrotic, adherent, collagen-rich and may be attached to the pial surface by glial bridges[67,68] (see Fig. 16.12). Demyelinated fibers are numerous and display some decrease in axonal diameter, a

phenomenon also noted in the PNS subsequent to demyelination.[64] There is more axonal sparing in the guinea pig model than in MS and much more than that encountered in mouse models (Fig. 16.3A). Ongoing myelin breakdown and removal is manifested by parenchymal and perivascular mononuclear cells containing recognizable myelin debris, most apparent at the lesion margin (Figs 16.2D and 16.3A). Mononuclear cells are the major inflammatory component in old lesions. Plasma cells are common and small lymphocytes are inconspicuous. In the guinea pig, a few PMNs are seen in early acute lesions but are rare in chronic lesions. The presence of abundant gliosis reaffirms the chronicity of the changes and oligodendroglial sparing has been noted.[69] Ultrastructurally, silent chronic lesions display the anticipated appearances, described in greater detail previously,[29,36] with naked axons embedded in a matrix of fibrillary astrogliosis (Fig. 16.3B). In these areas, demyelinated axons possess synapse-like axoglial membrane specializations (Fig. 16.3B, inset), a phenomenon also seen in MS.[70,71]

In mouse chronic relapsing EAE, lesions are usually intensely gliotic, depleted of axons and the extent of demyelination is less spectacular. Lesions from mice in which the disease was induced by active sensitization with CNS emulsions tend to be more destructive, less demyelinative and less widespread (Fig. 16.2A,C), than those occurring in the spinal cords of mice in which the disease was adoptively transferred with MBP-activated lymph node cells (Fig. 16.2B,D). Adoptively-transferred murine models invariably show more axonal sparing than after active sensitization (Fig. 16.2B,D), and old lesions display a proclivity to remyelinate (Fig. 16.2E). Recent forms of murine EAE utilizing MOG as the encephalitogen and active sensitization can display narrow subpial lesions with remarkable sparing of axons (Fig. 16.4A). Some lesions may exhibit widespread spontaneous remyelination (Fig. 16.4B). In addition to nerve fiber damage in murine EAE, vascular injury, hemorrhage, extracellular fibrin, disruption of normal architecture by invaginations of the glia limitans and an abundance of PMNs (neutrophils and eosinophils) are not uncommon appearances.[11,29,44] The latter characteristics are unusual to the MS lesion. However, these features are less prominent (or in the case of vascular damage, virtually absent) in the adoptively-transferred model.[12]

Present in many murine forms of EAE is the unusual phenomenon of heterotopic regeneration of PNS fibers into the subarachnoid space overlying the spinal cord. Many of these fibers probably emanate from regenerating sprouts from PNS fibers severed as they enter or leave the spinal cord at root entry zones.[72] Although axonal disease is not usually common in the guinea pig model, long-term animals frequently display axonal dystrophy and abortive regeneration[73] (see Fig. 16.12). Similar dystrophic axons are very common in MS plaques, particularly during acute and recurrent activity (see Ch. 11). An interesting historical note is that in one of the first ultrastructural studies of acute EAE in outbred guinea pigs,[74] axonal dystrophy was a prominent feature and, although it was raised as a possible component of the lesion, it was disregarded as significant in favor of EAE being purely demyelinative.[75]

THE ACTIVE PLAQUE IN CHRONIC EXPERIMENTAL AUTOIMMUNE ENCEPHALOMYELITIS

In a manner reminiscent of MS, CNS lesions in the EAE models reveal a constellation of active, chronic and reparatory events that complement the clinical picture. Examination of CNS lesions sampled during relapsing clinical disease will show large foci of chronic demyelination upon which intense inflammation

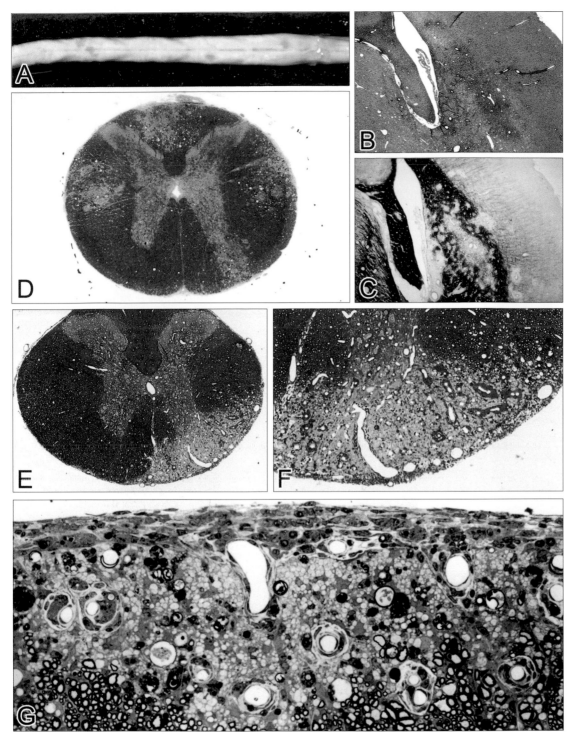

FIG. 16.1 A. Strain 13 guinea pig; chronic relapsing EAE, 20 weeks postinoculation (p.i.) with whole spinal cord/CFA; one relapse; gross specimen. Note the multiple darker-colored demyelinated plaques breaking through the white matter along the pial surface of this lower thoracic/lumbar spinal cord. Plaques are totally disseminated, as in MS (see Ch. 11). **B**. Paraffin section from the brain of another guinea pig at 16 weeks p.i., stained with hematoxylin–eosin (H&E). Note the large area of inflammation to right of the ventricle. Hippocampal fibrium hangs into the ventricle and anterior thalamus is to the left. **C**. An adjacent section to **B**, stained with Sudan black for myelin. Note the large demyelinated plaque to right of the ventricle, the association between areas of demyelination and perivascular infiltrates, and the punctate lesions in the gray matter (cortex) to the right. **D**. A section of thoracic spinal cord from a specimen similar to that in **A** reveals the presence of multiple demyelinated subpial and parenchymal lesions, particularly two large ones in the lateral columns. **E**. Lumbar spinal cord of a guinea pig sampled during a relapse 5 months p.i. reveals a large demyelinated plaque extending from anterior to lateral columns on right. Perivascular infiltrates are evident along margins of the expanding lesion, indicative of recent activity. **F**. Higher magnification from **E** shows extent of demyelination, perivascular cuffs of infiltrating cells and extensive infiltration within the subarachnoid space. **G**. A slightly more detailed image from a subpial lesion from an animal with chronic relapsing EAE sampled 18 weeks p.i. and 4 weeks after onset of signs shows masses of preserved, demyelinated axons with intervening fibrous astrocytes, the presence of infiltrating cells and scarring around some vessels and within the subarachnoid space, and macrophages containing myelin debris. ×300. **D–F)** are all from 1 μm epoxy sections; toluidine blue stain.

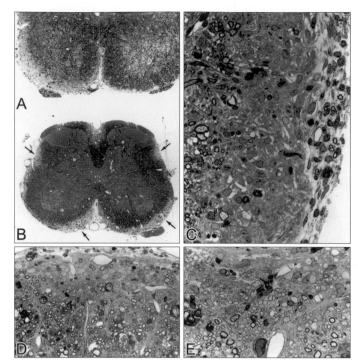

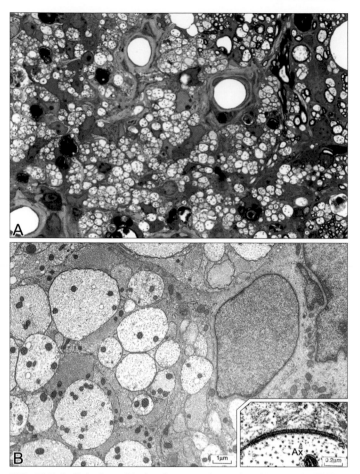

FIG. 16.2 A. SJL/J mouse; chronic relapsing EAE, induced by active sensitization with spinal cord tissue; 7 months p.i. A broad zone of subpial demyelination in lumbar spinal cord involves anterior and lateral columns, particularly on the left. Inflammatory cells are evident in subarachnoid space. **B**. SJL/J mouse; chronic relapsing EAE induced by adoptive transfer of bulk-isolated, MBP-stimulated lymph node cells; 3 months post-transfer. This section of lumbar spinal cord displays several well demarcated, demyelinated chronic lesions (arrows). **C**. SJL/J mouse; chronic relapsing EAE actively induced by CNS antigen in adjuvant; 7 months p.i. The subpial parenchyma is gliotic and severely depleted of nerve fibers. Some scattered CNS remyelinated fibers are apparent at the edge of the lesion and heterotopic PNS-myelinated fibers can be seen within the leptomeninges (right). ×750. **D**. PL/J mouse; chronic relapsing EAE; 5 months post-transfer of MBP-sensitized lymph node cells. A small subpial lesion from lumbar spinal cord is shown. Note many surviving, chronically demyelinated axons in the lesion area and the myelin debris and residual Wallerian degeneration in the adjacent white matter (lower left). **E**. PL/J mouse; chronic relapsing EAE; adoptive transfer; 9 months post-transfer. Remyelinated axons are seen throughout this subpial lesion. L7 spinal cord. ×550. 1 μm epoxy sections; toluidine blue stain.

FIG. 16.3 A. Spinal cord lesion from a guinea pig with chronic EAE for 5 months; no relapses. Note the large number of demyelinated axons within a fibrous astrogliotic parenchyma. Blood vessels are scarred and contain fibroblasts, collagen and macrophages within the Virchow–Robin space. The small dots in the axons are mitochondria. 1 μm epoxy section; toluidine blue; ×400. **B**. A typical silent chronic EAE lesion is shown by electron microscopy. Note the multinucleated fibrous astrocyte to the right and the gliotic background surrounding the many well-preserved demyelinated axons. **Inset**. An axoglial membrane specialization is shown between an axon (Ax) and an astrocyte (above) (see reference 70). ×8000 and ×50 000.

by large mononuclear cells has been superimposed[76] (Fig. 16.5A). Inflammatory changes also occur around marginal areas of chronic lesions where ongoing myelin damage once more becomes a major feature (Fig. 16.5B). Close packing of recently denuded axons predominates in these areas (Fig. 16.5A–C), readily distinguishing this stage of the disease from chronic silent phases where axons become separated by fibrous astrogliosis[36] (Fig. 16.3B) and small foci of perivascular cuffs surrounded by recently demyelinated axons.

The intense parenchymal and perivascular infiltration by small lymphocytes seen in active MS lesions is present but not as pronounced in chronic EAE and is best observed by immunocytochemistry.[1] Class II MHC expression plays an integral role in these inflammatory events and has been localized to both endothelial cells and macrophages.[77–79] T-cell invasion is more a feature of early stages of acute EAE. In areas of recurrent activity in the guinea pig, there is an abundance of mononuclear macrophages and plasma cells. PMNs are rare. Smaller active lesions in chronic animals are not entirely dissimilar to regions of demyelination occurring during acute EAE[36] where demyelin-

ated lesions consist of narrow rims of naked axons closely associated with inflammatory foci. The latter, as in MS, comprise small lymphocytes and some macrophages early on that eventually give way to macrophages and plasma cells.

THE PATTERN OF MYELIN BREAKDOWN

The mechanism of myelin breakdown in EAE lesions has been described previously and displays many similarities to active MS.[29] This process has been analyzed in a number of species and the various patterns of demyelination form the subject of a number of reviews.[1,23,80] The previously described phenomena of myelin stripping by macrophages,[81] myelin vesiculation[36,82] and receptor-mediated phagocytosis of myelin[83,84,85] are the common patterns of myelin breakdown in EAE. Both cell- and antibody-mediated demyelination are implicated, as is also the case in the acute MS lesion.[2] Longitudinal study of antibody titers in chronic relapsing EAE have shown fluctuations in antiglial antibodies that correlate with periods of disease worsening.[86] In addition, antibodies against oligodendroglial antigens have been implicated in the induction of relapses in EAE.[87]

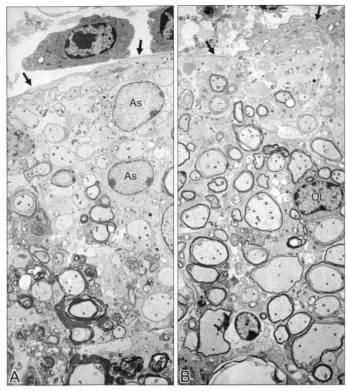

FIG. 16.4 A. BalbC mouse; MOG-induced chronic EAE; 7 weeks p.i. Ultrastructurally, a large subpial spinal cord lesion is chronically demyelinated with axons lying in a gliotic parenchyma (astrocytes at Ag), plasma cells and pial surface above (arrows), lesion edge (showing myelin debris) and normally myelinated white matter lie below. ×4000. **B**. Another lesion from a similar animal shows an extensively remyelinated subpial lesion (glia limitans at arrows) and an oligodendrocyte (OL). Note the uniformly thin myelin sheaths typical of remyelination. ×4000.

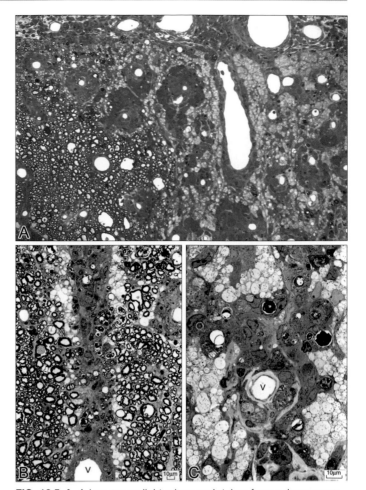

FIG. 16.5 A. A low-power light micrograph taken from a 1 μm epoxy section stained with toluidine blue, from the spinal cord of a guinea pig at 5 months p.i. which displayed a relapse prior to sampling. Note the abundance of recent perivascular cuffs of infiltrating cells in the heavily demyelinated white matter. The tightly packed axons are recently demyelinated. Normal white matter is to the lower left, meninges above. ×400. **B**. Strain 13 guinea pig; chronic EAE; 3 months postsensitization. Within this early lesion, note the association between perivascular inflammation and demyelination. Vessel lumen at (V). Macrophages contain recognizable myelin debris and lie along the perivascular sleeve of demyelination. ×400. **C**. Detail from a spinal cord lesion taken from an animal sampled during a clinical relapse. Vessel lumen at (V). Inflammation is superimposed upon recently demyelinated areas showing tight packing of axons and little astrogliosis, and macrophages contain myelin debris. ×700.

Chronic active lesions in mouse models are less extensive than those seen in the guinea pig. As in other species such as the rabbit (originally a much used species, now moved aside in favor of rodents) (Fig. 16.6A), undermining and stripping by macrophage processes leads to phagocytosis with dissociated myelin droplets becoming attached to clathrin-coated pits on the surface of macrophages (Fig. 16.6A, inset). The same histopathologic scenario is repeated during lesion expansion, albeit on a smaller scale, whereby fresh waves of infiltrating cells enter new and old lesion areas, demyelination of previously unaffected fibers occurs and lesions expand (Fig. 16.6B). Receptor-mediated phagocytosis of myelin is also seen in different models in the mouse (Fig. 16.6C–F). Therefore, at the level of myelin breakdown in the different species during EAE, patterns are identical. More significantly, that identical patterns are encountered in MS[88,89] renders these demyelinating models highly relevant to the human disease (see also below under Marmoset EAE). It needs to be emphasized, however, that this pattern of myelin degradation is very early, rapid and transient, lasting only for 1–2 days after the process has commenced. It is also related to the binding of IgG, after which the opsonized fragments of myelin associate with clathrin-coated pits on the macrophage surface, probably by binding to Fc receptors.[85]

MECHANISMS RELATED TO RECURRENCE OF DISEASE

Chronic active or relapsing activity in EAE has been assumed by some to be related to periodic antigen stimulation by antigen

depots persisting (loculated) at the site of injection. While this may be difficult to refute in models involving subcutaneous injection of antigenic emulsion, it does not explain why relapses (clinical and structural) occur in adoptively-transferred murine models which involves a single intravenous injection of sensitized cells. Therefore, one must seek other explanations. One could be that soon after injection, antigen becomes deposited (or bound) peripherally within draining lymph nodes. Many years ago, one of us (CSR) recalls Dr Byron Waksman (as in reference 45) describing experiments where rabbits were sensitized in a single digit with CNS emulsion and then at various timepoints shortly thereafter the digit was amputated. He found that amputation of the digit before 12 hours after sensitization led to no development of acute EAE, but amputation between 12 and 24 hours (and later) did not prevent disease outcome and animals developed EAE 12–16 days later. These unpublished observations would tend to support the concept of early and persistent antigen deposition in the draining lymphatics.

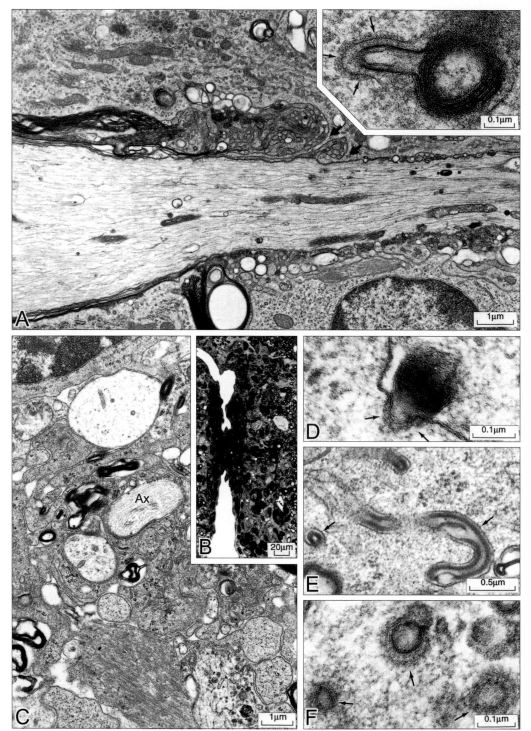

FIG. 16.6 A. Acute EAE; rabbit; 14 days p.i. whole WM in CFA; In this electron micrograph taken from tissue sampled on the day of onset of EAE, an image typical of immune-mediated myelin damage is shown. A longitudinally sectioned large-diameter myelinated nerve fiber in the lumbar spinal cord is undergoing demyelination. Processes from an investing macrophage (arrows) undermine layers of myelin, reducing them to vesicular droplets that are then internalized by the invading cell. Note the abrupt decrease in axonal diameter from the point at which myelin is lost from the fiber. ×11000. **Inset**. Detail from **A** showing an extracellular droplet of myelin being internalized by a macrophage following its attachment to a clathrin-coated pit (arrows) on the surface of the cell. ×100000. **B**. Mouse chronic relapsing EAE; actively induced; sampled during a relapse. A perivascular infiltrate of hematogenous cells, vessel lumen at (V), is superimposed upon chronic demyelination. **C**. Same lesion by electron microscopy. An axon (Ax) lies among a collection of mononuclear cell processes between which myelin droplets at different stages of internalization are located. Appearances such as these are supportive of recent demyelinative activity, occurring here 30 days p.i. **D**. PL/J mouse EAE; adoptive transfer; 9 months post-transfer; L7 spinal cord. Stages of receptor-mediated phagocytosis of myelin are shown in (**D–F**). In **D** an extracellular droplet of myelin has become associated with a clathrin-coated pit (arrows) on the surface of a macrophage. ×120000 **E**. PL/J mouse, chronic relapsing EAE; adoptive transfer, 9 days post-transfer. Vermiform droplets of myelin lie within channels in a macrophage that is engaged in myelin phagocytosis. The channels and adjacent rounded profiles are surrounded by clathrin-coated pit material (arrows). ×30000. **F**. PL/J mouse, chronic relapsing EAE; adoptive transfer, 7 months post-transfer. A glancing section across a macrophage surface shows several ring-like droplets of myelin lying within chambers (arrows) surrounded by coated-pit material. Elsewhere, the tangentially-sectioned subplasmalemmal web of actin filaments can be seen. ×110000.

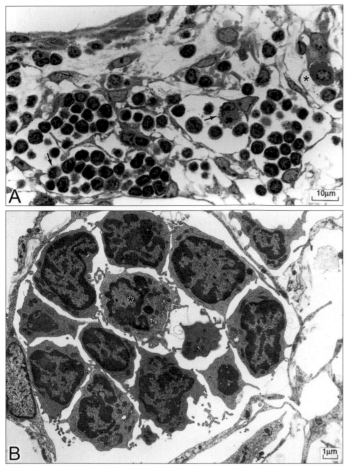

FIG. 16.7 A. SJL/J mouse; chronic relapsing EAE; adoptive transfer; 3 months post-transfer. Within the subependymal CNS parenchyma beneath the lateral ventricle of the cerebrum, infiltrates of lymphocytes are seen organized within sinusoids. Cells resembling dendritic cells (arrows) occur among the lymphocytes and, between the sinusoids, macrophages and a plasma cell (*) are found. This type of lymphoid organization within the CNS is reminiscent of lymph node medulla. 1 μm epoxy section; toluidine blue. **B**. Ultrastructurally, the same lymphoid deposits present as collections of small lymphocytes around cells with features of dendritic cells (*) within sinusoids. ×750 and ×3500.

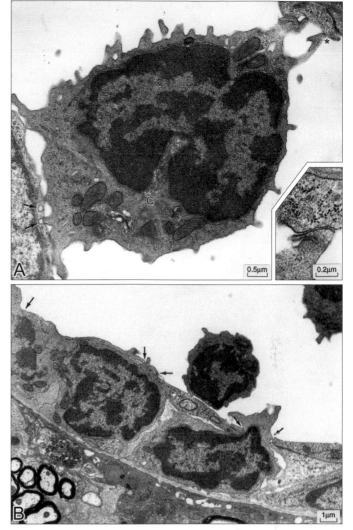

FIG. 16.8 A. SJL/J mouse; adoptive transfer of MBP[1] T cell line; onset of disease; 7 days post-transfer. A small lymphocyte spans a venule with pseudopodia contacting the endothelium on the left at coated pits (arrows), and on the right via a gap-junction-like contact. The cell contains centrioles (C), suggestive of recent or imminent mitosis. **Inset**: detail of the junction at the asterisk in **A**. The section has been tilted through 40° with a goniometer stage to resolve the membrane specialization. Note the extent of the membrane-membrane association between the lymphocyte (below) and the endothelial cell (above). ×10000 and ×25000. **B**. Same animal as **A**: lymphocytes are attached to and breach the wall of a venule, seen here at different stages of migration. Note how the cells have interrupted the endothelial lining (arrows) and pass directly through the vessel wall and, in the case of the migrating lymphocyte on the right, not along the endothelial cell tight junction. ×4000.

A second interesting line of evidence related to persistence of disease emerged from murine models in which collections of lymphoid elements were often encountered within the CNS of relapsing animals.[41,44] These consisted of collections of subependymal sinusoids containing small lymphocytes centered on cells with the appearance of dendritic cells, with plasma cells and macrophages between the sinusoids (Fig. 16.7A,B), – an appearance reminiscent of lymph node medulla, here occurring within the CNS. In some cases, the lymphoid collections comprised aggregates of macrophages containing myelin debris abutting small lymphocytes,[44] interactions suggestive of intercellular communication. These appearances support the concept[41] that extralymphoid system elements within the target organ, sensitized to CNS antigen, might play a role in the perpetuation of the autoimmune disease process, a concept of a later study which functionally associated the phenomenon with lymphotoxin β.[90] Such was perhaps also the implication of an earlier study on MS which described lymphoid elements in the CNS.[91]

The notion that lymphocytic deposits might become organized within a target organ is not a novel observation and is a feature of many chronic inflammatory conditions.[92] Interpreted in the context of lymphocyte homing, lymphocytic trafficking and adhesion molecule expression, the presence of collections of lymphoid elements in the CNS might denote a role for lymphocyte–endothelial cell interactions whereby high endothelial venules (HEVs) or other vascular molecules normally present only in lymphoid tissue become expressed in a nonlymphoid target organ, the CNS. The homing of lymphocytes (both CNS antigen-specific and non-CNS antigen-specific) to the CNS and their unusual affinity to associate with the endothelium of selected vessels in the white matter sometimes with the features of HEVs[93] via unique membrane associations (Fig. 16.8A), occurring concomitantly with the aberrant expression of lymph node markers and prior to the invasion of the CNS by lymphocytes (Fig. 16.8B), have been extensively studied.[94–97] Interestingly, this work showed that different populations of lymphocytes traversed the endothelium at different regions of the cell, with lymphocytes crossing in parajunctional areas, monocytes directly through the cell body and PMNs through tight junctions.[93,98] The unravelling of molecular interactions at the CNS endothelial interphase not only remains topical, recently revisited,[99] and of fundamental importance to CNS inflammation, but may also have important therapeutic ramifications for MS.[100,101]

MARMOSET MODEL OF EXPERIMENTAL AUTOIMMUNE ENCEPHALOMYELITIS

Common marmosets (*Callithrix jacchus*) are small New World monkeys (about the size of a guinea pig) that have been extensively used in research and are known to develop spontaneous autoimmunity (colitis, thyroiditis and wasting syndrome). A new model of relapsing–remitting MS has been successfully developed in these outbred primates over the last decade that has shed some light on mechanisms of demyelination and tissue destruction. The marmoset lesion comprises moderate inflammation but extensive concentric demyelination at an acute stage, a feature generally lacking from rodent models.

Whole white matter (WM)- and MOG-induced *C. jacchus* EAE are chronic, relapsing–remitting disorders with variable clinical severity, reminiscent of typical forms of human MS. Sensitive neurological examinations are possible for accurate clinical assessment of disease. The neuropathology of acute *C. jacchus* EAE reproduces MS pathology in many regards and partial remyelination and shadow plaques are observed in chronic cases. Serial paraclinical and laboratory studies, such as peripheral blood reactivity to myelin antigens, CSF sampling and in vivo magnetic resonance imaging (MRI) can be obtained during the course of the disease. Because they are outbred, marmosets exhibit a very broad immunological repertoire against myelin antigens, similar to humans. Diverse epitope recognition and T-cell receptor-α chain utilization are seen in the encephalitogenic repertoires against myelin proteins. The pathophysiology of MS-like lesions in *C. jacchus* marmosets involves both T-cell and antibody responses against diverse myelin antigens, a concept that is most probably applicable to MS. Finally, these monkeys show a very high degree of homology with humans for myelin and immune system genes, and thus are an attractive model for preclinical studies.

PRIMARY DEMYELINATING FORMS OF EXPERIMENTAL AUTOIMMUNE ENCEPHALOMYELITIS IN *CALLITHRIX JACCHUS*

Experimental autoimmune encephalomyelitis was first induced in *C. jacchus* by Massacesi et al[19] using active immunization with whole human WM homogenized in complete Freund's adjuvant (CFA) supplemented with 3 mg/ml killed *Mycobacterium tuberculosis* H37Ra and followed by intravenous injections of 1×10^{10} killed *Bordetella pertussis* organisms on the day of immunization and 48 h later (this adjuvant regimen is subsequently designated CFA/H37Ra/*B. pertussis*). This procedure reproducibly induced clinical signs of EAE. Although initial experiments employed 200 mg of WM, identical results could be obtained with 100 mg.[102,103] In over 100 animals immunized in this manner, EAE developed within 96 days of immunization

and, remarkable for an outbred species, 100% of immunized animals developed disease; in 70% of cases, onset was between days 14 and 28 after immunization. Typically, acute illness was characterized by mild or moderate neurological signs and a maximal clinical deficit that developed within 48 h of the clinical onset. In animals followed to assess the chronic course of disease, the first attack was noted to remit between 14 and 110 days after immunization and, in all, spontaneous relapses occurred within 3 weeks to 11 months of the initial attack.

Neuropathologically, the typical acute EAE lesion in *C. jacchus* is characterized by large foci of primary demyelination surrounding perivascular infiltrates comprising of mononuclear cells. Extensive demyelination is seen in association with dense collections of macrophages and the early development of astrocytic proliferation and gliosis. Animals studied to date rarely displayed the hemorrhagic–necrotic lesions or infiltration with PMNs, characteristics of other acute forms of primate or rodent EAE.[8,104–108] In animals examined during the chronic, relapsing–remitting phase of EAE, pathological findings reveal large, sharply defined areas of demyelination, minimal mononuclear cell infiltration and extensive astrogliosis reminiscent of MS plaques. Inflammatory demyelinating lesions are disseminated throughout the CNS white matter with great individual variations with respect to size and number. Plaques are frequently located in deep periventricular white matter of the frontal and the occipital lobes, optic tracts, chiasm and nerves, brainstem and posterior and lateral funiculi of the spinal cord (Fig. 16.9). Not infrequently, cerebellar white matter, cerebellar peduncles and corpus callosum are also involved. Despite the diversity in size, number and location of the lesions, in our experience there is always excellent correlation between clinical and pathological findings, in particular between paralysis and spinal cord involvement. Other characteristics of acute, whole-WM-induced EAE include mild infiltration of the subpial space by mononuclear cells with moderate underlying demyelination, and infiltration and demyelination in the proximal segments of spinal nerve roots. Involvement of cortical gray matter (which also contains myelin) is also a common finding.[109]

C. jacchus marmosets are equally susceptible to immunization with MOG. In studies of MOG-induced EAE, the protein employed for immunization was a recombinant protein containing the extracellular, Ig-like domain of rat MOG (residues 1–125, termed rMOG). MS-like features of the disease observed following immunization with whole WM were faithfully reproduced by a single immunization with 50–100 µg rMOG in CFA/H37Ra/*B. pertussis*. In some animals observed for extended periods (42–93 days), relapses were observed. However, cases that relentlessly progress towards severe clinical signs and extensive neuropathological involvement without remission are also observed. This form of EAE is reminiscent of primary progressive, severe or hyperacute forms of human MS. Several independent investigations have confirmed the widespread susceptibility of marmosets to myelin antigens,[108–112] including the recombinant Ig-like domain of human MOG.[113]

The ultrastructural features of the primary demyelinating lesions in *C. jacchus* EAE were analyzed and compared to lesions of human MS.[114] Lesions of acute EAE appear centered on blood vessels, with inflammatory changes involving small lymphocytes, monocytes and plasma cells (Fig. 16.10A,B). Within the surrounding parenchyma, a broad zone of demyelination with preserved denuded axons and macrophages containing myelin debris was present, as well as areas of ongoing demyelination characterized by the transformation of compact lamellar myelin sheaths into disorganized, vesiculated membranous networks (see Fig. 16.11F). At the periphery of lesions were broad zones where compact myelin appeared vacuolated

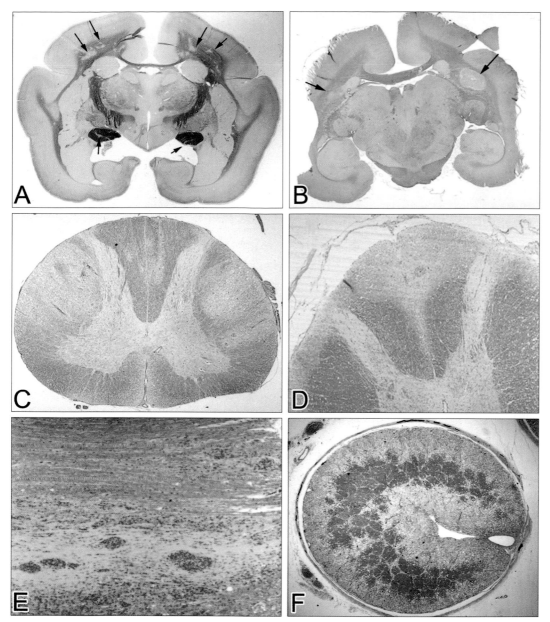

FIG. 16.9 Marmoset EAE. Neuropathology of acute and chronic *C. jacchus* EAE. **A**. Coronal brain section showing the presence of large and sharply demarcated plaques of demyelination subcortical, periventricular white matter and the optic tracts (arrows). Whole WM-induced EAE, day 28 p.i. **B**. Chronic EAE. Coronal brain section showing large and sharply demarcated plaques of demyelination and gliosis (arrows). RMOG-induced EAE, day 93 p.i.; three relapses. **C**. Transverse section of thoracic spinal cord, showing large inflammatory infiltrates accompanied by prominent demyelination in posterior and lateral funiculi. WM-induced EAE, 48 h after onset of clinical signs. **D**. Chronic WM-induced EAE, day 105 p.i. Transverse section of the spinal cord illustrating a large demyelinated plaque in the posterior funiculi. **E**. Chronic WM-induced EAE, day 105 p.i. spinal cord. A demyelinated lesion centered on a blood vessel is heavily infiltrated and extends longitudinally in an anterior column. **A–E** stained with Luxol fast blue/periodic acid Schiff (LFB/PAS). **F** 1 μm epoxy section, toluidine blue stain, of an optic nerve in cross section from a marmoset at 3 months p.i. showing extensive demyelination and gliosis around an area of preserved myelin (dense blue). ×30.

by intralamellar edema, with axons displaced laterally (Fig. 16.10C,D). The pattern of vacuolated myelin at the lesion edge was reminiscent of changes produced by proinflammatory cytokines,[115] was not associated with cell infiltration and may represent the initial stage of myelin injury mediated by soluble factors. These characteristic features were present throughout the entire CNS in marmoset EAE and appeared indistinguishable from acute, actively demyelinating lesions observed in acute MS.[114,116] Analysis of lesions from animals with chronic disease revealed extensive gliotic changes with significant loss of oligodendrocytes and axons, in addition to remyelination.[114]

THE DIFFERENT EXPERIMENTAL AUTOIMMUNE ENCEPHALOMYELITIS PHENOTYPES IN *CALLITHRIX JACCHUS*

Interesting features of the marmoset model became apparent as protocols to study immune responses were developed and implemented during the last decade. The ability to clone T cells (as in humans) with limited amounts of blood from repeated phlebotomy[102,117] and to dissect autoantibody responses[118,119] afforded quantum leap contributions to understanding the pathogenesis of the fully demyelinated lesion in acute and chronic MS using a single animal model where serial clinical

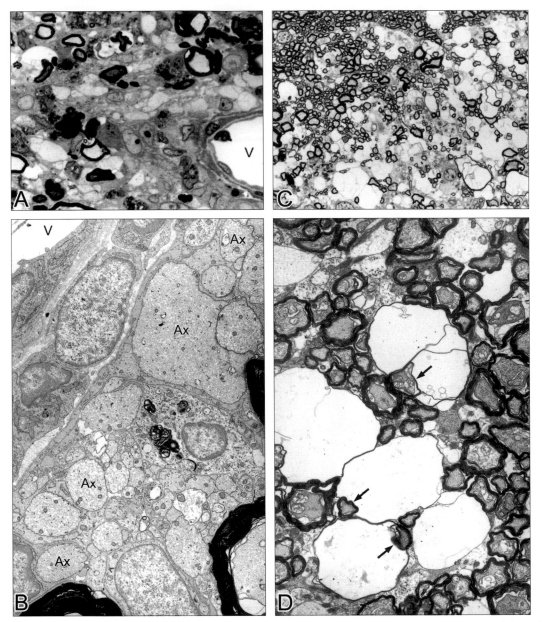

FIG. 16.10 Ultrastructural features of *C. jacchus* EAE. **A**. Acute *C. jacchus* EAE. 1 μm epoxy section of the spinal cord illustrating the center of a lesion with an inflammatory infiltrate with a broad zone of demyelination filled with naked axons, macrophages and myelin debris centered around a blood vessel (V). Toluidine blue. ×800. **B**. By EM, demyelinated axons (Ax) lie in a gliotic parenchyma. Vessel at (V) above. ×6000. **C**. At the leading edge of the marmoset lesion is a broad zone of nerve fibers showing intralamellar splitting of the compact myelin which form large edematous vacuoles pushing the axon to one side. Normal white matter, upper left. 1 μm epoxy section. ×750. **D**. By electron microscopy, the vacuolation of the myelin sheaths is shown to be due to intralamellar splitting, with the axon still surrounded by myelin displaced to one side (arrows). Note that this myelin vacuolation occurs in the absence of a cellular infiltrate ×5300.

and paraclinical observations could be made in the same animals. Adoptive T cell and passive antibody transfers, combined with the use of different myelin antigens, uncovered a major role for antibodies (against MOG) in producing CNS tissue damage. Later, it was the fractionation of antibodies against MOG, absorption studies and the use of short peptides versus folded MOG polypeptide as immunogens that demonstrated heterogeneity of antibodies against this sole and relatively small-size antigen and the link between epitope recognition and pathogenicity.[118,119] This conceptual framework will have extremely important implications for translation to human MS: current antibodies assays, and especially those involving poorly water-soluble antigens such as MOG, are unable to discriminate between the pathogenic and nonpathogenic antibodies in humans and a major effort is being committed to develop better

techniques that will achieve this differentiation in human anti-myelin antibody assays. Finally, molecular cloning that was first required to decipher the germline marmoset sequences,[120,121] allowed us to uncover the broad heterogeneity of TCR and B-cell receptor usage and repertoires with a high degree of homology and similarity with humans, both at the nucleic acid and protein/epitope conformation levels. It will become clear from the following sections that in many instances the information gleaned could not have been obtained from any of the rodent models available, unless one could find a way to combine them and reconstitute an 'artificial' outbred model. Finally, one key component that gives *C. jacchus* marmoset EAE a unique niche as a transitional tool between human MS and laboratory models is the availability of quality autopsy materials for studies that can be conducted by specialized neuropathologists.

ADOPTIVE T-CELL TRANSFER EXPERIMENTAL AUTOIMMUNE ENCEPHALOMYELITIS AND ROLE OF MYELIN-SPECIFIC T CELLS

Common marmosets are unique primates for the study of T-cell-mediated diseases because these monkeys are born as naturally-occurring bone marrow chimeras. While individual animals arise from separate ova that are fertilized independently, the placentae of the developing animals fuse, resulting in a cross-circulation of bone-marrow-derived elements between the fetuses. Thus, while animals are genetically distinct, they share, and are tolerant to, each other's bone-marrow-derived cell populations.[122] It is thus possible to perform adoptive T-cell transfer without risking allorejection. Several adoptive transfer experiments were performed using T-cell clones specific for MBP- and MOG-derived peptides, with the intention of elucidating the restriction of pathogenic of T cell repertoires claimed from rodent studies. Adoptive transfer EAE resulted in the appearance of clinical EAE, CSF pleocytosis (inflammation) and development of MRI abnormalities. Interestingly, T-cell clones derived from healthy, unimmunized animals were as efficient in transferring disease as were clones derived from animals with acute EAE.[117] Similar observations were reported in rodents,[123] and Rhesus macaques[124] receiving MBP-reactive T-cell clones from healthy donors. Clones reactive to different regions of MBP could efficiently mediate adoptive transfer of inflammatory EAE, indicating that, in *C. jacchus*, the encephalitogenic T-cell repertoire against MBP is diverse.

The pathology of adoptive transfer EAE in *C. jacchus* significantly differs from that in animals actively immunized with WM or rMOG, in that limited macrophage infiltration and demyelination are present. The disease transferred by MBP-reactive T-cell clones was characterized by meningeal and subpial inflammation, occasional areas of parenchymal inflammation, mononuclear cells (T cells) and areas of necrosis alone. Adoptive transfer of T-cell clones reactive to the immunodominant epitope of MOG_{21-40} resulted clinically in a monophasic and transient illness with mild CSF pleocytosis. Pathology obtained at the acute phase of disease was remarkable by rare perivascular infiltrates in the cervical spinal cord, with limited demyelination unless the animals developed antibodies against MOG (see below).[125]

EXPERIMENTAL AUTOIMMUNE ENCEPHALOMYELITIS INDUCED WITH OTHER MYELIN AUTOANTIGENS

In addition to adoptive T-cell transfer, models of nondemyelinating, inflammatory EAE can be produced in *C. jacchus* by active immunization against human MBP, MBP-derived peptides, PLP[102] or MOG-derived peptides. Immunization against MBP, PLP or MBP-derived peptides failed to reproduce the demyelinating disease to the extent of that following immunization with WM or rMOG. A separate investigation using a chimeric molecule comprising the entire sequence of MBP and the extramembranous domains of PLP (termed MP4) reported induction of mild to moderate EAE[126] with limited demyelination, unless antibody to MOG was introduced, a characteristic example of intermolecular humoral response spreading in EAE that may be highly relevant to MS.

We have studied the clinical and pathologic phenotypes of EAE induced in *C. jacchus* with linear peptides of human MOG encompassing the most frequently recognized epitopes. Active immunization with $100\,\mu g$ of MOG_{21-40}, combinations of equal amounts of peptides spanning residues aa_{51-90} and aa_{81-120}, or

combination of each of 11 overlapping peptides corresponding to the entire sequence of human rMOG, reproducibly induced mild, chronic EAE. Neuropathologically, rare inflammatory infiltrates were observed, accompanied by moderate, albeit significant demyelination. Reminiscent of adoptive transfer EAE, pathology remained scarce and mostly confined to the cervical spinal cord. No combination of peptides was capable of reproducing the protracted, multifocal disease associated with prominent demyelination that resulted from immunization with whole rMOG in this species.[118] Separate studies in C57/BL6 mice indicate that the phenotype of EAE induced with the immunodominant peptide of this protein (MOG_{35-55}) is not different in wild-type and B-cell-deficient mice, whereas the phenotype of whole MOG-induced EAE in the species is attenuated in the B-cell-deficient animals.[127,128] Although no detailed neuropathological studies were carried out, these observations suggest that B-cells and perhaps antibodies against the extended (and properly folded) polypeptide of MOG may be of importance in rodent EAE.

AUTOANTIBODIES DETERMINE THE PHENOTYPES OF EXPERIMENTAL AUTOIMMUNE ENCEPHALOMYELITIS IN *CALLITHRIX JACCHUS*

A role for antibody in plaque formation in *C. jacchus* was demonstrated using passive transfer of purified IgG antibodies into MBP-immunized recipients.[102] As described above, immunization of *C. jacchus* with MBP resulted in clinically mild EAE, low levels of CSF inflammation and no demyelination. However, in a manner similar to experiments in rat EAE,[129] passive transfer of purified IgG preparations from the plasma of animals with demyelinating forms of EAE (WM-induced) in MBP-immunized *C. jacchus* restored the demyelinating phenotype. Clinical deterioration and demyelination also followed the administration of IgG from rMOG-immunized animals or the murine MOG-specific monoclonal antibody 8–18-C5.

It is noteworthy that, in the study employing chimeric recombinant protein MP4 that does not contain any MOG sequence,[126] some animals developed an anti-MOG antibody response and clear demyelinating pathology. The methodology employed was ELISA, which detects some of the anti-MOG antibodies directed against conformational epitopes of the protein. Underscoring the importance of myelin autoantibodies in CNS demyelinating disease, this finding of intermolecular autoantibody spreading is widely known in diabetes and other disorders but has not been well investigated, if at all, in either EAE or MS because of the previously predominant belief from the lessons of rodent EAE that the human disorder is solely caused by cellular mechanisms and because of a related lack of adequate techniques to study the diversity of antibodies against soluble protein antigens in myelin, among other factors. In diabetes, however, the spreading of the antibody response has proved to be extremely useful as a paraclinical marker, both in terms of predicting onset and prognostic in already diagnosed patients. It is therefore possible to envision that, with time, such studies could be applied to human MS.

Using immunocytochemistry with gold-conjugated antigenic peptides of MOG, coupled with silver enhancement to detect antigen-specific autoantibodies in situ, we obtained direct evidence that MOG-specific antibodies were intimately associated with the networks of vesiculated myelin present in actively demyelinating lesions of *C. jacchus* EAE (Fig. 16.11A,B,F). Importantly, these MOG-specific antibodies were also identified in association with vesiculated myelin in actively demyelinating lesions of human MS[114,130] (Fig. 16.11C–E,G). These observations showed definitively that autoantibodies to MOG play a

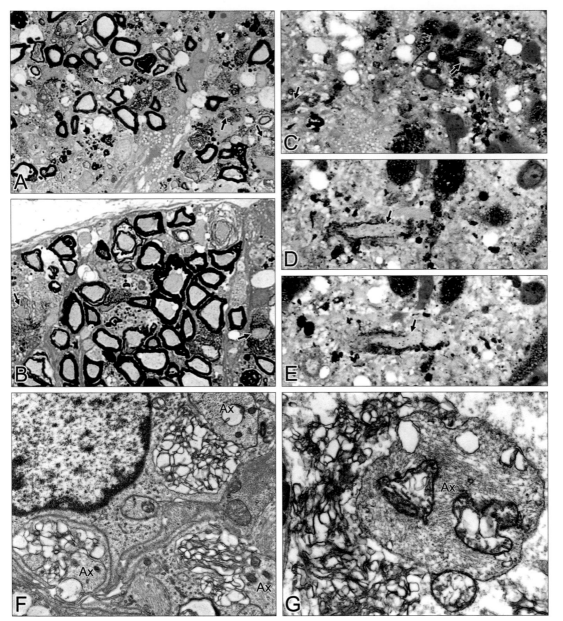

FIG. 16.11 Detection of MOG-specific autoantibodies in lesions of *C. jacchus* EAE and human MS. Immunostaining of epoxy-embedded thin sections of CNS tissue with gold-conjugated MOG$_{21-40}$ peptide to detect anti-MOG antibody in situ.[127] **A, B.** Acute marmoset EAE (spinal cord) showing the gold-conjugated peptide as a brown precipitate (silver enhancement) within networks of vesiculated myelin around axons (arrows). This immunoreactivity indicates the presence of specific MOG antibody on the disrupted myelin. Normally myelinated axons with thick myelin sheaths are also seen that do not stain brown. ×400 and ×800. **C.** Acute MS, biopsy. Staining for anti-MOG IgG is shown on vesiculated myelin around axons in cross section (arrows) and also in phagocytic cells (macrophages and microglia). ×800. **D.** In addition in MS, vesiculated myelin around an axon (in longitudinal section, arrow) stained positively for anti-MBP. ×800. **E.** Adjacent section to **D** immunoreacted with gold-conjugated anti-human IgG showing the same axon (arrow) and the localization of IgG on the degenerate myelin. ×800. See reference 114 for details. **F.** Electron micrograph from a marmoset 28 days to p.i. to show the ultrastructure of the vesiculated myelin sheaths. The myelin sheaths of three nerve fibers lie to one side of the axons (Ax) as membranous networks partially surrounded by the cytoplasm of a macrophage (upper left). ×16 000. **G.** Acute MS. An almost identical aggregate of vesiculated myelin to those shown in the marmoset in **F** lies to the left of a demyelinated axon (Ax). ×16 000.

causal role in the transformation of myelin into vesicular networks (Fig. 16.11F,G).

While they clearly demonstrated an important pathogenic role for myelin-reactive T-cells in *C. jacchus* EAE, these data also indicated that the multifocal, fully demyelinating CNS illness reminiscent of lesions of MS in WM- or rMOG-immunized marmosets was dependent on pathogenic autoantibody responses. The demyelinating properties of autoantibodies against MOG have also been demonstrated in rodent models of EAE (reviewed in reference 131). The magnitude of the MOG-specific autoantibody response directly influences the severity of clinical and pathological phenotypes in both rodents and primates.[126,129,130,132,133] The results also demonstrated a significant degree of heterogeneity in immune responses directed against MOG in outbred species. Finally, the development of severe demyelination appeared to require an antibody response that was induced by the whole rMOG polypeptide. Interestingly, the antibody response to myelin in situ in MS appeared to have a broader spectrum, in as much as antibody to peptides of both MOG and MBP could be localized (Fig. 16.11C–E), a feature perhaps of the longer duration or more extensive involvement of the human disease.[114]

IMMUNE REPERTOIRES AGAINST MYELIN PROTEINS IN *CALLITHRIX JACCHUS*

T-CELL REPERTOIRE

Myelin-reactive T cells can be cloned from blood, spleen and lymph nodes of marmosets, which permits studies of T-cell repertoire diversity against myelin antigens.[103,117] The repertoire of myelin-reactive T cells was elucidated for MBP and MOG by limiting dilution cloning in individual animals. The precursor frequency of circulating MBP-reactive clones, estimated at $0.3-1 \times 10^7$, was identical in *C. jacchus* and in humans.[117,134,135] Also similar to human MBP-reactive T cells, T-cell clones from *C. jacchus* were heterogeneous in their reactivity to different regions of MBP as defined by the use of synthetic peptides corresponding to overlapping amino acid sequences of the molecule. The T-cell immune response to MBP in *C. jacchus* was further characterized by study of the TCR repertoire of MBP-reactive T cells. Sequence analysis revealed the existence of two C genes with a high degree of homology to human counterparts (94.3% for C1 and 94.5% for C2), with each of the joining (J) chain elements described in humans. The variable (V) gene segment homologies to human counterparts ranged between 78–95% at the amino acid level and marmoset sequences corresponding to 18 human V families were identified. Analysis of TCRV usage by MBP-reactive T-cell clones revealed no preferential TCRVβ usage.[136]

The naive epitope repertoire of rMOG-reactive T-cells was similarly elucidated by limiting dilution cloning from peripheral blood mononuclear cells (PBMC) of healthy *C. jacchus* and mapping reactivity with overlapping synthetic peptides corresponding to the amino acid sequence of human rMOG. Compared to MBP, a surprisingly high frequency of rMOG-reactive precursor T cells (average 2.6 per 10^5 PBMC), was consistently observed in all animals studied. MOG-reactive T cells recognized diverse epitope sequences, with clustering around three main regions of the rMOG molecule, MOG_{1-40}, MOG_{51-70} and MOG_{81-110}.[125]

In animals actively immunized with rat rMOG, T-cell reactivity developed within 15 days and was found to be directed against peptides located between MOG_{21-40} in 100% of animals (fine mapping: MOG_{28-36}), MOG_{51-70} in 25% (MOG_{63-72}) and MOG_{81-110} in 35% (not refined, $n=17$). A similar analysis in marmosets immunized with human rMOG confirmed the existence of a major T-cell epitope within the MOG_{21-40} sequence.[113] This peptide appears to be presented to T cells in association with an MHC class II molecule with limited polymorphism that is unique to marmosets.[137] Thus, with the exception of MOG_{91-110}, encephalitogenic epitopes of MOG in marmosets are different from those reported in rodent species.[14,138–141]

ANTIBODY REPERTOIRE

Antibody responses against the immunizing antigen develop concomitantly to T-cell reactivity in *C. jacchus* and can be similarly mapped by ELISA using overlapping linear peptides. Because of the importance of the MOG antigen, we have studied the fine specificities of antibody responses to this protein. In contrast to T-cell reactivity, which can be detected in both naive and immunized monkeys, rMOG-specific antibodies are only detected in sera and cerebrospinal fluid of immunized animals. The polyclonal antibody response was primarily directed against MOG_{13-21} (100% of animals) and MOG_{63-75} (85%). Additional reactive peptides were identified at residues MOG_{28-35} and MOG_{40-4}.[5] It is not surprising that some of the B-cell epitopes

in marmosets match the location of T-cell epitopes, as has been shown for MOG in rodents,[138] and for an immunodominant epitope of MBP in humans.[142]

The diversity of the Ig repertoire in *C. jacchus* was analyzed by constructing an expression library of *C. jacchus* V_H genes using rapid amplification of 5′ cDNA ends (RACE) and degenerate primers constructed from the sequence of the human gene counterparts. Sequence analysis revealed a high homology to all seven human V_H subfamily genes (82–91% at the nucleotide level) with the exception of human V_H2, for which no counterpart was identified in *C. jacchus*. The sequences of individual *C. jacchus* V_H clones were compared to those of the most closely related human germline V_H segments.[120,121] At the protein expression level, and as discussed above, it has now become clear that the pathogenic anti-MOG antibodies are directed against the properly folded polypeptide.[118] This has important implications for studies of anti-MOG antibodies in human MS and more attention needs to be given to the technologies employed to detect those antibodies. It is critical to understand that, although anti-MOG antibodies against linear epitopes and those against conformational epitopes are functionally different, they may somewhat overlap and be simultaneously detected with existing methods. As said, major efforts are devoted to the refinement of such methods by several laboratories using cell-based assays[143] and other cutting-edge methods such as plasmon resonance spectroscopy. In addition, it is now demonstrated that liquid phase systems, unlike those using other antigens that are soluble, fail to display any of the relevant epitope of MOG and are inadequate for anti-MOG antibody detection in humans.[144]

Although we have not examined additional myelin proteins, these studies indicate that broad diversity is present in the T-cell and antibody repertoires against CNS autoantigens in *C. jacchus*. Therefore, this experimental system is likely to approximate the complexity of the same immune responses in humans.

REMYELINATION IN CHRONIC EXPERIMENTAL AUTOIMMUNE ENCEPHALOMYELITIS

What makes it a highly relevant model for therapeutic trials of relevance to MS is the fact that CNS remyelination to some degree always occurs in chronic EAE and that a number of experimental interventions are known to enhance the phenomenon.[83] A feature probably reflecting the smaller dimensions of lesions in chronic relapsing EAE (in comparison to MS), was the observation that, in the majority of established lesions in the guinea pig, remyelination was common, sometimes to the extent that the entire lesion was involved (Fig. 16.12). Remyelination was readily apparent structurally when one compared the large axonal diameter and the investing thin myelin sheaths of affected fibers with those of adjacent unaffected fibers. Blood vessels in these lesions retained evidence of chronic inflammatory activity, were hyalinized and usually increased in number (? neovascularization). Ultrastructurally, the morphological criteria of remyelination were readily satisfied (Fig. 16.13A). The myelin sheaths of large-diameter axons were disproportionately thin, contained varied amounts of oligodendroglial cytoplasm and were sometimes noncompacted. The areas were sometimes associated with increased numbers of oligodendroglial cells and remyelinated areas possessed a fibrous astrogliotic background, as is also the case in MS.[5] Such regions of CNS remyelination in EAE animals probably correspond to the shadow plaques of MS (Ch. 11). Remyelination was also a constant feature of the chronic murine models (Fig. 16.4B), although it was usually less

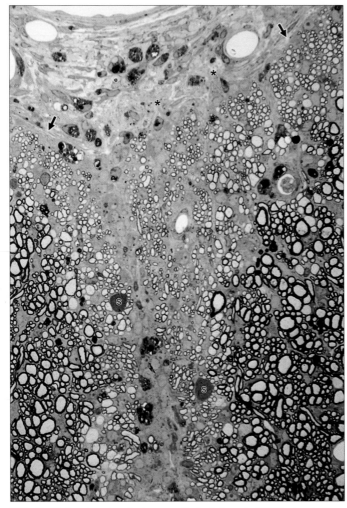

FIG. 16.12 An almost entirely remyelinated chronic EAE lesion in the anterior columns of the lumbar spinal cord (pial surface above, arrows) of a strain 13 guinea pig. The many large-diameter axons with disproportionately thin myelin sheaths are typical of remyelination. Note the normal thickness of myelin in the less-affected white matter (left and below), the chronic, scarring changes around blood vessels and the fibrous and collagen deposition in the meninges, above, as well as some adventitial gliosis where astrocytes extend bridges into the meningeal space.[68] Two axonal spheroids (S) are also visible ×500.

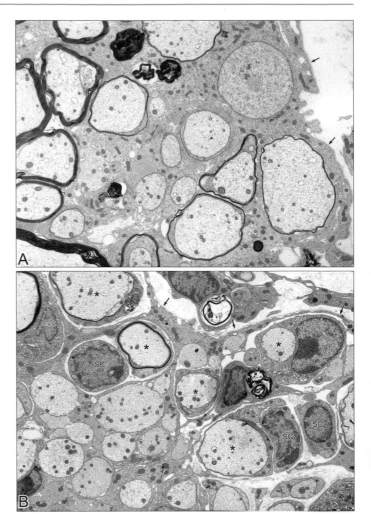

FIG. 16.13 A. By electron microscopy, CNS remyelination is typified by thin, sometimes uncompacted myelin sheaths around large axons, seen here in a lesion from the spinal cord of a guinea pig with chronic relapsing EAE for 5 months. Demyelinated axons are also present. Note the intense fibrous astrogliosis in the background tissue, a few myelin sheaths of normal thickness (left), the fibrous astroglial cell body (upper right), and the pial margin and glia limitans of the spinal cord (arrows, right). ×3500. **B**. The margin of this chronically demyelinated spinal cord lesion from a guinea pig with chronic relapsing EAE demonstrates Schwann cell invasion of the CNS and PNS myelination of demyelinated CNS axons, a phenomenon described in chronic EAE[76] and MS.[143] Note axons (*) undergoing early myelination by Schwann cells. Several uncommitted Schwann cells (SC) are also present. Note presence of basal lamina around each Schwann cell. Chronically demyelinated CNS axons are seen below and the basal lamina covering the pial surface of the spinal cord (glia limitans) lies above (arrows). ×4500.

extensive than in guinea pigs, probably because of smaller lesion diameter and greater axonal attrition.

Another phenomenon common to both chronic EAE and MS lesions was Schwann cell invasion (schwannosis) and PNS myelination of CNS axons.[76] Analysis of most established chronic EAE lesions within the spinal cord invariably revealed zones of PNS myelination, most noticeable towards subpial margins of the spinal cord, involving Schwann cell invasion and PNS myelination, sometimes accompanying or preceding CNS remyelination and intermixed with naked CNS axons embedded in a gliotic background (Fig. 16.13B). Many free (noncommitted) Schwann cells resided in these areas and one can only speculate that these cells might eventually have sought out and associated with naked segments of CNS axons. The route of entry of these PNS elements has been followed morphologically and attributed to an invasive process from root entry zones and the Virchow–Robin space of penetrating vessels.[145] As has been the experience in MS,[146] it appeared that PNS myelination of demyelinated CNS fibers in chronic EAE[76] did not correlate with functional improvement.

THERAPEUTIC APPLICATIONS OF THE MODELS TO MULTIPLE SCLEROSIS

The field of MS has profited enormously from the availability of chronic demyelinating models in a number of inbred animal species in which the disease process has a latent period and a protracted, chronic or relapsing course,[29,147] albeit not without limitations.[3,148] With an increasing interest in the administration to MS patients of a vast battery of compounds to thwart the aberrant immune response within the CNS (Chs 21 and 23), the above models might provide preclinical adjuncts for clinical trials in humans. With guinea pig EAE, a disease induced by injections of whole spinal cord in CFA, MBP was shown to be 100% efficacious and suppressed the clinical expression of both acute and chronic EAE when administered in IFA prior to onset of signs.[34] This procedure did not prevent initial lesion formation but, when examined later, CNS lesions displayed extensive remyelination. Thus it appeared that suppression with MBP prevented lesion progression and fostered remyelination. Later studies demonstrated that guinea pigs in which chronic relapsing disease was treated with MBP (i.e. MBP given after the establishment of relapsing disease) showed only transient improvement and disease activity eventually returned.[29] On the other hand, guinea pigs treated with a combination of MBP and GalC in IFA displayed long-lasting clinical stabilization and/or improvement that correlated histologically with oligodendroglial cell proliferation, widespread CNS remyelination and the downregulation of inflammation in the CNS (Fig. 16.14). The rationale for this MBP/GalC therapy was believed to be mechanistically related to the activation of the T-cell arm of the immune response to MBP and a B-cell response to GalC. It was suggested that the remyelination was effected both by local proliferating oligodendroglial cells and precursor cells which became differentiated during remyelination. A similar protocol described had beneficial effects in a murine viral-induced demyelinative disease caused by Theiler's murine encephalomyelitis virus (TMEV)[149] and an extension of this work[150] showed that IgG from animals sensitized with whole myelin had a remyelinating effect upon TMEV-induced lesions, particularly in chronic models. The latter phenomenon has since been extended to samples of normal human IgM of unknown specificity and to humanized monoclonal antibodies to the human IgM, but the mechanism remains to be elucidated.[151] Interestingly, and somewhat related to the guinea pig treatment experiments, in work on acute EAE in the rat induced adoptively, injection of antiserum to MOG intrathecally enhanced demyelination in an otherwise poorly demyelinating model.[129]

An excellent survey of many of the immunomodulatory-based therapeutic trials in EAE, their outcome and status as MS therapies has recently been presented.[148] Of potential relevance was the reported manipulation of acute EAE in the rat using, in a therapeutic mode, peptides homologous to TCR sequences derived from encephalitogenic T cells,[152,153] also under test in humans.[154] Anti-T-cell and anti-Ia (MHC II) monoclonal antibody therapy of chronic EAE in mice has also demonstrated clinical improvement.[155–157] In none of the latter TCR or monoclonal antibody approaches has material been analyzed neuropathologically, leaving the findings interesting at the clinical level only. Antibodies to proinflammatory cytokines in prevention and treatment of murine EAE have been tested, since cytokines play a major role in the regulation of most immune system molecules and two studies reported successful blocking of murine EAE with antibodies to the Th1-type proinflammatory cytokines TNFα and LT.[158,159] Inhibitors of TNFα also abrogated disease development.[160–162] Modulation of regulatory Th2-type cytokine levels has also been shown to have a beneficial outcome on EAE; this involved transforming growth factor β,[163] IL-10[164] and IL-4.[165] Therapeutic attempts to manipulate EAE with antibodies to adhesion molecules have yielded mixed results. An antibody to the α4β1 integrin (VLA-4) blocked murine EAE effectively,[100] while studies on antibodies to ICAM-1 and LFA-1 displayed differing effects.[101,166–168] The recent emphasis on the role of antibodies and B cells as mechanisms of CNS damage in EAE models, both rodent and primates, has opened a door for the use of new therapeutic avenues for human MS and similar disorders that have been traditionally considered to be T-cell-mediated. For example, B-cell depletion achieved with anti-CD20 has now been tried in the prototypical antibody-mediated MS variant neuromyelitis optica.[169] Preliminary results with ongoing and completed trials in relapsing-remitting MS, albeit involving relatively small numbers of

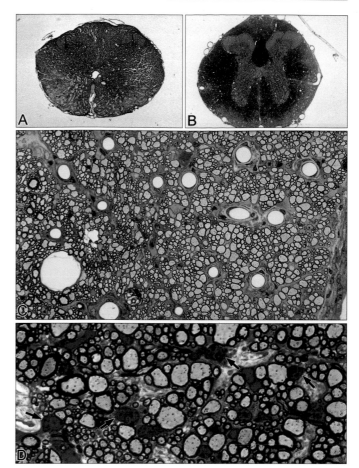

FIG. 16.14 Remyelination after treatment of chronic relapsing EAE has been shown after many different regimens, here after a combination of MBP/GalC in the guinea pig.[29] In this model, CNS inflammation and demyelination was reversed. **A.** LFB-stained paraffin section of upper lumbar cord showing diffuse staining for myelin over two lesions in the anterior columns, which are also heavily vascularized, perhaps as a result of angiogenesis. ×25. **B.** A 1 µm epoxy section of the same lumbar spinal cord shows a broad zone of myelin pallor (remyelination) around the entire margin of the cord. ×30. **C.** At higher magnification, the broad zone of CNS remyelination is seen in detail. This animal had chronic relapsing EAE for 5 months that was then treated for 1 month with injections of MBP/GalC/IFA. Note the remyelination of virtually every fiber in the lesioned areas, the lack of inflammatory activity and, for comparison, the greater thickness of the normal myelin sheaths to the left. There is also an increase in the number of blood vessels (angiogenesis?). The subpial surface of the spinal cord is to the right. ×400. **D.** This 1 µm section comes from the spinal cord of a guinea pig with chronic relapsing EAE for 24 months that was then treated for 1 month with MBP/GalC/IFA and sampled 2 months later (27 mo p.i.), after the animal had displayed clinical improvement. A lesion shows widespread CNS remyelination and proliferation of oligodendrocytes (arrows). Some unaffected fibers with myelin sheaths of normal thickness can also be seen. ×800.

subjects, show promising results for this type of approach. Finally, a recent investigation[170] showing an anti-inflammatory and protective effect of αB-crystalline (CRYAB) was conducted in CRYAB$^{-/-}$ mice with EAE. Apparently, since CRYAB is a primary target of the immunologic assault on the CNS during EAE, its deletion led to disease worsening and administration of recombinant CRYAB ameliorated the disease. It was suggested that since CRYAB is a potent negative regulator of the inflammatory pathway, it holds promise as a therapy in MS.

The ability to conduct preclinical trials in the marmoset outbred model with its good approximation of clinical, immunological and neuropathological features reminiscent of MS and similarity of genes with the human counterpart has made this model attractive for preclinical trials, especially with modern drugs (including large antibodies) that are identical to the actual clinical compounds and cannot be tested in rodents.

Rolipram is a well characterized selective inhibitor of type IV phosphodiesterases (PDE-IV) that suppresses release of TNF-α from macrophages and monocytes, two cell types that express primarily the type IV isoenzyme. Treatment with rolipram beginning 7 days after immunization with WM resulted in sustained protection from clinical EAE, marked reduction or disappearance in CSF and MRI indices of disease, and complete inhibition of demyelination on pathological examination. The high levels of TNF-α in brain tissue, characteristic of EAE in *C. jacchus*, were suppressed in protected animals. Although these data argue for a role of TNF-α in plaque formation in *C. jacchus*, other effects of rolipram may explain the observed efficacy.[162,171]

Interferon (IFN)β-1b, an approved therapy for MS, decreases attack rate and subclinical MRI activity in relapsing–remitting forms of the disease. Interestingly, in a limited pilot trial of marmoset EAE, we observed that IFNβ-1b administered prior to, or at onset of clinical signs aggravated the disease in approximately half the treated animals (Genain and Hauser, unpublished data). This complication has also been reported in Lewis rat EAE upon discontinuation of treatment with IFNβ[172] and is to be placed in perspective with the observation that initiation of treatment with IFNβ is often followed by an increase in the frequency of IFNγ-producing T- cells in the peripheral blood of patients with MS.[173] The mechanism(s) of action of interferons in MS is poorly understood and it is not entirely surprising that IFNβ therapy was found to worsen acute EAE in marmosets and rodents. Alternative explanations for the lack of benefit of IFNβ in marmosets are quality control in the preparations, dosing regimen and the rapid production of neutralizing antibodies in marmosets.

In rodents, administration of myelin antigens in nonimmunogenic form results in specific immunological tolerance and can prevent or reverse EAE. Several approaches were employed in order to induce immunological tolerance to MBP in *C. jacchus*. In the first, we used an attenuated strain of vaccinia virus genetically engineered to contain either the entire coding sequence for human MBP (vT15) or the equine herpes virus glycoprotein gH gene (vAbT249) under the control of the vaccinia virus 40K early/late promoter. Vaccination with vT15 was followed by transient expression of MBP reactivity by circulating mononuclear cells and markedly delayed onset of clinical EAE. Proliferative T-cell responses against MBP were present in PBMC of control animals but suppressed in protected animals.[174] Immunological tolerance was achieved in *C. jacchus* marmosets immunized with rMOG with intraperitoneal injections of soluble rMOG (300 μg) every 48 h from day 7 to day 18 after immunization.[132] T-cell reactivity against rMOG was suppressed and the onset of clinical disease significantly delayed. Surprisingly, however, following cessation of tolerization treatment the disease developed into a lethal and hyperacute form associated with restored proliferative T-cell responses against rMOG, immune deviation towards Th2-type cytokines and increased autoantibody production against rMOG. This complication was not observed in a separate study where animals were immunized and treated with a chimeric MBP/PLP protein.[175]

These experiments show that induction of immunological tolerance in outbred species may be more difficult than initially thought on the basis of experiments in rodent EAE. Furthermore, these strategies have the potential to exacerbate diseases where pathogenic antibodies play a role, via elaboration of factors that promote B-cell differentiation and antibody produc-

tion.[129] This unexpected complication had not been predicted from experiments in rodent EAE. Additional studies of tolerance induction are being conducted in *C. jacchus*, using MOG-derived peptides and intravenous and mucosal routes of administration. A more recent – and different – version of immunological tolerance using DNA vaccination containing MBP, PLP and other constructs has been proved effective in rodents[16,176] and is being pursued in human clinical trials.[177] However, the approach may not be immune from the type of complication observed using soluble MOG in marmosets.[178]

Costimulation is an essential mechanism for the differentiation of pathogenic Th1 cells, and blocking the CD40–CD40 ligand (CD40L) interaction inhibited the development of EAE in rodents.[179] A preliminary report indicated that marmosets sensitized with MOG and treated with chimeric antagonist anti-CD40 monoclonal antibody were protected from EAE.[113] A clinical trial based on this approach is currently planned for human MS. Finally, anti-IL12p40 antibody has proved to be effective in this model.[180]

Nerve growth factor (NGF) is a cytokine with pleiotropic effects on the immune system and a growth factor for neurons, oligodendrocytes and Schwann cells. To test its remyelinating properties in *C. jacchus* EAE, NGF was administered intracerebroventricularly to marmosets 7 days after immunization with rMOG. Interestingly, administration of NGF significantly attenuated clinical and histological signs of EAE. The mechanism for this unexpected anti-inflammatory property of NGF in EAE involved suppression of proinflammatory Th1-type cytokines (IFN-γ) in inflammatory infiltrates and tissue-specific stimulation of the suppressive Th2-type cytokine IL-10 by astrocytes.[181] In the mouse system, the glial growth factor GGF2 was found to significantly improve clinical outcome, lower relapse rate and induce remyelination in the presence of a shift towards a Th2-type phenotype.[182]

Despite the limitations on the use of nonhuman primates, marmoset EAE is perhaps the closest model of MS that we have with respect to its clinical and neuropathological features and it offers many advantages over other species. These animals are easy to maintain and breed in captivity, and EAE can be monitored noninvasively by MRI and immunological studies. The respective roles of cellular and humoral immunity against myelin antigens can be studied in *C. jacchus* using the T-cell adoptive transfer and antibody passive transfer systems. In addition, this experimental system can be manipulated to reliably produce inflammatory and/or demyelinating forms of EAE, which are analogous to the different phenotypes encountered in MS. Because of unique similarities to *C. jacchus* EAE, the MOG protein is now one of the top candidate antigens and most widely used for EAE studies in primates and rodents, a shift from the past focus on MBP and PLP. By analogy, MOG has been proposed to be a likely target for pathogenic autoantibodies in human CNS demyelinating disorders,[183] although more recent studies have failed to confirm this.[184] Marmosets are small animals, which reduces the amount needed of compounds that are only testable in nonhuman primates because of interspecies differences. Perhaps more relevant to therapeutic success, studies of marmoset EAE support the concept that MS probably represents a group of heterogeneous disorders with a common lesion but diverse etiologies and pathophysiologies.

CONCLUSIONS AND FUTURE PERSPECTIVES

What started out as an attempt to reproduce in animals, clinical and structural likenesses to ADEM, became the basis for most of today's research on MS and what we now recognize as molecular neuroimmunology, along with a veritable armamentarium of models of EAE. It has been our purview to compare objectively the various attributes and the CNS lesions associated with these forms of EAE and to relate them to events occurring in MS.

It will be clear from the images presented and their comparison with Chapter 11 that, regardless of our skills in the laboratory, a lesion identical in scale and texture to that of MS has not yet been realized. One reason for this lies in our inability to simulate in a laboratory setting the time-frame associated with the development of the chronic MS lesion (usually measured in decades) or the voracity of the acute MS lesion, sometimes occurring along with remyelination.[185,186] Furthermore, although yet to be confirmed, the possibility proposed by some workers[187] of the existence in MS of heterogeneous types of lesions may prove a significant hurdle for the experimentalist. However, the concept of different types of heterogeneous lesions has been challenged by studies claiming overlap between types,[188] and absence of heterogeneity and failure to confirm criteria for lesion segregation.[189] Nevertheless, faithful reproductions of selected facets of stages of the typical MS lesion can be reproduced with models, feats sufficient to convince us that the MS lesion has a significant immunogenic basis.

One myth commonly permeating the literature is that demyelinated axons are largely spared in MS and that forms of EAE with lesions displaying fiber depletion are not appropriate – a major criticism of early studies in guinea pigs.[74,75] Thus, criticism of mouse models on the grounds that they display unacceptable degrees of Wallerian degeneration was invalid in the context of the present updated image of the typical MS lesion.[2,38] In MS, widespread axonal sparing is typically not the case and most authors couch their evaluation of axonal involvement in the phrase 'relative sparing'. It is a fact of life that large numbers of axons are lost from the acute MS lesion and that the number remains depleted thereafter. It is also a fact of life that, despite the axonal loss and the intensity of the disease process, remyelination frequently prevails. The striving, therefore, of researchers to produce toxin-induced models of demyelination with total preservation of axons has probably been a goal with limited relevance to the human condition, in which significant axonal loss is typical. When the above observations are set alongside the fact that MS frequently remits clinically, it is clear that compensatory mechanisms must reside in the CNS that permit some functional recovery in the face of axonal loss. These are but a few of the many paradoxes that continue to render MS a fascinating challenge.

The often heated debates on the relative attributes and limitations of the various animal models of MS, particularly the many forms of EAE,[3,27,148,190] pale in comparison with the questions yet unanswered in MS. More important perhaps is the bounty of information emanating from the many seminal studies on immune-mediated demyelination showing the exquisite selectivity of the inflammatory or humoral response for the CNS in EAE. It is in this arena that much progress has been made in recent years, even though many of the molecules tested have had limited success in MS.[148] Furthermore, the immunological terrain in EAE is clearly more complex than we first imagined, with even the CD4/Th1 dependence being challenged by studies showing effector pathogenic roles for CD8+ T cells[191] and Th2-type cytokines.[192]

Overall, progress in the analysis of pathogenetic events underlying the establishment of the demyelinated lesion in MS has been slow and sporadic. Subsequent to the pens of Charcot (1868) and Dawson (1916) (see reference 5), relatively little new has been added to the pathological picture of MS despite the addition of vast tomes to the literature. Anecdotally, with regard to EAE, there has been a Darwin-like pattern in the evolution of thinking and that hypotheses on the mechanism of demyelination have tended to last about a decade before being recycled

in fresh clothing. Hence, ideas promulgated by pioneers like Rivers, Freund, Waksman, Kabat, Patterson, Levine and McFarlin, inter alia, continue to provide intellectual fodder. In recent years, the pre-eminent position of the neuropathologist in MS research has been usurped somewhat as more multidisciplinary approaches have evolved, and has been replaced by the molecular neurobiologist/immunologist.[193] EAE today straddles neurology, pathology, neuroscience, biochemistry, immunology, virology and molecular biology. In the light of the enormous degree of informational maturation that has developed amongst these disciplines, it is now possible to arrange in rank order significant features of the MS lesion that relate to its genesis.[2] Some of these are the subject of the preceding paragraphs, others are discussed in detail in Chapter 11.

Historically, difficulties in the analysis of clinical, structural and immunological events in MS with suitably preserved human tissue caused investigators to search for alternative systems. The novice entering the field today is faced with a healthy choice of models – immunological, virological and toxic, acute and chronic, and in vivo and in vitro. While the search for new systems has sometimes fuzzied our focus on the human condition, it has been gratifying to witness the emergence of valid therapies in MS emanating from pilot work on EAE – all, take note, based on immunological rationales! As an adjunct to studies on the pathogenesis of MS, this laboratory and others have developed over the past decades a number of models of chronic relapsing EAE, models that have proved to share features in common with MS. The expansion in the 1980s of our EAE expertise to the mouse (through collaborations with the late Dale McFarlin), a species for which there was a wealth of well defined markers, and in the 1990s to the marmoset, which shares many immunological markers with humans, propelled us forward after many years with guinea pigs and rabbits in which the immunological terrain was muddy and not well mapped. Chronic relapsing EAE has been shown to simulate MS in being age-, sex- and strain-dependent, often with a latent period prior to onset, a progressive, protracted and sometimes fatal course that displays relapses, and lesions that are disseminated, demyelinative, sometimes large and of different ages. Other parameters of relevance to MS include the requirement for most models of chronic relapsing EAE of a single sensitization only, neuropathological similarities, immunogenetic requirements for susceptibility, the observation of immunological changes in blood and CSF, and its potential as a therapeutic tool, particularly with our access today to technologies that have followed the sequencing of the human genome.

In a manner paralleling CNS lesion activity, circulating lymphocyte values fluctuate with clinical disease in both MS and EAE, as do most other immunological parameters, and in EAE the first cells to arrive in the CNS appear to be CNS antigen-specific.[94,194,195] Furthermore, lymphocyte trafficking molecules[196] interact in the CNS with adhesion molecules on endothelial cells[94–98] and expression of these molecules waxes and wanes as the disease evolves. It is also recognized that, at the blood–brain barrier, lymphocytes and endothelial cells 'are dynamic partners in multiple, complex interactions involving macromolecular and cellular constituents of blood as well as vessel wall components'.[197] Future progress in a number of known or suspected autoimmune conditions will come from understanding the functional status of this interphase as well as the inducibility of the CNS to serve as an adjunct to the immune system. Indeed this thinking was central to the development of the drug Tysabri for MS (see Ch. 21), based on an antibody against VLA-4, a lymphocyte receptor specific for CNS-antigen specific T-cells,[195] the blocking of which presumably prevents such cells from entering the CNS. This therapy stemmed directly from work on EAE.[100]

However, a word of caution is needed as we are reaching a stage of 'too well' understood immunology in models and still poorly understood mechanisms in human MS. The remarkably effective new therapies are extremely specific but also induce broad immune suppression, which unfortunately has led to lethal complications such as progressive multifocal leukoencephalopathy in the case of natalizumab.[193,194] On the bright side, this kind of rare, but unacceptable risk for a lifetime disease that is usually not lethal represents a tremendous opportunity for many (neuroscientists, immunologists, virologists to name a few) to learn more about etiopathogeny of MS and related white and gray matter, disease, opportunistic infections and how they may interact with the course of MS. Other laboratories are turning their attention towards the further characterization of cytokines, growth factors and developmental pathways and their effects upon cells (especially oligodendrocytes) of the nervous system.[200–202] In the context of EAE, animals possessing a deletion of one of these molecules, LINGO-1, a negative regulator of oligodendrocyte differentiation and myelination, displayed functional recovery, improved axonal integrity and remyelination after induction of EAE.[203] Families of adhesion molecules such as the integrins, immunoglobulins and selectins, plus a whole bevy yet to be identified (including their respective immune modulators) and stem cell transplantation in EAE[204–206] (not to mention associated upstream and downstream pathways), will provide additional major areas of activity in MS well into the 21st century.

Finally, we know that, in the case of the MS lesion, more often than not we are looking at the footprints of a disease process long since passed by. We also know that, by the application of appropriate immunological models, we may come to understand better the mechanisms responsible for these footprints. Perhaps an overuse of short experiments with acute EAE has led to an excessive level of confidence and has limited the successful translation of many new therapies that showed promising experimental preclinical data but failed in clinical trials. Experimentation with chronic relapsing EAE continues to target the development of protocols capable of arresting disease progression and fostering repair (remyelination) in MS, the central goal of many laboratories. With this in mind, and already with about a dozen treatments (drugs) out there specific for MS (versus none in 1992) and the knowledge that remyelination of a demyelinated lesion is feasible, the future is bright for the MS patient.

ACKNOWLEDGMENTS

Drs Robert D. Terry, William T. Norton, Celia F. Brosnan, John W. Prineas, G.R. Wayne Moore, Krzysztof Selmaj, Anne H. Cross, Barbara Cannella, Kakuri Omari, Michael K. Racke, Stephen L. Hauser and Henry F. McFarland had substantial input into the work described. The late Drs Dale E. McFarlin, Sanford H. Stone and Murray B. Bornstein played significant roles in the development and analyses of the EAE models. To all of these colleagues, to CSR's faithful, long-established technical team of Everett Swanson, Howard Finch and Miriam Pakingan, to Patricia Cobban-Bond who painstakingly assembled this chapter, and to others too numerous to name, the authors extend their sincere thanks.

Supported in part by NIH grants NS 08952, NS 11920 and NS 07098 (CSR); NS 46678 and AIAI 43073 (CPG); by grants RG 1001-K-11 (CSR), RG 3370-A-3, 3438-A-7 and JF 2087-A-2 (CPG) from the National Multiple Sclerosis Society; the Wollowick Family Foundation (CSR); the Cure MS Now Fund (CPG); and the Lunardi Fdn. (CPG).

REFERENCES

1. Raine CS. Experimental allergic encephalomyelitis and experimental allergic neuritis. In: Vinken PJ, Bruyn GW, Klawans HL, eds. Handbook of clinical neurology, vol 47. Amsterdam: North-Holland; 1985: 429–466.

2. Frohman EM, Racke MK, Raine CS. Multiple sclerosis: the plaque and its pathogenesis. N Engl J Med 2006; 54: 942–955.

3. Gold R, Linington C, Lassmann H. Understanding pathogenesis and therapy of multiple sclerosis via animal models: 70 years of merits and culprits in experimental autoimmune encephalomyelitis research. Brain 2006; 129: 1953–1971.

4. Rivers T, Sprunt DH, Berry GP. Observations on attempts to produce acute disseminated encephalomyelitis in monkeys. J Exp Med 1933; 58: 39–53.

5. Raine, CS. Demyelinating diseases. In: Davis RL, Robertson DM, eds. Textbook of neuropathology, 3rd ed. Baltimore: Williams & Wilkins; 1997: 243–286.

6. Stone SH, Lerner EM. Chronic disseminated allergic encephalomyelitis in guinea pigs. Ann NY Acad Sci 1965; 122: 227–241.

7. Raine C, Stone SH. Animal model for multiple sclerosis. Chronic experimental allergic encephalomyelitis in inbred guinea pigs. NY State J Med 1977; 77: 1693–1696.

8. Raine CS, Barnett LB, Brown A et al. Neuropathology of experimental allergic encephalomyelitis in inbred strains of mice. Lab Invest 1980; 43: 150–157.

9. Lassmann H, Kitz, K, Wisniewski HM. Structural variability of demyelinating lesions in different models of subacute and chronic experimental allergic encephalomyelitis. Acta Neuropathol (Berlin) 1980; 51: 191–201.

10. Brown AM, McFarlin DE. Relapsing experimental allergic encephalomyelitis in the SJL/J mouse. Lab Invest 1981; 45: 278–284.

11. Brown A, McFarlin DE, Raine CS. Chronologic neuropathology of relapsing experimental allergic encephalomyelitis in the mouse. Lab Invest 1982; 46: 171–185.

12. Mokhtarian F, McFarlin D, Raine CS. Adoptive transfer of myelin basic protein-sensitized T cells produces chronic relapsing demyelinating disease in mice. Nature 1984; 309: 356–358.

13. Tabira T, Sakai K. Demyelination induced by T cell lines and clones specific for myelin basic protein in mice. Lab Invest 1987; 56: 518–525.

14. Mendel I, Kerlero de Rosbo N, Ben-Nun A. A myelin oligodendrocyte glycoprotein peptide induces typical chronic experimental autoimmune encephalomyelitis in H-2b mice: fine specificity and T cell receptor Vβ expression of encephalitogenic T cells. Eur J Immunol 1995; 1951–1959.

15. Miller SD, Eagan TN. Functional role of epitope spreading in the chronic pathogenesis of autoimmune and virus-induced demyelinating diseases. Adv Exp Med Biol 2001; 490: 99–107.

16. Selmaj K, Kowal C, Walczak A et al. Naked DNA vaccination differentially modulates autoimmune responses in experimental autoimmune encephalomyelitis. J Neuroimmunol 2000; 111: 34–44.

17. Amor S, Smith PA, Baker D. Biozzi mice: of mice and human diseases. J Neuroimmunol 2005; 165: 1–10.

18. Pender MP, Stanley GP, Yoong G, Nguyen KB. The neuropathology of chronic relapsing experimental allergic encephalomyelitis induced in the Lewis rat by inoculation with spinal cord and treatment with cyclosporine A. Acta Neuropathol (Berlin) 1990; 80: 172–183.

19. Massacesi L, Genain CP, Lee-Parritz D et al. Active and passively induced experimental autoimmune encephalomyelitis in common marmosets: a new model for multiple sclerosis. Ann Neurol 1995; 37: 519–530.

20. Adams RD. A comparison of the morphology of the human demyelinating diseases and experimental allergic encephalomyelitis. In: Alvord EC, ed.

Allergic encephalomyelitis. Springfield, IL: Charles C Thomas; 1959: 183–209.

21. Levine S. Hyperacute, neutrophilic, and localized forms of experimental allergic encephalomyelitis: a review. Acta Neuropathol (Berlin) 1974; 28: 179–189.

22. Paterson PY. Experimental autoimmune (allergic) encephalomyelitis. Induction, pathogenesis and suppression. In: Mueller-Eberhard J, ed. Textbook of immunopathology. New York: Grune & Stratton; 1976: 179–213.

23. Lampert PW. Fine structure of the demyelinating process. In: Hallpike J, Adams CWM, Tourtelotte W, eds. Multiple sclerosis. London: Chapman & Hall; 1983: 29–46.

24. Goverman J, Woods A, Larson L et al. Transgenic mice that express a myelin basic protein-specific T cell receptor develop spontaneous autoimmunity. Cell 1993; 72: 551–560.

25. Lafaille JJ, Nagashima K, Katsuki M, Tonegawa S. High incidence of spontaneous autoimmune encephalomyelitis in immunodeficient anti-myelin basic protein T cell receptor transgenic mice. Cell 1994; 78: 399–408.

26. Bettelli E, Pagany M, Weiner HL et al. Myelin oligodendrocyte glycoprotein-specific T cell receptor transgenic mice develop spontaneous autoimmune optic neuritis. J Exp Med 2003; 197: 1073–1081.

27. Sriram S, Steiner I. Experimental allergic encephalomyelitis: a misleading model for multiple sclerosis. Ann Neurol 2005; 58: 939–945.

28. Steinman L. Assessment of animal models for MS and demyelinating disease in the design of rational therapy. Neuron 1999; 24: 511–514.

29. Raine CS. Biology of disease. Analysis of autoimmune demyelination: its impact upon multiple sclerosis. Lab Invest 1984; 50: 608–635.

30. Wisniewski HM, Keith AB. Chronic relapsing experimental allergic encephalomyelitis: an experimental model of multiple sclerosis. Ann Neurol 1977; 1: 144–147.

31. Lassmann H. Chronic relapsing experimental allergic encephalomyelitis: its value as an experimental model for multiple sclerosis. J Neurol 1983; 229: 207–220.

32. Raine CS, Traugott U, Farooq M et al. Augmentation of immune-mediated demyelination by lipid haptens. Lab Invest 1981; 45: 174–182.

33. Raine CS, Johnson AB, Marcus DM et al. Demyelination in vitro. Absorption studies demonstrate that galactocerebroside is a major target. J Neurol Sci 1981; 52: 117–131.

34. Raine CS, Traugott U, Stone SH. Suppression of chronic allergic encephalomyelitis: relevance to multiple sclerosis. Science 1978; 201: 445–448.

35. Raine CS, Moore GR, Hintzen R, Traugott U. Induction of oligodendrocyte proliferation and remyelination after chronic demyelination. Relevance to multiple sclerosis. Lab Invest 1988; 59: 467–476.

36. Raine CS, Snyder DH, Valsamis MP, Stone SH. Chronic experimental allergic encephalomyelitis in inbred guinea pigs. An ultrastructural study. Lab Invest 1974; 369–380.

37. Stone SH, Snyder DH, Raine CS. Adoptive transfer of experimental allergic encephalomyelitis from immature guinea pig donors. J Neurol Sci 1983; 60: 401–409.

38. Trapp BD, Peterson J, Ransohoff RM et al. Axonal transaction in the lesions of multiple sclerosis. N Engl J Med 1998; 338: 323–325.

39. Pettinelli CB, McFarlin DE. Adoptive transfer of experimental allergic encephalomyelitis in SJL/J mice after in vitro activation of lymph node cells by myelin basic protein: requirement for Lyt 1⁺ 2⁻ T lymphocytes. J Immunol 1981; 127: 1420–1423.

40. Voskuhl RR, Pitchekian-Halabi H, MacKenzie-Graham A et al. Gender differences in autoimmune demyelination in the mouse: Implications for multiple sclerosis. Ann Neurol 1996; 39: 724–733.

41. Raine CS, Mokhtarian F, McFarlin DE. Adoptively transferred chronic relapsing experimental autoimmune encephalomyelitis in the mouse. Neuropathologic analysis. Lab Invest 1984; 51: 534–546.

42. Smith ME, Eller NL, Racke MK et al. Age dependence of clinical and pathologic manifestations of autoimmune demyelination: implication for multiple sclerosis. Am J Pathol 1999; 155: 1147–1161.

43. Sakai K, Tabira T, Endoh M, Steinman L. Ia expression in chronic relapsing experimental allergic encephalomyelitis induced by long-term cultured T cell lines in mice. Lab Invest 1986; 54: 345–352.

44. Cross AH, McCarron R, McFarlin DE, Raine CS. Adoptively transferred acute and chronic relapsing autoimmune encephalomyelitis in the PL/J mouse and observations on altered pathology by intercurrent virus infection. Lab Invest 1987; 57: 499–512.

45. Waksman BH, Porte, H, Lees MD et al. A study of the chemical nature of components of bovine white matter effective in producing allergic encephalomyelitis in the rabbit. J Exp Med 1954; 100: 451–471.

46. Yoshimura T, Kunishita T, Sakai K et al. Chronic experimental allergic encephalomyelitis in guinea pigs induced by proteolipid protein. J Neurol Sci 1985; 69: 47–58.

47. Yamamura T, Namikawa T, Endoh M et al. Experimental allergic encephalomyelitis induced by proteolipid apoprotein in Lewis rats. J Neuroimmunol 1986; 12: 143–153.

48. Endoh M, Tabira T, Kunishita T et al. DM-20, a proteolipid apoprotein, is an encephalitogen of acute and relapsing autoimmune encephalomyelitis in mice. J Immunol 1986; 137: 3832–3835.

49. Trotter JL, Clark HB, Collins KG et al. Myelin proteolipid protein induces demyelinating disease in mice. J Neurol Sci 1987; 79: 173–188.

50. Satoh J, Sakai K, Endo M et al. Experimental allergic encephalomyelitis mediated by murine encephalitogenic T cell lines specific for myelin proteolipid apoprotein. J Immunol 1987; 138: 179–184.

51. Fallis RJ, Raine CS, McFarlin DE. Chronic relapsing experimental allergic encephalomyelitis in SJL mice following

the adoptive transfer of an epitope-specific T-cell line. J Neuroimmunol 1989; 22: 93–106.

52. Cross AH, Tuohy VK, Raine CS. Development of reactivity to new myelin antigens during chronic relapsing autoimmune demyelination. Cell Immunol 1993; 146: 261–269.

53. McRae BL, Kennedy MK, Tan LJ et al. Induction of active and adoptive relapsing experimental autoimmune encephalomyelitis (EAE) using an encephalitogenic epitope of proteolipid protein. J Neuroimmunol 1992; 38: 229–240.

54. McMahon EJ, Bailey SL, Castenada CV, Miller SD. Epiotope spreading initiates in the CNS in two models of multiple sclerosis. Nat Med 2005; 11: 335–339.

55. Amor S, O'Neill J, Morris M et al. Encephalitogenic epitopes of myelin basic protein, proteolipid protein, myelin oligodendrocyte glycoprotein for experimental allergic encephalomyelitis induction in Biozzi ABH (H-2Ag7) mice share an amino acid motif. J Immunol 1996; 156: 3000–3008.

56. Johns TG, Rosbo NK, Menon KK et al. Myelin oligodendrocyte glycoprotein induces a demyelinating encephalomyelitis resembling multiple sclerosis. J Immunol 1995; 154: 5536–5541.

57. Adelmann M, Wood J, Benzel I et al. The N-terminal domain of the myelin oligodendrocyte glycoprotein (MOG) induces acute demyelinating experimental autoimmune encephalomyelitis in the Lewis rat. J Neuroimmunol 1995; 63: 17–27.

58. Cross AH, Ishikawa, S, Raine CS, Diamond B. Autoimmune demyelination in transgenic Eᵘ-alpha positive A.CA mice: comparison with E-negative A.CA mice. Lab Invest 1991; 66: 598–607.

59. Power C, Kong PA, Trapp BD. Major histocompatibility complex class 1 expression in oligodendrocytes induces hypomyelination in transgenic mice. J Neurosci Res 1996; 44: 165–175.

60. Furtado GC, Pina B, Tacke F et al. A novel model of demyelinating encephalomyelitis induced by monocytes and dendritic cells. J. Immunol 2006; 177: 6871–6879.

61. Liedtke W, Edelmann W, Chiu FC et al. EAE in mice lacking glial fibrillary acidic protein is characterized by a more severe clinical course and an infiltrative central nervous system lesion. Am J Pathol 1998; 152: 251–259.

62. Yin X, Crawford TO, Griffin JW et al. Myelin-associated glycoprotein is a myelin signal that modulates the caliber of myelinated axons. J Neurosci 1998; 18: 1953–1962.

63. Raine CS, Traugott U, Nussenblatt RB, Stone SH. Optic neuritis and chronic relapsing experimental allergic encephalomyelitis: relationship to clinical course and comparison with multiple sclerosis. Lab Invest 1980; 42: 327–335.

64. Raine CS, Wisniewski H, Prineas J. An ultrastructural study of experimental demyelination and remyelination. Part II. Chronic experimental allergic encephalomyelitis in the peripheral nervous system. Lab Invest 1969; 21: 316–327.

65. Prineas J, Raine CS, Wisniewski H. An ultrastructural study of experimental demyelination and remyelination. Part III.

257

Chronic experimental allergic encephalomyelitis in the central nervous system. Lab Invest 1969; 21: 472–483.

66. Snyder D, Hirano A, Raine CS. Fenestrated CNS blood vessels in chronic experimental allergic encephalomyelitis. Brain Res 1975; 100: 645–649.

67. Moore GRW, Traugott U, Farooq M et al. Experimental autoimmune encephalomyelitis: Augmentation of demyelination by different myelin lipids. Lab Invest 1984; 51: 416–424.

68. Moore GRW, Raine CS. Leptomeningeal and adventitial gliosis as a consequence of chronic inflammation. Neuropathol Appl Neurobiol 1986; 12: 371–378.

69. Moore GRW, Traugott U, Raine CS. Survival of oligodendrocytes in chronic relapsing autoimmune encephalomyelitis. J Neurol Sci 1984; 65: 137–145.

70. Raine CS. Membrane specializations between demyelinated axons and astroglia in chronic EAE lesions and multiple sclerosis plaques. Nature 1978; 225: 326–327.

71. Soffer D, Raine CS. Morphologic analysis of axo-glial membrane specializations in the demyelinated central nervous system. Brain Res 1980; 186: 301–313.

72. Raine CS, Brown AM, McFarlin DE. Heterotopic regeneration of peripheral nerve fibres into the subarachnoid space. J Neurocytol 1982; 11: 109–118.

73. Raine CS, Cross AH. Axonal dystrophy as a consequence of long-term demyelination. Lab Invest 1989; 60: 714–725.

74. Field EJ, Raine CS. Experimental allergic encephalomyelitis: an electron microscopic study. Am J Pathol 1966; 49: 537–553.

75. Lampert P, Kies MW. Mechanism of demyelination in allergic encephalomyelitis of guinea pigs – an EM study. Exp Neurol 1967; 18: 210–223.

76. Snyder DH, Valsamis MP, Stone SH, Raine CS. Progressive demyelination and reparative phenomena in chronic experimental allergic encephalomyelitis. J Neuropathol Exp Neurol 1975; 34: 209–221.

77. Sobel R, Blanchette B, Bhan A, Colvin R. The immunopathology of experimental allergic encephalomyelitis. II. Endothelial cell Ia increases prior to inflammatory cell infiltration. J Immunol 1984; 132: 2402–2407.

78. Sobel R, Natal B, Schneeberger E. The immunopathology of acute experimental allergic encephalomyelitis. IV. An ultrastructural immunocytochemical study of class II major histocompatibility complex molecule (Ia) expression. J Neuropathol Exp Neurol 1987; 46: 239–249.

79. Lassmann H, Vass K, Brunner C, Seitelberger F. Characterization of inflammatory infiltrates in experimental allergic encephalomyelitis. Prog Neuropathol 1986; 6: 33–62.

80. Brosnan CF, Raine CS. Mechanisms of immune injury in multiple sclerosis. Brain Pathol 1996; 6: 243–257.

81. Lampert P, Carpenter S. Electron microscope studies on the vascular permeability and the mechanisms of demyelination in experimental allergic encephalomyelitis. J Neuropathol Exp Neurol 1965: 11–24.

82. DalCanto MC, Wisniewski HM, Johnson AB et al. Vesicular disruption of myelin in autoimmune demyelination. J Neurol Sci 1975; 24: 313–319.

83. Raine CS. The lesion in multiple sclerosis and chronic relapsing EAE – a structural comparison. In: Raine CS, McFarland HF, Tourtellotte WW, eds. Multiple sclerosis: clinical and pathogenetic basis. London: Chapman & Hall; 1997: 243–286.

84. Epstein LG, Prineas JW, Raine CS. Attachment of myelin to coated pits on macrophages in experimental allergic encephalomyelitis. J Neurol Sci 1983; 61: 341–348.

85. Moore GRW, Raine CS. Immunogold localization and analysis of IgG during immune-mediated demyelination. Lab Invest 1988; 59: 641–648.

86. Pekovic D, Raine CS, Traugott U. Increase in anti-astrocyte antibodies in the serum of guinea pigs during active stages of experimental autoimmune encephalomyelitis. J Neuroimmunol 1990; 26: 251–259.

87. Schluesener HJ, Sobel RA, Linington C, Weiner HL. A monoclonal antibody against a myelin oligodendrocyte glycoprotein induces relapses and demyelination in central nervous system autoimmune disease. J Immunol 1987; 139: 4016–4021.

88. Prineas JW, Connell F. The fine structure of chronically active multiple sclerosis plaques. Neurology 1978: 68–75.

89. Raine CS, Scheinberg LC. On the immunopathology of plaque development and repair in multiple sclerosis. J Neuroimmunol 1988; 20: 189–201.

90. Koni PA, Sacca R, Lawton P et al. Distinct roles in lymphoid organogenesis for lymphotoxins alpha and beta revealed in lymphotoxin beta-deficient mice. Immunity 1997; 6: 491–500.

91. Prineas J. Multiple sclerosis: presence of lymphatic capillaries and lymphoid tissue in the brain and spinal cord. Science 1979; 203: 1123–1125.

92. Yednock T, Rosen S. Lymphocyte homing. Adv Immunol 1989; 44: 313–378.

93. Raine CS, Cannella B, Duijvestijn AM, Cross AH. Homing to central nervous system vasculature by antigen-specific lymphocytes: II. Lymphocyte/ endothelial cell adhesion during the initial stages of autoimmune demyelination. Lab Invest 1990; 63: 476–483.

94. Cross AH, Cannella B, Brosnan CF, Raine CS. Homing to central nervous system vasculature by antigen specific lymphocytes: I. Localization of ^{14}C-labeled cells during acute, chronic and relapsing experimental allergic encephalomyelitis. Lab Invest 1990; 63: 162–170.

95. Cannella B, Cross AH, Raine CS. Upregulation and coexpression of adhesion molecules correlate with relapsing autoimmune demyelination in the central nervous system. J Exp Med 1990; 172: 1521–1524.

96. Cannella B, Cross AH, Raine CS. Adhesion-related molecules in the central nervous system. Upregulation correlates with inflammatory cell influx during relapsing experimental autoimmune encephalomyelitis. Lab Invest 1991; 65: 23–31.

97. Skundric DS, Kim C, Tse HY, Raine CS. Homing of T cells to the central nervous system throughout the course of relapsing experimental autoimmune

encephalomyelitis in Thy-1 congenic mice. J Neuroimmunol 1993; 46: 113–121.

98. Cross AH, Raine CS. Central nervous system endothelial cell/polymorphonuclear leukocyte interactions during autoimmune demyelination. Am J Pathol 1991; 139: 1401–1409.

99. Engelhardt B. Regulation of immune cell entry into the central nervous system. Probl Cell Differ 2006; 43: 259–280.

100. Yednock T, Cannon C, Fritz L et al. Prevention of experimental autoimmune encephalomyelitis by antibodies against alpha 4 beta 1 integrin. Nature 1992; 356: 63–66.

101. Cannella B, Cross AH, Raine CS. Anti-adhesion molecule therapy in experimental autoimmune encephalomyelitis. J Neuroimmunol 1993; 46: 43–56.

102. Genain CP, Nguyen MH, Letvin NL et al. Antibody facilitation of multiple sclerosis-like lesions in a non human primate. J Clin Invest 1995; 96: 2966–2974.

103. Genain CP, Hauser SL. Allergic encephalomyelitis in common marmosets: pathogenesis of a multiple sclerosis-like lesion. Methods 1996; 10: 420–434.

104. Alvord EC, Shaw J, Hruby CM. Myelin basic protein treatment of experimental allergic encephalomyelitis in monkeys. Ann Neurol 1979; 6: 467–473.

105. Massacesi L, Josh N, Lee-Parritz D et al. Experimental allergic encephalomyelitis in cynomolgus monkeys. Quantitation of T-cell responses in peripheral blood. J Clin Invest 1992; 90: 399–404.

106. McFarlin DE. Murine experimental allergic encephalomyelitis. Acta Neuropathol (Berlin) 1983; Suppl IX: 39–46.

107. Shaw CM, EC Alvord J, Hruby S. Chronic remitting-relapsing experimental allergic encephalomyelitis induced in monkeys with homologous myelin basic protein. Ann Neurol 1988; 24: 738–748.

108. Jordan E, McFarland H, Lewis B et al. Serial magnetic resonance imaging of experimental autoimmune encephalomyelitis induced by human white matter or by chimeric myelin basic protein-proteolipoprotein in the common marmoset. Am J Neuroradiol 1999; 20: 965–976.

109. Pomeroy IM, Matthews PM, Frank JA et al. Demyelinated neocortical lesions in marmoset autoimmune encephalitis mimic those in multiple sclerosis. Brain 2005; 128: 2713–2721.

110. T'Hart B, Bauer J, Muller H-J et al. Animal model. Histopathological characterization of magnetic resonance imaging-detectable brain white matter lesions in a primate model of multiple sclerosis. Am J Pathol 1998; 153: 649–663.

111. Poliani PL, Brok H, Furlan R et al. Delivery to the central nervous system of a nonreplicative herpes simplex type 1 vector engineered with the interleukin 4 gene protects rhesus monkeys from hyperacute autoimmune encephalomyelitis. Hum Gene Ther 2001; 12: 905–920.

112. Mancardi G, t'Hart B, Roccatagliata L et al. Demyelination and axonal damage in a non-human primate model of multiple sclerosis. J Neurol Sci 2001; 184: 41–49.

113. Brok H, Uccelli A, Kerlero De Rosbo N et al. Myelin/oligodendrocyte glycoprotein-induced autoimmune encephalomyelitis in common marmosets: the encephalitogenic

SECTION 2

T cell epitope pMOG24–36 is presented by a monomorphic MHC class II molecule. J Immunol 2000; 165: 1093–1101.

114. Raine CS, Cannella B, Hauser S, Genain C. Demyelination in non-human primate autoimmune encephalomyelitis and acute multiple sclerosis lesions: a case for antigen-specific antibody mediation. Ann Neurol 1999; 46: 144–160.

115. Selmaj K, Raine CS. Tumor necrosis factor mediates myelin and oligodendrocyte damage in vitro. Ann Neurol 1988; 23: 339–346.

116. Lee SC, Moore GRW, Golenwsky G, Raine CS. A role for astroglial in active demyelination suggested by class II MHC expression and ultrastructural study. J Neuropath Exp Neurol 1990; 49: 122–136.

117. Genain CP, Lee-Parritz D, Nguyen MH et al. In healthy primates, circulating autoreactive T cells mediate autoimmune disease. J Clin Invest 1994; 94: 1339–1345.

118. Von Budingen HC, Hauser SL, Ouallet JC et al. Frontline: epitope recognition on the myelin/oligodendrocyte glycoprotein differentially influences disease phenotype and antibody effector functions in autoimmune demyelination. Eur J Immunol 2004; 34: 2072–2083.

119. Mathey E, Breithaupt C, Schubart AS, Linington C. Commentary: Sorting the wheat from the chaff: identifying demyelinating components of the myelin oligodendrocyte glycoprotein (MOG)-specific autoantibody repertoire. Eur J Immunol 2004; 34: 2065–2071.

120. Von Büdingen H-C, Hauser S, Nabavi C, Genain C. Characterization of the expressed immunoglobulin IGHV repertoire in the New World marmoset Callithrix jacchus. Immunogenetics 2001; 53: 557–563.

121. Von Büdingen H-C, Hauser S, Fuhrmann A et al. Molecular characterization of antibody specificities against myelin oligodendrocyte glycoprotein in autoimmune demyelination. Proc Natl Acad Sci USA 2002; 99: 8207–8212.

122. Watkins D, Chen Z, Hughes A et al. Genetically distinct cell populations in naturally occurring bone marrow-chimeric primates express similar MHC class I gene products. J Immunol 1990; 144: 3726–3735.

123. Schluesener HJ, Wekerle H. Autoaggressive T lymphocyte lines recognizing the encephalitogenic region of myelin basic protein: in vitro selection from unprimed rat T lymphocyte populations. J Immunol 1985; 135: 3128–3133.

124. Meinl E, Hoch R, Dornmair K et al. Encephalitogenic potential of myelin basic protein-specific T cells isolated from normal rhesus macaques. Am J Pathol 1997; 150: 445–453.

125. Villoslada P, Abel K, Heald N et al. Frequency, heterogeneity and encephalitogenicity of T cells specific for myelin oligodendrocyte glycoprotein in naive outbred primates. Eur J Immunol 2001; 31: 2942–2950.

126. McFarland H, Lobito A, Johnson M et al. Determinant spreading associated with demyelination in a nonhuman primate model of multiple sclerosis. J Immunol 1999; 162: 2384–2390.

127. Lyons J, San M, Happ M, Cross A. B cells are critical to induction of experimental allergic encephalomyelitis by protein but not by a short encephalitogenic peptide. Eur J Immunol 1999; 29: 3432–3439.

128. Lyons JA, Ramsbottom MJ, Cross AH. Critical role of antigen-specific antibody in experimental autoimmune encephalomyelitis induced by recombinant myelin oligodendrocyte glycoprotein. Eur J Immunol 2002; 32: 1905–1913.

129. Linington C, Engelhardt B, Kapoes G, Lassmann H. Induction of persistently demyelinated lesions in the rat following the repeated adoptive transfer of encephalitogenic T cells and demyelinating antibody. J Neuroimmunol 1992; 40; 219–224.

130. Genain C, Cannella B, Hauser S, Raine CS. Identification of autoantibodies associated with myelin damage in multiple sclerosis. Nat Med 1999; 5: 170–175.

131. Von Büdingen H-C, Tanuma N, Villoslada P et al. Immune responses against the myelin/oligodendrocyte glycoprotein in experimental autoimmune demyelination. J Clin Immunol 2001; 21: 155–170.

132. Genain CP, Abel K, Belmar N et al. Late complications of immune deviation therapy in a nonhuman primate. Science 1996; 274: 2054–2057.

133. Litzenburger T, Fassler R, Bauer J et al. B lymphocytes producing demyelinating autoantibodies: development and function in gene-targeted transgenic mice. J Exp Med 1998; 188: 169–180.

134. Jingwu ZR, Madaer R, Hashim GA et al. Myelin basic protein-specific T lymphocytes in multiple sclerosis and controls. Precursor frequency, fine specificity and cytotoxicity. Ann Neurol 1992; 32: 330–338.

135. Joshi N, Usuku K, Hauser SL. The T-cell response to myelin basic protein in familial multiple sclerosis: Diversity of fine specificity restricting elements, and T-cell receptor usage. Ann Neurol 1993; 34: 385–393.

136. Uccelli A, Oksenberg JR, Jeong MC et al. Characterization of the TCRB chain repertoire in the New World Monkey Callithrix jacchus. J Immunol 1997; 158: 1201–1207.

137. Uccelli A, Giunti D, Caroli F et al. Responses to myelin basic protein in an outbred non human primate model for multiple sclerosis. Eur J Immunol 2001; 31: 474–479.

138. Antunes S, de Groot N, Brok H et al. The common marmoset: a new world primate species with limited Mhc class II variability. Proc Natl Acad Sci USA 1998; 95: 11745–11750.

139. Linington C, Berger T, Perry L et al. T cells specific for the myelin oligodendrocyte glycoprotein, mediate an unusual autoimmune inflammatory response in the central nervous system. Eur J Immunol 1993; 23: 1364–1373.

140. Bernard C, Johns T, Slavin A et al. Myelin oligodendrocyte glycoprotein: a novel candidate autoantigen in multiple sclerosis. J Mol Med 1997; 75: 77–88.

141. Ichikawa M, Johns TG, Liu J, Bernard CCA. Analysis of the fine B-cell specificity during the chronic/relapsing course of a multiple sclerosis-like disease in Lewis rats injected with the encephalitogenic myelin oligodendrocyte glycoprotein peptide 35–55. J Immunol 1996; 157: 919–926.

142. Wucherpfennig KW, Catz I, Hausmann S et al. Recognition of the immunodominant myelin basic protein peptide by autoantibodies and HLA-DR2-restricted T cell clones from multiple sclerosis patients. Identity of key contact residues in the B-cell and T-cell epitopes. J Clin Invest 1997; 100: 1114–1122.

143. Lalive PH, Menge T, Delarasse C et al. Antibodies to native myelin oligodendrocyte glycoprotein are serologic markers of early inflammation in multiple sclerosis. Proc Natl Acad Sci USA 2006; 103: 2280–2285.

144. Menge T, Budingen H-C, Lalive P et al. Relevant antibody subsets against MOG recognize conformational epitopes exclusively exposed in solid-phase ELISA. Eur J Immunol 2007; 37: 3229–3239.

145. Raine CS. On the occurrence of Schwann cells in the normal central nervous system. J Neurocytol 1976; 5: 371–380.

146. Ghatak H, Hirano A, Doron Y, Zimmerman H. 1973. Remyelination in MS with peripheral type myelin. Ann Neurol 1973; 29: 262–127.

147. Tabira T. Cellular and molecular aspects of the pathomechanisms and therapy of murne experimental allergic encephalomyelitis. Crit Rev Neurobiol 1989; 55: 113–142.

148. Friese MA, Montalban X, Willcox N et al. The value of animal models for drug development in multiple sclerosis. Brain 2006; 129: 1940–1952.

149. Lang W, Rodriguez M, Lennon VA, Lampert PW. Demyelination and remyelination in murine viral encephalomyelitis. Ann NY Acad Sci 1984; 436: 98–102.

150. Rodriguez M, Lennon VA. Immunoglobulins promote remyelination in the central nervous system. Ann Neurol 1990; 27: 12–17.

151. Pirko I, Ciric B, Gomez J et al. A human antibody that promotes remyelination enters the CNS and decreases lesion load as detected by T1-weighted spinal cord MRI in a virus-induced model of MS. FASEB J 2004; 18: 1577–1579.

152. Howell M, Winters S, Olee T et al. Vaccination against experimental allergic encephalomyelitis with T cell receptor peptides. Science 1989; 246: 668–670.

153. Vandenbark AA, Hashim G, Offner H. Immunization with a synthetic T-cell receptor V-region peptide protects against experimental autoimmune encephalomyelitis. Nature 1989: 341; 541–544.

154. Vandenbark AA, Chou YK, Whitham R et al. Treatment of multiple sclerosis with T-cell receptor peptides: results of a double-blind pilot trial. Nat Med 1996; 2: 11009–1115.

155. Sriram S, Roberts C. Treatment of established chronic relapsing experimental allergic encephalomyelitis with anti-L3T4 antibodies. J Immunol 1986; 136: 4404–4409.

156. Sriram S, Steinman L. Anti-I-A antibody suppresses active encepahlomyelitis: treatment model for diseases linked to IR genes. J Exp Med 1983; 158: 1362–1367.

157. Waldor M, Mitchell D, Kipps R et al. Importance of immunoglobulin isotype in therapy of experimental autoimmune encephalomyelitis with monoclonal anti-CD4 antibody. J Immunol 1987; 139: 3660–3664.

158. Ruddle NH, Bergman CM, McGrath KM et al. An antibody to lymphotoxin and tumor necrosis factor prevents transfer of experimental allergic encephalomyelitis. J Exp Med 1990; 172: 1193–1200.

159. Selmaj K, Raine CS, Cross AH. Anti-tumor necrosis factor therapy abrogates autoimmune demyelination. Ann Neurol 1991; 30: 694–700.

160. Monastra G, Cross AH, Bruni A, Raine CS. Phosphatidylserine, a putative inhibitor of tumor necrosis factor, prevents autoimmune demyelination. Neurology 1993; 43: 153–163.

161. Sommer N, Loschmann P, Northoff G et al. The antidepressant rolipram suppresses cytokine production and prevents autoimmune encephalomyelitis. Nat Med 1995; 1: 244–248.

162. Genain CP, Roberts T, Davis RL et al. Prevention of autoimmune demyelination by a cAMP-specific phosphodiesterase inhibitor. Proc Natl Acad Sci USA 1995; 92: 3601–3605.

163. Racke MK, Cannella B, Albert P et al. Evidence of endogenous regulatory function of transforming growth factor-beta 1 in experimental allergic encephalomyelitis. Int Immunol 1992.4: 615–620.

164. Rott O, Fleischer,B, Cash E. Interleukin-10 prevents experimental allergic encephalomyelitis in rats. Eur J Immunol 1994; 24: 1434–1440.

165. Racke MK, Bonomo A, Scott DE et al. Cytokine-induced immune deviation as a therapy for inflammatory autoimmune disease. J Exp Med 1994; 180: 1961–1966.

166. Welsch C, Rose J, Hill K, Townsend J. Augmentation of adoptively transferred EAE by administration of a monoclonal antibody specific for LFA-1 alpha. J Neuroimmunol 1993; 43: 161–168.

167. Willenborg DO, Simmons R, Tamatami T, Miyasaka M. ICAM-1 dependent pathway is not critically involved in the inflammatory process of autoimmune encephalomyelitis or in cytokine-indiced inflammation of the central nervous system. J Neuroimmunol 1993; 45: 147–154.

168. Archelos J, Hartung H. The role of adhesion molecules in multiple sclerosis: biology, pathogenesis and therapeutic implications. Mol Med Today 1997; 3: 310–321.

169. Cree BA, Lamb S, Morgan K et al. An open label study of the effects of rituximab in neuromyelitis optica. Neurology 2005; 64: 1270–1272.

170. Ousman SS, Tomooka BH, van Noort JM et al. Protective and therapeutic role of αB-crystallin in autoimmune demyelination. Nature 2007; 448: 474–479.

171. Folcik V, Smith T, O'Bryant S et al. Treatment with BBB022A or rolipram stabilizes the blood–brain barrier in experimental autoimmune encephalomyelitis: an additional mechanism for the therapeutic effect of type IV phosphodiesterase inhibitors. J Neuroimmunol 1999; 97: 119–128.

172. Van der Meide P, de Labie M, Ruuls S et al. Discontinuation of treatment with IFN-beta leads to exacerbation of experimental autoimmune encephalomyelitis in Lewis rats. Rapid reversal of the antiproliferative activity of IFN-beta and excessive expansion of autoreactive T cells as disease promoting mechanisms. J Neuroimmunol 1998; 84: 14–23.

173. Dayal A, Jensen M, Lledo A, Arnason B. Interferon-gamma-secreting cells in multiple sclerosis patients treated with interferon beta-1b. Neurology 1995; 45: 2173–2177.

174. Genain CP, Gritz L, Joshi N et al. Inhibition of allergic encephalomyelitis in marmosets by vaccination with recombinant vaccinia virus encoding for myelin basic protein. J Neuroimmunol 1997; 79: 119–128.

175. McFarland H, Lobito A, Johnson M et al. Effective antigen-specific immunotherapy in the marmoset model of multiple sclerosis. J Immunol 2001; 166: 2116–2121.

176. Ho PP, Fontoura P, Platten M et al. A suppressive oligodeoxynucleotide enhances the efficacy of myelin cocktail/IL-4-tolerizing DNA vaccination and treats autoimmune disease. J Immunol 2005; 175: 6226–6234.

177. Bar-Or A, Vollmer T, Antel J et al. Induction of antigen-specific tolerance in multiple sclerosis after immunization with DNA encoding myelin basic protein in a randomized, placebo-controlled phase $\frac{1}{2}$ trial. Arch Neurol 2007; 64: 1407–1415.

178. Bourquin C, Iglesias A, Berger T et al. Myelin oligodendrocyte glycoprotein-DNA vaccination induces antibody-mediated autoaggression in experimental autoimmune encephalomyelitis. Eur J Immunol 2000; 30: 3663–3671.

179. Gerritse K, Laman JD, Noelle RJ et al. CD40-CD40 ligand interactions in experimental allergic encephalomyelitis and multiple sclerosis. Proc Natl Acad Sci USA 1996; 93: 2499–2504.

180. T'Hart BA, Brok HP, Remarque E et al. Suppression of ongoing disease in a nonhuman primate model of multiple sclerosis by a human-anti-human IL-12p40 antibody. J Immunol 2005; 175: 4761–4768.

181. Villoslada P, Hauser S, Bartke I et al. Human nerve growth factor protects common marmosets against autoimmune encephalomyelitis by switching the balance of T helper type 1 and 2 cytokines within the central nervous system. J Exp Med 2000; 191: 1799–1806.

182. Cannella B, Hoban C, Gao YL et al. The neuregulin, GGF2, diminishes autoimmune demyelination and enhances remyelination in a model for multiple sclerosis. Proc Natl Acad Sci USA 1998; 95: 10100–10105.

183. Berger T, Rubner P, Schautzer F et al. Antimyelin antibodies as a predictor of clinically definite multiple sclerosis after a first demyelinating event. N Engl J Med 2003; 349: 139–145.

184. Kuhle J, Pohl C, Mehling M et al. Lack of association between antimyelin antibodies and progression to multiple sclerosis. N Engl J Med 2007; 356: 371–378.

185. Prineas JW, Barnard RO, Kwon EE et al. Multiple sclerosis: remyelination of nascent lesions. Ann Neurol 1993; 33: 137–151.

186. Raine CS, Wu E. Multiple sclerosis: remyelination in acute lesions. J Neuropath Exp Neurol 1993; 52: 199–205.

187. Lucchinetti C, Bruck W, Parisi J et al. Heterogeneity of multiple sclerosis lesions: implications for the pathogenesis of demyelination. Ann Neurol 2000; 47: 707–717.

188. Barnett MH, Prineas JW. Relapsing and remitting multiple sclerosis: Pathology of newly forming lesion. Ann Neurol 2004; 55: 458–468.

189. Breij ECW, Brink BP, Veerhuis R et al. Homogeneity of active demyelinating lesions in established multiple sclerosis. Ann Neurol 2008; 193: 12–23.

190. Steinman L, Zamvil S. How to successfully apply animal studies in experimental allergic encephalomyelitis to research in multiple sclerosis. Ann Neurol 2006; 60: 12–21.

191. Sun D, Whitaker JN, Huang Z et al. Myelin antigen-specific CD8+ T cells are encephalitogenic and produce severe disease in C57BL/6 mice. J Immunol 2001; 166: 7579–7587.

192. Lafaille JJ, Van de Keere F, Hsu A et al. Myelin basic protein-specific Th2 cells cause experimental autoimmune encephalomyelitis in immunodeficient hosts rather than protect them from the disease. J Exp Med 1997; 186: 307–312.

193. Lock C, Hermans G, Pedotti R et al. Harvest of gene microarray analysis of multiple sclerosis lesions yields new targets validated in the experimental autoimmune encephalomyelitis model. Nat Med 2002; 8: 500–508.

194. Cross AH, O'Mara T, Raine CS. Chronologic localization of myelin-reactive cells in the lesions of relapsing EAE. Implications for the study of multiple sclerosis. Neurology 1993; 43: 1028–1033.

195. Baron JL, Madri JA, Ruddle NH et al. Surface expression of alpha 4 integrin by CD4 T cells is required for their entry into brain parenchyma. J Exp Med 1993; 177: 57–68.

196. Stoolman LM. Adhesion molecules controlling lymphocyte migration. Cell 1989; 56: 907–910.

197. Gimbrone M, Bevilacqua M. Vascular endothelium. Functional modulation at the blood interface. In: Simionescu N, Simionescu M, eds. Endothelial cell biology. New York: Plenum; 1988: 255–273.

198. Berger JR, Koralnik IJ. Progressive multifocal leukoencephalopathy and natalizumab–unforeseen consequences. N Engl J Med 2005; 353: 414–416.

199. Ransohoff RM. Natalizumab and PML. Nat Neurosci 2005; 8: 1275.

200. John GR, Shankar SL, Shafit-Zagardo B et al. Multiple sclerosis: re-expression of a developmental pathway that restricts remyelination. Nat Med 2002; 8: 1115–1121.

201. Juryneczk M, Jurewicz A, Bielecki B et al. Inhibition of Notch signaling enhances tissue repair in an animal model of multiple sclerosis. J Neuroimmunol 2005; 170: 3–10.

202. Zhang Y, Taveggia C, Melendez-Vasquez C et al. Interleukin-11 potentiates oligodendrocyte survival and maturation and myelin formation. J Neurosci 2006; 26: 12174–12185.

203. Mi S, Hu B, Hahm K et al. LINGO-1 antagonist promotes spinal cord remyelination and axonal integrity in MOG-induced experimental autoimmune encephalomyelitis. Nature Med 2007; 13: 1228–1233.

204. Zappia E, Casazza S, Pedemonte E et al. Mesenchymal stem cells ameliorate experimental autoimmune encephalomyelitis inducing T-cell anergy. Blood 2005; 106: 1755–1761.

205. Pluchino S, Martino G. The therapeutic use of stem cells for myelin repair in autoimmune demyelinating disorders. J Neurol Sci 2005; 233: 117–119.

206. Matysiak M, Stasiolek M, Orlowski W et al. Stem cell ameliorate (EAE) via an indoleamine 2,3-dioxygenase (IDO) mechanism. J Neuroimmunol 2008; 193: 12–23.

CHAPTER 17

Genetic manipulations of experimental autoimmune encephalomyelitis in the mouse

S. P. Zehntner and T. Owens

INTRODUCTION

The ability to manipulate gene expression in animals provides an opportunity to dissect the mechanism of pathogenesis as well as to explore etiology of disease. Experimental autoimmune encephalomyelitis (EAE), as has been described in Chapter 16, can be induced in any mammalian species. Chapter 16 described the relative suitability of, for instance, guinea pig, rat and marmoset as EAE models for selected aspects of human disease. But, for now and in the immediate future, the species of choice for genetic manipulations of EAE is the mouse.

The focus on the mouse derives from this being the species with the widest application of both immunological reagents and genetic manipulations. As a specific example, the mouse pronucleus is more accessible than that of the rat and so more amenable to microinjection of DNA constructs. Also, embryonic stem cell lines with potential for germline transmission are (to date) uniquely available in mouse. This is not to say that comparable studies could not be performed in other species (e.g. transgenic rats have been described[1]) but the ease of manipulation and access to gene libraries and other databases is greater for the mouse.

The most direct goal of genetic manipulation is to ask whether a targeted gene contributes to the pathological process. What has emerged from many of the studies that have been done are new insights into the pathological process, sometimes from unexpected observations. Considerations that must be taken into account in interpreting results of genetic manipulations include the underlying genetics of the mouse (strain background) and specific examples of the effects of this are discussed. Indirect effects of transgenesis or gene disruption must also be considered, one example being that knockout of CD4+ cells affects the CD8+ T-cell repertoire, so complicating interpretation (see reference 2 for a fuller analysis of this particular point).

The focus of this review will be on genetic manipulations that were then applied to EAE. These include over expression via transgenesis and viral vector gene delivery, and gene deficiency in knockouts. This focus unfortunately does not permit coverage of the many genetic models that have resulted in spontaneous pathology, from which much has been learned about the pathophysiology of central nervous system (CNS) inflammatory and degenerative diseases. These genetic models have been the subject of numerous reviews (e.g. by Owens et al[3]).

Similarly, a number of 'core' observations to which genetic models made significant contributions have stood the test of time and have not required re-examination in recent years. These are summarized in Table 17.1 and the reader is referred to reviews rather than the primary papers, but they are not dealt with in any more detail. On the other hand, wherever recent studies have added to or modified conclusions made earlier, we have recapitulated previously reviewed material in order to provide context for the update. Given this, and as an organizational device, the chapter sets out to examine precepts that have been tested or established using genetically modified mice.

EXPERIMENTAL AUTOIMMUNE ENCEPHALOMYELITIS IS A T-HELPER-1 DISEASE REGULATED BY COMPLEX CYTOKINE NETWORKS

Inflammatory processes generally tend to involve Th1 immune responses. This is especially true for the CNS. The immunization strategies that induce EAE are themselves T-helper (Th)1-promoting. However, observations have been made that suggest that the CNS microenvironment itself predisposes to Th1 cytokine production, once the prerequisite entry of immune cells and antigen recognition has taken place.[4] Transgenic and knockout approaches have thrown new light on these issues, focusing attention to the antigen-presenting cells with the CNS and the cytokines that they express. This research parallels increased understanding of the regulation of Th1 and Th2 responses, which has brought to our attention the role of

TABLE 17.1 Molecules implicated in experimental autoimmune encephalomyelitis through genetic manipulations

Molecule	References
Cytokines	
IFNγ, TNFα, IL6, IL4, IL10	3, 54, 125–128
Chemokines	
CCL2, CCL5	129–133
Receptors	
IFNγR, TNFRI TNFRII	3; 129–131; 134

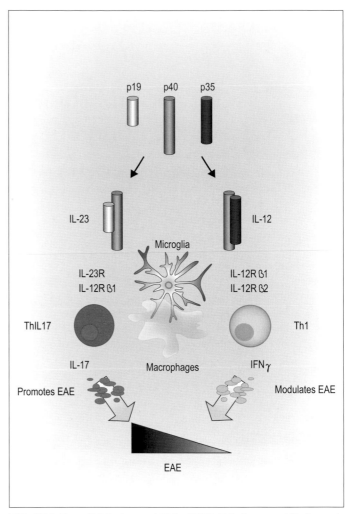

FIG. 17.1 Essential features of ThIL-12/23 dichotomy and its impact on generation of Th1 and ThIL-17 cells in EAE.

complex cytokines and networks. Current research focuses on whether CNS glial cells selectively express or respond to specific cytokines and whether this is critical to defining the CNS microenvironment.

CD4⁺ VERSUS CD8⁺ T CELLS AS MEDIATORS OF EXPERIMENTAL AUTOIMMUNE ENCEPHALOMYELITIS

That EAE is a CD4⁺ T-cell-mediated disease has remained a core tenet, with ample evidence from antibody depletion and gene knockout studies. However, the role of CD8⁺ T cells was obscured partly by the strength of the evidence for CD4⁺ T cells, partly because of difficulty of transferring disease with CD8⁺ T cells and partly because of knockout studies that suggested, if anything, a regulatory role for CD8⁺ T cells. The latter is probably correct, but for a subset of, and not all CD8⁺ T cells. More recent analyses of myelin/oligodendrocyte glycoprotein (MOG)-induced EAE in DBA/1-background CD8⁻ and CD4-deficient mice showed that CD8⁺ T cells may indeed play a propathological role.[5] Taken together with demonstrations of the presence of CD8⁺ T cells at consistent proportions[6] and more recent demonstrations that CD8⁺ T cells could transfer EAE,[7–9] this shines new light on CD8⁺ T cells in EAE, as has been authoritatively reviewed by Friese and Fugger.[2]

INTERLEUKIN-12 VERSUS INTERLEUKIN-23

Earlier observations that interleukin (IL)-12 was required for EAE had to be reinterpreted in light of findings that mice lacking the p35 subunit of IL-12 were susceptible to disease, and that IL-23 shares the p40 subunit, itself homologous to the IL-6 receptor, coupled to a p19 subunit. This family of cytokines shares features with other heterodimeric cytokines that use nonsignaling chains to facilitate secretion.[10] It was subsequently shown in p19 knockouts that IL-23 is the critical cytokine in EAE. Whereas IL-12 is critical for immune responses to infection, once a Th1 response has been induced in lymphoid tissue EAE is relatively IL-12-independent. Use of chimeric mice made with IL-12 receptor-deficient bone marrow showed that IL-12 response was not required for pathogenesis of inflammatory demyelination.[11] Gene delivery to p40- and p35-deficient mice using adenoviral vectors confirmed that IL-12 was required in the periphery for induction of the immune response but was inadequate to restore pathogenesis if delivered to the CNS, whereas IL-23 could fulfill this role.[12] A pivotal observation was that CNS microglia and infiltrating macrophages differ in their IL-12 and IL-23 responses. Microglia respond preferentially to IL-12, whereas macrophages respond to both IL-12 and IL-23. Both microglia and macrophages express IL-12 and IL-23, so regulation of response within the CNS appears to be mediated at the level of the functional IL-12 receptor (Fig. 17.1).

INTERLEUKIN-17

Related to the emergence of IL-23 as a key player in the CNS immune response was the identification of IL-17-producing T cells as critical for EAE.[13] IL-17 has been implicated in arthritis and other inflammatory autoimmune diseases.[14] To date, no transgenic approaches to direct investigation of its role in EAE have been published. However, mice deficient in IL-17, whether through direct gene targeting or as an indirect consequence, were resistant to EAE.[15,16]

OSTEOPONTIN AND GRANULOCYTE–MACROPHAGE COLONY STIMULATING FACTOR

A nonbiased array study identified a number of candidate cytokines in multiple sclerosis (MS).[17] Two of these, osteopontin and granulocyte–macrophage colony stimulating factor (GM-CSF), were further examined by investigating the effect of their deficiency on MOG-induced EAE in knockout mice. Both were shown to be critical for EAE. Osteopontin, named originally for its implication in bone development, regulates the Th1 response by controlling the IL-10/interferon (IFN) ratio, and is itself induced by IFNγ. In the case of GM-CSF, knockout studies were complemented by results from over-expression via gene delivery using retrovirally transfected T cells, which exacerbated disease.[18] This illustrates the power of coupling genetic analyses of human disease with genetic manipulation in animal models.

CYTOKINE REGULATION BY PROTEASES: TUMOR NECROSIS FACTOR-α

Cytokine regulation can also be effected by proteases. One very good example of this is tumor necrosis factor (TNF)α. The cytokine TNFα has been extensively studied in EAE as well as in MS, with confusing and disappointing therapeutic results. The complex activities of this cytokine in EAE have been reviewed recently.[3] Its activities include promotion of chemokine expression at the blood–brain barrier[19] as well as action as a survival/proliferation factor for oligodendrocyte precursor cells that can mediate remyelination,[20] depending on which receptor it acts through. TNFα has also been implicated, through antibody blocking, in the exacerbated MOG-induced EAE that is induced in C57Bl/6 mice that lack the cytokine/neurotrophin ciliary neurotrophic factor (CNTF).[21] CNTF overexpression induces a glial response similar to that associated with protection from lesions or injury.[22] Inflammatory activities of TNFα require that it be released from its membrane-associated form; mice in which this was disallowed by knock-in of a modified gene construct showed reduced susceptibility to EAE.[23] Cleavage of TNFα from the membrane is mediated by a disintegrin and metalloprotease (ADAM)-17, a member of the broader metalloproteinase family.[24] Another protease, the enzyme matrixmetalloprotease-12, has been shown to inhibit EAE through an effect on the Th1/Th2 balance, but it is unclear whether this reflects direct protease activity[25] (see below). One needs to understand what regulates the regulator in order to understand the regulation of response.

INTERFERON-β

Interferon-β is used as an immunomodulatory therapy in the treatment of MS. The mechanism(s) of action are unclear. It has been reported to have antiproliferative effects on T cells, reduce the production of IL12, which inhibits Th1 development, and induce production of IL10.[26,27] Analysis of IFNβ knockout animals during EAE has led to a revision of its proposed role as a T-cell modulator.[28] In IFNβ-deficient animals EAE is more severe and chronic. Lack of IFNβ had no impact on peripheral encephalitogenic T-cell development or proliferation, or on antibody production, thus implying a role for IFNβ in the effector phase of disease. This study and others showed that IFNβ is produced by microglia-like cells in the CNS.[29–31] Whereas IFNβ deficiency did not skew the Th1/Th2 balance, there were dramatic differences in IFNβ-deficient mice in the Mac-1/CD11b expression levels on microglia and macrophages. Elevated levels of TNFα were observed, potentially as a secondary response to elevated Mac-1/CD11b. Use of the IFNβ-deficient mouse in this EAE model helps to illustrate the role of IFNβ in a physiological situation, suggesting that IFNβ plays a significant role in regulation of myeloid cells.

TRANSCRIPTIONAL REGULATION

Specific transcription factors are associated with control of Th1 and Th2 responses. Thus, Th1 cells express T-bet while Th2 T cells express GATA-3.[32–34] Both have defined binding sites in promoter regions of Th1- and Th2-associated cytokines, respectively. Similarly, action of many cytokines through their receptors is mediated via phosphorylation of STAT proteins, which then dimerize and migrate to the nucleus where they interact with promoter regions of target genes. This couples receptor-associated signaling to gene transcription. Specific STAT proteins are implicated in responses to cytokine-inducing factors such as IL-12, as well as in response to selected Th1 and Th2 cytokines. Administration of T-bet-specific antisense oligonucleotides or small interfering RNA (siRNA) at the time of immunization inhibited MOG-induced EAE in C57Bl/6 mice.[35] Mice that lack T-bet or STAT4, which are associated to IFNγ production and IL-12 response respectively,[36,37] are resistant to MOG-induced EAE, whereas mice lacking STAT6, which normally drives the Th2 cytokine IL-4, and STAT1, which is associated to signaling by a number of cytokines, including IFNγ, IL-6, CNTF and type I interferons, showed exacerbated EAE.[36,37] The STAT1 result identifies the need for caution in prediction of the effects of targeting a gene that encodes a multifunctional protein. The cytokines whose responses are signaled by STAT1 exert opposing effects in inflammatory demyelination and the result shows that protective effects predominate over pathology in this case.

The transcription factor NF-κB is fundamental to many physiological and pathological responses, including regulation of costimulatory molecules, cytokines, chemokines inflammatory enzymes and adhesion molecules. Originally implicated in regulation of Ig light chain, NF-κB is expressed by a variety of cell types. The five most prominent NF-κB family members are NF-κB1, NF-κB2, Rel-A, Rel-B and c-rel. RelA-deficient mice die in utero and NF-κB2-deficient mice show developmental defects. Mice deficient in Rel-B and c-rel develop severe immunological disorders postnatally. By contrast, NF-κB1-deficient mice develop normally and do not show significant defects as adults. A recent study in NF-κB1 knockout mice showed that NF-κB1 plays a crucial role in the activation and differentiation of autoreactive T cells, since MOGp35–55-induced EAE was markedly less severe with decreased infiltration to CNS in NF-κB-deficient C57Bl/6-crossed mice. This study did not allow for the dissection of the role of NF-κB in the effector phase, since mice that did develop disease showed similar infiltration and therefore unaltered CNS pathology local to those infiltrates.

Bone marrow chimeras or adoptive transfers using the knockout as host may help elucidate answers to these questions. An alternative approach that may be useful in such analyses is to specifically downregulate NF-κB by cell-specific transgenic expression of a dominant negative I-κBα. I-κBα is a natural regulator of NF-κB, dissociating from it to allow translocation to the nucleus upon phosphorylation. The dominant negative construct prevents this and so blocks the mobilization and translocation of NF-κB. This has been applied to analysis of the role of NF-κB using GFAP promoters in astrocytes in responses to spinal cord injury.[38] Findings that an NF-κB-driven astrocyte response plays some role in inhibiting white matter preservation and recovery in that model have been complemented in MOG-induced EAE, where the IκBα-dominant negative mice developed EAE slightly later but then showed a reduction in severity that was not seen in wild-type mice.[39] This complements the earlier finding that mice deficient in GFAP showed more severe EAE.[40] These elegant genetic manipulations open new perspectives on the role of astrocytes in EAE, which will probably influence our thinking on these glial cells as potential targets for therapy in MS.

EPITOPE SPREADING IS DRIVEN BY ANTIGEN PRESENTATION WITHIN THE CENTRAL NERVOUS SYSTEM

As EAE progresses, the breadth of the T cell response increases to include recognition of antigens that were not targeted by the initial immunization, a process known as epitope spreading. This also occurs in MS, as reviewed in Chapter 13. One of the core questions about this development of a more diverse and ultimately more pathogenic response in the CNS is whether novel T-cell reactivities originate within the CNS or whether they reflect peripheral activation in lymphoid organs. The issue is central to understanding neuroinflammation and neuroinflammatory disease, because it turns on whether endogenous antigen-presenting cells within the CNS have the ability to induce a primary immune response or whether CNS antigens can leak or be transported across the blood–brain barrier. There is evidence for and against both, depending on the nature of experimental antigens and on conditions used for assay of antigen presentation (reviewed in reference 41). A recent study made use of transgenic expression of herpes simplex thymidine kinase (TK) as a device to deplete cells that express it when challenged with the drug ganciclovir. By coupling CD11b-promoter-driven TK expression with reconstitution of peripheral CD11b+ cells in bone marrow chimeras, mice whose microglia could be targeted were generated. In conjunction with Flt3-treatment to promote growth of dendritic cells (DC), DC-specific expression of MHC II using a CD11c promoter, and bone marrow chimeras that did not express MHC II in CNS parenchyma, the authors were able to show that perivascular DCs in CNS are a critical component of the immune response in EAE.[42] This complements a study using CFSE-labeled TCR transgenic T cells, whose proliferation could be followed in otherwise genetically unmodified mice, that showed that CNS DCs were critical antigen-presenting cells (APCs) for epitope spreading and Th17 response.[43,44] These studies illustrate the power of genetic modification in addressing mechanistic questions in EAE and, taken together with demonstrations of DCs in germinal centers in MS CNS,[44] make a strong case for intra-CNS antigen presentation as a primary basis for epitope spreading.

COSTIMULATOR LIGANDS ON ANTIGEN-PRESENTING CELLS CONTROL INFLAMMATION IN THE CENTRAL NERVOUS SYSTEM

Allied to demonstrations that intra-CNS APCs are critical for development and progression of EAE are a series of studies showing that expression of costimulator and regulatory ligands by APCs also control disease. The classical B7/CD28 ligand/counterligand axis was shown by gene knockout to be critical for induction of EAE, as expected, because of its central role in the induction of most T-cell immune responses.[46,47] However, subsequent studies showed that this was dependent on the strain background on which the gene knockout was expressed.[48] Further studies showed that by adoptive transfer or more aggressive immunization, resistance could be overcome even in C57Bl/6-background CD28-deficient mice.[49] The CD28 receptor binds both costimulatory and regulatory ligands. Notable among the latter is CTLA-4. Mice lacking this molecule develop a fatal lymphoproliferative disease.[50] Deficiency in CD28 would therefore result in loss not only of costimulatory B7.1 or B7.2 signals but also of regulatory CTLA4 signals. Consistent with this, it has been noted that B7-deficient animals are more consistently affected with regards to EAE induction (being resistant) than are CD28-deficient mice.[49] The homologous ligand BTLA-4, expressed on activated T cells and binding to a B7 family member (B7.x), regulates T cell activation similarly to CTLA4. Mice lacking BTLA4 show enhanced susceptibility to EAE.[51] Deficiency in another T-cell-expressed receptor, PD-1, also enhances susceptibility to EAE.[52] PD-1 is an apoptosis-inducing receptor whose ligand PDL-1 is expressed in the CNS at increased levels

in mice with MOG-induced EAE. These systemic knockouts make important points regarding the role of costimulator and regulatory systems in the autoimmune T-cell response but they do not provide detailed information regarding whether such regulation occurs within the CNS. It would be expected that they might, given that DCs can induce T-cell responses in the CNS, and the adoptive transfer experiments in CD28-deficient mice[49] speak to this possibility. This is at the same time an important question with regard to the etiology of MS, for which EAE is a model, since CNS infections would be expected to induce costimulator expression on endogenous APCs and thus promote T-cell responses in the CNS (Fig. 17.2). A more direct indication for an intra-CNS role for costimulation in EAE came from the spontaneous encephalomyelitis that develops in transgenic mice that express B7.2/CD86 on microglia,[53] although the peripheral dysregulation that also occurs in these mice obscures the exact role of intra-CNS costimulation (Fig. 17.3).

INTERFERON-γ IS A KEY REGULATORY T-HELPER-1 CYTOKINE

It has become a truism that interferon makes EAE better but makes MS worse.[54] The discrepancy between the effects of this cytokine in the two diseases remains unresolved. It was significant that adenoviral-encoded IFNγ could cure ongoing EAE when administered intrathecally to mice,[55] thus getting past potential complications resulting from lifelong and developmental expression, as had been obtained previously in transgenic mice, and incidental effects of needle trauma from intra-CNS administration. One potential cause of the severe and nonremitting EAE that occurs in IFNγ-deficient mice was the abrogation of a regulatory loop involving infiltrating neutrophils and macrophages and their production of NO.[56,57] It is not clear that this can explain all effects of IFNγ, since there has not been reported universal observation of neutrophils in EAE and the role of NO in neuroinflammation is itself unresolved (see below). Nevertheless, it is clear that IFNγ can exert a profound regulatory role in inflammatory responses and that genetic interventions involving IFNγ in EAE tend to favor regulation over inflammation. It is not obvious why all of the transgenic models described to date have shown exacerbation of, or even spontaneous EAE, whereas other interventions have had opposite effects. One possibility is that expression of IFNγ from birth (MBP or GFAP promoters were used in all transgenics) generates a different response from at the time of intervention. This was not supported by studies in conditional promoter-driven transgenic mice, where adult-onset IFNγ in CNS impaired clinical recovery from EAE and prevented oligodendrocyte repopulation.[58] Alternatively, it cannot be excluded that IFNγ has different effects in humans versus rodents.

Attention has shifted recently to those cytokines that induce IFNγ. The case of IL12/23 has been discussed already. Another potent IFNγ-inducing cytokine with potential regulatory effects in EAE is IL-18. It had previously been shown that mice deficient in IL-18 were resistant to MOG-induced EAE, and that subsequent administration of IL-18 to IL-18-deficient CNS induced an EAE-like disease, consequent to IFNγ activation of NK cells.[59] More recently, it was reported that whereas the IL-18R was critical for EAE, IL-18 itself was not.[60] This member of the IL-1 family requires post-translational processing via proteolytic cleavage by caspase-1 for biological activity, which hinders use of conventional mRNA analysis to dissect its role. Expression of a natural inhibitor, IL-18 binding protein (IL-18BP) in the CNS via transfection of antigen-specific T cells has been shown to perturb Th1/Th2 regulation so that tolerance-inducing IL-4-production was promoted.[61]

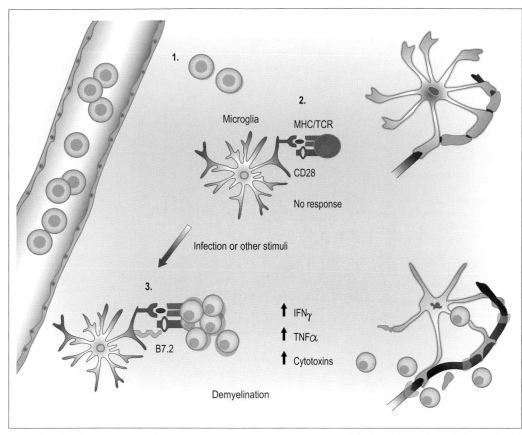

FIG. 17.2 Costimulatory ligand expression by central nervous system (CNS) resident microglia is required for spontaneous development of autoimmune demyelinating disease. **1.** T cells enter the healthy CNS to perform immune surveillance. **2.** In the healthy CNS, T cells that interact with microglia are anergized as a result of a lack of costimulation. **3.** Activation of microglia as it occurs during infection, upregulates costimulatory ligands such as B7.2. T cells specific for myelin peptides presented in the context of B7.2 by activated microglial cells, are reactivated leading to destructive autoimmunity. With permission from Zehntner et al 2003.[53]

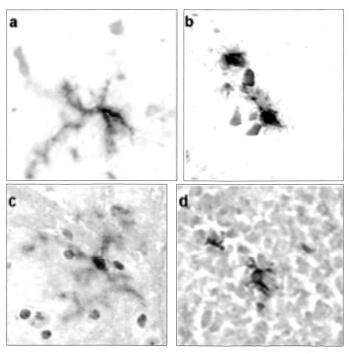

FIG. 17.3 Constitutive B7.2 expression in the nervous tissue of Line 31 mice. B7.2 expression on isolated cells with microglial morphology in the spinal cord and macrophage-like morphology in spinal roots of symptomatic (**a, b**) and TCRβ$^{-/-}$ (**c, d**) Line 31 mice. Adapted with permission from Zehntner et al 2003.[53]

INDUCIBLE NITRIC OXIDE SYNTHASE

Inducible nitric oxide synthase (iNOS or NOS2) is an IFNγ-inducible enzyme that is a major source of high-level NO production during inflammation. The role of this enzyme and of the NO that it drives remain an enigma. On the one hand, levels of iNOS in the CNS are significantly reduced during EAE in IFNγ-deficient mice, and this correlates both with reduced T cell-suppressive effect of infiltrating myeloid cells[62,63] and with the fact that EAE is exacerbated in iNOS-deficient mice (reviewed by Willenborg et al[64]). Accelerated disease has been described in iNOS-deficient mice and was associated with increased infiltration of IFNγ-producing Th1 T cells[65,66] that was further amplified by failure of apoptotic mechanisms.[66] On the other hand, nitric oxide has been implicated in oligodendrocyte and axonal pathology in MS and EAE.[64] The enzyme has many cell sources (Fig. 17.4) and selective depletion from CNS or blood-derived sources in bone-marrow chimeras produced a delay in EAE onset that was independent of cellular source and was not replicated in global knockouts.[57] On balance, it seems that iNOS-induced NO plays a regulatory role in EAE. Nevertheless, NO is a critical component of peroxynitrite, formed by the immediate associate of NO and O_2^- radicals, and peroxynitrite is implicated as a highly oxidative cytopathic mediator in EAE. Mice that lack the superoxide-generating enzyme NADPH-oxidase are resistant to EAE and this reflects its lack in blood cells.[57] This is difficult to reconcile with the exacerbation of EAE in mice lacking iNOS, and points to the operation of other NOS isoforms in generation of peroxynitrite.

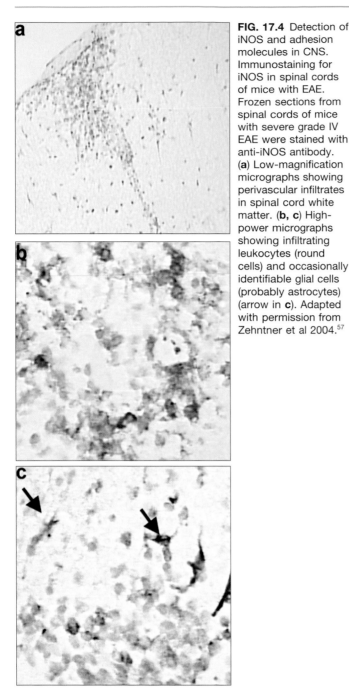

FIG. 17.4 Detection of iNOS and adhesion molecules in CNS. Immunostaining for iNOS in spinal cords of mice with EAE. Frozen sections from spinal cords of mice with severe grade IV EAE were stained with anti-iNOS antibody. (**a**) Low-magnification micrographs showing perivascular infiltrates in spinal cord white matter. (**b, c**) High-power micrographs showing infiltrating leukocytes (round cells) and occasionally identifiable glial cells (probably astrocytes) (arrow in **c**). Adapted with permission from Zehntner et al 2004.[57]

INNATE CENTRAL NERVOUS SYSTEM IMMUNITY IS CRITICAL FOR EXPERIMENTAL AUTOIMMUNE ENCEPHALOMYELITIS

The concept of innate immunity has received much attention in recent years. The term can be somewhat loosely employed to describe those immune responses that do not involve antigen receptor-bearing cells (the adaptive response), and risks being defined more by what it is not than what it is. The clearest definitions are those deriving from immune responses to pathogens that express pathogen-associated molecular pattern (PAMP) antigens, which are recognized by innate receptors and so induce immune responses through broad recognition of 'pathogen' as opposed to 'self'. This basic concept of innate responsiveness to pathogens has obvious evolutionary advantage and is easily understood as a modification of classical immunological self–

non-self concepts. In the context of EAE, CNS innate immunity extends to include responses of glial cells, which parallels the greater complexity now appreciated for other tissues, where innate responses are understood to be induced not only by infection but also by inflammation and injury. The latter stimulus introduces the concept that there may be endogenous, non-pathogen-derived ligands for innate receptors and thus the simple self–vs-non-self distinction becomes blurred. This also widens the definition of an innate receptor to include cell surface receptors that bind ligands produced in response to loss of homeostasis and so allows use of definitions such as innate cytokines or chemokines. Cytokines and chemokines, whether induced by antigen recognition or not, are dealt with in a separate section. Here we will consider genetic approaches to dissection of the role of receptors and enzymes that operate independently of adaptive responses, whether or not they may be involved in adaptive responses, and so fall into the broad category of innate mediators.

What emerges from these studies is that innate mechanisms operate as often as not to downregulate the inflammatory response, exposing a complex control network that must be overcome in order to induce EAE. The need for aggressive adjuvants likely has as much to do with circumventing innate regulation as with the traditional 'breaking of tolerance' that is usually suggested as its role.

TOLL-LIKE RECEPTORS

The toll-like receptors (TLRs) are mammalian homologs of receptors first described in *Drosophila*. A total of 11 TLRs have been defined at time of writing. They recognize categories of PAMPs, including dsRNA, flagellin, bacterial CpG DNA motifs and bacterial and fungal cell wall components such as lipoproteins and petidoglycans.[67] Many of the TLRs function as dimers, either as homodimers or as heterodimers with other TLRs. TLR2 and TLR4 can also associate with CD14, which functions as a receptor for lipopolysaccharide with TLR4.[68] It is frequently observed that, in EAE, or even when lipopolysaccharide is the stimulus, the rodent CNS shows a predisposition for upregulation of TLR2.[69] Nevertheless, both rodent and human glial cells have been shown to be capable of expressing a wide range of TLRs in vivo and in vitro.[70,71] In the first direct test of TLR involvement in EAE, TLR4 was implicated in MOG-induced EAE by use of TLR4-deficient mice, which show reduced response to pertussis toxin, a commonly used adjuvant, and reduced leukocyte interaction with cerebrovascular endothelium.[72,73] In contradiction to this, Prinz and colleagues did not observe any effect of TLR2- or TLR4-deficiency on susceptibility to MOG-induced EAE in C57Bl/6 mice. However, their study noted a dependence on TLR9.[74] This was not ascribable to response to bacterial CpGs in adjuvant but appeared to reflect a requirement for innate response within the CNS. It is expected that similar studies of this and other TLRs will appear in the near future. In particular, the observation that TLR2 is required for the microglial response to axonal injury that leads to chemokine expression and leukocyte infiltration[75] points to a role for this TLR member in inflammation.

INNATE SIGNALING

An alternative approach to dissection of the role of innate responsiveness in EAE has been to target signaling pathways. The tyrosine kinase receptor RON is expressed on selected subpopulations of tissue macrophages and engages the ligand macrophage-stimulating protein MSP. RON levels are reduced in MS and EAE. Mice deficient in RON showed reduced IL-4 production when EAE was induced by immunization with MOG peptide, and EAE was exacerbated, with increased demyelination and gliosis.[76] Treatment with MSP itself reduces release of proinflammatory cytokines by human and rodent monocytoid cells, and RON-deficient mice showed a significant increase in IL-1β, IL-12, MMP-12 and TNF in spinal cord in EAE. Interestingly, unmanipulated RON knockout animals did not show any differences from wild-type controls as regards cytokine and chemokine levels, arguing that the RON receptor differs from, for example, the TREM receptor, deficiency in which is associated with spontaneous microglial activation and neurodegenerative disease.[77] RON appears to act as a regulator of innate inflammatory response rather than of normal function.

COMPLEMENT

Complement proteins also appear to mediate innate regulation. A recent study showed that the complement binding/inhibitory protein DAF or CD55 downregulates T-cell responses and, when knocked out, reveals higher basal T-cell responses to mitogenic or antigenic stimulation. Correspondingly, mice deficient in DAF showed exacerbated MOG-induced EAE.[78] Mice deficient in another complement binding protein, CD59a, were similarly more susceptible to MOG-induced EAE and developed more severe disease.[79] Identification of a role for complement as a repressor of T cell response is of interest, since complement is synthesized in the CNS[80] and activation of the alternative pathway has been proposed to play a role in the effector phase of EAE.[81] For instance, overexpression of the complement inhibitor sCrry in the CNS made mice resistant to EAE.[82] DAF/CD55 has been reported to be upregulated on neurons in chronic (but not acute) EAE in marmosets and Rhesus monkeys, and to protect them against complement attack.[83] Mice deficient in the C5 complement component showed reduced remyelination, increased axonal depletion and increased gliosis in EAE, suggesting a protective role for C5.[84] It was also recently reported that C4-deficient C57Bl/6 mice show no difference in susceptibility to MOG-induced EAE,[85] arguing against a role for either the classical or mannose-binding lectin pathway of complement activation in EAE and indirectly supporting the proposition that the alternative pathway operates in the CNS.

MATRIX METALLOPROTEINASES

Interest in these zinc-containing cellular proteases in EAE grew initially from their implication in metastasis of cancer cells, thus directing attention to their potential role in degradation of the extracellular matrix during leukocyte infiltration to and within the CNS. MMPs and the related ADAMs are also of interest for their activity in cleaving membrane-associated molecules, notably TNFα, the soluble form of which is generated by ADAM-17 (TACE), and modulation of the biological activity of chemokines. A variety of other roles for MMPs in CNS inflammation have been proposed.[86] Expression of many MMPs and ADAMs are up- and downregulated in CNS inflammation in MS and EAE, with evidence for immune and neural cell sources.[87,88] Functionally active enzyme requires post-translational modification of precursor proteins but correspondence between RNA and protein, or substrate degradation, has been shown[88] (Fig. 17.5). Inhibitor studies suggested that MMPs

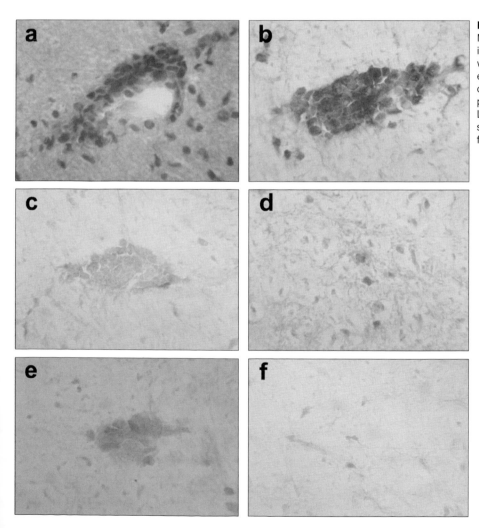

FIG. 17.5 In situ hybridization for TIMP-1 and MMP-10 expression in EAE. (a) Perivascular infiltrates in cerebellar white matter of mice with EAE were identified using hematoxylin–eosin staining. (b, d) Infiltrates were hybridized on separate sections with (b) TIMP-1 antisense probe and (d) MMP-10 antisense probe. (c, e) Lack of hybridization with TIMP-1 and MMP-10 sense probes, respectively. With permission from Toft-Hansen et al 2004.[88]

would play a propathological role in EAE,[89] and this has been supported by reduced EAE susceptibility in analyses of young MMP-9-deficient mice[90] and indirectly by enhanced susceptibility in MMP-2-deficient mice,[91] which was attributed to increased levels of MMP-9, or by overexpressing MMP-2 using viral vectors to down-regulate MMP-9 and confer resistance.[92] More recent analysis of older MMP-12-deficient mice reveals a regulatory role, in that these mice were more susceptible to EAE.[24] Weaver et al's data show, therefore, that upregulation of an MMP can be protective in EAE, and specifically that MMP-12 functions in part by modulating the Th1/Th2 effector cytokine balance. Although the mechanism involves differential regulation of critical transcription factors, the complexity of MMP interactions so far suggests that this may not be the whole story. What is clear is that MMPs may direct conflicting outcomes in EAE and, until more selective inhibitors become available, targeting them to control inflammatory demyelinating disease seems a distant prospect.

T-CELL APOPTOSIS IS A NATURAL REGULATOR OF EXPERIMENTAL AUTOIMMUNE ENCEPHALOMYELITIS

A characteristic aspect of many EAE models, as of MS, is remission from active disease, frequently followed by relapses, depending on specifics of the model used. It has been shown that T cells in the CNS apoptose and that this is associated to remission from EAE.[93,94] Apoptosis is mediated by a cascade of enzyme activations, notably the effector or death caspases. These differ from regulatory caspases such as caspase-1, which is implicated in post-translational processing of cytokines such as IL-1 and IL-18. Deletion, inhibition or blockade of caspase-1 had previously been shown to inhibit MOG-induced EAE, in caspase-1-deficient or wild-type C57Bl/6 mice.[95] The death cascade not only acts to terminate the T cell response but is also implicated in oligodendrocyte loss and demyelination. Effects of its inhibition would therefore be expected to vary with the cell source that is targeted. Thus, targeting a baculovirus p35 caspase inhibitor to oligodendrocytes in transgenic mice protected those mice against MOG-induced EAE.[96] Correspondingly, over-expression of the anti-apoptotic protein Bcl-2 in neurons was also protective.[97] By contrast, transgenic overexpression of Bcl-2 in T cells, while having no effect on initial disease onset or severity nor on first recovery from disease, did lead to more severe symptoms in chronic MOG-induced EAE.[98] Bcl-2 acts at the level of mitochondria, where it inhibits the release of cytochrome c, a normal part of the apoptotic cascade. The caspase cascade is initiated by caspase-3, or FADD-like IL-1β-converting enzyme (FLICE). FLICE is regulated by a natural inhibitor, cellular FLICE inhibitory protein or c-FLIP. FLIP is a potent inhibitor of death-receptor-induced apoptosis, and effects of its overexpression have been examined in MOG-induced EAE. In one study, the long form of human c-FLIP was expressed by retroviral transfer in hemopoietic stem cells to express it in the CNS in EAE. This resulted in exacerbation of infiltration and symptoms in acute EAE and prolongation of chronic EAE, consistent with a protective effect on otherwise apoptosing T cells.[99] A different effect was obtained when c-FLIP was expressed in T cells using a CD2 promoter. In this study, Th2 polarization was affected, so that a Th2 response was induced rather than the usual Th1 response and animals were resistant to EAE.[100] Transfer of c-FLIP-transgenic T cells could ameliorate established EAE in wild-type mice. Reasons for the different outcomes could include the different cell source of c-FLIP, and whether or not expression in the CNS was actually achieved. This highlights the need for caution in interpretation of gene overexpression, in that outcomes may not always reflect the primary activity of the gene-encoded protein or enzyme.

Another class of apoptosis inhibitors are the inhibitors of apoptosis (IAPs). These intracellular proteins act as natural caspase inhibitors and their expression is increased in MS.[101] It has been reported that targeting one of the IAPs, the X-linked IAP (XIAP), using antisense has beneficial effects on EAE, as a consequence of amplification of T cell apoptosis in the CNS.[102] Conversely, apoptosis-inducing factor (AIF) has been implicated through antisense inhibition in TNFα-mediated apoptotic death of oligodendrocytes in EAE.[103]

CHEMOKINES AND ADHESION MOLECULES DRIVE IMMUNE CELL ENTRY TO THE CENTRAL NERVOUS SYSTEM

Entry of leukocytes to the CNS is a critical step in the initiation of EAE. Many experimental models include animals in which an autoimmune response is induced but that do not develop CNS disease. This has in many cases been shown to reflect a defect in immune cell entry and, although the exact causes remain uncertain, it illustrates the importance of cellular entry for CNS inflammation. For example, the principal consequence of lack of TNFα or its receptor TNFR1 is a delay in onset of EAE, which is characterized by a build-up of leukocytes in perivascular space in spinal cord blood vessels. Murphy et al analyzed the mechanism underlying this build-up and identified a TNF-induced chemokine response that was critical for initiation of parenchymal invasion and disease. The chemokines CCL2/MCP-1, CCL8/TCA3 and CXCL10/IP10 were particularly implicated. Mice that were deficient in the receptor for CCL8, normally expressed by microglia, showed a similar delay in onset.[18] In the absence of TNFα or CCL8, EAE eventually ensued, probably indicating redundancy with other chemokines and cytokines. It had previously been reported by a number of labs that C57Bl/6 mice deficient in CCL2 or its receptor CCL2 were resistant to EAE.[104–106] This may turn out to be another instance where strain background influences the outcome of a gene deficiency, because in BALB/c and C57Bl/6×129J mice, EAE can be induced in the absence of CCL2.[107] In fact, this study also showed that C57Bl/6 CCR2-deficient mice were susceptible, albeit with reduced frequency. EAE induced in the absence of CCR2 was characterized by a neutrophil infiltration rather than macrophages, a feature shared with IFNγ-deficient mice[63,108] and probably reflecting similar chemokine disruption[109] (Fig. 17.6).

Overexpression of CCL2/MCP-1 in the CNS had previously been reported to induce a nonsymptomatic perivascular leukocyte accumulation,[110] which could be converted to frank encephalopathy by systemic administration of pertussis toxin.[111] Elhofy et al have shown that such mice are resistant to EAE, showing reduced clinical symptoms despite equivalent infiltration by T cells and macrophages. Protection reflected reduced Th1 response in the CNS, as a result of reduced IL-12 receptor expression on T cells.[112]

ADHESION MOLECULES

Adhesion molecules as a broad group participate in the infiltration of leukocytes into the CNS at many levels, participating in the rolling (E-selectin, P-selectin, L-selectin CD62-L), adhesion (ICAM-1, β7 integrin) and extravasation through the endothelium (PECAM); there are also numerous roles reported for adhesion molecules not directly involving cellular traffic, rather directly impacting them in the roles of cell activation

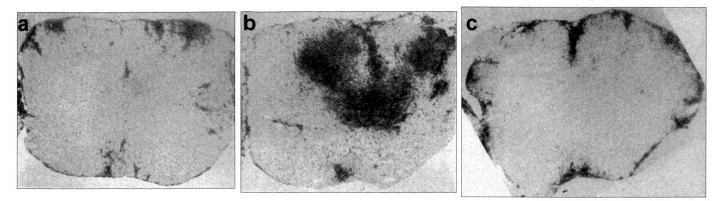

FIG. 17.6 Distribution of infiltrates in spinal cords from three models of EAE. Cross-sections of frozen spinal cords from perfused misce with severe EAE were stained with anti-CD11b, which visualizes macrophages, activated microglia and granulocytes. **Left-hand panel**: SJL/J mouse with MBP-induced EAE. Middle panel: IFNγ-deficient BALB/c mouse with MBP-inducing EAE; **right-hand panel**: C57B1/6 mouse with MIG-induced EAE. MBP-EAE sections courtesy of Elise Tran.

and effector function. L-selectin is expressed on leukocytes, while P- and E- selectin are expressed on endothelium. Brocke et al had suggested that L-selectin is not required for development of EAE based on antibody blockade.[113] However, L-selectin[-/-] MBP TCR transgenic mice do not develop EAE.[114] Interestingly Grewal et al suggest that L-selectins are not essential for the adhesion and extravasation into the CNS, as lack of L-selectin did not prevent infiltration into the perivascular tissue. Their analysis showed that L-selectin does not effect activation of T cells but rather plays an essential role in the effector function of the macrophage. Using chimeras, L-selectin expression on macrophages was determined to be essential for induction of EAE. L-selectin has also been shown to directly interact with oligodendrocytes, placing selectins at the immune–glial interface of effector function rather than just 'at the front door'. It has been shown using antibody blockade that P-selectin inhibits onset of EAE[115] and that selectins and their ligands are important for recruitment of antigen specific T cells to the CNS.[116] In contrast to P-selectin, mice lacking the L- and P-selectin ligand PSGL-1 showed no apparent deficit in either induction or progression of EAE.[117] It was proposed from these findings that PSGL-1 is only important in very early trafficking events and that in chronic disease other adhesion pathways play a role. The beauty of adhesion molecule biology, as for chemokines but less for cytokines, is that there is a lot of redundancy built into the system. An instance where redundancy did not overcome the lack of an adhesion molecule is in the lack of the B7 integrin. The A4β7 integrin very late antigen (VLA)4 has been implicated in adhesion of T cells to CNS endothelia, and antibody blockade prevented EAE.[118,119] This adhesion system has been targeted for MS therapy. Kanwar et al showed that mice deficient in β7 integrin were partially resistant to EAE. T cells from these mice were poor encephalitogens and adoptive transfer of β7-deficient lymphocytes to wild-type, or of wild-type immune cells to β7-deficient, recipients led to delayed development of EAE.[120]

The adhesion molecule ICAM-1 (CD54) is a ligand for the integrins LFA-1 (CD11a/CD18) and Mac-1 (CD11b/CD18). Both P-selectin and ICAM-1 have also been implicated in the development of effector function of regulatory T cells in individual knockout mice, irrespective of their role in trafficking.[121] Consistent with this, ICAM-1-deficient mice develop more severe MOG- or MBP-induced EAE in C57Bl/6-crossed mice, and this was shown to reflect a lack of Th2 cytokines rather than having any effect on infiltration of immune cells to the CNS.[122]

CD43 or leukosialin is a large sialoglycoprotein that is broadly expressed on bone-marrow-derived cells, including CD4[+] and CD8[+] T cells. CD43 has been implicated, by antibody blockade, in entry of T cells to secondary lymphoid organs and to tissues. Mice deficient in the CD43 gene fail to express either of the two isoforms that are differentially expressed by CD4[+] and CD8[+] T cells.[123] These mice are resistant to actively induced and adoptively transferred MOGp35–55-induced EAE. Histopathological analysis suggests that resistance was due to blockade of T cell entry to the CNS, although there was also a shift away from Th1 towards Th2 immune response (reduced IFNγ and increased IL-4), opposite to the effect seen in ICAM-1-deficient mice.

An interesting contrast to the pattern whereby removal of an adhesion ligand impedes inflammation is provided by mice lacking PECAM/CD31. This molecule is expressed on platelets, monocytes, granulocytes, lymphocytes and endothelium. Staining for PECAM can be used for dramatic highlighting of endothelia in inflamed CNS.[109] PECAM-directed interaction with lymphocytes via either homophilic (PECAM) or heterophilic (glucosaminoglycans) ligand binding mediates specific inflammatory infiltration to tissues but antibody blocking showed that it is not absolutely required for development of EAE. Mice that lack PECAM/CD31 unexpectedly showed accelerated onset of EAE.[124] The likely explanation for this relates to the role of PECAM in promoting endothelial integrity, which would not be affected by antibody blockade.

SUMMARY AND CONCLUSIONS

The mammalian genome contains approximately 30 000 genes. It is interesting to note that the effects on EAE of genetic manipulations that range from complete ablation of expression through to widespread upregulation of a variety of genes converge to three broad immune consequences. These are the Th1/Th2 balance, entry of cells to the CNS and the activation and regulation of effector functions within the CNS (Fig. 17.7). There may be isolated instances where the mechanistic consequence of a genetic manipulation do not easily fit to this triad, but the ability to fit most of them is impressive. The power of genetic manipulation in this mouse model is therefore revealed through an impressive consensus of effects. They in turn reveal fundamental control steps in the disease. These become rational targets for therapy in clinical diseases that are modelled in whole or in part by EAE, the most obvious example being MS.

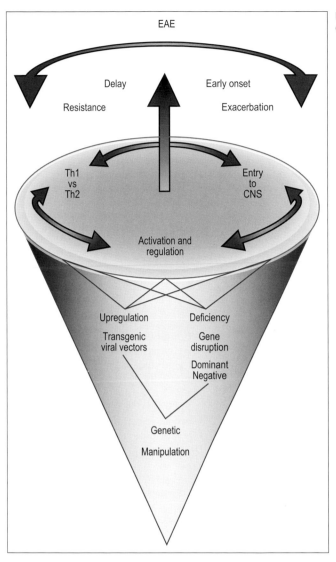

FIG. 17.7 Schematic to illustrate the Th1/Th2 balance, entry of cells to the CNS and the activation and regulation of effector functions within the CNS.

REFERENCES

1. Bradl M, Bauer J, Inomata T et al. Transgenic Lewis rats overexpressing the proteolipid protein gene: myelin degeneration and its effect on T cell-mediated experimental autoimmune encephalomyelitis. Acta Neuropathol (Berl) 1999; 97: 595–606.
2. Friese MA, Fugger L. Autoreactive CD8+ T cells in multiple sclerosis: a new target for therapy? Brain 2005; 128: 1747–1763.
3. Owens T, Wekerle H, Antel J. Genetic models for CNS inflammation. Nat Med 2001; 7: 161–166.
4. Krakowski ML, Owens T. The central nervous system environment controls effector CD4+ T cell cytokine profile in experimental allergic encephalomyelitis. Eur J Immunol 1997; 27: 2840–2847.
5. Abdul-Majid KB, Wefer J, Stadelmann C et al. Comparing the pathogenesis of experimental autoimmune encephalomyelitis in CD4−/− and CD8−/− DBA/1 mice defines qualitative roles of different T cell subsets. J Neuroimmunol 2003; 141: 10–19.
6. Zeine R, Owens T. Loss rather than downregulation of CD4+ T cells as a mechanism for remission from experimental allergic encephalomyelitis. J Neuroimmunol 1993; 44: 193–198.
7. Huseby ES, Liggitt D, Brabb T et al. A pathogenic role for myelin-specific CD8+ T cells in a model for multiple sclerosis. J Exp Med 2001; 194: 669–676.
8. Sun D, Whitaker JN, Huang Z et al. Myelin antigen-specific CD8+ T cells are encephalitogenic and produce severe disease in C57BL/6 mice. J Immunol 2001; 166: 7579–7587.
9. Ford ML, Evavold BD. Specificity, magnitude, and kinetics of MOG-specific CD8+ T cell responses during experimental autoimmune encephalomyelitis. Eur J Immunol 2005; 35: 76–85.
10. Wheeler RD, Brough D, Le Feuvre RA et al. Interleukin-18 induces expression and release of cytokines from murine glial cells: interactions with interleukin-1 beta. J Neurochem 2003; 85: 1412–1420.
11. Zhang GX, Yu S, Gran B et al. Role of IL-12 receptor beta 1 in regulation of T cell response by APC in experimental autoimmune encephalomyelitis. J Immunol 2003; 171: 4485–4492.
12. Cua DJ, Sherlock J, Chen Y et al. Interleukin-23 rather than interleukin-12 is the critical cytokine for autoimmune inflammation of the brain. Nature 2003; 421: 744–748.
13. Langrish CL, Chen Y, Blumenschein WM et al. IL-23 drives a pathogenic T cell population that induces autoimmune inflammation. J Exp Med 2005; 201: 233–240.
14. Aggarwal S, Gurney AL. IL-17: prototype member of an emerging cytokine family. J Leukoc Biol 2002; 71: 1–8.
15. Mendel I, Natarajan K, Ben-Nun A, Shevach EM. A novel protective model against experimental allergic encephalomyelitis in mice expressing a transgenic TCR-specific for myelin oligodendrocyte glycoprotein. J Neuroimmunol 2004; 149: 10–21.
16. Komiyama Y, Nakae S, Matsuki T et al. IL-17 plays an important role in the development of experimental autoimmune encephalomyelitis. J Immunol 2006; 177: 566–573.
17. Lock C, Hermans G, Pedotti R et al. Gene-microarray analysis of multiple sclerosis lesions yields new targets validated in autoimmune encephalomyelitis. Nat Med 2002; 8: 500–508.

18. Marusic S, Miyashiro JS, Douhan J III et al. Local delivery of granulocyte macrophage colony-stimulating factor by retrovirally transduced antigen-specific T cells leads to severe, chronic experimental autoimmune encephalomyelitis in mice. Neurosci Lett 2002; 332: 185–189.

19. Murphy CA, Hoek RM, Wiekowski MT et al. Interactions between hemopoietically derived TNF and central nervous system-resident glial chemokines underlie initiation of autoimmune inflammation in the brain. J Immunol 2002; 169: 7054–7062.

20. Arnett HA, Mason J, Marino M et al. TNFα promotes proliferation of oligodendrocyte progenitors and remyelination. Nat Neurosci 2001; 4: 1116–1122.

21. Linker RA, Maurer M, Gaupp S et al. CNTF is a major protective factor in demyelinating CNS disease: a neurotrophic cytokine as modulator in neuroinflammation. Nat Med 2002; 8: 620–624.

22. Winter CG, Saotome Y, Levison SW, Hirsh D. A role for ciliary neurotrophic factor as an inducer of reactive gliosis, the glial response to central nervous system injury. Proc Natl Acad Sci USA 1995; 92: 5865–5869.

23. Ruuls SR, Hoek RM, Ngo VN et al. Membrane-bound tnf supports secondary lymphoid organ structure but is subservient to secreted tnf in driving autoimmune inflammation. Immunity 2001; 15: 533–543.

24. Zheng Y, Saftig P, Hartmann D, Blobel C. Evaluation of the contribution of different ADAMs to tumor necrosis factor alpha (TNFα) shedding and of the function of the TNFα ectodomain in ensuring selective stimulated shedding by the TNFα convertase (TACE/ADAM17). J Biol Chem 2004; 279: 42898–42906.

25. Weaver A, Goncalves da Silva A, Nuttall RK et al. An elevated matrix metalloproteinase (MMP) in an animal model of multiple sclerosis is protective by affecting Th1/Th2 polarization. FASEB J 2005; 19: 1668–1670.

26. Arnason BG. Immunologic therapy of multiple sclerosis. Annu Rev Med 1999; 50: 291–302.

27. Keegan BM, Noseworthy JH. Multiple sclerosis. Annu Rev Med 2002; 53: 285–302.

28. Teige I, Treschow A, Teige A et al. IFN-beta gene deletion leads to augmented and chronic demyelinating experimental autoimmune encephalomyelitis. J Immunol 2003; 170: 4776–4784.

29. Akiyama H, Ikeda K, Katoh M et al. Expression of MRP14, 27E10, interferon-alpha and leukocyte common antigen by reactive microglia in postmortem human brain tissue. J Neuroimmunol 1994; 50: 195–201.

30. Yamada T, Horisberger MA, Kawaguchi N et al. Immunohistochemistry using antibodies to alpha-interferon and its induced protein, MxA, in Alzheimer's and Parkinson's disease brain tissues. Neurosci Lett 1994; 181: 61–64.

31. Theofilopoulos AN, Baccala R, Beutler B, Kono DH. Type I interferons (alpha/beta) in immunity and autoimmunity. Annu Rev Immunol 2005; 23: 307–336.

32. Zheng W, Flavell RA. The transcription factor GATA-3 is necessary and sufficient for Th2 cytokine gene expression in CD4 T cells. Cell 1997; 89: 587–596.

33. Szabo SJ, Kim ST, Costa GL et al. A novel transcription factor, T-bet, directs Th1 lineage commitment. Cell 2000; 100: 655–669.

34. Agnello D, Lankford CS, Bream J et al. Cytokines and transcription factors that regulate T helper cell differentiation: new players and new insights. J Clin Immunol 2003; 23: 147–161.

35. Lovett-Racke AE, Rocchini AE, Choy J et al. Silencing T-bet defines a critical role in the differentiation of autoreactive T lymphocytes. Immunity 2004; 21: 719–731.

36. Chitnis T, Najafian N, Benou C et al. Effect of targeted disruption of STAT4 and STAT6 on the induction of experimental autoimmune encephalomyelitis. J Clin Invest 2001; 108: 739–747.

37. Bettelli E, Sullivan B, Szabo SJ et al. Loss of T-bet, but not STAT1, prevents the development of experimental autoimmune encephalomyelitis. J Exp Med 2004; 200: 79–87.

38. Brambilla R, Bracchi-Ricard V, Hu WH et al. Inhibition of astroglial nuclear factor kappaB reduces inflammation and improves functional recovery after spinal cord injury. J Exp Med 2005; 202: 145–156.

39. Bethea JR, Bracchi-Ricard V, Brambilla R. Inhibition of astroglial NF-kB reduces inflammation and improves functional recovery following spinal cord injury and EAE. Immunology 2005; 116: abstract OP78 19.

40. Liedtke W, Edelmann W, Chiu FC et al. Experimental autoimmune encephalomyelitis in mice lacking glial fibrillary acidic protein is characterized by a more severe clinical course and an infiltrative central nervous system lesion. Am J Pathol 1998; 152: 251–259.

41. Owens T, Tran ET, Hassan-Zahraee M et al. The pathogenesis of encephalitis. Amsterdam: Elsevier; 2001.

42. Greter M, Heppner FL, Lemos MP et al. Dendritic cells permit immune invasion of the CNS in an animal model of multiple sclerosis. Nat Med 2005; 11: 328–334.

43. McMahon EJ, Bailey SL, Castenada CV et al. Epitope spreading initiates in the CNS in two mouse models of multiple sclerosis. Nat Med 2005; 11: 335–339.

44. Bailey SL, Schreiner B, McMahon EJ, Miller SD. CNS myeloid DCs presenting endogenous myelin peptides 'preferentially' polarize CD4+ T(H)-17 cells in relapsing EAE. Nat Immunol 2007; 8: 172–180.

45. Serafini B, Rosicarelli B, Magliozzi R et al. Detection of ectopic B-cell follicles with germinal centers in the meninges of patients with secondary progressive multiple sclerosis. Brain Pathol 2004; 14: 164–174.

46. Chang TT, Jabs C, Sobel RA et al. Studies in B7-deficient mice reveal a critical role for B7 costimulation in both induction and effector phases of experimental autoimmune encephalomyelitis. J Exp Med 1999; 190: 733–740.

47. Girvin AM, Dal Canto MC, Rhee L et al. A critical role for B7/CD28 costimulation in experimental autoimmune encephalomyelitis: a comparative study using costimulatory molecule-deficient mice and monoclonal antibody blockade. J Immunol 2000; 164: 136–143.

48. Jabs C, Greve B, Chang TT et al. Genetic background determines the requirement for B7 costimulation in induction of autoimmunity. Eur J Immunol 2002; 32: 2687–2697.

49. Chitnis T, Najafian N, Abdallah KA et al. CD28-independent induction of experimental autoimmune encephalomyelitis. J Clin Invest 2001; 107: 575–583.

50. Chambers CA, Sullivan TJ, Allison JP. Lymphoproliferation in CTLA-4-deficient mice is mediated by costimulation-dependent activation of CD4+ T cells. Immunity 1997; 7: 885–895.

51. Watanabe N, Gavrieli M, Sedy JR et al. BTLA is a lymphocyte inhibitory receptor with similarities to CTLA-4 and PD-1. Nat Immunol 2003; 4: 670–679.

52. Salama AD, Chitnis T, Imitola J et al. Critical role of the programmed death-1 (PD-1) pathway in regulation of experimental autoimmune encephalomyelitis. J Exp Med 2003; 198: 71–78.

53. Zehntner SP, Brisebois M, Tran E et al. Constitutive expression of a costimulatory ligand on antigen-presenting cells in the nervous system drives demyelinating disease. FASEB J 2003; 17: 1910–1912.

54. Muhl H, Pfeilschifter J. Anti-inflammatory properties of pro-inflammatory interferon-gamma. Int Immunopharmacol 2003; 3: 1247–1255.

55. Furlan R, Brambilla E, Ruffini F et al. Intrathecal delivery of IFN-gamma protects C57BL/6 mice from chronic-progressive experimental autoimmune encephalomyelitis by increasing apoptosis of central nervous system-infiltrating lymphocytes. J Immunol 2001; 167: 1821–1829.

56. Dalton DK, Haynes L, Chu CQ et al. Interferon gamma eliminates responding CD4 T cells during mycobacterial infection by inducing apoptosis of activated CD4 T cells. J Exp Med 2000; 192: 117–122.

57. Zehntner SP, Bourbonniere L, Hassan-Zahraee M et al. Bone marrow-derived versus parenchymal sources of inducible nitric oxide synthase in experimental autoimmune encephalomyelitis. J Neuroimmunol 2004; 150: 70–79.

58. Lin W, Harding HP, Ron D, Popko B. Endoplasmic reticulum stress modulates the response of myelinating oligodendrocytes to the immune cytokine interferon-gamma. J Cell Biol 2005; 169: 603–612.

59. Shi FD, Takeda K, Akira S et al. IL-18 directs autoreactive T cells and promotes autodestruction in the central nervous system via induction of IFN-gamma by NK cells. J Immunol 2000; 165: 3099–3104.

60. Gutcher I, Urich E, Wolter K et al. Interleukin 18-independent engagement of interleukin 18 receptor-alpha is required for autoimmune inflammation. Nat Immunol 2006; 9: 946–953.

61. Schif-Zuck S, Westermann J, Netzer N et al. Targeted overexpression of IL-18 binding protein at the central nervous system overrides flexibility in functional polarization of antigen-specific Th2 cells. J Immunol 2005; 174: 4307–4315.

62. Chu CQ, Wittmer S, Dalton DK. Failure to suppress the expansion of the activated CD4 T cell population in interferon gamma-

deficient mice leads to exacerbation of experimental autoimmune encephalomyelitis. J Exp Med 2000; 192: 123–128.

63. Zehntner SP, Brickman C, Bourbonniere L et al. Neutrophils that infiltrate the central nervous system regulate T cell responses. J Immunol 2005; 174: 5124–5131.

64. Willenborg DO, Staykova MA, Cowden WB. Our shifting understanding of the role of nitric oxide in autoimmune encephalomyelitis: a review. J Neuroimmunol 1999; 100: 21–35.

65. Kahl KG, Schmidt HH, Jung S et al. Experimental autoimmune encephalomyelitis in mice with a targeted deletion of the inducible nitric oxide synthase gene: increased T-helper 1 response. Neurosci Lett 2004; 358: 58–62.

66. Dalton DK, Wittmer S. Nitric-oxide-dependent and independent mechanisms of protection from CNS inflammation during Th1-mediated autoimmunity: evidence from EAE in iNOS KO mice. J Neuroimmunol 2005; 160: 110–121.

67. Medzhitov R. Toll-like receptors and innate immunity. Nat Rev Immunol 2001; 1: 135–145.

68. Akira S, Takeda K. Toll-like receptor signalling. Nat Rev Immunol 2004; 4: 499–511.

69. Zekki H, Feinstein DL, Rivest S. The clinical course of experimental autoimmune encephalomyelitis is associated with a profound and sustained transcriptional activation of the genes encoding toll-like receptor 2 and CD14 in the mouse CNS. Brain Pathol 2002; 12: 308–319.

70. Olson JK, Girvin AM, Miller SD. Direct activation of innate and antigen-presenting functions of microglia following infection with Theiler's virus. J Virol 2001; 75: 9780–9789.

71. Bsibsi M, Ravid R, Gveric D, van Noort JM. Broad expression of Toll-like receptors in the human central nervous system. J Neuropathol Exp Neurol 2002; 61: 1013–1021.

72. Kerfoot SM, Long EM, Hickey MJ et al. TLR4 contributes to disease-inducing mechanisms resulting in central nervous system autoimmune disease. J Immunol 2004; 173: 7070–7077.

73. Racke MK, Hu W, Lovett-Racke AE. PTX cruiser: driving autoimmunity via TLR4. Trends Immunol 2005; 26: 289–291.

74. Prinz MF, Garbe H, Schmidt A et al. Innate immunity mediated by TLR9 modulates pathogenicity in an animal model of multiple sclerosis. J Clin Invest 2006; 116: 456–464.

75. Babcock A, Wirenfeldt M, Toft-Hansen H et al. Toll-like receptor 2 signaling in response to brain injury: an innate bridge to neuroinflammation. J Neurosci 2006; 26: 12826–12837.

76. Tsutsui S, Noorbakhsh F, Sullivan A et al. RON-regulated innate immunity is protective in an animal model of multiple sclerosis. Ann Neurol 2005; 57: 883–895.

77. Takahashi K, Rochford CDP, Neumann H. Clearance of apoptotic neurons without inflammation by microglial triggering receptor expressed on myeloid cells-2. J Exp Med 2005; 201: 647–657.

78. Liu J, Miwa T, Hilliard B et al. The complement inhibitory protein DAF (CD55) suppresses T cell immunity in vivo. J Exp Med 2005; 201: 567–577.

79. Mead RJ, Neal JW, Griffiths MR et al. Deficiency of the complement regulator CD59a enhances disease severity, demyelination and axonal injury in murine acute experimental allergic encephalomyelitis. Lab Invest 2004; 84: 21–28.

80. Nadeau S, Rivest S. The complement system is an integrated part of the natural innate immune response in the brain. FASEB J 2001; 15: 1410–1412.

81. Nataf S, Carroll SL, Wetsel RA et al. Attenuation of experimental autoimmune demyelination in complement-deficient mice. J Immunol 2000; 165: 5867–5873.

82. Davoust N, Nataf S, Reiman R et al. Central nervous system-targeted expression of the complement inhibitor sCrry prevents experimental allergic encephalomyelitis. J Immunol 1999; 163: 6551–6556.

83. Van Beek J, van Meurs M, t'Hart BA et al. Decay-accelerating factor (CD55) is expressed by neurons in response to chronic but not acute autoimmune central nervous system inflammation associated with complement activation. J Immunol 2005; 174: 2353–2365.

84. Weerth SH, Rus H, Shin ML, Raine CS. Complement C5 in experimental autoimmune encephalomyelitis (EAE) facilitates remyelination and prevents gliosis. Am J Pathol 2003; 163: 1069–1080.

85. Boos LA, Szalai AJ, Barnum SR. Murine complement C4 is not required for experimental autoimmune encephalomyelitis. Glia 2005; 49: 158–160.

86. Yong VW, Power C, Forsyth P, Edwards DR. Metalloproteinases in biology and pathology of the nervous system. Nat Rev Neurosci 2001; 2: 502–511.

87. Bar-Or A, Nuttall RK, Duddy M et al. Analyses of all matrix metalloproteinase members in leukocytes emphasize monocytes as major inflammatory mediators in multiple sclerosis. Brain 2003; 126: 2738–2749.

88. Toft-Hansen H, Nuttall RK, Edwards DR, Owens T. Key metalloproteinases are expressed by specific cell types in experimental autoimmune encephalomyelitis. J Immunol 2004; 173: 5209–5218.

89. Hewson AK, Smith T, Leonard JP, Cuzner ML. Suppression of experimental allergic encephalomyelitis in the Lewis rat by the matrix metalloproteinase inhibitor Ro31–9790. Inflamm Res 1995; 44: 345–349.

90. Dubois B, Masure S, Hurtenbach U et al. Resistance of young gelatinase B-deficient mice to experimental autoimmune encephalomyelitis and necrotizing tail lesions. J Clin Invest 1999; 104: 1507–1515.

91. Esparza J, Kruse M, Lee J et al. MMP-2 null mice exhibit an early onset and severe experimental autoimmune encephalomyelitis due to an increase in MMP-9 expression and activity. FASEB J 2004; 18: 1682–1691.

92. Nygardas PT, Gronberg SA, Heikkila J et al. Treatment of experimental autoimmune encephalomyelitis with a neurotropic alphavirus vector expressing

tissue inhibitor of metalloproteinase-2. Scand J Immunol 2004; 60: 372–381.

93. Schmied M, Breitschopf H, Gold R et al. Apoptosis of T lymphocytes in experimental autoimmune encephalomyelitis. Evidence for programmed cell death as a mechanism to control inflammation in the brain. Am J Pathol 1993; 143: 446–452.

94. Pender MP. Genetically determined failure of activation-induced apoptosis of autoreactive T cells as a cause of multiple sclerosis. Lancet 1998; 351: 978–981.

95. Furlan R, Martino G, Galbiati F et al. Caspase-1 regulates the inflammatory process leading to autoimmune demyelination. J Immunol 1999; 163: 2403–2409.

96. Hisahara S, Araki T, Sugiyama F et al. Targeted expression of baculovirus p35 caspase inhibitor in oligodendrocytes protects mice against autoimmune-mediated demyelination. EMBO J 2000; 19: 341–348.

97. Offen D, Kaye JF, Bernard O et al. Mice overexpressing Bcl-2 in their neurons are resistant to myelin oligodendrocyte glycoprotein (MOG)-induced experimental autoimmune encephalomyelitis (EAE). J Mol Neurosci 2000; 15: 167–176.

98. Okuda Y, Okuda M, Bernard CC. The suppression of T cell apoptosis influences the severity of disease during the chronic phase but not the recovery from the acute phase of experimental autoimmune encephalomyelitis in mice. J Neuroimmunol 2002; 131: 115–125.

99. Djerbi M, Abdul-Majid KB, Abedi-Valugerdi M et al. Expression of the long form of human FLIP by retroviral gene transfer of hemopoietic stem cells exacerbates experimental autoimmune encephalomyelitis. J Immunol 2003; 170: 2064–2073.

100. Tseveleki V, Bauer J, Taoufik E et al. Cellular FLIP (long isoform) overexpression in T cells drives Th2 effector responses and promotes immunoregulation in experimental autoimmune encephalomyelitis. J Immunol 2004; 173: 6619–6626.

101. Sharief MK, Semra YK. Upregulation of the inhibitor of apoptosis proteins in activated T lymphocytes from patients with multiple sclerosis. J Neuroimmunol 2001; 119: 350–357.

102. Zehntner SP, Bourbonniere L, Morris SJ et al. Apoptosis induction as a therapeutic intervention in a murine model of multiple sclerosis. J Immunol 2007, submitted.

103. Jurewicz A, Matysiak M, Tybor K et al. Tumour necrosis factor-induced death of adult human oligodendrocytes is mediated by apoptosis inducing factor. Brain 2005; 128: 2675–2688.

104. Fife BT, Huffnagle GB, Kuziel WA, Karpus WJ. CC chemokine receptor 2 is critical for induction of experimental autoimmune encephalomyelitis. J Exp Med 2000; 192: 899–906.

105. Izikson L, Klein RS, Charo IF et al. Resistance to experimental autoimmune encephalomyelitis in mice lacking the CC chemokine receptor (CCR)2. J Exp Med 2000; 192: 1075–1080.

106. Huang D, Wang J, Kivisakk P et al. Absence of monocyte chemoattractant

protein 1 in mice leads to decreased local macrophage recruitment and antigen-specific T helper cell type 1 immune response in experimental autoimmune encephalomyelitis. J Exp Med 2001; 193: 713–726.

107. Gaupp S, Pitt D, Kuziel WA et al. Experimental autoimmune encephalomyelitis (EAE) in CCR2$^{-/-}$ mice: susceptibility in multiple strains. Am J Pathol 2003; 162: 139–150.

108. Willenborg DO, Fordham S, Bernard CC et al. IFN-gamma plays a critical down-regulatory role in the induction and effector phase of myelin oligodendrocyte glycoprotein-induced autoimmune encephalomyelitis. J Immunol 1996; 157: 3223–3227.

109. Tran EH, Prince EN, Owens T. IFN-gamma shapes immune invasion of the central nervous system via regulation of chemokines. J Immunol 2000; 164: 2759–2768.

110. Fuentes ME, Durham SK, Swerdel MR et al. Controlled recruitment of monocytes and macrophages to specific organs through transgenic expression of monocyte chemoattractant protein-1. J Immunol 1995; 155: 5769–5776.

111. Huang D, Tani M, Wang J et al. Pertussis toxin-induced reversible encephalopathy dependent on monocyte chemoattractant protein-1 overexpression in mice. J Neurosci 2002; 22: 10633–10642.

112. Elhofy A, Wang J, Tani M et al. Transgenic expression of CCL2 in the central nervous system prevents experimental autoimmune encephalomyelitis. J Leukoc Biol 2005; 77: 229–237.

113. Brocke S, Piercy C, Steinman L et al. Antibodies to CD44 and integrin α4, but not L-selectin, prevent central nervous system inflammation and experimental encephalomyelitis by blocking secondary leukocyte recruitment. Proc Natl Acad Sci USA 1999; 96: 6896–6901.

114. Grewal IS, Foellmer HG, Grewal KD et al. CD62L is required on effector cells for local interactions in the CNS to cause myelin damage in experimental allergic encephalomyelitis. Immunity 2001; 14: 291–302.

115. Kerfoot SM, Kubes P. Overlapping roles of P-selectin and alpha 4 integrin to recruit leukocytes to the central nervous system in experimental autoimmune encephalomyelitis. J Immunol 2002; 169: 1000–1006.

116. Piccio L, Rossi B, Scarpini E et al. Molecular mechanisms involved in lymphocyte recruitment in inflamed brain microvessels: critical roles for P-selectin glycoprotein ligand-1 and heterotrimeric G$_i$-linked receptors. J Immunol 2002; 168: 1940–1949.

117. Osmers I, Bullard DC, Barnum SR. PSGL-1 is not required for development of experimental autoimmune encephalomyelitis. J Neuroimmunol 2005; 166: 193–196.

118. Yednock TA, Cannon C, Fritz LC et al. Prevention of experimental autoimmune encephalomyelitis by antibodies against alpha 4 beta 1 integrin. Nature 1992; 356: 63–66.

119. Baron JL, Madri JA, Ruddle NH et al. Surface expression of alpha 4 integrin by CD4 T cells is required for their entry into brain parenchyma. J Exp Med 1993; 177: 57–68.

120. Kanwar JR, Harrison JE, Wang D et al. Beta7 integrins contribute to demyelinating disease of the central nervous system. J Neuroimmunol 2000; 103: 146–152.

121. Kohm AP, Carpentier PA, Anger HA, Miller SD. Cutting edge: CD4+CD25+ regulatory T cells suppress antigen-specific autoreactive immune responses and central nervous system inflammation during active experimental autoimmune encephalomyelitis. J Immunol 2002; 169: 4712–4716.

122. Samoilova EB, Horton JL, Chen Y. Experimental autoimmune encephalomyelitis in intercellular adhesion molecule-1-deficient mice. Cell Immunol 1998; 190: 83–89.

123. Ford ML, Onami TM, Sperling AI et al. CD43 modulates severity and onset of experimental autoimmune encephalomyelitis. J Immunol 2003; 171: 6527–6533.

124. Graesser D, Solowiej A, Bruckner M et al. Altered vascular permeability and early onset of experimental autoimmune encephalomyelitis in PECAM-1-deficient mice. J Clin Invest 2002; 109: 383–392.

125. Popko B, Corbin JG, Baerwald KD et al. The effects of interferon-gamma on the central nervous system. Mol Neurobiol 1997; 14: 19–35.

126. Campbell IL, Stalder AK, Akwa Y et al. Transgenic models to study the actions of cytokines in the central nervous system. Neuroimmunomodulation 1998; 5: 126–135.

127. Moore KW, de Waal Malefyt R, Coffman RL, O'Garra A. Interleukin-10 and the interleukin-10 receptor. Annu Rev Immunol 2001; 19: 683–765.

128. Ransohoff RM, Trapp BD. Taking two TRAILS. Neuron 2005; 46: 355–356.

129. Campbell IL. Transgenic mice and cytokine actions in the brain: bridging the gap between structural and functional neuropathology. Brain Res Brain Res Rev 1998; 26: 327–336.

130. Elhofy A, Kennedy KJ, Fife BT, Karpus WJ. Regulation of experimental autoimmune encephalomyelitis by chemokines and chemokine receptors. Immunol Res 2002; 25: 167–175.

131. Wang J, Asensio VC, Campbell IL. Cytokines and chemokines as mediators of protection and injury in the central nervous system assessed in transgenic mice. Curr Top Microbiol Immunol 2002; 265: 23–48.

132. Mahad DJ, Ransohoff RM. The role of MCP-1 (CCL2) and CCR2 in multiple sclerosis and experimental autoimmune encephalomyelitis (EAE). Semin Immunol 2003; 15: 23–32.

133. Ransohoff RM, Kivisakk P, Kidd G. Three or more routes for leukocyte migration into the central nervous system. Nat Rev Immunol 2003; 3: 569–581.

134. Probert L, Eugster HP, Akassoglou K et al. TNFR1 signalling is critical for the development of demyelination and the limitation of T-cell responses during immune-mediated CNS disease. Brain 2000; 123: 2005–2019.

Biology of myelin

B. Zalc and C. Lubetzki

INTRODUCTION

Myelin is a biological membrane, which enwraps axons and is deposited along axons, interrupted at regular intervals by nodes of Ranvier.[1] Myelin-forming cells in the peripheral nervous system (PNS) are Schwann cells and oligodendrocytes in the central nervous system (CNS).[2] Myelin is an electrical insulator that facilitates the rapid propagation of nerve impulses. Myelin has unique ultrastructural and biochemical characteristics.[3] With the electron microscope, it appears as a double membrane leaflet formed by the apposition of processes of the myelin-producing cells (Fig. 18.1). These membranous extensions wrap tightly in a spiral fashion around segments of axons to form internodes, delimited at each extremity by nodes of Ranvier. Therefore, the axonal membrane has access to the extracellular milieu only at the node of Ranvier. The electrical resistance of the myelin sheath is much higher than that of the axonal membrane. When a depolarization event occurs at a node of Ranvier, the local current reflecting the high local concentration of voltage-gated sodium channels at the node of Ranvier cannot reach the nearby area, which is covered by myelin, and therefore propagates only at the following node. This type of conduction of the influx is called saltatory conduction.[4,5] The biological consequence of saltatory conduction is that propagation of the nerve impulse is much faster (about 50–100 times faster) in myelinated axons compared with nonmyelinated axons of the same diameter, in which the succession of polarization–depolarization events occurs along the entire axonal membrane. The node of Ranvier is flanked by paranodal regions, interposed between the node and the juxtaparanode, and where the myelin loops are anchored to the axon. New insights into the molecular organization of these domains has emerged during the last few years (see reviews by Peles and Salzer[6] and Poliak and Peles[7]) and it was recently shown[8] that two isoforms of the cell adhesion molecule neurofascin play key roles in assembling the nodal and paranodal domains of myelinated axons and are essential for the transition to saltatory conduction in developing vertebrate nerves.

The myelin sheath has been a crucial acquisition of vertebrates, its major function being to increase the velocity of propagation of nerve impulses. The speed of propagation of action potentials along axons can be increased in two ways: either by increasing axonal diameter or by ensheathing axons with a membrane, the myelin sheath. Invertebrate axons are ensheathed by glial cells but lack a compact myelin. As a consequence, action potentials along invertebrate axons propagate at about 1 m/s or less. This is sufficient, however, for the survival of small animals (between 0.1 and 30 cm). Among invertebrates, only cephalopods have larger axons. By increasing their axonal diameter from 1 μm or less to 1 mm or more, cephalopods have been able to increase the speed of propagation of the action potential and have therefore adapted nerve conduction to their larger body size. However, because of the physical constraints imposed by the skull and vertebrae, vertebrates had to find an alternative solution. This was achieved by introducing the myelin sheath, which allows action potentials to propagate at speeds of 50–100 m/s without increasing the diameter of axons.[9] It is of note that there have been attempts during evolution to generate the equivalent of the myelin sheath in some invertebrates. This is the case in some crustaceans and annelids. In the central nerve of the shrimp or of the copepod, the ensheathing glial cells make a series of concentric wraps around the axons of the central nerve. This creates a pseudomyelin-like structure, which is not as compact as in the vertebrate but which nevertheless is sufficient to increase the speed of propagation of the action potential.[10,11]

The successive spiral wrapping of the oligodendroglial membrane extensions around axons explains the polystratified structure of myelin, which at the ultrastructural level is viewed as the succession of clear and dense lines, with a periodicity of 15 nm in the CNS (Fig. 18.1). The clear lines are formed by the lipid bilayers of the oligodendroglial membrane, while the dense lines correspond to the electron dense proteins of the membranes. There are two types of dark line: the major dense line is formed by the apposition of the internal face of the membrane and the intraperiodic dense line corresponds to the apposition

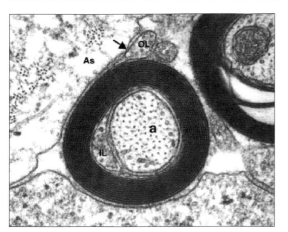

FIG. 18.1 An electron micrograph shows a central nervous system myelinated axon in cross section. The myelin sheath is formed by a cell process from an oligodendrocyte, elaborated in a spiral around the axon (a) and from which cytoplasm has been extruded. An inner loop of cytoplasm (IL) lies adjacent to the axon, and an outer loop (OL), connected elsewhere to an oligodendrocyte, is seen to the upper left. Note the gap junction (arrow) between the outer loop and an adjacent astrocyte (As). The compacted myelin sheath comprises a succession of clear and dense lines, the latter consisting of a major dense line (the fused inner leaflets of the unit oligodendroglial membrane) and a less dense intraperiod line (the juxtaposed outer leaflets of the unit membrane), see Figure 18.2. (Courtesy of Dr Cedric S. Raine.)

of external faces and is continuous with the extracellular space.[12]

THE BIOCHEMICAL COMPOSITION OF MYELIN

Myelin has peculiar and specific biochemical characteristics. With a water content of 40%, myelin renders white matter relatively dehydrated compared to gray matter (82%). The lipid : protein ratio of myelin is 70 : 30, which is inverted compared with any other membrane in the organism. This relative lipid enrichment, compared to other membranes, allowed for the early purification of highly purified myelin fractions and therefore the analysis of its biochemical content.[13,14]

LIPIDS OF MYELIN

The three major groups of myelin lipids are cholesterol, phospholipids and glycolipids. The major characteristic of myelin lipid composition is its high content of glycolipids and in particular galactolipids: galactosylceramide (GalC) and its sulfated derivative, sulfatide. GalC represents 20–25% of the total myelin lipids and is used as a selective marker of myelin and oligodendrocytes.[15–17]

PROTEINS OF MYELIN

We will here review only the major CNS myelin proteins. For a more detailed review see Baumann and Pham-Dinh.[18]

Proteolipid protein

The proteolipid protein (PLP) of myelin originally described by Folch and Lees[19] represents 50% of myelin proteins (Fig. 18.2). PLP comes in two forms -PLP itself (25 kDa) and DM-20 (20 kDa), which are produced by alternative splicing of the single *plp* gene product localized on the X chromosome.[20] This protein is highly conserved among myelinated species, as illustrated by the 90% homology at the amino-acid level between human and mouse. The *plp–DM-20* transcripts have been

detected very early during embryogenesis and have been shown to define a subpopulation of oligodendrocyte progenitor cells that do not depend on PDGFRα signaling for their proliferation and survival.[21,22] (see below). Despite numerous attempts, it has not been possible to attribute to PLP any function other than a structural protein of myelin. The different forms of Pelizaeus–Merzbacher disease, including X-linked spastic paraparesia (SGP2), are caused by mutations of *plp*.[23–25] The alterations described include point mutations, gene deletion or gene duplication. Point mutations are the cause of naturally-occurring animal mutants: the jimpy mouse[26] and its allele jimpy[msd],[27] the myelin deficient rat,[28] the shaking pup[29] and the paralytic tremor rabbit.[30] In addition, genetically engineered deletions or duplications have been generated, and represent animal models of the human diseases.

Myelin basic protein

Myelin basic protein (MBP) is the second most abundant protein of myelin, accounting for 30% of total myelin proteins in the CNS[31] (Fig. 18.2). At least four isoforms have been described in humans, with a molecular weight ranging between 14 and 21.5 kDa. These isoforms are produced by alternative splicing of the *mbp* gene, which in humans and mice is localized on chromosome 18.[32,33] The *mbp* gene is included in a larger (105 kb) transcriptional unit named *Golli–mbp*.[34] The role played by MBP in the compaction of myelin sheath has been illustrated by the dysmyelinated phenotype of *mbp* mutants, the shiverer and its allele shiverer[mld] mice.[35,36] In these mutants the myelin formed is devoid of major dense lines, and this defect has been corrected by addition through transgenesis of one or two copies of the *mbp* gene in the shiverer background.[37,38] MBP has been extensively used to induce experimental allergic encephalomyelitis (EAE), a model of multiple sclerosis (see Ch. 16). It is of note that, while immunization with MBP produces clinical symptoms of EAE, the pathology of these animals shows mostly signs of inflammation and very little demyelination.[39]

2',3'-cyclic nucleotide 3'-phosphodiesterase

2',3'-cyclic nucleotide 3'-phosphodiesterase (CNP) accounts for 5% of myelin proteins and is encoded by the *cnp* gene localized on chromosome 21[40,41] (Fig. 18.2). The *cnp* gene is transcribed in two mRNAs produced by alternative splicing and encoding two proteins of 46 and 48 kDa.[42] The name of this protein is misleading. Although it was initially described by its enzymatic activity, it is clear that this is not the main function of this protein, since 2',3'-cyclic nucleotides are not naturally occurring substrates. Several lines of evidence suggest a role for CNP in mediating process formation in oligodendrocytes. Based on the demonstration that tubulin is a major CNP-interacting protein, it has been proposed that CNP is an important component of the cytoskeletal machinery that directs process outgrowth in oligodendrocytes.[43]

Myelin associated glycoprotein and myelin-associated inhibitors of axonal growth

Myelin associated glycoprotein (MAG) is a transmembrane protein, a member of the immunoglobin family, and represents 1% of total myelin proteins.[44–46] (Fig. 18.2). MAG presents two isoforms of 64 and 69 kDa (before glycosylation) produced by alternative splicing of the *mag* gene localized on chromosome 19 in humans.[47] MAG is one of the myelin-associated factors (together with Nogo-A, oligodendrocyte–myelin glycoprotein (OMgp) and semaphorin 4D) responsible for the lack of axonal growth after injury in the adult central nervous system.[48,49] MAG inhibits axonal regeneration by high affinity interaction with the Nogo66 receptor (NgR) and activation of a p75 neurotrophin receptor-mediated signaling pathway.

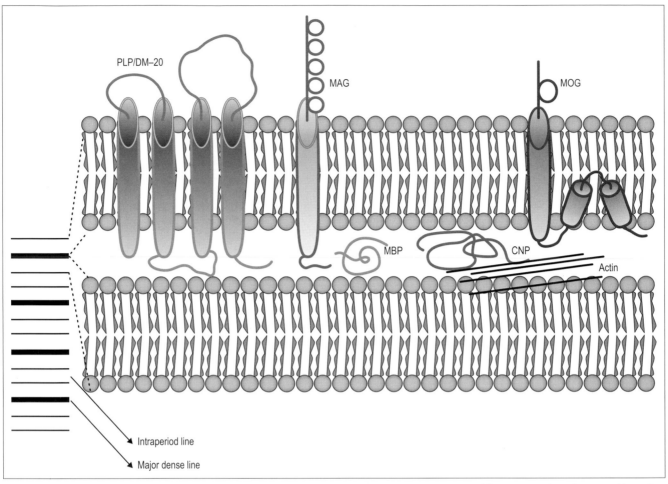

FIG. 18.2 Schematic representation of the major myelin protein inserted in the double lipid bilayer. After compaction, the apposition of two cytoplasmic faces of the membrane results in the formation of the major dense line. The apposition of the two external faces forms the intraperiod line. Only the major myelin proteins are represented either embedded in the lipid bilayer (PLP, MAG, MOG) or in the cytoplasm (MBP, CNP). (Modified with permission from Baumann & Pham-Dinh 2001.[18])

Myelin oligodendrocyte glycoprotein

Myelin oligodendrocyte glycoprotein (MOG) is a relatively minor component of myelin since it accounts for 0.01–0.05% of total myelin proteins (Fig. 18.2). MOG is a transmembrane protein, a member of the immunoglobulin family, with a molecular weight of 26–28 kDa.[50,51] The *mog* gene has been localized to chromosome 17.[52] MOG is expressed in the myelin only of mammals, not of other vertebrates. Immunization with MOG or MOG peptides induces a form of EAE associated with inflammation and demyelination in rat and mouse. For some, it is the molecule of choice for the induction of EAE.[53]

ORIGIN OF OLIGODENDROCYTES

The question of how neurons and macroglial cells are generated during development in ventricular proliferative zones of the neural tube has occupied the scientific world for years. His suggested the existence of two cell lines in the ventricular zone, one giving rise to neurons ('germinal cells'), the other to glia ('spongioblasts').[54] In the early embryo, the primitive neural tube is composed of neuroepithelial cells, which contact both the ventricular and pial surfaces. It is generally agreed that, directly or indirectly, neurons and glia are derived from neuroepithelial cells. As development proceeds, it has been suggested that neuroepithelial cells might transform into radial glial cells.[55] The term 'radial glia' was introduced by Rakic[56] to des-

ignate cells that have their soma in the ventricular zone, where they contact the lumen of the ventricles, and possess a long process that extends towards the pial surface. It has for long been accepted that radial glia are astroglial progenitors.[57–59] It has also been proposed that radial glia serve as oligodendrocyte progenitors.[60,61] Finally, recent evidence from several laboratories has demonstrated that radial glia can also produce neurons.[62–65] Therefore, there is agreement that both neurons and glia are the progeny of neuroepithelial cells and radial glia. However, the question as to whether neurons and glia are derived from separate neuroepithelial cells and/or separate radial glia (segregating model) or if there is a continuum from neuroepithelial cells generating neurons and radial glia, which in turn give rise by asymmetric division to neurons and glia (switching model), remains unresolved.

In the spinal cord, it has also been shown that neurons and glia arise sequentially from the same neuroepithelial domain. For example, the pMN domain generates first motoneurons and then oligodendrocytes.[66–68] The basic helix–loop–helix (bHLH) transcription factor Olig2 is selectively expressed in this pMN, and these authors have demonstrated that Olig2 functions sequentially in motoneuron and oligodendrocyte fate specification. It could therefore have been postulated that the same set of neuroepithelial progenitors (or stem cells) first generates motoneurons and then switches to the production of oligodendrocytes, as suggested by the fact that neurospheres generated from clonally isolated Olig2-expressing cells, following FGF2 treatment, behave as tripotent neural stem cells.[69] However, using a conditional cell-ablation approach, Wu et al[70] have provided evidence that, in vivo, motoneurons and oligodendrocytes are sequentially generated and do not share a common lineage-restricted progenitor. Similarly, in the diencephalon, plp/DM-20 transcripts are expressed in the laterobasal plate between E9.5 and E13.5, where they label first neuroepithelial cells and later radial glial cells (Fig. 18.3). Cre/loxP fate mapping has shown that plp/DM-20-expressing cells give rise to all three types of neural cell. In vitro clonal analysis revealed that their potentiality of differentiation is restricted towards either a neuronal or a glial fate when isolated at E9.5 or E13.5, respectively. This stage-dependent restriction in their fate of differentiation was confirmed in vivo, using inducible cre/loxP fate mapping and the demonstration that plp/DM-20 expressing cells recombining at E13.5 are not the progeny of neuroepithelial cells expressing plp/DM-20 at E9.5. All these findings lead to the conclusion that, in the embryonic diencephalon, neurons and glial cells are generated by distinct progenitors, which segregate shortly after the closure of the neural tube and have different intrinsic commitments, thereby supporting the model of segregation.[71]

MULTIPLE ORIGINS OF OLIGODENDROCYTES

The oligodendrocyte was first described by Del Rio-Hortega[72] and further examined by Penfield.[73] On the basis of morphological criteria (size of the cell body, number of myelinated internodes, diameter of myelinated axons), these authors distinguished four subgroups of oligodendrocytes. More recently, other subpopulations have been described on the basis of biochemical criteria: expression of carbonic anhydrase II, or P2 protein, or a member of the collapsin response mediator protein family.[74–76] It has also been observed that subsets of oligodendrocytes are not equally resistant to toxic agents such as hexachlorophene or cuprizone.[77–79] However, despite indications that oligodendrocytes form a heterogeneous family, it has long been believed that there is a single source of oligodendrocytes or, more precisely, that all along the neural tube generation of oligodendrocyte precursor cells responds to the same molecular mechanisms and that oligodendrocytes form a homogeneous population.

Two potential markers have been proposed to define the restricted territories of oligodendrogliogenesis. It has been suggested that oligodendrocyte precursors can be distinguished from other neuroepithelial cells by their expression of platelet derived growth factor alpha-receptor (PDGFRα) transcripts.[80] A second possible marker is plp/DM-20 mRNA, an alternatively spliced product of the plp gene. During mouse embryonic development, only DM-20 transcript has been detected, whereas plp mRNA has been found postnatally, probably concomitant with the deposition of the first myelin sheaths.[21,81,82] However, trace amounts of plp message have also been detected during embryonic development.[83] Using in situ hybridization, plp/DM-20 message has been detected in the CNS, beginning at E9.5. The first evidence in favor of a multiple origin of oligodendrocytes has been proposed based on the observation that early plp/DM-20-expressing precursors appear to be a separate population from PDGFRα oligodendrocyte precursors, as shown by the striking differences in their patterns of distribution[22] (Fig. 18.3). The different responsiveness of these cells to PDGF-AA has been a strong argument to demonstrate that they constitute two different oligodendrocyte lineages. Indeed, it has been shown that oligodendrocytes in the olfactory bulb are generated within

the rostral pallium from ventricular progenitors characterized by the expression of plp/DM-20, and these plp/DM-20 oligodendrocyte progenitors do not depend on signal transduction mediated by platelet-derived growth factor receptors for their survival and proliferation.[84] More recently, several groups have reported other sources of oligodendrocytes expressing different types of transcription factor in the spinal cord[85–87] and also in the telencephalon.[88] Recently, Richardson et al[89] have published a very elegant and comprehensive review on the multiple origins of oligodendrocytes.

FACTORS CONTROLLING OLIGODENDROCYTE DEVELOPMENT

Although the early segregation of neuronal and glial lineages appears to be largely intrinsic, all further stages of progression, from specification towards an oligodendrocyte fate to the maturation of a myelin-forming oligodendrocyte, have been shown to involve different morphogens and growth factors. Induction of ventrally born oligodendrocytes depends on sonic hedgehog (Shh) signaling, while those generated dorsally seem to be dependent on FGF-2.[90–93] The importance of growth factors on the development of oligodendrocytes stems from the observation that, in the optic nerve, 50% of oligodendrocyte precursor cells (OPCs) that have migrated and proliferated into the nerve will die, and only those that have established contact with nearby axons survive.[94] The survival and proliferation of OPCs have been shown to depend on different growth factors, mostly PDGF-AA,[95,96] FGF-2[97] and IGF-1.[98] Thyroid hormones, NT3 and CNTF have also been shown to act on oligodendrocyte survival, at least under certain culture conditions.[99] More recently, it has been shown that VEGF-C is a survival and mitogen for a subpopulation of OPCs in the optic nerve.[100]

MIGRATION OF OLIGODENDROCYTES

Oligodendrocytes are generated in the ventricular layer from discrete foci scattered along the neural tube. From their site of emergence towards their final destination (mainly the white matter tracts), OPCs need to migrate more or less long distances. Their migration pathways towards the presumptive white matter tracts and the gray matter have been analyzed, notably in birds, where long distances and tangential migrations have been described in the forebrain.[101,102] In contrast, in the chick rhombencephalon, OPCs adopt a radial type of migration, which is restricted to their rhombomer of origin.[102] The molecular mechanisms guiding OPCs during their migration remain an active domain of research. Contact-mediated cues have been implicated, notably cell adhesion molecules and components of the extracellular matrix such as integrins,[103,104] the polysialylated form of NCAM[105] and tenascin-C.[106,107] Interaction of ephrins, expressed by OPCs, with their Eph receptors, expressed at the axonal surface, has been shown to segregate subpopulations of oligodendrocytes entering the optic nerve along certain subpopulations of retinal ganglion cell axons and have been suggested to act as a potential stop signal of migration.[108] Growth factors such as FGF-2 and PDGF-AA, secreted along their migratory pathways, may also promote the migration of OPCs.[109,110] These growth factors seem to act more as chemokinetic factors, i.e. inducing the motility of OPCs, rather than on the directional guidance of oligodendrocytes.

A series of reports suggests that the migration of OPCs in the embryonic optic nerve is modulated by a balance of effects mediated by members of the semaphorin and netrin families. It has been shown, using different functional migration assays, that Sema 3A on the one hand and netrin-1 and sema 3F on the other exert opposite chemotactic effects, repulsive or attractive respectively, on embryonic OPCs. In the embryonic spinal cord it has been shown that netrin-1 acts as a chemo-repulsive factor. These apparent discrepancies are easily explained by the different types of receptor to netrin expressed by OPCs, depending on their localization and the time in development.[111-113]

PROGRESSION IN THE OLIGODENDROCYTE LINEAGE

Many studies on the development of oligodendrocytes have been conducted in the optic nerve. The optic nerve is formed by the axons of retinal ganglion cells, the cell bodies of which are in the retina. Therefore, the optic nerve is a structure free of neuronal cell bodies. It has been shown in the rat that, before E16,

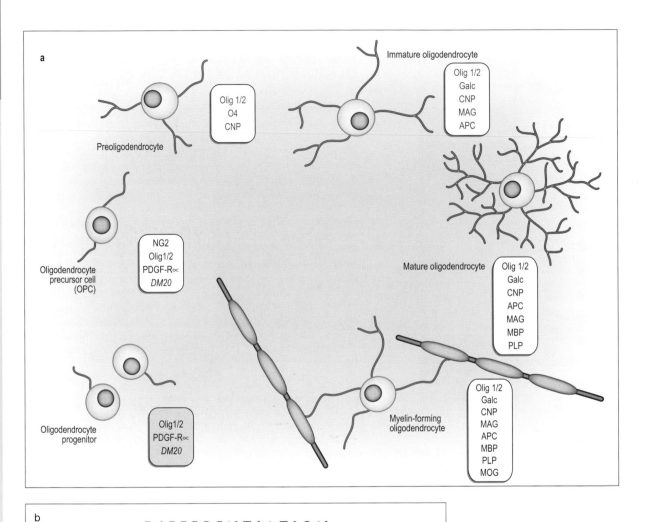

FIG. 18.3 A. Schematic representation of the successive developmental stages leading an oligodendrocyte progenitor to become a myelinating oligodendrocyte. The most frequently-used markers that permit to identify each stage are indicated in the boxes. **B**. These different stages can be observed either in vivo (oligodendrocyte progenitor) or in culture. Oligodendrocyte progenitor cells in the ventricular layer are seen by detection of the β-galactosidase activity by means of Bluo-gal substrate on a coronal section of an E12.5 *plp-lacZ* transgenic embryo.[22] The oligodendrocyte precursor cell is immunolabeled with anti-NG2 mAb. The preoligodendrocyte in culture is immunolabeled with O4 mAb, the immature oligodendrocyte with an anti-Galc mAb, and the mature oligodendrocyte with an anti-MBP mAb. The myelin-forming oligodendrocyte stained with an anti-PLP mAb is observed in a neuron/oligodendrocyte co-culture.[119]

the optic nerve can generate only astrocytes. After E16 (E14.5 in the mouse) precursors of oligodendrocyte start to invade the optic nerve from the chiasm end.[114] Although there may be other sources, some of these precursors originate from progenitors located in the nearby supra-chiasmatic area.[101] When OPCs finish migrating, they divide and, at the same time, start to acquire a more complex morphology, typical of the preoligodendrocyte stage. Preoligodendrocytes, which are still mitotic, are recognized by the O4 mAb.[115] The preoligodendrocyte then enters the stage of the immature oligodendrocyte, a post-mitotic, highly-branched cell. Immature oligodendrocytes express GalC, CNP, MOG and also the tumor suppressor protein APC (adenomatous polyposis coli), recognized by the CC1 mAb[116] (Fig. 18.3).

After having exited the cell cycle, the immature oligodendrocyte matures. This phase lasts approximately 3–5 days. The maturation period is characterized by the expression (or increase of level of expression) of most of the major myelin proteins such as MBP, PLP and MAG. At this stage, the cell presents an extremely rich array of processes corresponding to the mature nonmyelinated oligodendrocyte. This is the stage when the oligodendrocyte starts to establish contacts with nearby axons, and to express MOG. Simultaneously with the establishment of contact with the axonal membrane, a dramatic simplification in the morphology occurs. Only processes having reached an axon will be maintained, all others being pruned (Fig. 18.3).

SIGNALS AND MECHANISMS OF MYELINATION

In spite of the increasing knowledge of the mechanisms involved in the successive steps of myelinating cell development, little was known until recently about the molecular basis of cell–cell interaction leading to the process of myelination by Schwann cells or oligodendrocytes. Progress has been made that opens new perspectives in our understanding of the cellular and molecular basis of myelination. The influence of different axonal signals in the myelination process has been demonstrated, as has the role of non-axonally-derived growth factors (see review by Sherman and Brophy[117]). In addition, several studies have indicated that, while some myelination signals are shared between the CNS and PNS, others have opposite or at least different influences. Finally, the intracellular pathways elicited in the myelinating cell by either axonal or nonaxonal myelination signals represent a new and as yet poorly explored field of research.

AXONAL SIGNALS OF MYELINATION

Different axonal signals act on the myelination step, which can be divided into successive phases: 1) the phase of adhesion between the myelinating cell membrane and the axon and 2) the wrapping process leading to the formation of the myelin sheath.

AXONAL SIGNALS IN THE EARLY STAGES OF MYELINATION

The early stages of adhesion of the myelination process on the axonal surface do not correspond to nonspecific apposition between two membranes. Such nonspecific apposition has been reported in cultures where oligodendrocytes are put in contact with artificial fibres mimicking axons such as carbon fibres.[118] The specificity of the interaction between axonal and oligodendroglial membranes is strengthened by the fact that, in vitro in CNS myelinating cocultures, oligodendroglial processes form a myelin sheath along axons only, never around dendrites or astrocytic processes.[119] This restricted myelination around axons detected in vitro suggests a specific interaction between the two membranes, as if there was an axonal recognition signal, triggering targeted alignment (not only apposition) of the oligodendroglial process along the axon.

Adhesion molecules, with their potential not only to bring the axon and glial cell into close apposition but also to transduce the signals between these cells, are most probably involved in the early phase of myelination. Among the candidates, L1 cell adhesion molecule and PSA-NCAM (the sialylated form of the neural cell adhesion molecule), have been shown to act in opposite ways, at least in the CNS. Other candidates for sensing axonally presented molecules on Schwann cells or oligodendrocytes include the integrins and N-cadherin, and the jagged/Notch pair.

Adhesion molecules

L1 cell adhesion molecule L1 is a cell adhesion molecule expressed at the axonal surface.[120–124] In the PNS, it has been shown that L1 is involved in the myelination process, as antibodies against L1 inhibit Schwann cell myelination of dorsal root ganglia axons.[125] In addition, it has been shown that electrical stimulation of DRG neurons at a frequency of 0.1 Hz, i.e. corresponding to the firing frequency of neurons during the premyelinating period, reduces the number of myelinated profiles.[126] Interestingly enough, such inhibition of myelin formation has been linked to a downregulation of L1 neural cell adhesion molecule, suggesting a specific molecular mechanism relating an appropriate rate of firing to the myelinating activity of Schwann cells.[127] In myelinating CNS cocultures, whereas L1 is diffusely expressed on nonmyelinated axons, the onset of myelination is associated with a drastic reduction of L1 immunoreactivity on myelinated axons. In addition, antibodies directed against the extracellular domain of L1, as well as fusion protein containing the extracellular domain of L1 fused to the Fc fragment of human immunoglobulins, strongly inhibit myelination in vitro.[128] These data are suggestive of a positive role of L1 in the early stage of myelination, L1 being necessary for the early apposition of the myelinating cell/axon membranes but not for the subsequent steps of the myelination process.

The polysialylated form of cell adhesion molecule (PSA-NCAM) The neural cell adhesion molecule (NCAM), a member of the immunoglobulin superfamily, is involved in many different processes during development such as cell–cell adhesion and migration. There are several isoforms of this molecule, which result from differential splicing and post-translational modifications. Expression of the different NCAM isoforms is developmentally regulated and all are capable of bearing long homopolymers of α-2,8-linked sialic acid, attached to the fifth Ig domain. Polysialic acid (PSA) moieties on NCAM not only prevent homophilic NCAM–NCAM adhesion but also serve more generally as negative regulators of cell–cell interactions.[129,130] In a myelinating coculture system, PSA-NCAM disappearance from the axonal surface during development is coincident with the initiation of myelin deposition. In cocultures of DRG neurons and oligodendrocytes, cleavage of PSA residues by endoneuraminidase induces alignment of the oligodendroglial processes along axons.[131] Furthermore, in CNS myelinating cocultures, as well as in vivo in the optic nerve, suppression of sialylated determinants by specific antibodies, or enzymatic cleavage, increases myelination (or speeds up its initiation).[132] Therefore, in the CNS, expression of PSA-NCAM at the surface of axons could act as an inhibitor of myelination, presumably by preventing myelin-forming cells from attaching to the axon. Removal of PSA-NCAM from the axonal surface is a necessary prerequisite to rendering the axon permissive to myelination.

Nonmembers of the adhesion molecule family

N-cadherin Expressed by Schwann cells and axons, N-cadherin mediates axon-aligned process outgrowth and cell–cell interactions in rat Schwann cells.[133] All blocking agents of N-cadherin (antibodies and cyclic pentapeptides) reduced the number of Schwann cell/Schwann cell junctions and perturbed axon-aligned growth of Schwann cell processes in cocultures of Schwann cells and DRG neurons.[133] Other studies have shown that N-cadherin is also involved in axon/oligodendrocyte contacts and myelination, in cultures of DRG neurons and CG4 oligodendroglial cell line.[134]

Laminin and integrins Whether laminin is involved in the process of myelination itself or, more probably, influences this process through maturation of the myelinating cells, remains uncertain. α_2 chains containing laminin are found within axonal tracts and can control and regulate growth factor influence on oligodendrocytes and Schwann cells,[135,136] inducing, depending on the stage of development, proliferation, differentiation or survival. Laminin ligands interact on the glial surface with different sets of α and β integrins. In the PNS, the suppression of integrins, either by antibodies against β_1 integrin[137] or by conditional knock-out,[135] interferes with myelination. This delay of myelination is related to the failure of Schwann cells both to subdivide bundles of axons and to progress past the promyelinating stage. In addition, immature Schwann cells may require β_1 integrins to adhere to their basal lamina and initiate the formation of a myelin sheath. In oligodendrocytes, suppression of α integrin results in fewer myelin-forming oligodendrocytes, suggesting that axon-associated laminin might interact with integrin receptors on oligodendrocytes providing a mechanism for target-dependent survival during development of the CNS.

The Notch/Jagged pathway In the rat optic nerve it has been shown that, during development, activation of the Notch pathway is inhibitory to oligodendrocyte differentiation. Oligodendrocytes and OPCs express Notch receptor, while Jagged, which is a Notch ligand, is expressed by retinal ganglion cells.[138] Jagged is downregulated with a time course that parallels myelination in the optic nerve, suggesting that myelination is controlled via the Notch pathway by axonally expressed Jagged. The influence of Notch activation on the myelination process is most probably related to its effect on the maturation of oligodendrocytes rather than to a direct effect on the myelination process. The influence of a reactivation of Notch pathway on OPCs in multiple sclerosis lesions, through re-expression of Jagged by astrocytes, has been proposed to be one of the factors impairing the remyelination process.[139] Experimental nonimmune models of demyelination have failed to confirm the involvement of the Notch pathway in myelin repair.[140]

AXONAL SIGNALS AND THE WRAPPING PROCESS

The signals that determine whether axons are myelinated have long been elusive. Electrical activity of neurons, possibly through activation of purinergic receptors on myelinating cells, has been shown to be needed for the initiation of myelination, at least in the CNS. In the PNS, important advances have been made recently, with reports of the key roles of axonally-derived NRG 1 type III and nerve growth factor (NGF) on PNS myelination.

Electrical activity and the promyelinating role of adenosine

The influence of neuronal electrical activity has been shown to be critical, early in development, for the proliferation of the progenitors of oligodendrocytes.[96] The possibility that electrical impulses could also influence myelination has been suggested by different studies on the optic nerve. Mice reared in the dark developed fewer myelinated axons in the optic nerve compared with normally reared mice.[141] Myelination is highly decreased in the optic nerve of blind cape mole rats,[142] whereas premature opening of eyelids accelerated the process of myelination in the optic nerve of the rabbit.[143] To evaluate the role of electrical activity on the process of myelination, we have used specific neurotoxins either blocking, like tetrodotoxin (TTX), or stimulating, like α-scorpion toxin, electrical activity of axons. Binding of TTX to Na_v channels blocks the channel and thus inhibits the propagation of the action potential. In contrast, binding of α-scorpion toxin to Na_v channels increases the probability of opening of the channel and thus induces repetitive firing. Neurotoxins were added to the culture medium of myelinating cultures prior to the initiation of myelination. Blockade of electrical activity with 10^{-6} mol/l TTX drastically inhibited myelination without impairing the viability of either oligodendrocytes or neurons. In contrast, addition of α-scorpion toxin induced a strong increase in the number of myelinated segments. The effect of TTX has been confirmed in vivo in the optic nerve by intravitreous injections of TTX, enabling the blockade of electrical activity of retinal ganglion cells, the axons of which form the optic nerve. When TTX was injected intravitreously at 4 days postnatally (P4), i.e. 2 days prior to the onset of myelination in the optic nerve, a 60% decrease in the number of myelinating oligodendrocytes was observed at P6 in TTX-injected mice compared to sham-injected animals.[144] Altogether, these results indicate that electrical activity plays a key role in central nervous system myelination.

Interestingly enough, since this work was published, experimental data have added a major brick to our understanding of the mechanisms involved in this promyelinating effect of electrical activity.[145] Indeed, these authors have shown that, in cocultures of murine dorsal root ganglia neurons and oligodendrocytes, the promyelinating efficacy of electrical activity is related to the extrasynaptic release of the mediator adenosine, which acts on purinergic receptors expressed at the surface of OPCs. Whether this promyelinating effect is related to an influence on maturation of oligodendrocytes or is involved in the early contact between oligodendrocytes and axons remains elusive.

The situation is different in the peripheral nervous system, where action-potential-mediated release of adenosine triphosphate (ATP) acting on purinergic receptors expressed by Schwann cells inhibits myelination by delaying terminal differentiation of Schwann cells.[127,146] Therefore, it appears that different mediators released by electrically active axons may mediate opposite effects in regard to the terminal differentiation of myelinating cells in the PNS or CNS during development.

Type III neuregulin-1

Recently, it has been shown that the threshold levels of neuregulin (NRG)-1 type III, independent of axon diameter, determines the fate of ensheathment. NRG-1 type III is the major isoform expressed by neurons that project into the PNS. NRG-1 interactions with ErbB receptor influence most of the stages of Schwann cell development, including commitment of neural crest cells to the glial lineage and the proliferation, survival and maturation of Schwann cells.

Recent studies have demonstrated that NRG 1 also has a major influence on the myelination process. A role in the regulation of axonal thickness has been suggested by analysis of mice haplo-insufficient for NRG-1, which exhibit a thinner peripheral myelin sheath than wild-type mice, whereas transgenic overexpression in neurons of the cDNA encoding for

NRG-1 type III showed that it was active in regulating myelin thickness.[147] In addition, recent data have suggested that, in the PNS, the NRG-1 level dictates the myelinating fate of an axon. In the PNS, ensheathed nonmyelinated axons within Remak bundles express low levels of NRG-1 type III, whereas myelinated fibres express high levels. Expression of NRG-1 type III also converts the normally unmyelinated axons to myelinated.[148] These data are in agreement with the study of Michailov et al,[147] showing that myelin thickness is graded to the amount of NRG-1 type III. It has long been shown that axon diameter and surface area are strongly correlated to the number of myelin lamellae generated. These recent data indicate that large axons not only have increased surface area but also express greater amounts of NRG-1 type III per unit membrane area. In addition, NRG-1 type III activates the PI3 kinase pathway (see below), which is required for Schwann cell myelination. Whether this mechanism is also involved in CNS myelination remains to be shown.

NGF/TrkA

It has been reported that neurotrophins regulate the development of myelinating glia. Neurotrophin (NT)3 helps to promote the proliferation of purified OPC[149] and the survival of oligodendrocytes.[150] In addition, NT3 acting through glial TrkC inhibits myelination by Schwann cells.[151] Recent data demonstrate that neurotrophins also profoundly influence oligodendrocytes and Schwann cells indirectly by regulating the axonal signals that control their development. Indeed, in DRG neurons, NGF, acting through TrkA receptors expressed on the axonal surface, promotes myelination by Schwann cells and reduces myelination by oligodendrocytes. These effects are mediated by changes in the axonal signals that control myelination rather than by a direct action on myelinating glia.[151] These results indicate a novel role for growth factors in regulating the receptivity of axons to myelination. They also imply, in agreement with other lines of evidence, that distinct, differentially regulated axonal signals promote myelination by oligodendrocytes and Schwann cells.

NONAXONAL SIGNALS OF MYELINATION

Different growth factors have been shown, besides their neurotrophic activity, to promote myelination, either directly or through promotion of the maturation of myelinating cells. This effect may vary between PNS and CNS myelination. In the CNS, these factors are mostly derived from astrocytes but can also be secreted by inflammatory cells. In this context, several reports have demonstrated that, in experimental models of demyelination, the reduction of the inflammatory component impairs the remyelination capacity and, in contrast, that inducing inflammation in the vicinity of a demyelinated lesion increased the extent of the remyelinated area from transplanted cells.[152,153]

GDNF

Whereas GDNF has no effect on CNS myelination in vitro,[154] recent data have shown that it increases myelination by Schwann cells, which express the GDNF receptor GDR1.[155]

CNTF

In addition to the role of CNTF in early oligodendroglial development, CNTF, but also other members of the CNTF family such as leukemia inhibiting factor (LIF), cardiotrophin (CT)1 and oncostatin M, induce a strong promyelinating effect in vitro, in cocultures of neurons and oligodendrocytes. This effect is related to an increased maturation of oligodendrocytes and is mediated through the gp130 kDa glycoprotein receptor common

to the CNTF family and transduced through the Janus kinase pathway.[154]

BDNF

In the PNS, BDNF, acting through the neurotrophic receptor p75, is an endogenous regulator of myelination. Elevation of BDNF levels in BDNF transgenic mice produced an increase in both the rate and extent of myelination.[156] In CNS myelination, BDNF has no reported promyelinating effect.[154]

SIGNALING PATHWAYS IN OLIGODENDROCYTES LEADING TO MYELINATION

The molecular mechanisms associated with the initiation of myelination, and hence controlling the coordinated induction or upregulation of myelin protein synthesis necessary for the elaboration of myelin membranes, is still poorly understood. To date, a few intracellular signaling pathways have been reported to be activated during the myelination process.

Fyn

The Src family kinases (SFKs) are nonreceptor tyrosine kinases that integrate external signals received through both integrins and growth factor receptors and are thus good candidates to transduce signals that regulate both integrin- and growth-factor-driven phases of oligodendrocyte development. One of these, Fyn, is expressed throughout the brain, in both neurons and glia, but the peak of its activity during development can be correlated with myelination.[157,158] Fyn may be involved in the oligodendrocyte differentiation process, because mice lacking Fyn are hypomyelinated,[157] and cultured oligodendrocytes from Fyn-deficient mice show defects in the number of newly formed oligodendrocytes as well as in the formation of complex branches of myelin membranes.[158,159]

Furthermore, mice deficient for laminin α_2 chains have a similar region-specific hypomyelination, suggesting that Fyn and laminin may operate in the same signaling pathway and that integrin receptors may contribute to this pathway.[160] Fyn is activated through stimulation of cell surface receptors such as L-MAG. In addition, in maturing oligodendrocytes, Fyn is associated in raft microdomains with NCAM 120 and F3/contactin, which are GPI-anchored proteins. Fyn activation in oligodendrocytes blocks activation of Rho as well as MBP expression. Recently, the transmembrane molecule LINGO 1 has been shown to inhibit Fyn phosphorylation in oligodendrocytes. LINGO 1 is selectively expressed in the brain and spinal cord and functions as a component of the NgR1/p75 and Troy signaling complexes that regulated axon growth.[161] Recently, it has been shown that LINGO 1 is expressed by oligodendrocytes. Attenuation of LINGO 1 function promotes oligodendroglial differentiation, with an increase in the number of mature oligodendrocytes in vitro and increased synthesis of myelin proteins. This promyelinating effect of LINGO 1 attenuation is mediated through increased Fyn phosphorylation and down-regulation of RhoA-GTP (see below).[162,163] Taken together, these results suggest that the intraoligodendroglial Fyn signaling pathway plays a key role in oligodendrocyte maturation and in myelination.

Rho pathway

Rho GTPases RhoA, Rac1 and cdc42 are a family of small GTP-binding proteins that are important candidates to coordinate remodeling of the actin cytoskeleton during myelination. ROCK is a downstream effector of Rho and has been shown to play a key role in the coordinated progression of the Schwann cell membrane around the axon during myelination by regulating the phosphorylation of myosin light chains and the assembly of actomyosin.[164] In oligodendrocytes, it has been shown that the introduction of Rho blocks oligodendrocyte differentiation and that RhoGTPases are downregulated during oligodendrocyte development. Fyn activation (see above) in oligodendrocytes blocks activation of Rho GTPases. Taken together, the linear signal transduction pathway of integrin–Fyn–Rho family GTPases is most probably a key player in the control of the morphology and differentiation of oligodendrocytes.[165] In oligodendrocytes, LINGO 1 antagonists reduce Rho A-GTP amounts to promote oligodendrocyte differentiation and myelination.[166]

PI3 kinase/Akt

The PI3 kinase pathway likely mediates some steps of the myelination process. PI3 kinase has been implicated in the reorganization of the actin cytoskeleton required for cell mobility and lamellipodia formation in other cell types.[167] Selective activation or inactivation of the PI3 kinase/Akt pathway in Schwann cells, through adenoviral vectors, has been shown to modulate myelination, and GSK3β, a modulator of glycogen synthase kinase 3β, has been shown to be a downstream regulator of the pI3 kinase pathway promoting Schwann cell differentiation. Recently, the PI3 kinase pathway, via phosphorylation of Akt, a key effector of PI3 kinase, has been shown to be involved in the Schwann cell promyelinating effect induced by NRG-1 type III.[148]

In addition to these pathways, signaling cascades induced by some growth factors with promyelinating activity, such as the Janus kinase pathway, also play a role in the initiation of myelination (see above).

CONCLUDING REMARKS

These data underline the major influence of axonal signals on myelination. It is thus hypothesized that, during development, myelination depends on a balance between negative signals, which need to be downregulated for the myelination process to occur, and positive signals, which have to be activated in order to allow the initiation of the wrapping process. Some are shared by the PNS and CNS, such as the 'myelin-promoting' axonal adhesion molecule L1 or the extracellular matrix molecule laminin, interacting with integrins. Others have only been shown (or studied) in the PNS, such as neuregulins NRG-1 type III, or in the CNS, such as axonally expressed PSA-NCAM or the Notch differentiation pathway. In addition, some signals, such as neurotrophin/TrkA activation or electrical-activity-induced release of purinergic ligands, appear to have opposite effects in the CNS and PNS.

In addition, growth factors, released either by astrocytes or under pathological conditions by inflammatory cells, also regulate the process of myelination. Finally, the intracellular oligodendroglial signaling cascade leading to upregulation of myelin protein synthesis is beginning to be elucidated, with the demonstration of the key roles for Fyn, Rho and PI3 kinase pathways. Interestingly enough, the recent demonstration of oligodendroglial molecules involved in this cascade, such as LINGO-1, is opening new avenues to promote remyelination in demyelinating conditions such as multiple sclerosis. In this respect, the recent demonstration of the multiplicity of origins of oligodendrocytes may explain the partial or limited response to different insults or treatments in the demyelination process or during attempts to remyelinate. This, in turn, may lead to the development of more targeted treatments influencing one subtype of oligodendrocyte, depending on the localization of the lesion and therefore the origin of the damaged and remyelinating oligodendrocyte.

ACKNOWLEDGMENTS

We are greatly indebted to Dr Cedric S. Raine for the gift of the photograph shown in Figure 18.1. Work from the authors cited in this paper has benefited from the support of INSERM, ELA and ARSEP.

REFERENCES

1. Ranvier LA. Contributions à l'histologie et à la physiologie des nerfs périphériques. C R Acad Sci 1871; 73: 1168–1187.

2. Bunge MB, Bunge RP, Pappas GD. Electron microscopic demonstration of connections between glia and myelin sheaths in the developing mammalian central nervous system. J Cell Biol 1962; 12: 448–453.

3. Raine CS. Morphological aspects of myelin and myelination. In: Morell P, ed. Myelin. New York: Plenum Press; 1977: 1–50.

4. Huxley AF, Sämpfli R. Evidence for saltatory conduction in peripheral myelinated nerve fibres. J Physiol (Lond) 1949; 108: 315–339.

5. Rasminsky M, Sears TA. Internodal conduction in undissected demyelinated nerve fibres. J Physiol 1972; 227: 323–350.

6. Peles E, Salzer JL. Molecular domains of myelinated axons. Curr Opin Neurobiol 2000; 10: 558–565.

7. Poliak S, Peles E. The local differentiation of myelinated axons at nodes of Ranvier. Nat Rev Neurosci 2003; 4: 968–980.

8. Sherman DL, Tait S, Melrose S et al. Neurofascins are required to establish axonal domains for saltatory conduction. Neuron 2005; 48: 737–742.

9. Zalc B, Colman DR. Origins of vertebrate success. Science 2000; 288: 271–272.

10. Roots BI, Cardone B, Pereyra P. Isolation and characterization of the myelin-like membranes ensheathing giant axons in the earthworm nerve cord. Ann NY Acad Sci 1991; 633: 559–561.

11. Davis AD, Weatherby TM, Hartline DK, Lenz PH. Myelin-like sheaths in copepod axons. Nature 1999; 398: 571.

12. Robertson JD. The ultrastructure of adult vertebrate peripheral myelinated fibers in relation to myelinogenesis. J Biophys Biochem Cytol 1955; 1: 271–278.

13. Autilio LA, Norton WT, Terry RD. The preparation and some properties of purified myelin from the central nervous system. J Neurochem 1964; 11: 17–27.

14. Norton WT, Autilio LA. The lipid composition of purified bovine brain myelin. J Neurochem 1966; 13: 213–222.

15. Dupouey P, Zalc B, Lefroit-Joly M, Gomes D. Localization of galactosylceramide and sulfatide at the surface of the myelin sheath: an immunofluorescence study in liquid medium. Cell Mol Biol 1979; 25: 269–272.

16. Raff MC, Fields KL, Hakomori S et al. Cell type specific markers for distinguishing and studying neurons and the major classes of glial cells in culture. Brain Res 1979; 174: 283–308.

17. Zalc B, Monge M, Dupouey P et al. Immunohistochemical localization of galactosyl and sulfogalactosylceramide in the brain of the 30 day-old mouse. Brain Res 1981; 211: 341–354.

18. Baumann N, Pham-Dinh D. Biology of oligodendrocyte and myelin in the mammalian central nervous system. Physiol Rev 2001; 81: 871–927.

19. Folch J, Lees M. Proteolipides, a new type of tissue lipoproteins; their isolation from brain. J Biol Chem 1951; 191: 807–817.

20. Willard HF, Riordan JR. Assignment of the gene for myelin proteolipid protein to the X chromosome: implications for X-linked myelin disorders. Science 1985; 230: 940–942.

21. Timsit SG, Bally-Cuif L, Colman D, Zalc B. DM20 messenger RNA is expressed during the embryonic development of the nervous system of the mouse. J Neurochem 1992; 58: 1172–1175.

22. Spassky N, Goujet-Zalc C, Parmantier E et al. Multiple restricted origin of oligodendrocytes. J Neurosci 1998; 18: 8331–8343.

23. Boulloche J, Aicardi J. Pelizaeus–Merzbacher: clinical and nosological study. J Child Neurol 1986; 1: 233–239.

24. Hudson LD, Nadon NL. Amino acid substitutions in proteolipid protein that cause dysmyelination. In: Martenson R, ed. Myelin: a treatise. Caldwell, NJ: Telford Press, 1991.

25. Saugier-Veber P, Munnich A, Bonneau D et al. X linked spastic paraplegia (SPG2) and PM disease are allelic disorder at the proteolipid protein (PLP) locus on chromosome Xq21-q22. Nat Genet 1994; 6: 257–261.

26. Morello D, Dautigny A, Pham-Dinh D, Jolles P. Myelin proteolipid protein (PLP and DM-20) transcripts are deleted in jimpy mutant mice. EMBO J 1986; 5: 3489–3493.

27. Gencic S, Hudson LD. Conservative amino acid substitution in the myelin proteolipid protein of *jimpy^msd* mice. J Neurosci 1990; 10: 117–124.

28. Boison D, Stoffel W. Myelin-deficient rat: a point mutation in exon III of the myelin proteolipid protein causes dysmyelination and oligodendrocyte death. EMBO J 1989; 8: 3295–3302.

29. Nadon NL, Duncan ID, Hudson LD. A point mutation in the proteolipid protein gene of the 'shaking pup' interrupts oligodendrocyte development. Development 1990; 110: 529–537.

30. Tosic M, Dolivo M, Domanska-Janik K, Matthieu J-M. Paralytic tremor (*pt*) a new allele of the proteolipid protein gene in rabbit. J Neurochem 1994; 63: 2210–2216.

31. Kies MW, Murphy JB, Alvord EC. Studies of the encephalitogenic factor in guinea pig central nervous system. In: Folch-Pi J, ed. Chemical pathology of the nervous system. Oxford: Pergamon Press; 1961: 197–206.

32. De Ferra F, Engh H, Hudson L et al. Alternative splicing accounts for the four forms of myelin basic protein. Cell 1985; 43: 721–727.

33. Saxe DF, Takahashi N, Hood L, Simon MI. Localization of the human myelin basic protein gene (MBP) to region 18q22→qter by *in situ* hybridization. Cytogenet Cell Genet 1985; 39: 246–249.

34. Campagnoni AT, Pribyl TM, Campagnoni CW et al. Structure and developmental regulation of *Golli-mbp*, a 105-kilobase gene that encompasses the myelin basic protein gene and is expressed in cells in the oligodendrocyte lineage in the brain. J Biol Chem 1993; 268: 4930–4938.

35. Kimura M, Inoko H, Katzuki M et al. Molecular genetic analysis of *myelin-deficient* mice: shiverer mutant mice show deletion in gene(s) coding for myelin basic protein. J Neurochem 1985; 44: 692–696.

36. Roch JM, Tosic M, Roach A, Matthieu JM. Myelin basic protein transcriptional activity in myelin deficient mice.Schweiz Arch Neurol Psychiatr 1989; 140: 6–9.

37. Privat A, Jacque C, Bourre JM et al. Absence of major dense line in the myelin of the mutant mouse *shiverer*. Neurosci Lett 1979; 12: 107–112.

38. Readhead C, Popko B, Takahaski N et al. Expression of myelin basic protein gene in transgenic *shiverer* mice: correction of the dysmyelinating phenotype. Cell 1987; 48: 703–712.

39. Moore GR, Traugott U, Farooq M et al. Experimental autoimmune encephalomyelitis. Augmentation of demyelination by different myelin lipids. Lab Invest 1984; 51: 416–424.

40. Olafson RW, Drummond GI, Lee JF. Studies on 2'-3' cyclic nucleotide 3'-phosphohydrolase from brain. Can J Biochem 1969; 47: 961–966.

41. Bernier L, Colman DR, D'Eustachio P. Chromosonal locations of genes encoding 2', 3' cyclic nucleotide 3'-phosphodiesterase and glial fibrillary acidic protein in the mouse. J Neurosci Res 1988; 20: 201–211.

42. Kurihara T, Fowler AV, Takahashi Y. cDNA cloning and amino acid sequence of bovine brain 2', 3'-cyclic nucleotide 3'-phosphodiesterase. J Biol Chem 1987; 262: 3256–3261.

43. Lee J, Gravel M, Zhang R et al. Process outgrowth in oligodendrocytes is mediated by CNP, a novel microtubule assembly myelin protein. J Cell Biol 2005; 170: 661–673.

44. Quarles RH. Glycoproteins in myelin and myelin-related membranes. In: Margolis RV, Margolis RK, eds. Complex carbohydrates of nervous tissue. New York: Plenum Press; 1979: 209–233.

45. Arquint M, Roder J, Chia LS et al. Molecular cloning and primary structure of myelin associated glycoprotein. Proc Natl Acad Sci USA 1987; 84: 600–604.

46. Salzer JL, Holmes WP, Colman DR. The amino acid sequences of myelin associated glycoproteins: homology to the immunoglobin gene family. J Cell Biol 1987; 104: 957–965.

47. Sutcliffe JG. The genes for myelin. Trends Genet 1987; 3: 73–76.

48. Filbin MT. Myelin-associated inhibitors of axonal regeneration in the adult mammalian CNS. Nat Rev Neurosci 2003; 4: 703–713.

49. Schwab ME. Nogo and axon regeneration. Curr Opin Neurobiol 2004; 14: 118–124.

50. Linington C, Webb M, Woodhams PL. A novel myelin-associated glycoprotein defined by a mouse monoclonal antibody. J.Neuroimmunol 1984; 6: 387–396.

51. Gardinier MV, Amiguet P, Linington C, Matthieu JM. Myelin/oligodendrocyte glycoprotein is a unique member of the immunoglobulin superfamily. J Neurosci Res 1992; 33: 177–187.

52. Pham-Dinh D, Mattei MG, Nussbaum JL et al. Myelin/oligodendrocyte glycoprotein is a member of a subset of the immunoglobulin superfamily encoded within the major histocompatibility complex. Proc Natl Acad Sci USA 1993; 90: 7990–7994.

53. Linington C, Lassmann H. Antibody responses in chronic relapsing experimental allergic encephalomyelitis: correlation of serum demyelinating activity with antibody titre to the myelin/oligodendrocyte glycoprotein (MOG). J Neuroimmunol 1987; 17: 61–69.

54. His W. Die Neuroblasten und deren Entstehung im embryonalen Mark. Arch Anat Physiol Anat Abt 1889: 249–300/Abh Sächs Ges Wiss Math Phys Kl 1889; 15: 311–372.

55. Alvarez-Buylla A, Garcia-Verdugo JM, Tramontin AD. A unified hypothesis on the lineage of neural stem cells. Nat Rev Neurosci 2001; 2: 287–293.

56. Rakic P. Neuron-glia relationship during granule cell migration in developing cerebellar cortex. A Golgi and electronmicroscopic study in *Macacus rhesus*. J Comp Neurol 1971; 141: 283–312.

57. Levitt P, Cooper ML, Rakic P. Coexistence of neuronal and glial precursor cells in the cerebral ventricular zone of the fetal monkey: an ultrastructural immunoperoxidase analysis. J Neurosci 1981; 1: 27–39.

58. Schmechel DE, Rakic P. A Golgi study of radial glial cells in developing monkey telencephalon: morphogenesis and transformation into astrocytes. Anat Embryol (Berl) 1979; 156: 115–152.

59. Voigt T. Development of glial cells in the cerebral wall of ferrets: direct tracing of their transformation from radial glia into astrocytes. J Comp Neurol 1989; 289: 74–88.

60. Choi BH, Kim RC. Expression of glial fibrillary acidic protein by immature oligodendroglia and its implications. J Neuroimmunol 1985; 8: 215–235.

61. Hirano M, Goldman JE. Gliogenesis in rat spinal cord: evidence for origin of astrocytes and oligodendrocytes from radial precursors. J Neurosci Res 1988; 21: 155–167.

62. Malatesta P, Hartfuss E, Gotz M. Isolation of radial glial cells by fluorescent-activated cell sorting reveals a neuronal lineage. Development 2000; 127: 5253–5263.

63. Hartfuss E, Galli R, Heins N, Gotz M. Characterization of CNS precursor subtypes and radial glia. Dev Biol 2001; 229: 15–30.

64. Noctor SC, Flint AC, Weissman TA et al. Neurons derived from radial glial cells establish radial units in neocortex. Nature 2001; 409: 714–720.

65. Miyata T, Kawaguchi A, Okano H, Ogawa M. Asymmetric inheritance of radial glial fibers by cortical neurons. Neuron 2001; 31: 727–741.

66. Novitch BG, Chen AI, Jessell TM. Coordinate regulation of motor neuron subtype identity and pan-neuronal properties by the bHLH repressor Olig2. Neuron 2001; 31: 773–789.

67. Lu QR, Sun T, Zhu Z et al. Common developmental requirement for Olig function indicates a motor neuron/oligodendrocyte connection. Cell 2002; 109: 75–86.

68. Zhou Q, Anderson DJ. The bHLH transcription factors OLIG2 and OLIG1 couple neuronal and glial subtype specification. Cell 2002; 109: 61–73.

69. Gabay L, Lowell S, Rubin LL, Anderson DJ. Deregulation of dorsoventral patterning by FGF confers trilineage differentiation capacity on CNS stem cells in vitro. Neuron 2003; 40: 485–499.

70. Wu S, Wu Y, Capecchi MR. Motoneurons and oligodendrocytes are sequentially generated from neural stem cells but do not appear to share common lineage-restricted progenitors in vivo. Development 2006; 133: 581–590.

71. Delaunay D, Heydon K, Cumano A et al. Early neuronal and glial fate restriction of embryonic neural stem cells. J Neurosci 2007, submitted.

72. Del Rio-Hortega P. Tercera aportacion al conocimiento morfologica e interpretacion funcional de la oligodendroglia. Mem R Soc Expan His Nat 1928; 14: 5–122.

73. Penfield W. Neuroglia: normal and pathological. In: Cytology and cellular pathology of the nervous system, vol 2. New York: Hoeber, 1932: 437–443.

74. Trapp BD, Itoyama Y, MacIntosh TD, Quarles RH. P2 protein in oligodendrocytes and myelin of the rabbit central nervous system. J Neurochem 1983; 40: 47–54.

75. Butt AM, Ibrahim M, Ruge FM, Berry M. Biochemical subtypes of oligodendrocyte in the anterior medullary velum of the rat as revealed by the monoclonal antibody Rip. Glia 1995; 14: 185–197.

76. Honnorat J, Aguerra M, Zalc B et al. POP66 A paraneoplastic encephalomyelitis related antigen homologous to Unc33 protein is specifically expressed by a subpopulation of oligodendrocytes in the adult brain. J Neuropathol Exp Neurol 1998; 57: 311–322.

77. Cammer W, Rose AL, Norton WT. Biochemical and pathological studies of myelin in hexachlorophene intoxication. Brain Res 1975; 27: 547–559.

78. Ludwin SK. Central nervous system demyelination and remyelination in the mouse: an ultrastructural study of cuprizone toxicity. Lab Invest 1978; 3: 597–612.

79. Komoly S, Jeyasingham MD, Pratt OE, Lantos PL. Decrease in oligodendrocyte carbonic anhydrase activity preceding myelin degeneration in cuprizone induced demyelination. J Neurol Sci 1989; 79: 141–149.

80. Pringle NP, Richardson WD. A singularity of PDGF alpha-receptor expression in the dorso-ventral axis of the neural tube may define the origin of the oligodendrocyte lineage. Development 1993; 117: 525–533.

81. Ikenaka K, Kagawa T, Mikoshiba K. Selective expression of DM-20, an alternatively spliced myelin proteolipid gene product, in developing nervous system of the mouse. J Neurochem 1992; 58: 2248–2253.

82. Timsit S, Martinez S, Allinquant B et al. Oligodendrocytes originate in a restricted zone of the embryonic ventral neural tube defined by DM-20 mRNA expression. J Neurosci 1995; 15: 1012–1024.

83. Dickinson PJ, Fanarraga ML, Griffiths IR et al. Oligodendrocyte progenitors in the embryonic spinal cord express DM-20. Neuropathol Appl Neurobiol 1996; 22: 188–198.

84. Spassky N, Heydon K, Mangatal A et al. Sonic hedgehog-dependent emergence of oligodendrocytes in the telencephalon: evidence for a source of oligodendrocytes in the olfactory bulb that is independent of PDGFRalpha signaling. Development 2001; 128: 4993–5004.

85. Cai J, Qi Y, Hu X et al. Generation of oligodendrocyte precursor cells from mouse dorsal spinal cord independent of Nkx6 regulation and Shh signaling. Neuron 2005 6; 45: 41–53.

86. Vallstedt A, Klos JM, Ericson J. Multiple dorsoventral origins of oligodendrocyte generation in the spinal cord and hindbrain. Neuron 2005 6; 45: 55–67.

87. Fogarty M, Richardson WD, Kessaris N. A subset of oligodendrocytes generated from radial glia in the dorsal spinal cord. Development 2005; 132: 1951–1959.

88. Kessaris N, Fogarty M, Iannarelli P et al. Competing waves of oligodendrocytes in the forebrain and postnatal elimination of an embryonic lineage. Nat Neurosci 2006; 9: 173–179.

89. Richardson WD, Kessaris N, Pringle N. Oligodendrocyte wars. Nat Rev Neurosci 2006; 7: 11–18.

90. Trousse F, Giess MC, Soula C et al. Notochord and floor plate stimulate oligodendrocyte differentiation in cultures of the chick dorsal neural tube. J Neurosci Res 1995; 41: 552–560.

91. Orentas DM, Miller RH. The origin of spinal cord oligodendrocytes is dependent on local influences from the notochord. Dev Biol 1996; 177: 43–53.

92. Pringle NP, Yu WP, Guthrie S et al. Determination of neuroepithelial cell fate: induction of the oligodendrocyte lineage by ventral midline cells and sonic hedgehog. Dev Biol 1996; 177: 30–42.

93. Orentas DM, Hayes JE, Dyer KL, Miller RH. Sonic hedgehog signaling is required during the appearance of spinal cord oligodendrocyte precursors. Development 1999; 126: 2419–2429.

94. Barres BA, Hart IK, Coles HS et al. Cell death and control of cell survival in the oligodendrocyte lineage. Cell 1992; 70: 31–46.

95. Richardson WD, Pringle N, Mosley MJ et al. A role for platelet-derived growth factor in normal gliogenesis in the central nervous system. Cell 1988; 53: 309–319.

96. Barres BA, Raff MC. Proliferation of oligodendrocyte precursor cells depends on electrical activity in axons. Nature 1993; 361: 258–260.

97. Eccleston PA, Silberberg DH. Fibroblast growth factor is a mitogen for oligodendrocytes in vitro. Brain Res 1985; 353: 315–318.

98. McMorris FA, Smith TM, DeSalvo S, Furlanetto RW. Insulin-like growth factor I/somatomedin C: a potent inducer of oligodendrocyte development. Proc Natl Acad Sci USA 1986; 83: 822–826.

99. Raff MC, Barres BA, Burne JF et al. Programmed cell death and the control of cell survival. Philos Trans R Soc Lond B Biol Sci 1994; 345: 265–268.

100. Le Bras B, Barallobre MJ, Homman-Ludiye J et al. VEGF-C is a trophic factor for neural progenitors in the vertebrate embryonic brain. Nat Neurosci 2006; 9: 340–348.

101. Ono K, Yasui Y, Rutishauser U, Miller RH. Focal ventricular origin and migration of oligodendrocyte precursors into the chick optic nerve. Neuron 1997; 19: 283–292.

102. Olivier C, Cobos I, Perez Villegas EM et al. Monofocal origin of telencephalic oligodendrocytes in the anterior entopeduncular area of the chick embryo. Development 2001; 128: 1757–1769.

103. Payne HR, Lemmon V. Glial cells of the O-2A lineage bind preferentially to N-cadherin and develop distinct morphologies. Dev Biol 1993; 159: 595–607.

104. Milner R, ffrench-Constant C. A developmental analysis of oligodendroglial integrins in primary cells: changes in alpha v-associated beta subunits during differentiation. Development 1994; 120: 3497–3506.

105. Wang C, Rougon G, Kiss JZ. Requirement of polysialic acid for the migration of the O-2A glial progenitor cell from neurohypophyseal explants. J Neurosci 1994; 14: 4446–1457.

106. Kiernan BW, Gotz B, Faissner A, ffrench-Constant C. Tenascin-C inhibits oligodendrocyte precursor cell migration by both adhesion-dependent and adhesion-independent mechanisms. Mol Cell Neurosci 1996; 7: 322–335.

107. Garcion E, Faissner A, ffrench-Constant C. Knockout mice reveal a contribution of the extracellular matrix molecule tenascin-C to neural precursor proliferation and migration. Development 2001; 128: 2485–2496.

108. Prestoz L, Chatzopoulou E, Lemkine G et al. Control of axonophilic migration of oligodendrocyte precursor cells by Eph/ephrin interaction. Neuron Glia Biol 2004; 1: 74–85.

109. Armstrong RC, Harvath L, Dubois-Dalcq ME. Type 1 astrocytes and oligodendrocyte-type 2 astrocyte glial progenitors migrate toward distinct molecules. J Neurosci Res 1990; 27: 400–407.

110. Milner R, Anderson HJ, Rippon RF et al. Contrasting effects of mitogenic growth factors on oligodendrocyte precursor cell migration. Glia 1997; 19: 85–90.

111. Spassky N, de Castro F, Le Bras B et al. Directional guidance of oligodendroglial migration by class 3 semaphorins and netrin-1. J Neurosci 2002; 22: 5992–6004.

112. Sugimoto Y, Taniguchi M, Yagi T et al. Guidance of glial precursor cell migration by secreted cues in the developing optic nerve. Development 2001; 128: 3321–3330.

113. Tsai HH, Tessier-Lavigne M, Miller RH. Netrin 1 mediates spinal cord oligodendrocyte precursor dispersal. Development 2003; 130: 2095–2105.

114. Small RK, Riddle P, Noble M. Evidence for migration of oligodendrocyte-type-2 astrocyte progenitor cells into the developing rat optic nerve. Nature 1987; 328: 155–157.

115. Bansal R, Steffanson K, Pfeiffer SE. POA, a developmental antigen expressed by A007/O4-positive oligodendrocyte progenitors prior to the appearance of sulfatide and galactocerebroside. J Neurochem 1992; 58: 2221–2229.

116. Bhat RV, Axt KJ, Fosnaugh JS et al. Expression of the APC tumor suppressor protein in oligodendroglia. Glia 1996; 17: 169–174.

117. Sherman DL, Brophy PJ. Mechanisms of axon ensheathment and myelin growth. Nat Rev Neurosci 2005; 6: 683–690.

118. Althaus HH, Montz H, Neuhoff V, Schwartz P. Isolation and cultivation of mature oligodendroglial cells. Naturwissenschaften 1984; 71: 309–315.

119. Lubetzki C, Demerens C, Anglade P et al. Even in culture, oligodendrocytes myelinate solely axons. Proc Natl Acad Sci USA 1993; 90: 6820–6824.

120. Rathjen FG, Schachner M. Immunocytological and biochemical characterization of a new neuronal cell surface component (L1 antigen) which is involved in cell adhesion. EMBO J 1984; 3: 1–10.

121. Martini R, Schachner M. Immunoelectron microscopic localization of neural cell adhesion molecules (L1, N-CAM, and MAG) and their shared carbohydrate

epitope and myelin basic protein in developing sciatic nerve. J Cell Biol 1986; 103: 2439–2448.

122. Persohn E, Schachner M. Immunohistological localization of the neural adhesion molecules L1 and N-CAM in the developing hippocampus of the mouse. J Neurocytol 1990; 19: 807–819.

123. Hortsch M. The L1 family of neural cell adhesion molecules: old proteins performing new tricks. Neuron 1996; 17: 587–593.

124. Hortsch M. Structural and functional evolution of the L1 family: are four adhesion molecules better than one? Mol Cell Neurosci 2000; 15: 1–10.

125. Wood PM, Schachner M, Bunge RP. Inhibition of Schwann cell myelination in vitro by antibody to the L1 adhesion molecule. J Neurosci 1990; 10: 3635–3645.

126. Itoh K, Stevens B, Schachner M, Fields RD. Regulated expression of the neural cell adhesion molecule L1 by specific patterns of neural impulses. Science 1995; 270: 1369–1372.

127. Stevens B, Tanner S, Fields RD. Control of myelination by specific patterns of neural impulses. J Neurosci 1998; 18: 9303–9311.

128. Barbin G, Charles P, Foucher A et al. Axonal cell adhesion molecule L1 in central nervous system myelination. Neuron Glia Biol 2004; 1: 65–73.

129. Doherty P, Fruns M, Seaton P et al. A threshold effect of the major isoforms of NCAM on neurite outgrowth. Nature 1990; 343: 464–466.

130. Kiss JZ, Wang C, Olive S et al. Activity-dependent mobilization of the adhesion molecule polysialic NCAM to the cell surface of neurons and endocrine cells. EMBO J 1994; 13: 5284–5292.

131. Meyer-Franke A, Shen S, Barres BA. Astrocytes induce oligodendrocyte processes to align with and adhere to axons. Mol Cell Neurosci 1999; 14: 385–397.

132. Charles P, Hernandez MP, Stankoff B et al. Negative regulation of central nervous system myelination by polysialylated-neural cell adhesion molecule. Proc Natl Acad Sci USA 2000; 97: 7585–7590.

133. Wanner IB, Wood PM. N-cadherin mediates axon-aligned process growth and cell–cell interaction in rat Schwann cells. J Neurosci 2002; 22: 4066–4079.

134. Schnadelbach O, Ozen I, Blaschuk OW et al. N-cadherin is involved in axon-oligodendrocyte contact and myelination. Mol Cell Neurosci 2001; 17: 1084–1093.

135. Feltri ML, Graus Porta D, Previtali SC et al. Conditional disruption of beta 1 integrin in Schwann cells impedes interactions with axons. J Cell Biol 2002; 156: 199–209.

136. Colognato H, MacCarrick M, O'Rear JJ, Yurchenco PD. The laminin α2-chain short arm mediates cell adhesion through both the α1β1 and α2β1 integrins. J Biol Chem 1997; 272: 29330–293306.

137. Fernandez-Valle C, Gwynn L, Wood PM et al. Anti-beta 1 integrin antibody inhibits Schwann cell myelination. J Neurobiol 1994; 25: 1207–1226.

138. Wang S, Sdrulla AD, diSibio G et al. Notch receptor activation inhibits oligodendrocyte differentiation. Neuron 1998; 21: 63–75.

139. John GR, Shankar SL, Shafit-Zagardo B et al. Multiple sclerosis: re-expression of a developmental pathway that restricts oligodendrocyte maturation. Nat Med 2002; 8: 1115–1121.

140. Stidworthy MF, Genoud S, Li WW et al. Notch1 and Jagged1 are expressed after CNS demyelination, but are not a major rate-determining factor during remyelination. Brain 2004; 127(Pt 9): 1928–1941.

141. Gyllensten L, Malmfors T. Myelinization of the optic nerve and its dependence on visual function–a quantitative investigation in mice. J Embryol Exp Morphol 1963; 11: 255–266.

142. Omlin FX. Optic disc and optic nerve of the blind cape mole-rat (Georychus capensis): a proposed model for naturally occurring reactive gliosis. Brain Res Bull 1997; 44: 627–632.

143. Tauber H, Waehneldt TV, Neuhoff V. Myelination in rabbit optic nerves is accelerated by artificial eye opening. Neurosci Lett 1980; 16: 235–238.

144. Demerens C, Stankoff B, Logak M et al. Induction of myelination in the central nervous system by electrical activity. Proc Natl Acad Sci USA 1996; 93: 9887–9892.

145. Stevens B, Porta S, Haak LL et al. Adenosine: a neuron-glial transmitter promoting myelination in the CNS in response to action potentials. Neuron 2002; 36: 855–868.

146. Stevens B, Fields RD. Response of Schwann cells to action potentials in development. Science 2000; 287: 2267–2271.

147. Michailov GV, Sereda MW, Brinkmann BG et al. Axonal neuregulin-1 regulates myelin sheath thickness. Science 2004; 304: 700–703.

148. Taveggia C, Zanazzi G, Petrylak A et al. Neuregulin-1 type III determines the ensheathment fate of axons. Neuron 2005; 47: 681–694.

149. Barres BA, Raff MC, Gaese F et al. A crucial role for neurotrophin-3 in oligodendrocyte development. Nature 1994; 367: 371–375.

150. Barres BA, Schmid R, Sendnter M, Raff MC. Multiple extracellular signals are required for long-term oligodendrocyte survival. Development 1993; 118: 283–295.

151. Chan JR, Watkins TA, Cosgaya JM et al. NGF controls axonal receptivity to myelination by Schwann cells or oligodendrocytes. Neuron 2004; 43: 183–191.

152. Kotter MR, Zhao C, van Rooijen N, Franklin RJ. Macrophage-depletion induced impairment of experimental CNS remyelination is associated with a reduced oligodendrocyte progenitor cell response and altered growth factor expression. Neurobiol Dis 2005; 18: 166–175.

153. Foote AK, Blakemore WF. Inflammation stimulates remyelination in areas of chronic demyelination. Brain 2005; 128: 528–539.

154. Stankoff B, Aigrot MS, Noel F et al. Ciliary neurotrophic factor (CNTF) enhances myelin formation: a novel role for CNTF and CNTF-related molecules. J Neurosci 2002; 22: 9221–9227.

155. Iwase T, Jung CG, Bae H et al. Glial cell line-derived neurotrophic factor-induced signaling in Schwann cells. J Neurochem 2005; 94: 1488–1499.

156. Tolwani RJ, Cosgaya JM, Varma S et al. BDNF overexpression produces a long-term increase in myelin formation in the peripheral nervous system. J Neurosci Res 2004; 77: 662–669.

157. Umemori H, Sato S, Yagi T et al. Initial events of myelination involve Fyn tyrosine kinase signalling. Nature 1994; 367: 572–576.

158. Osterhout DJ, Wolven A, Wolf RM et al. Morphological differentiation of oligodendrocytes requires activation of Fyn tyrosine kinase. J Cell Biol 1999; 145: 1209–1218.

159. Sperber BR, McMorris FA. Fyn tyrosine kinase regulates oligodendroglial cell development but is not required for morphological differentiation of oligodendrocytes. J Neurosci Res 2001; 63: 303–312.

160. Chun SJ, Rasband MN, Sidman RL et al. Integrin-linked kinase is required for laminin-2-induced oligodendrocyte cell spreading and CNS myelination. J Cell Biol 2003; 163: 397–408.

161. Mi S, Lee X, Shao Z et al. LINGO-1 is a component of the Nogo-66 receptor/p75 signaling complex. Nat Neurosci 2004; 7: 221–228.

162. Shao Z, Browning JL, Lee X et al. TAJ/TROY, an orphan TNF receptor family member, binds Nogo-66 receptor 1 and regulates axonal regeneration. Neuron 2005; 45: 353–359.

163. Park JB, Yiu G, Kaneko S et al. A TNF receptor family member, TROY, is a coreceptor with Nogo receptor in mediating the inhibitory activity of myelin inhibitors. Neuron 2005; 45: 345–351.

164. Melendez-Vasquez CV, Einheber S, Salzer JL. Rho kinase regulates schwann cell myelination and formation of associated axonal domains. J Neurosci 2004; 24: 3953–3963.

165. Liang X, Draghi NA, Resh MD. Signaling from integrins to Fyn to Rho family GTPases regulates morphologic differentiation of oligodendrocytes. J Neurosci 2004; 24: 7140–7149.

166. Mi S, Miller RH, Lee X et al. LINGO-1 negatively regulates myelination by oligodendrocytes. Nat Neurosci 2005; 8: 745–751.

167. Nagata-Ohashi K, Ohta Y, Goto K et al. A pathway of neuregulin-induced activation of cofilin-phosphatase Slingshot and cofilin in lamellipodia. J Cell Biol 2004; 165: 465–471.

New tools for investigating the immunopathogenesis of multiple sclerosis: principles and applications

M. Bradl, K. Dornmair and R. Hohlfeld

INTRODUCTION

The past few years have witnessed the arrival of many novel biomedical techniques, which are likely to greatly improve our knowledge of the molecular and cellular pathways involved in the immunopathogenesis of multiple sclerosis (MS). In this chapter, we will discuss the strengths and limitations of these techniques and show their potential for studying such a complex disease as MS. Among other topics, we discuss the analysis of antigen-specific T-cell receptors from individual infiltrating T cells found in MS plaques, show how it is possible to trace such cells over many years in different anatomical locations and demonstrate that it is now even possible to watch in real time how disease-inducing cells behave in the central nervous system (CNS) target organ. We also address 'unbiased' microarray studies of expression profiles of thousands of genes in peripheral blood or MS lesions. Such analyses could have great potential for identifying new therapeutic targets, and for monitoring disease activity and therapeutic responsiveness. Further, we describe tools for the high-throughput screening of proteins, which may eventually lead to the identification of CNS antigens targeted by the autoantibodies found in the serum or the cerebrospinal fluid (CSF) of MS patients.

CHARACTERIZATION OF AUTOREACTIVE T AND B CELLS IN CENTRAL NERVOUS SYSTEM TISSUES

MICRODISSECTION OF T CELLS FROM MULTIPLE SCLEROSIS LESIONS

Much work has been done over the years to characterize immune cells in blood and cerebrospinal fluid (CSF). It is relatively easy to obtain fresh samples, and living cells from blood or CSF can be directly analyzed ex vivo or can be studied in vitro in cell culture. Another advantage of this 'peripheral cell sampling' approach is that at least blood samples can be taken repeatedly over time. One obvious problem with this approach, however, is that the cells present in blood and CSF may be quite different from those attacking the CNS target tissue. It has, therefore,

become increasingly appreciated that techniques allowing the characterization of inflammatory cells directly in target tissues would be very useful and are in fact badly needed. One of the major hurdles is that specimens of human brain or spinal cord are usually fixed or frozen, so that it is impossible to extract living cells from these tissues. Another important consideration relates to the stage of disease as it is reflected in biopsy and autopsy samples: biopsies are often obtained from early and/or unusual cases, whereas autopsy material usually comes from patients with long-standing, chronic MS.

It has long been known that T and B cells represent important components of inflammatory infiltrates in MS lesions. However, very little is known about their properties, let alone their pathogenic contribution. Regarding T-cell infiltrates, for example, it would be important to know whether they represent a small number of T-cell clones or a broad range of polyclonal T cells. A complicating factor is that the nature of the T-cell infiltrates may differ in relation to the anatomical location: for example, T cells deep in the CNS parenchyma, T cells in perivascular locations and T cells trapped in the vasculature are likely to be different.[1] Analysis of tissue homogenates, e.g. by reverse-transcriptase polymerase chain reaction (RT-PCR), does not allow any distinction between these different T lymphocytes. However, this problem can be overcome by the isolation of morphologically characterized T cells prior to further analysis.

Simple mechanical microdissection techniques rely on the dissection of the intact tissue with fine needles to separate the cells of interest from adjacent cells prior to polymerase chain reaction (PCR) analysis. Faster and more efficient and precise techniques rely on laser-mediated manipulation of single cells or cell clusters from tissue sections mounted on slides. To date, two different laser-mediated procedures are available for microdissection of tissues (Fig. 19.1A): laser-capture microdissection (LCM)[2] and a combination of laser microbeam microdissection (LMM) and laser pressure catapulting (LPC).[3] LCM uses a transparent thermoplastic foil that is coated on to the surface of a microfuge cap. This foil is brought in direct contact with the entire tissue section on a glass support. A heat-generating infrared laser is then used to melt the foil and to fuse the selected areas of the tissue section with the foil. Afterwards, the cap is

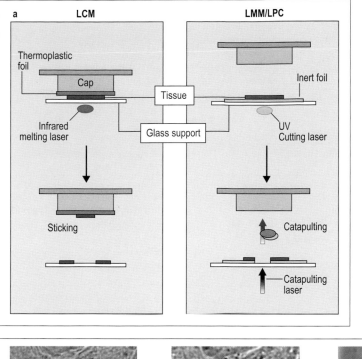

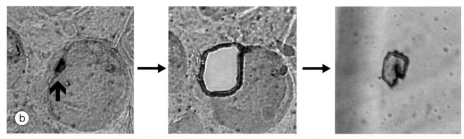

FIG. 19.1 Laser microdissection. **A.** Two different laser-assisted microdissection techniques available today. For laser-capture microdissection (LCM), a heat-generating infrared laser is used to fuse selected areas of a tissue section with a temperature-sensitive transfer membrane mounted on to a microfuge cap. Afterwards, the cap is removed and the selected tissue components on its temperature-sensitive membrane can be processed for further analysis. The combination of laser microbeam microdissection (LMM) and laser pressure catapulting (LPC) avoids mechanical contact with the entire histological tissue. Instead, single cells or cell clusters are first circumscribed with a focused laser beam and the excised tissue piece is then catapulted into the cap of a microfuge tube. **B.** Single cell isolation by LMM/LPC from a polymyositis muscle biopsy sample. A T cell in direct contact with a muscle fiber was labeled with a specific antibody and stained by alkaline phosphates (arrow). The T cell was excised by a laser beam and catapulted into the lid of a PCR tube. With permission from Hofbauer et al 2003.[15]

removed, together with the molten foil and the selected tissue components, which adhere to their temperature-sensitive membrane and can be processed for further analysis. The second method, LMM/LPC, avoids mechanical contact with the entire histological tissue, further enhancing the purity of the isolates. Instead, single cells or cell clusters are precisely circumscribed with a focused ultraviolet laser beam that isolates the selected specimen from the surrounding tissue. Cutting is accomplished by a photophysical process called ablation that does not produce heat. Then, the high photon density of a focused laser beam is used to create pressure forces that catapult the excised tissue piece into the cap of a microfuge tube that is several millimeters away from the tissue section (Fig. 19.1B).

The first published report using microdissection techniques to study the clonality of T cells in MS lesions was the paper by Babbe and colleagues.[4] They stained frozen tissue sections of MS lesions with antibodies to clearly identify CD4+ or CD8+ T cells and then used a micromanipulator to mobilize single T cells and separate them from the surrounding tissue. Because T-cell receptors (TCRs) are the most discriminating feature of different T-cell clones, and because only the clonal descendants of the same cell share the same TCR, Babbe et al[4] proceeded to analyze the TCRs of the microdissected lymphocytes by single-cell PCR. They observed that infiltrating CD8+ T cells represented the descendants of only a few different T-cell clones, although they dominated in MS lesions. In contrast, the CD4+ T cells were much more heterogenous and represented the progeny of many different T-cell clones, even though they were much less numerous in the lesions.[4]

The pioneering paper by Babbe and colleagues[4] paved the way for further microdissection analyses of individual cells in complex lesions or of single lesions in complex anatomical structures. However, there is an important limitation to these microdissection analyses: they are incompatible with the widely used paraformaldehyde fixation of biopsy or postmortem material because this may lead to irreversible damage of DNA and RNA and may thus interfere with subsequent molecular analyses.[5] Instead, frozen tissue blocks remain the material of choice for this type of analysis. With this type of specimen, the microdissected areas are ideally suited for further analysis, as demonstrated by recent comparable analysis of T cells in the CNS and cerebrospinal fluid (CSF) of MS patients.[6]

CLONAL PERSISTENCE OF CD8+ T CELLS IN MULTIPLE SCLEROSIS PATIENTS

The work by Babbe and coworkers[4] showed that oligoclonal CD8+ T cells might be the dominant T-cell population in MS lesions, which suggested that CD8+ T cells could play a more important role in the disease process than previously thought (see reference 7 for a comprehensive review of the role of CD8+ T cells in MS). But does the dominance of CD8+ T-cell clones in inflammatory lesions really reflect a true preferential recruitment of certain clones into the affected area? Or does it reflect random migration of clones that are overrepresented in the peripheral immune repertoire? There are several possible approaches to address these questions (Table 19.1). A more conventional way would involve the isolation of the cells from the CNS and from the blood, cellular cloning and characterization of these T cells in vitro and then, finally, molecular cloning and characterization of the TCRs carried by these cells by sequencing analyses.

TABLE 19.1 Overview on some recent techniques to T cells in MS

Method	Material	Sensitivity	Comments
Functional tests (proliferation and Elispot, cytotoxicity assays, limited dilution assays, CSFE)	Living cells	Variable (e.g. antigen-induced proliferation: low sensitivity; Elispot: potentially high sensitivity	Classical techniques for detection of antigen-specific T-cell responses
MHC–peptide multimers	TCR surface proteins	Theoretically unlimited (may detect single cells)	T cells with downregulated TCRs might escape detection; antigen and MHC restriction must be known
Clone-specific quantitative PCR	mRNA/cDNA	≈ 1 cell in 10^5–10^6	TCR sequence of target T-cell clone must be known
CDR3 spectratyping	mRNA/cDNA	$\approx 5 \times 10^4$ cells for a complete β-chain spectratype	Unbiased screening technique; can detect clonal expansions of T-cells with unknown TCR sequence and antigen specificity
Single-cell PCR	mRNA/cDNA or genomic DNA of single cells (by limiting dilution, sorted or from tissue sections)	Unlimited (detects single cells)	Can relate morphological information (pathogenic relevance!) to clonal TCR sequence
Microarrays (expression profiles)	cDNA	Variable	Can provide a global overview of gene expression in a defined population of T cells or even a single cell
Live imaging	GFP transfected cells	Large populations only	Applicable only in animal models

Obviously, this is a laborious task. A novel, more efficient method takes advantage of a different technique, which is especially suitable for the screening of TCR repertoires. The method is called CDR3 spectratyping or immunoscope. It allows a semiquantitative measure of the clonal distribution of particular T-cell populations. In other words, CDR3 spectratyping may identify polyclonal or monoclonal populations and it may as well detect particular expanded clones on a polyclonal background (reviewed by Pannetier et al[8]).

CDR3 spectratyping is based on the fact that individual T cells and their clonal descendants carry unique heterodimeric TCRs, which are composed both of an α and a β chain. The high degree of diversity of these receptors is caused by peculiarities shared by TCRs and antibodies. First, each α or β chain is composed of different genetic elements, termed variable (V), joining (J) and constant (C). There are about 50 different V elements for α and β chains, and 13 J-β and 50 J-α elements. Each individual α or β chain is composed of one V, one J and the constant element. Permutation of these arrangements already yields a considerable heterogeneity. Secondly, α and β chains may be combined arbitrarily. Thirdly, and most importantly, random (N) nucleotides may be added between the V and the J elements during rearrangement of the chains. Further, some nucleotides of the germline elements may be removed, and the β chains contain further 'diversity' elements. Therefore, each TCR α or β chain contains sequence segments that are hypervariable both in their length and in their precise nucleotide sequence. It has been estimated that theoretically 10^{15} different TCR molecules may exist.[9] The hypervariable region between V and J elements is called a complementarity-determining region (CDR)3 and is known to play a pivotal role in antigen recognition (reviewed by Rudolph et al[10]). Amplification of this region by PCR yields a spectrum of PCR products of different lengths (the spectra type): polyclonal populations show typical gaussian distributions whereas monoclonal populations yield distinct peaks (Fig. 19.2).[11] Thus, prominent peaks, even if they are superimposed on to a gaussian distribution, strongly suggest expansions of particular T-cell clones. For definite proof, the nucleotide sequence of such dominant peaks may be determined.[12,13,14]

The diagnostic brain biopsy of the MS patient studied by Babbe et al[4] revealed the presence of a putatively pathogenic, oligoclonal CD8+ T-cell infiltrate in the MS plaque. In a follow-up of this patient, these clones were then tracked in two additional compartments: in the peripheral blood, and in the CSF.[6] It turned out that the CD8+ T-cell clones that infiltrated the CNS, and had been initially found in the biopsied lesion, persisted for more than 5 years in the CSF and in the blood of this patient (Fig. 19.3). Clonal persistence was also observed in a second patient available for this study: again, this patient had a diagnostic brain biopsy, which helped to establish the diagnosis of MS. More importantly, also in this patient, oligoclonal CD8+ T cells were found in the CNS lesions. When his CSF and peripheral blood were reexamined 6 months later, CD8+ T cells with exactly the same TCR V-β CDR3 sequence were found in both compartments.[6] These findings indicate that the clonal persistence of CD8+ T cells in the peripheral blood and the CSF is not a unique feature of one singular patient but is probably common to a larger number of MS patients. For this reason it was suggested that surveying these cells in the peripheral immune repertoire could provide a powerful means to monitor disease activity and assess the response to immunosuppressive and immunomodulatory therapies.[6] Unfortunately, spectratyping cannot provide any further information about the T-cell clones identified. Hence it remains open whether these clones play a role in the progression of the disease or whether they have important regulatory functions. Similarly, the reasons for the skewing of the T-cell repertoire observed in MS patients remain unresolved.

IDENTIFICATION OF PAIRED T-CELL RECEPTOR α AND β CHAINS FROM INDIVIDUAL TISSUE-INFILTRATING T CELLS

In animal models, the relevance of T-cell clones for disease initiation and progression can be directly tested.[1] In human

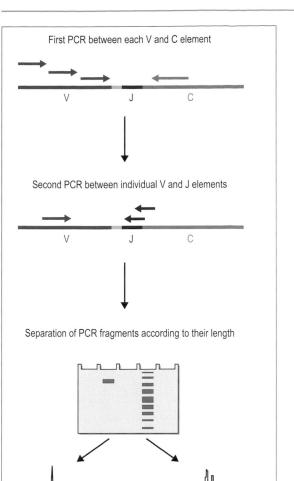

FIG. 19.2 CDR3 spectratyping measures the length distribution of the hypervariable regions of TCR β-chains (shown in red). The length and sequence is characteristic for individual clones. cDNA of T cells is amplified using primers specific for the constant region (C) (brown) or for specific V-β regions (green) of the T-cell receptor (TCR). A specific primer is used for each of the V-β family (typically 25 families). In a second PCR reaction each individual Vβ-C PCR product is amplified using Vβ and typically 13 specific Jβ primers (blue). All 325 PCR products are then individually analyzed by high-resolution polyacrylamide gel electrophoresis (PAGE), which separates the fragments according to their length. The size of the products is determined by the length of the hypervariable CDR3 region (red). For analysis the bands are scanned and plotted. Monoclonal T-cell populations have, by definition, identical CDR3 regions. Therefore only a single peak appears. Polyclonal populations show gaussian length distributions. The distance between individual peaks corresponds to three nucleotides, which code for one amino acid.

diseases, however, the putative pathogenic role of T-cell clones cannot be demonstrated directly but needs to be deduced from indirect evidence. This includes, for example, morphological criteria (e.g. juxtaposition of T cells with their target structures[15]) or suggestive temporal variations (e.g. emergence or expansion of T-cell clones immediately before a clinical disease relapse.[16]

How can one investigate the antigen specificity of brain-infiltrating T cells of MS patients? The basic approach to experimentally addressing this problem seems relatively straightforward: if it were possible to characterize TCR of single lymphocytes in MS lesions, then it should be possible to 'revive' the T cells found in histological sections of MS lesions and study their antigen recognition in vitro. The prerequisites for such a study are 1) identification of paired α and β TCR chains from expanded, putatively pathogenic, CNS-infiltrating T lymphocytes, and 2) expression of these TCR in T-hybridoma cell lines that contain the complete machinery for signaling through TCR but lack their own endogenous TCR. When such cells are then challenged with different antigens, they secrete cytokines and possibly even proliferate after they recognize 'their' antigen (i.e. the antigen specifically recognized by the cloned TCR.[17]

The feasibility of such an approach was recently demonstrated with an autoreactive γδ T-cell clone derived from polymyositis lesions. Although the repertoire of CD8+ T cells in polymyositis is usually oligo- or polyclonal,[18] a monoclonal expansion of tissue-invasive γδ TCR-positive T cells has been observed in a unique case.[19,20] Therefore is was possible to clone the α and β chains by conventional PCR techniques, i.e. without the need of single-cell PCR (see below). Both chains were then functionally expressed in the T hybridoma cell line 58α⁻β⁻,[21] which has the major advantage of lacking both endogenous TCR chains as compared to other possible recipient cell lines (discussed by Dornmair et al[17]). These transfectants were used to investigate the antigen of the autoaggressive γδ TCR. The 'resurrected' γδ TCR recognized not only an autoantigen expressed in human muscle but also an antigen of bacterial origin. Although the precise chemical nature of both antigens is not yet known, both antigens were recognized specifically. This was shown by introducing defined amino acid substitutions in the CDR3 regions of both TCR chains, which abrogated the antigen recognition completely.[22,23]

Unfortunately, it is even more difficult to identify the target antigens of tissue-infiltrating αβ T cells in MS lesions. For a long time, research along this line has been hindered by the fact that a functional TCR is composed of two different chains, an α and a β chain, but only tools for investigating the β chain repertoire were available.[17] Firstly, antibodies that recognize particular TCR V regions can be used to monitor T-cell populations by immunohistochemistry or flow cytometry. There are many antibodies that recognize about 70% of the spectrum of V-β regions but only three antibodies may detect particular V-α chains. Secondly, the much greater number of J-α regions compared to J-β regions impedes α-chain spectratyping. Thirdly, single cell analysis is required because often several different T-cell clones are expanded in the tissue. Although bulk analysis by conventional PCR methods may detect expanded clones, they may not correlate particular α to particular β chains. Fourthly, many other irrelevant T cells are present in the tissue that may only be distinguished by morphology. This also requires analysis by single cell PCR, which is notoriously difficult because of the extremely low amount of template RNA/cDNA. In the past, β chains were therefore commonly used to monitor the expansion of T-cell clones[6] but α chains are only poorly characterized.[17] Therefore, it is technically highly demanding to characterize and clone TCR α and β chains from single T cells microdissected from CNS lesions of MS patients. We have recently developed a multiplex PCR method that allows concomitant amplification of TCR α and β chains.[24] Because the β-chain sequences were previously known from CDR3 spectratyping, the intricate multiplex format was only required for the α chains. We succeeded in detecting several matching TCR α and β chains from microdissected single cells. These chains can be reconstituted in the mouse T hybridoma cell line 58α⁻β⁻ and can be used for searching their target antigens.

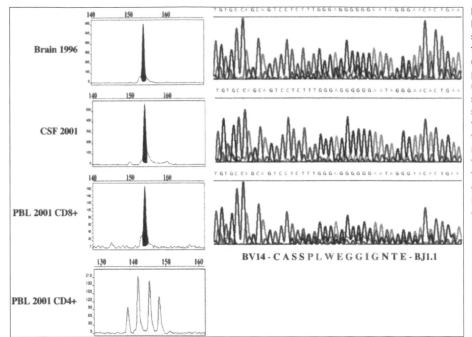

FIG. 19.3 Expanded CD8+ T cells persist in brain, CSF and blood of an MS patient. CDR3 spectratype analysis was performed on T cells from brain tissue (biopsied 1996), from CSF (2001) and from the CD8 compartment of peripheral blood (2001) of a patient who had undergone diagnostic brain biopsy. CDR3 spectratypes showed strong single peaks in all samples. True monoclonal expansions were verified by sequencing of the PCR products, which all yielded identical sequences. This means that the same expanded TCR β-chain was present in all samples. For comparison, the CD4 compartment of blood yielded a gaussian distribution typical for polyclonal populations. With permission from Skulina et al 2004.[6]

STRATEGIES FOR SEARCHING THE TARGET ANTIGENS OF 'RECONSTRUCTED' T-CELL RECEPTORS

An intrinsic property of αβ TCR molecules is that they recognize specific complexes of major histocompatibility complex (MHC) molecules (human MHC molecules are also termed human leukocyte antigens (HLA)) and short peptides bound in a groove at the MHC surface (reviewed by Rudolph et al[10]). Thus, for each T-cell clone actually two antigens have to be revealed: the restriction element (i.e. the HLA molecule) and its bound antigenic peptide. After an autoaggressive T-cell clone has been characterized, at first neither its restricting HLA allele nor the antigenic peptide is known. Although there is a statically relevant genetic link of MS to particular HLA alleles (see Ch. 14), such links need not to be predictive for individual clones.

First of all, T cells need antigen-presenting cells (APCs) that expose peptides bound to HLA molecules on their surface. Basically there are two types of APC that may be employed. One possibility is to use autologous cells of the particular patient. For practical reasons, an Epstein–Barr virus (EBV) transformed B-cell line may be established from the patient's blood. Such immortalized APC lines carry all relevant HLA alleles, including the particular HLA allele to which the respective T cell is specific. This approach may allow the testing of peptide antigens without prior knowledge of the restriction element. Alternatively, the HLA spectrum of the patient may be determined by classical HLA typing in a preliminary experiment. Then each allele can be transfected individually into an APC line such as mouse fibroblasts or COS cells. If it is unknown a priori which of the patients HLA alleles is the restriction element for a certain T-cell clone, then several transfectants have to be generated and tested individually.

Two types of library may be used for determining the nature of the antigenic peptide: cDNA libraries and synthetic peptide libraries. cDNA libraries represent the entire spectrum of transcribed genes of the particular tissue. Ideally this would be the brain tissue of the respective patient. Considerable amounts of fresh or frozen tissue are necessary for establishing such a library, because long, full-length transcripts are required that translate into complete proteins. Therefore, formaldehyde-fixed tissue cannot be used. Powerful, although quite demanding, techniques are the 'linear transcriptome amplification' methods that are based either on in vitro transcription by T7 RNA polymerase[25] or on sophisticated PCR procedures.[26–28] These methods amplify the entire spectrum of mRNA so that the relative relation between different mRNA species is preserved. Such techniques might in future enable us to significantly reduce the amount of required tissue for generating cDNA libraries, perhaps to the single-cell level. Alternatively, brain tissue of unrelated donors might be used, although this approach bears some risks. Thus, the antigenic protein may be specific for the particular patient and therefore not be contained in the library, or the cells used for antigen presentation may not generate the appropriate peptides from the parent protein. However, the concept of screening cDNA libraries has already been used successfully in determining T-cell antigens from tumors,[29] although experiences in autoimmunity are still limited to model systems.[30]

Another, completely different, type of library comprises the positional scanning synthetic combinatorial libraries (PS-SCL) (reviewed by Sospedra et al[31]). They are based on the observation that TCR molecules show some degeneracy in their antigen recognition, i.e. they recognize motifs rather than defined structures. Therefore, particular amino acids may often be replaced by similar ones without loss of recognition. The PS-SCL libraries are designed to measure the relative importance of particular amino acids at a given position in the peptide. This will reveal the motif recognized by the TCR. Then protein databases are searched for peptide sequences from real proteins that represent such a motif. In a final step the suggested candidate peptides are synthesized in vitro and tested for recognition by the TCR molecules.

Other libraries, such as the serological identification by recombinant expression cloning (SEREX) libraries or phage display libraries, are designed to identify (auto)antibodies. Although they have proved useful in MS research,[32] they are not suited for determining T-cell epitopes.

CLONAL ANALYSIS OF B CELLS

B cells long ago reappeared center stage in MS pathogenesis research (see Meinl et al[33] for review). Similar strategies as described above for T cells have also been applied for the analysis of B cells, not only in blood and CSF but also in CNS lesions of MS patients. Increased synthesis of intrathecal IgG and its distribution as oligoclonal bands have long been recognized as diagnostic hallmarks of MS. However, the antigen specificity of these oligoclonal bands has remained a mystery. On the other hand, there are several clues suggesting that antibodies directed against myelin–oligodendrocyte glycoprotein (MOG) have pathogenic and prognostic relevance. These antibodies have been detected in tissue of MS patients, using immunogold-labeled peptides of myelin antigens and high-resolution microscopy.[34] Regarding their prognostic relevance, initial studies indicated that circulating anti-MOG antibodies can serve as predictors of clinically definite MS after a first demyelinating event but these findings have not been universally confirmed.[35,36]

Several studies have demonstrated clonally expanded B cells in the CNS and CSF of MS patients.[37–41] Single-cell strategies as described for T cells can be used for the identification of the pairing light and heavy immunoglobulin chains from individual infiltrating B cells. The paired chains can be incorporated into recombinant antibodies, which can be used in the search for target antigens. This search will be facilitated by the rapid progress in protcomics techniques (see below), including miniaturized autoantigen arrays for large-scale multiplex characterization of autoantibody responses directed against diverse autoantigens.[42] At the present time these protein arrays are best suited for the detection of antibodies directed against conformation-independent epitopes but future progress in this area will help to identify new antibody targets.

CLONAL TRACKING OF ANTIGEN-SPECIFIC T CELLS USING MHC–PEPTIDE TETRAMERS AND CLONE-SPECIFIC POLYMERASE CHAIN REACTION

T-cell responses can be studied by a variety of techniques, each with their respective advantages and disadvantages (Table 19.1). Once the antigen is known, soluble MHC–peptide tetramers, oligomers or multimers can be constructed to find and trace the antigen-specific T cells in various locations. Because the affinity of TCR to MHC-peptide complexes is low, the MHC–peptide complexes are oligomerized (best known are tetramers) to compensate for their low affinity by high avidity.[43] Soluble MHC tetramers are synthetic structures that behave similarly to the natural MHC–peptide complexes found on the surface of antigen presenting cells: They are recognized by T cells carrying the corresponding antigen-specific TCR. Principally, tetramers can be constructed using MHC class I[44,45] or MHC class II[46,47] molecules and peptides, or CD1 molecules and glycolipids,[48] thus allowing the tracking of CD8+ and CD4+ T lymphocytes or natural killer (NK) T cells. This approach works well with flow cytometry (FACS) analyses of peripheral blood cells, where it has been used to visualize antigen-specific T cells, e.g. in cancer patients,[49,50] or in EBV-[45] or HIV-infected patients.[51] It was also applied in experimental autoimmune encephalomyelitis (EAE), the animal model of MS.[52] In this model, MHC class II tetramers were used in FACS analyses to assess the expansion and differentiation of self-reactive T cells[53] or to trace T cells specific for the myelin-derived glycolipid sulfatide in lymphatic organs and in the CNS.[48] Unfortunately, tetramers do not yet work reliably on histological sections. However, since there are ongoing efforts in many different laboratories to optimize

MHC–peptide tetramer techniques,[54,55] it is probably just a matter of time until this problem is solved.

In a recent study, Muraro and colleagues[56] combined the MHC-tetramer technique with clone-specific PCR for the tracking of single clones of (auto-) antigen-specific T-cells in three patients with different immunological or infectious neurological diseases – multiple sclerosis, HTLV-I-associated myelopathy (HAM) and chronic Lyme neuroborreliosis. Real-time (quantitative) RT-PCR[57] allowed the authors to amplify mRNA transcripts of the TCR chains of the investigated T-cell clones. By designing CDR3-specific (and hence clone-specific) oligonucleotide primers suitable for RT-PCR, the authors were able to track a T-cell clone that recognized myelin basic protein (MBP) in the patient with multiple sclerosis, a second one that recognized an HTLV-I antigen in the patient with HAM/TSP and a third clone that recognized *Borrelia burgdorferi* in the patient with chronic Lyme disease. This approach was combined with the MHC tetramer technique.[58] The known antigen (in this case a peptide of the HTLV-I Tax antigen) was coupled to the same HLA molecule that normally presents this antigen on the surface of an APC. Such soluble HLA–peptide multimer complexes can bind directly to the TCR. If the multimeric HLA–peptide complexes are labeled, e.g. with a fluorescent dye, the T cells to which they bind will also be labeled and thus can be analyzed by FACS. This combination of quantitative PCR and TCR staining with HLA–peptide multimeric complexes provides an extremely powerful tool for assessing the clonal dynamics of antigen-specific T-cells in neuroimmunological diseases. One of the most intriguing findings of Muraro and colleagues was that the frequency of the investigated T-cell clones increased during periods of clinical exacerbation. The course of their MS patient strikingly illustrated this. Some 5 weeks after beginning treatment with an altered peptide ligand (APL) related to MBP, he had a severe clinical relapse. One week before the relapse, the frequency of the investigated MBP-specific T-cell clone, which cross-reacted with the therapeutic APL peptide, had increased fivefold. After clinical remission, the frequency of the clone returned to baseline. This observation supports both the validity of the techniques and the pathogenic relevance of this particular T-cell clone.

This elegant approach has an obvious limitation: it requires prior knowledge of the antigen specificity and TCR sequence of the T cells being tracked. Additional techniques are necessary to obtain this information, for example, in this case, the classic cloning of antigen-specific T-cell lines and subsequent sequencing of their antigen-specific receptors. If nothing is known a priori about the antigen specificity of the T cells of interest, CD3 spectratype analysis combined with in situ identification and single-cell PCR analysis of putatively autoaggressive T cells might help to identify their target antigen(s) (see above).

IN VIVO STUDIES OF AUTOREACTIVE T CELLS USING HUMANIZED ANIMAL MODELS

Mostly for ethical reasons, the experimental possibilities for studying human autoreactive T cells in vivo are very limited. An alternative approach, which is increasingly applied, is to use transgenic technology to introduce molecular components of the human T-cell response into living animals, usually mice (reviewed by Gregersen et al[59]). Regarding MS research, the first successful study of this kind was published in 1999.[60,61] The authors constructed transgenic mice that expressed three human components involved in T-cell recognition of an MS-relevant autoantigen, MBP, presented by the HLA-DR2 molecule: DRA*0101/DRB1*1501 (HLA-DR15), an MHC class II MS susceptibility gene; a TCR from an MS-patient-derived T-cell clone specific for the HLA-DR15 bound immunodominant

MBP$_{84-102}$ peptide; and the human CD4 co-receptor. The amino acid sequence of the MBP$_{84-102}$ peptide is the same in both human and mouse MBP. Following administration of the MBP peptide, together with adjuvant and pertussis toxin, transgenic mice developed focal CNS inflammation and demyelination that led to clinical manifestations and disease courses resembling those seen in MS. Spontaneous disease was observed in 4% of mice.[60] When DR15 and TCR double-transgenic mice were backcrossed twice to Rag2 (recombination-activating gene 2)-deficient mice, the incidence of spontaneous disease increased, demonstrating that T cells specific for the HLA-DR15 bound MBP peptide are sufficient and necessary for development of disease. For a similar model, humanized transgenic mice were constructed that expressed the HLA-DR DRA*0101/DRB1*1501 molecule together with an MS-derived MBP$_{85-99}$-specific TCR.[62] Even on a Rag-2 wild-type background, these mice spontaneously developed paralysis. Clinical disease correlated with inter- and intramolecular spreading of the T-cell response to HLA-DR15-restricted epitopes of MBP, MOG and αB-crystallin.[62]

Yet another humanized transgenic model focused on a different myelin epitope and HLA restriction molecule. Amino acid residues 111–129 represent an immunodominant epitope of MBP in humans with human leukocyte antigen (HLA)-DRB1*0401 allele(s). An MBP$_{111-129}$-specific T-cell clone was repeatedly isolated from a patient with MS, indicating an involvement of this clone in the pathogenesis. To address the pathogenic potential of this T-cell clone, transgenic mice expressing the relevant TCR and restriction element, HLA-DRB1*0401, were generated.[63] The mice were used to examine the pathogenic characteristics of the T cells by adoptive transfer into HLA-DRB1*0401 transgenic mice. In addition to the ascending paralysis typical of experimental autoimmune encephalomyelitis, mice displayed dysphagia and abnormal gait. In accordance with the clinical phenotype, T-cell infiltrates were predominantly located in the brainstem and the cranial nerve roots in addition to the spinal cord and spinal nerve roots. These observations might help to understand the clinical and pathological heterogeneity of MS.

LIVE IMAGING OF ENCEPHALITOGENIC T CELLS IN THE CNS: 'VISUALIZING IMMUNITY IN CONTEXT'

Recent advances in imaging techniques have empowered immunologists to investigate fundamental questions in living animals by 'visualizing immunity in context'. Using intravital microscopy, investigators are gaining unprecedented insights into basic cellular and molecular mechanisms controlling cell motility and interactions in tissues. This has been greatly facilitated by the explosion of fluorescence imaging techniques, which are revolutionizing microscopy (see reviews by Lichtman and Conchello[64] and Helmchen and Denk[65]).

One of the first applications of live imaging to neuroinflammatory disease was reported by Kawakami and colleagues,[66] who combined two-photon imaging and fluorescence video microscopy to track pathogenic MPB-specific CD4$^+$ effector T cells in early (CNS) lesions of EAE. As a first step, the authors labeled encephalitogenic, MBP-specific rat T cells by retroviral transduction with green fluorescent protein (GFP) according to a previously established protocol.[67] Next, they injected the GFP-labeled T cells into naive recipient animals and imaged the behavior of these autoreactive T cells in live spinal cord slices.[66] The majority of the cells (65%) moved fast (maximum speed 25 μm/min) and apparently randomly through the compact tissue, whereas a smaller group of effector T cells (35%) appeared to be tethered to a fixed point (Fig. 19.4). Polarization of TCR and adhesion molecules towards this fixed point suggested the formation of functional immune synapses. In control experiments, nonpathogenic, ovalbumin-specific T cells did not form synapse-like contacts but moved steadily through the tissue.

Live confocal imaging was applied to investigate degenerative and regenerative processes in the CNS.[68] The authors monitored individual fluorescent axons in the spinal cords of living transgenic mice over several days after spinal injury. They observed that, within 30 min after trauma, axons died back hundreds of micrometers, indicating a newly observed, acute form of axonal degeneration, similar in mechanism to the more delayed, well established wallerian degeneration of the disconnected distal axon. However, in contrast to the asymmetric character of wallerian degeneration, acute degeneration affects the proximal and distal axon ends equally. In vivo imaging further showed that many axons attempted regeneration within 6–24 h after lesion.[68] This growth response, however, seemed to fail because of the inability of the regenerating axons to navigate in the proper direction. This model system can now be applied to study axonal regeneration in inflammatory lesions.[69]

'UNBIASED' APPROACHES FOR TRANSCRIPTIONAL PROFILING: APPLICATION TO MULTIPLE SCLEROSIS

AN ARRAY OF POSSIBILITIES FOR THE STUDY OF AUTOIMMUNITY: TOOLS TO ENHANCE SERENDIPITY?

Central nervous system inflammation in MS patients is a very complex process that requires not only the spatial and temporal interaction between T cells and local glial cells but also the interactions between many different genes and gene products of individual cell populations.[11,70] In an attempt to study these interactions and to identify novel molecules and pathways involved in the different phases of neuroinflammation, many groups are trying to characterize gene expression patterns in MS patients, either concentrating on the target tissue – the MS plaque – or peripheral compartments such as blood and CSF. Conventional methods of studying these patterns would involve in situ hybridization or northern blotting, probing one gene at a time. Obviously, this is a difficult task and would require an enormous coordinated effort from many investigators, similar to the one undertaken when linkage analysis was used to search for candidate genes involved in MS predisposition and progression.[71-74] A much faster, state-of-the-art technique is the gene expression profiling with DNA microarrays, which indeed offer an impressive 'array of possibilities' for MS research[75] and have very aptly been called 'tools to enhance serendipity'.[76]

DNA microarrays (also called DNA chips) consist of hundreds to thousands of DNA sequences representing defined genes, which are attached to a glass surface (the 'platform'). To analyze the spectrum of transcribed genes (the 'transcriptome'), mRNA is isolated from tissue or the cells of interest. For amplification and to introduce photolabels, mRNA is transcribed (via cDNA) to cRNA, which is finally used for hybridization to the DNA on the platform. Thus, the labeled cRNA probes bind to matching gene spots on the DNA microarray and identify all expressed genes of a given sample. Two samples (or a sample and a control) may be compared directly (Fig. 19.5). With such microarray experiments, the expression of many thousands of genes can be simultaneously monitored in one single hybridization experiment (for review see reference 77.)

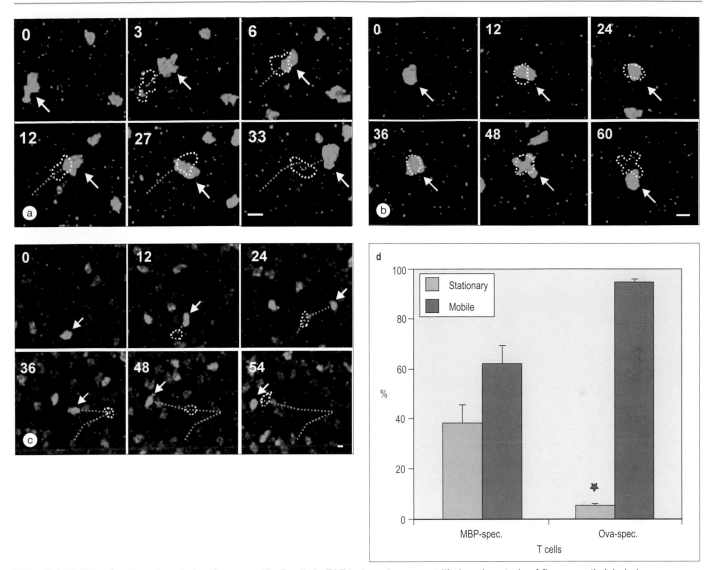

FIG. 19.4 Motility of auto and control antigen specific T cells in EAE lesions. In a recent life-imaging study of fluorescently labeled, encephalitogenic T cells in acute spinal cord slices, Kawakami and his colleagues[66] observed that the disease-inducing T cells move freely and with great speed through the CNS (**A**), apparently in search of 'their specific' target antigens. At certain intervals, these cells temporarily stick to and tether around still undefined structures in the CNS, which could represent antigen-presenting cells (**B**). Most interestingly, highly encephalitogenic T cells seem to have many more of these stop-and-go phases than T lymphocytes with lower encephalitogenic potential or T cells that do not recognize CNS antigens. Such ovalbumin-specific control cells are shown in **C**. Dotted lines indicate trajectories and the cell shape of the preceding picture. The time after start of observation is indicated. In **D** the relative proportions of motile and stationary cells are given for encephalitogenic T_{MBP} and control cells T_{OVA}. It is evident that T_{MBP} are more often stationary than the control cells, indicating that they interact specifically with antigen-presenting cells. Reproduced from Kawakami et al[66] by copyright permission of the Rockefeller University Press.

SEARCH FOR MOLECULES AND DISEASE PATHWAYS IN THE CENTRAL NERVOUS SYSTEM

One of the earliest studies of a human neurological disease with custom printed microarrays was published by Whitney and colleagues.[78] In their search for genes contributing to lesion pathology, these researchers compared the gene expression in normal white matter with that in acute lesions of the same MS patient and found many genes that were either downregulated or upregulated in the MS plaques.[78] Examples of such differentially expressed gene products are 5-lipoxygenase, a key enzyme in the biosynthesis of proinflammatory leukotrienes,[79] the Duffy chemokine receptor, interferon regulatory factor-2 and tumor necrosis factor α receptor-2.[78] These findings convincingly demonstrated that the cDNA microarray technology is a powerful

tool for the identification of novel genes associated with the MS disease process[78] but it remained open whether similar changes were also found in other MS patients, or how these changes are functionally related to the disease.[77]

Other studies were to follow soon. Unfortunately, these studies did not reveal a consistent pattern of up- or downregulated gene products.[78–82] The first differences in gene expression between plaques representing defined phases of lesion formation were observed by Lock and colleagues.[80] Their microarrays revealed an upregulation of the immunoglobulin Fc receptor in chronic inactive lesions and of the granulocyte colony stimulating factor in acute lesions. Further studies of MS lesions with pathologically proven different activity showed that even within one single plaque differences in gene expression exist between the lesion edge and the lesion center,[83] which essentially corroborated older pathological findings.[84] Of note, a large number of genes belonging to the family of inflammatory/immune-related proteins showed higher expression levels at the margin of active lesions than in the corresponding lesion centers, which could indicate that the expansion of active MS lesions might depend on immune-mediated mechanisms,[83] as suggested by the presence of T cells and macrophages/activated microglia cells in these areas.[84] The most interesting transcripts upregulated at the lesion edge were the FMS-related tyrosine kinase 3 ligand (FLT3-L), a potent hematopoietic cytokine known to recruit dendritic cells,[85] and the epithelial discoidin receptor (EDDR)-1, a protein that is upregulated in dendritic cells derived from CD14+ monocytes[86] and had been identified earlier by genome screen analysis as associated with MS.[71-73] More recently, microarrays were instrumental to the observation that, in MS patients, normal-appearing white matter and plaques show a continuum of differential gene regulation instead of forming discrete compartments. Remarkably, over 70% of all up- or downregulated genes in one location showed similar changes in the other site. The most discriminating genes, however, were those involved either directly or indirectly in humoral immune responses. These genes were much more expressed in the lesions than in the normal-appearing white matter.[87]

A meta-analysis collected information for all genome-wide genetic screens performed to date in MS and EAE and integrated these results with those from all high-throughput gene expression studies in humans and mice.[82] The authors analyzed a total of 55 studies. Disturbingly, in no less than 149 instances the same gene was reported as both upregulated and downregulated by different studies with human samples. This discrepancy also occurred in mouse experiments. These contradictory findings underscore heterogeneity not only on the clinicopathological but also on the experimental level when different samples, methods and statistical methods were used. Platform choice, ambiguity in probe annotation and statistical processing all may significantly alter the reported results in similar or sometimes even the same dataset.[82]

So what have we learned so far from the microarray studies performed on human MS lesions? Skeptics might say, not very much (yet). Presently there is a collection of up- and down-regulated genes. Some of the contradictory findings might be explained by the facts that many studies were based on the analysis of lesions at different stages of plaque formation, were restricted to just one or only very few patients and/or included patients suffering from different types of MS (relapsing–remitting, secondary progressive or primary progressive).[78–81] In addition, the most discriminating of the differentially expressed genes detected so far are those involved in immune responses already known to play a role in the formation of MS lesions. The discrepancy between the high expectations aroused by this technology and the actual findings is at least in part due to the limited availability of suitable material: fresh biopsy specimens can only rarely be obtained and autopsy material is often only available from patients with end-stage disease.

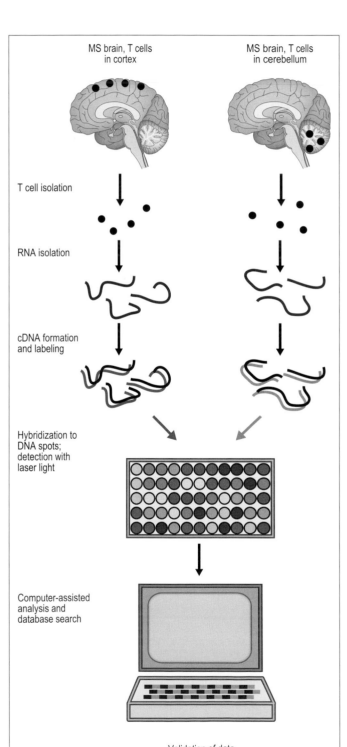

FIG. 19.5 DNA microarrays. mRNA is isolated from T cells found, for example, within the cortex or cerebellum of MS patients and is converted to fluorescence-labeled, hence colored cDNA. The cDNA of cortex-derived T cells is labeled red, the cDNA of cerebellum-derived T cells green. The two different sets of cDNA are mixed and hybridized to the microarray. A microarray (also called DNA chip) contains spots of thousands of DNA sequences, which all represent different genes and which can be simultaneously tested with the labeled cDNA. If the cDNA finds corresponding sequences on the microarray, it will bind to it. Unbound cDNA is washed off. The microarray is analyzed with laser light (red and green). The resulting images are analyzed. Green spots represent genes that are expressed in cerebellum-derived T cells only; red spots represent genes that are only expressed in T cells isolated from the cortex; yellow spots represent genes that are expressed in both sets of T cells, and the absence of colored spots indicates that a particular gene is not expressed at all. Using appropriate computer software, the relative expression levels of the different cDNAs are measured. Afterwards, the data must be validated by independent techniques.

SEARCH FOR MOLECULES AND DISEASE PATHWAYS IN BLOOD CELLS

As mentioned, the availability of suitable study material has been a major limitation in the search of disease pathways in the MS plaque. Therefore, a number of research groups have concentrated on the peripheral blood of MS patients, with the aim of identifying molecular markers indicative of disease progression and activity state. In an early study,[88] cDNA arrays were used to search for differences in gene expression between healthy controls and patients with relapsing–remitting MS. It was observed that only 34 genes of more than 4000 tested were significantly different in relapsing–remitting MS patients and showed either increased or decreased levels of expression. Of these genes, 12 had inflammatory and/or immunological functions that could be relevant to the MS disease process. Hence, this study indicated that cDNA microarrays can indeed help to identify abnormal gene expression patterns in the peripheral blood of patients with relapsing–remitting MS.

Bomprezzi and colleagues extended these studies.[89] They used somewhat larger cDNA microarrays for gene expression profiling of peripheral blood mononuclear cells of MS patients and healthy controls, and could identify two groups of informative genes that were differentially expressed in MS patients. Interestingly, nine of the over- or underexpressed genes mapped to chromosome 6p21, a chromosome region that has shown the strongest association with MS and other autoimmune diseases[89] and that also harbors the MHC locus and the *EDDR1* gene identified by Mycko and colleagues as upregulated at the edge of chronically active MS lesions.[83]

Significant differences in gene expression patterns between peripheral blood mononuclear cells from MS patients and healthy subjects were also observed by Achiron et al,[90] using microarrays that carry probes for approximately 12 000 genes. Again, discriminating transcriptional signatures were found that clearly distinguished between MS patients and healthy controls. The differentially expressed gene products encoded proteins involved in T-cell activation, T-cell expansion, inflammation and apoptosis. In addition, the authors were able to differentiate between MS patients in relapse and those in remission. The differentially expressed genes encoded proteins involved in cellular recruitment, epitope spreading and escape from regulatory immune surveillance.[90]

Taken together, these studies on peripheral blood mononuclear cells identified several genes that were differentially expressed in the blood of MS patients and healthy controls. Many of these genes have immunological functions, which is not surprising considering the important role of T cells and antibodies in the disease process. However, the diagnostic and/or prognostic value of such under- or overexpressed gene products needs to be confirmed in larger, appropriately controlled, prospective studies.

SEARCH FOR MOLECULES AND DISEASE MECHANISMS OPERATING AT THE BLOOD–BRAIN BARRIER

It is thought that one of the primary events in lesion formation is the migration of activated, autoimmune T cells across the endothelial blood–brain barrier.[1] Once inflammation is initiated, the blood–brain barrier is impaired. This leads to an increased traffic of leukocytes into the CNS, and to edema formation. The molecular mechanisms involved in blood–brain barrier disruption were recently studied in the animal model of EAE. Alt and colleagues[91] isolated microvessels from the brains of C57Bl/6 and SJL mice with EAE, and from brains of corresponding healthy controls, and studied the gene expression profiles in these two different compartments with oligonucleotide microarrays. They found a large number of differentially expressed genes, including adhesion molecules, cytokines and chemokines along with cytokine and chemokine receptors, extracellular matrix proteins and tissue inhibitor of matrix metalloproteases. Interestingly, some genes were only differentially expressed in C57Bl/6 mice with EAE, not in SJL mice with EAE. One of these genes is the ganglioside GM3 synthase, which may modify the expression of adhesion molecules at the blood–brain barrier endothelium and could thus alter leukocyte adhesion and infiltration into the CNS.[91] It remains to be seen whether the ganglioside GM3 synthase plays also an important role in the lesion formation of MS patients.

IDENTIFICATION OF THERAPEUTIC BIOMARKERS USING MICROARRAY TECHNOLOGY

Multiple sclerosis is not only a disease with variable clinical and pathological patterns[92,93] but also a disease with heterogeneity in the response to treatment.[94] There has been increasingly intense effort to develop biomarkers for these different aspects of the disease.[95] Stürzebecher and colleagues[96] analyzed the RNA expression profile of peripheral blood mononuclear cells derived from MS patients under interferon (IFN)β therapy by cDNA microarrays. Their cohort consisted of patients with clinically definite, relapsing–remitting multiple sclerosis. Based on clinical and MRI findings, these patients were categorized into three different groups. The first group contained treatment responders, who were clinically stable and showed a reduction of more than 60% in mean number of gadolinium-enhancing lesions compared with baseline. The second group included patients who developed high titers of neutralizing antibodies to IFNβ, and the third group consisted of patients who failed to respond to initiation of IFNβ therapy. Microarray analysis of the peripheral blood mononuclear cells from these three groups of patients revealed that treatment responders had much more genes regulated by IFNβ than the treatment nonresponders.[96] What mechanisms underlie the heterogeneic response to IFNβ therapy? To answer this question, Weinstock-Guttman et al[97] studied the transcription rates of many different RNAs in the peripheral blood from relapsing–remitting MS patients just before and at different time points after IFNβ treatment. Their transcriptional profiling revealed that IFNβ induces or enhances the expression of genes implicated in antiviral responses (e.g. the double stranded RNA-dependent protein kinase), in IFNβ-signaling (e.g. the αβ IFN receptor 2 and Stat1) and in lymphocyte activation (e.g. β_2 microglobulin and CD69). Hence, these specific and time-dependent changes in multiple mRNAs could provide a framework for rapid monitoring of the response to therapy.[97] In the future, microarray analyses will increasingly become an integral part of MS therapeutic studies.[98]

ADVANTAGES, DISADVANTAGES AND PITFALLS OF MICROARRAY TECHNOLOGY

There is little question that microarrays are important tools for overcoming many problems intrinsic to the analysis of complex diseases such as MS, provided that the experiments are carefully planned, optimal tissue specimens are used and patient cohorts are appropriately composed and controlled. Under these conditions, this technology will have its place in the search for disease pathways, in the hunt for new targets for therapeutic intervention and in the monitoring of treatment. But even under ideal experimental conditions, data obtained by microarray analyses must be critically interpreted.[99]

Firstly, the definition of 'differentially regulated genes' obviously relies on the set threshold. Microarrays can only reliably detect gene expression changes greater than twofold.[100] Such changes in expression levels are rarely seen in the CNS.[101] On the other hand, small changes in expression levels below the factor 2 could already be critical for the function of entire regions or neural cell types, as seen in transgenic mice[102,103] and rats overexpressing the proteolipid protein gene.[104] Such subtle changes could already profoundly affect T-cell infiltration into the CNS[105,106] but would not show up in the microarray analysis. In addition, de novo gene expression or mRNA shutdowns rarely occur in the CNS.[101] Secondly, even when several genes in a particular pathway show changes at the RNA level, the actual function of the pathway may not be affected if none of these genes is the rate-limiting factor.[77]

Thirdly, cDNA microarrays from different commercial sources yield significantly different experimental outcomes. Many different microarray platforms are currently available but these platforms differ in a number of variables, for example the numbers of probes used to detect a given gene, the length of the probes, and the required procedures to label and amplify the probes, translate the array images into digital data and analyse the data obtained (for overview see reference 100). Just how much such factors may influence the outcome of experiments is seen in the work of Hollingshead and her coworkers.[100] This group used human brain samples derived from a schizophrenic patient and a healthy control to study differences in gene expression with three different microarray platforms: single-color gel matrix deposited CodeLink© oligonucleotide arrays (Amersham Biosciences) containing a single 30-base probe for each of the investigated genes; photolithographically synthesized short oligonucleotide GeneChips© (Affymetrix) containing multiple probes and intrinsic controls; and 200–1000 bp cDNA microarrays containing dual-fluorescence from Vanderbilt Microarray Shared Resource. All these platforms had a good range, yielded highly reproducible data and identified differentially expressed genes. However, not a single one of these differentially expressed genes was identified by all three platforms and there was even very little overlap between just two different platforms.[100] A similar discrepancy between different platforms had been reported before.[107] These observations are rather disturbing. On the one hand, they show that different microarray platforms measure different things. This can be explained by differences in the design and function of the platforms used. On the other hand, these observations also reveal a very high probability of false-negative data, which means that a large number of differentially expressed genes are simply missed.[100]

Fourthly, since there is also a possibility for false-positive results, array data have to be validated by immunohistochemistry, by real-time qPCR, by in situ hybridization, by RNAse protection assays or in animal models. When this has been done so far, investigators concentrated on the most robust expression changes and could validate the microarray findings.[80,100] It remains to be seen whether a systematic validation of genes with much smaller expression changes gives similar results. However, recent attempts to standardize microarray hardware, hybridization technology and data analysis will surely increase reliability and reproducibility.[108,109]

PROTEOMICS TECHNIQUES AS NEW TOOLS FOR MULTIPLE SCLEROSIS RESEARCH

LARGE-SCALE ANALYSIS OF PROTEINS

Following completion of the Human Genome Project, attention has begun to shift to deciphering the networks of proteins within cells and tissues. Proteins are much more complex than

genes and more difficult to study. Proteomics, the large-scale analysis of proteins, will contribute greatly to the understanding of gene function in the postgenomic era. Proteomics can be divided into three main areas: 1) protein microcharacterization for large-scale identification of proteins and their post-translational modifications; 2) 'differential display' proteomics for comparison of protein levels with potential application in a wide range of diseases; and 3) studies of protein–protein interactions using techniques such as mass spectrometry or the yeast two-hybrid system.[110] Because it is often difficult to predict the function of a protein based on homology to other proteins or even their three-dimensional structure, a central part of functional analysis by proteomic studies is the determination of components of a protein complex or of a cellular structure.[110] After the revolution in molecular biology exemplified by DNA cloning methods, proteomics is expected to add to our understanding of the biochemistry of proteins, processes and pathways. An excellent review of proteomic tools and applications can be found in reference 111.

INVESTIGATION AND CHARACTERIZATION OF DISEASE-RELEVANT PROTEINS IN THE CEREBROSPINAL FLUID AND SERUM OF MULTIPLE SCLEROSIS PATIENTS

Powerful as DNA microarray technology is, it is obviously inadequate to study the proteins contained in cell-free CSF and serum samples. The protein profiles of both types of body fluid are altered in more or less typical ways in many diseases.[112] To identify and characterize disease relevant proteins in these fluids, high-throughput proteome analysis ('proteomics') is the tool of choice. The classical tool for displaying the proteome is still two-dimensional gel electrophoresis. This technique separates proteins by two-dimensional SDS-polyacrylamide gel electrophoresis(PAGE) according to their size and charge. Proteins found in patient samples but not in the corresponding control samples (or vice versa) are then isolated for identification and further analyses by mass spectrometry (Fig. 19.6). Recent technical innovations have introduced alternative techniques such as liquid chromatography tandem mass spectrometry (LC-MS-MS) or matrix-assisted laser desorption/ionization (MALDI) in conjunction with time of flight (TOF) spectrometry.[113] Such new technologies allowed investigation of mouse brain plasma membrane proteins that would not have been feasible by classical two-dimensional methods.[114]

SEARCH FOR DISEASE RELEVANT PROTEINS IN THE CEREBROSPINAL FLUID BY PROTEOME ANALYSIS

In the past, numerous studies have attempted to identify protein markers of MS in the CSF, but most of these earlier attempts were unsuccessful. More recently, researchers have shown renewed interest in this type of study, hoping that the progress in protein and proteome analysis provides a basis for more successful studies. For example, Dumont et al[112] used proteome analysis to search for protein markers of MS in the CSF. They separated CSF proteins from four relapsing–remitting and one secondary progressive MS patient by two-dimensional gel electrophoresis, isolated protein spots from these gels and identified the proteins by mass spectroscopy. With this approach, they were able to identify 65 different proteins. Of these, 47 were also found in the CSF of non-MS patients, while the other 18 were specific for MS CNS samples and included S100A7, cystatin A, superoxide dismutase 3, glutathione peroxidase and tetranectin,[107] a protein that is secreted by many different

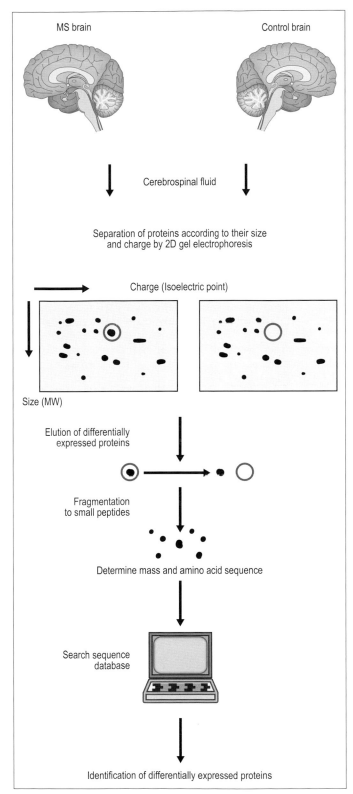

FIG. 19.6 Proteomics. Proteins, for example from the cerebrospinal fluid of MS patients or healthy controls are separated by two-dimensional (2D) SDS-PAGE gel electrophoresis according to their size and charge. Proteins that show differences in their expression pattern are isolated for identification and further analysis.

tissues[115] and binds to hepatocyte growth factor and plasminogen activator.

The presence of tetranectin in the CSF of MS patients was also observed by Hammack and colleagues,[116] who used a similar approach to compare proteins found in the pooled CSF from three MS patients with those found in the pooled CSF from an equal number of patients with non-MS inflammatory CNS disease. Other proteins unique to the MS CSF were autotaxin t (a phosphodiesterase), SPARC-like protein (a calcium binding cell signaling glycoprotein) and CRTAC-1B (cartilage acidic protein).[116] Whether any of these proteins play a role in the initiation and/or progression of MS remains to be seen.

SEARCH FOR TARGET ANTIGENS OF CEREBROSPINAL FLUID OLIGOCLONAL IgG BANDS USING PROTEIN CHIPS

Similar to the chips used for DNA microarrays, protein analysis can also be miniaturized by using 'protein chips'.[117] Briefly, proteins are spotted on to chemically derivatized glass slides at extremely high spatial densities. The proteins are covalently attached to the slide surface but still able to interact with other proteins/molecules in solution. Hence, it is possible to screen samples for protein–protein interactions and identify protein substrates and protein targets of small molecules.[117] Protein chips were used to study the oligoclonal IgG bands in the CSF of MS patients.[118] The authors used separate arrays of 37 000 tagged proteins and probed them with CSF samples from MS patients and controls. The results indicated that EBV proteins might by targeted by at least some of the oligoclonal IgG bands. The implications of these findings for the immunopathogenesis of MS are uncertain.

PROFILING OF SERUM AUTOANTIBODY RESPONSES USING PROTEOME MICROARRAYS

A similar approach was used by Robinson and colleagues,[42] who profiled the evolution of serum autoantibody responses in EAE with myelin proteome microarrays. These authors used a robotic arrayer to spot and attach myelin proteins and synthetic peptides to poly-L-lysine-coated slides. The spotted molecules on these 'protein chips' or 'proteome arrays' included proteins and peptides from MBP, proteolipid protein (PLP), MOG, myelin-associated oligodendrocytic basic protein (MBOP), αB crystallin, cyclic nucleotide phosphodiesterase (CNPase), peripheral myelin protein 2 (P2), acetylcholine receptor and other nonmyelin peptides or proteins. This myelin proteome array was then probed with serum of two animals with relapsing EAE induced by immunization with PLP (animal 1) and MBP (animal 2) peptides. Both animals showed antibody responses not only to the peptides used for immunization but also to peptides derived from other myelin proteins, indicating that epitope spreading occurred during the course of the disease. These array data were then validated in two different ways. First, it was analyzed whether antibodies with known peptide specificity detect their corresponding target structures on the myelin proteome array. This was the case. In a second validation approach, the data obtained from the array were compared with data obtained from conventional enzyme-linked immunosorbent assays (ELISA) of EAE serum. This approach also confirmed the array data, and revealed an additional strength of the myelin proteome arrays: they were four- to eightfold more sensitive than conventional ELISA and provided consistent intra- and interassay results.[42]

The authors then investigated whether it is possible to predict disease severity based on the autoantibody reactivity pattern. This seemed indeed to be the case. Differences in the diversity of the autoantibody responses helped to identify distinct subclusters of mice with increased relapse rates. Animals from all of these subclusters were similar to each other in that they had a more severe disease course and a dominant autoreactive antibody response against the peptide used for immunization.

However, they differed from each other in the fine specificity of the other myelin antibodies found in the serum. For example, mice immunized with $PLP_{139-151}$ also responded to MBP_{71-89}, while mice immunized with MBP_{85-99} also produced antibodies against $MBP_{141-159}$.[42] This finding pointed to an extensive intra- and intermolecular spreading of autoantibody responses to sets of myelin epitopes that differed between groups of mice.[42] Hence, myelin protein arrays seem to be useful tools to reveal the antigen specificity of autoantibodies found in the serum of experimental animals with EAE, and possibly also in the serum of patients with MS.

SEARCH FOR MYELIN TARGET ANTIGENS OF AUTOANTIBODIES IN SERUM OF MULTIPLE SCLEROSIS PATIENTS

In the study described in the previous section, serum antibodies against myelin targets were detected by their ability to bind to their specific protein on a protein chip. Alternatively, the specificity of such autoantibodies can be revealed by their ability to bind to selected bands or spots on one-dimensional or two-dimensional gels. This approach was used by Almeras and colleagues[119] when they defined myelin antigen targets of the global IgG antibody response in the serum of patients with clinically definite MS. A total of 18 MS patients were investigated: seven of these patients had relapsing/remitting type MS, four had secondary progressive MS, and the remaining seven primary progressive MS. All patients were free of relapse at the time of blood collection and had not been treated with immunomodulating or immunosuppressive drugs before serum collection.[119] The serum of these patients was used to probe one-dimensional and two-dimensional gels prepared from protein extracts of a healthy brain. The bands or dots recognized by serum antibodies were then excised from the gels and identified by mass spectroscopy. One of the recognized bands represented neurofilament protein. Interestingly, the presence of antibodies against this protein clearly discriminated between MS patients and healthy controls. Another recognized band was identified as a particular isoform of glial fibrillary acidic protein. Antibodies against this isoform seem to distinguish between relapsing–remitting, primary progressive and secondary progressive MS.[119] The results of this pilot study need to be confirmed in much larger cohorts of patients.

ADVANTAGES AND DISADVANTAGES OF PROTEOME ANALYSES

Obviously, the data of Robinson and colleagues,[42] Almeras et al[119] and Cepok and coworkers[118] provide only a first glimpse of what might eventually be achievable with proteomics techniques in MS research. These early studies suggest that, for example, proteome analysis could indeed be a powerful tool to identify target antigens of CNS-specific antibodies in MS patients and to screen protein profiles of tissues, cells and body fluids in a reasonably short period of time. However, as seen before with DNA microarrays, proteome analysis has limitations as well, especially when used for the characterization of cells and tissues. For example, very large and very small proteins, as well as membrane-bound and secreted proteins, are often lost or missed during protein preparation from cells. This limitation is of special concern for MS studies: basically all cell types isolated from MS lesions probably produce cytokines or chemokines but these proteins will almost certainly be lost for proteomics because they are secreted and not retained within the cell. Just how much protein secretion could influence the outcome of proteome studies can be easily deduced from T-cell analysis in vitro, where cytokine detection by immunohistochemistry or FACS analysis crucially depends on the pretreatment of cells with protein transport blockers,[120] a procedure that by itself would already significantly interfere with proteomics studies.

CORRELATION BETWEEN DNA AND PROTEOME ARRAYS

The correlation between protein and gene expression profiling is rather low.[121] The most likely explanation is that changes in mRNA levels below a factor of 2 cannot be reliably detected in DNA microarrays and are usually discarded, although such changes might very well translate into much higher protein concentrations. Another possible reason for low correlation between transcriptomics and proteomics data is the fact that very few proteins are regulated only at the transcriptional level. In contrast, the vast majority of proteins are post-translationally modified or processed and the resulting individual protein products of the same gene will migrate to different locations on 2D-PAGE-gels, where they could easily be missed.[122] In addition, there could be negative feedback regulatory mechanisms between any expressed protein and its corresponding gene transcripts.[121] On a more technical side, further problems relate to the stability and/or proteolytic degradation of proteins.

CONCLUDING REMARKS

The animal models of MS, collectively referred to as EAE, have reached an unprecedented level of complexity and sophistication (Ch. 16). On the other hand, as we have emphasized in this chapter, a growing number of novel techniques for analysis of human tissue samples are beginning to provide fascinating and unprecedented insights. For example, molecular analyses of the antigen receptor repertoire of pathogenic T and B cells can be combined with immunocytochemistry and single-cell microdissection techniques to identify paired TCR α and β chains directly from tissue-infiltrating cells. Human TCR chains can be expressed in cell lines for in vitro studies and in transgenic animals for in vivo analysis. 'Unbiased' transcriptomics and proteomics technologies are beginning to provide new insights into disease heterogeneity, and should help to identify diagnostic and prognostic biomarkers, as well as biomarkers of the therapeutic response. These are exciting times in MS research, and we can be optimistic that ever-advancing scientific technology will help to translate hopes into reality.

ACKNOWLEDGMENTS

The authors were supported by the Hermann and Lilly Schilling Foundation, Deutsche Forschungsgemeinschaft (DFG-SFB 571, A1) and Fonds zur Förderung der wissenschaftlichen Forschung (FWF, project P16047-B02).

REFERENCES

1. Bradl M, Flugel A. The role of T cells in brain pathology. Curr Top Microbiol Immunol 2002; 265: 141–162.

2. Emmert-Buck MR, Bonner RF, Smith PD et al. Laser capture microdissection. Science 1996; 274: 998–1001.

3. Schütze K, Lahr G. Identification of expressed genes by laser-mediated manipulation

of single cells. Nat Biotech 1998; 16: 737–742.

4. Babbe H, Roers A, Waisman A et al. Clonal expansions of CD8+ T cells dominate the T cell infiltrate in active multiple sclerosis lesions as shown by micromanipulation and single cell polymerase chain reaction. J Exp Med 2000; 192: 393–404.

5. Karsten SL, Van Deerlin VMD, Sabatti C et al. An evaluation of tyramide signal amplification and archived fixed and frozen tissue in microarray gene expression analysis. Nucleic Acids Res 2002; 30: e4.

6. Skulina C, Schmidt S, Dornmair K et al. Multiple sclerosis: brain-infiltrating CD8+ T cells persist as clonal expansions in the cerebrospinal fluid and blood. Proc Natl Acad Sci USA 2004; 101: 2428–2433.

7. Friese MA, Fugger L. Autoreactive CD8+ T cells in multiple sclerosis: a new target for therapy? Brain 2005; 128: 1747–1763.

8. Pannetier C, Even J, Kourilsky P. T-cell repertoire diversity and clonal expansions in normal and clinical samples. Immunol Today 1995; 16: 176–181.

9. Davis MM, Bjorkman PJ. T-cell antigen receptor genes and T-cell recognition. Nature 1988; 334: 295–402.

10. Rudolph MG, Luz JG, Wilson IA. Structural and thermodynamic correlates of T cell signaling. Annu Rev Biophys Biomol Struct 2002; 31: 121–149.

11. Bradl M, Hohlfeld R. Neuroscience for neurologists: molecular pathogenesis of neuroinflammation. J Neurol Neurosurg Psychiatr 2003; 74: 1364–1370.

12. Derfuss T, Segerer S, Herberger S et al. Presence of HSV-1 immediate early genes and clonally expanded T cells with a memory effector phenotype in human trigeminal ganglia. Brain Pathol 2007; DOI 10.1111/j.1750-3639.2007.00088.x

13. Junker A, Ivanidze J, Malotka J et al. Multiple sclerosis: T-cell receptor expression in distinct brain regions. Brain 2007; DOI 10.1093/brain/awm214

14. Grundtner R, Dornmair K, Dahm R et al. Transition from enchanced T cell infiltration to inflammation in the myelin-degenerative central nervous system. Neurobiol Dis 2007; DOI 10.1016/j.nbd.2007.05.006

15. Hofbauer M, Wiesener S, Babbe H et al. Clonal tracking of autoaggressive T cells in polymyositis by combining laser microdissection, single-cell PCR, and CDR3-spectratype analysis. Proc Natl Acad Sci USA 2003 100: 4090–4095.

16. Tuohy VK, Yu M, Yin L et al. Spontaneous regression of primary autoreactivity during chronic progression of experimental autoimmune encephalomyelitis and multiple sclerosis. J Exp Med 1999; 189: 1033–1042.

17. Dornmair K, Goebels N, Weltzien HU et al. T-cell-mediated autoimmunity. Novel techniques to characterize autoreactive T-cell receptors. Am J Pathol 2003 163: 1215–1226.

18. Bender A, Ernst N, Iglesias A et al. T cell receptor repertoire in polymyositis: clonal expansion of autoaggressive CD8+ T cells. J Exp Med 1995; 181: 1863–1868.

19. Hohlfeld R, Engel AG, Ii K, Harper MC. Polymyositis mediated by T lymphocytes that express the gamma/delta receptor. N Engl J Med 1991; 324: 877–881.

20. Pluschke G, Ruegg D, Hohlfeld R, Engel AG. Autoaggressive myocytotoxic T lymphocytes expressing an unusual gamma/delta T cell receptor. J Exp Med 1992; 176: 1785–1789.

21. Blank U, Boitel B, Mege D et al. Analysis of tetanus toxin peptide/DR recognition by human T cell receptors reconstituted into a murine T cell hybridoma. Eur J Immunol 1993; 23: 3057–3065.

22. Wiendl H, Malotka J, Holzwarth B et al. An autoreactive gamma delta TCR derived from a polymyositis lesion. J Immunol 2002; 169: 515–521.

23. Dornmair K, Schneider CK, Malotka J et al. Antigen recognition properties of a Vγ1.3 Vδ2-T-cell receptor from a rare variant of polymyositis. J Neuroimmunol 2004; 152: 168–175.

24. Seitz S, Schneider CK, Malotka J et al. Reconstitution of paired T cell receptor alpha- and beta-chains from microdissected single cells of human inflammatory tissues. Proc Natl Acad Sci USA 2006; 103: 12057–12062.

25. Van Gelder RN, von Zastrow ME, Yool A et al. Amplified RNA synthesized from limited quantities of heterogeneous cDNA. Proc Natl Acad Sci USA 1990; 87: 1663–1667.

26. Iscove NN, Barbara M, Gu M et al. Representation is faithfully preserved in global cDNA amplified exponentially from sub-picogram quantities of mRNA. Nat Biotechnol 2002; 20: 940–943.

27. Klein CA, Seidl S, Petat-Dutter K et al. Combined transcriptome and genome analysis of single micrometastatic cells. Nat Biotechnol 2002; 20: 387–392.

28. Tietjen I, Rihel JM, Cao Y et al. Single-cell transcriptional analysis of neuronal progenitors. Neuron 2003; 38: 161–175.

29. Van den Eynde B, Peeters O, De Backer O et al. A new family of genes coding for an antigen recognized by autologous cytolytic T lymphocytes on a human melanoma. J Exp Med 1995; 182: 689–698.

30. Wong FS, Karttunen J, Dumont C et al. Identification of an MHC classI-restricted autoantigen in type 1 diabetes by screening an organ-specific cDNA library. Nat Med 1999; 5: 1026–1031.

31. Sospedra M, Pinilla C, Martin R. Use of combinatorial peptide libraries for T-cell epitope mapping. Methods 2003; 29: 236–247.

32. Cortese I, Tafi R, Grimaldi LM et al. Identification of peptides specific for cerebrospinal fluid antibodies in multiple sclerosis by using phage libraries. Proc Natl Acad Sci USA 1996; 93: 11063–11067.

33. Meinl E, Krumbholz M, Hohlfeld R. B lineage cells in the inflammatory central nervous system environment: migration, maintenance, local antibody production, and therapeutic modulation. Ann Neurol 2006; 59: 880–892.

34. Genain CP, Cannella B, Hauser SL, Raine CS. Identification of autoantibodies associated with myelin damage in multiple sclerosis. Nat Med 1999; 5: 170–175.

35. Berger T, Rubner P, Schautzer F et al. Antimyelin antibodies as predictor of clinically definite multiple sclerosis after a first demyelinating event. N Engl J Med 2003; 349: 139–145.

36. Lim ET, Berger T, Reindl M et al. Anti-myelin antibodies do not allow earlier diagnosis of multiple sclerosis. Mult Scler 2005; 11: 492–494.

37. Qin Y, Duquette P, Zhang Y et al. Clonal expansion and somatic hypermutation of V(H) genes of B cells from cerebrospinal fluid in multiple sclerosis. J Clin Invest 1998; 102: 1045–1050.

38. Owens GP, Kraus H, Burgoon MP et al. Restricted use of VH4 germline segments in an acute multiple sclerosis brain. Ann Neurol 1998; 43: 236–243.

39. Baranzini SE, Jeong MC, Butunoi C et al. B cell repertoire diversity and clonal expansion in multiple sclerosis brain lesions. J Immunol 1999; 163: 5133–5144.

40. Owens GP, Ritchie AM, Burgoon MP et al. Single-cell repertoire analysis demonstrates that clonal expansion is a prominent feature of the B cell response in multiple sclerosis cerebrospinal fluid. J Immunol 2003; 171: 2725–2733.

41. Haubold K, Owens GP, Kaur P et al. B-lymphocyte and plasma cell clonal expansion in monosymptomatic optic neuritis cerebrospinal fluid. Ann Neurol 2004; 56: 97–107.

42. Robinson WH, Fontoura P, Lee BJ et al. Protein microarrays guide tolerizing DNA vaccine treatment of autoimmune encephalomyelitis. Nat Biotech 2003; 21: 1033–1039.

43. Bakker AH, Schumacher TN. MHC multimer technology: current status and future prospects. Curr Opin Immunol 2005; 17: 428–433.

44. Altman JD, Moss PA, Goulder PJ et al. Phenotypic analysis of antigen-specific T lymphocytes. Science 1996; 274: 94–96.

45. Callan MF, Tan L, Annels N et al. Direct visualization of antigen-specific CD8+ T cells during the primary immune response to Epstein–Barr virus in vivo. J Exp Med 1998; 187: 1395–1402.

46. Crawford F, Kozono H, White J et al. Detection of antigen-specific T cells with multivalent soluble class II MHC covalent peptide complexes. Immunity 1998; 8: 675–682.

47. Reddy J, Bettelli E, Nicholson L et al. Detection of autoreactive myelin proteolipid protein 139–151-specific T cells by using MHC II (IAs) tetramers. J Immunol 2003; 170: 870–877.

48. Jahng A, Maricic I, Aguilera C et al. Prevention of autoimmunity by targeting a distinct, noninvariant CD1d-reactive T cell population reactive to sulfatide. J Exp Med 2004; 199: 947–957.

49. Pittet MJ, Speiser DE, Valmori D et al. Ex vivo analysis of tumor antigen specific CD8+ T cell responses using MHC/peptide tetramers in cancer patients. Int Immunophamacol 2001; 1: 1235–1247.

50. Cerundolo V. Use of major histocompatibility complex class I tetramers to monitor tumor-specific cytotoxic T lymphocyte response in melanoma patients. Cancer Chemother Pharmacol 2000; 46: S83–S85.

51. McCloskey TW, Haridas V, Pahwa R, Pahwa S. T cell receptor V beta repertoire of the antigen specific CD8 T lymphocyte subset of HIV infected children. AIDS 2002; 16: 1459–1465.

52. Lassmann H. Experimental autoimmune encephalomyelitis. In: Lazzarini RA, ed. Myelin biology and disorders. London: Elsevier Academic Press; 2004: 1039–1071.

53. Bischof F, Hofmann M, Schumacher TN et al. Analysis of autoreactive CD4 T cells in experimental autoimmune encephalomyelitis after primary and secondary challenge using MHC class II tetramers. J Immunol 2004; 172: 2878–2884.

54. Sato Y, Sahara H, Tsukahara T et al. Improved generation of HLA class I/peptide tetramers. J Immunol Methods 2002; 271: 177–184.

55. Cunliffe SL, Wyer JR, Sutton JK et al. Optimization of peptide linker length in production of MHC classII/peptide tetrameric complexes increases yield and stability, and allows identification of antigen-specific CD4+ T cells in peripheral blood mononuclear cells. Eur J Immunol 2002; 32: 3366–3375.

56. Muraro PA, Wandinger KP, Bielekova G et al. Molecular tracking of antigen-specific T cell clones in neurological immune-mediated disorders. Brain 2003; 126: 20–31.

57. Walker J. A technique whose time has come. Science 2002; 296: 557–559.

58. Klenerman P, Cerundolo V, Dunbar PR. Tracking T cells with tetramers: new tales from new tools. Nat Rev Immunol 2002; 2: 263–272.

59. Gregersen JW, Holmes S, Fugger L. Humanized animal models for autoimmune diseases. Tissue Antigens 2004; 63: 383–394.

60. Madsen LS, Andersson EC, Jansson L et al. A humanized model for multiple sclerosis using HLA-DR2 and a human T-cell receptor. Nat Genet 1999; 23: 343–347.

61. Ebers G. Modelling multiple sclerosis. Nat Genet 1999; 23: 258–259.

62. Ellmerich S, Mycko M, Takacs K et al. High incidence of spontaneous disease in an HLA-DR15 and TCR transgenic multiple sclerosis model. J Immunol 2005; 174: 1938–1946.

63. Quandt JA, Baig M, Yao K et al. Intravital microscopy: visualizing immunity in context. Immunity 2004; 21: 315–329.

64. Lichtman JW, Conchello JA. Fluorescence microscopy. Nat Methods 2005; 2: 910–919.

65. Helmchen F, Denk W. Deep tissue two-photon microscopy. Nat Methods 2005; 2: 932–940.

66. Kawakami N, Nagerl UV, Odoardi F et al. Live imaging of effector cell trafficking and autoantigen recognition within the unfolding autoimmune encephalomyelitis lesion. J Exp Med 2005; 201: 1805–1814.

67. Flügel A, Willem M, Berkowicz T, Wekerle H. Gene transfer into CD4+ T lymphocytes: green fluorescent protein-engineered, encephalitogenic T cells illuminate brain autoimmune responses. Nat Med 1999; 5: 843–847.

68. Kerschensteiner M, Schwab ME, Lichtman JW, Misgeld T. In vivo imaging of axonal degeneration and regeneration in the injured spinal cord. Nat Med 2005; 11: 572–577.

69. Misgeld T, Kerschensteiner M. In vivo imaging of the diseased nervous system. Nat Rev Neurosci 2006; 7: 1–16.

70. Dyment DA, Ebers GC, Sadovnick AD. Genetics of multiple sclerosis. Lancet Neurol 2004; 3: 104–110.

71. Ebers GC, Kukay K, Bulman DE et al. A full genome search in multiple sclerosis. Nat Genet 1996; 13: 472–476.

72. Chataway J, Feakes R, Coraddu F et al. The genetics of multiple sclerosis: principles, background and updated results of the United Kingdom systematic genome screen. Brain 1998; 121: 1869–1887.

73. Multiple Sclerosis Genetics Group. A complete genomic screen for multiple sclerosis underscores a role for the major histocompatibility complex. Nat Genet 1996; 13: 469–471.

74. Sawcer S, Jones HB, Feakes R et al. A genome screen in multiple sclerosis reveals susceptibility loci on chromosome 6p21 and 17q22. Nat Genet 1996; 13: 464–468.

75. Fathman CG, Soares L, Chan SM, Utz PJ. An array of possibilities for the study of autoimmunity. Nature 2005; 435: 605–611.

76. Steinman L. Gene microarrays and experimental demyelinating disease: a tool to enhance serendipity. Brain 2001; 124: 1897–1899.

77. Geschwind DH. DNA microarrays: translation of the genome from laboratory to clinic. Lancet Neurol 2003; 2: 275–282.

78. Whitney LW, Becker KG, Tresser NJ et al. Analysis of gene expression in multiple sclerosis lesions using cDNA microarrays. Ann Neurol 1999; 46: 425–428.

79. Whitney LW, Ludwin SK, McFarland HF, Biddison WE. Microarray analysis of gene expression in multiple sclerosis and EAE identifies 5-lipoxygenase as a component of inflammatory lesions. J Neuroimmunol 2001; 212: 40–48.

80. Lock C, Hermans G, Pedotti R et al. Gene-microarray analysis of multiple sclerosis lesions yields new targets validated in autoimmune encephalomyelitis. Nat Med 2002; 8: 500–508.

81. Tajouri L, Mellick AS, Ashton KJ et al. Quantitative and qualitative changes in gene expression patterns characterize the activity of plaques in multiple sclerosis. Mol Brain Res 2003; 119: 170–183.

82. Fernald GH, Yeh RF, Hauser SL et al. Mapping gene activity in complex disorders: Integration of expression and genomic scans for multiple sclerosis. J Neuroimmunol 2005; 167: 157–169.

83. Mycko MP, Papoian R, Boschert U et al. cDNA microarray analysis in multiple sclerosis lesions: detection of genes associated with disease activity. Brain 2003; 126: 1048–1057.

84. Lassmann H. Cellular damage and repair in multiple sclerosis. In: Lazzarini RA, ed. Myelin biology and disorders. London: Elsevier Academic Press; 2004: 733–762.

85. Karsunky H, Merad M, Cozzio A et al. Flt3 ligand regulates dendritic cell development from flt3+ lymphoid and myeloid-committed progenitors to flt3+ dendritic cells in vivo. J Exp Med 2003; 198: 305–313.

86. Lapteva N, Ando Y, Nieda M et al. Profiling of genes expressed in human monocytes and monocyte-derived dendritic cells using cDNA expression array. Br J Haematol 2001; 114: 191–197.

87. Lindberg RLP, De Groot CJ, Certa U et al. Multiple sclerosis as a generalized CNS disease – comparative microarray analysis of normal appearing white matter and lesions in secondary progressive MS. J Neuroimmunol 2004; 152: 154–167.

88. Ramanathan M, Weinstock-Guttman B, Nguyen LT et al. In vivo gene expression revealed by cDNA arrays: the pattern in relapsing–remitting multiple sclerosis patients compared with normal subjects. J Neuroimmunol 2001; 116: 213–219.

89. Bomprezzi R, Ringner M, Kim S et al. Gene expression profile in multiple sclerosis patients and healthy controls: identifying pathways relevant to disease. Hum Mol Genet 2003; 12: 2191–2199.

90. Achiron A, Gurevich M, Friedman N et al. Blood transcriptional signatures of multiple sclerosis: unique gene expression of disease activity. Ann Neurol 2004; 55: 410–417.

91. Alt C, Duvefelt K, Franzen B et al. Gene and protein expression profiling of the microvascular compartment in experimental autoimmune encephalomyelitis in C57Bl/6 and SJL mice. Brain Pathol 2005; 15: 1–16.

92. Lucchinetti C, Bruck W, Rodrigues M, Lassmann H. Distinct patterns of multiple sclerosis pathology indicates heterogeneity on pathogenesis. Brain Pathol 1996; 6: 259–274.

93. Lucchinetti C, Bruck W, Parisi J et al. Heterogeneity of multiple sclerosis lesions: implications for the pathogenesis of demyelination. Ann Neurol 2000; 47: 707–717.

94. Hohlfeld R. Biotechnological agents for the immunotherapy of multiple sclerosis. Principles, problems and perspectives. Brain 1997; 120: 865–916.

95. Bielekova B, Richert N, Howard T et al. Humanized anti-CD25 (daclizumab) inhibits disease activity in multiple sclerosis patients failing to respond to interferon beta. Proc Natl Acad Sci USA 2004; 101: 8705–8708.

96. Stürzebecher S, Wandinger KP, Rosenwald A et al. Expression profiling identifies responder and non-responder phenotypes to interferon-b in multiple sclerosis. Brain 2003; 126: 1419–1429.

97. Weinstock-Guttman B, Badgett D, Patrick K et al. Genomic effects of IFN-beta in multiple sclerosis patients. J Immunol 2003; 171: 2694–2702.

98. Kappos L, Achtnichts L, Dahlke F et al. Genomics and proteomics: role in the management of multiple sclerosis. J Neurol 2005; 252(Suppl 3): iii21–iii27.

99. Fathallah-Shaykh HM. Microarrays: applications and pitfalls. Arch Neurol 2005; 62: 1669–1672.

100. Hollingshead D, Lewis DA, Mirnics K. Platform influence on DNA microarray data in postmortem brain research. Neurobiol Dis 2004; 18: 649–655.

101. Mirnics K, Pevsner J. Progress in the use of microarray technology to study the neurobiology of disease. Nat Neurosci 2004; 7: 434–439.

102. Kagawa T, Ikenaka K, Inoue Y et al. Glial cell degeneration and hypomyelination caused by overexpression of myelin proteolipid protein gene. Neuron 1994; 13: 427–442.

103. Readhead C, Schneider A, Griffiths IR, Nave KA. Premature arrest of myelin formation in transgenic mice with increased proteolipid protein gene dosage. Neuron 1994; 12: 583–595.

104. Bradl M, Bauer J, Inomata T et al. Transgenic Lewis rats overexpressing the

proteolipid protein gene: myelin degeneration and its effect on T cell-mediated experimental autoimmune encephalomyelitis. Acta Neuropathol (Berl) 1999; 97: 595–606.

105. Aboul-Enein F, Bauer J, Klein M et al. Selective and antigen-dependent effects of myelin degeneration on central nervous system inflammation. J Neuropathol Exp Neurol 2004; 63: 1284–1296.

106. Bradl M, Bauer J, Flugel A et al. Complementary contribution of CD4 and CD8 T lymphocytes to T-cell infiltration of the intact and the degenerative spinal cord. Am J Pathol 2005; 166: 1441–1450.

107. Tan PK, Downey TJ, Spitznagel EL et al. Evaluation of gene expression measurements from commercial microarray platforms. Nucleic Acids Res 2003; 31: 5676–5684.

108. Larkin JE, Frank BC, Gavras H et al. Independence and reproducibility across microarray platforms. Nat Methods 2005; 2: 337–344.

109. Irizarry RA, Warren D, Spencer F et al. Multiple-laboratory comparison of microarray platforms. Nat Methods 2005; 2: 345–350.

110. Pandey A, Mann M. Proteomics to study genes and genomes. Nature 2000; 405: 837–846.

111. Banks RE, Dunn MJ, Hochstrasser DF et al. Proteomics: new perspectives, new biomedical opportunities. Lancet 2000; 356: 1749–1756.

112. Dumont D, Noben J-P, Raus J et al. Proteomic analysis of cerebrospinal fluid from multiple sclerosis patients. Proteomics 2004; 4: 2117–2124.

113. Steen H, Mann M. The ABC's (and XYZ's) of peptide sequencing. Nat Rev Mol Cell Biol 2004; 5: 699–711.

114. Nielsen PA, Olsen JV, Podtelejnikov AV et al. Proteomic mapping of brain plasma membrane proteins. Mol Cell Proteomics 2005; 4: 402–408.

115. Cunningham TJ, Hodge L, Speicher D et al. Identification of a survival-promoting peptide in medium conditioned by oxidatively stressed lines of nervous system origin. J Neurosci 1998; 18: 7047–7060.

116. Hammack BN, Fung KY, Hunsucker SW et al. Proteomic analysis of multiple sclerosis cerebrospinal fluid. Mult Scler 2004; 10: 245–260.

117. MacBeath G, Schreiber SL. Printing proteins as microarrays for high-throughput function determination. Science 2000; 289: 1760–1763.

118. Cepok S, Zhou D, Srivastava R et al. Identification of Epstein-Barr virus proteins as putative targets of the immune response in multiple sclerosis. J Clin Invest 2005; 115: 1352–1360.

119. Almeras L, Lefranc D, Drobecq H et al. New antigenic candidates in multiple sclerosis: identification by serological proteome analysis. Proteomics 2004; 4: 2184–2194.

120. Hill T, Galatowicz G, Akerele T et al. Intracellular T lymphocyte cytokine profiles in the aqueous humour of patients with uveitis and correlation with clinical phenotype. Clin Exp Immunol 2005; 139: 132–137.

121. Chen G, Gharib TG, Huang C-C et al. Discordant protein and mRNA expression in lung adenocarcinomas. Mol Cell Proteomics 2002; 1: 304–313.

122. Anderson NL, Anderson NG. Proteome and proteomics: new technologies, new concepts, and new words. Electrophoresis 1998; 19: 1853–1861.

- Natalizumab classified as a immunomodulator.
- Cannot anticipate a progressive course, until irreversible clinical disability has developed.
- Optimal opportunity may have passed! The optimal opportunity for the use of Tysabri is early in the disease.

CHAPTER 20

Immunomodulatory therapy: critical appraisal of trial results and marketing claims

J. H. Noseworthy

INTRODUCTION AND BACKGROUND

This chapter will primarily address the results of published, full-scale, phase III controlled trials of immunomodulatory agents performed with the purpose of altering the natural history of multiple sclerosis (MS). The results of these trials will be largely familiar to the readership. The discussion will emphasize the likelihood that these data represent important steps in altering aspects of the disease course. As such, how certain are we that the results are definitive (e.g. convincing), robust (e.g. durable) and, therefore, likely to matter for individual patients and groups of patients with similar demographic findings?

The term 'immunomodulatory therapies' has been applied loosely to MS agents that have one or more effects on immune function and have been tested for and shown to alter one or more features of the disease course. Five are currently approved by the Food and Drug Administration (FDA) for use in North America (three beta interferons (IFNs), glatiramer acetate (GA) and mitoxantrone). A sixth agent (natalizumab; see below) was transiently approved in 2004 but later disapproved because of important safety concerns.[1] A small number of other 'immunomodulatory therapies' that are now either infrequently used, not recently critically studied or not FDA-approved for use in MS (cyclophosphamide, azathioprine, plasma exchange, bone marrow transplantation) will be discussed in Chapters 21–23.

It has been repeatedly emphasized in this text that there is considerable uncertainty about the factors that initiate and perpetuate this illness. There is still much to learn about the primary mechanism(s) of tissue injury in MS and the factors that govern and limit repair. Is there one dominant initiating event (immune-mediated, triggered by infection, modified by genetic influences, etc.) or are there either a finite number[2] or multiple mechanisms of tissue injury that occur during the course of this chronic disease?[3,4] There are no precise predictive factors that will inform on short- and long-term prognosis or likelihood of response to treatment. Truly, we are uncertain who will do well and avoid progressive disability during their lifetime until at least a decade has passed since the onset of symptoms and, even then, late progression may occur. In addition, we often cannot adequately anticipate a progressive course until irreversible clinical disability has developed. By that time,

there is considerable evidence that the optimal opportunity for treatment with the currently approved agents may have passed. Without a better understanding of what triggers and perpetuates the illness, it remains difficult to design trials and select patients most suited for putative therapeutic interventions. These uncertainties impose considerable limitations on our current ability to impact the course of MS.

That said, for the last three decades we have been following ever-evolving guidelines for trial design in attempts to optimize the uniformity of study populations in order to permit conclusions from completed trials. The nuances of trial design are reviewed in Chapter 29 but a few points will be emphasized in this chapter as these features each importantly influence interpretation of trials and our willingness to extend these findings into our practice (Table 20.1).

PUBLISHED LARGE-SCALE TRIALS

This last decade has seen a sea change in our attitude to the treatment of this disease. There is now a sense that it is possible to alter the short-term course of MS and we anticipate that more meaningful progress is imminent. Since the licensure of IFNβ-1b (Betaseron) in 1993, the number of trials and reports of the IFNs and other agents has increased exponentially[5] with a corresponding increase in activity from the pharmaceutical industry. Each month there are nearly too many reports to read describing additional insights into potential mechanisms of action of these and other putative therapies for MS, findings from case series and pilot studies and the application of magnetic resonance techniques to the study of models of MS and patients with the disorder.

In a recently completed monograph,[6] several of us reviewed and reported the last two decades of MS trials in considerable detail. In this chapter I propose to deal with the 'big picture' only and refer the readers to this other text for further details. In short, there is evidence that the immunomodulatory drugs reduce clinical and magnetic resonance imaging (MRI) evidence of disease activity in patients at high risk of developing MS (this is true for IFNβ-1a in clinically isolated syndromes (CIS)[7,8] and in those with actively relapsing forms of the disease (relapsing–

TABLE 20.1 Appraisal of trial results: factors to consider in reviewing trial design

Factor	Comments
Diagnostic precision	Diagnosis of PPMS in PROMISE (e.g. inclusion of CSF normal patients)
Classification of course	'Relapsing MS' in North American IFNβ-1a trial
Selection of control group	Increasing number of direct 'head-to-head' trials Disappearance of placebo-control groups
Sample size and power	Properly powered trial to avoid a type 2 error (false negative trial)?
Randomization	Was this done? Was this concealed?
Balance of demographic variables	Balance of predictive indices
Blinding: single, double; success?	Inability to blind patients to side effects of IFN
Safety of intervention	Important, common concern (linomide, natalizumab)
'Predetermined' outcome measures • Subjective or objective? • Validated? • Confirmed observation? Biologically meaningful?	No clinical or MRI outcomes validated to predict long-term disability Known tendency for relapse-related worsening to be temporary, reversible 'Disability' in North American IFNβ-1a trial did not require that EDSS change reflected consistent worsening within same Functional Systems category In European mitoxantrone trial, unblended evaluator determined presence of clinical relapse Unclear understanding of meaning and relevance of Z-scores in IMPACT trial
Interim analysis	Early termination of North American IFNβ-1a trial predicated by few drop-outs
Duration of follow-up	Trend to shorter trials
Behavior of control group	Did control group in CHAMPS do worse than predicted?
Drop-outs: number, management	Continues to be a major confounder
Correction for multiple comparisons?	Often not reported in manuscript
Time lapse between initial report and publication	Publication of European mitoxantrone trial delayed for 4 years
Were negative data published?	Oral myelin trial still unpublished
Did investigators have access to primary data?	This seems to be a pervasive problem in MS trials sponsored by the pharmaceutical industry
Was trial registered before completed?	See editorial by De Angelis, 2005[83]
What long-term safety and efficacy surveillance mechanisms are in place?	FDA has not tied continued approval to demonstration of continued benefit
Repeated, confirmed phase III trial results (grade I recommendation)	Remains essential

CSF, cerebrospinal fluid; EDSS, Expanded Disability Status Score; FDA, Food and Drug Administration; IFN, interferon; MS, multiple sclerosis; PPMS, primary progressive multiple sclerosis.

remitting MS, RRMS).[9-14] There remains no certain evidence that these drugs provide long-term protection against relapses or progression but this vital question has not been adequately studied. Extension trials suggest that patients tolerating treatment and doing well may continue to do well for prolonged periods of observation but there are methodological problems with this approach.[15-17] The IFNs seem also to favorably modify these same hallmarks of disease activity (relapses and MRI) in secondary progressive MS (SPMS) without significantly slowing the course of progression significantly as measured by the Expanded Disability Status Score (EDSS).[18-25] There is increasing understanding of how these drugs may work in vitro but only indirect evidence of their mechanisms of their action in MS patients.[26-29]

EVIDENCE-BASED MEDICINE VARIABLES

The magnitude of benefit from these treatments can be shown if one calculates the absolute risk reduction (ARR) and numbers needed to treat (NNT)[30] from the major, definitive phase III trials. With this knowledge and with an understanding of the important adverse effects of treatment, the treating physician can involve patients and their families in making a shared, informed decision

on the timing and type of treatment. Authors and sponsors often publish the relative risk reduction (RRR) to summarize the size of benefit from intervention (see footnotes to Tables 20.3, 20.5 and 20.7). A second metric is the absolute risk reduction. As noted in Tables 20.3, 20.5 and 20.7, the RRR generally exceeds the ARR and is, therefore, frequently used in promotional materials. The ARR is preferred, however, as it weighs the frequency of the event (e.g. how often an event occurs in the control group) and thereby informs on the absolute magnitude of effect. As such, the RRR may be impressive (e.g. 50% benefit) but if the outcome measure occurs infrequently the metric may be clinically meaningless.[30] The concept of risk reduction necessitates comparisons of proportions (ratios). As such, RRR, ARR and NNT can only be calculated when the reports of trial results present proportion data or provide sufficient detail to allow these ratios to be calculated. It is possible to make these calculations using the odds ratio (OR) if one can accurately calculate the patient's expected event rate (PEER), e.g. $(1-(PEER(1-OR)))/((1-PEER)(PEER)(1-OR))$. A common primary outcome measure in MS trials is relapse frequency (annualized relapse rate). Regrettably, this metric cannot be used to calculate the change in risk (RRR, ARR), however, as individual patients may have widely variable numbers of relapses.

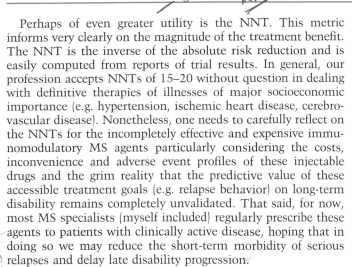

Perhaps of even greater utility is the NNT. This metric informs very clearly on the magnitude of the treatment benefit. The NNT is the inverse of the absolute risk reduction and is easily computed from reports of trial results. In general, our profession accepts NNTs of 15–20 without question in dealing with definitive therapies of illnesses of major socioeconomic importance (e.g. hypertension, ischemic heart disease, cerebrovascular disease). Nonetheless, one needs to carefully reflect on the NNTs for the incompletely effective and expensive immunomodulatory MS agents particularly considering the costs, inconvenience and adverse event profiles of these injectable drugs and the grim reality that the predictive value of these accessible treatment goals (e.g. relapse behavior) on long-term disability remains completely unvalidated. That said, for now, most MS specialists (myself included) regularly prescribe these agents to patients with clinically active disease, hoping that in doing so we may reduce the short-term morbidity of serious relapses and delay late disability progression.

The evidence-based medicine (EBM) numbers in Tables 20.3, 20.5 and 20.7 have been calculated from published data. A recent report from an employee at Serono Inc. presents more extensive EBM calculations based on data available from the sponsor.[31]

CLINICALLY ISOLATED SYNDROMES

There are two definitive trials of IFNβ-1a in CIS with high risk for developing MS (e.g. abnormal head MRI scans with multiple asymptomatic lesions; Table 20.2[7,8]). These trials differ in important ways. The inclusion criteria of CHAMPS insured that true CIS patients were preferentially enrolled whereas ETOMS probably included many more patients with early RRMS. Additionally, the dose of IFNβ-1a (Rebif) used in the ETOMS trial is now known to be suboptimal (OWIMS trials[32]). As illustrated in Table 20.2, treatment with IFNβ-1a significantly impacted the primary outcome of each of these trials (proportion of patients converting to clinically definite MS). These findings were soon followed by licensure and widespread use in CIS patients, presumably sharing clinical and MRI features of the study groups (particularly the need for several asymptomatic MRI lesions).

It bears mention, however, that treated patients were probably incompletely blinded to their treatment and that this may have impacted the interpretation by the blinded evaluator of the 'soft outcome' of a perceived relapse used therein for this primary outcome (e.g. IFN-treated patients may have under-reported relapse symptoms, attributing these to adverse effects of IFN). There was limited clinical follow-up of these patients, hence leaving unanswered the question of the clinical relevance of delaying the first relapse. In CHAMPS, only one-third of patients remained in the study beyond 2 years and MRIs were only obtained in stable patients (e.g. the MRI data was not collected on those failing because of a clinical relapse to compare with those apparently benefiting from IFN treatment). Approximately 50% of IFN-treated patients either experienced a clinical relapse or showed MRI evidence of disease activity within 18 months of starting treatment, indicating an incomplete degree of protection by the IFNs in CIS.[33] Some 44% of IFN-treated patients and 56% of placebo-treated patients either had a relapse or dropped out of the study; this finding in a trial setting (presumably constructed to optimize compliance) suggests that similar behavior (failure to comply with prolonged treatment) may diminish the benefits realized by CIS patients in a practice setting. As illustrated in Table 20.3, the ARR is only 11–14% and the NNT is 7–9 patients for up to 2 years to prevent one patient converting to MS. In summary, there is likely to be a benefit in treating CIS patients with IFNs but the benefits appear to be modest and of uncertain duration.

The management of CIS patients is discussed in detail in Chapter 21. Suffice it to say that these patients are generally young and early on in the psychological adjustment to what may be a chronic illness. The treating physician should be

TABLE 20.2 Primary outcome results of trials of immunomodulatory agents in patients with clinically isolated syndromes

Trial (no. enrolled)	Treatment	Primary outcome	Design	Duration of follow-up
CHAMPS (383)	Corticosteroids, then: IFN-β1a 30 μg by intramuscular injection weekly versus placebo	Delayed conversion to clinically definite multiple sclerosis (38% placebo vs 24% IFN-β1a; p=0.002)	RBPC	71% 1 year, 34% 2 year, 16% 3 year
ETOMS (309)	IFNβ1a 22 μg by subcutaneous injection once weekly versus placebo	Delayed conversion to clinically definite multiple sclerosis (45% placebo vs 34% IFN-β1a)	RBPC	2 year

IFN, interferon; RBPC, randomized, double-blinded (but patients unlikely to be blinded because of side effects), placebo-controlled.
Source: modified from Noseworthy & Hartung 2003.[85]

TABLE 20.3 Evidence-based medicine results of 'positive' trials of immunomodulatory agents in patients with clinically isolated syndromes

Trial	Outcome used for NNT calculations	Duration of follow-up	RRR	ARR	NNT
CHAMPS	Delayed conversion to clinically definite multiple sclerosis (38% placebo vs 24% IFN-β1a; p=0.002)	34% 2 years	2 year data: 38%	2 year data: 14.6%	7 patients – 2 years to prevent one converting to clinically definite MS
ETOMS	Delayed conversion to clinically definite multiple sclerosis (45% placebo vs 34% IFN-β1a)	2 years	24%	11%	9 patients – 2 years to prevent one converting to clinically definite MS

ARR, absolute risk reduction; IFN, interferon; NNT, numbers needed to treat; RBPC, randomized, double-blinded (but patients unlikely to be blinded because of side effects), placebo-controlled; RRR, relative risk reduction. RRR is calculated as (CER−EER)/CER where CER is the clinical event rate and EER is the experimental event rate. ARR is calculated as the difference between the CER and the EER (e.g. CER−EER). NNT is calculated as 1/ARR.

particularly patient and supportive as the implications of these first neurological symptoms are enormous and require a period of adjustment for patients and their families. In practice, an informed decision with regard to starting treatment in CIS is often largely influenced by the patient's inherent personality features. Admittedly, these features are important with all patients with regard to their willingness or need to be in control or to optimize healthy living behaviors (treat early).

RELAPSING–REMITTING MULTIPLE SCLEROSIS

Shortly after the North American trial was reported (Table 20.4), the FDA approved IFNβ-1b (Betaseron) as the first licensed treatment for MS (1993). This landmark decision was heavily influenced by the apparent benefit of treatment with IFN on the 'objective' measures of disease activity reflected by MR imaging.[9-11] As such, the FDA elected to license a treatment based on relatively 'soft' findings in, largely (my view), unblinded patients derived from a short period of observation of an unvalidated clinical outcome measure (e.g. relapses have not been shown to accurately predict long-term disability) buttressed by the findings of an equally unvalidated biomarker (e.g. MRI activity has not been shown to be a powerful predictor of long-term disability). This decision opened the door to countless studies

and enormous investment of resources by the pharmaceutical industry. As such, there were more than 1500 papers on the study of IFN and GA in multiple sclerosis during the decade 1995–2004. Only the reports that particularly inform on treatment decisions will be highlighted here. I will highlight a few observations from these published trials that may not be immediately apparent from a casual review of these tables or the abstracts of these reports.

The salient message from this literature is as follows. For periods of at least 1 year (perhaps longer) the β IFNs and GA modestly reduce clinical relapses (frequency and, perhaps, severity) and MRI evidence of inflammatory activity in RRMS patients. As summarized in Tables 20.4 and 20.5, the magnitude of the treatment effect varies widely across studies. Important differences in the design of these trials severely limit the ability to make comparisons across studies. In principle, however, it is wise to recall that experimental trials enroll patients with recently active disease who are highly motivated to realize a benefit from their participation. Trials are constructed to optimize compliance (reduce drop-outs) and safety; patients in trials may have an enhanced degree of access to study nurses and their treating physicians. In most trials patients are seen or, at the very least, interviewed every 3 months in order to capture clinical behavioral changes that may indicate an on-study relapse. Presumably patients with frequent

TABLE 20.4 Primary outcome results of trials of immunomodulatory agents in patients with relapsing-remitting multiple sclerosis

Trial (no. enrolled)	Treatment	Primary outcome	Design	Duration of follow-up
North American IFNβ-1b trial (Betaseron; 372)	8 MIU (0.25 mg) IFNβ-1b s.c. alternate days (1.6 MIU also tested) vs placebo	Relapse frequency: 1.27 placebo vs 0.84 for 8 MIU at 2 years	RBPC	2–3 years
MSCRG IFNβ-1a trial (Avonex; 301)	6 MIU (30 μg) IFNβ-1a i.m. once weekly vs. placebo	Time to EDSS change: Patients completing 2 years (57%): 33.3% placebo vs 21.1% IFN All patients: 34.9% placebo vs 21.9% IFN	RBPC	Up to 2 years
IFNβ-1a PRISMS trial (Rebif; 560)	12 MIU (44 μg) IFNβ-1a s.c. three times weekly (22 μg also tested) vs placebo	Relapse frequency: 2.56 placebo vs. 1.73 12 MIU IFNβ-1a	RBPC	2 years
North American GA trial (Copaxone; 251)	GA 20 mg s.c. daily vs placebo	Relapse frequency: 1.68 placebo vs 1.19 GA	RBPC	2 years
European–Canadian GA trial (239)	GA 20 mg s.c. daily injection	Total number of Gd+ lesions (29% reduction, $p=0.003$)	RBPC	9 months
INCOMIN trial (188)	IFN-β1a 30 μg i.m. once-weekly injection vs 9 MIU IFN-β1b s.c. alternate days	Months 6–12, IFN-β1b superior reduction in relapse rate, proportion relapse-free and EDSS	R	1 year
EVIDENCE trial (677)	IFN-β1a 30 μg i.m. once weekly vs 44 μg s.c. three times a week	Proportion relapse-free favors high dose s.c. three times a week (75% versus 63%)	R	6–12 months
Natalizumab (213)	Natalizumab 3 or 6 mg/kg i.v. monthly vs placebo	Fewer Gd+ lesions seen in active treatment group ($p<0.0001$); more patients relapse-free	RBPC	6 months
AFFIRM (942)	Natalizumab 300 mg i.v. monthly vs placebo	Reduced relative annualized relapse rate at 1 year by 68% ($p<0.0001$) with natalizumab; see Table 20.5	RBPC	1 year
SENTINEL (1,171)	6 MIU (30 μg) IFNβ-1a (Avonex) i.m. once weekly alone (placebo) or with natalizumab 300 mg i.v. monthly	Reduced relative annualized relapse rate at 1 year by 53% ($p<0.0001$) with combination treatment; see Table 20.5	RBPC	1 year

EDSS, Expanded Disability Status Scale; GA, glatiramer acetate; Gd+, gadolinium enhancing MRI lesions; IFN, interferon; MIU, million international units; MSCRG, MS Collaborative Research Group; RBPC, randomized, double-blinded (but patients unlikely to be blinded because of side effects), placebo-controlled; TIW, three times per week. Natalizumab=humanized monoclonal anti-α4 integrin antibody.
Source: modified from Noseworthy & Hartung 2003.[85]

TABLE 20.5 Evidence-based medicine results of 'positive' trials of immunomodulatory agents in patients with relapsing-remitting multiple sclerosis

Trial	Outcome used for NNT calculations	Duration of follow-up	RRR (%)	ARR (%)	NNT
North American IFNβ-1b (Betaseron) trial	Proportion relapse free: 16% placebo vs. 31% 8 MIU IFN (relapse frequency was primary outcome); EBM calculations done for proportion with relapses	3 years	18	15	7 for 3 years to increase by one the number relapse free
MSCRG IFNβ-1a (Avonex) trial	Time to EDSS progression (primary outcome)	2 years – patients completing 2 years of trial	37	13	8 for 2 years
		All patients in trial	37	12	8 for 2 years
	Proportion relapse free: 26% placebo vs 38% IFN 30 µg; EBM calculations done for proportion with relapses	Data presented only for all patients in trial	16	12	8 for up to 2 years to increase by one the number relapse free
IFNβ-1a PRISMS trial (Rebif)	Proportion relapse free: 16% placebo vs 32% IFN (relapse frequency was primary outcome); EBM calculations done for proportion with relapses	2 years	19	16	6 for 2 years to increase by one the number relapse free
North American GA (Copaxone)	Proportion relapse free: 27% placebo vs 34% GA (relapse frequency was primary outcome); EBM calculations done for proportion with relapses	2 years	10	7	14 for 2 years to increase by one the number relapse free
INCOMIN	Proportion relapse free: 51% IFNβ-1b vs 36% IFNβ-1a; EBM calculations done for proportion with relapses	1 year	23	15	7 for 2 years to increase by one the number relapse free
EVIDENCE	Proportion relapse free: 63% IFN IFNβ-1a (Avonex) vs 75% IFNβ-1a (Rebif); EBM calculations done for proportion with relapses	6 months	32	12	8 for 6 months to increase by one the number relapse free
Natalizumab	Proportion with relapses (38% placebo vs 19% natalizumab)	6 months	50	19	5 to increase the proportion relapse free at 6 months
AFFIRM	Proportion with relapses (47% placebo vs 24% natalizumab)	1 year	49	23	4 for 1 year to increase the proportion relapse free
SENTINEL	Proportion with relapses (54% IFNβ-1a+placebo vs 37% IFNβ-1a+natalizumab)	1 year	31	17	6 for 1 year to increase the proportion relapse free

ARR=absolute risk reduction; IFN=interferon; MSCRG, MS Collaborative Research Group; NNT=numbers needed to treat; RBPC, randomized, double-blinded (but patients unlikely to be blinded because of side effects), placebo-controlled; RRR=relative risk reduction. RRR is calculated as (CER−EER)/CER where CER is the clinical event rate and EER is the experimental event rate. ARR is calculated as the difference between the CER and the EER (i.e. CER−EER). NNT is calculated as 1/ARR.

recent relapses (for example) are more likely to demonstrate benefit (fewer relapses) in a short period of observation (1–2 years) than are patients treated in a practice setting with an 'average' degree of disease activity. Hence, efficacy in a trial may not invariably predict a similar degree of effectiveness in practice.

As shown in Tables 20.4 and 20.5, multiple IFN and GA trials have shown favorable primary outcomes in RRMS. As mentioned earlier, approval of IFNβ-1b (Betaseron) set the stage for accepting changes in relapse frequency coupled with a parallel influence on measures of MRI activity as sufficient evidence of treatment benefit to consider drug approval. Throughout the observation period of the North American IFNβ-1b (Betaseron) trial there was an apparent benefit from the higher dose of IFN and this has become the standard dose of this preparation. The MS Collaborative Research Group trial of IFNβ-1a (Avonex) was terminated by the investigators when an interim analysis found benefit on the risk of 'confirmed progression' (worsening of at least 1.0 EDSS[34] for 6 months) sooner than expected because fewer patients than predicted dropped out of the study. This outcome measure did not require that the Functional Systems scores contributing to the calculated EDSS change were consis-

tent across visits. These reports were followed by FDA approval in 1996 'to slow the accumulation of physical disability and to decrease the frequency of clinical exacerbations'. This trial has had its critics. The trial demonstrated less convincing evidence of an effect on relapses and MRI metrics than had been reported for IFNβ-1b and the degree of certainty that treatment with IFNβ-1a favorably impacted EDSS change was eroded by the short duration of follow-up (43% were evaluated for less than 24 months when the trial was stopped). Nonetheless, this agent has held market share for most of the time since approval presumably because of the convenience of the once-weekly IM schedule, the putative disability effect, a low rate of reported neutralizing antibody formation and strong marketing support.

Three-times-weekly subcutaneous IFNβ-1b (Rebif) was shown in the PRISMS trial to favorably effect relapse and MRI outcomes with evidence-based metrics similar to the IFNβ-1b findings (Table 20.5).[14] Upon completion, PRISMS was extended for 2 additional years (total 4 years) with volunteers from the placebo group randomized to one of the active doses of subcutaneous IFNβ-1b.[17] The primary outcome of this extension trial was relapse count over 4 years. This seems a somewhat suspect metric, again not accounting for variable relapse rates across individuals and not providing a chance for the patients originally randomized to placebo to 'catch up' with those first randomized to IFN. These analyses reported a benefit for IFN treatment ($p<0.001$). The largest drop-out rate was in the high-dose group (44 µg subcutaneously twice weekly) and no statistical adjustments were made for multiple comparisons. These findings received editorial support for early treatment despite these caveats.[35] In 2002 the FDA approved subcutaneous IFNβ-1b (Rebif) for use in relapsing forms of MS.

Glatiramer acetate (Copaxone) was licensed by the FDA in 1996 for 'the reduction in the frequency of relapses in patients with relapsing–remitting multiple sclerosis' based on the results of the North American GA trial. In this trial, the primary outcome (relapse frequency) reached statistical significance although RRR and NNT are less robust than comparable metrics for the β IFNs (Table 20.5). When considering these EBM metrics, one should also review the results of a recent systematic review of the evidence that GA is effective in RRMS and the heated correspondence engendered by this essentially negative meta-analysis report.[36–41] This phase III trial did not collect MRI outcomes. A subsequent MRI study (the European–Canadian GA trial[42]), however, demonstrated that GA reduced the total number of gadolinium-enhancing lesions by 29% compared with placebo at 9 months. The MRI benefit was not apparent until patients had been treated for 6 months. Prior to that time, many new MRI lesions developed in the GA-treated patients. The analysis did not suggest a benefit of treatment on the proportion of patients with gadolinium-enhancing lesions; the volume of T1 'black holes' and T2 volumes continued to increase in treated patients. These data suggest that GA may be less effective than the β IFNs in rapidly influencing MRI measures of disease activity. Subsequent extension study results have been reported at 2-year intervals, demonstrating continued benefit for the volunteers who elected for long-term GA treatment.[15,16] These extension trials are without the benefit of a comparison group, however, and are enriched by patients with fewer relapses and disability worsening than nonparticipants. The first report of the GA extension trials included an inappropriate comparison with a published, population-based historical control group that contained patients with progressive MS.[15]

The next era of RRMS trials compared 'active' agents head to head, forgoing placebo controls. The INCOMIN trial reported superiority of subcutaneous IFNβ-1b on alternate days to once-weekly intramuscular IFNβ-1a.[43] In this trial, only the radiologist was blinded to the results of randomization (e.g. the physicians determining the presence of relapses were not blinded). In the EVIDENCE trial, superiority in the proportion of relapse-free patients emerged for three-times weekly subcutaneous IFNβ-1a compared with once weekly intramuscular IFNβ-1b.[44] Efforts were made to blind the evaluators of this shortest of all 'definitive' MS trials.

We should briefly mention the trial results and marketing claims for the humanized monoclonal antibody, natalizumab. This antibody blocks α4 integrin adhesion molecules on lymphocytes and monocytes, thereby reducing migration of activated immune cells into the central nervous system (CNS).[45–52] In a randomized phase II trial ($n=213$ RRMS), patients treated intravenously once monthly for 6 months with natalizumab experienced fewer gadolinium-enhancing lesions and were more likely to be free of relapses (81% vs 62%) than placebo-treated patients although the benefit was short-lived, reversing within a few months of stopping treatment. Within 6 months after discontinuing treatment, the two groups were comparable for these outcome measures. These early results led to the launch of two phase III studies (SENTINEL trial: 1200 RRMS patients

randomized to IFNβ-1a (Avonex) and natalizumab or IFNβ-1a (Avonex) with placebo; AFFIRM trial: 900 RRMS patients randomized to placebo or natalizumab) and a phase II trial of GA alone or with natalizumab (110 RRMS patients). Early results suggested both benefit and safety, leading to FDA approval late in the fall of 2004 after there was a median of 13 months of safety data for the 'reduction of clinical exacerbations in patients with relapsing forms of multiple sclerosis' (primary data, including NNTs, are shown in Tables 20.4 and 20.5).[53] Within weeks, however, on 28 February 2005, the sponsors of these trials (Biogen IDEC and Elan Pharmaceuticals) removed natalizumab from the market[1] and these studies were stopped when progressive multifocal leukoencephalopathy was reported to have developed in two patients receiving the combination of natalizumab and IFNβ-1a and in one patient with Crohn's disease who had been treated with azathioprine and other immunosuppressants prior to being started on natalizumab.[54–58] There are now unconfirmed reports of an additional two cases of progressive multifocal leukoencephalopathy. This tragic lesson informs on the potential for harm in all clinical trials of experimental agents[59] and, perhaps, especially when combinations of powerful immune active agents are used in a disease in which the cause and the factors sustaining disease activity are incompletely understood. It also clearly illustrates that 'many years of patient safety' can be sadly misleading when the experience is limited to a short duration of treatment in many experimental subjects.

Finally, a brief look at the NNT for the drugs used in the RRMS population reminds us that we need to treat at least six patients (and as many as 14) for up to 3 years to reduce the likelihood of one patient receiving a clinical benefit. These numbers are much smaller than those required to show a difference in other non-neurological illnesses but are not trivial considering the costs involved and the misperceptions in patients' minds about the benefit they expect (see below).

SECONDARY PROGRESSIVE MULTIPLE SCLEROSIS

The results of the pivotal SPMS trials are summarized in Tables 20.6 and 20.7. GA has not been studied extensively in SPMS. As such, it seems that GA should not be started de novo in patients with SPMS and its use should probably be discontinued in GA-treated patients with RRMS who develop secondary progression. The IFNs and GA are not approved by the FDA for use in SPMS. Only mitoxantrone (discussed below) has been approved for use in progressive forms of MS.

There remains some considerable uncertainty about whether the IFNS should be used in patients with SPMS despite the absence of FDA approval. As noted in the summary tables, results have differed significantly across the four pivotal SPMS IFN trials. The European trial of IFNβ-1b (Betaseron) was completed first and was followed by approval in Europe for use in SPMS.[18,19,21] Both the primary and secondary outcome measures showed a treatment benefit. Within 1 year of starting treatment, the investigators noted that IFNβ-1b enhanced the probability of patients remaining progression-free. Subsequently, however, a report was published that MRI T2 volumes increased in year 3 in treated patients.[60] IFNβ-1b treatment had only a minor effect on preventing progressive cerebral atrophy as measured by serial MRI studies.[61] The published survival curves suggested that progression was delayed for less than 1 year, calling into question the value of IFNβ-1b in these patients. Additionally, the study patients were sometimes intolerant of treatment because of enhanced spasticity.

These early findings of a benefit on progression rates were not corroborated by the SPECTRIMS trial of subcutaneous

TABLE 20.6 **Primary outcome results of trials of immunomodulatory agents in patients with secondary progressive MS**

Trial (no. enrolled)	Treatment	Primary outcome	Secondary outcome	Design	Duration of follow-up
European IFN-β1b (718)	8 MIU IFN-β1b s.c. alternate days versus placebo	Time to EDSS worsening confirmed at 3 months (39% IFN-β1b v.s. 50% placebo; $p=0.0048$). Probability of remaining progression-free noted by 1 year	Time to become wheelchair-bound, hospitalizations, annual relapse rate, effect on MRI T2 volume and activity. Time to 1.0 and 2.0 point EDSS change. Proportion with either relapses or progression	RBPC	2–3 years
SPECTRIMS (618)	22 μg or 44 μg IFNβ-1a s.c. q.2 d. vs placebo	No effect on time to 3 months confirmed EDSS worsening ($p=0.88$)	Treatment reduced relapse rate Delayed progression in women at both doses. MRI effect seen on number of active lesions / patient / scan, combined unique activity and T2 volume	RBPC	3 years
IMPACT (436)	IFNβ-1a s.c. 60 μg i.m. once weekly vs placebo	Benefit on MSFC noted in year 2	No effect on EDSS	RBPC	2 years
North American IFN-β1b (939)	IFNβ-1b s.c. 8 MIU or 5 MIU/m² q 2 d vs placebo	No effect on proportion with confirmed EDSS worsening	Positive effect on relapse rate, MRI activity and T2 volume	RBPC	3 years
European mitoxantrone (188)	5 or 12 mg/m² mitoxantrone i.v. q 12 weeks vs placebo (methylene blue)	Benefit on composite measure (EDSS, AI, SNS, time to first attack needing steroids, time to attack)	Number of patients with with EDSS progression. Fewer new T2 and Gd⁺ lesions	RBPC	2 years

AI, Ambulation index; EDSS, Expanded Disability Status Scale; GA, glatiramer acetate; Gd+, gadolinium enhancing MRI lesions; IFN, interferon; MIU, million international units; MSFC, MS Functional Composite score RBPC, randomized, double-blinded (but patients unlikely to be blinded because of side effects), placebo-controlled; SNS, Scripps Neurologic Scale.
Source: modified from Noseworthy & Hartung 2003.[85]

TABLE 20.7 **Evidence-based medicine results of 'positive' trials of immunomodulatory agents in patients with secondary progressive multiple sclerosis**

Trial	Outcome used for NNT calculations	Duration of follow-up	RRR (%)	ARR (%)	NNT
European IFN-β1b	Primary outcome was time to EDSS worsening confirmed at 3 months (39% IFN-β1b vs 50% placebo; $p=0.0048$)	≤3 y	22	11	11 for up to 3 years to prevent one patient from worsening on EDSS
SPECTRIMS	Data not presented to permit EBM results based on proportions				
IMPACT	Proportion of relapse free: 63% placebo vs 74% IFN-β1b; EBM calculations done for proportion with relapses	2 years	30	11	9 for 2 years to increase by one the number of patients relapse free
North American IFN-β1b	Proportion relapse-free 62% placebo vs 71% 8 MIU IFN-β1b; EBM calculations done for proportion with relapses	3 years	24	9	11 for 3 years to increase by one the number of patients relapse free
European mitoxantrone	Proportion with EDSS worsening >1.0: 25% placebo vs 16% mitoxantrone	2 years	36	9	11 for 2 years to prevent one patient from worsening by 1.0 EDSS

AI, Ambulation index; ARR, absolute risk reduction; EDSS, Expanded Disability Status Scale; GA, glatiramer acetate; Gd+, gadolinium enhancing MRI lesions; IFN, interferon; MIU, million international units; MSCRG, MS Collaborative Research Group; NNT, numbers needed to treat; RBPC, randomized, double-blinded (but patients unlikely to be blinded because of side effects), placebo-controlled; RRR=relative risk reduction; SNS=Scripps Neurologic Scale. RRR is calculated as (CER−EER)/CER where CER is the clinical event rate and EER is the experimental event rate. ARR is calculated as the difference between the CER and the EER (i.e. CER−EER). NNT is calculated as 1/ARR.

IFNβ-1a (Rebif) administered three times weekly.[20,62] An unexplained gender effect was seen in this trial with male patients (but not females) showing partial apparent benefit.

In SPECTRIMS, neutralizing antibodies blocked any MRI benefit. The IMPACT trial showed a second year (and overall) benefit of treatment with once-weekly IM IFNβ-1a (Avonex) on the predetermined primary outcome measure (MS Functional Composite Scale (MSFC)[63]) but not on EDSS.[22] The FDA did not grant approval to IFNβ-1a (Avonex) for use in SPMS.

The results of the long-completed North American IFNβ-1b (Betaseron) SPMS trial were recently published and also failed to substantiate the findings of the European IFNβ-1b (Betaseron) trial, although, again, a benefit was reported for the secondary outcomes of relapse and MRI behavior.[23–25]

In 1998, the positive results of the large European mitoxantrone study were first presented in abstract form.[64] Despite the absence of a peer-reviewed, published manuscript (this surfaced in 2002[65]), in 2000 the FDA approved mitoxantrone for 'reducing neurologic disability and/or the frequency of clinical relapses in patients with secondary (chronic) progressive, progressive relapsing, or worsening relapsing-remitting multiple sclerosis (i.e. patients whose neurologic status is significantly abnormal between relapses)'. As summarized in Table 20.6, mitoxantrone seemed to benefit the composite (and not validated) outcome measure selected by the investigators. If one examines this short report carefully, however, one is struck by a few concerns. The EDSS benefit was seen for only the first of 3 years of surveillance. The higher dose (12 mg/m² every 3 months) was generally the more effective dose yet only the low dose (5 mg/m²) reduced gadolinium enhancements and neither dose influenced MRI T2 volumes. Measures of cerebral volume were not reported and, at the time of writing, there has not been a full report of the MRI behavior from this trial. As noted below, mitoxantrone has important safety concerns, limiting its widespread use.

With these results, the practicing neurologist must advise SPMS patients about the best treatment for them. The situation that occurs most commonly is the RRMS patient who has been on long-term IFN treatment and who is now experiencing slow progressive disability. The dearth of evidence suggesting that IFNs slow progression independent of relapses suggests that any benefit from continued IFN treatment in this setting will be minimal and probably measured only by the hoped-for benefit of reducing future relapses. As discussed above, patients bring their own desires and personality-dependent preferences to this decision making setting – some preferring to remain on treatment to risk the frequency and severity of future relapses and others selecting to stop further treatment because of the scarcity of published evidence of benefit. There is certainly very little, if any, evidence that patients with SPMS should be started de novo on IFN therapy in the absence of a history of ongoing relapses. Natural history data suggest that progression of EDSS is largely independent of relapse in both SPMS and PPMS patients once a fixed deficit (EDSS 3.0 or 4.0) has developed.[66,67] This is not to say that there is no possibility that IFN treatment could slow progression in any given patient; the evidence for such an effect is unfortunately limited.

PRIMARY PROGRESSIVE MULTIPLE SCLEROSIS

In short, there is no convincing evidence that these agents influence the course of primary progressive MS. A randomized trial of 50 PPMS patients randomized to placebo or either 30 μg or 60 μg IM IFNβ-1a (Avonex) weekly[68] suggested a trend to reduce the accumulation of T2 lesion load in the 30 μg patients whereas the high-dose group demonstrated greater brain atrophy. This trial was clearly underpowered to show clinical benefit. The

preliminary report from one recent trial involving 73 PPMS or transitional MS patients suggested that IFNβ-1b may favorably affect the MSFC and MRI lesion volumes in PPMS patients although the full report has not been published at the time of writing.[69]

The PROMISE trial randomized 943 PPMS patients to either placebo or GA.[70] Although the full report has not yet been published, this trial was terminated when an interim analysis projected a negative primary outcome.

As noted above, studies of natural history suggest that the rate of clinical decline (progression) is similar in untreated SPMS and PPMS patients with or without occasional relapses.[66,67] In SPMS, the findings of treatment trials have not supported the idea that suppressing relapses impacts clinical progression to a meaningful extent. It will be virtually impossible to determine whether the story differs in PPMS as few with this variant (perhaps 15%) have one or more relapses during their illness.

ADVERSE EFFECTS OF IMMUNOMODULATORY AGENTS

There is now a decade of experience with the β IFNs and several years with GA and mitoxantrone. Again, it seems highly improbable that efforts to blind patients receiving these agents could be successful, despite early claims to the contrary. Perhaps a minority of patients truly could not tell that they were receiving active drug. Few trials in recent years have reported an assessment of the success of these efforts. Presumably evaluator blinding is often possible; the importance of this step in trial design is well known and necessary.[71]

Most patients have access to educational materials either from their primary physician, on line, through local MS chapters or at a specialty clinic. Side effects are common but often reasonably well tolerated with time and with one or more approaches to symptomatic care (see Chapters 21 and 25).

BETA INTERFERONS

In general, MS patients tolerate treatment with the β IFNs reasonably well. Most accommodate to the inconvenience and discomfort of administering intramuscular or subcutaneous injections, although some prefer to have a care-giver do this. Some patients prefer one route of injection to another and this preference may influence their choice of agent. Severe injection site reactions (encountered primarily with the subcutaneous route of administration) that persist despite proper technique may necessitate changing treatment. The majority of patients who experience flu-like symptoms have found one or more anti-inflammatory medications (acetaminophen/paracetamol or ibuprofen, for example) that ameliorate these symptoms if taken concomitantly. Systemic effects and injection site reactions may improve with time. The β IFNs may worsen symptoms of spasticity, particularly in patients with PPMS,[72] although this has not been found in all reports.[73] A few will be intolerant because of headaches and, rarely, depression. Most will comply with the inconvenience of contraception and scheduled blood work (complete blood count, liver profile and periodic tests of thyroid function) to optimize the safety of these agents. There are isolated reports of induced autoimmunity and, although apparently infrequent, this possibility must be kept in mind for individual cases. These reports include the development or worsening of pre-existing thyroid dysfunction, myasthenia gravis, systemic lupus erythematosus, rheumatoid arthritis and other inflammatory arthritis, urticaria, Raynaud's syndrome, psoriasis and a severe capillary leak syndrome in patients with a coexisting monoclonal gammopathy. Patients who develop neutralizing antibodies to the β IFNs appear to achieve less therapeutic benefit.[74–76] In this situation, there appears little rationale for continuing with this form of treatment[77] (see Ch. 21).

GLATIRAMER ACETATE

This agent is generally more easily tolerated than the β IFNs and does not require monitoring of blood tests. In a few, injection-associated burning pain seems to be independent of technique and necessitates stopping treatment. The much discussed occasional development of a postinjection 'systemic reaction' characterized by nearly immediate symptoms of facial flushing, anxiety, palpitations, dyspnea and chest pressure syndrome lasting up to 30 minutes seems to be uncommonly experienced in practice. A minority of women will experience injection-site focal lipoatrophy, sometimes associated with regional lymphadenopathy, and in some patients this is sufficiently bothersome to stop treatment. Other GA adverse effects appear to be infrequent.

MITOXANTRONE

The potential for this cytotoxic agent to cause harm should not be forgotten. Mitoxantrone should be administered only by experienced personnel trained in the administration of chemotherapeutic agents. Extravasation causes staining of the subcutaneous tissues that may be permanent (tattooing). Gastrointestinal symptoms (nausea and vomiting) are rarely severe but bone marrow suppression may increase the risk of infection. Hair loss is rarely noticeable but menstrual dysfunction (irregularity or premature menopause) occurs in up to 25% of premenopausal patients.[65] The potential for treatment-related myocardial injury is well known and is felt to be dose-dependent. The concern that cardiac comorbidity (existing or future events) may compound any treatment-related myocardial toxicity should not be taken lightly[78] and may be delayed by several years.[79] There are several reports of mitoxantrone-induced leukemia in the literature (estimated frequency is estimated to be 0.05–0.1%[80,81]). Although uncommon, this possibility must be kept in mind when administering this agent to young patients with a nonmalignant disorder.

PERCEPTIONS OF EFFICACY

Patients, and many neurologists, often hold unrealistic expectations for these agents. Some of this is understandable. Human nature is such that optimistic patients will assume the best for themselves and the reverse is true of those possessed of a less positive outlook. Physicians prefer to err on the side of being overly optimistic with their patients. When asked, many patients will offer the claim that these agents reduce relapse frequency 'by one-third' despite the published evidence of a more modest effect; some may have heard this from their neurologist. Many patients will ask to be changed to another agent after their first or second on-treatment relapse, again despite being told that these treatments may reduce but do not prevent further attacks. Many hold to the hope that early treatment will prevent, or at least reduce or delay, disability. Physicians should continue to provide hope for their patients and encourage a positive outlook but not at the expense of clarity, candor and truth. The pharmaceutical industry may contribute to these misperceptions through their aggressive marketing strategies.

FUTURE STRATEGIES

This is a rapidly changing landscape. There is an increasing sense that progress is being made in understanding the mechanisms of axonal injury, demyelination and repair. As outlined previously, increasingly sophisticated MRI-based strategies may inform on neuronal and axonal health and the early mechanisms of injury and aborted attempts at repair (Chs 10, 12 and 24). Resolution of the working hypothesis that there are a limited number of dominant mechanisms of active inflammatory injury in MS that remain consistent for the patient throughout the course of the illness will determine if biomarkers of these subtypes should be validated and then used to be more selective in designing treatment strategies and enrollment criteria for future trials.[2] We must achieve consensus on 'how much time is enough' to determine that a treatment has altered disease course and adopt ways to secure long-term follow-up on treated patients to insure both continued safety and efficacy. It is likely that drug discovery will parallel these fundamental events and that the practice of MS therapy will undergo significant change in the coming decade.

ACCESS TO TRIAL DATA

In the interim, what additionally can clinician-investigators do to contribute to this progress? It is essential that we fully appreciate both the progress that has been made and the limitations that need to be redressed. The pharmaceutical industry has provided resources to get us to the point where there are approved treatments for our patients, but more is needed. It is likely that the tension between protecting the assets of the sponsor (data) and full access to data will continue and needs to be actively managed. It is also highly likely, however, that sponsors will be required by the federal US government to be more transparent. The editors of the major biomedical journals have taken two steps to advance this process. In the fall of 2001[82] they first required that authors sign a letter indicating that they had been granted access to the primary data from the trial. In the late spring of 2005, editors gave notice that they would now require that clinical trials be fully registered at inception for the results to be published.[83] In my view, these are both important steps but probably insufficient to change the behavior of the pharmaceutical industry.

Despite this first step (acknowledgment of access to data), every indication suggests that academic investigators are not given access to unprocessed primary trial data for ongoing and completed MS trials. Journal editors have admitted that this first step has gone largely unnoticed by their staff with the exception of mandating one additional piece of correspondence in the submission of manuscripts (personal communication). It seems, at least within the MS trial community, that a 'don't ask, don't tell' culture of silence persists in the relationship of lead investigators with sponsors. There are probably several factors behind this willingness of leading MS investigators to accept restricted access to data. Many do not have access to independent statisticians for additional analyses; those that do have staff willing to do this work may not have funding to support an independent analysis. Most presumably feel the pressure to retain a good working relationship with the sponsor to secure continued funding. Presumably, most investigators trust the sponsor, believe that FDA will adequately review the statistical analyses and are interested in getting their work published.

In recent months there have been a number of well publicized examples of incomplete disclosure by sponsors of clinical trial result that have compromised patient safety and seemingly obscured the degree of treatment benefit. The efforts to encourage more open disclosure and access to data from pharmaceutical studies seems to be gaining considerable momentum. It seems likely that, as these individual examples are brought to public attention, federal legislation may one day be enacted to mandate a change in how US clinical trials are conducted.

There are several examples of restricted access to important MS data that are known by many who have been active in this field. Perhaps the best known is the early and prolonged reluctance of sponsors to facilitate the many questions underlying the neutralizing antibody issue in the interferon trials. Additionally, however, and perhaps of greater importance, is the complete gap in our understanding of what distinguishes a 'treatment responder' from one who presumably will not benefit from treatment. This question would lead every list of 'next analysis steps' by virtually every informed professional or lay person reading each of the published studies proclaiming a partial benefit from treatment. An equally pressing and obvious question is whether these treatments delay disability and, if so, in what percentage of what type of patient? It is absolutely beyond explanation how these first of many 'next steps' have been ignored in the now 14 years since the first MS drug was approved for use. A disciplined approach to these and other questions by investigators and sponsors working together would have led to focused experimental studies and data analyses to the benefit of persons with MS.

Investigators have addressed these unmet needs in a number of ways. As discussed in Chapter 29, some have offered continued participation in 'extension trials'. In these extension trials, study participants are given the opportunity to remain on (or switch to) active treatment beyond the completion of the initial trial. The advantages gained by this design (prolonged follow-up) must be balanced by the bias introduced by the change in the study population resulting from those patients who dropped out because of perceived failure to respond, adverse effects or other reasons. Several countries (Denmark, Spain, the UK and Canada) have created registries to optimize access to these expensive treatments and to facilitate data collection and future analyses. Repeated discussions with FDA on issues of longer duration trials and more complete long-term surveillance (durability of benefit) have, to date, not borne results.

The Sylvia Lawry MS Research Centre (SLCMSR; Munich) was founded in 2001 to redress a number of these issues. The fundamental idea behind this initiative was the ever-diminishing role of academic neurologists in hypothesis-testing research (especially trial design and analysis) and the complete exclusion of investigators from access to trial data.[84] This idea initially met with limited interest from funding agencies but was transformed to a reality when Professor W. Ian McDonald convinced the MS International Federation to help raise private funds to allow this to proceed. Between 1999 and 2001, several leading MS clinical investigators (Christian Confavreux, George Ebers, Ludwig Kappos, Jurg Kesselring, Fred Lublin, David Miller, Chris Polman, Jerry Wolinsky) kindly agreed to assist Henry McFarland and me in drafting a charter and overseeing early efforts to create an independent data analysis centre. This centre would access clinical and laboratory (primarily MRI) data from completed and ongoing trials and natural history studies to mathematically model the disease course and thereby better understand the variables that determine disease activity. Once funds were obtained to support this effort, a request for proposals was promulgated in the spring of 2000 and the contract was awarded to a team of mathematicians associated with the Technical University of Munich. With the scientific direction initially by Professor Albrecht Neiss and now by Dr Martin Daumer, the centre has now collected natural history data sets from leading academic centers and most of the control group data from completed definitive trials (45 data sets, 20 000 patients and 81 000 patient-years of follow-up). The centre's superb staff use sophisticated information technology methods to anonymize the data to avoid attributing specific outcomes to individual trials. The centre has created two data sets – one 'open' and available for hypothesis-testing and the second 'closed' and available for validation of preliminary findings. This brilliant concept of two data sets will lead to new insights into an expanding number of questions, including: What are the clinical and MRI predictors of disease activity? What are the best measures of short-term clinical worsening? The centre is actively partnering with investigators and sponsors to design future trials and provide accurate sample size estimates.

It is telling, however, that despite continued, concentrated efforts, pharmaceutical sponsors of MS trials have refused to provide the SLCMSR with active treatment data from completed trials despite the steps taken voluntarily by the center to anonymize all data donated to it. This single step demonstrates that the SLCMSR will not be evaluating the relative efficacies of experimental agents but rather will focus on the indicators of treatment response. The SLCMSR was established with the hope that academics and sponsors would collaborate to advance knowledge of MS and hasten the discovery of effective therapies. Active treatment data would allow investigators to address the fundamental issues of what determines response to treatment and thereby optimize the care of our patients. Again, the stance taken by sponsors has not helped to address these key unanswered questions.

Other steps are taking place simultaneously to identify and ultimately reduce the influence of the pharmaceutical industry within the health care profession. The Accreditation Council for Graduate Medical Education guidelines now requires more complete disclosure of potential competing interests in research studies. Academic centers have largely embraced the American Association of Medical Colleges guidelines for disclosure. Increasingly, academic societies are requiring participants at their meetings to fully disclose their personal relationships with sponsors and not simply those that appear to apply to the specific work being presented. The American Academy of Neurology (AAN) in 2005 adopted a stringent disclosure policy for all presenters and co-authors at each AAN event and has made this information available to attenders at these meetings.

Steady progress is being made in understanding this complex and often unpredictable disease. MS investigators are partnering effectively with basic discovery scientists to identify and address the fundamental questions that will reveal what causes MS and what factors contribute to disease onset (prevention strategies) and recovery (treatment strategies). The MS clinical trial community is working well with the statistical community to apply increasingly effective trial design strategies to address the relative merits of each putative new therapy. It is my fervent hope that the near future will see increasing disclosure of the data from clinical trials by all sponsors with the research community in a manner that will clearly help us to understand the progress that has been made and the gaps that need to be filled as we try to advise on the best treatment approach for each of our patients.

REFERENCES

1. Steinman L. Blocking adhesion molecules as therapy for multiple sclerosis: natalizumab. Nat Rev Drug Discov 2005; 4: 510–518.

2. Lucchinetti CF, Bruck W, Lassmann H. Evidence for pathogenic heterogeneity in multiple sclerosis. Ann Neurol 2004; 56: 308.

3. Noseworthy JH, Lucchinetti C, Rodriguez M et al. Multiple sclerosis. N Engl J Med 2000; 343: 938–952.

SECTION 3

4. Barnett MH, Prineas JW. Relapsing and remitting multiple sclerosis: pathology of the newly forming lesion. Ann Neurol 2004; 55: 458–468.

5. Hohlfeld R, Wiendl H. The ups and downs of multiple sclerosis therapeutics. Ann Neurol 2001; 49: 281–284.

6. Noseworthy JH, Miller D, Compston A. Disease-modifying treatments in multiple sclerosis. In: Compston DAS, ed. McAlpine's multiple sclerosis, 4th ed. Edinburgh: Elsevier Churchill Livingstone; 2006.

7. Jacobs LD, Beck RW, Simon JH et al. Intramuscular interferon beta-1a therapy initiated during a first demyelinating event in multiple sclerosis. CHAMPS Study Group. N Engl J Med 2000; 343: 898–904.

8. Comi G, Filippi M, Barkhof F et al. Effect of early interferon treatment on conversion to definite multiple sclerosis: a randomised study. Lancet 2001; 357: 1576–1582.

9. IFNB Multiple Sclerosis Study Group. Interferon beta-1b is effective in relapsing-remitting multiple sclerosis. I. Clinical results of a multicenter, randomized, double-blind, placebo-controlled trial. Neurology 1993; 43: 655–661.

10. Paty DW, Li DKB, the UBC MS/MRI Study Group and the IFNB Multiple Sclerosis Study Group. Interferon beta-1b is effective in relapsing-remitting multiple sclerosis. II. MRI analysis results of a multicenter, randomized, double-blind, placebo-controlled trial. Neurology 1993; 43: 662–667.

11. IFNB Study Group and the University of British Columbia MS/MRI Analysis Group. Interferon beta-1b in the treatment of multiple sclerosis: final outcome of the randomized, controlled trial. Neurology 1995; 45: 1277–1285.

12. Johnson KP, Brooks BR, Cohen JA et al. Copolymer 1 reduces relapse rate and improves disability in relapsing-remitting multiple sclerosis: results of a phase III multicenter, double-blind placebo-controlled trial. The Copolymer 1 Multiple Sclerosis Study Group. Neurology 1995; 45: 1268–1276.

13. Jacobs LD, Cookfair DL, Rudick RA et al. Intramuscular interferon beta-1a for disease progression in relapsing multiple sclerosis. The Multiple Sclerosis Collaborative Research Group (MSCRG). Ann Neurol 1996; 39: 285–294.

14. PRISMS (Prevention of relapses and disability by interferon beta-1a subcutaneously in multiple sclerosis) Study Group. Randomised double-blind, placebo-controlled study of interferon beta-1a in relapsing-remitting multiple sclerosis. Lancet 1998; 352: 1498–1504.

15. Johnson KP, Brooks BR, Cohen JA et al. Extended use of glatiramer acetate (Copaxone) is well tolerated and maintains its clinical effect on multiple sclerosis relapse rate and degree of disability. Copolymer 1 Multiple Sclerosis Study Group. Neurology 1998; 50: 701–708.

16. Johnson KP, Brooks BR, Ford CC et al. Sustained clinical benefits of glatiramer acetate in relapsing multiple sclerosis patients observed for 6 years. Mult Scler 2000; 6: 255–266.

17. Prisms Study Group, University of British Columbia MS MRI Analysis Group.

18. Kappos L and the European Study Group on Interferon beta-1b in secondary-progressive MS. Placebo-controlled multicentre randomised trial of interferon beta-1b in treatment of secondary progressive multiple sclerosis. Lancet 1998; 352: 1491–1497.

19. Kappos L, Polman C, Pozzilli C et al. Final analysis of the European multicenter trial on IFNβ-1b in secondary-progressive MS. Neurology 2001; 57: 1969–1975.

20. Secondary Progressive Efficacy Clinical Trial of Recombinant Interferon-beta-1a in MS Study Group. Randomized controlled trial of interferon-beta-1a in secondary progressive MS – clinical results. Neurology 2001; 56: 1496–1504.

21. Li DK, Zhao GJ, Paty DW et al. Randomized controlled trial of interferon-beta-1a in secondary progressive MS: MRI results. Neurology 2001; 56: 1505–1513.

22. Cohen J, Goodman A, Heidenreich F et al. Results of IMPACT, a phase 3 trial of interferon beta-1a in secondary progressive multiple sclerosis. Neurology 2001; 56: A148–A149.

23. MS TNASGoIb-biSP. Interferon beta-1b in secondary progressive MS: results from a 3-year controlled study. Neurology 2004; 63: 1788–1795.

24. Kappos L, Weinshenker B, Pozzilli C et al for the European (EU-SPMS) and North American (NA-SPMS) Interferon beta 1-b in Secondary Progressive Multiple Sclerosis Trial Steering Committees and Independent Advisory Boards. Interferon beta-1b in secondary progressive MS: a combined analysis of the two trials. Neurology 2004; 63: 1779–1787.

25. Cohen J, Antel J. Does interferon beta help in secondary progressive MS? Neurology 2004; 63: 1768–1769.

26. Zang Y, Hong J, Robinson R et al. Immune regulatory properties and interactions of copolymer-I and beta-interferon 1a in multiple sclerosis. J Neuroimmunol 2003; 137: 144–153.

27. Yong VW. Differential mechanisms of action of interferon-beta and glatiramer aetate in MS. Neurology. 2002; 59: 802–808.

28. Dhib-Jalbut S. Mechanisms of action of interferons and glatiramer acetate in multiple sclerosis. Neurology 2002; 58(suppl 4): S3–S9.

29. Zhang J, Hutton G, Zang Y. A comparison of the mechanisms of action of interferon beta and glatiramer acetate in the treatment of multiple sclerosis. Clin Ther 2002; 24: 1998–2021.

30. Sackett DL, Straus SE, Richardson WS et al. Evidence-based medicine. how to practice and teach EBM, 2nd ed. Toronto: Churchill Livingstone; 2000.

31. Francis GS. Importance of benefit-to-risk assessment for disease-modifying drugs used to treat MS. J Neurol 2004; 251(suppl 5): v42–v49.

32. Freedman MS, Francis GS, Sanders EA et al. Randomized study of once-weekly interferon beta-1a therapy in relapsing multiple sclerosis: three-year data from the OWIMS study. Mult Scler 2005; 11: 41–45.

33. Beck RW, Chandler DL, Cole SR et al. Interferon beta-1a for early multiple sclerosis: CHAMPS trial subgroup analyses. Ann Neurol 2002; 51: 481–490.

34. Kurtzke JF. Rating neurological impairment in multiple sclerosis: an expanded disability status scale (EDSS). Neurology 1983; 33: 1444–1452.

35. Schwid SR, Bever CT Jr. The cost of delaying treatment in multiple sclerosis: what is lost is not regained. Neurology 2001; 56: 1620.

36. Munari L, Lovati R, Boiko A. Therapy with glatiramer acetate for multiple sclerosis. In: Cochrane Database of Systematic Reviews 2004: CD004678.

37. Munari LM, Filippini G. Lack of evidence for use of glatiramer acetate in multiple sclerosis. Lancet Neurol 2004; 3: 641.

38. Caramanos Z, Arnold DL. Evidence for use of glatiramer acetate in multiple sclerosis. Lancet Neurol 2005; 4: 74–75; discussion 76–77.

39. Comi G, Hartung H. Evidence for use of glatiramer acetate in multiple sclerosis. Lancet Neurol 2005; 4: 75–76; discussion 76–77.

40. Munari L, Filippini G. Evidence for use of glatiramer acetate in multiple sclerosis. Lancet Neurol 2005; 4: 76–77.

41. De Jong BA, Engelen M, van Schaik IN et al. Confusing Cochrane reviews on treatment in multiple sclerosis. Lancet Neurol 2005; 4: 330–331.

42. Comi G, Filippi M, Wolinsky JS. European/Canadian multicenter, double-blind, randomized, placebo-controlled study of the effects of glatiramer acetate on magnetic resonance imaging-measured disease activity and burden in patients with relapsing multiple sclerosis. Ann Neurol 2001; 49: 290–297.

43. Durelli L, Verdun E, Barbero P et al. Every-other-day interferon beta-1b versus once-weekly interferon beta-1a for multiple sclerosis: results of a 2-year prospective randomised multicentre study (INCOMIN). Lancet 2002; 359: 1453–1460.

44. Panitch H, Goodin DS, Francis G et al. Randomized, comparative study of interferon beta-1a treatment regimens in MS: the EVIDENCE Trial. Neurology 2002; 59: 1496–1506.

45. Yednock TA, Cannon C, Fritz LC et al. Prevention of experimental autoimmune encephalomyelitis by antibodies against alpha 4 beta 1 integrin. Nature 1992; 356: 63–66.

46. Tubridy N, Behan PO, Capildeo R et al. The effect of anti-α4 integrin monoclonal antibody (Antegren©) on brain lesion activity in multiple sclerosis. Neurology 1999; 53: 466–472.

47. Miller DH, Khan OA, Sheremata WA et al. A controlled trial of natalizumab for relapsing multiple sclerosis. N Engl J Med 2003; 348: 15–23.

48. Dalton CM, Miszkiel KA, Barker GJ et al. Effect of natalizumab on conversion of gadolinium enhancing lesions to T1 hypointense lesions in relapsing multiple sclerosis. J Neurol 2004; 251: 407–413.

49. Vollmer TL, Phillips JT, Goodman AD et al. An open-label safety and drug interaction study of natalizumab (Antegren) in combination with interferon-beta (Avonex) in patients with multiple sclerosis. Mult Scler 2004; 10: 511–520.

50. Rudick RA, Sandrock A. Natalizumab: α4-integrin antagonist selective adhesion

molecule inhibitors for MS. Expert Rev Neurother 2004; 4: 571–580.

51. O'Connor PW, Goodman A, Willmer-Hulme AJ et al. Randomized multicenter trial of natalizumab in acute MS relapses. Clinica and MRI effects. Neurology 2004; 62: 2038–2043.

52. Rice GP, Hartung HP, Calabresi PA. Anti-α4 integrin therapy for multiple sclerosis: mechanisms and rationale. Neurology 2005; 64: 1336–1342.

53. Noseworthy JH, Kirkpatrick P. Natalizumab. Nat Rev Drug Discov 2005; 4: 101–102.

54. Van Assche G, Van Ranst M, Sciot R et al. Progressive multifocal leukoencephalopathy after natalizumab therapy for Crohn's disease. N Engl J Med 2005; 353: 362–368.

55. Kleinschmidt-Demasters BK, Tyler KL. Progressive multifocal leukoencephalopathy complicating treatment with natalizumab and interferon beta-1a for multiple sclerosis. N Engl J Med 2005; 353: 369–374.

56. Berger JR, Koralnik IJ. Progressive multifocal leukoencephalopathy and natalizumab – unforeseen consequences. N Engl J Med 2005; 353: 414–416.

57. Langer-Gould A, Atlas SW, Bollen AW et al. Progressive multifocal leukoencephalopathy in a patient treated with natalizumab. N Engl J Med 2005; 353: 375–381.

58. Adelman B, Sandrock A, Panzara MA. Natalizumab and progressive multifocal leukoencephalopathy. N Engl J Med 2005.

59. Drazen JM. Patients at risk. N Engl J Med 2005; 353: 417.

60. Miller D, Molyneux P, Barker G et al. Effect of interferon b-1b on magnetic resonance imaging outcomes in secondary progressive multiple sclerosis: Results of a European Multicenter, randomized, double-blind, placebo-controlled trial. Ann Neurol 1999; 46: 850–859.

61. Molyneux PD, Kappos L, Polman C et al. The effect of interferon beta-1b treatment on MRI measures of cerebral atrophy in secondary progressive multiple sclerosis. European Study Group on Interferon beta-1b in secondary progressive multiple sclerosis. Brain 2000; 123: 2256–2263.

62. Li DK, Zhao GJ, Paty DW et al. Randomized controlled trial of interferon-beta-1a in secondary progressive MS: MRI results. Neurology 2001; 56: 1505–1513.

63. Cutter GR, Baier ML, Rudick RA et al. Development of a multiple sclerosis functional composite as a clinical trial outcome measure. Brain 1999; 122: 871–882.

64. Hartung H, Gonsette R. Mitoxantrone in progressive multiple sclerosis (MS): a placebo-controlled, randomized, observer-blind European phase III multicenter study – clinical results. Mult Scler 1998; 4: 325.

65. Hartung HP, Gonsette R, Konig N et al. Mitoxantrone in progressive multiple sclerosis: a placebo-controlled, double-blind, randomised, multicentre trial. Lancet 2002; 360: 2018–2025.

66. Kremenchutzky M, Cottrell D, Rice G et al. The natural history of multiple sclerosis: a geographically based study 7. Progressive-relapsing and relapsing-progressive multiple sclerosis: a re-evaluation. Brain 1999; 122: 1941–1949.

67. Confavreux C, Vukusic S, Moreau T et al. Relapses and progression of disability in multiple sclerosis. N Engl J Med 2000; 343: 1430–1438.

68. Leary SM, Miller DH, Stevenson VL et al. Interferon beta-1a in primary progressive MS: an exploratory, randomized, controlled trial. Neurology 2003; 60: 44–51.

69. Montalban X. Overview of European pilot study of interferon β-1b in primary progressive multiple sclerosis. Mult Scler 2004; 10(suppl 1): S62–S64.

70. Wolinsky JS. The PROMiSe trial: baseline data review and progress report. Mult Scler 2004; 10(suppl 1): S65–S71; discussion S71–S72.

71. Noseworthy JH, Ebers GC, Vandervoort MK et al. The impact of blinding on the results of a randomized, placebo-controlled multiple sclerosis clinical trial. Neurology 1994; 44: 16–20.

72. Bramanti P, Sessa E, Rifici C et al. Enhanced spasticity in primary progressive MS patients treated with interferon beta-1b. Neurology 1998; 51: 1720–1723.

73. Leary SM, Thompson AJ. The effect of interferon beta-1a on spasticity in primary progressive multiple sclerosis. J Neurol Neurosurg Psychiatr 2004; 75: 508–509.

74. Francis GS, Rice GP, Alsop JC. Interferon beta-1a in MS: results following development of neutralizing antibodies in PRISMS. Neurology 2005; 65: 48–55.

75. Kappos L, Clanet M, Sandberg-Wollheim M et al. Neutralizing antibodies and efficacy of interferon beta-1a: a 4-year controlled study. Neurology 2005; 65: 40–47.

76. Sorensen PS, Koch-Henriksen N, Ross C et al. Appearance and disappearance of neutralizing antibodies during interferon-beta therapy. Neurology 2005; 65: 33–39.

77. Giovannoni G, Goodman A. Neutralizing anti-IFN-beta antibodies: how much more evidence do we need to use them in practice? Neurology 2005; 65: 6–8.

78. Ghalie RG, Edan G, Laurent M et al. Cardiac adverse effects associated with mitoxantrone (Novantrone) therapy in patients with MS. Neurology 2002; 59: 909–913.

79. Goffette S, van Pesch V, Vanoverschelde JL et al. Severe delayed heart failure in three multiple sclerosis patients previously treated with mitoxantrone. J Neurol 2005; 252: 1217–1222.

80. Ghalie RG, Mauch E, Edan G et al. A study of therapy-related acute leukemia after mitoxantrone therapy for multiple sclerosis. Mult Scler 2002; 8: 441–445.

81. Voltz R, Starck M, Zingler V et al. Mitoxantrone therapy in multiple sclerosis and acute leukaemia: a case report of 644 treated patients. Mult Scler 2004; 10: 472–474.

82. Davidoff F, DeAngelis CD, Drazen JM et al. Sponsorship, authorship, and accountability. N Engl J Med 2001; 345: 825–826; discussion 826–827.

83. De Angelis CD, Drazen JM, Frizelle FA et al. Is this clinical trial fully registered? – A statement from the International Committee of Medical Journal Editors. N Engl J Med 2005; 352: 2436–2438.

84. Noseworthy John H, Kappos L, Daumer M. Competing interest in multiple sclerosis research (correspondence). Lancet 2003; 361: 350.

85. Noseworthy, JH, Hartung HP. Multiple sclerosis and related conditions. In: Noseworthy JH, ed. Neurological therapeutics: principles and practice. London: Martin Dunitz; 2003.

D. S. Goodin and L. Kappos

INTRODUCTION

Multiple sclerosis (MS) is an inflammatory disorder of the central nervous system (CNS), which results in injury to the myelin sheaths, to the oligodendrocytes and to the nerve axons.[1–6] The clinical onset of the disease is usually between 20 and 40 years of age, although it can start either earlier or later in life.[1–4] Women are affected twice as often as men. Although the primary cause of MS is not known, the immune system is clearly involved (either primarily or secondarily) and all of our current therapeutic approaches to MS have been focused on immunological mechanisms. Pathologically, MS is characterized by multifocal patches of demyelination (plaques), which are found principally in the central white matter and are often in a perivenular distribution. In MS, it is thought that autoreactive CD4+ T cells proliferate, cross the blood–brain barrier, and enter the CNS under the influence of cellular adhesion molecules and proinflammatory cytokines.[5,6] In addition to these T cells, however, it has become increasingly clear that other mononuclear cells, such as macrophages and B cells, also play an important role in MS pathogenesis. It has also become increasingly clear that these pathological processes can combine to produce irreversible axonal injury or transsection[7,8] and to lead, thereby, to permanent neurological disability.

Four different clinical courses of MS have been defined.[9] Relapsing–remitting MS (RRMS) accounts for approximately 85–90% of cases at onset and is characterized by self-limiting attacks of neurological dysfunction (typically lasting days to weeks). Secondary progressive MS (SPMS) begins as RRMS but at some point the clinical course changes such that the attacks become less frequent and are replaced by a slow deterioration in function. This type of MS, which ultimately occurs in the majority of patients, causes the greatest amount of neurological disability. However, some patients with RRMS have a very benign course without disability, a circumstance that deserves consideration when treatment options are contemplated for individual patients. Primary progressive MS (PPMS) accounts for about 10% of cases at onset and is characterized by a slow decline in function without any acute attacks. Progressive–relapsing MS (PRMS) begins as PPMS although these patients will ultimately experience occasional attacks superimposed upon their progressive disease course.

In judging the effectiveness of different therapies, it is important to consider which outcome measure, or measures, should be used for this purpose. Clearly, the most important goal of disease-modifying therapy is to prevent or postpone long-term disability. However, this disability tends to evolve slowly over many years[1–4] whereas, by comparison, clinical trials are necessarily short and, therefore, our current outcomes are only short-term measures. Ideally, in such circumstances we would want to choose only those short-term measures that had been validated by their correlation with long-term outcome. Regrettably, however, this kind of data is not yet available. Consequently, most clinical trials have tended to use a combination of short-term measures (both clinical and MRI) to establish that treatment at least has a favorable impact on the biology of MS. For example, the short-term activity of the disease can be assessed by various clinical and MRI measures such as the clinical attack rate, the time to first attack, the attack-free status, the number of new lesions, enhancing lesions or combined unique active lesions. Similarly, the severity of the disease can be assessed by various clinical and MRI measures such as confirmed progression on the Expanded Disability Status Scale (EDSS), changes in the total T2 disease burden seen on magnetic resonance imaging (MRI), cerebral atrophy or T1 black holes.[10,11] In assessing the effectiveness of therapy on these two constructs (inflammatory activity in MRI and clinical relapses or progression over time), the MRI and clinical measures provide important complementary evidence of efficacy. Thus, together, they provide considerably stronger support for therapeutic claims when the findings on MRI and clinical measures are consistent with each other.[12–38]

It is the purpose of this chapter to review the data supporting the use of different therapeutic agents for MS. Specifically, the impact on disease activity and severity of the currently approved therapies such as IFNβ-1a (Avonex, Rebif), IFNβ-1b (Betaseron), glatiramer acetate (Copaxone), mitoxantrone (Novantrone) and natalizumab (Tysabri) will be considered. In addition, evidence about the use of other nonapproved agents or promising new therapies will be discussed.

DISEASE-MODIFYING THERAPY IN MULTIPLE SCLEROSIS (APPROVED AGENTS)

In assembling the evidence for the use of IFNβ (either IFNβ-1a or IFNβ-1b) in MS, there are seven randomized controlled trials (RCTs) involving over 300 patients each.[10–21] Three of these trials[12–14,17,18,21,22] involved RRMS patients and four[15,16,19,20,23] studied patients with SPMS. In addition to these RCTs, there have been two randomized head-to-head trials in RRMS patients comparing high-dose (more frequently administered) IFNβ with low-dose, once-weekly IFNβ.[24–26] Because SPMS always begins as RRMS, and because RRMS typically evolves into SPMS, it seems reasonable to consider both RRMS and SPMS as part of the same underlying disease process (e.g. to assume that a therapeutic benefit on MS attacks in one setting would translate to a similar benefit in the other). In addition, because the in vivo and in vitro biological effects of both IFNβ-1a and IFNβ-1b are quite similar[39,40] it also seems reasonable to consider all the IFNβ data in aggregate. In assembling the evidence for the use of glatiramer acetate, there are four studies that involve more than 150 patients,[27–31] but only two of these were RCTs.[27–29] In the case of mitoxantrone there are considerably fewer data available. There are only three randomized trials of 40 or more patients (including both RRMS and SPMS) for analysis.[32–35] In assembling the evidence for natalizumab, there have been three RCTs of over 200 patients, with two of these including over 2000 patients in total.[36,37,41]

For the purpose of this chapter, studies have been classified according to the four-tiered system used by the American Academy of Neurology (AAN) and recommendations derived according to the AAN guidelines, as shown in Table 21.1.[42]

Because the minimum type I (α) error rate (post-hoc) for an observation with a p-value of 0.05 is actually 13%,[43–46] observations with p-values between 0.01 and 0.05 have been considered to be only marginally significant.

The classification of the different clinical trials of IFNβ, glatiramer acetate, mitoxantrone and natalizumab is shown in Table 21.2. As mentioned earlier, all the IFNβ trials were placebo-controlled RCTs and all therefore provided class I data with respect to both activity and severity measures of efficacy. In the case of glatiramer acetate, only two of the trials were RCTs[27–29] and neither of these was as large as the smallest of the IFNβ trials. Moreover, the first RCT did not include any MRI outcomes.[27,28] The 'extended' trial of glatiramer acetate[30] is an open-label (nonblinded) trial without any concurrent control group. This trial would, therefore, provide either class III or class IV data depending upon whether or not a control group derived from a natural history cohort is considered adequate. The study of Kahn et al[31] was nonrandomized and nonblinded and, therefore, provides only class III data. In the case of mitoxantrone, all the trials were RCTs but two were quite small[32,33] and, in all three, blinding was maintained for only some (not all) outcomes. Consequently, the trials of Edan[32] and Millifiorini[33] provide a mixture of class II and class III data (downgraded to class II because of the small sample size). By contrast, the MIMS trial[34,35] provides a mixture of class I and class III data. It is important to note, however, that the composite primary outcome of the MIMS trial included nonblinded assessments so that observations on this composite measure are class III. The results of the different clinical trials for IFNβ, glatiramer acetate, mitoxantrone and natalizumab are shown in Tables 21.3–21.5.

TABLE 21.1 Scheme for classification of the evidence and translation of evidence into recommendations

Study characteristics for classification	Classification of study			
	I	II	III	IV
Control group present	✓	✓	✓	✗
Representative population (i.e. not a highly selected sample)	✓	✓	✓	✗
Outcome assessment independent of treatment (does not need to be a blinded assessment)	✓	✓	✓	✗
Outcome assessment blinded	✓	✓	✗	✗
Prospective design	✓	✓	✗	✗
Randomized trial*	✓	✗	✗	✗
Translation into recommendations and conclusions	**Level†**			
	A	B	C	U
Two or more class I studies (or one convincing‡ class I study)	✓			
One class I study	✓			
Two or more class II studies (or one convincing‡ class II study)	✓			
One class II study	✓			
Two or more class III studies	✓			
Data inadequate or results conflicting	✓			

*Also meets standard of:
1. Primary outcomes clearly defined
2. Exclusion/Inclusion criteria clearly defined
3. Dropout rate low (generally <20%), with an accounting for dropouts
4. Baseline characteristics detailed and substantially equivalent between groups or important covariates were specified in the a priori statistical analysis plan.
†A, Established as effective, ineffective or harmful; B, Probably effective, ineffective, or harmful; C, Possibly effective, ineffective or harmful; U, Data inadequate or conflicting.
‡Lower limit of the 95% confidence interval for the odds ratio ≥2.0, if a single study.
✓, Yes; ✗, No.

TABLE 21.2 Classification of the evidence for the various clinical trials of interferon-β, glatiramer acetate and mitoxantrone in the treatment of multiple sclerosis

	n	Controls	Randomized	Prospective	Blinded	Class
IFNβ						
Betaseron, RRMS[12–14]	372	✓	✓	✓	✓	I
Avonex, RRMS[21,22]	301	✓	✓	✓	✓	I
Rebif, RRMS[17,18]	560	✓	✓	✓	✓	I
Betaseron, SPMS (E)[15]	718	✓	✓	✓	✓	I
Betaseron, SPMS (NA)[16]	939	✓	✓	✓	✓	I
Avonex, SPMS[23]	436	✓	✓	✓	✓	I
Rebif, SPMS[19,20]	506	✓	✓	✓	✓	I
Glatiramer acetate						
Copaxone, RRMS[27,28]	251	✓	✓	✓	✓	I
Copaxone, RRMS (9 months)[29]	249	✓	✓	✓	✓	I
Copaxone, Extended[30]	152	?✓	✗	✓	✗	III/IV
Copaxone, Comparative[31]	156	✓	✗	✓	✗	III
Mitoxantrone						
Mitoxantrone, RRMS[32]	42	✓	✓	✓	✓/✗	II/III
Mitoxantrone, RRMS[33]	51	✓	✓	✓	✓/✗	II/III
MIMS trial, RRMS/SPMS[34,35]	188	✓	✓	✓	✓/✗	I/III
Natalizumab						
Phase II Trial, RRMS[36]	213	✓	✓	✓	✓	I
AFFIRM, RRMS[37]	942	✓	✓	✓	✓	I
SENTINEL, RRMS[38]	1171	✓	✓	✓	✓	I

✓, Yes; ✗, No; ?✓, uncertain; ✓/✗, blinded for some outcomes but not others.

Interferon β

Interferon (IFN)β is a naturally occurring human protein that has important antiproliferative, antiviral and immunomodulatory properties. Its mechanism of action in MS is unknown but could relate to any of a number of mechanisms, including interfering with the transmigration of T cells across the blood–brain barrier, altering the expression of class II molecules on antigen-presenting cells within the CNS, inhibition of T-cell proliferation and IFNγ release, and the alteration of cytokine expression patterns.[47] It is generally well tolerated and safe, although many patients experience transient flu-like side effects at the start of therapy and injection site reactions (with subcutaneous administration) that tend to persist. Elevations in liver enzymes are common, although liver failure is quite rare. In each of the RCTs of IFNβ in MS, a beneficial effect on clinical attack rates was reported and in six of the seven this benefit was statistically convincing (Table 21.3). Similarly, for MRI activity measures, each of the trials reported a benefit and, again, in six of the seven this effect was statistically convincing (Table 21.3). Consequently, there is a very consistent and convincing evidence for a benefit of IFNβ on MS disease activity, regardless of whether this is measured clinically or by MRI.

By contrast, the evidence for a beneficial effect of treatment on confirmed progression was less convincing. Thus, only three of the seven trials reported a benefit and in only one trial[15] was this benefit statistically convincing. Moreover, the result of this one SPMS trial was not confirmed on this same outcome when another SPMS trial was undertaken in North America.[16] Nevertheless, despite the less robust findings for IFNβ on this outcome, it seems likely that disease severity is also benefited by IFNβ therapy. Thus, even in the original IFNβ-1b trial, there was a nonsignificant trend in favor of therapy of similar magnitude to that found in the other RRMS trials (Table 21.4). Also, in the nonsignificant SPMS trials of Betaseron and Rebif[16,19,20] there seemed to be a benefit of therapy in the subgroup of patients who continued to experience relapses or had a more than average pretreatment progression.[48] This suggests that patients who are still in the active inflammatory phase of their disease may continue to derive benefit (on this measure) from IFNβ therapy. Importantly also, when disease severity was assessed by MRI, a statistically convincing benefit from therapy was reported in six of the seven trials.

Three clinical trials[49–51] have also addressed the use of IFNβ in the treatment of clinically isolated syndromes (CIS). In fact, at this early stage of disease, the effect of treatment seems, in general, to be considerably more robust than that reported in the later stages (Table 21.5). For example, IFNβ-1a (Avonex; 30 μg i.m. once weekly) resulted in a 44% reduction in the likelihood of a second clinical episode (hazard model) in a group of monosymptomatic CIS patients.[49] Similarly, IFNβ-1a (Rebif), at a dose found to be ineffective in RRMS (22 μg s.c. once weekly), reduced the hazard of a second clinical episode in a mixed group of mono- and polysymptomatic CIS patients by 35%.[50] Most recently, IFNβ-1b (Betaseron; 250 μg s.c. every other day), resulted in a 50% reduction in the hazard of a second clinical episode, also in a mixed group of mono- and polysymptomatic CIS patients.[51] These results, together with the largely negative results in late-stage SPMS patients, suggest that IFNβ has a

SECTION 3

TABLE 21.3 Results (improvement) in different outcomes found in the trials of interferon-β, glatiramer acetate and mitoxantrone in the treatment of multiple sclerosis

	Clinical attack rate	MRI activity	Clinical severity	MRI severity
IFNβ				
Betaseron, RRMS[12–14]	✓	✓	n.s.	✓
Avonex, RRMS[21,22]	○	○	○	n.s.
Rebif, RRMS[17,18]	✓	✓	○	✓
Betaseron, SPMS (E)[15]	✓	✓	✓	✓
Betaseron, SPMS (NA)[16]	✓	✓	n.s.	✓
Avonex, SPMS[23]	✓	✓	n.s.	✓
Rebif, SPMS[19,20]	✓	✓	n.s.	✓
Glatiramer acetate				
Copaxone, RRMS[27,28]	✓		n.s.	
Copaxone, RRMS (9 months)[29]	○	✓	n.s.	✓
Copaxone, extended[30]	?✓		?✓	
Copaxone, comparative[31]	✓			
Mitoxantrone				
Mitoxantrone, RRMS[32]	○	✓	○	
Mitoxantrone, RRMS[33]	✓	○	○	
MIMS trial, RRMS/SPMS[34,35]	✓	○	○	
Natalizumab				
Phase II Study, RRMS[36]	○	✓		
AFFIRM, RRMS[37]	✓	✓	✓	✓
SENTINEL, RRMS[38]	✓	✓	✓	

✓, Significant (p<0.01); ○, Marginally significant (p=0.01–0.05); n.s., not significant; ?✓, Uncertain; blank cells, not reported.

progressively greater clinical impact earlier in the course of MS and is particularly effective at the time of its earliest clinical manifestations. Such a circumstance may be applicable to all our currently available therapies, although to date this has only been studied for IFNβ. Nevertheless, a trial addressing this possibility for glatiramer acetate is currently under way.

With regard to the possible role of IFNβ dose in the treatment of MS, there are four lines of evidence suggesting that the total weekly dose, the frequency of administration or both are important factors in determining the efficacy of treatment. First, it is clear (from both in vitro and in vivo evidence) that higher doses of IFNβ have greater biological effects.[47] Second, as shown in Table 21.4 (where the IFNβ columns have been arranged in approximate order of increasing dose), a cross-trial comparison of the results of the pivotal trials generally supports the notion that higher dose, or more frequently administered, IFNβ has greater efficacy than once-weekly IFNβ. Third, in both of the two pivotal clinical trials that compared two different doses of IFNβ within the same trial,[12–14,17,18] the higher dose arm did consistently better than the lower dose for almost all outcomes (Table 21.4). Despite the fact that only some between-group comparisons were statistically significant in these trials, the consistency of this apparent dose-effect is notable (Table 21.4). However, in contrast to the notion that dosage alone is the critical factor, the European dose comparison study of IFNβ-1a 30 versus 60 μg once weekly i.m. (a randomized double-blind 3-year study of 804 patients with relapsing MS) found no difference between groups either for the primary outcome of disability progression or for secondary outcomes such as steroid treated relapses, number and volume of Gd-enhancing lesions, T2-lesion volume, and brain parenchymal fraction.[52,53] Fourth, and most importantly, there have now been two randomized head-to-head trials that directly compared these two high-dose (more frequent) preparations to once-weekly IFNβ-1a.[24–26] As is shown in Table 21.6, the INCOMIN trial[24] compared standard-dose Betaseron (250 μg s.c. every other day) to standard dose Avonex (30 μg i.m. once weekly), and the EVIDENCE trial[25,26] compared standard high-dose Rebif (44 μg s.c. three times a week) to standard dose Avonex (30 μg i.m. once weekly). The INCOMIN trial was blinded for MRI but not for clinical assessments and, as a result, provides a mixture of class I data (MRI outcomes) and class III data (clinical outcomes). By contrast, the EVIDENCE trial used blinded outcome assessment for both clinical and MRI measures and thus provides class I data for each (Table 21.6). In both trials, the high-dose (more frequent) IFNβ was superior to once-weekly IFNβ on several outcome measures of disease activity and disease severity (Table 21.6). The only nonsignificant difference was in the EVIDENCE trial for the outcome of confirmed EDSS progression and may have been due in part to the short duration of prospectively planned follow-up in this trial.

Most patients treated with IFNβ will develop antibodies to the molecule and two different classes of antibody are recognized.[54–66] The first, the so-called binding antibodies (BAbs), are the most prevalent and do not necessarily interfere with the receptor-mediated functions of IFNβ. The second, the so-called neutralizing antibodies (NAbs), are a subset of the BAbs, do interfere with receptor-mediated functions and are associated

TABLE 21.4 Principal outcomes in the randomized, placebo-controlled trials of interferon-β, glatiramer acetate, mitoxantrone and natalizumab in relapsing–remitting multiple sclerosis

	IFNβ-1b[a]	IFNβ-1a[b]	IFNβ-1a[c]	IFNβ-1b[a]	IFNβ-1a[c]	GA[d]	MTX[e]	NTZ[f]
Dosing and other information								
Dosage	50 μg	30 μg	22 μg	250 μg	44 μg	20 mg	12 mg/m^2	300 mg
Schedule	q.o.d.	q.w.	t.i.w.	q.o.d.	t.i.w.	q.d.	q. 3 mo.	q. mo.
Route	s.c.	i.m.	s.c.	s.c.	s.c.	s.c.	i.v.	i.v.
Weekly dose, MIU[3]	5.6	6	18	28	36	n.a.	n.a.	n.a.
Mean EDSS at entry	2.9	2.4	2.5	3.0	2.5	2.6	4.5	2.3
EDSS range	0–5.5	1–3.5	0–5.0	0–5.5	0–5.0	0–5.0	3–6.0	0–5.5
Mean age (SD), years	35 (8)	37 (7)	35 (8)	35 (7)	35 (8)	35 (6)	40 (7)	36 (9)
Female, %	68	75	67	69	66	70	47	72
Outcome measures (%)								
Relapse rate (ITT), 2 years	−13[†]	−18*	−29[†]	−34[‡]	−32[‡]	−29[†]	−66[‡]	−68[‡]
MRI activity[2], median								
New T2 lesions	−67*	n.r.	−67[‡]	−83[†]	−78[‡]	−38[†]	−79*	−83[‡]
Gd[+] or CU lesions	n.r.	−33*	−81[†*]	n.r.	−88[‡]	−33[†]	+7	−92[‡]
Sustained EDSS progression	−0	−37*	−19*	−29	−30*	−12	−75*	−42[‡]
MRI △ BOD, median	−5	−7	−12[‡]	−17[‡]	−15[‡]	−8[†]	n.r.	−18[‡]

1. *Percentage reductions (or increases) have been calculated by dividing the reported rates in the treated group by the comparable rates in the placebo group, except for MRI disease burden (BOD), which was calculated as the difference in the median% change between the treated and placebo groups.*
2. *MRI attack rate (activity) was measured differently in different trials. The Betaseron trial[12–14] included the number of new, recurrent and enlarging T2 lesions but not gadolinium (Gd) enhancement; the Rebif trial,[17,18] the Copaxone trial,[27,28] the Novantrone trial[34,35] and the Tysabri trial[37] included both; the Avonex[21,22] trial used only the number of Gd-enhancing lesions. In the Copaxone trial data is from only 9 months, rather than 2 years as in the other trials. In the Mitoxantrone trial the mean (not the median) is reported for Gd-enhancing lesions because the median was 0 in both groups.*
3. *MIU scales not exactly comparable between products because each company used a different reference standard for the assay.*
a, *Betaseron Trial[12–14]; b, Avonex Trial[21,22]; c, Rebif Trial[17,18]; d, Glatiramer Acetate Trials[27,28]; e, Mitoxantrone trial[34,35]; f, Natalizumab Trial.[37]*
*, p≤0.05; [†], p≤0.01; [‡], p≤0.001.
△ *BOD, change in burden of disease; CU, combined unique lesions[18,20]; EDSS, Kurtzke Expanded Disability Status Scale; Gd[+], gadolinium-enhancing lesions; i.m., intramuscular; ITT, intention to treat analysis; i.v., intravenous; MRI, magnetic resonance imaging; MIU, millions of international units of IFNβ activity as reported; n.a., not applicable; n.r., not reported; q.o.d., every other day; q. mo., once per month; q. 3mo., once every 3 months; q.w., once per week; s.c., subcutaneous; SD, standard deviation; t.i.w., three times per week.*

TABLE 21.5 Comparison of outcomes for three interferon-β trials in patients with clinically isolated syndromes

Outcomes	Clinical studies		
	ETOMS (IFNβ-1a) (22 μg s.c. q.w.) n=309	CHAMPS (IFNβ-1a) (30 μg i.m. q.w.) n=383	BENEFIT (IFNβ-1b) (250 μg s.c. e.o.d.) n=468
Risk of CDMS			
Active drug	0.34	0.24	0.28
Placebo	0.45	0.37	0.45
Relative risk of CDMS (RR) (risk active drug/risk placebo)	0.76	0.65	0.62
Risk reduction (i.e. 1−RR)	0.24	0.35	0.38
Absolute risk reduction (ARR)	0.11	0.13	0.17
Number needed to treat (NNT) to prevent 1 CDMS conversion	9.1	7.7	5.9

with a reduction in the biological activity of IFNβ. For example, several recent reports have found that the in vivo and in vitro responses to IFNβ are markedly attenuated in the presence of NAbs.[67–70] Given this evidence, it is somewhat surprising perhaps that the impact of NAbs has been so difficult to establish, particularly with respect to clinical measures of disease activity and severity. There are many potential reasons for this, including the variability of the assay used to determine NAb-

positivity, the tendency of NAb-status to change over time, the unclear relationship between the functions assayed and the clinical effect of IFNβ, the potentially greater impact of high-titer compared to low-titer NAbs, the variable duration of follow-up and the small number of patients typically included in the published reports. In addition, other potential sources of variability are difficult to exclude completely. For example, despite the fact that the evidence regarding NAbs is often derived

TABLE 21.6 Classification of the evidence and results of the head-to-head trials assessing the role of interferon-β dose in the treatment of multiple sclerosis

Classification	n	Controls	Randomized	Prospective	Blinded	Class
INCOMIN, RRMS[22]	188	✓	✓	✓	✓/✗	I/III
EVIDENCE, RRMS[23,24]	677	✓	✓	✓	✓	I

✓, Yes; ✗, No; ?✓, uncertain; ✓/✗, blinded for some outcomes but not others.

Results*	Attack-free status	MRI activity	Clinical severity	MRI severity
INCOMIN, RRMS[22]	○	✓	✓	✓
EVIDENCE, RRMS[23,24]	○	✓	ns	

✓, Significant (p<0.01); ○, Marginally significant (p=0.01–0.05); ns, not significant; Blank cells, not reported.
INCOMIN compared Betaseron and Avonex; EVIDENCE compared Rebif and Avonex.
*Statistical significance indicates a better outcome for the Betaseron or Rebif arms compared to the Avonex arm in each trial.

from RCTs, it is impossible to randomize patients with respect to their ultimate NAb status (i.e. the data is at best only class II or III). Consequently, it is impossible to exclude the possibility that patient-specific factors both predispose a person to the development of NAbs and, in an unrelated manner, make them either more or less likely to experience MS attacks. Such a circumstance (if applicable) will make NAbs artificially appear to increase (or decrease) the attack rate.

Regardless of these complexities, however, it seems probable that persistently high NAb titers to IFNβ will have a deleterious effect on the clinical and radiographic efficacy of IFNβ. In fact, when all of the evidence on NAbs is assembled, efficacy does seem to be impacted, especially with respect to MRI outcomes (Table 21.1). Even for clinical measures of disease activity (i.e. attack rate), the majority of studies with follow up of two years or more found an increased attack rate in NAb-positive patients compared to NAb-negative controls (Table 21.1). Thus, trials such as the PRISMS,[17,18,65] the European SPMS,[15,56] and the North American SPMS studies[16] demonstrated a significant NAb-associated increase in relapse rate (p=0.05–0.01). Therefore, it seems reasonable to conclude that the presence of NAbs is probably deleterious. Surprisingly, however, in a recent study of 6,698 MS patients on IFNb-1b,[71] two cohorts were selected specifically because patients had continued relapses or clinical deterioration while on therapy and, in these two cohorts, the prevalence of NAbs (21.3% in North America and 27.6% in Europe) was very significantly lower (p<10⁻¹¹) compared to the prevalence of NAbs in an unselected cohort (37% in Australia). In addition, NAbs were less prevalent in these two cohorts at every titer level evaluated. If confounding factors with an impact on observed prevalence rates can be excluded,[71] this observation is exactly opposite to a priori expectations, by which these two cohorts would be expected to be enriched for NAb positivity. The fact that NAb prevalence was actually less in these two cohorts indicates that NAbs cannot be responsible for the poor clinical response seen in these patients. Moreover, it raises the question of what factor or factors might account for the apparent association between NAb positivity and reduced clinical efficacy in other circumstances.

It is a consistent finding in the available literature that NAbs are more likely to be present following treatment with Rebif and Betaseron (≈20–40%) than following treatment with Avonex as it is currently formulated (<5%). However, it is still uncertain how these considerations should alter therapeutic decisions. For example, it is uncertain from this evidence whether the presence of NAbs is associated merely with an attenuation of the beneficial effects of IFNβ as opposed to a complete elimination of these effects. For example, in a longitudinal study of patients who had

monthly MRIs both before and after beginning treatment with IFNβ-1b, there were several individuals who still seemed to have a continuing IFNβ benefit, despite having high NAb titers and despite there being an overall negative impact of NAbs in this study.[56] Thus, over the 36 months following the start of IFNβ-1b, the patient with the second highest NAb titer (1044 NU/ml) had a stable EDSS and a 97% suppression of MRI activity.[56] Also, in a recent study of IFNβ bioactivity,[70] the authors reported that, despite the observation of a marked reduction of the normalized ratio (NR) for in vivo IFNβ-induced MxA production in NAb-positive (>20 NU/ml) patients, the NR was still greater than the normal mean in 82% of the NAb-positive patients studied and in 65% the NR was more than three times the normal mean, even in the presence of NAb titers up to 800 NU/ml. Thus it seems that, although MxA induction by IFNβ is markedly attenuated by NAbs, it is not completely eliminated. Whether such a low level of MxA induction is associated with any residual clinical benefit of IFNβ is unknown. However, because of this uncertainty, it is unclear under what circumstances it might be advisable to switch NAb-positive patients to a non-interferon product when they are otherwise doing well clinically. The apparent abolition or marked attenuation of MxA induction in the presence of NAbs[67–70] might be taken to suggest such a course of action. However, because of our uncertainty about the relationship of MxA induction to the mechanisms of IFNβ benefit, because of the variability of the clinical data (Table 21.7) and because there seems to be persistent MxA mRNA expression or MxA induction in at least some persistently NAb-positive individuals,[66–68] this course of action cannot be recommended. By contrast, in a NAb-positive patient who is not doing well on IFNβ an alternative therapy should be considered regardless of the antibody status.

It is also uncertain whether the apparently deleterious effect of NAbs (which are more prevalent following treatment with Betaseron and Rebif than after treatment with Avonex) is offset by the improved efficacy reported with high-dose (more frequently administered) IFNβ. Neither of the two randomized, head-to-head comparative trials that might conceivably be used to address this question – the 63-week EVIDENCE trial[25,26] and the 2-year INCOMIN trial[24] – provides a definitive answer. Both trials, particularly EVIDENCE, are too short for such a purpose. It is nevertheless noteworthy that, in both of these trials, the NAb-positive patients in the high-dose (more frequent) IFNβ arms had fewer relapses and less MRI activity (reported only in EVIDENCE) than the arm receiving low-dose (once-weekly) IFNβ, regardless of their antibody status.[24–27] Consequently, at least over the initial year and perhaps up to 2 years of therapy, the available randomized head-to-head evidence favors the use

TABLE 21.7 Effect of neutralizing antibodies on clinical and MRI outcomes in multiple sclerosis therapeutic trials[†]

Study	n	Year	Clinical activity	Clinical severity	MRI activity	MRI severity	Class
IFNβ-1b MS Study Group (high dose)[†12–14,54,59]	53	1996	+ (*)	− (n.s.)	+ (n.s.)	+ (n.s.)	II
MSCRG[21,22,55]	23	1998	− (n.s.)	+ (n.s.)	+ (n.s.)		II
PRISMS (both doses)[†17,18,65]	90	2001	+ (*)	+ (*)[‡]	+ (***)	+ (***)	II
SPECTRIMS (low dose)[†19,20]	43	2001	− (n.s.)	− (n.s.)			II
SPECTRIMS (high dose)[†19,20]	30	2001	+ (n.s.)	− (n.s.)			II
INCOMIN[24,64]	28	2002	− (n.s.)		+ (n.s.)		II
EVIDENCE[25,26]	91	2002	+ (n.s.)		+ (***)		II
European SPMS IFNβ-1b[†15,54]	95	2003	+ (**)			+ (**)	II
Sorensen et al[†57]	169	2003	+ (**)	+ (n.s.)			III
Frank et al[†58]	11	2004			+ (**)	+ (**)	II
North American SPMS IFNβ-1b Study Group[†14]	174	2004	+ (*)		? (n.s.)	? (n.s.)	II
Malucchi et al[61]	13	2004	+ (*)[§]	+ (*)[§]			III
Perini et al[62]	22	2004	+ (n.s.)[§]	? (n.s.)[§]			III
European Dose Comparison Study (both doses)[†64]	26	2005	+ (*)	+ (n.s.)	+ (n.s.)		II

Clinical activity was assessed by attack rate or attack-free status. MRI activity was assessed by Gd-enhancement, new T2 lesions, or both. Clinical severity was assessed by confirmed EDSS progression. MRI severity was assessed by total T2 volume (burden) of disease.
Statistical significance is given in parentheses: n.s., not significant; *, $p<0.05$; **, $p<0.01$; ***, $p<0.001$.
[†] Trials of more than 2 years duration. [‡] Significant only on 'interval analysis' method ($p=0.03$); not significant on the 'any time positive' method. [§] Analysis using combined data from Avonex-, Betaseron- and Rebif-treated patients.
n, number of NAb-positive patients studied of IFN treated; +, outcome worse in NAb-positive group than NAb-negative group; −, outcome worse in NAb-negative group than NAb-positive group; ?, actual outcome not reported; Blank cells, no information provided.

of the more effective therapy, even if this therapy has a greater propensity to produce NAbs. Whether this relative advantage of high-dose therapy is sustained over the long term (>2 years) is unknown. Any consideration of the long-term impact needs to take account of the fact that NAbs to IFNβ often disappear spontaneously, even with continued therapy either using the same IFNβ product or switching between products.[24,58,59,64,72,73]

On the basis of this evidence, therefore, IFNβ seems to be established as an effective treatment for reducing MS disease activity (level A conclusion) and as a probably effective treatment for reducing MS disease severity (level B conclusion). In addition, there is probably a dose-response to the clinical use of IFNβ for reducing MS activity (level B conclusion). However, because the effects of dose are confounded with the effects of the frequency it is not possible to separate which factor is most important. In addition, it is very probable that the presence of NAbs, especially in persistently high titer, is associated with a reduction in both the clinical and radiographic effectiveness of IFNβ treatment (level B conclusion). Also, it seems clear that IFNβ-1a (as currently formulated for intramuscular injection) is less immunogenic than the current IFNβ preparations (either IFNβ-1a or IFNβ-1b) given multiple times per week subcutaneously (level A conclusion). However, over the first 1–2 years of therapy the increased efficacy of the high-dose (high-frequency) formulations seems to offset the greater immunogenicity of these products. Whether this relative advantage is maintained over the longer term is unknown.

Glatiramer acetate

Glatiramer acetate (Copaxone) is a random polypeptide made up of four amino acids (L-tyrosine, L-glutamic acid, L-lysine and L-alanine) in a specific molar ratio (1.0, 1.4, 3.4 and 4.2 respectively). Its mechanism of action is unknown but possibly relates to immunological effects such as the induction of antigen-specific suppressor T cells, inhibition of antigen presentation,

displacing bound myelin basic protein or causing a deviation in the phenotype of CD4+ T cells from a Th1 to a Th2 pattern.[74–76] Glatiramer acetate is generally well tolerated, although a few patients may experience a brief postinjection reaction and a few may develop lipoatrophy at injection sites. In all of the trials of Copaxone in MS, clinical attacks were reduced in the treated group compared to controls (Table 21.3). This apparent benefit was statistically convincing in two of the trials (including one of RCTs). MRI activity was prospectively assessed in only one of the trials.[29] Nevertheless, in this single MRI class I study there was a statistically convincing benefit of therapy reported. The potential benefit of therapy with respect to confirmed progression, as with the IFNβ trials, was less convincing. In fact, neither of the class I studies demonstrated a significant benefit on this measure (Tables 21.3–21.5). The only trial to suggest a benefit was the 'extended Copaxone' study, which is difficult to evaluate because it lacks any concurrent control group, because the subgroup included for long-term follow-up was not representative of the entire study cohort and because the patients who dropped out were those who were doing poorly.[46]

On the basis of this evidence, therefore, glatiramer acetate seems to be established as an effective treatment for reducing MS disease activity (type A recommendation). On the basis of the currently available data, however, the benefit of glatiramer acetate treatment for reducing MS disease severity is only possible (type C recommendation).

Mitoxantrone

Mitoxantrone (Novantrone) is an immunosuppressive agent (an anthracenedione) that intercalates into DNA and produces both DNA strand breaks and interstrand cross-links; it also interferes with RNA synthesis and inhibits topoisomerase II, an enzyme that aids in the DNA repair process. Despite the small amount of data available for mitoxantrone, the findings have been relatively consistent. Thus, in the trials of mitoxantrone in MS, clinical attacks were reduced in all three of the studies; the results being statistically convincing in two of them (Table 21.3). In considering this potential effect, however, it is important to note that the assessment of clinical attacks was not blinded in any of these trials. MRI activity was also reduced in all three trials, although this effect was statistically convincing only in one of the small class II studies. In addition, in the only class I study of MRI parameters using mitoxantrone, the primary MRI outcome was not significantly improved with therapy.[35] Confirmed EDSS progression was also improved by treatment in all three trials, although this effect was statistically marginal in each (Table 21.3). Moreover, this outcome was assessed in a blinded fashion in only one of the three trials.[34] MRI severity was either not measured or has not been reported.

On the basis of this evidence, therefore, mitoxantrone is probably an effective treatment for reducing MS disease activity (type B recommendation) and may also reduce MS disease severity (type B recommendation). Nevertheless, the risks of cardiac toxicity and probably the increased risk of long-term malignancy associated with this agent limit its use as first-line therapy.[77] An antagonist of the cardiotoxic but not the immunosuppressive effects (dexrazoxane) is currently being tested as adjunctive treatment in MS after first promising results in experimental models.[78,79] Most neurologists will use mitoxantrone as a second-line agent in patients unresponsive to treatment with IFNβ or glatiramer acetate and in patients with unusually active relapsing–remitting or secondary progressive disease. Interestingly two of the three available randomized studies have included patients with lower rates of progression as shown by the behavior of their placebo groups; therefore the evidence supporting this specific indication is relatively weak.

Natalizumab

Natalizumab (Tysabri) is a humanized monoclonal antibody that binds to the α4 subunit of α4β1 and α4β7 integrins, which are expressed on the surface of activated T cells, and blocks binding to their endothelial receptors (vascular cellular adhesion molecule (VCAM)-1 and mucosal addressin (CAM-1), respectively), which is a necessary step in T-cell transmigration through the blood–brain barrier into the CNS. Natalizumab may also suppress ongoing inflammatory reactions by inhibiting the binding of α4-positive leukocytes to osteopontin and fibronectin.[80–84]

All three of the natalizumab trials showed a significant benefit of treatment on both clinical and MRI measures of disease activity.[36–38] Moreover, in both of the two larger (and longer) trials there was a significant reduction in disease severity measures as well (Table 21.3). In fact, these trials have a highly significant benefit ($p < 0.001$) demonstrated for each of the four principal outcomes (i.e. disease activity and severity assessed both clinically and by MRI) and it is the only agent to date to achieve this result (Tables 21.3 and 21.4). In addition, the effect size was generally larger using this agent than using any of the other agents, particularly with respect to clinical outcome measures (Table 21.4). In each of these trials, also, these therapeutic benefits seemed to be conferred with few notable side effects of therapy. However, after the completion of the clinical trial, two patients on combined natalizumab and IFNβ-1a treatment developed progressive multifocal leukoencephalopathy (PML) and one of them died. In reviewing the previous experience of using natalizumab in Crohn's disease, a third case of PML was identified in a patient receiving natalizumab alone. Nevertheless, this patient had previously been immunosuppressed and was still lymphopenic at the time natalizumab was restarted prior to the development of PML. Thus, the basis for this complication is not clear. However, the possibility that concurrent immunosuppression contributes to the development of PML in patients on natalizumab cannot be excluded. Nevertheless, because extensive studies on the patients in these clinical trials failed to reveal viremia in two of the three patients prior to the onset of clinical symptoms, it seems that there will not be laboratory tests to monitor for this potential complication of therapy.

When considering the use of this agent, practitioners need to face the difficult task of assessing accurately both the risks and the benefits of therapy. Although, on the basis of the available data, Yousry and colleagues[41] have estimated the risk of PML as 1 per 1000 patients treated for an average of 17.9 months (95% confidence interval 0.2–2.8/1000), this estimate is almost certainly inaccurate. For example, if concomitant IFNβ therapy predisposes to PML, the risk for patients on monotherapy will probably be much lower and possibly nonexistent. Conversely, if this complication is due to natalizumab alone, the risk will probably increase with increased exposure time so that the actual risk to patients (expected to be on treatment for many years) will probably be substantially greater. Only time and future experience will tell. In the absence of a clear understanding of the actual risk, however, many practitioners will err on the side of caution, especially for a nonfatal disease and a partially effective therapy with potentially fatal complications, For these physicians, treatment will probably be considered only in patients with particularly aggressive presentations (or in those apparently failing other therapies). Naturally, not all physicians will be so cautious and, over the next several years, the patients of these practitioners will provide the data we need to give future patients a more informed choice than we can give them at the moment.

On the basis of this evidence, therefore, natalizumab is a proven effective treatment for reducing MS disease activity (type A conclusion) and also for reducing MS disease severity (type A conclusion). However, despite this strong evidence for the efficacy of natalizumab therapy, the risk of PML will probably limit the use of this agent early in the disease course, especially when safer options are available.

DISEASE-MODIFYING THERAPY IN MULTIPLE SCLEROSIS (NONAPPROVED AGENTS)

AGENTS FOR THE TREATMENT OF ACUTE ATTACKS

Glucocorticoids

Glucocorticoids are a class of naturally occurring steroids that are known to have important anti-inflammatory and immunomodulatory effects. Following the early trial of adrenocorticotropic hormone (ACTH) in the treatment of acute MS attacks,[85] there have been 15 articles using synthetic glucocorticoids in the management of MS that provide either class I or class II evidence. Of these, a third relate to the optic neuritis treatment trial (ONTT), which was begun in 1988.[86–91] In this trial, 457 patients received placebo or active treatment with either 1 g of intravenous methylprednisolone daily for 3 days followed by 11 days of oral prednisone (1 mg/kg/day) or a 14-day course of oral prednisone alone. Both steroid courses were followed by a very rapid taper over 4 days. The primary endpoints of the trial were visual field and contrast sensitivity and the secondary outcomes were visual acuity and color vision. With respect to these endpoints, the ONTT results were disappointing. Thus, although initially the IVMP group recovered visual function more quickly than the placebo group, by 6 months there was no statistical difference in visual recovery between the two groups. The outcome in the oral prednisone group was intermediate between the other two groups and was not statistically different from either. This trial also reported that recurrent optic neuritis was more common following oral prednisone treatment than it was in either of the two other treatment groups.[87] Despite this report, however, the observation is unreliable. Thus, the statistical significance of this unexpected finding was only marginal ($p=0.02$), this outcome was not one of the preplanned primary or secondary aims of the ONTT and the a priori assumptions of the trial required modification to include this observation as meaningful.[92] In an additional analysis of the raw data, the ONTT investigators reported that the time to development of CDMS was lengthened by treatment with IVMP.[90] In both cases, however, because of serious methodological problems the reported findings of the ONTT regarding the effects of glucocorticoids on both recurrent optic neuritis and the development of MS have been challenged.[92–95]

In a 1987 study,[96] 22 patients with acute relapses were treated with either IVMP (500 mg/d for 5 d) or placebo and a marginal benefit of active treatment was reported on EDSS and functional scores at 1 and 4 weeks ($p=0.04$). Another class II study with 23 patients having MS attacks[97] also showed short-term benefit from IVMP (with an oral prednisone taper) compared to placebo.

The total dose of glucocorticoid administered and the need for a taper following treatment may be important considerations. For example, the use of high-dose steroid treatment accelerates resolution of gadolinium enhancement on MRI scanning.[98–101] One study[99] investigated two 5-day courses of IVMP in patients with RRMS (0.5 g/d compared to 2 g/d) and reported fewer new enhancing lesions on MRI at 30 and 60 days following onset of therapy in the higher-dose group.[102] Following the discontinuation of steroid treatment, a second burst of gadolinium enhancement has been reported to occur.[103–105] This finding could be explained by a rebound in disease activity following a rapid steroid taper – a circumstance for which there is other experimental evidence.[106]

Unfortunately, however, there are only limited clinical data available regarding these points. In a one-center study,[107] 35 MS patients with acute relapses were randomized to receive either IVMP (500 mg for 5 d plus an oral placebo) or oral methylprednisolone (500 mg for 5 d plus an i.v. placebo). In both groups, EDSS improved equally following therapy. In another study,[108] 79 relapsing MS patients received either IVMP at 1 g/d or low-dose oral methylprednisolone (<48 mg/d) for 3 days and no difference on EDSS was found between groups. Two placebo-controlled studies of high-dose oral methylprednisolone (500 mg for 5 d followed by a 10 d taper) in patients with RRMS or with monosymptomatic optic neuritis reported a significant short-term benefit of treatment.[109,110]

Another provocative single-blind, randomized, controlled, single center trial of glucocorticoids in 88 patients with RRMS was recently published.[111] This trial compared regular treatment with pulse IVMP to IVMP administered only during acute relapses. After 5 years of treatment, the group receiving regular pulses of IVMP had a smaller T1-weighted black hole volume on MRI ($p<0.0001$), less brain atrophy ($p=0.003$), and a longer time to EDSS worsening ($p<0.0001$) compared to patients who received IVMP only for acute attacks. Even though this is only a single trial, the reported findings suggest that this therapeutic approach deserves further investigation.

In summary, these studies provide consistent class I and class II evidence that glucocorticoids have a short-term benefit on the speed of neurological recovery from acute MS attacks (level A conclusion). However, there does not seem to be any long-term benefit of such treatment with respect to the degree of functional recovery from an attack (type B recommendation). Moreover, these results do not provide convincing guidance with

regard to the optimal total glucocorticoid dose or route of administration (level C conclusion). On the basis of a single class II study, it seems possible that regular pulse glucocorticoids may be beneficial for the long-term outcome of patients with RRMS (level C conclusion).

Plasma exchange

Plasma exchange has been used successfully in the management of several different neurological disorders that seem to involve the humoral immune system. Its use in the treatment of MS has also been investigated. As discussed below, neither the class III Harvard trial[112] nor the class I Canadian cooperative trial[113] provided evidence for the use of plasma exchange in the treatment of progressive MS. In a pilot trial,[114] 20 chronically progressive definite MS patients were randomized in a double-blind, placebo-controlled study of plasma exchange versus sham exchange. There were no apparent differences between the groups with respect to EDSS, whether measured in the interval between pre-exchange and postexchange or after 6 months of follow-up.

In 1985 another study[115] evaluated the use of plasma exchange in 55 patients with progressive MS randomized to receive plasma exchange or sham exchange once weekly for 20 weeks. All patients also received oral cyclophosphamide, prednisone and intravenous immune globulin (IVIg) with each exchange for 21 weeks. Although plasma exchange was reported to produce a significantly better outcome at 5 and 11 months ($p<0.007$), the statistical methods used to arrive at this observation are unclear and the authors performed multiple between-group statistical comparisons without any adjustment being made. More importantly, a chi-square analysis of the results presented in their Table 21.4a yields a p-value of only 0.12 (not the reported 0.007) at each of these time points. Consequently, even though this study is class I, it cannot be used to support any therapeutic benefit from plasma exchange.

In 1989,[116] a randomized, double-blind trial of plasma exchange in 116 MS patients (40 with a progressive course and 76 with a relapsing course) was reported. All patients received ACTH and cyclophosphamide in addition to plasma exchange or sham exchange. Despite numerous statistical comparisons, no statistically significant differences were seen on any of the outcome measures.

Recently, a class I sham-controlled, randomized clinical trial[117] reported that patients with a severe episode of demyelination unresponsive to intravenous glucocorticoids within the prior 2 months (not necessarily from MS) seemed to benefit from a course of plasma exchange. Thus, clinical improvement was noted in 42% of patients who received plasma exchange compared to only 5.9% of patients who received sham exchange ($p<0.05$).

Thus, on the basis of consistent class I, II and III evidence, plasma exchange is of little or no value in the treatment of progressive MS (level A conclusion). Conversely, on the basis of a single small class I study, it seems possible that plasma exchange may be helpful in the management of severe, acute demyelinating events (level C conclusion).

Intravenous immune globulin

Intravenous immune globulin has also been successfully applied in the management of disorders of the humoral immune system and in peripheral demyelinating disorders (e.g. Guillain–Barré syndrome) it has been used as an alternative to plasma exchange. Following a number of preliminary studies, the results of a randomized, multicenter, double-blind, placebo-controlled study (class I) of IVIg in 148 RRMS patients was reported.[118] Patients received either monthly IVIg (0.15–0.2 g/kg) or placebo for 2 years. These authors reported that treatment with IVIg reduced the clinical attack rate (−49%; $p=0.006$). There was no significant difference in (unconfirmed) EDSS progression at the end of the trial. The study was criticized for lacking a placebo effect and because of incomplete blinding.[119]

A small crossover study of IVIg in 26 RRMS patients (class II evidence) has also been reported.[120] In this trial patients received either IVIg (1 g/kg/d for 2 d) or placebo every month for 6 months. For patients who completed both treatment arms ($n=18$), the total number of enhancing lesions seen on MRI (−64%; $p=0.03$) and the number of new lesions (−60%; $p=0.01$) were reduced in patients treated with IVIg. This study, however, found no differences in T2 lesion load, clinical attack rate or EDSS progression. Also there was a high drop-out rate, which makes interpretation of the results difficult.

In 1998,[121] IVIg (0.4 g/kg/d for 5 d and then monthly for 1 d) was compared with placebo over a period of 2 years. This trial (class II) found reductions in the clinical attack rate but no between-group differences on other outcomes, including EDSS and MRI. Moreover, an original investigator on this trial has raised serious concerns with regard to the conduct of this study.[122]

Recently, the results of a large randomized multicenter European/Canadian study of IVIg in 318 patients with SPMS were reported.[123,124] In this study, patients received either IVIg (1 g/kg) or placebo (albumin) monthly for 27 months. No difference was found between groups for either clinical or MRI parameters except for a modest reduction in the accumulation of brain atrophy in the IVIg group.

In another recent double-blind, placebo-controlled study,[125] IVIg (1 g/kg) was compared to placebo (albumin) as add-on therapy given 24 hours prior to IVMP in 76 patients with acute MS attacks. Over the 6 months of follow-up no difference was observed between groups on any outcome measure. Similarly, a recent double-blind, placebo-controlled trial of IVIg (0.4 g/kg or placebo given on days 0, 1, 2, 30 and 60) in 68 patients with optic neuritis,[126] failed to demonstrate any difference between treatment groups in terms of relapses or MRI lesions over the 6 months of follow-up.

In summary, the studies of IVIg, to date, have, in general, been disappointing and, moreover, the better-designed studies have been negative. Consequently, it seems that IVIg provides little or no benefit either in reducing the number of clinical attacks or the slowing of disease progression (level C conclusion).

IMMUNOSUPPRESSIVE AGENTS OTHER THAN MITOXANTRONE

Cyclophosphamide

Cyclophosphamide (Cytoxan) is an alkylating agent with potent immunosuppressive and cytotoxic effects. Often it has prominent side effects such as alopecia, nausea, vomiting and hemorrhagic cystitis. Other side effects include sterility, myelosuppression and a long-term risk of malignancy. In 1983, the first randomized, controlled trial of this agent in 58 patients with chronic progressive MS (SPMS and PPMS) was published.[112] Patients were assigned to one of three treatment groups: 1) i.v. ACTH for 21 days; 2) ACTH and i.v. cyclophosphamide (400–500 mg/d for 10–14 d); and 3) ACTH and low-dose oral cyclophosphamide in addition to five courses of plasma exchange over 2 weeks. Grouping patients who improved and those who remained stable into a 'stabilized' subgroup, these authors found a benefit to therapy at both 6 and 12 months ($p<0.002$). The study, however, was unblinded and no true placebo group was included (class III evidence). More importantly, another small, but randomized and blinded, class I study in the same patient population (undertaken by the Kaiser physicians

in an attempt to replicate this earlier result) was completely unsuccessful.[127]

In 1987, the results of a nonrandomized trial of cyclophosphamide in 27 treated and 24 untreated patients with chronic progressive MS (SPMS and PPMS) were reported.[128] Patients either received intravenous cyclophosphamide (500 mg/d for 10–14 d) in addition to intravenous ACTH or oral prednisone, or oral cyclophosphamide (700 mg/m²/week for 6 weeks) in addition to oral prednisone. The authors reported a benefit to treatment at both the 1- and 2-year time-points ($p=0.002$ and $p=0.009$). This study, however, was not randomized, the treatment regimen varied considerably and the outcome assessment was not carried out by blinded observers. Consequently, this study provides only weak (class III) evidence for any treatment effect.

By far the best study was the multicenter Canadian trial of cyclophosphamide and plasma exchange in the treatment of patients with either SPMS or PPMS.[113] This trial involved 168 patients who were randomized to one of four treatment arms: 1) i.v. cyclophosphamide (1000 mg) on alternate days until either the white blood cell count dropped to below 4500/µl or the patient had received nine courses of treatment; 2) 40 mg/day of oral prednisone for 10 d; 3) oral cyclophosphamide (1.5–2.0 mg/kg) and oral prednisone on alternate days for 22 weeks (with the dose of cyclophosphamide adjusted to achieve a white blood cell count of 4000–5000/µl) and plasma exchange weekly for 20 weeks; and 4) an oral cyclophosphamide placebo, a prednisone placebo and a sham plasma exchange on the same schedule. Patients were followed for up to 3 years and at no time was a significant difference in outcome noted between the different treatment groups. After 3 years, the cumulative failure rate was actually less in the placebo arm than in the two active treatment arms. This study provides class I evidence that neither pulse cyclophosphamide treatment nor plasma exchange alters the course of progressive MS.

In 1993, the use of regular pulse cyclophosphamide therapy in 256 progressive MS patients (SPMS and PPMS) was evaluated.[129] Patients were randomized to receive an induction treatment with intravenous cyclophosphamide, either 500 mg/d for 8–18 d until the white blood cell count dropped below 4000/µl (groups 1 and 2) or 600 mg/m² given on days 1, 2, 4, 6 and 8 (groups 3 and 4). All groups were also given ACTH. Groups 2 and 4 subsequently received boosters of intravenous cyclophosphamide (700 mg/m²) every other month for 2 years whereas groups 1 and 3 were not given booster treatment. Assessment of outcome assessment was not blinded (class III). After 3 years, Kaplan–Meyer analysis for treatment failure showed no significant benefit from booster treatment ($p=0.18$). A subgroup analysis, by contrast, suggested a benefit of treatment in patients younger than 41 years ($p=0.003$) but no such benefit in the older population. However, this subgroup was not prospectively identified so that the validity of the observation is uncertain. Also, because all patients received induction with cyclophosphamide, the value of induction or the benefit of therapy compared to no therapy cannot be assessed.

Consequently, based on consistent class I evidence, cyclophosphamide treatment does not seem to alter the course of progressive MS (level B recommendation). However, based on a single class III study, it is uncertain whether younger patients with progressive MS might benefit from pulse plus booster cyclophosphamide treatment (level U recommendation).

Methotrexate

Methotrexate (Rheumatrex) is an inhibitor of dihydrofolate. It has anti-inflammatory properties, decreases proinflammatory cytokines and augments suppressor cell function, and it is in widespread use for other inflammatory disorders, especially rheumatoid arthritis. Following prolonged treatment (>2 years), some patients get liver damage and some experts recommend a percutaneous liver biopsy after 2 years of treatment to detect drug-related hepatic toxicity. The long-term risk of developing non-Hodgkin's lymphoma following therapy is slightly increased. In 1993, the results of an 18-month, double-blind, randomized, placebo-controlled pilot study of low-dose methotrexate (7.5 mg/week) in MS were reported.[130] The study population, however, was small (45 individuals) and was not focused on any specific disease category (class II evidence). The results of this trial suggested a possible benefit to treatment in RRMS but not in progressive MS.

In 1995, the effect of low-dose oral methotrexate (7.5 mg/week) in 60 MS patients with either SPMS or PPMS treated for 2 years was assessed.[131] Treatment failure (defined using a composite outcome measure) was reported to be less common with active treatment ($p=0.011$). This result, however, was driven entirely by the findings on the nine-hole peg test ($p=0.007$). None of the other components of the composite measure showed any significant benefit of treatment. Outcome was also assessed by MRI scans in 56 of the 60 patients, including measures of T2 lesion burden, gadolinium enhancement and new T2 lesions.[132] A subgroup analysis of 35 patients (not prospectively defined) with scans performed every 6 weeks suggested a reduction in T2 disease burden favoring treatment with methotrexate ($p=0.036$) although, considering the entire cohort, no significant difference was noted between the placebo and treated groups with respect to any MRI outcome measure. In summary, this trial provides equivocal evidence of a treatment effect for methotrexate in progressive MS. The subgroup analysis of those patients classified as primary progressive did not reveal any therapeutic benefit on the primary outcome.

Based on limited, and somewhat conflicting, class II evidence, it is possible that methotrexate favorably alters the disease course in patients with secondary progressive MS (level C recommendation).

Azathioprine

Azathioprine (Imuran) is a nucleoside analogue of 6-mercaptopurine that impairs DNA and RNA synthesis. The clinical benefits may be delayed and expected changes such as lymphopenia or an increase in the mean corpuscular volume may not be observed for 3–6 months.[133] Side effects of treatment include lymphopenia, anemia, elevated liver enzymes, pancreatitis, alopecia and the reactivation of latent viral infections including warts and herpetic infections. There is concern regarding the possible long-term risk of developing malignancy (particularly lymphoma) in those treated with this agent.[134] Studies of this agent in MS have produced mixed results, probably related to differences in trial design, study duration and the number of patients studied. A meta-analysis of all randomized, blinded, controlled trials of azathioprine in MS included seven studies (793 patients) and reported an odds ratio of 2.04 for remaining relapse-free after 2 years of azathioprine therapy compared to placebo.[135,136]

In 1988, the British and Dutch Multiple Sclerosis Azathioprine Trial Group reported the results of a 3-year randomized, double-blind trial of azathioprine (2.5 mg/kg daily) or placebo[137] in 354 MS patients (class I evidence). After three years, the mean EDSS score was slightly better in the azathioprine-treated patients compared to controls. By contrast, there was no difference in attack rate between groups.[137]

In 1989, a three-arm placebo-controlled, randomized, double-blind trial including 98 MS patients with progressive MS (SPMS and PPMS) evaluated the clinical impact of azathioprine.[138] Patients were treated with: 1) oral azathioprine (beginning at 2.2 mg/kg increasing as necessary to achieve a white blood cell count of 3000–4000/µl) in addition to a course of IVMP; 2) oral azathioprine (as in the first arm) plus an intravenous placebo instead of IVMP; and both oral and intravenous placebo. Patients were followed over 36 months of treatment. There was no statistically significant difference in the rates of EDSS progression among the three treatment arms, although the azathioprine treatment groups had half the relapse rate of the placebo group. In an open-label study to demonstrate efficacy of azathioprine on paraclinical markers of MS disease activity including 14 patients, azathioprine at lymphocyte-suppressing dosage showed a reduction in the development of new inflammatory brain lesions as assessed by MRI.[139]

On the basis of several, but somewhat conflicting, class I and II studies, it is possible that azathioprine reduces the relapse rate in patients with MS (level C conclusion). By contrast, its effect on disability progression is unproven (level U conclusion).

Mycophenolate mofetil

Mycophenolate mofetil (Cellcept) belongs to the antimetabolite group and is a product of the active metabolite mycophenolic acid. The drug is administered orally at a usual dose of 2 g/d, has a good adverse effect profile and thus is convenient for the patient. Its use in neuroimmunological autoimmune disorders is becoming increasingly popular, despite the fact that almost all applications are unsupported by quality clinical trial data.[140–142] With regard to its use in MS, only very few reports or open-label studies currently exist. A small open-label trial using mycophenolate mofetil as monotherapy in various progressive MS cases suggests efficacy in this patient population while, overall, few patients complained about side effects, e.g. diarrhea.[143] A total of 30 patients suffering from RRMS were enrolled in an open-label phase II clinical trial testing the combination of mycophenolate mofetil with IFNβ-1a.

On the basis of this evidence, the use of mycophenolate mofetil in MS is of unproven efficacy (level U conclusion).

Ciclosporin

Ciclosporin (Sandimmune) is a calcineurin inhibitor that blocks the production of the cytokines interleukin (IL)-2 and IL-4 by T lymphocytes. Common serious side effects associated with this drug are nephrotoxicity and neurotoxicity, which affect 25–60% of transplant patients.[144] Others include hypertension, diabetes and hyperlipidemia. Thus, the overall risk:benefit ratio seems unfavorable. In a double-blind, multicenter trial comparing ciclosporin with azathioprine in patients with MS, patients in the ciclosporin group were more than twice as likely to report side effects as patients in the azathioprine arm.[145] In 1990 the results from a 2-year randomized, double-blind, placebo-controlled study including 547 patients with chronic progressive MS were published.[146] Patients in the treated group experienced a statistically significant but modest delay of disease progression while the overall lesion load was not affected, as revealed by a subsequent MRI study.[147]

On the basis of a single class I study, therefore, it is possible that ciclosporin provides some therapeutic benefit in progressive MS (level C conclusion). Nevertheless, because adverse reactions to treatment, especially nephrotoxicity, occur frequently and because the magnitude of the potential benefit is small, the risk:benefit of this therapeutic option is quite low (level B conclusion).

Cladribine

Cladribine (Leustatin) is an adenosine-deaminase-resistant purine nucleoside. It is a potent immunosuppressive agent that is relatively selective for lymphocytes and affects blast cells as well as mature cells. Therefore it can induce a very prolonged state of immunosuppression. It has been used to treat a variety of lymphoid malignancies but seems to be especially effective in the treatment of hairy-cell leukemia. The first randomized trial of cladribine in 51 chronic progressive MS patients (SPMS and PPMS) was reported in 1994 from the Scripps Clinic.[148] Patients were treated with either cladribine (0.01 mg/kg/d i.v. for 7 days in 4-monthly courses) or placebo. Patients were followed for a year and then crossed over.[149] The investigators reported significant benefit in EDSS outcome between the cladribine and placebo groups ($p=0.004$ and $p=0.001$ respectively). They also noted a beneficial effect on the outcomes of total MRI lesion volume ($p<0.002$) and gadolinium-enhancing lesion volume ($p<0.001$). There are concerns, however, about this trial because of its small size and other methodological issues.[92] Also, the MRI lesion volume data is not easily interpreted because of the fact that the largest difference in lesion volume between groups was seen at baseline. Following treatment the two groups were not statistically different; in fact, the lesion volume was slightly greater in the cladribine-treated group.[148] This trial provides some class II data that cladribine favorably affects the course of progressive MS.

In another small trial from the Scripps Clinic,[150] these same authors examined the value of cladribine treatment in 52 patients with RRMS. Patients were randomized to receive either cladribine (0.07 mg/kg/d for 5 days in 6-monthly courses) or placebo and they were followed for 18 months (class I). These authors found a nonsignificant reduction in relapse rate in the treated group compared to controls and no difference between groups on the EDSS. By contrast, MRI measures were favorably affected by treatment. Indeed, enhancing lesions were completely suppressed in the cladribine-treated group at 6 months. At 7 months, the frequency of enhancing lesions was significantly greater in the placebo group ($p=0.0001$) and remained so at the end of the trial ($p=0.002$).

A multicenter placebo-controlled trial of cladribine in 159 progressive MS patients (SPMS and PPMS) from North America was also reported recently.[151] Patients were randomized to receive either cladribine (0.07 mg/kg/d for 5 days in 2- or 6-monthly cycles) or placebo, and they were followed for 12 months. At the end of the trial there was no difference in mean EDSS change between groups. As before, however, MRI measures were dramatically affected by treatment. Thus, there was a greater than 90% reduction in the number of gadolinium-enhancing lesions ($p<0.003$) and a minimal reduction in the T2 volume of disease (-4%; $p=0.029$) in the high-dose group compared to placebo.

Consequently, on the basis of consistent class I and class II evidence, it is concluded that cladribine reduces gadolinium enhancement in patients with both relapsing and progressive forms of MS (level A recommendation). Cladribine treatment does not, however, appear to alter the course of the disease, with respect to either disease activity or disease severity measures (level C conclusion). Nevertheless, interest in the possible role of this agent in the treatment of MS has increased as an oral preparation has become available. This led to the initiation of a randomized, double-blind, placebo-controlled phase III study planned to include 1290 patients with active inflammatory RRMS. This trial was launched in April 2005 to further test the safety and effectiveness of oral cladribine (10 mg cladribine or placebo is given orally over 5 days per month, administered in 2–4 cycles per year). Outcomes include relapse rate, EDDS progression and MRI activity.

DISEASE-MODIFYING THERAPY IN MULTIPLE SCLEROSIS (CURRENTLY UNDER INVESTIGATION IN PHASE II OR III TRIALS)

Several novel agents are currently under active investigation for their potential use in the treatment of MS. These include oral agents, monoclonal antibodies and other immunomodulatory approaches directed at a variety of targets in the immune system (Tables 21.8–21.11).

Sirolimus

Sirolimus (rapamycin) is a potent antiproliferative agent with a specific mechanism of action. Sirolimus forms a complex with the intracellular protein FKBP12 that blocks the activation of a kinase cascade essential for cell-cycle progression. This novel macrocyclic compound is derived from the bacterium *Streptomyces hygroscopius* and specifically inhibits mTOR (mammalian target of rapamycin) kinase, an enzyme required to control a cell's life cycle, preventing cell division into new cells. Sirolimus thus inhibits antigen-induced proliferation of T and B cells and antibody production.[152] In addition, the agent probably induces persisting regulatory T cells. One major side effect is the consistent elevation of blood lipids (hypercholesterinemia).

TABLE 21.8 Components of multiple sclerosis pathogenesis and currently available interventions

Systemic
Immune dysfunction (IFNβ, glatiramer acetate, steroids, natalizumab, immunosuppressants)
Blood–brain barrier
Increased permeability (steroids, IFNβ, glatiramer acetate, natalizumab, immunosuppressants)
Dysfunction?
Central nervous system
Inflammation (IFNβ, glatiramer acetate, immunosuppressants)
Demyelination?
Axonal loss?
Scar formation/gliosis?

TABLE 21.9 Components of multiple sclerosis pathogenesis and some evolving interventions

Systemic
Immune dysfunction (immunosuppressants, new immunomodulators: natalizumab, fingolimod, teriflunomide, laquinimod, temsirolimus, statins . . .)
Blood–brain barrier
Increased permeability/dysfunction (natalizumab, chemokine antagonists, metalloprotease inhibitors . . .)
Central nervous system
Inflammation (immunosuppressants, new immunomodulators, altered peptide ligands (APLs) and APL-producing plasmids, vaccination . . .)
Demyelination (neuroprotectants . . .)
Axonal loss (neuroprotectants: AMPA antagonists, calcium channel blockers . . .)
Scar formation/gliosis?
Remyelination/regeneration (growth factors, pre-oligos, stem-cell transplants . . .)

TABLE 21.10 Humanized monoclonal antibodies under investigation in multiple sclerosis

Cell-type-specific	
Alemtuzumab (Campath) phase II/III ongoing	++
Anti-CD20, Rituximab (Rituxan) phase I/II	(+)
Targeting the immunological synapse	
CTLA4-Ig (BMS188667) phase II interrupted	–
Anti-IL-2R, Daclizumab (Zenapax) phase I/II	(+)
Anti-CD40L/-CD154 (IDEC-131) phase I	n.d.
Anti IL12p40 (J695)/anti IL23 phase I/II	n.d.
Others	
Selective adhesion molecule (SAM) inhibitors	
Anti-VLA-4 – α4-integrin, natalizumab (Tysabri)	++

+, denotes positive result for primary MRI outcome in phase II studies; ++, both MRI and clinical outcome met; (+), phase I/II study result; –, negative outcome; n.d., not done/completed.

TABLE 21.11 New oral immunomodulators/suppressants in phase II and III studies, 2005/2006

Teriflunomide (leflunomide metabolite)	+
Laquinimod	+
CCI-779 (Temsirolimus)	(+)
Fingolimod (FTY720)	++
CCR1-antagonist	–
Fumaric acid (BG12)	+
Xaliproden	–
Statins	(+) n.d.
Others	
Statins	(+)
Rosiglitazone (anti-inflammatory, PPARγ agonist)	–
Minocycline (MMP-antagonism)	(+)
Oral integrin antagonists (small molecules) Anti VLA4 Anti LFA-1	 n.d. n.d.

+, positive result for primary outcome in phase II studies, usually MRI; ++, both MRI and clinical outcome met; (+), phase I/II study result; –, negative outcome; n.d., not done/completed.

Temsirolimus

Temsirolimus (CCI-779) is a newly developed ester analog (formulated for improved oral absorption) of sirolimus. Several studies are currently investigating the safety and effectiveness of this substance in breast and renal cancer and rheumatoid arthritis. Fast-track approval has been received for the treatment of renal cancer. In addition, a phase II study has been completed in MS. The substance was tested with three different doses against placebo in 296 individuals with RRMS and active SPMS for a period of 9 months.[153] At the end of the study patients on the highest dose had significantly fewer contrast-enhancing MRI lesions (48% reduction) and 51% fewer relapses than those on placebo. Side effects occurred more frequently in the high-dose subgroup and included menstrual dysfunction, mouth ulceration or inflammation, hyperlipidemia and rashes.

Fingolimod

Fingolimod (FTY720) is an oral sphingosine-1-phosphate receptor modulator. After rapid phosphorylation, fingolimod-P acts as a 'super agonist' of the sphingosine-1-phosphate-1 receptor on thymocytes and lymphocytes and induces aberrant internalization of this receptor, thereby depriving these cells of a signal necessary to egress from secondary lymphoid tissues. The majority of circulating lymphocytes are thus sequestered in lymph nodes, reducing peripheral lymphocyte counts and the recirculation of lymphocytes to the central nervous system.[154–156] Lymphocytes in secondary lymphoid organs and those remaining in blood continue to be functional. In animal experiments, fingolimod did not impair T-cell activation, expansion or memory to systemic viral infection.[157] In animal models of multiple sclerosis, fingolimod prevented disease onset and reduced established neurological deficits.[154,158–160]

In a randomized, placebo-controlled phase II study (level I evidence) 255 of 281 patients completed 6 months' treatment[161] The median total number of gadolinium-enhancing lesions per patient was lower with both doses tested (1.25 mg and 5 mg) versus placebo. The annualized relapse rate was reduced by over 50% in the FTY720 groups (0.77 with placebo versus 0.35 with 1.25 mg ($p=0.009$) and 0.36 with 5 mg ($p=0.014$)). A high proportion (98%) of patients decided to continue with dose-blinded FTY720 treatment after month 6. Among the 226 patients who completed the 12-month extension, the number of gadolinium-enhanced lesions and relapse rates remained low in the continuous fingolimod groups, while both measures decreased in patients switching from placebo to fingolimod.[162] Adverse events included nasopharyngitis, dyspnea, headache, diarrhea, nausea and clinically asymptomatic liver enzyme (alanine aminotransferase) elevations. One case of posterior reversible encephalopathy occurred. Fingolimod also was associated with an initial reversible reduction in heart rate and a mild increase in airway resistance.[161] Phase III studies are currently ongoing and will determine the place this compound might take in the therapeutic armamentarium against MS.

Teriflunomide

Teriflunomide is a purine analog that exerts immunosuppressive properties. It is an analog of leflunomide, which in some countries is approved for the therapy of rheumatoid arthritis. Teriflunomide belongs to the group of malononitrilamide agents, which block the mitochondrial enzyme dihydroorotate-dehydrogenase and inhibit T- and B-cell proliferation.[163,164] Teriflunomide has been found to suppress experimental autoimmune encephalomyelitis, probably via the suppression of TNFα and IL-2 production.[165,166] The results from a clinical phase II study testing teriflunomide in patients with relapsing RRMS and SPMS have recently been published.[167] Two different teriflunomide doses (7 and 14 mg once-daily) were compared to placebo over an observation period of 36 weeks. The primary endpoint of the study was met, since subjects receiving feriflunomid had significantly fewer active MS lesions and reduced numbers of new lesions on MRI. EDSS progression was delayed in the high-dose arm and a trend towards reduction in relapses was observed. Overall, teriflunomide was well tolerated, with upper respiratory tract infections and headache as the most common adverse effects. However, serious adverse events, including toxic liver necrosis and pancytopenia, have been described in relation to treatment of rheumatoid arthritis with leflunomide. The safety and efficacy of the drug in MS is being further investigated in an ongoing phase III trial.

Laquinimod

Laquinimod is a new, orally active immunomodulator that was shown to be approximately 20 times more potent than its 'ancestor' roquinimex (linomide) in experimental autoimmune encephalomyelitis.[168] The synthetic compound has an excellent oral bioavailability and serves as an immunoregulatory drug without general immunosuppressive properties. Its sustained inhibitory activity has been shown in other autoimmune and inflammatory diseases in several animal models.[169–171] Roquinimex (linomide) efficiently reduced active MRI lesions in phase II and III clinical studies of MS but a large phase III program in MS had to be stopped prematurely because of unexpected severe side effects (serositis, myocardial infarction).[172,173] The results from a double-blind, randomized, multicenter proof-of-concept study testing two different doses of oral laquinimod (0.1 mg/d and 0.3 mg/d) versus placebo in 180 patients with RRMS have recently been published.[174] The duration of the study was 24 weeks. Taken together, a significant difference between 0.3 mg laquinimod and placebo was observed for the primary outcome measure, i.e. the mean cumulative number of active MRI lesions (5.24 versus 9.44; 44% reduction). This effect was even more pronounced in those patients with at least one active lesion at baseline (52% reduction). Clinical outcome parameters (relapse rate, disability) were not different between the groups. The overall safety profile was favorable, with no signs of undesired tissue inflammation. A further phase II study is ongoing.

Fumaric acid

Fumaric acid is an immunomodulator used for the treatment of psoriasis. Because of gastrointestinal side effects, novel fumaric acid esters (BG12, fumarate) have been developed with better tolerability. An exploratory, prospective, open-label study of fumaric acid esters (Fumaderm) was conducted in 10 patients with RRMS and indicated an attenuating effect of the drug on contrast-enhancing MRI lesions.[175] A double blind, placebo-controlled, phase II study was launched in November 2005 to further test the drug's safety and effectiveness in controlling disease course and development of MS brain lesions. In January 2006, the product sponsor announced that the study had met its primary endpoint by reducing the number of active MRI lesions within 6 months of treatment (http://wwww.FDA.org). Details of the secondary outcome measures had not been released at the time of writing.

Statins

Statins are lipid-lowering drugs approved for the therapy of hyperlipidemia. They act on the enzyme 3-hydroxy-3-methylglutaryl coenzyme A (HMG-CoA) reductase, which converts HMG-CoA to L-mevalonate, a key intermediate in cholesterol biosynthesis. In recent years evidence has accumulated that statins have potent immunomodulatory properties.[176,177] Accordingly, statins have demonstrated beneficial effects in different experimental autoimmune encephalomyelitis models.[178–180] Relevant immunomodulatory properties that might be of benefit in the treatment of MS include: 1) inhibition of the proliferative activity of T and B cells; 2) reduction of the secretion of matrix metalloprotease (MMP)-9; 3) reduction of the expression of activation-induced adhesion molecules on T cells; 4) downregulation of chemokine receptors on B and T cells; 5) inhibition of IFNγ-inducible major histocompatibility complex (MHC) class II expression on various types of nonprofessional antigen-presenting cell; 6) suppression of the upregulation of costimulatory molecules required for antigen presentation; 7) inhibition of secretion of proinflammatory cytokines; and 8) promotion of the secretion of anti-inflammatory cytokines.[181]

Beneficial effects of oral simvastatin (80 mg daily) in MS have first been demonstrated in a small, multicenter, open-label, 6-month cohort study involving 28 patients with RRMS where the number and volume of gadolinium-enhancing lesions were reduced by 44% and 41%, respectively.[182] Although these results are promising, the lack of a placebo arm in the study limits interpretation. Currently a larger, placebo-controlled trial in patients with clinically isolated syndrome suggestive of MS is under way (treatment for 12 months with 80 mg atorvastatin or placebo). Both the pharmacological profile and its assumed mechanisms of action make statins attractive candidates for combination studies. A small clinical trial is currently testing the combination of high-dose IFNβ-1a (44 μg three times a week) with atorvastatin in RRMS. In addition, based on promising results in the animal model experimental autoimmune encephalomyelitis,[183] a trial testing atorvastatin in combination with GA is being planned.

MONOCLONAL ANTIBODIES

Alemtuzumab (Campath) is a humanized monoclonal IgG1κ antibody directed against the CD52 cell-surface antigen expressed mainly on B cells, T cells, natural killer (NK) cells and monocytes. It induces a profound lymphocyte depletion and is approved for the treatment of B-cell chronic lymphocytic leukemia in patients not responding to treatment with alkylating agents or fludarabine. After positive results in open-label-treated patients with active RR disease,[184] a 3-year comparative trial against IFNβ-1a subcutaneously three times weekly was initiated that, according to a press release from the sponsor, yielded clear indication of superiority both on clinical and MRI outcomes. Unfortunately the drug seems also to induce adverse (so-called 'Th2-driven') autoimmune events, including antithyroid autoimmunity[185] but also cases of autoimmune thrombocytopenia with fatal outcome that led to suspension of dosing in this trial.

Rituximab (Rituxan) is a chimeric monoclonal antibody directed against the CD20 cell-surface antigen on B-lymphocytes. It is currently under investigation in a controlled study in primary progressive MS under the assumption of an important role of B cells in this course of the disease.[186,187]

Daclizumab is a humanized monoclonal antibody, which blocks IL-2 signaling by means of its high-affinity receptor (CD-25) that is expressed on activated T cells. Here again positive results have been reported from open label Phase I/II trials and more advanced Phase II/III trials are planned.

CONCLUSION

In recent years the neurological community has witnessed a change in the attitude towards treatment of MS. Currently available disease-modifying drugs have impressive effects on inflammatory measures of disease activity (both clinical and MRI) and are associated with a reduction in relapse frequency of about 30%, a reduction in attack severity and limitation of the sequelae of acute relapses. Their effect on disease progression (as currently measured) has been more modest and their impact on long-term function is still largely unstudied. More intensive immunosuppressive regimens, either with cytostatic agents or with monoclonal antibodies, have the potential for significantly increased efficacy but we still have a lot to learn about how to control the potential for additional risks (both overt and hidden) that all these therapies have. Several new potentially more effective and convenient immunosuppressants and immunomodulators are now in phase II and phase III clinical trials and promise further advances in our therapeutic approach to MS. However, there is still much work to be done to treat effectively the neurodegenerative aspect of MS, which characterizes both the primary progressive disease and, ultimately, also the later stages of most patients with relapsing–remitting disease.

REFERENCES

1. Weinshenker BG, Bass B, Rice GPA et al. The natural history of multiple sclerosis: a geographically based study: I. clinical course and disability. Brain 1989; 112: 133–146.

2. Weinshenker BG, Bass B, Rice GPA et al. The natural history of multiple sclerosis: a geographically based study: II. predictive value of the early clinical course. Brain 1989; 112: 1419–1428.

3. Weinshenker BG. The epidemiology of multiple sclerosis. Neurol Clin 1996; 14: 291–308.

4. Compston DA, ed. McAlpine's multiple sclerosis, 4th ed. Edinburgh: Churchill Livingstone; 2006.

5. Bar-Or A, Oliviera EML, Anderson DE, Hafler DA. Molecular pathogenesis of multiple sclerosis. J Neuroimmunol 1999; 100: 252–259.

6. Conlon P, Oksenberg JR, Zhang J. The immunobiology of multiple sclerosis: an autoimmune disease of the central nervous system. Neurobiol Dis 6; 1999: 149–166.

7. Ferguson B, Matyszak MK, Esiri MM, Perry VH. Axonal damage in acute multiple sclerosis lesions. Brain 1997; 120: 393–399.

8. Trapp BD, Bo L, Mork S, Chang A. Pathogenesis of tissue injury in MS lesions. J Neuroimmunol 1999; 98: 49–56.

9. Lublin FD, Reingold SC. Defining the clinical course of multiple sclerosis. Neurology 1996; 46: 907–911.

10. McFarland H, Barkhof F, Antel J, Miller DH. The role of MRI as a surrogate outcome measure in multiple sclerosis. Mult Scler 2002; 8: 40–51.

11. Goodin DS. MRI as a surrogate outcome measure of disability in multiple sclerosis: Have we been overly harsh in our assessment? Ann Neurol 2006; 59: 597–605.

12. The IFNB Multiple Sclerosis Study Group. Interferon beta-1b is effective in relapsing-remitting multiple sclerosis: I. Clinical results of a multicenter, randomized, double blind, placebo-controlled trial. Neurology 1993; 43: 655–661.

13. Paty DW, Li DKB, the UBC MS/MRI Study Group, the IFNB Multiple Sclerosis Study Group. Interferon beta-1b is effective in remitting and relapsing multiple sclerosis: II. MRI analysis results of a multicenter, randomized, double-blind, placebo-controlled trial. Neurology 1993; 43: 662–667.

14. The IFNB Multiple Sclerosis Study Group and the UBC MS/MRI Analysis Group. Interferon beta-1b in the treatment of MS: final outcome of the randomized controlled trial. Neurology 1995; 45: 1277–1285.

15. European Study Group on Interferon beta-1b in Secondary Progressive MS. Placebo-controlled multicentre randomized trial of interferon β-1b in treatment of secondary progressive multiple sclerosis. Lancet 1998; 352: 1491–1497.

16. Panitch H, Miller A, Paty D et al, and the North American Study Group on Interferon beta-1a in Secondary Progressive MS. Interferon beta-1b in secondary progressive MS: results from a 3-year controlled study. Neurology 2004; 63: 1788–1795.

17. PRISMS Study Group. Randomized double-blind placebo-controlled study of interferon β-1a in relapsing/remitting multiple sclerosis. Lancet 1998; 352: 1498–1504.

18. Li DK, Paty DW, UBC MS/MRI Analysis Research Group, PRISMS Study Group. Magnetic resonance imaging results of the PRISMS trial: a randomized, double-blind, placebo-controlled study of interferon-beta1a in relapsing-remitting multiple sclerosis. Prevention of relapses and disability by interferon-beta1a subcutaneously in multiple sclerosis. Ann Neurol 1999; 46: 197–206.

19. SPECTRIMS Study Group. Randomized controlled trial of interferon-beta-1a in secondary progressive MS: clinical results. Neurology 2001; 56: 1496–1504.

20. Li DK, Zhao GJ, Paty DW, the University of British Columbia MS/MRI Analysis Research Group and the SPECTRIMS Study Group. Randomized controlled trial of interferon-beta-1a in secondary progressive MS: MRI results. Neurology 2001; 56: 1505–1513.

21. Jacobs LD, Cookfair DL, Rudick RA et al. Intramuscular interferon beta-1a for disease progression in exacerbating-remitting multiple sclerosis. Ann Neurol 1996; 39: 285–294.

22. Simon JH, Jacobs LD, Campion M et al. and the Multiple Sclerosis Collaborative Research Group (MSCRG). Magnetic resonance studies of intramuscular interferon β-1a for relapsing multiple sclerosis. Ann Neurol 1996; 43: 79–87.

23. Cohen JA, Cutter GR, Fischer JS et al and the IMPACT Investigators. Benefit of interferon β-1a on MSFC progression in secondary progressive MS. Neurology 2002; 59: 679–687.

24. Durelli L, Verdun E, Barbero P et al and the Independent Comparison of Interferon (INCOMIN) Trial Study Group. Every-other-day interferon beta-1b versus once-weekly interferon beta-1a for multiple sclerosis: results of a 2-year prospective randomised multicentre study (INCOMIN). Lancet 2002; 359: 1453–1460.

25. Panitch H, Goodin DS, Francis G et al, the EVIDENCE Study Group and the UBC MS/MRI Research Group. A randomized, comparative study of interferon beta dose in MS: the EVIDENCE trial. Neurology 2002; 59: 1496–1506.

26. Panitch H, Goodin DS, Francis G et al, the EVIDENCE Study Group and the UBC MS/MRI Research Group. Benefits of high-dose, high-frequency interferon beta-1a in relapsing MS are sustained to 16 months: final comparative results of the EVIDENCE trial. J Neurol Sci 2005; 239: 67–74.

27. Johnson KP, Brooks BR, Cohen JA et al. Copolymer 1 reduces relapse rate and improves disability in relapsing-remitting multiple sclerosis: results of a phase III multicenter, double-blind, placebo-controlled trial. Neurology 1995; 45: 1268–1276.

28. Johnson KP, Brooks BR, Cohen JA et al. Extended use of glatiramer acetate (Copaxone) is well tolerated and maintains its clinical effect on multiple sclerosis relapse rate and degree of disability. Neurology 1998; 50: 701–708.

29. Comi G, Filippi M, Wolinsky JS et al. European/Canadian multicenter, double-blind, randomized, placebo-controlled study of the effects of glatiramer acetate on magnetic resonance imaging-measured disease activity and burden in patients with relapsing multiple sclerosis. Ann Neurol 2001; 49: 290–297.

30. Johnson KP, Brooks BR, Ford CC et al. and the Copolymer 1 Multiple Sclerosis Study Group. Sustained clinical benefits of glatiramer acetate in relapsing multiple sclerosis patients observed for 6 years. Multi Scler 2000; 6: 255–266.

31. Khan OA, Tselis AC, Kamholz JA et al. A prospective, open-label treatment trial to compare the effect of IFN beta-1a (Avonex), IFN beta-1b (Betaseron), and glatiramer acetate (Copaxone) on the relapse rate in relapsing-remitting multiple sclerosis. Eur J Neurol 2001; 8: 141–148.

32. Edan G, Miller D, Clanet M et al. Therapeutic effect of mitoxantrone combined with methylprednisolone in multiple sclerosis: a randomised multicentre study of active disease using MRI and clinical criteria. J Neurol Neurosurg Psychiatr 1997; 62: 112–118.

33. Millefiorini E, Gasperini C, Pozzilli C et al. Randomized placebo-controlled trial of mitoxantrone in relapsing-remitting multiple sclerosis: 24-month clinical and MRI outcome. J Neurol 1997; 244: 153–159.

34. Hartung HP, Gonsette R, König N et al. Mitoxantrone in progressive multiple sclerosis: a placebo-controlled, double-blind, randomised, multicentre trial. Lancet 2002; 360: 2018–2025.

35. Krapf H, Morrissey SP, Zenker O et al and the MIMS Study Group. Effect of mitoxantrone on MRI in progressive MS: results of the MIMS trial. Neurology 2005; 65: 690–695.

36. Miller DH, Khan OA, Sheremata WA et al and the International Natalizumab Multiple Sclerosis Trial Group. A controlled trial of natalizumab for relapsing multiple sclerosis. N Engl J Med 2003; 348: 15–23.

37. Polman CH, O'Connor PW, Hardova E et al. A randomized, placebo-controlled trial of natalizumab for relapsing multiple sclerosis. N Engl J Med 2006; 354: 899–910.

38. Rudick RA, Stuart WH, Calabresi PA et al. Natalizumab plus interferon beta-1a for relapsing multiple sclerosis. N Engl J Med 2006; 354: 911–923.

39. Williams GJ, Witt PL. Comparative study of the pharmacodynamic and pharmacologic effects of Betaseron and Avonex. J Interferon Cytokine Res 1998; 18: 967–975.

40. Stürzebecher S, Maibauer R, Heuner A et al. Pharmacodynamic comparison of single doses of IFN-β1a and IFN-β1b in healthy volunteers. J Interferon Cytokine Res 1999; 19: 1257–1264.

41. Yousry TA, Major EO, Ryschkewitsch C et al. Evaluation of patients treated with natalizumab fro progressive multifocal leukloencephalopathy. N Engl J Med 2006; 354: 924–933.

42. Goodin DS, Frohman EM, Garmany GP Jr et al. Disease modifying therapies in multiple sclerosis: Report of the Therapeutics and Technology Assessment Subcommittee of the American Academy of Neurology and the MS Council for Clinical Practice Guidelines. Neurology 2002; 58: 169–178.

43. Goodman SN. Reviews and commentary: p values, hypothesis tests, and likelihood: implications for epidemiology of a neglected historical debate. Am J Epidemiol 1993; 137: 485–496.

44. Bellhouse DR. Invited commentary: p values, hypothesis tests, and likelihood. Am J Epidemiol 1993; 137: 497–499.

45. Goodman SN. Author's response to: invited commentary: p values, hypothesis tests, and likelihood. Am J Epidemiol 1993; 137: 500–501.

46. Goodin DS. Disease-modifying therapy in MS: a critical review of the literature. Part I: Analysis of clinical trial errors.. J Neurology 2004; 251(suppl 5): v3–v11.

47. Goodin DS. Interferon-β therapy in multiple sclerosis: evidence for a clinically relevant dose response. Drugs 2001; 61: 1693–1703.

48. Kappos L, Weinshenker B, Pozzilli C et al. Interferon beta-1b in secondary progressive MS: a combined analysis of the two trials. Neurology 2004; 63: 1779–1787.

49. Jacobs LD, Beck RW, Simon JH et al and the CHAMPS Study Group. Intramuscular interferon beta-1a therapy initiated during a first demyelinating event in multiple sclerosis. N Engl J Med 2000; 343: 898–904.

50. Comi G, Filippi M, Barkhof F et al. Effect of early interferon treatment on conversion to definite multiple sclerosis: a randomised study, Lancet 2001; 357: 1576–1582.

51. Kappos L, Polman CH, Freedman MS et al. Treatment with interferon beta-1b delays conversion to clinically definite and McDonald MS in patients with clinically isolated syndromes. Neurology 2006; 67: 1242–1249.

52. Clanet M, Radue EW, Kappos L et al. A randomized, double-blind, dose-comparison study of weekly Interferon beta-1a (Avonex) in relapsing-remitting MS. Neurology 2002; 249: 1088–1097.

53. Clanet M, Kappos L, Hartung HP, Hohlfeld R and the European IFN Beta-1a Dose Comparison Study Investigators. Interferon beta-1a in relapsing multiple sclerosis: four-year extension of the European IFN beta-1a dose-comparison study. Mult Scler 2004; 10: 139–144.

54. The IFNB Multiple Sclerosis Study Group and the UBC MS/MRI Analysis Group. Neutralizing antibodies during treatment of multiple sclerosis with interferon beta-1b. Neurology 1996; 47: 889–894.

55. Rudick RA, Simonian NA, Alam JA et al. Incidence and significance of neutralizing antibodies to interferon beta-1a in multiple sclerosis. Multiple Sclerosis Collaborative Research Group (MSCRG). Neurology 1998; 50: 1266–1272.

56. Polman C, Kappos L, White R et al and the European Study Group in Interferon Beta-1b in Secondary Progressive MS. Neutralizing antibodies during treatment of secondary progressive MS with interferon beta-1b. Neurology 2003; 60: 37–43.

57. Sorensen PS, Ross C, Clemmesen KM et al and the Danish Multiple Sclerosis Study Group. Clinical importance of neutralising antibodies against interferon beta in patients with relapsing-remitting multiple sclerosis. Lancet 2003; 362: 1184–1191.

58. Frank JA, Richert N, Bash C et al. Interferon-beta-1b slows progression of atrophy in RRMS: Three-year follow-up in NAb⁻ and NAb⁺ patients. Neurology 2004; 62: 719–725.

59. Petkau AJ, White RA, Ebers GC et al and the IFNB Multiple Sclerosis Study Group. Longitudinal analyses of the effects of neutralizing antibodies on interferon beta-1b in relapsing-remitting multiple sclerosis. Mult Scler 2004; 10: 126–138.

60. Panitch H, Miller A, Paty D et al and the North American Study Group on Interferon beta-1a in Secondary Progressive MS. Interferon beta-1b in secondary progressive MS: results from a 3-year controlled study. Neurology 2004; 63: 1788–1795.

61. Malucchi S, Sala A, Gilli F et al. Neutralizing antibodies reduce the efficacy of βIFN during treatment of multiple sclerosis. Neurology 2004; 62: 2031–2037.

62. Perini P, Calabrese M. The clinical impact of interferon beta antibodies in relapsing-remitting MS. J Neurol 2004; 251: 305–309.

63. Sorensen PS, Koch-Henriksen N, Ross C et al and the Danish Multiple Sclerosis Study Group. Appearance and disappearance of neutralizing antibodies during interferon-beta therapy. Neurology 2005; 65: 33–39.

64. Kappos L, Clanet M, Sandberg-Wollheim et al and the European Interferon Beta-1a IM Dose-Comparison Study Investigators. Neutralizing antibodies and efficacy in interferon β-1a: A 4-year controlled study. Neurology 2005; 65: 40–47.

65. Francis GS, Rice GPA, Alsop JC and the PRISMS Study Group. Interferon β-1a in MS: Results following development of neutralizing antibodies in PRISMS. Neurology 2005; 65: 48–55.

66. Barbero P, Bergui M, Versino E et al and the INCOMIN Trial Study Group. Every-other-day interferon beta-1a versus once-weekly interferon beta-1a for multiple sclerosis (INCOMIN Trial) II: Analysis of MRI responses to treatment and correlation with NAb. Multi Scler 2006; 12: 72–76.

67. Khan QA, Xia Q, Bever CT et al. Interferon beta-1b serum levels in multiple sclerosis patients following subcutaneous administration. Neurology 1996; 46: 1639–1643.

68. Bertolotto A, Gilli F, Sala A et al. Persistent neutralizing antibodies abolish the interferon β bioavailability in MS patients. Neurology 2003; 60: 634–639.

69. Bertolotto A. Neutralizing antibodies to interferon beta: implications for the management of multiple sclerosis. Curr Opinion Neurol 2004; 17: 241–246.

70. Pachner AR, Dail D, Pak E, Narayan K. The importance of measuring IFNβ bioactivity: monitoring in MS patients and the effect of anti-IFNβ antibodies. J Neuroimmunol 2005; 166: 180–188.

71. Goodin DS, Hurwitz B, Noronha A. Neutralizing antibodies to interferon beta-1b are not associated with disease worsening in multiple sclerosis. J Int Med Res 2007; 35: 173–187.

72. Rice GP, Paszner B, Oger J et al. The evolution of neutralizing antibodies in multiple sclerosis patients treated with interferon β-1b. Neurology 1999; 52: 1277–1279.

73. Herndon RM, Rudick RA, Munschauer FE et al. Eight-year immunogenicity and safety of interferon beta-1a-Avonex treatment in patients with multiple sclerosis. Mult Scler 2005; 11: 409–419.

74. Teitelbaum D, Aharoni R, Sela M, Arnon R. Cross-reactions and specificities of monoclonal antibodies against myelin basic protein and against the synthetic copolymer-1. Proc Natl Acad Sci USA 1991; 88: 9528–9532.

75. Teitelbaum D, Milo R, Arnon R, Sela M. Synthetic copolymer-1 inhibits human T-cell lines specific for myelin basic protein. Proc Natl Acad Sci USA 1992; 89: 137–141.

76. Neuhaus O, Farina C, Wekerle H, Hohlfeld R. Mechanisms of action of glatiramer acetate in multiple sclerosis. Neurology 2001; 56: 702–708.

77. Goodin DS, Arnason BG, Coyle PK et al. The use of mitoxantrone (Novantrone) for the treatment of multiple sclerosis. Report of the Therapeutics and Technology Assessment subcommittee of the American Academy of Neurology. Neurology 2003; 61: 1332–1338.

78. Bernitsas E, Wei W, Mikol DD. Suppression of mitoxantrone cardiotoxicity in multiple sclerosis patients by dexrazoxane. Ann Neurol 2006; 59: 206–209.

79. Weilbach FX, Chan A, Toyka KV, Gold R. The cardioprotector dexrazoxane augments therapeutic efficacy of mitoxantrone in experimental autoimmune encephalomyelitis. Clin Exp Immunol 2004; 135: 49–55.

80. Davis LS, Oppenheimer-Marks N, Bednarczyk JL et al. Fibronectin promotes proliferation of naive and memory T cells by signaling through both the VLA-4 and VLA-5 integrin molecules. J Immunol 1990; 145: 785–793.

81. Chan PY, Aruffo A. VLA-4 integrin mediates lymphocyte migration on the inducible endothelial cell ligand VCAM-1 and the extracellular matrix ligand fibronectin. J Biol Chem 1993; 268: 24655–24664.

82. O'Regan AW, Chupp GL, Lowry JA et al. Osteopontin is associated with T cells in sarcoid granulomas and has T cell adhesive and cytokine-like properties in vitro. J Immunol 1999; 162: 1024–1031.

83. Chabas D, Baranzini SE, Mitchell D et al. The influence of the proinflammatory cytokine, osteopontin, on autoimmune demyelinating disease. Science 2001; 294: 1731–1735.

84. Yednock TA, Cannon C, Fritz LC et al. Prevention of experimental autoimmune encephalomyelitis by antibodies against α4β1 integrin. Nature 1992; 356: 63–66.

85. Rose AS, Kuzma JW, Kurtzke JF et al. Cooperative study in the evaluation of therapy in multiple sclerosis. ACTH vs. placebo-final report. Neurology 1970; 20: 1–59.

86. Beck RW. The optic neuritis treatment trial. Arch Opthalmol 1988; 106: 1051–1053.

87. Beck RW, Cleary PA, Anderson MM Jr et al. A randomized, controlled, trial of corticosteroids in the treatment of acute optic neuritis. N Engl J Med 1992; 326: 581–588.

88. Beck RW. Corticosteroid treatment of optic neuritis: a need to change treatment practices. The Optic Neuritis Study Group. Neurology 1992; 42: 1133–1135.

89. Beck RW, Cleary PA. Optic neuritis treatment trial. One-year follow-up results. Arch Opthalmol 1993; 111: 773–775.

90. Beck RW Clearly PA, Trobe JD et al. The effect of corticosteroids for acute optic neuritis on the subsequent development of

multiple sclerosis. N Engl J Med 1993; 329: 1764–1769.

91. Optic Neuritis Study Group. The 5-year risk of MS after optic neuritis: the experience of the optic neuritis treatment trial. Neurology 1997; 49: 1404–1413.

92. Goodin DS. Perils and pitfalls in the interpretation of clinical trials: a reflection on the recent experience in multiple sclerosis. Neuroepidemiol 1999; 18: 53–63.

93. Achiron A, Djaldetti R, Ziv I. Corticosteroids in the treatment of optic neuritis. N Engl J Med 1992; 327: 281–282.

94. Silberberg DH. Corticosteroids and optic neuritis. N Engl J Med 1993; 329: 1808–1810.

95. Olek MJ, Kahn OA. Corticosteroids, optic neuritis, and multiple sclerosis. N Engl J Med 1994; 330: 1238.

96. Milligan NM, Newcombe R, Compston DA. A double-blind controlled trial of high dose methyprednisolone in patients with multiple sclerosis: 1. Clinical effects. J Neurol Neurosurg Psychiatr 1987; 50: 511–516.

97. Durelli L, Cocito D, Riccio A et al. High-dose intravenous methylprednisolone in the treatment of multiple sclerosis: clinical-immunologic correlations. Neurology 1986; 36: 238–243.

98. Barkhof F, Hommes OR, Scheltens P, Valk J. Quantitative MRI changes in gadolinium-DPTA enhancement after high-dose intravenous methylprednisolone in multiple sclerosis. Neurology 1991; 41: 1219–1222.

99. Barkhof F, Scheltens P, Frequin ST et al. Relapsing-remitting multiple sclerosis: sequential enhanced MR imaging vs clinical findings in determining disease activity. Am J Roentgeonol 1992; 159: 1041–1047.

100. Kappos L, Staedt D, Rohrbach E et al. Time course of gadolinium enhancement in MRI of patienst with multiple sclerosis: effects of corticosteroid treatment. J Neurol 1988; 235: 10.

101. Burnham JA, Wright RR, Dreisbach J, Murray RS. The effect of high-dose steroids on MRI gadolinium enhancement in acute demyelinating lesions. Neurology 1991; 41: 1349–1354.

102. Oliveri RL, Valentino P, Russo C et al. Randomized trial comparing two different high doses of methylprednisolone in MS. Neurology 1998; 50: 1833–1836.

103. Miller DH, Thompson AJ, Morrissey SP et al. High dose steroids in acute relapses of multiple sclerosis: MRI evidence for a possible mechanism of therapeutic effect. J Neurol Neurosurg Psychiatr 1992; 55: 450–453.

104. Barkhof F, Tas MW, Frequin STFM et al. Limited duration of the effect of methylprednisolone on changes on MRI in multiple scleros1one. Neuroradiology 1994; 36: 382–387.

105. Smith ME, Stone LA, Albert PS et al. Clinical worsening in multiple sclerosis is associated with increased frequency and area of gadopentate dimeglumine-enhancing magnetic resonance imaging lesions. Ann Neurol 1993; 33: 480–489.

106. Reder AT, Thapar M Jensen MA. A reduction in serum glucocorticoids provokes experimental allergic encephalomyelitis: implications for treatment of inflammatory brain disease. Neurology 1994; 44: 2289–2294.

107. Alam SM, Kyriakides T, Lawden M, Newman PK. Methylprednisolone in multiple sclerosis: a comparison of oral with intravenous therapy at equivalent high dose. J Neurol Neurosurg Psychiatr 1993; 56: 1219–1220.

108. Barnes MP, Hughes RA, Morris RW et al. Randomized trial of oral and intravenous methylprednisolone in acute relapses of multiple sclerosis. Lancet 1997; 349: 902–906.

109. Sellebjerg F, Frederiksen JL, Nielsen PM, Olesen J. Double-blind, randomized, placebo-controlled study of oral, high-dose methylprednisolone in attacks of MS. Neurology 1998; 51: 529–534.

110. Sellebjerg F, Nielsen HS, Frederiksen JL, Olesen J. A randomized, controlled trial of oral high-dose methylprednisolone in acute optic neuritis. Neurology 1999; 52: 1479–1484.

111. Zivadinov R Rudick RA, DeMasi R et al. Effects of IV methylprednisolone on brain atrophy in relapsing-remitting MS. Neurology 2001; 57: 1239–1247.

112. Hauser SL, Dawson DM, Lehrich JR et al. Intensive immunosuppression in progressive multiple sclerosis. A randomized, three-arm study of high-dose intravenous cyclophosphamide, plasma exchange, and ACTH. N Engl J Med 1983; 308: 173–180.

113. Canadian Cooperative Multiple Sclerosis Study Group. The Canadian cooperative trial of cyclophosphamide and plasma exchange in progressive multiple sclerosis. Lancet 1991; 337: 441–446.

114. Gordon PA, Carroll DJ, Etches WS et al. A double-blind controlled pilot study of plasma exchange versus sham pharesis in chronic progressive multiple sclerosis. Can J Neurol Sci 1985; 12: 39–44.

115. Khatri BO, McQuillen MP, Harrington GJ et al. Chronic progressive multiple sclerosis: double-blind controlled study of plasmapheresis in patients taking immunosuppressive drugs. Neurology 1985; 35: 312–319.

116. Weiner HL, Dau PC, Khatri BO et al. Double-blind study of true vs. sham plasma exchange in patients treated with immunosuppression for acute attacks of multiple sclerosis. Neurology 1989; 39: 1143–1149.

117. Weinshenker BG, O'Brien PC, Petterson TM et al. A randomized trial of plasma exchange in acute central nervous system inflammatory demyelinating disease. Ann Neurol 1999; 46: 878–886.

118. Fazekas F, Deisenhammer F, Strasser-Fuchs S et al. Randomized placebo-controlled trial of monthly intravenous immunoglobulin therapy in relapsing-remitting multiple sclerosis. Austrian immunoglobulin in Multiple Sclerosis Study Group. Lancet 1997; 349: 589–593.

119. Kappos L. Critical comment: Randomized placebo-controlled trial of monthly intravenous immunoglobulin therapy in relapsing-remitting multiple sclerosis, by Fazekas et al. in Lancet 1997; 349: 589–593. Int Mult Scler J 1997; 4: 43.

120. Sorensen PS, Wanscher B, Schreiber K et al. A double-blind, cross-over trial of intravenous immunoglobulin G in multiple sclerosis: preliminary results. Mult Scler 1997; 3: 145–148.

121. Achiron A, Gabbay U, Gilad R et al. Intravenous immunoglobulin treatment in multiple sclerosis. Effect on relapses. Neurology 1998; 50: 398–402.

122. Gadoth N, Melamed E, Miller A et al. Intravenous immunoglobulin treatment in multiple sclerosis Neurology 1999; 52: 214–215.

123. Hommes OR, Sorensen PS, Fazekas F, et al. Intravenous immunoglobulin in secondary progressive multiple sclerosis: randomised placebo-controlled trial. Lancet 2004; 364: 1149–1156.

124. Fazekas F, Sorensen PS, Filippi M et al and the ESIMS Study Group. MRI results from the European Study on Intravenous Immunoglobulin in Secondary Progressive Multiple Sclerosis (ESIMS). Mult Scler 2005; 11: 433–440.

125. Sorensen PS, Haas J, Sellebjerg F et al and the TARIMS Study Group. IV immunoglobulins as add-on treatment to methylprednisolone for acute relapses in MS. Neurology 2004; 63: 2028–2033.

126. Roed HG, Langkilde A, Sellebjerg F et al. A double-blind, randomized trial of IV immunoglobulin treatment in acute optic neuritis. Neurology 2005; 64: 804–810.

127. Likosky WH, Fireman B. Intense immunosuppression in chronic progressive multiple sclerosis: the Kaiser study. J Neurol Neurosurg Psychiatr 1991; 54: 1055–1060.

128. Goodkin DE, Plencer S, Palmer-Saxreud J et al. Cyclophosphamide in chronic progressive multiple sclerosis. Neurology 1987; 44: 823–827.

129. Weiner HL, Mackin GA, Orav EJ et al. Intermittent cyclophosphamide pulse therapy in progressive multiple sclerosis: final report of the Northeast Cooperative Multiple Sclerosis Treatment Group. Neurology 1993; 43: 910–918.

130. Currier RD, Haerer AF, Meydrech EF. Low dose oral methotrexate treatment of multiple sclerosis: a pilot study. J Neurol Neurosurg Psychiatr 1993; 56: 1217–1218.

131. Goodkin DE, Rudick RA, VanderBrug-Medendorp S et al. Low-dose (7.5mg) oral methotrexate reduces the rate of progression in chronic progressive multiple sclerosis. Ann Neurol 1995; 37: 30–40.

132. Goodkin DE, Rudick RA, VanderBrug Meendorp S et al. Low-dose oral methotrexate in chronic progressive multiple sclerosis: analysis of serial MRIs. Neurology 1996; 47: 1153–1157.

133. Witte AS, Cornblath DR, Schatz NJ, Lisak RP. Monitoring azathioprine therapy in myasthenia gravis. Neurology 1986; 36: 1533–1534.

134. Confavreux C, Saddier P, Grimaud J et al. Risk of cancer from azathioprine therapy in multiple sclerosis: a case-control study. Neurology 1996; 46: 1607–1612.

135. Yudkin PL, Ellison GW, Ghezzi A et al. Overview of azathioprine treatment in multiple sclerosis. Lancet 1991; 338: 1051–1055.

136. Palace J, Rothwell P. New treatments and azathioprine in multiple sclerosis. Lancet 1997; 350: 261.

137. British and Dutch Multiple Sclerosis Azathioprine Trial Group. Double-masked trial of azathioprine in multiple sclerosis. Lancet 1988; 2: 179–183.

138. Ellison GW, Myers LW, Mickey MR et al. A placebo-controlled, randomized, double-masked, variable dosage, clinical trial of azathioprine with and without methylprednisolone in multiple sclerosis. Neurology 1989; 39: 1018–1026.

139. Massacesi L, Parigi A, Barilaro A et al. Efficacy of azathioprine on multiple sclerosis new brain lesions evaluated using magnetic resonance imaging. Arch Neurol 2005; 62: 1843–1847.

140. Schneider-Gold C, Hartung HP, Gold R. Mycophenolate mofetil and tacrolimus: new therapeutic options in neuroimmunological diseases. Muscle Nerve 2006; 34: 284–291.

141. Frohman EM, Brannon K, Racke MK et al. Mycophenolate mofetil in multiple sclerosis. Clin Neuropharmacol 2004; 27: 80–83.

142. Vermersch P, Stojkovic T, de Seze J. Mycophenolate mofetil and neurological diseases. Lupus 2005; 14(suppl 1): s42–s45.

143. Ahrens N, Salama A, Haas J. Mycophenolate-mofetil in the treatment of refractory multiple sclerosis. J Neurol 2001; 248: 713–714.

144. Serkova NJ, Christians U, Benet LZ. Biochemical mechanisms of cyclosporine neurotoxicity. Mol Interv 2004; 4: 97–107.

145. Kappos L, Patzold U, Dommasch D et al. Cyclosporine versus azathioprine in the long-term treatment of multiple sclerosis-results of the German multicenter study. Ann Neurol 1988; 23: 56–63.

146. The Multiple Sclerosis Study Group. Efficacy and toxicity of cyclosporine in chronic progressive multiple sclerosis: a randomized, double-blinded, placebo-controlled clinical trial. Ann Neurol 1990; 27: 591–605.

147. Zhao GJ, Li DK, Wolinsky JS et al. Clinical and magnetic resonance imaging changes correlate in a clinical trial monitoring cyclosporine therapy for multiple sclerosis. The MS Study Group. J Neuroimaging 1997; 7: 1–7.

148. Sipe JC, Romine JS, Koziol JA et al. Cladribine in treatment of chronic progressive multiple sclerosis. Lancet 1994; 344: 9–13.

149. Beutler E, Sipe J, Romine JS et al. Treatment of chronic progressive multiple sclerosis with cladribine. Proc Natl Acad Sci USA 1996; 93: 1716–1720.

150. Romine JS, Sipe JC, Koziol JA, Beutler E. A double-blind, placebo-controlled, randomized trial of cladribine in relapsing-remitting multiple sclerosis. Proc Assoc Am Physicians 1999; 111: 35–44.

151. Rice GP, Filippi M, Comi G and the Cladribine Study Group. Cladribine and progressive MS: clinical and MRI outcomes of a multicenter controlled trial. Neurology 2000; 54: 1145–1155.

152. Sehgal SN. Sirolimus: its discovery, biological properties, and mechanism of action. Transplant Proc 2003; 35: 7S–14S.

153. Kappos L, Barkhof F, Desmet A. The effect of oral temsirolimus on new magnetic resonance imaging scan lesions, brain atrophy, and the number of relapses in multiple sclerosis: results from a randomised, controlled clinical trial. J Neurol 2005; 252: S46.

154. Mandala S, Hajdu R, Bergstrom J et al. Alteration of lymphocyte trafficking by sphingosine-1-phosphate receptor agonists. Science 2002; 296: 346–349.

155. Brinkmann V, Cyster JG, Hla T. FTY720: Sphingosine 1-phosphate receptor-1 in the control of lymphocyte egress and endothelial barrier function. Am J Transplant 2004; 4: 1019–1025.

156. Matloubian M, Lo CG, Cinamon G et al. Lymphocyte egress from thymus and peripheral lymphoid organs is dependent on S1P receptor 1. Nature 2004; 427: 355–360.

157. Pinschewer DD, Ochsenbein AF, Odermatt B et al. FTY720 immunosuppression impairs effector T cell peripheral homing without affecting induction, expansion, and memory. J Immunol 2000; 164: 5761–5770.

158. Webb M, Tham C-S, Lin F-F et al. Sphingosine 1-phosphate receptor agonists attenuate relapsing-remitting experimental autoimmune encephalitis in SJL mice. J Neuroimmunol 2004; 153: 108–121.

159. Fujino M, Funeshima N, Kitazawa Y et al. Amelioration of experimental autoimmune encephalomyelitis in Lewis rats by FTY720 treatment. J Pharmacol Exp Ther 2003; 305: 70–77.

160. Webb M, Tham CS, Lin FF et al. Sphingosine 1-phosphate receptor agonists attenuate relapsing-remitting experimental autoimmune encephalitis in SJL mice. J Neuroimmunol 2004; 153: 108–121.

161. Kappos L, Radu E, Antel J et al. Promising results with a novel oral immunomodulator-FTY720-in relapsing multiple sclerosis. Mult Scler 2005; 11: S13.

162. O'Connor PW, Antel J, Comi G. Oral FTY720 in relapsing MS: Results of the dose blinded, active drug extension phase of a phase II study. Neurology 2006; 66: A123.

163. Korn T, Magnus T, Toyka K et al. Modulation of effector cell functions in experimental autoimmune encephalomyelitis by leflunomide–mechanisms independent of pyrimidine depletion. J Leukoc Biol 2004; 76: 950–960.

164. Nakajima A, Yamanaka H, Kamatani N. [Leflunomide: clinical effectiveness and mechanism of action]. Clin Calcium 2003; 13: 771–775.

165. Korn T, Toyka K, Hartung HP et al. Suppression of experimental autoimmune neuritis by leflunomide. Brain 2001; 124: 1791–1802.

166. Smolen JS, Emery P, Kalden JR et al. The efficacy of leflunomide monotherapy in rheumatoid arthritis: towards the goals of disease modifying antirheumatic drug therapy. J Rheumatol Suppl 2004; 71: 13–20.

167. O'Connor PW, Li D, Freedman MS et al. A Phase II study of the safety and efficacy of teriflunomide in multiple sclerosis with relapses. Neurology 2006; 66: 894–900.

168. Brunmark C, Runstrom A, Ohlsson L et al. The new orally active immunoregulator laquinimod (ABR-215062) effectively inhibits development and relapses of experimental autoimmune encephalomyelitis. J Neuroimmunol 2002; 130: 163–172.

169. Jonsson S, Andersson G, Fex T et al. Synthesis and biological evaluation of new 1,2-dihydro-4-hydroxy-2-oxo-3-quinolinecarboxamides for treatment of autoimmune disorders: structure–activity relationship. J Med Chem 2004; 47: 2075–2088.

170. Runstrom A, Leanderson T, Ohlsson L et al. Inhibition of the development of chronic experimental autoimmune encephalomyelitis by laquinimod (ABR-215062) in IFN beta k.o. and wild type mice. J Neuroimmunol 2006; 173: 69–78.

171. Yang JS, Xu LY, Xiao BG et al. Laquinimod (ABR-215062) suppresses the development of experimental autoimmune encephalomyelitis, modulates the Th1/Th2 balance and induces the Th3 cytokine TGF-beta in Lewis rats. J Neuroimmunol 2004; 156: 3–9.

172. Andersen O, Lycke J, Tollesson PO et al. Linomide reduces the rate of active lesions in relapsing–remitting multiple sclerosis. Neurology 1996; 47: 895–900.

173. Karussis DM, Meiner Z, Lehmann D et al. Treatment of secondary progressive multiple sclerosis with the immunomodulator linomide: a double-blind, placebo-controlled pilot study with monthly magnetic resonance imaging evaluation. Neurology 1996; 47: 341–346.

174. Polman C, Barkhof F, Sandberg-Wollheim M et al. Treatment with laquinimod reduces development of active MRI lesions in relapsing MS. Neurology 2005; 64: 987–991.

175. Schimrigk K, Brune N, Hellwig K et al. An open-label, prospective study of oral fumaric acid therapy for the treatment of relapsing–remitting multiple sclerosis (RRMS). Neurology 2005; 64: A392.

176. Kwak B, Mulhaupt F, Myit S et al. Statins as a newly recognized type of immunomodulator. Nat Med 2000; 6: 1399–1402.

177. Menge T, Hartung HP, Stuve O. Statins–a cure-all for the brain? Nat Rev Neurosci 2005; 6: 325–331.

178. Aktas O, Waiczies S, Smorodchenko A et al. Treatment of relapsing paralysis in experimental encephalomyelitis by targeting Th1 cells through atorvastatin. J Exp Med 2003; 197: 725–733.

179. Paintlia AS, Paintlia MK, Khan M et al. HMG-CoA reductase inhibitor augments survival and differentiation of oligodendrocyte progenitors in animal model of multiple sclerosis. FASEB J 2005; 19: 1407–1421.

180. Youssef S, Stuve O, Patarroyo JC et al. The HMG-CoA reductase inhibitor, atorvastatin, promotes a Th2 bias and reverses paralysis in central nervous system autoimmune disease. Nature 2002; 420: 78–84.

181. Rizvi SA, Bashir K. Other therapy options and future strategies for treating patients with multiple sclerosis. Neurology 2004; 63: S47–S54.

182. Vollmer T, Key L, Durkalski V et al. Oral simvastatin treatment in relapsingremitting multiple sclerosis. Lancet 2004; 363: 1607–1608.

183. Stuve O, Youssef S, Weber MS et al. Immunomodulatory synergy by combination of atorvastatin and glatiramer acetate in treatment of CNS autoimmunity. J Clin Invest 2006; 116: 1037–1044.

184. Coles AJ, Cox A, Le Page E et al. The window of therapeutic opportunity in multiple sclerosis Evidence from monoclonal antibody therapy. J Neurol 2006; 253: 98–108.

185. Coles AJ, Wing M, Smith S et al. Pulsed monoclonal antibody treatment and autoimmune thyroid disease in multiple sclerosis. Lancet 1999; 354: 1691–1695.

186. Monson NL, Cravens PD, Frohman EM et al. Effect of rituximab on the peripheral blood and cerebrospinal fluid B cells in patients with primary progressive multiple sclerosis. Arch Neurol 2005; 62: 258–264.

187. Pender MP. The pathogenesis of primary progressive multiple sclerosis: antibody-mediated attack and no repair? J Clin Neurosci 2004; 11: 689–692.

SECTION 3

Escape therapies and management of multiple sclerosis

H. El-Moslimany and A. E. Miller

INTRODUCTION

Based on the conviction that multiple sclerosis (MS) is an autoimmune disease, primarily cell-mediated, nonspecific immunosuppressants have long been used in an attempt to halt or slow disease progression. Because current disease-modifying agents are only moderately successful at preventing further exacerbations and persistent neurological deterioration, neurologists continue to resort to the use of nonspecific immunosuppressants while seeking newer more effective agents. Currently, class I evidence of benefit exists only for interferon (IFN)β,[1–3] glatiramer acetate,[4] natalizumab, and mitoxantrone.[5] Although some other agents, particularly the nonspecific immunosuppressants, have been the subject of extensive research, none has been clearly determined to provide benefit in double-blinded, randomized, placebo-controlled trials. The newer agents still require study for safety as well as efficacy, a concern intensified after the occurrence of progressive multifocal leukoencephalopathy associated with natalizumab.[6] This chapter will review a variety of drugs or procedures that have been studied for the treatment of MS and suggest a context for their use. Before the agents are discussed individually, however, one must consider the circumstances that would prompt their use.

TREATMENT FAILURE

Multiple sclerosis is a chronic inflammatory disease of the central nervous system (CNS) in which immune-mediated events result in demyelination and also probably lead to axon damage, ultimately causing neurological disability. Inflammatory events are recognized more frequently in the early stages both as clinical attacks and MRI disease activity. Often, over time, inflammatory events diminish in frequency. Progressive neurological disability may also result from neurodegeneration.

Controversy exists over whether inflammation or neurodegeneration is the primary pathological process in MS[7] but most investigators agree that inflammation plays an important role in the eventual development of neurological disability. Trapp et al found that axon destruction occurs in active lesions.[8] IFNβ treatment has decreased clinical disease activity and, more strikingly, lesions that are evident on magnetic resonance imaging (MRI).[1,2,9–12] Hence, reduction of inflammation may potentially limit subsequent disability, as has been demonstrated, for example, in some of the trials of IFNβ.[1,3]

The clinical trials of various immunomodulatory drugs for the treatment of MS have demonstrated a modest reduction in the relapse rate and limited effects on disability. Relatively few patients were completely free of disease activity in each study ranging in duration from 24 weeks to 6 years. Thus, for most patients the treatment was only partially effective in controlling the clinical expressions of disease.

Establishing precise definitions of treatment failure is difficult. Rio et al[13] examined different criteria for treatment failure in a cohort of relapsing–remitting MS (RRMS) patients treated with IFNβ. They noted that determinations of progression that rely on a certain degree of deterioration on clinical rating scales sustained for 3 or 6 months may include a significant proportion of erroneously categorized treatment failures because of delayed improvement after exacerbations. In an extension of their work, Rio et al[14] concluded, after applying various criteria for nonresponsiveness after 2 years of IFN treatment, that the development of disability (confirmed after 6 months) was more sensitive, specific and accurate in predicting progression to considerable disability (median Expanded Disability Status Scale (EDSS) 6.5) after 6 years than measures that relied totally or in part on relapses.[14] The Multiple Sclerosis Therapy Consensus Group determined that no recommendations regarding the optimal total duration of treatment with any immunomodulatory regimen in MS can be considered to be evidence-based.[15] Patients should be evaluated every 3–6 months using the EDSS and the Multiple Sclerosis Functional Composite score (MSFC). If worsening is apparent on clinical examination, as determined by the EDSS and MSFC, the patient should undergo an MRI of the brain with gadolinium. If clinical worsening is present, escalation of treatment with either a different disease-modifying agent or a nonspecific immunosuppressant for the management of disease may be considered at this stage.

Clearly, clinical relapses often produce a sustained effect on disability. Lublin et al found residual deficit months after the first in-study relapse among placebo-treated patients who participated in the trials of the disease-modifying agents.[16] Also, evidence suggests that inflammation contributes to cumulative neurological impairment,[17,18] e.g. the observation by Weinshenker et al that patients who have an increased frequency of relapses in the first years of MS have a higher risk of later disability.[17] In the CHAMPS trial of patients who had a positive MRI at the time of their initial neurological event, the best predictors of the development of clinically definite MS over a short interval were the presence of gadolinium-enhancing lesions and satisfaction of the Barkhof MRI criteria[19] for dissemination in space.[20]

Recent functional MRI studies have suggested that relapse recovery involves adaptive recruitment of networks of additional brain regions to restore function.[21–23] Therefore, multiple attacks may gradually erode the reserve available for recruitment and, consequently, some might consider that any attack is an indication of suboptimal treatment response. Most neurologists would agree that patients who are still having frequent attacks on disease-modifying therapy are suboptimal responders, especially if serial examinations demonstrate progression of neurological impairment. Insidious progression also indicates a suboptimal treatment response but, in the absence of signs of active inflammation, has negative implications for a response to any immunosuppressive agent. An important issue is whether to use MRI findings alone to determine suboptimal response. New enhancing lesions are associated with increased relapse rates and increased T2 lesion burden, and may be associated with progression of disability in the short term in patients with RRMS.[24–28] Since the disease-modifying agents, particularly the IFNs, reduce the number of new T2 lesions, an increasing T2 lesion burden in a patient on therapy might be considered indicative of a suboptimal response.[28–30] However, because existing US Food and Drug Administration (FDA)-approved disease-modifying therapies are only moderately effective in reducing MRI activity and because the correlation of T2 disease burden on brain MRI with clinical activity is weak, using change in MRI alone as a basis for changing treatment is problematic.

A task force of MS specialists convened by the National Multiple Sclerosis Society of the USA recently recommended criteria for determining suboptimal response to therapy and changing treatment. The task force advised that patients remain on a medication for at least a year before a judgment of suboptimal response is made.[31] Suboptimal responders would then be patients who had experienced more than one attack per year or had failed to show a reduction from the pretreatment relapse rate. The patient can also be considered a suboptimal responder if there has been an increase in the EDSS of 1 point from a baseline score of 3.0–5.5 or a 0.5 point increase from a baseline score of 6.0 or greater. The task force cautioned, however, about basing a decision to change treatment on deterioration in EDSS score that was associated with an acute exacerbation, because of the potential for recovery.

Although new activity on the MRI is a cause for concern, the task force opposed switching therapy on the basis of changes on regularly scheduled or periodic MRIs alone, in the absence of clinical activity. However, ongoing MRI activity after an attack

has occurred could support a decision to change treatment. While a significant increase of T2 disease burden is a cause for concern, the extent of change that is considered significant was not established. While current agents do not completely suppress new lesion activity, Cohen et al stated that brainstem and spinal cord lesions are more worrisome and that the presence of new lesions in those regions is sufficient reason to alter therapy.[32]

The frequency at which the physician should obtain MRIs also remains controversial. The Multiple Sclerosis Treatment Consensus Group advises obtaining MRI scans only if there is any change in EDSS or MSFC.[15] Cohen et al suggest that MRIs should be obtained when treatment is changed, in order to provide an updated baseline to determine the effectiveness of the new therapy.[32] If surveillance scans are to be done, the studies are helpful only in the first few years of disease and not after 5 years if there is little change clinically.[32] According to the NMSS task force, all patients should have a baseline brain MRI, and spinal cord MRI if the patient has myelopathic symptoms.[31] The patients should report any suspected relapse, which would then require prompt neurological examination.[31] MRI scans should be obtained in suspected suboptimal responders to support decisions to change therapy and should be obtained to establish a new baseline if change of therapy occurs.[31] If patients are developing progressive impairment, with subtle relapse activity, a follow-up MRI is needed.

Subtle symptoms affecting activities of daily living, even in the absence of a change on examination, can also be indicative of a suboptimal response to treatment if the symptom accumulation is stepwise.[32] However, potential effects of medications, sedation, increased spasticity, sleep disturbances and comorbid medical conditions must be excluded before attributing changes to a suboptimal response. Cohen et al[32] also suggested that patients developing multifocal disease affecting multiple neurological systems while on therapy could be considered suboptimal responders. A patient who experiences progressive motor or cognitive impairment sufficient to disrupt daily activities could be regarded as a suboptimal responder.

Río and his group re-examined in 2006 the question of suboptimal response to IFNβ.[33] They followed 393 patients with RRMS who were treated with IFNβ. Various criteria were examined in an attempt to define nonresponse to IFNβ, including number of relapses, disability progression or both. They found that the most clinically relevant criterion of response to IFNβ is disability progression. Disability progression was defined as an increase in the EDSS of 1.5 points for patients with a baseline EDSS of 0; an increase of 1 point for scores from 1.0–5.0, and an increase of 0.5 points for scores equal to or higher than 5.5.

Natalizumab, which is discussed in Chapter 21, was reintroduced to the market in July 2005 with a risk management program, known as TOUCH®, to minimize the potential of harm from the development of PML. Two cases of that opportunistic viral infection of the brain had occurred in patients who had received a combination of natalizumab and weekly interferon β-1a for more than 2 years.[34,35] Now, natalizumab, which reduced relapse rate by 68% and slowed EDSS progression in the monotherapy AFFIRM trial,[36] is a reasonable option for patients who are having an inadequate response to interferon or glatiramer and are willing to accept the uncertain level of risk associated with the use of that monoclonal antibody against the adhesion molecule, α4β1 integrin (VLA-4).

Irrespective of the specific criteria applied, the physician who decides a patient is failing currently approved disease-modifying therapy faces a bewildering number of agents that might be potentially beneficial. The rest of this chapter will focus on the individual drugs and procedures that are currently available. These drugs can be classified in a variety of ways, including their route of administration (Table 22.1), whether they are used alone or in combination (Table 22.2), or by their class (Table 22.3).

TABLE 22.1 Drugs for the management of multiple sclerosis, by route of administration

Drugs taken orally	Drugs taken by injection	Nonpharmacological approaches
Azathioprine	Mitoxantrone	Plasma exchange
Cyclophosphamide	Cyclophosphamide	Bone marrow transplantation
Mycophenolate mofetil	Steroids	
Methotrexate	Intravenous immunoglobulin	
Cladribine	Alemtuzumab	
Tacrolimus	Rituximab	
Ciclosporin	Daclizumab	
Sulfasalazine		

TABLE 22.2 Therapies for the management of multiple sclerosis, by method of use

Therapies used by themselves	Therapies used in combination with interferon-β
Azathioprine	Azathioprine
Ciclosporin	Ciclosporin
Mitoxantrone	Methotrexate
Methotrexate	Mycophenolate mofetil
Mycophenolate mofetil	Alemtuzumab
Intravenous immunoglobulin	Daclizumab
Plasma exchange	
Tacrolimus	
Ciclosporin	
Sulfasalazine	
Alemtuzumab	
Rituximab	
Daclizumab	
Bone marrow transplantation	

TABLE 22.3 Classes of drug studied in the management of multiple sclerosis

Antineoplastic agents	Immunosuppressants
Mitoxantrone	Cyclophosphamide
Methotrexate	Azathioprine
Rituximab	Steroids
	Mycophenolate mofetil
	Cladribine
	Intravenous immunoglobulin
	Tacrolimus
	Ciclosporin
	Alemtuzumab
	Daclizumab

MITOXANTRONE

Mitoxantrone (Novantrone) was the first drug approved by the FDA for treatment of patients with secondary progressive MS (SPMS) or with a worsening relapsing disease course.[37] This approval was based on the results of a multicenter, randomized, placebo-controlled phase III trial.[5] Like Adriamycin and daunorubicin, mitoxantrone is an anthracenedione, which is used as an antineoplastic agent alone or in combination therapy for the treatment of prostate cancer, non-Hodgkin's lymphoma and acute nonlymphocytic leukemia.[38–40]

Mitoxantrone intercalates into DNA through hydrogen bonding, causing crosslinks and strand breaks.[38] It also interferes with DNA topoisomerase II.[38] When DNA is replicated or transcribed, the topological formation of DNA is altered, resulting in a DNA molecule that is not in the correct formation, making it impossible to undergo further transcription or replication.[41] DNA topoisomerase II is an enzyme that helps in the separation of two intertwined daughter DNA molecules after DNA replication by the transient formation of double-strand breaks.[42] The transient breaks allow the DNA molecules to separate and then rewind into the correct topological formation prior to ligation. Mitoxantrone affects replication by inhibiting

topoisomerase II in dividing and nondividing cells. Most pharmacokinetic data in humans were generated through its use in cancer patients receiving daily doses of this drug.[43,44]

Mitoxantrone is 80% plasma-protein-bound and its half-life is approximately 1–3 hours. The drug is extensively distributed in various tissues and metabolized primarily in the liver. In MS, some of its beneficial clinical effects are believed to be attributable to the suppression of replication of autoreactive T cells, B cells and macrophages.[42] In vitro studies demonstrated that mitoxantrone impairs antigen presentation and the secretion of inflammatory cytokines, including IFNγ, tumor necrosis factor (TNF)α, and interleukin (IL)-2.[45,46]

Mitoxantrone can cause cardiotoxicity, which may manifest as tachycardia and arrhythmia, asymptomatic decrease in measures of left ventricular ejection fraction, or symptomatic congestive heart failure.[47] An increased risk of cardiotoxicity is also associated with higher cumulative doses of mitoxantrone, prior treatment with anthracyclines, prior mediastinal radiotherapy and pre-existing cardiovascular disease. It is therefore mandatory that patients undergo evaluation of their cardiac output before initiation of therapy, if they develop signs and symptoms of congestive heart failure, and before each dose when the drug is administered every 3 months, as currently recommended.[48] MS patients with a left ventricular ejection fraction of less than 50% or signs of congestive heart failure should not be treated with this drug.[47] Patients should also be asked if they have ever been treated with mitoxantrone or one of the anthracyclines. Factors resulting in mitoxantrone-induced cardiotoxicity are not entirely understood but may include formation of reactive oxygen intermediates that lead to damage of myocardial tissue. Another explanation for cardiotoxicity is that the impairment of DNA repair by mitoxantrone's inhibition of topoisomerase II may exert a cytocidal effect on myocardial cells by chelating with iron and forming complexes. The myocardial damage is due to intracellular generation of reactive oxygen intermediates via iron- or enzyme-mediated oxidation–reduction reactions.[49] Myocytes appear to be selectively susceptible to the formation of reactive oxygen intermediates because of their relative lack of defense mechanisms such as catalase and superoxide dismutase.[49] Dexrazoxane is an iron chelator that can prevent iron–mitoxantrone complex formation, potentially inhibiting the generation of reactive oxygen intermediates.[50] It may be a potential cardioprotectant, but more investigation is necessary.[51] A study analyzing the long-term safety and tolerability of mitoxantrone in MS patients is expected to be completed in 2007.[49]

Leukemia, albeit rare, is another serious adverse effect of mitoxantrone.[49] Topoisomerase II inhibitors are associated with characteristic toxic acute myelogenous leukemias (AMLs) that differ from those reported with alkylating agents.[49] Topoisomerase-II-related AMLs exhibit shorter latency (median 2 years), absence of a myelodysplastic phase and characteristic chromosomal aberrations.[49] An increased risk for leukemia has been observed in breast cancer patients when mitoxantrone was used in combination with other alkylating agents and radiotherapy.[52] In a series of breast cancer patients, the prognosis for toxic AML was poorer than for those with de novo cases of AML.[52,53] At least seven cases of toxic AML and two cases of promyelocytic leukemia have been reported in association with mitoxantrone therapy for MS.[52–60] In contrast to the experience with breast cancer patients, most of the MS cases had a favorable response to therapy for leukemia.[61] Previous exposure to alkylating agents may increase the risk for mitoxantrone-associated leukemia and may account for some of the difference in the two populations. The cancer patients may also have received higher doses. Mitoxantrone should be used with caution in patients who have received previous cytotoxic therapy (e.g. cyclophosphamide). Because the total number of MS patients treated with mitoxantrone is unknown, it is difficult to determine an accurate incidence rate.[62] Ongoing registries will help to further determine the frequency of toxic leukemias in association with mitoxantrone monotherapy for MS. An estimate of 0.07% has been reported based on a review of three series comprising over 1300 patients.[49]

Patients treated with mitoxantrone usually develop transitory leukopenia and neutropenia, with the nadir typically occurring 10–14 days postinfusion.[49] Mitoxantrone should not be used in patients who are otherwise immunosuppressed.[58] Treatment with mitoxantrone can cause uremia and may lead to acute attacks of gout.[49,63] Thrombocytopenia may also occur.[49,63] Other less serious adverse effects include reversible alopecia, temporary discoloration of sclera and urine, sinus congestion, constipation, diarrhea, nausea, vomiting, headaches, dysmenorrhea and cervical lymphadenopathy.[49]

Mitoxantrone may cause birth defects if either the female or the male partner was being treated at the time of conception or during pregnancy.[49] Sterility, sometimes permanent, has been reported when the drug was used alone or in combination with other antineoplastic agents.[63] Permanent amenorrhea occurs in about 14% of women over the age of 35.[49] Female patients should not breast-feed.

The FDA has approved the use of mitoxantrone in SPMS and worsening relapsing MS when administered at $12\,mg/m^2$ once every 3 months until the lifetime cumulative dose of $140\,mg/m^2$ is met, based on the phase II safety trial[64,65] and the phase III randomized, placebo-controlled, double blind trial (MIMS trial).[5] The phase II trial included 42 MS patients with very active disease by clinical and MRI criteria who were randomized to

receive monthly intravenous pulse doses of either 20 mg mitoxantrone plus 1 g methylprednisolone or 1 g methylprednisolone alone for 6 months. In the methylprednisolone alone group, five patients dropped out because of severe clinical exacerbations.[65] Blinded analysis of MRI data showed significantly fewer new enhancing lesions in the mitoxantrone group.[65] Unblinded clinical assessments showed a significant improvement in clinical disability and a significant reduction in the number of relapses at months 2–6 in the mitoxantrone-treated group.[65]

The MIMS trial included 194 patients who had relapsing–progressive MS (i.e. relapsing disease with incomplete recovery between relapses) or SPMS.[5] Patients were randomized to receive either placebo, low-dose intravenous mitoxantrone ($5\,mg/m^2$), or high-dose mitoxantrone ($12\,mg/m^2$) every 3 months for 24 months. The total follow-up time was 36 months. The primary efficacy outcome consisted of five clinical measures tested in one composite of stochastic ordered alternatives: change from baseline EDSS at 24 months, change from baseline ambulation index at 24 months, number of relapses treated with corticosteroids, time to first treated relapse, and change from baseline standardized neurological status at 24 months.[5] Secondary endpoints included the proportion of patients with deterioration of at least 1 EDSS point, proportion of patients with such EDSS deterioration confirmed after 3 months and 6 months, time to first sustained EDSS deterioration, time to first relapse, number and annual rate of relapses, proportion of patients without relapse, number of days in hospital, use of wheelchair assistance, and quality of life assessed by the Stanford Health Assessment Questionnaire.[5] The high-dose ($12\,mg/m^2$) mitoxantrone-treated group showed a 64% reduction in sustained disease progression and a 69% reduction in the number of treated relapses compared with the placebo control group.[5] Blinded evaluations of brain MRI scans from a subgroup of patients showed a decrease of gadolinium-enhancing lesions and T2-weighted lesion load in the high-dose mitoxantrone-treated group compared with the placebo treatment group.[5] The correlation of improvement in the clinical outcome measures with diminished CNS inflammation as measured by brain MRI suggests that broad-spectrum immunosuppression is of some benefit in patients with progressive MS.[5]

Gonsette noted that an induction phase with 3-monthly administrations of $12\,mg/m^2$ of mitoxantrone followed by a maintenance phase every 3 months seems to be a good compromise, allowing treatment for at least 2 years with an acceptable lifetime dose. An induction phase may be helpful in the control of rapidly progressive disease, but then a rapid switch to maintenance therapy would allow a longer period of treatment for a chronic disease.[66] Mitoxantrone has been shown to be effective in patients with active inflammatory disease in a randomized, double blind trial comparing it to methylprednisolone.[67] Despite Gonsette's suggestion, opinion differs about the dose regimen and whether to use mitoxantrone alone or with methylprednisolone. However, practice recommendations for the use of mitoxantrone state that the medication should be used in patients with rapidly advancing disease who have failed other therapies, and that patients can receive a dose every 3 months. Cardiac, liver and kidney function should be regularly monitored in patients taking mitoxantrone.[68]

SUMMARY

Mitoxantrone is the only medication approved by the FDA for severe relapsing disease (both RRMS and SPMS). Side effects, particularly cardiotoxicity, limit the lifetime dosage of the medication, thereby limiting the length of time during which a patient can be treated with it. Issues such as optimal dosage and frequency of administration still need to be resolved.

AZATHIOPRINE

Azathioprine is cleaved to 6-mercaptopurine, which in turn is converted to additional metabolites that inhibit de novo purine synthesis.[69,70] The metabolite is incorporated into DNA and gene translation is inhibited.[69,71] Azathioprine may reduce levels of TNFα and increase suppressor–inducer lymphocytes.[72] The side effects include bone marrow suppression with leukopenia, thrombocytopenia and/or anemia.[72] An increased susceptibility to infections, hepatotoxicity, alopecia, gastrointestinal toxicity, pancreatitis and increased risk of neoplasia may occur.[73] Patients who take azathioprine may also develop an idiosyncratic hypersensitivity reaction.[74] This reaction has been reported in about 2% of patients with inflammatory bowel disease[75] and ranges in occurrence from 11–15% in rheumatoid arthritis[76] and myasthenia gravis.[77] In one report of azathioprine intolerance in MS, many patients had nausea, myalgia and arthralgia, which manifests early in the course of therapy, with most of the patients withdrawing from therapy within 2 months of initiation.[75] Patients could also have vomiting, diarrhea, rash, purpura, fever, dermatitis and malaise.[78] The symptoms disappear upon withdrawal of the drug and re-emerge when the patient is rechallenged.[78]

In a British and Dutch prospective, double-blind, placebo-controlled, randomized trial, patients with RRMS and SPMS[79] were treated for 3 years with either azathioprine 2.5 mg/kg/d or placebo. No difference between the treatment and placebo groups was seen in the first 3 years after the start of the trial, so follow-up was continued up to 4.5 years. After the first year, the EDSS score had worsened slightly more in the azathioprine group compared to placebo but the ambulation index was better in the azathioprine group. In subsequent years, the patients in the azathioprine group deteriorated slightly less than the patients taking placebo. The only statistically significant difference was a reduction in the deterioration of the ambulation index of the patients taking azathioprine compared to those taking placebo after 3 years of study.

At the last follow-up, in July 2002, of the 149 patients who had received active drug, 34 had died and 12 had diagnosed cancers.[80] In the placebo group, 40 had died and seven had diagnosed cancers. The increase in cancer and deaths in patients with a diagnosis of cancer in those taking azathioprine was not statistically significant.[80] However, another study examining the risk of cancer in patients treated with azathioprine showed an increased risk of cancer after 10 years of continuous therapy.[81]

Another prospective, double-blind, placebo-controlled trial randomized 59 patients who had experienced at least two exacerbations in the 18 months prior to the beginning of the study to receive either 3 mg/kg/day of azathioprine or placebo for 2 years.[82] Results suggested that azathioprine may reduce rates of relapse in patients with relapsing forms of MS. However, side effects are common, particularly gastrointestinal disorders and hematological disorders, which may affect drug adherence.[82]

A meta-analysis of published blinded, placebo-controlled trials showed that azathioprine significantly increases the likelihood of remaining relapse-free and marginally decreases progression of disability after 2–3 years of treatment, but not after the first year.[83,84] However, whether the slight clinical benefits of azathioprine outweigh the risks is debatable.

COMBINATION WITH INTERFERON

The combination of azathioprine with IFNβ-1b was evaluated in an open-label pilot study of six RRMS patients with continuing disease activity despite IFNβ-1b treatment.[85] The addition of azathioprine to IFNβ-1b decreased the number of contrast-enhancing lesions by 69% after a period of 15 months compared to the IFNβ-1b only group. Azathioprine with IFNβ-1a was evaluated in another open-label study in RRMS patients who were not responsive to either IFNβ-1a or azathioprine as monotherapy, or who had never been previously treated.[86]

The dose of azathioprine was adjusted to reduce lymphocyte count to 1000/µl in association with IFNβ-1a at a dose of 6 MIU every other day. The number of new lesions was decreased on MRI and the number of relapses and change in EDSS was less on the combined therapy when compared to the observations in the same patients prior to combined therapy.

SUMMARY

In the blinded, placebo-controlled trials for the treatment of MS with azathioprine, one trial showed a possible benefit of azathioprine in the reduction of relapses in MS while the other trial showed no benefit for the treatment of MS. These studies, as well as published meta-analysis, suggest that azathioprine as monotherapy has, at best, marginal benefit in MS. The combination of azathioprine with IFNβ has only been evaluated in open-label studies, which showed some benefit, but until the combination is studied in rigorous, double-blinded trials, the results are not very helpful. Consideration of the use of azathioprine should be further tempered by its adverse effect profile, including a probable increased risk of cancer with long-term use.

CYCLOPHOSPHAMIDE

Cyclophosphamide is an alkylating agent that is chemically related to the nitrogen mustards. The drug undergoes metabolic activation (hydroxylation) by the cytochrome P450 system, with transport of the activated intermediate to sites of action,[87] where it forms covalent linkages by alkylation of various nucleophilic moieties. The cytotoxic effects are directly related to the alkylation of DNA. Cyclophosphamide is used for the treatment of many autoimmune disorders, including Wegener's granulomatosis, polyarteritis nodosa, polymyositis, peripheral neuropathies[88] and lupus nephritis.[89,90] Toxicity includes myelosuppression with platelet sparing, alopecia, nausea, vomiting, mucosal ulcerations, interstitial pulmonary fibrosis, sterile hemorrhagic cystitis (reduced by MESNA[90]), the syndrome of inappropriate antidiuresis, amenorrhea and gonadal failure.[91]

IMMUNOLOGIC EFFECTS OF CYCLOPHOSPHAMIDE

Cyclophosphamide suppresses experimental autoimmune encephalomyelitis (EAE).[92] In humans, it enters the CNS and reduces cerebrospinal fluid (CSF) myelin basic protein (MBP) and IgG.[93–96] The drug causes lymphopenia involving T and B cells, with a more pronounced effect on CD4+ cells,[97–99] which usually resolves 4 months after treatment is stopped. It increases the anti-inflammatory cytokines IL-4, IL-5, IL-10 and transforming growth factor (TGF)β and is associated with eosinophilia.[100–102] Cyclophosphamide also decreases IL-12, which has been linked to its therapeutic response.[103] The levels of IL-12 pretreatment may have predictive value, as patients who have higher levels of IL-12 pretreatment do not respond as well.[104] Cyclophosphamide preferentially induces antigen Th2 responses to myelin autoantigens[102] and shifts immune responses from T helper (Th)1 towards Th2.[103]

USE IN MULTIPLE SCLEROSIS

Cyclophosphamide has been used for the treatment of MS since 1966.[90] Open-label studies of short duration demonstrated positive effects in small populations of both RRMS and progressive patients.[105–107] Hommes[108] studied a group of 32 progressive patients who were treated in an uncontrolled open-label trial with 100 mg oral cyclophosphamide four times daily and 50 mg prednisone twice daily.[108] The patients received a total of 8 g cyclophosphamide over 20 days. The authors reported stabilization in 69% of patients over a period of 1–5 years. Hommes[109] studied 39 patients with chronic progressive disease in another open-label, uncontrolled trial, which also showed stabilization in 69% of the patients over a period of 1–5 years.[109] Factors that predicted a good response to therapy included disease onset before 28 years of age, short duration of disease prior to treatment, rapid progression of disease, low initial disability and HLA-DRw2 positivity.[102] Hommes[110] also reported six patients with chronic progressive MS who had been treated with oral cyclophosphamide plus prednisone in order to induce leukopenia below 2000/mm^3.[110] The authors found that CSF and serum levels of cyclophosphamide were in the same range, indicating that cyclophosphamide crosses the blood–brain barrier and, perhaps, is effective in the CNS.

In a retrospective study, Theys and colleagues, on the other hand, reported that patients with moderately advanced MS experienced no benefit from treatment with 6–8 g of cyclophosphamide given over 3–4 weeks compared to patients with similar disability scores who were not treated with cyclophosphamide.[111] Gonsette and colleagues reported on 110 patients in an open-label study, with follow up for 2–6 years.[112] Patients were treated with 1–2 g intravenous cyclophosphamide without corticosteroids over a 1–2-week period, with dosage adjusted to maintain a leukopenia of 2000 and lymphopenia of 1000 for 2–3 weeks. The annual relapse rate decreased by 75% compared to the relapse rate 1–2 years prior to treatment in 70% of patients. The most pronounced effects occurred in those patients with the shortest duration of disease. Patients who were already severely handicapped experienced no benefit. Some 30% of patients failed to respond to cyclophosphamide.

Open-label studies with cyclophosphamide have shown positive results in patients refractory to currently approved disease-modifying therapies.[113,114] Weinstock-Guttman reported 75% improved or stable at 12 months following induction therapy with intravenous cyclophosphamide followed by maintenance therapy with cyclophosphamide and either methotrexate, methylprednisolone or IFNβ-1b in an open-label study involving 17 patients.[115] Of these, 13 either improved or were stable at 12 months, and nine of the 13 remained stable at 24 months. Khan reported clinical improvement or stability in an open-label study of 14 consecutive patients with clinically definite MS who had severe clinical deterioration during the 12 months prior to treatment with cyclophosphamide.[116] The patients received monthly cyclophosphamide pulses for 6 months with doses adjusted to achieve a leukocyte nadir of 2000–2200 cells/mm^3 followed by resumption of one of the approved disease-modifying therapies. All patients were followed for at least 18 months after the first dose of cyclophosphamide.

Gobbini and colleagues treated five patients with RRMS not responsive to immunomodulatory therapies with monthly pulses of cyclophosphamide (1000 mg/m^2), in an open-label study.[113] Patients were followed with monthly MRI and clinical evaluation for a mean of 28 months. All patients showed a rapid reduction in contrast-enhancing lesion frequency and three patients experienced a decrease in T2 lesion load within 5 months of starting therapy.

A randomized double-blind placebo-controlled trial evaluated 14 RRMS patients, six of whom were treated with monthly pulses of 750 mg/m^2 intravenous cyclophosphamide for 1 year.[117] Although fewer relapses occurred in the treated patients than in the placebo patients after 1 year of treatment, the results were not statistically significant. A Canadian study evaluating cyclophosphamide and plasma exchange in 168 patients with progressive disease in a randomized, double-blind, placebo-controlled study found no difference between the treatment and the placebo groups.[118] Patients with progressive MS received either active drug treatment consisting of 1 g of cyclophosphamide on alternate days until the leukocyte count fell below 4.5 or until 9 g had been administered plus 40 mg prednisone orally for 10 days, placebo, or plasma exchange. Of the cyclophosphamide-treated patients, 60% were classified as chronic–progressive whereas 40% were relapsing–progressive. Although a positive trend early in the study favored the cyclophosphamide-treated patients, subsequently the cyclophosphamide group fared worse than the placebo group. Notably, though, the Canadian study reported stable disease in two-thirds of their placebo patients. The study results suggest that cyclophosphamide is not effective in later stages of progressive MS, when inflammation is probably playing a lesser role in the disease process.[102]

In a randomized, single-blind, placebo-controlled study in 22 progressive patients, Likosky and colleagues found no difference between cyclophosphamide-treated patients and the placebo group over a 24-month treatment period.[119]

In a multicenter study of 489 patients, Zephir and colleagues found that, after 12 months of pulse cyclophosphamide, 78.6% of the SPMS and 73.5% of the primary progressive MS (PPMS) patients had stabilized or had an improved EDSS.[120] In this study, for patients with an EDSS score of 5 or less, improvement or worsening was defined as at least a 1 point variation on EDSS. For patients with an EDSS score of 5.5, improvement was defined as at least a one point improvement, and worsening was at least 0.5 point worsening. For patients with an EDSS of 6 or over, improvement or worsening corresponded to at least a 0.5 point variation. There was no difference in treatment response among the groups. The apparent beneficial response to cyclophosphamide in SPMS patients was linked to the presence of superimposed relapses during the year prior to treatment, supporting the hypothesis that cyclophosphamide is most effective when there is an inflammatory component to the disease. Perini and colleagues reported development of fewer T2 lesions and gadolinium-enhancing lesions on MRI in 26 secondary progressive patients given monthly intravenous cyclophosphamide at 800–1250 mg/m^2 for 1 year and then every 8 weeks the second year.[121]

The safety and tolerability of cyclophosphamide pulse therapy was further evaluated by Portaccio et al in primary progressive or SPMS patients who had experienced deterioration of at least 0.5 points on the EDSS in the year prior to treatment and in RRMS patients who had a high relapse rate with incomplete remission.[122] A total of 112 patients received monthly pulses of 700 mg/m^2 of cyclophosphamide for 12 months followed by a bimonthly administration at the same dosage for an additional 12 months. Side effects included urinary tract infections (56.3%), nausea and vomiting (38.4%), amenorrhea (33.3%), lymphopenia (15%), increase of hepatic enzymes (10.8%), hypogammaglobulinemia 6.3%, respiratory tract infections (6%), alopecia, hemorrhagic cystitis, macroscopic hematuria, microscopic hematuria, hypersensitivity reaction and leukopenia. Four patients (3.6%) had developed malignancies but three of these had previously been treated with azathioprine.

TREATMENT REGIMENS

A variety of regimens for intravenous cyclophosphamide for the treatment of MS have been suggested (Table 22.4).[102] In one 8-day induction protocol, 600 mg/m^2 of cyclophosphamide is given on days 1, 2, 4, 6 and 8 along with daily methylprednisolone. In another protocol, 1 g of methylprednisolone is

TABLE 22.4 Regimens for intravenous cyclophosphamide for the treatment of multiple sclerosis

Protocol	Administration route	Dosage	Frequency	Duration	Adjuvant therapy
1	Intravenous	600 mg/m^2	Day 1, 2, 4, 6, 8	8 d	i.v. methylprednisolone
2	Intravenous	800 mg/m^{2*}	q.4 weeks	12 cycles	i.v. methylprednisolone†
3	Intravenous	800 mg/m^{2*}	q.6 weeks	12 cycles	i.v. methylprednisolone†
4	Intravenous	800 mg/m^{2*}	q.8 weeks	12 cycles	i.v. methylprednisolone†
5	Intravenous	800–1000 mg/m^2	q.4–8 weeks	12–24 months	None

*Variable dosage to maintain a leucopenia of 2000/mm^3, maximum dosage 1600 mg/mm^3. †Initially 5 days of 1 g of i.v. methylprednisolone, then 1 g of i.v. methylprednisolone administered at the same time as the cyclophosphamide.
Source: Adapted from reference 102.

administered daily for 5 days, followed by intravenous pulses of cyclophosphamide with 1 g of methylprednisolone. The cyclophosphamide pulses begin at 800 mg/m^2 and the dose is escalated to produce a leukopenia of 2000/mm^3. The cyclophosphamide and methylprednisolone can be given every 4 weeks for 12 cycles, every 6 weeks for 12 cycles or every 2 months for 12 cycles. The maximum cyclophosphamide dose for this protocol is 1600 mg/m^2.

If one does not want to deal with variable doses of cyclophosphamide, one can give intravenous pulse therapy of cyclophosphamide, either with or without methylprednisolone, at a fixed dose of 800–1000 mg/m^2 every 4–8 weeks for 12–24 months. If patients are not responding well to IFNβ or glatiramer acetate, some authors suggest the use of intravenous pulse cyclophosphamide therapy using one of the above protocols, in combination with an approved disease-modifying agent.

COMBINATION WITH INTERFERON

The addition of a cyclophosphamide regimen to IFNβ treatment has been reported to show benefit in small open-label studies of patients with rapidly 'transitional' MS,[123–125] a stage during which a RRMS patient may be converting to a secondary progressive course. In some, this transition is associated with rapidly progressive deterioration unresponsive to steroid therapy.[123] In one open-label, unblinded trial of consecutive patients with clinically definite MS that became rapidly progressive following an initial relapsing–remitting course, 10 patients were treated with cyclophosphamide and methylprednisolone followed by IFNβ maintenance therapy.[123] Two of the 10 patients had become rapidly progressive while taking IFN therapy for 1 year or more. Treatment consisted of cyclophosphamide 500 mg/m^2 and 1000 mg daily methylprednisolone by intravenous infusion for 5 days. Then 6 weeks after cyclophosphamide/methylprednisolone induction, patients were started on either IFNβ-1b or IFNβ-1a. At 3 months, seven patients were improved by 1.0 EDSS and three remained stable. At 12 months, five of seven remained improved and two of seven were stable. No serious complications of treatment occurred.

Patti and colleagues reported on the effectiveness of a combination of cyclophosphamide and IFNβ in patients with rapidly progressive or 'transitional' MS characterized by frequent and severe attacks plus worsening on the disability status scale.[124] A total of 10 patients underwent monthly pulses of intravenous cyclophosphamide to obtain a lymphopenia of between 600 and 900/mm^3 for 12 consecutive months and then at 2-month intervals for a further 6 months. The authors reported a significant reduction of the number of relapses, progression, disability and T2 MRI burden of disease. Leukopenia and nausea were the most frequent side effects.

Patti and colleagues reported 36-month clinical and MRI follow-up on the patients reported in their 2001 study who had received 18 months of combination therapy with IFNβ and cyclophosphamide.[125] The patients were found to have stable relapse rates, EDSS, T2 MRI burden and lesion number. No gadolinium-enhancing lesions had appeared.

Patti's group looked at another ten patients with rapidly transitional MS (extremely active with very frequent and severe attacks, which produced a dramatic increase on the EDSS), who were treated with IFNβ without benefit (six on intramuscular IFNβ-1a, four on IFNβ-1b).[126] Monthly treatment with intravenous cyclophosphamide from 500–1500 mg/m^2 was titrated to produce a chronic lymphocytopenia. Patients experienced a marked and significant reduction in the number of relapses, disability accumulated and T2 MRI lesion burden. The EDSS was stable in all patients 1 year after the treatment course and relapses occurred with very low frequency. Side effects, including leukopenia and nausea, were mild. One patient developed a peripheral neuropathy. Weiner and colleagues analyzed the data from multiple trials involving cyclophosphamide and concluded that its use can be effective in MS during the active inflammatory component of the disease.[102]

SUMMARY

Many, but not all, unblinded studies of cyclophosphamide appear to show a benefit of the drug, used alone or in combination with IFN. Unfortunately, double-blind studies have generally failed to prove a benefit. Cyclophosphamide tends to show an effect in patients who are earlier in their disease process, with a recent history of multiple relapses and multiple gadolinium enhancing lesions on MRI.[127–129] Once the disease enters the later, progressive stages, with less accumulation of T2 lesions, the drug is not effective.[102,127] The use of cyclophosphamide is worth considering for patients with very aggressive disease or rapidly progressive disease with a high frequency of relapses and a rapid accumulation of disability, particularly after a suboptimal response to high dose IFNβ therapy. Patients should be informed of the absence of convincing blinded, placebo-controlled data substantiating its benefit, and adequately educated about its risks.

MYCOPHENOLATE MOFETIL

Mycophenolate mofetil is a prodrug rapidly hydrolyzed to the active drug, mycophenolic acid, which is a selective, uncompetitive and reversible inhibitor of inosine monophosphate dehydrogenase, an important enzyme in the de novo pathway of guanine nucleotide synthesis.[130] B or T lymphocytes are highly dependent on the inosine monophosphate dehydrogenase pathway for cell proliferation, whereas other cell types use salvage pathways. Thus, mycophenolate mofetil inhibits lymphocyte proliferation and functions. The addition of guanosine or deoxyguanosine to the cells can reverse the effects of myco-phenolic acid on lymphocytes. Side effects of mycophenolate mofetil include leukopenia, diarrhea, vomiting and increased incidence of some infections, especially cytomegalovirus.[131,132]

IMMUNOLOGICAL EFFECTS OF MYCOPHENOLATE MOFETIL

Mycophenolate mofetil almost completely inhibits antibody formation and inhibits superantigen induction of IL-1, IL-2, IL-3, IL-4, IL-5, IL-6, IL-10, TNFα, TGFβ and granulocyte–macrophage colony-stimulating factor (GM-CSF) but not mitogen induction.[133] Mycophenolate also impairs the synthesis of adhesion molecules, which facilitate the attachment of leu-kocytes to endothelial cells and target cells.[134] Its use in MS is based on studies in experimental allergic encephalomyelitis, where treatment with mycophenolate at the onset of clinical symptoms resulted in a more rapid recovery than in control or ciclosporin-treated mice.[135] Oral treatment with mycophenolate mofetil from the day of immunization for 2 weeks both signifi-cantly delayed the development of active experimental allergic encephalomyelitis in Lewis rats and reduced the antibody response to MBP. Rats treated with mycophenolate mofetil had less infiltration of T cells, B cells, macrophages and dendritic cells into brainstems than either the control or ciclosporin-treated rats. The brainstems of mycophenolate-mofetil-treated rats also had lower levels of mRNA for Th1 (IL-2, IL-12Rβ2, IFNγ), Th2 (IL-4, IL-10) cytokines and TNFα and TGFβ than ciclosporin-treated and control groups.

Frohman et al[133] reviewed their experience with the use of mycophenolate mofetil in 79 patients (14 with RRMS, 61 with SPMS, four with PPMS) who were not responsive to currently approved disease-modifying therapy.[136] Patients were started on mycophenolate mofetil at 250 mg b.i.d. for 1 week, then 500 mg b.i.d. for 1 week, then 750 mg b.i.d. for 1 week and 1000 mg b.i.d. thereafter. Of the patients, 15 used mycophenolate as monotherapy while the rest took it as an adjunctive treatment with glatiramer acetate or IFNβ. A total of 70% of the patients continued mycophenolate mofetil for an average of 12 months. Eight patients discontinued therapy because of side effects, most commonly diarrhea, one of which was secondary to cytomega-lovirus. One stopped because of abnormal liver function studies that resolved upon drug discontinuation. Seven patients discon-tinued mycophenolate because of clinical deterioration. Subjec-tive clinical improvement was experienced by 12 patients, characterized by reduction or absence of relapse, stabilization or improvements in activities of daily living, marked reductions in daily chronic fatigue, improved ambulation, less dependency on assistive devices and greater exercise tolerance.

SUMMARY AND RECOMMENDATIONS

There are few data on the management of MS with mycophe-nolate mofetil. Available data are unblinded and without placebo control. However, because of its substantial immunosuppres-sant activity, its strong benefit in other clinical situations such as organ transplantation, its oral route of administration and its relatively good tolerability, mycophenolate mofetil seems worth trying in MS patients who are failing conventional disease-modifying therapy and may not be candidates for intra-venous immunosuppressant agents such as mitoxantrone or cyclophosphamide.

METHOTREXATE

Methotrexate, an inhibitor of dihydrofolate reductase, directly interferes with the folate-dependent enzymes of de novo purine

and thymidylate synthesis, and inhibits cell mediated immune reactions.[87] Methotrexate affects all rapidly dividing cells, so toxicity includes mucositis, myelosuppression and thrombocy-topenia. Pneumonitis characterized by patchy inflammatory infiltrates, which rapidly regresses upon discontinuation of the drug, may occur, as well as hepatic fibrosis and cirrhosis.[87]

Methotrexate was considered to be a potential treatment for MS because of its success in the treatment of rheumatoid arthri-tis, a disorder that has some immunological similarities with MS (e.g. reduced number of suppressor–inducer cells, increased ratio of helper–inducer to suppressor–inducer cells in blood).[137,138] Additionally, methotrexate inhibits the development of experi-mental allergic encephalomyelitis.[139]

An early trial suggested a reduction in exacerbation rates for RRMS patients treated with methotrexate but not for chronic progressive MS.[140] Goodkin et al treated clinically definite chronic progressive patients with weekly, oral, low-dose (7.5 mg) methotrexate for 2 years, followed by observation for an addi-tional year, in a placebo controlled, randomized, double-blinded clinical trial.[141] The improvement in the EDSS scale was not statistically significant; however, the improvement in upper extremity function as evaluated with the nine-hole peg test (16.1% failing with methotrexate treatment vs 48% failing with placebo: $n=31$) and the box and block test (12.9% failing with methotrexate vs 34.5% failing with placebo: $n=29$) was statisti-cally significant. Analysis of serial MRIs revealed a slight drop in the number of enlarging and active lesions in the methotrex-ate-treated group compared to the placebo group.[142] The change in the lesion load was related significantly to sustained change in the nine-hole peg test. Side effects, including upper respira-tory tract infection, urinary tract infection, nausea, headache, fever, mucocutaneous herpes, sore muscles, back ache, indiges-tion and diarrhea), were similarly distributed between the treat-ment and placebo group. Only three of the 31 patients in the study had to stop therapy.

COMBINATION WITH INTERFERONS

In an open-label pilot study, 21 patients who had continued to experience exacerbations while taking weekly IFNβ-1a were treated with methotrexate in addition to IFN.[143] The combina-tion was safe and well tolerated, with nausea as the major side effect (12 of 15 patients). There was a 44% reduction in the number of gadolinium-enhancing lesions (done with triple-dose gadolinium) in patients treated with methotrexate and IFN compared to those noted during treatment with IFN alone.

In another open-label study, 15 patients with relapsing MS who were worsening while on once-weekly IFNβ-1a therapy were treated with high dose intravenous methotrexate at 2 g/m² followed by leucovorin rescue.[144] Treatment was administered every 2 months for a total of six treatments. Once-weekly IFNβ-1a therapy was continued throughout the study. MSFC scores and MRIs were determined at baseline and every 4 months. Among the four patients who completed six treatments, three had an improved MSFC score and one was unchanged. Among the four patients who completed three treatments, all had posi-tive changes in MSFC. No significant hematological, renal or other toxicity occurred.

SUMMARY AND RECOMMENDATIONS

The very limited available studies on methotrexate provide little basis for enthusiasm about the use of this medication for manage-ment of MS. In particular, one double-blind, placebo-controlled study in progressive MS showed only marginal benefit.[141] Use of the drug should probably be reserved for circumstances in which other alternatives have either failed or cannot be used.

CLADRIBINE

Cladribine, an adenosine-deaminase-resistant purine analog, is converted to cladribine triphosphate and incorporated into DNA. It causes DNA strand breaks and NAD and ATP depletion, as well as apoptosis in some cell lines.[145,146] Although its mechanism of action is not entirely understood, the drug does not require cell division to be cytotoxic.[87] Cladribine's toxicity includes myelosuppression, thrombocytopenia, infections including opportunistic infections associated with low CD4+ cell counts, nausea, high fever, headache, fatigue and skin rashes.

In one study, 51 patients with MS (mostly secondary progressive) were randomized to cladribine treatment consisting of four monthly, 7-day infusions (0.1 mg/kg/d) or placebo.[147] During the second year, blinding was maintained but patients who had received placebo were given active drug at half the total dose given the drug-treated patients in the first year. In the first year of the study, the average EDSS scores and Scripps Neurologic Rating Scale (Scripps NRS) scores of patients on cladribine improved modestly while patients on placebo continued to deteriorate. Differences at 1 year were significant using both the EDSS scores and the Scripps NRS. The scores were at their best level about 18 months after beginning treatment. The patients were able to maintain their improved EDSS and SNRS scores for the 24 months of follow-up.

After 2 years, unblinded observations revealed a decline in the average scores. This suggested a dose–response effect with cladribine and a wearing off of improvement, with resumption of progressive MS symptoms in some patients 2 years after discontinuation of treatment. The number of enhancing lesions was much less in the cladribine group. Toxicity observed in this study included thrombocytopenia, leukopenia and mild dermatomal herpes zoster.

In a subsequent multicenter, double blind, placebo-controlled trial done to evaluate the safety and efficacy of cladribine in progressive MS,[148] no significant treatment effects were found for cladribine, using the Expanded Disability Status Scale scores. In this study, 159 patients, with a median Expanded Disability Status Scale of 6.0, were randomly assigned to receive either cladribine or placebo. The patients who received cladribine took 0.07 mg/kg/d for 5 consecutive days every 4 weeks for either two or six cycles (total dose 7 mg/kg or 2.1 mg/kg), followed by placebo for 8 weeks. Of these patients, 30% had PPMS while 70% had SPMS. The EDSS scores and the Scripps NRS scores were assessed bimonthly. MRIs were performed every 6 months. Even though no difference was achieved in the primary outcome measure of disability change, fewer patients receiving cladribine at either dose developed gadolinium-enhancing lesions. Patients in the cladribine group had a reduction in the number and volume of gadolinium-enhancing T1 lesions when compared to the placebo group, which was statistically significant at 6 months through month 18. The T2 burden of disease improved in the cladribine-treated group and worsened in the placebo group. Patients in the cladribine-treated group were more likely to have upper respiratory tract infections, muscle weakness, purpura, injection site reactions, hypertonia, back pain, urinary tract infections, depression, arthralgias, rhinitis, ataxia and pharyngitis. None of the side effects were treatment-limiting.

SUMMARY AND RECOMMENDATIONS

Initial trials with cladribine showed promise in the treatment of SPMS but these results were not seen in the subsequent blinded, randomized, placebo-controlled trial. Furthermore, studies of cladribine continue to show an enigmatic dissociation between positive effects on MRI and unconvincing clinical benefit. Another drawback to the use of cladribine is the pro-

found and very long-lasting lymphopenia induced by the drug. This may preclude the use of other immunosuppressant agents and administration of cladribine almost invariably disqualifies a patient from consideration for other clinical trials. At this point, it seems prudent to await the results of a prospective, randomized, blinded trial of oral cladribine before recommending its use in patients with MS.

STEROIDS

Glucocorticoids affect the immune system by inhibiting or increasing transcription of selected genes by acting through the glucocorticoid receptor.[149] The binding of the hormone to the receptor causes it to activate and translocate to the nucleus. Glucocorticoids increase the transcription of specific genes either by stabilizing the transcription preinitiation complexes at the TATA box of gene promoters or by distorting chromatin structure and unmasking binding sites for factors that facilitate initiation of transcription. They also cause repression of genes for certain inflammatory cytokines, including IL-1, IL-2–6, IL-8 and IFNγ.[150] Glucocorticoids have also been shown to inhibit mRNA translation of IL-1b.[151]

In MS, steroids decrease E selectin and ICAM-1 expression in vitro.[152] They inhibit inflammatory edema by reducing capillary permeability, resulting in a reduction of gadolinium enhancement on MR imaging.[153–155] They also inhibit metalloproteases.[156]

Steroids decrease the number of circulating CD4+ T cells and B lymphocytes, but not CD8+ cells, within 4 hours by redistribution.[157] They decrease lymphocyte proliferation to lectins and antigen, mixed lymphocyte responses and cytokine release, including IFNγ.[158] Steroids also upregulate expression of IL-10 and TGFβ.[159,160] Glucocorticoid administration leads to apoptosis of T cells activated against MBP and protects oligodendrocytes from cytokine-induced death.[161]

The Optic Neuritis Treatment Trial studied the effects of steroid treatment in monosymptomatic optic neuritis.[162,163] Patients treated with intravenous methylprednisolone had greater recovery of visual acuity, visual fields, contrast sensitivity and color vision by 2 weeks. The treatment effect on visual acuity was no longer evident at 6 months, at which time 94% of the study subjects had recovered visual acuity to 20/40 or better. Surprisingly, patients who received oral prednisone at a dose of 1 mg/kg had a higher rate of recurrence of optic neuritis.

Chronic use of corticosteroids has not been convincingly demonstrated to slow progression of disability. However, rigorously controlled phase III clinical trials have not addressed the question.[164] In a double blind, dose comparison phase II study in SPMS, Goodkin et al gave intravenous methylprednisolone every other month for up to 2 years to 109 patients.[165] Patients were randomly assigned to receive intravenous pulses of either 500 mg or 10 mg methylprednisolone in lieu of placebo, on 3 consecutive days, every 8 weeks for 2 years. Each bimonthly pulse was followed by a tapering course of methylprednisolone administered orally, starting on day 4 and concluding on day 14. The primary outcome measure for the study was a comparison of the proportion of sustained treatment failures in each treatment arm during the 2-year treatment phase.

Patients were considered to be at risk for sustained treatment failure if any of the components of the primary composite outcome were satisfied. The primary composite outcome included worsening of the entry EDSS score by 1.0 or more points for patients with an entry score of 4.0–5.0, or by 0.5 or more points for patients with an entry score of 5.5–6.5; worsening of the entry ambulation index score by 1.0 or more points;

CHAPTER 22

worsening of 20% or more from the baseline value on the best performance of two box and block tests or nine-hole peg tests obtained with either hand; or two exacerbations treated with unscheduled doses of methylprednisolone within 11 successive months.

Patients who experienced worsening of any of the components of the primary composite outcome and sustained the worsening for 5 or more months or experienced three exacerbations treated with unscheduled doses of methylprednisolone during 12 successive months met criteria for sustained treatment failure. Patients were evaluated within a 1-month window of scheduled 6-month visits or upon report of clinical deterioration by an examining neurologist, who was blinded to treatment assignment and treating neurologist.

No significant difference in efficacy was demonstrated between groups receiving high- or low-dose intravenous methylprednisolone on sustained progression of disability at the end of 2 years; however, patients who were treated with high doses had a delay in the onset of sustained treatment failure.[165,166]

In a randomized, controlled, single-blind phase II clinical trial, 126 patients with clinically definite RRMS were randomly assigned to receive either regular pulses of intravenous methylprednisolone (1 g/d for 5 d) with an oral prednisone taper as well as steroid treatment for relapses, or steroid treatment for relapses only, using the same treatment regimen of 1 g/d for 5 d with an oral prednisone taper.[167] Treatment was administered every 4 months for 3 years and then every 6 months for the next 2 years. The primary outcome measure was the treatment effect on quantitative MRI parameters (T2 and T1 lesion volume) and brain parenchymal volume changes. There were no significant differences in T2 lesion volume between the two treatment arms at the 5-year follow up. Although both groups demonstrated significant increases in T1 lesion volumes over the course of the study, the increase in lesion volume was less in the pulsed methylprednisolone group. Patients in the pulsed methylprednisolone arm did not develop brain atrophy during the study, whereas patients in the control group had significant brain atrophy by the end of the study. The patients treated with the pulse steroids had lower disability scores compared to patients receiving steroids only for relapses.

SUMMARY AND RECOMMENDATIONS

At this point, intravenous steroids have shown proven benefit in the management of acute exacerbations by achieving clinical benefit faster than if the patient was left untreated. Administration of regularly scheduled intermittent doses of pulse steroids has not been established as effective therapy for the prevention of clinical worsening in MS. Nonetheless, perhaps because the regimen is inexpensive and generally well tolerated, the practice continues to be fairly widespread among clinicians dealing with patients with worsening MS. Suggestion of possible benefit comes from the 5-year study by Zivadinov and colleagues[167] and a hint of at least transient success in the earlier study by Goodkin et al.[165] Physicians who consider the use of intermittent pulse steroid regimens should recognize the fact that no data support the use of monthly single-day high doses of intravenous methylprednisolone and should perhaps opt instead for multiday regimens similar to those cited above.

INTRAVENOUS IMMUNOGLOBULIN

Although the mechanism of action of polyclonal immunoglobulin is unknown, its beneficial effects in the treatment of neurological disease may include inhibition of complement binding and prevention of membrane attack complex formation, neutralization of certain pathogenic cytokines, downregulation of antibody production and modulation of Fc-receptor-mediated phagocytosis.[168] Additional actions include an effect on superantigens, modulation of T-cell function and antigen recognition, and enhancement of remyelination.

In experimental allergic encephalomyelitis, prophylactic treatment with intravenous immunoglobulin (IVIg) is effective if it is administered at the time of induction. When given in this manner, immunoglobulin significantly reduces the symptoms of disease as well as the underlying CNS pathology.[169] Therapeutic IVIg treatment of established experimental allergic encephalomyelitis did not prove effective.

Fazekas et al conducted a randomized, double-blind, placebo-controlled study in which 75 patients with RRMS received 1 g/kg IVIg once a month for 2 years and were compared with 73 patients receiving placebo.[170] The IVIg group experienced 62 relapses compared to 116 in the placebo group. A total of 40 IVIg patients remained relapse-free during the 2-year study compared to 26 in the placebo group. The annual relapse rate reduction was similar during year 1 and year 2 in the IVIg-treated group, whereas in the placebo group some reduction was noted only in year 2. The time from baseline to first relapse did not differ significantly between the groups. However, the interval between relapses during the study period was significantly longer among patients in the IVIg group than among those in the placebo group. The severity of relapses during the study, as measured by the change in EDSS, did not differ significantly between the groups. A slight improvement in clinical disability occurred in the IVIg group, compared to no significant change in clinical disability in the placebo group. Adverse events were reported by three IVIg-treated patients and four patients in the placebo group. Cutaneous reactions were reported by two IVIg-treated patients; symptoms consisted of a short-lived rash, which developed a few days after the infusion but was not seen by the treating physician.

In the first year of an open-label trial with IVIg in a small number of RRMS patients, the exacerbation rate dropped post-treatment when compared to pretreatment exacerbation rates in the same patients.[171] In another small, open-label trial, IVIg patients showed a greater drop in the mean annual exacerbation rate after being on treatment both for 2 years and for 3 years, compared to their exacerbation rates in the years prior to being treated with immunoglobulin.[172] The adverse event rate inversely correlated with duration of IVIg treatment. Also, the severity of acute exacerbations was favorably influenced by treatment. The majority of exacerbations in the IVIg group were mild to moderate, while in untreated controls most of the acute exacerbations were moderate to severe. The mean change in neurological disability was significantly different after 3 years.

In another study by Sorensen et al, 20 RRMS patients and five SPMS patients were randomly assigned to receive either infusions of IVIg at 1.0 g/kg/d for 2 consecutive days at intervals of 4 weeks or placebo, for 2 years.[173] A total of 17 patients (11 treated, six placebo) completed the study. The relapse rate was lower in the treated group than in the placebo group. The total number of acute exacerbations in the IVIg treatment group was 11 compared to 15 in the placebo group. Severe acute exacerbations requiring treatment with intravenous methylprednisolone occurred in four cases during IVIg treatment and in six cases on placebo. However, neurological disability did not change significantly from baseline in either group. Adverse effects included eczema (most common), urticaria, headache, hepatitis C (the most severe), fever and nausea. The urticaria and headaches were mild and subsided within hours or a few days. Two patients withdrew because of severe eczema; one died from a pulmonary embolism occurring 2 weeks after infusion.

A recent European study evaluated IVIg in SPMS (ESIMS).[174] A total of 318 patients with clinically definite SPMS were randomly assigned to receive IVIg 1 g/kg per month or an equivalent volume of placebo for 27 months. Patients were assessed clinically every 3 months and with MRI every 12 months. No difference between the IVIg- and placebo-treated groups occurred for the primary outcome of confirmed worsening of disability, as defined by the time to first confirmed progression on EDSS. Similarly no significant differences occurred for the secondary outcome measures of the annual relapse rate and change in lesion load on T2-weighted MRI.[175]

SUMMARY AND RECOMMENDATIONS

The ESIMS study has clearly demonstrated a lack of benefit in SPMS[174] and no justification exists for use of this treatment in such patients. While one might consider that 'the jury is still out' on the question of the efficacy of IVIg in RRMS, the answer may come when the results of a prospective, randomized clinical trial sponsored by Bayer Pharmaceuticals are revealed.

PLASMA EXCHANGE

Plasma exchange has been used to treat many neuroimmunological diseases. In the process of removing a patient's plasma by continuous flow centrifugation and replacing it with saline and albumin, antibodies are eliminated, presumably thereby mitigating the immunological attack against the nervous system.[176] Plasmapheresis has been used successfully in myasthenia gravis,[177] Guillain–Barré syndrome[176] and chronic inflammatory demyelinating polyneuropathy.

Weinshenker et al treated 22 patients who had experienced a severe inflammatory attack (not all patients had MS)[178] Patients chosen for this study had either clinically definite or laboratory-supported definite MS by the Poser criteria, or other idiopathic inflammatory demyelinating diseases, which had caused an acute severe neurological deficit affecting consciousness, language, brainstem function or spinal cord function.[180] Patients had previously been treated with high-dose intravenous corticosteroids for a minimum of 5 days with minimal improvement at most. The deficit must have been present for at least 21 days from onset of symptoms and 14 days from onset of treatment with intravenous methylprednisolone. If the deficit had continued to worsen after 5 days of intravenous corticosteroid treatment, plasma exchange could be initiated 12 days after the onset of symptoms. Half the patients initially received active exchange while half received sham exchange, for a total of seven treatments. Then the groups were crossed over to the other treatment. After the first cycle, five of the actively treated patients improved to a marked or moderate degree compared to only one who received sham treatment. When the patients were crossed over to the other group, three who received active treatment in the second treatment period improved moderately to markedly, compared with none who received sham. Responders tended to be male and younger. Nonresponders tended to have a worse baseline deficit. However, neither the type of demyelinating disease nor the interval from onset to enrollment was significantly associated with outcome. Plasma exchange was tolerated well, although anemia occurred in most patients. Improvement during treatment was sustained during follow-up, whereas moderate improvement occurred over the course of follow-up in only two of 12 patients who were treatment failures.

In a follow-up to the previous study, Keegan et al looked at predictors of response to plasma exchange treatment for severe attacks of CNS demyelination.[176] Male sex, preserved reflexes and early initiation of treatment were associated with moderate or marked improvement. Successfully treated patients improved rapidly following plasma exchange and improvement was sus-

tained for at least 1 year post treatment. Even though early initiation of treatment was associated with greater improvement, some patients who were treated as long as 60 days after the onset of symptoms also experienced a favorable response. The authors suggest that such patients should not be excluded from treatment if the onset of the neurological event was acute.

Keegan and colleagues studied treatment success and failure with plasmapheresis, in the four immunopathological patterns of demyelination.[180] Looking at 19 patients treated with therapeutic plasma exchange, only patients with pattern II MS pathology, characterized by immunoglobulin deposition and complement activation, responded. This selective response caused the authors to theorize that the mechanism of action of plasma exchange in the successful treatment of patients with pattern II MS pathology is the removal of pathogenic humoral and plasma factors. The authors also theorized that cellular components probably do not account for the recorded differences in response to plasma exchange.

SUMMARY AND RECOMMENDATIONS

At the present time, plasmapheresis should be reserved for patients with poor recovery from severe attacks. No evidence currently exists to support the use of plasma exchange in chronic treatment of MS.

TACROLIMUS

Tacrolimus, a macrolide antibiotic produced by *Streptomyces tsukubaensis*,[181] inhibits T-cell activation by inhibiting calcineurin.[182] The drug binds to an intracellular protein, FK506-binding protein (FKBP)-12, an immunophilin structurally related to cyclophilin. A complex of tacrolimus-FKBP-12, calcium, calmodulin and calcineurin then forms, and calcineurin phosphatase activity is inhibited, leading to inhibition of T-cell activation.[69]

Tacrolimus has been tested in MS because it markedly protects against demyelination and axonal loss in an EAE animal model.[183] Treatment failed to modify either acute or chronic disease activity and its use was limited by the side effects of nephrotoxicity, hypertension and hyperlipidemia.[184]

SUMMARY AND RECOMMENDATION

Data do not support the use of tacrolimus for the treatment of MS at this time, especially in view of the occurrence of potentially serious adverse events.

CICLOSPORIN

Ciclosporin suppresses humoral immunity to some extent but is more effective against T-cell-dependent immune mechanisms such as those underlying transplant rejection and some forms of autoimmunity.[185] It preferentially inhibits antigen-triggered signal transduction in T lymphocytes, blunting expression of many lymphokines, including IL-2, as well as expression of antiapoptotic proteins. Ciclosporin forms a complex with cyclophilin, a cytoplasmic receptor protein present in target cells. Calcineurin enzymatic activity is inhibited following physical interaction with the ciclosporin/cyclophilin complex. This results in the blockade of nuclear factor of activated T cells(NFAT) dephosphorylation; thus, the cytoplasmic component of NFAT does not enter the nucleus, gene transcription is not activated and the T lymphocyte fails to respond to specific antigenic stimulation.[69] Ciclosporin also increases expression of TGFβ, a potent inhibitor of IL-2-stimulated T-cell proliferation and generation of cytotoxic T lymphocytes.[186]

The drug has been compared with azathioprine as a long-term immunosuppressive treatment for patients with MS in a randomized drug comparison study.[187] A total of 31 patients were randomized to complete 12 months' treatment with either ciclosporin (5 mg/kg/d)[17] or azathioprine (2 mg/kg/d). The ciclosporin treatment group improved in the mean EDSS score and remained more or less stable for the remaining 9 months, while no change could be observed in the azathioprine treatment group. There was no significant difference between the treatment groups in terms of the disability status score or Ambulation Index, although the azathioprine group scored slightly higher throughout the 12-month study on both scores.

The frequencies of concomitant corticosteroid treatment were not significantly different between the two treatment groups. The total frequency of clinical side effects was significantly higher in the ciclosporin treatment group, mainly because of hypertrichosis and headache. There was no significant difference for the CD4 inducer/CD8suppressor, cytotoxic mean ratio. This study suggested a trend for improvement in MS by ciclosporin but the effect was by no means as dramatic as that in reported studies in kidney transplant or type I diabetes. Because of its narrow risk : therapeutic ratio, due to its dose-dependent nephrotoxicity, long-term administration of larger doses of ciclosporin would be unsafe.

A large randomized, double-blind, placebo-controlled trial evaluated the use of ciclosporin in chronic progressive MS. A total of 577 patients were randomized to receive either ciclosporin (273) or placebo (274).[188] Ciclosporin dosage was adjusted for toxicity. The primary combined outcome measure included time to become wheelchair-bound, time to sustained progression and effect on activities of daily living. Ciclosporin delayed the time to becoming wheelchair-bound, but the effects seen in the time to sustained progression and effect on activities of daily living were not statistically significant. A large number of patients from the ciclosporin arm had to drop out of the study because of nephrotoxicity or hypertension.

SUMMARY AND RECOMMENDATIONS

Given its success in the therapy of other autoimmune disorders, ciclosporin seemed a promising candidate for the treatment of MS. However, a large prospective trial in chronic progressive MS showed little, if any, benefit and certainly not enough to warrant its use considering the significant risks of hypertension or renal damage. Other studies have not emerged to justify reconsideration of this verdict. At this point, ciclosporin should not be considered part of the therapeutic armamentarium for the treatment of MS.

SULFASALAZINE

Sulfasalazine, widely used in the treatment of inflammatory bowel disease, is metabolized to its active components, sulfapyridine and mesalamine, by bacteria in the colon.[189] When given as sulfasalazine, a larger quantity of sulfapyridine and mesalamine reach the colon than when these agents are administered as single agents. Once sulfapyridine and mesalamine reach the colon, the beneficial effects result primarily from the anti-inflammatory properties of mesalamine. The anti-inflammatory mechanism of mesalamine is believed to occur, at least in part, through the inhibition of arachidonic acid metabolism in the bowel mucosa by inhibition of cyclooxygenase. This effectively diminishes the production of prostaglandins, thereby reducing colonic inflammation. Production of arachidonic metabolites appears to be increased in patients with inflammatory bowel disease. Mesalamine also inhibits leukotriene synthesis, possibly through the inhibition of lipoxygenase.

This action has been suggested as a major component of the drug's anti-inflammatory effects. Inhibition of colonic mucosal sulfidopeptide leukotriene synthesis and chemotactic stimuli for polymorphonuclear leukocytes may also occur.[189]

Side effects of sulfasalazine are common.[189] Several of these are dependent on plasma levels of sulfapyridine and are therefore related to both dose and acetylation status of the patient. They include fever and malaise, nausea, vomiting, headaches, epigastric discomfort and diarrhea and may be partially overcome by gradual increments of the dose. Megaloblastic anemia and low sperm counts, believed to be due to impaired folic acid absorption, can also occur, and some physicians advocate the routine coadministration of folate supplements. Allergic reactions (not related to plasma levels) can include arthralgias, hemolysis, agranulocytosis, thrombocytopenia, red cell aplasia and a variety of skin manifestations such as rash, urticaria and a bluish discoloration. Most serious, but rare, are toxic epidermal necrolysis and Stevens–Johnson syndrome, pancreatitis, eosinophilic pneumonia, bronchospasm, fibrosing alveolitis, drug-induced lupus and neurotoxicity.

Noseworthy et al conducted a placebo-controlled, randomized, double-blind phase III trial of sulfasalazine in MS.[190] A total of 199 patients with RRMS (151) and progressive (48) MS were evaluated at 3-month intervals for a minimum of 3 years. MRI studies were performed at 6-month intervals on a subset of 89 patients.

By the end of the study, sulfasalazine had failed to slow or prevent disability progression as measured on EDSS. However, during the first 18 months of the trial, the annualized relapse rate, proportion of relapse-free patients, rate of EDSS progression at 1 and 2 years in the progressive subgroup only, and median time to EDSS progression were all better in the treatment group compared to placebo. The positive findings observed in the first half of the trial were not sustained, however.

SUMMARY AND RECOMMENDATIONS

The major prospective trial of sulfasalazine emphasizes the important point that short-term results can be misleading in this chronic disease. At the present time, this drug should not be considered a useful agent for the treatment of MS.

ALEMTUZUMAB

The monoclonal antibody alemtuzumab targets the CD52 antigen, present on T and B cells and macrophages.[191] It causes a sustained depletion of T-cells.[192] Alemtuzumab was first used in patients with MS in 1991 with the hope that the T-cell repertoire regenerated after lymphocyte depletion by the antibody would no longer exert the aberrant autoimmune responses characteristic of MS.[192] By 1999, 36 patients had been treated; all had SPMS with an EDSS of 6.0 or less.[193] Enhancing lesions were present on an MRI done 3 months prior to treatment in all patients. Alemtuzumab was administered as an intravenous infusion of 100 mg over 5 consecutive days as a daily 20 mg infusion over 4 h, every 12 months. Treated patients experienced a systemic response accompanied by a transient, often severe but reversible reactivation of neurological disease activity that lasted for a few hours. This was thought to be due to the release of mediators that impede conduction at previously demyelinated sites. The reaction could be prevented by pretreatment with methylprednisolone. Radiological markers of cerebral inflammation persisted for several weeks after treatment but thereafter radiological markers of cerebral inflammation were suppressed for at least 18 months during which patients remained asymptomatic. Some 6 years after treatment a subgroup of patients underwent MRI, which showed no appreciable increase in the T1-hypointense, or T2-lesion volume in these patients. However, approximately half the patients continued to experience progressive disability and increasing brain atrophy, thought to be secondary to axonal degeneration, which correlated with the extent of cerebral inflammation in the pretreatment phase. Because of the observations in SPMS, the emphasis was switched to studying patients with active RRMS. Some 22 patients with active RRMS whose disease was not controlled by currently approved DMAs or in whom a high relapse rate was seen early in the disease were treated with alemtuzumab. The patients who received the monoclonal antibody had a 94% reduction in relapse rate. However, accumulation of disability continued despite suppression of inflammation. There was a reduction in new lesion incidence rates.[184] Use of alemtuzumab is also characterized by a markedly increased risk for autoimmune thyroiditis.[184,194]

A recent trial of alemtuzumab in comparison to IFN β-1a (subcutaneous) intended for 3 years, showed a 75% relapse rate reduction for the monoclonal antibody compared to IFNβ at the end of 2 years. However, six cases (one fatal) of idiopathic thrombocytopenic purpura developed in the alemtuzumab group, so the trial was stopped prematurely.[195] A Phase III trial will include a risk management plan with very close surveillance to reduce the risk of severe ITP.

SUMMARY AND RECOMMENDATIONS

Although alemtuzumab appears to be a drug of continuing interest for MS, the occurrence of thrombocytopenic purpura requires further clarification.

RITUXIMAB

Rituximab, the first monoclonal antibody approved by the FDA,[196] is a genetically engineered, chimeric murine/human monoclonal antibody containing IgG$_1$ heavy-chain and κ light-chain constant region sequences and murine variable region sequences.[197] It binds specifically to the CD20 antigen, a 35 kDa transmembrane protein that is involved in cell cycle progression and differentiation.[198,199] The CD20 is expressed on normal B lymphocytes, from pre-B cells to activated B cells, but not on differentiated plasma cells, T cells, hematopoietic stem cells or nonhematopoietic normal tissues.[200] Rituximab causes rapid depletion of CD20$^+$ B cells in the peripheral blood.[201] However, antibody production is still maintained by plasma cells, and normal peripheral B cells are subsequently replenished by hematopoietic stem cells in most patients 3–12 months after therapy.[200] Mechanisms of action may include inhibition of antibody-dependent cellular cytotoxicity, complement-mediated cell lysis, induction of apoptosis, inhibition of cell growth and sensitization to chemotherapy.[197,202,203]

Use of rituximab was initially reported in neuromyelitis optica and rapidly worsening MS.[204] Four patients with progressive relapsing myelitis each received 4-weekly intravenous infusions of rituximab (375 mg/m^2) and were followed for lymphocyte subset counts, adverse events and neurological disability. B-cell counts dropped to zero and remained undetectable 6 months after the infusions ended. Two of the four MS patients experienced an improvement in ambulation and fatigue following treatment. All four patients remained relapse-free for the duration of follow-up, which was an average of 6 months.[204] Other lymphocyte subsets were not affected, except for a transient drop in CD4$^+$ T cells in some patients.

A phase II trial in relapsing-remitting MS was recently completed. The results showed statistically significant benefit on both new gadolinium-enhanced lesions and relapse rate. Phase III trials in both RRMS and PPMS are planned.

Pender[205] proposed two different hypotheses to explain how progression of neurological impairment in PPMS could occur.[205] The first hypothesis postulates that neurological impairment is due to a rapid and relentless immune attack on CNS myelin and axons by T cells and antibody. The alternative is by prolonged slow immune attack on myelin and axons without CNS repair. This is more likely to occur when antibodies constitute the main mechanism of attack because of circulating antigen-specific T cells. A failure of CNS repair could be due to immune attack preventing remyelination or because of immune-medicated destruction of axons, which cannot regenerate in the human CNS. Antibodies are effective inhibitors of remyelination because of their persistence and ability to spread diffusely through the CNS parenchyma. Progressive MS could be due to a predominantly antibody-mediated immune attack that causes demyelination and inhibits remyelination or that causes axonal destruction. Relapses, on the other hand, may be due to T-cell immune attack on the CNS. Because of the possibility of antibody-mediated attack on the CNS in PPMS, an agent such as rituximab, which can cause depletion of B cells, might be beneficial in this form of the disease.

For the most part, the side effects of rituximab are mild, such as fever, chills and nausea, but hypersensitivity reactions can occasionally be severe or even fatal. Patients who receive this therapy must be monitored very carefully during infusion, particularly the second infusion.[206] Patients may need to be pretreated with diphenhydramine and steroids.[207] The infusion may need to run very slowly or even be stopped to prevent the occurrence of the hypersensitivity reaction.

SUMMARY AND RECOMMENDATIONS

Rituximab is a monoclonal antibody that remains of significant interest for its potential use in MS. It is currently undergoing randomized, placebo-controlled trials in both RRMS and PPMS. Pending results of these studies, very few data exist to support its use in worsening MS, although uncontrolled studies suggest a benefit in neuromyelitis optica. Since no controlled studies exist for treatment of neuromyelitis optica, rituximab may be a reasonable choice for this often devastating condition.

DACLIZUMAB

Daclizumab is a monoclonal antibody directed against the α chain (CD25), a component of the high-affinity IL-2 receptor. After demonstration that the drug inhibits experimental auto-immune encephalomyelitis models,[208–210] 10 patients with RRMS or SPMS were treated with the combination of daclizumab and IFNβ after suboptimal response to the latter alone.[211] The patients had experienced at least one exacerbation or progression of disability by at least 1 point on the EDSS during the preceding 18 months on therapy. Patients were treated with intravenous daclizumab at 1 mg/kg/dose 2 weeks apart for the first two doses and once every 4 weeks thereafter for a total of seven infusions (6 months). Patients were followed with monthly clinical and MRI examinations. Primary outcome measures were new contrast-enhancing lesions and total number of contrast-enhancing lesions on IFNβ versus combination therapy of IFNβ and daclizumab. The 10 patients with relapsing forms of MS treated with the combination of IFNβ and daclizumab had a 78% reduction in new contrast-enhancing lesions and a significant improvement in the nine-hole peg test, Scripps NRS and the exacerbation rate. There were also positive trends for EDSS, the timed 25-foot walk, changes in T2 lesion volume and black hole volume, and the ambulation index.

The reduction in contrast-enhancing lesions occurred gradually over 1.5–2 months, unlike that seen with IFN[212] or natalizumab.[213] The authors postulate that, instead of targeting the blood–brain barrier, daclizumab induces a gradual immunomodulatory change that is responsible for the observed decrease in brain inflammation.

In another open-label study, 19 patients with relapsing forms of MS were treated.[214] Of these patients, 17 had not responded well to conventional therapy. Most of the patients received daclizumab as monotherapy but two received both IFN and daclizumab and then were switched to daclizumab monotherapy. Clinical improvement occurred in 10 patients and the other nine had stabilization of disease and reduction of MRI activity during the mean treatment period of 14 months. Patients experienced minimal adverse events. A recently completed Phase II trial, in which daclizumab or placebo was added in patients taking weekly intramuscular IFNB-1a, showed a statistically significant benefit for the monoclonal antibody on the primary endpoint of new MRI activity. A reduction in relapse rate did not reach statistical significance.[215]

SUMMARY AND RECOMMENDATIONS

Daclizumab is another monoclonal antibody of substantial interest as a potential treatment for MS. Additional randomized clinical trials are planned or in progress, but, pending their conclusion, use of this agent off label (as it is approved for other purposes) seems unwarranted because of the limited data on efficacy and safety in MS, as well as its very high cost.

BONE MARROW TRANSPLANTATION

Autologous hematopoietic stem cell transplantation was introduced as a treatment for patients with MS after animal studies showed that the course of experimental allergic encephalomyelitis could be modified by high-dose immunosuppression causing hematolymphatic ablation, and subsequent bone marrow transplantation.[216–219] Further support for the idea resulted from the observations that some patients who were treated with hematopoietic stem cell transplantation for concurrent malignancies were found to have prolonged remissions of their MS.[220–222]

European studies of hematopoietic stem cell transplantation have been conducted in all types of MS.[223] In the largest European study, seven of 85 treated patients died.[218] The patients who died had high EDSS scores, were older and had received intensely T-cell-purged grafts. Still, the authors reported 74% progression-free survival for all patients after 3 years, 78% for SPMS. Clinical improvement was noted in 21%.

Originally conducted as single-center trials, the study of bone marrow transplantation in MS expanded to multicenter safety clinical trials. In one such trial the median EDSS was 4.5–8.[218,224] All patients had failed a number of standard therapies and had progressing disease, with a worsening EDSS over the past year. Patients were treated with immunosuppression, and peripheral blood stem cells were mobilized using cyclophosphamide and granulocyte colony-stimulating factor (G-CSF). Transient neurological deterioration often occurred after patients had received G-CSF.[225] Progression-free survival was 81% for SP and RRMS and 67% for PPMS. Pathological MRI activity was suppressed but brain atrophy continued to occur.[226]

Wolinsky outlined the obstacles to the use of hematopoietic stem cell therapy for patients with MS at a conference on the subject in 2001.[227] He felt that this treatment modality would need to effect a reduction in the level of morbidity and mortality, a drop in attack frequency of at least 70% and a drop in sustained EDSS score progression of 1.0 point to 8% of patients at 2 years and 17% at 3 years after therapy in order to demonstrate effectiveness comparable to that of mitoxantrone. Also,

hematopoietic stem cell therapy must have a durable response lasting beyond 3 years in order to warrant its use instead of mitoxantrone.

Stem cell transplantation can be used to treat MS in two different manners. The first method is to suppress disease activity with immunosuppressive agents without killing all immune cells.[228] The stem cells would then act as a rescue to overcome immunodeficiency. The other way is to cause total immune ablation, with the infusion of stem cells intended to completely renew the immune system. Hintzen noted that unsatisfactory results with the use of conventional immunosuppressants in autoimmune disease could be secondary to the incomplete removal of autoreactive lymphocytes.[228] However, he also acknowledged that increasing the intensity of immunosuppression will lead to higher morbidity.

Many obstacles must be overcome to develop a randomized clinical trial with bone marrow transplantation, and so far none have been done. Multiple variables are involved in the implementation of hematopoietic stem cell therapy, including the choices of tissue source of the graft, donor source of the graft and mobilization procedures, as well as different graft manipulations and the different methods of myeloablation. Patients selected for the procedure should have rapidly progressive disease without diffuse irreversible white matter disease. There must be a standardized protocol in order to conduct a controlled trial. Issues with the selection of an appropriate placebo therapy and with the establishment of effective blinding are also important. It would also be difficult to match the patients in both arms of the study. Nonetheless, Hintzen suggested that these obstacles could all be overcome, allowing the conduct of a blinded, placebo-controlled, randomized clinical trial.

SUMMARY AND RECOMMENDATIONS

Hematopoietic stem cell transplantation continues to garner much attention and patients frequently ask their clinicians about it. The treatment remains an interesting but very risky procedure the efficacy of which has not been clearly established. Patients who seek this treatment are generally unaware of the number of deaths, as well as other serious morbidity, that have been reported with the treatment. The barriers to the successful design of a properly controlled clinical trial have so far been formidable and have prevented such a much-needed study. In the interim, performance of this procedure should be restricted to centers with a high degree of experience, where investigators using well defined research protocols enroll only those patients who have failed more conventional therapy and fully understand the significant risks and lack of established benefit.

WHAT TO DO IF THE PATIENT DOES NOT RESPOND TO STANDARD THERAPY: A SYSTEMATIC APPROACH

Currently approved immunomodulatory medications are, at best, only moderately effective in preventing relapses. Furthermore, all currently available agents, including those immunosuppressive agents used 'off-label' for the treatment of MS, apparently target the inflammatory process. It is not clear that any currently available drug significantly affects the neurodegenerative process that seems to characterize most progressive cases.

No specific approach has yet been widely accepted for a patient who is failing conventional therapy. However, it is possible for clinicians to develop a strategy with which they are comfortable to deal with such situations. This will at least allow for consistency and the avoidance of agonizing indecision each time one confronts the issue.

In most RRMS patients who are continuing to experience attacks, logic suggests (and insurance often mandates) that the currently approved treatments remain the primary option. If a patient has been treated with weekly IFNβ-1a, a reasonable first approach would be to switch to an IFN preparation administered multiple times per week. The physician may wish to verify the absence of neutralizing antibodies before undertaking this option. If a patient has already been taking multiple weekly doses of IFN, a trial of glatiramer acetate might be considered next. Conversely, if glatiramer acetate had been the first agent prescribed, a switch to IFN would be appropriate. Today, many MS specialists might instead switch from the initial immunomodulatory agent to natalizumab.

In patients for whom the FDA-approved immunomodulatory drugs have failed and natalizumab is not going to be used, two potential approaches are available. The first would be to try a combination of IFN plus glatiramer. However, it must be emphasized that, while some data suggest that the combination of glatiramer acetate and IFNβ-1a (Avonex) is safe, no useful information is currently available to indicate added efficacy with the combination. Furthermore, cost considerations may be prohibitive for many patients, and third-party payers may be very reluctant to cover both drugs. The alternative approach of initiating therapy with immunosuppressive medication probably conveys a greater risk of potentially serious toxicity. Nonetheless, an evidence-based medicine paradigm would dictate the use of mitoxantrone, currently the only FDA-approved drug for SPMS (with the exception of IFNβ-1b, which has an indication in SPMS patients who are continuing to experience relapses). Mitoxantrone is also approved for the treatment of worsening forms of relapsing MS. Some experts consider the use of intravenous cyclophosphamide as equal or preferable to mitoxantrone but the evidence remains controversial.

For patients who are unwilling to use these intravenous immunosuppressive medications or are deemed by their physicians to be inappropriate candidates, the oral immunosuppressive agents may be considered. Many MS specialists currently consider mycophenolate mofetil as the first choice. This preference is probably based more on the positive effects of the drug in the prevention of organ rejection and on the general lack of enthusiasm for azathioprine (at least in the USA) and methotrexate than on currently available data supporting its benefit in MS. Rituximab and daclizumab are other options, but costs are much higher and definitive evidence of benefit is not yet available.

Patients who are failing approved therapy should be offered the opportunity to participate in properly designed clinical trials, if such are available. Clinicians should take ample time to explain the potential risks and benefits of unproved therapies, always offering hope while establishing realistic expectations for patients and their families.

REFERENCES

1. PRISMS Study Group. Randomised double-blind placebo-controlled study of interferon beta-1a in relapsing/remitting multiple sclerosis. PRISMS (Prevention of Relapses and Disability by Interferon beta-1a Subcutaneously in Multiple Sclerosis) Study Group. Lancet 1998; 352: 1498–1504.

2. IFN Beta Multiple Sclerosis Study Group. Interferon beta-1b is effective in relapsing-remitting multiple sclerosis. I. Clinical results of a multicenter, randomized, double-blind, placebo-controlled trial. The IFNB Multiple Sclerosis Study Group. Neurology 1993; 43: 655–661.

3. Jacobs LD, Cookfair DL, Rudick RA et al. Intramuscular interferon beta-1a for disease progression in relapsing multiple sclerosis. Ann Neurol 1996; 39: 285–294.

4. Johnson KP, Brooks BR, Cohen JA et al. Copolymer 1 reduces relapse rate and improves disability in relapsing-remitting multiple sclerosis: results of a phase III multicenter, double-blind placebo-controlled trial. The Copolymer 1 Multiple Sclerosis Study Group. Neurology 1995; 45: 1268–1276.

5. Hartung H-P, Gonsette R, Konig N et al. Mitoxantrone in progressive multiple sclerosis: a placebo-controlled, double-blind, randomised, multicentre trial. Lancet 2002; 360: 2018–2025.

6. Kleinschmidt-DeMasters BK, Tyler KL. Progressive multifocal leukoencephalopathy complicating treatment with natalizumab and interferon beta-1a for multiple sclerosis. N Engl J Med 2005; 353: 369–374.

7. Barnett MH, Prineas JW. Relapsing and remitting multiple sclerosis: pathology of the newly forming lesion. Ann Neurol 2004; 55: 458–468.

8. Trapp BD, Peterson J, Ransohoff RM et al. Axonal transection in the lesions of multiple sclerosis. N Engl J Med 1998; 338: 278–285.

9. PRISMS Study Group and the University of British Columbia MS/MRI Analysis Group. PRISMS-4: Long-term efficacy of interferon-beta-1a in relapsing MS. Neurology 2001; 56: 1628–1636.

10. Zhao GJ, R. A. Koopmans RA, Li DKB et al. Effect of interferon β-1b in MS: assessment of annual accumulation of PD/T2 activity on MRI. Neurology 2000; 54: 200–206.

11. Jacobs LD, Beck RW, Simon JH et al. Intramuscular interferon beta-1a therapy initiated during a first demyelinating event in multiple sclerosis. CHAMPS Study Group. N Engl J Med 2000; 343: 898–904.

12. Paty DW, Li DK. Interferon beta-1b is effective in relapsing-remitting multiple sclerosis. II. MRI analysis results of a multicenter, randomized, double-blind, placebo-controlled trial. UBC MS/MRI Study Group and the IFNB Multiple Sclerosis Study Group. Neurology 1993; 43: 662–667.

13. Rio J, Nos C, Tintore M et al. Assessment of different treatment failure criteria in a cohort of relapsing-remitting multiple sclerosis patients treated with interferon β: Implications for clinical trials. Ann Neurol 2002; 52: 400–406.

14. Rio J, Nos C, Tintore M et al. Defining the response to interferon-β in relapsing-remitting multiple sclerosis patients. Ann Neurol 2006; 59: 344–352.

15. Multiple Sclerosis Therapy Consensus Group. Escalating immunotherapy of multiple sclerosis. J Neurol 2004; 251: 1329–1339.

16. Lublin FD, Baier M, Cutter G. Effect of relapses on development of residual deficit in multiple sclerosis. Neurology 2003; 61: 1528–1532.

17. Weinshenker BG, Bass B, Rice GP et al. The natural history of multiple sclerosis: a geographically based study. 2. Predictive value of the early clinical course. Brain 1989; 112: 1419–1428.

18. Confavreux C, Vukusic S, Moreau T et al. Relapses and progression of disability in multiple sclerosis. N Engl J Med 2000; 343: 1430–1438.

19. Barkhof F, Filippi M, Miller DH et al. Comparison of MRI criteria at first presentation to predict conversion to clinically definite multiple sclerosis. Brain 1997; 120: 2059–2069.

20. CHAMPS study group. MRI predictors of early conversion to clinically definite MS in the CHAMPS placebo group. Neurology 2002; 59: 998–1005.

21. Reddy HS, Narayanan SR, Arnoutelis R et al. Evidence for adaptive functional changes in the cerebral cortex with axonal injury from multiple sclerosis. Brain 2000; 123: 2314–2320.

22. Cifelli A, Matthews PM. Cerebral plasticity in multiple sclerosis: insights from fMRI. Mult Scler 2002; 8: 193–199.

23. Filippi M, Rocca MA. Disturbed function and plasticity in multiple sclerosis as gleaned from functional magnetic resonance imaging. Curr Opin Neurol 2003; 16: 275–282.

24. European Study Group on Interferon beta-1b in Secondary Progressive MS. Placebo-controlled multicentre randomised trial of interferon beta-1b in treatment of secondary progressive multiple sclerosis. Lancet 1998; 352: 1491–1497.

25. Ciccarelli O, Giugni E, Paolillo A et al. Magnetic resonance outcome of new enhancing lesions in patients with relapsing-remitting multiple sclerosis. Eur J Neurol 1999; 6: 455–459.

26. Weiner H, Guttmann CR, Khoury SJ. Serial magnetic resonance imaging in multiple sclerosis: correlation with attacks, disability, and disease stage. J Neuroimmunol 2000; 104: 164–173.

27. Brex, P. A., Ciccarelli O., O'Riordan JI et al. A longitudinal study of abnormalities on MRI and disability from multiple sclerosis. N Engl J Med 2002; 346: 158–164.

28. Rovaris M, Comi G, Ladkani D et al. Short-term correlations between clinical and MR imaging findings in relapsing-remitting multiple sclerosis. Am J Neuroradiol 2003; 24: 75–81.

29. The IFNB Multiple Sclerosis Study Group and the University of British Columbia MS/MRI Analysis Group. Interferon beta-1b in the treatment of multiple sclerosis: final outcome of the randomized controlled trial. Neurology 1995; 45: 1277–1285.

30. PRISMS Study Group and the University of British Columbia MS/MRI Analysis Group. PRISMS-4: Long-term efficacy of interferon-beta-1a in relapsing MS. Neurology 2001; 56: 1628–1636.

31. Cohen J, Garmany G, Goodman A et al. Expert opinion paper. changing therapy in relapsing multiple sclerosis from the Medical Advisory Board of the National Multiple Sclerosis Society 2004; 1–8 Available on line at: http://www.nationalmssociety.org/pdf/forpros/Exp_ChangTherapy.pdf.

32. Cohen BA Khan O, Jeffery DR et al. Identifying and treating patients with suboptimal responses Neurology 2004; 63(suppl 6): S33–S40.

33. Río J, Nos C, Tintoré M et al. Defining the response to interferon-β in relapsing-remitting multiple sclerosis patients. Ann Neurol 2006; 59: 344–352.

34. Kleinschmidt-DeMasters BK, Tyler KL. Progressive multifocal leukoencephalopathy complicating treatment with natalizumab and interferon beta-1a for multiple sclerosis. N Engl J Med 2005; 353: 369–374.

35. Langer-Gould A, Atlas SW, Bollen AW, Pelletier D. Progressive multifocal leucoencephalopathy in a patient treated with natalizumab. N Engl J Med 2005; 353: 375–381.

36. Polman CH, O'Connor PW, Havrdova E et al. A randomized, placebo-controlled trial of natalizumab for relapsing multiple sclerosis. N Engl J Med 2006; 354: 899–910.

37. Polman CH, Uitdehaag BMJ. New and emerging treatment options for multiple sclerosis. Lancet Neurol 2003; 2: 563–566.

38. Durr FE, Wallace RE, Citarella RV. Molecular and biochemical pharmacology of mitoxantrone. Cancer Treat Rev 1983; 10(suppl B): 3–11.

39. Alberts DS, Peng YM, Bowden GT et al. Pharmacology of mitoxantrone: mode of action and pharmacokinetics. Invest New Drugs 1985; 3: 101–107.

40. Ehninger G, Proksch B, Heinzel G et al. Clinical pharmacology of mitoxantrone. Cancer Treat Rep 1986; 70: 1373–1378.

41. Granmer DK, Weil PA. DNA organization, replication, and repair. In: Murray RK, Daryl K, Granner DK et al, eds. Harper's illustrated biochemistry, 26th ed. New York: McGraw-Hill; 2003: 314–341.

42. Harkins TT, Lewis TJ, Lindsley, JE. A chemical kinetic model for the activity of DNA topoisomerase II. Biochemistry 1998; 37: 7299–7312.

43. Savaraj N, Lu K, Manuel V, Loo TL. Clinical kinetics of 1, 4-dihydroxy-5,8-bis [[2-[(2-(2-hydroxyethyl) amino] ethyl] amino]-9, 10-anthracenedione. Cancer Chemother Pharmacol 1982; 8: 113–117.

44. Wiseman LR, Spencer CM. Mitoxantrone. A review of its pharmacology and clinical efficacy in the management of hormone-resistant advanced prostate cancer. Drugs Aging 1997; 10: 473–485.

45. Fidler JM, DeJoy SQ, Gibbons JJ Jr. Selective immunomodulation by the antineoplastic agent mitoxantrone. II. Nonspecific adherent suppressor cells derived from mitoxantrone-treated mice. J Immunol 1986; 136: 2747–2754.

46. Wang BS, Lumanglas AL, Silva J et al. Inhibition of the induction of alloreactivity with mitoxantrone. Int J Immunopharmacol 1986; 8: 967–973.

47. Ghalie RG, Edan G, Laurent M et al. Cardiac adverse effects associated with mitoxantrone (Novantrone) therapy in patients with MS. Neurology 2002; 59: 909–913.

48. Dukart G, Barone JS. An overview of cardiac episodes following mitoxantrone administration. Cancer Treat Symp 1984; 3: 35–41.

49. Cohen BA, Mikol DD. Mitoxantrone treatment of multiple sclerosis: safety considerations. Neurology 2004; 63(suppl 6): S28–S32.

50. Herman EH, Zhang J, Hasinoff BB et al. Comparison of the structural changes induced by doxorubicin and mitoxantrone in the heart, kidney and intestine and characterization of the Fe(III)-mitoxantrone complex. J Mol Cell Cardiol 1997; 29: 2415–2430.

51. Speyer J, Wasserheit C. Strategies for reduction of anthracycline cardiac toxicity. Semin Oncol 1998; 25: 525–537.

52. Linassier C, Barin C, Calais G et al. Early secondary acute myelogenous leukemia in breast cancer patients after treatment with mitoxantrone, cyclophosphamide, fluorouracil and radiation therapy. Ann Oncol 2000; 11: 1289–1294.

53. Hagemeister FB. Are alkylating agents a necessary component in the therapy of Hodgkin's disease? Leuk Lymphoma 1993; 10(suppl): 91–97.

54. Chaplain G, Milan C, Sgro C et al. Increased risk of acute leukemia after adjuvant chemotherapy for breast cancer: a population-based study. J Clin Oncol 2000; 18: 2836–2842.

55. Goodkin DE. Therapy-related leukemia in mitoxantrone treated patients. Mult Scler 2003; 9: 426.

56. Cattaneo C, Almici C, Borlenghi E et al. A case of acute promyelocytic leukaemia following mitoxantrone treatment of multiple sclerosis. Leukemia 2003; 17: 985–986.

57. Mogenet I, Simiand-Erdociain E, Canonge JM et al. Acute myelogenous leukemia following mitoxantrone treatment for multiple sclerosis. Ann Pharmacother 2003; 37: 747–748.

58. Ghalie RG, Mauch E, Edan G et al. A study of therapy-related acute leukaemia after mitoxantrone therapy for multiple sclerosis. Mult Scler 2002; 8: 441–445.

59. Heesen C, Bruegmann M, Gbdamosi J et al. Therapy-related acute myelogenous leukaemia (t-AML) in a patient with multiple sclerosis treated with mitoxantrone. Mult Scler 2003; 9: 213–214.

60. Brassat D, Recher C, Waubant E et al. Therapy-related acute myeloblastic leukemia after mitoxantrone treatment in a patient with MS. Neurology 2002; 59: 954–955.

61. Vicari AM, Ciceri F, Folli F et al. Acute promyelocytic leukemia following mitoxantrone as single agent for the treatment of multiple sclerosis. Leukemia 1998; 12: 441–442.

62. Voltz R, Starck M, Zingler V et al. Mitoxantrone therapy in multiple sclerosis and acute leukaemia: a case report out of 644 treated patients. Mult Scler 2004; 10: 472–474.

63. Stüve O, Kita M, Pelletier D et al. Mitoxantrone as a potential therapy for primary progressive multiple sclerosis. Mult Scler 2004; 10(suppl 1): S58–S61.

64. Gonsette RE. Mitoxantrone immunotherapy in multiple sclerosis. Mult Scler 1996; 1: 329–332.

65. Edan G, Miller D, Clanet M et al. Therapeutic effect of mitoxantrone combined with methylprednisolone in multiple sclerosis: a randomised multicentre study of active disease using MRI and clinical criteria. J Neurol Neurosurg Psychiatr 1997; 62: 112–118.

66. Gonsette RE. Mitoxantrone in progressive multiple sclerosis: when and how to treat? J Neurol Sci 2003; 206: 203–208.

67. Van de Wyngaert FA, Beguin C, D'Hooghe MB et al. A double-blind clinical trial of mitoxantrone versus methylprednisolone in relapsing, secondary progressive multiple sclerosis. Acta Neurol Belg 2001; 101: 210–216.

68. Goodin DS, Arnason BG, Coyle PK et al. The use of mitoxantrone (Novantrone) for the treatment of multiple sclerosis: report of the Therapeutics and Technology Assessment Subcommittee of the American Academy of Neurology. Neurology 2003; 61: 1332–1338.

69. Krensky AM, Strom TB, Bluestone JA. Immunomodulators. immunosuppressive agents, tolerogens, and immunostimulants: section X – drugs used for immunomodulation. In: Hardman JG, Limbird LE, Goodman Gilman A, eds. Goodman & Gilman's the pharmacological basis of therapeutics 10th ed. New York: McGraw-Hill; 2001: 1461–1485.

70. Bertino JR. Chemical action and pharmacology of methotrexate, azathioprine and cyclophosphamide in man. Arthritis Rheum 1973; 16: 79–83.

71. Chan GL, Canafax DM, Johnson CA. The therapeutic use of azathioprine in renal transplantation. Pharmacotherapy 1987; 7: 165–177.

72. Elion GB. Symposium on immunosuppressive drugs. Biochemistry and pharmacology of purine analogues. Fed Proc 1967; 26: 898–904.

73. Salmaggi A, Corsini E, La Mantia L. Immunological monitoring of azathioprine treatment in multiple sclerosis patients. J Neurol 1997; 244: 167–174.

74. Sinico RA, Sabadini E, Borlandelli S et al. Azathioprine hypersensitivity: report of two cases and review of the literature. J Nephrol 2003; 16: 272–276.

75. Calbo Mayo JM, Blasco Colmenarejo M, Rivera Vaquerizo PJ et al. Hypersensitivity reaction to azathioprine in a patient with

SECTION 3

ulcerative colitis. infrequent manifestations. Inflamm Bowel Dis 2004; 10: 700.

76. Singh G, Fries JF, Spitz P et al. Toxic effecrs of azathioprine in rheumatoid arthritis. Arthritis Rheum 1989; 32: 837–843.

77. Hohlfeld R, Michels M, Heininger K et al. Azathioprine toxicity during long-term immunosuppression of gerneralized myasthenia gravis. Neurology 1988; 38: 258–261.

78. Craner MJ, Zajicek JP. Immunosuppressive treatments in MS – side effects from azathioprine. J Neurol 2001; 248: 625–626.

79. British and Dutch Multiple Sclerosis Azathioprine Trial Group. Double-masked trial of azathioprine in multiple sclerosis. Lancet 1988; 2: 179–183.

80. Taylor, L. Hughes RA, McPherson K et al. The risk of cancer from azathioprine as a treatment for multiple sclerosis. Eur J Neurol 2004; 11: 141.

81. Confavreux C, Saddier P, Grimaud J et al. Risk of cancer from azathioprine therapy in multiple sclerosis: a case-control study. Neurology 1996; 46: 1607–1612.

82. Goodkin D, Bailly RC, Teetzen ML. The efficacy of azathioprine in relapsing-remitting multiple sclerosis. Neurology 1991; 41: 20–25.

83. Yudkin, PL Ellison GW, Ghezzi A et al. Overview of azathioprine treatment in multiple sclerosis. Lancet 1991; 338: 1051–1055.

84. Confavreux C, Moreau T. Emerging treatment in multiple sclerosis: azathioprine and mofetil. Mult Scler 1996; 1: 379–384.

85. Markovic-Plese S, Bielekova B, Kadom N et al. Longitudinal MRI study: the effects of azathioprine in MS patients refractory to interferon β-1b. Neurology 2003; 60: 1489–1451.

86. Lus G, Romano F, Scuotto A et al. Azathioprine and interferon beta$_{1a}$ in relapsing–remitting multiple sclerosis patients: increasing efficacy of combined treatment. Eur Neurol 2004; 51: 15–20.

87. Chabner BA, Ryan DP, Paz-Ares L et al. Antineoplastic agents: section x – drugs used for immunomodulation. In: Hardman JG, Limbird LE, Goodman Gilman A, eds. Goodman & Gilman's the pharmacological basis of therapeutics 10th ed. New York: McGraw-Hill; 2001: 1381–1460.

88. Martin RHR, McFarland HF. Neurologic disorders: course and treatment. San Diego, CA: Academic Press; 1996: 497–499.

89. Zimmerman R, Radhakrishnan J, Valeri A et al. Advances in the treatment of lupus nephritis. Annu Rev Med 2001; 52: 63–78.

90. Brock N, Pohl J. Prevention of urotoxic side effects by regional detoxification with increased selectivity of oxazaphosphorine cytostatics., IARC Sci Publ 1986; 78: 269–279.

91. Aimard G, Girard PF, Raveau J. Multiple sclerosis and the autoimmunization process. Treatment by antimitotics. Lyon Med 1966; 215: 345–352.

92. Padmanabhan BKA, Karni A, Hancock WW et al. AAN 53rd Annual Meeting Program, Philadelphia, PA. Neurology 2001; 56(suppl 3): A226.

93. Hommes OR, Aerts F, Bahr U et al. Cyclophosphamide levels in serum and spinal fluid of multiple sclerosis patients treated with immunosuppression. J Neurol Sci 1983; 58: 297–303.

94. Bahr U, Schulten HR, Hommes OR et al. Determination of cyclophosphamide in urine, serum and cerebrospinal fluid of multiple sclerosis patients by field desorption mass spectrometry. Clin Chim Acta 1980; 103: 183–192.

95. Wender M, Tokarz E, Michalowska G et al. Therapeutic trials of multiple sclerosis and intrathecal IgG production. Ital J Neurol Sci 1986; 7: 205–208.

96. Lamers KJ, Uitdehaag BM, Hommes OR et al. The short-term effect of an immunosuppressive treatment on CSF myelin basic protein in chronic progressive multiple sclerosis. J Neurol Neurosurg Psychiatr 1988; 51: 1334–1337.

97. Ten Berge RJ, van Walbeek HK, Schellekens PT. Evaluation of the immunosuppressive effects of cyclophosphamide in patients with multiple sclerosis. Clin Exp Immunol 1982; 50: 495–502.

98. Brinkman CJ, Nillesen WM, Hommes OR. The effect of cyclophosphamide on T lymphocytes and T lymphocyte subsets in patients with chronic progressive multiple sclerosis. Clin Immunol Immunopathol 1983; 29: 341–348.

99. Strauss K, Hulstaert F, Deneys V et al. The immune profile of multiple sclerosis: T-lymphocyte effects predominate over all other factors in cyclophosphamide-treated patients. J Neuroimmunol 1995; 63: 133–142.

100. Smith DR, Balashov KE, Hafler DA et al. Immune deviation following pulse cyclophosphamide/methylprednisolone treatment of multiple sclerosis: increased interleukin-4 production and associated eosinophilia. Ann Neurol 1997; 42: 313–318.

101. Paterson PY, Drobish DG. Cyclophosphamide: effect on experimental allergic encephalomyelitis in Lewis rats. Science 1969; 165: 191–192.

102. Weiner HL, Cohen JA Treatment of multiple sclerosis with cyclphosphamide: critical review of clinical and immunologic effects. Mult Scler 2002; 8: 142–154.

103. Comabella M, Balashov K, Issazadeh S et al. Elevated interleukin-12 in progressive multiple sclerosis correlates with disease activity and is normalized by pulse cyclophosphamide therapy. J Clin Invest 1998; 102: 671–678.

104. Van boxel-Dezaire AH, Hoff SC, van Oosten BW et al. Contrasting responses to interferon beta-1b treatment in relapsing-remitting multiple sclerosis: does baseline interleukin-12p35 messenger RNA predict the efficacy of treatment? Ann Neurol 2000; 48: 313–322.

105. Hommes OR, Prick JJ, Lamers KJ. Treatment of the chronic progressive form of multiple sclerosis with a combination of cyclophosphamide and prednisone. Clin Neurol Neurosurg 1975; 78: 59–72.

106. Theys P, Gosseye-Lissoir F, Ketelaer P et al. Short-term intensive cyclophosphamide treatment in multiple sclerosis. A retrospective controlled study. J Neurol 1981; 225: 119–133.

107. Hommes OR et al. Prognostic factors in intensive immunosuppression on the course of chronic progressive multiple sclerosis. In: Bauer HJ, Poser S, Ritter G, eds. Progress in MU research. Berlin: Springer Verlag; 1980: 396–400.

108. Hommes OR, Prick JJ, Lamers KJ. Treatment of the chronic progressive form of multiple sclerosis with a combination of cyclophosphamide and prednisone. Clin Neurol Neurosurg 1975; 78: 592–597.

109. Hommes OR, Lamers KJB, Reekers P. Effect of intensive immunosuppression on the course of chronic progressive multiple sclerosis. J Neurol 1980; 223: 177–190.

110. Hommes OR, Aerts F, Bahr U et al. Cyclophosphamide levels in serum and spinal fluid of multiple sclerosis patients by field desoprtion mass spectrometry. J Neurol Sci 1983; 85: 297–303.

111. Theys P, Gosseye-Lissoir F, Ketelaer P et al. Short-term intensive cyclophosphamide treatment in multiple sclerosis. A retrospective controlled study. J Neurol 1981; 225: 119–133.

112. Gonsette RE, Demonty L, Delmotte P. Intensive immunosuppression with cyclophosphamide in multiple sclerosis. Follow up of 110 patients for 2–6 years. J Neurol 1977; 214: 173–181.

113. Gobbini MI, Smith ME, Richert ND et al. Effect of open label pulse cyclophosphamide therapy on MRI measures of disease activity in five patients with refractory relapsing-remitting multiple sclerosis. J Neuroimmunology 1999; 99: 142–149.

114. Patti F, Cataldi ML, Nicoletti F et al. Combination of cyclophosphamide and interferon-beta halts progression in patients with rapidly transitional multiple sclerosis. J Neurol Neurosurg Psychiatr 2001; 71: 404–407.

115. Weinstock-Guttmann B, Kinkel RP, Cohen JA et al. Treatment of fulminant multiple sclerosis with intravenous cyclophosphamide. Neurologist 1997; 3: 178–185.

116. Khan OA, Zvartau-Hind M, Caon C et al. Effect of monthly intravenous cyclophosphamide in rapidly deteriorating multiple sclerosis patients resistant to conventional therapy. Mult Scler 2001; 7 185–188.

117. Killian JM, Bressler RB, Armstrong RM et al. Controlled pilot trial of monthly intravenous cyclophosphamide in multiple sclerosis. Arch Neurol 1988; 45: 27–30.

118. Canadian Cooperative Multiple Sclerosis Study Group. The Canadian cooperative trial of cyclophosphamide and plasma exchange in progressive multiple sclerosis. Lancet 1991; 337: 441–446.

119. Likosky WH, Fireman B, Elmore R et al. Intense immunosuppression in chronic progressive multiple sclerosis: the Kaiser study. J Neurol Neurosurg Psychiatr 1991; 54: 1055–1060.

120. Zephir H, de Seze J, Duhamel A et al. Treatment of progressive forms of multiple sclerosis by cyclophosphamide: a cohort study of 490 patients. J Neurol Sci 2004; 218: 73–77.

121. Perini P, Marangoni M, Tzinteva E et al. Two years therapy of secondary progressive multiple sclerosis (SPMS) with pulse intravenous cyclophosphamide/ methylprednisolone. Clinical and MRI data. Mult Scler 2001; 7: S62.

122. Portaccio E, Zipoli V, Siracusa G et al. Safety and tolerability of cyclophosphamide 'pulses' in multiple sclerosis: a prospective study in a clinical cohort. Mult Scler 2003; 9: 446–450.

123. Weinstock-Guttman B, Kinkel RP, Cohen JA et al. Treatment of 'transistional MS' with cyclophosphamide and methylprednisolone (CTX/MP) followed by interferon β. Neurology 1997; 48(suppl 2): A341.

124. Patti F, Cataldi ML, Nicoletti F et al. Combination of cyclophosphamide and interferon-beta halts progression in patients with rapidly transitional multiple sclerosis. J Neurol Neurosurg Psychiatr 2001; 7: 404–407.

125. Patti F, Reggio E, Fiorilla T, et al. Rapidly transitional multiple sclerosis patients treated with combination of cyclophosphamide and interferon beta: follow-up 36 months after discontinuation of therapy. Neurology 2003; 60(suppl 1): A148.

126. Patti F, Reggio E, Palermo F et al. Stabilization of rapidly worsening multiple sclerosis for 36 months in patients treated with interferon beta plus cyclophosphamide followed by interferon beta. J Neurol 2004; 251: 1502–1506.

127. Hauser SL, Dawson DM, Lehrich JR et al. Intensive immunosuppression in progressive multiple sclerosis. A randomized, three-arm study of high-dose intravenous cyclophosphamide, plasma exchange, and ACTH. N Engl J Med 1983; 308: 173–180.

128. Carter JL, Hafler DA, Dawson DM et al. Immunosuppression with high-dose i.v. cyclophosphamide and ACTH in progressive multiple sclerosis: cumulative 6-year experience in 164 patients. Neurology 1988; 38(7 Suppl 2): 9–14.

129. Weiner HL, Mackin GA, Orav EJ et al. Intermittent cyclophosphamide pulse therapy in progressive multiple sclerosis: final report of the Northeast Cooperative Multiple Sclerosis Treatment Group. Neurology 1993; 43: 910–918.

130. Natsumeda Y, Carr SF. Human type I and II IMP dehydrogenases as drug targets. Ann NY Acad Sci 1993; 696: 88–93.

131. Fulton B, Markham A. Mycophenolate mofetil. A review of its pharmacodynamic and pharmacokinetic properties and clinical efficacy in renal transplantation. Drugs 1996; 51: 278–298.

132. Bardsley-Elliot A, Noble S, Foster RH. Mycophenolate mofetil: a review of its use in the management of solid organ transplantation. BioDrugs 1999; 12: 363–410.

133. Nagy SE, Andersson JP, Andersson UG. Effect of mycophenolate mofetil (RS-61443) on cytokine production: inhibition of superantigen-induced cytokines. Immunopharmacology 1993; 26: 11–20.

134. Eugui EM, Allison AC. Immunosuppressive activity of mycophenolate mofetil. Ann NY Acad Sci 1993; 685: 309–329.

135. Tran GT, Carter N, Hodgkinson SJ. Mycophenolate mofetil treatment accelerates recovery from experimental allergic encephalomyelitis. Int Immunopharmacol 2001; 1: 1709–1723.

136. Frohman EM, Brannon K, Racke MK et al. Mycophenolate mofetil in multiple sclerosis. Clin Neuropharmacol 2004; 27: 80–83.

137. Reynolds WJ, Perera M, Yoon SJ et al. Evaluation of clinical and prognostic significance of T-cell regulatory subsets in rheumatoid arthritis. J Rheumatol 1985; 12: 49–56.

138. Goto M, Miyamoto T, Nishioka K et al. T cytotoxic and helper cells are markedly increased and T suppressor and inducer cells are markedly decreased in rheumatoid synovial fluids. Arthritis Rheum 1987; 30: 737–743.

139. Lisak RP, Falk GA, Heinze RG et al. Dissociation of antibody production from disease suppression in the inhibition of allergic encephalomyelitis by myelin basic protein. J Immunol 1970; 104: 1435–1446.

140. Currier RD, Haerer AF, Maydrech EF. Low-dose oral methotrexate treatment of multiple sclerosis: a pilot study. J Neurol Neurosurg Psychiatr 1993; 56: 1217–1218.

141. Goodkin DE, Rudick RA, VanderBrug Medendorp S et al. Low-dose (7.5 mg) oral methotrexate reduces the rate of progression in chronic progressive multiple sclerosis. Ann Neurol 1995; 37: 30–40.

142. Goodkin D, Rudick RA, VanderBrug Medendorp S et al. Low-dose oral methotrexate in chronic progressive multiple sclerosis: analyses of serial MRIs. Neurology 1996; 47: 1153–1157.

143. Calabresi PA, Wilterdink JL, Rogg JM et al. An open-label trial of combination therapy with interferon β-1a and oral methotrexate in MS. Neurology 2002; 58: 314–357.

144. Rowe VD, Wang D, John HA et al. Rescue therapy with high dose intravenous methotrexate in MS patients worsening despite avonex therapy. 55th Annual Meeting Program. Neurology 2003; 60(suppl 1): A149–A150.

145. Piro LD. 2-Chlorodeoxyadenosine treatment of lymphoid malignancies. Blood 1992; 79: 843–845.

146. Beutler E. Cladribine (2-chlorodeoxyadenosine). Lancet 1992; 340: 952–956.

147. Sipe JC, Romine JS, Koziol JA et al. Development of cladribine treatment in multiple sclerosis. Mult Scler 1996; 1: 343–347.

148. Rice GP, Filippi M, Comi G. Cladribine and progressive MS: Clinical and MRI outcomes of a multicenter controlled trial. Neurology 2000; 54: 1145–1155.

149. Andersson PB, Goodkin DE. Glucocorticosteroid therapy for multiple sclerosis: a critical review. J Neurol Sci 1998; 160: 16–25.

150. Barnes PJ, Adcock I. Anti-inflammatory actions of steroids: molecular mechanisms. Trends Pharmacol Sci 1993; 14: 436–441.

151. Kern JA, Lamb RJ, Reed JC et al. Dexamethasone inhibition of interleukin 1 beta production by human monocytes. Posttranscriptional mechanisms. J Clin Invest 1988; 81: 237–244.

152. Cronstein BN, Kimmel SC, Levin RI et al. A mechanism for the antiinflammatory effects of corticosteroids: the glucocorticoid receptor regulates leukocyte adhesion to endothelial cells and expression of endothelial-leukocyte adhesion molecule 1 and intercellular adhesion molecule 1. Proc Natl Acad Sci USA 1992; 89: 9991–9995.

153. Barkhof F, Hommes OR, Scheltens P et al. Quantitative MRI changes in gadolinium-DTPA enhancement after high-dose intravenous methylprednisolone in multiple sclerosis. Neurology 1991; 41: 1219–1222.

154. Troiano RA, Hafstein MP, Zito G et al. The effect of oral corticosteroid dosage on CT enhancing multiple sclerosis plaques. J Neurol Sci 1985; 70: 67–72.

155. Troiano RA, Hafstein M, Ruderman M et al. Effect of high-dose intravenous steroid administration on contrast-enhancing computed tomographic scan lesions in multiple sclerosis. Ann Neurol 1984; 15: 257–263.

156. Rosenberg GA, Dencoff JE, Correa, Jr N et al. Effect of steroids on CSF matrix metalloproteinases in multiplesclerosis: relation to blood–brain barrier injury. Neurology 1996; 46: 1626–1632.

157. Fauci AS, Dale DC. The effect of in vivo hydrocortisone on subpopulations of human lymphocytes. J Clin Invest 1974; 53: 240–246.

158. Panitch HS, Bever CT. Clinical trials of interferons in multiple sclerosis. What have we learned? J Neuroimmunol 1993; 46: 155–164.

159. Ossege LM, Sindern E, Voss B et al. Corticosteroids induce expression of transforming-growth-factor-beta1 mRNA in peripheral blood mononuclear cells of patients with multiple sclerosis. J Neuroimmunol 1998; 84: 1–16.

160. Gelati M, Lamperti E, Dufour A et al. IL-10 production in multiple sclerosis patients, SLE patients and healthy controls: preliminary findings. Ital J Neurol Sci 1997; 18: 191–194.

161. Melcangi RC, Cavarretta I, Magnaghi V et al. Corticosteroids protect oligodendrocytes from cytokine-induced cell death. NeuroReport 2000; 11: 3969–3972.

162. Beck RW, Cleary PA, Anderson MM et al. A randomized, controlled trial of corticosteroids in the treatment of acute optic neuritis. The Optic Neuritis Study Group. N Engl J Med 1992; 326: 581–588.

163. Beck RW, Cleary PA, Trobe JD et al. The effect of corticosteroids for acute optic neuritis on the subsequent development of multiple sclerosis. N Engl J Med 1993; 329: 1764–1766.

164. Myers LW, Rudick R, Goodkin DE, eds. Multiple sclerosis. New York: Springer Verlag; 1992: 135–156.

165. Goodkin DE, Kinkel RP, Weinstock-Guttman B et al. A Phase II study of IV methylprednisolone in secondary progressive multiple sclerosis. Neurology 1998; 51: 239–245.

166. Weiss W, Stadlan EM, Goodkin DE, Rudick RA, eds. Treatment of multiple sclerosis. Trial design, results and future perspectives. New York: Springer Verlag; 1992: 91–122.

167. Zivadinov R, Rudick RA, De Masi et al. Effects of IV methylprednisolone on brain atrophy in relapsing–remitting multiple sclerosis. Neurology 2001; 5: 1239–1247.

168. Dalakas MC. Mechanism of action of intravenous immunoglobulin and therapeutic considerations in the treatment of autoimmune neurologic diseases. Neurology 1998; 51: 2–8.

169. Jorgensen SH, Sorensen PS. Intravenous immunoglobulin treatment of multiple sclerosis and its animal model, experimental autoimmune encephalomyelitis. J Neurol Sci 2005; 233: 61–65.

170. Fazekas F, Deisenhammer F, Strasser-Fuchs Siegrid et al. Randomized placebo controlled trial of monthly intravenous immunoglobulin therapy in relapsing–remitting multiple sclerosis. Lancet 1997; 349: 589–593.

171. Achiron A, Barak Y, Goren M et al. Intravenous immune globulin in multiple sclerosis: clinical and neuroradiological results and implications for possible mechanisms of action. Clin Exp Immunol 1996; 104(suppl 1): 67–70.

172. Achiron A, Rotstein Z, Barak Y et al. Intravenous immunoglobulin in multiple sclerosis and experimental autoimmune encephalomyelitis – the Israeli experience. Mult Scler 1997; 3: 142–144.

173. Sørensen PS, Wanscher B, Schreiber K et al. A double-blind, cross-over trial of intravenous immunoglobulin G in multiple sclerosis: preliminary results. Mult Scler 1997; 3: 145–148.

174. Hommes OR, Sørensen PS, Fazekas F et al. Intravenous immunoglobulin in secondary progressive multiple sclerosis: randomized placebo-controlled trial. Lancet 2004; 364: 1149–1156.

175. Fazekas F, Sørensen PS, Filippi M et al. MRI results from the European Study on Intravenous Immunoglobulin in Secondary Progressive Multiple Sclerosis. Mult Scler 2005; 11: 433–440.

176. Hughes RAC, Wijdicks EFM, Barohn R et al. Practice parameter: immunotherapy for Guillain–Barré syndrome: report of the Quality Standards Subcommittee of the American Academy of Neurology. Neurology 2003; 61: 736–740.

177. Blom RJ, Kuks JB, Westerterp-Maas A et al. Favorable results of plasmapheresis in severe myasthenia gravis. Ned Tijdschr Geneeskd 1997; 141: 381–384.

178. Weinshenker BG, O'Brien PC, Petterson TM et al. A Randomized trial of plasma exchange in acute central nervous system inflammatory demyelinating disease. Ann Neurol 1999; 46: 878–886.

179. Keegan M, Pineda AA, McClelland RL et al. Plasma exchange for severe attacks of CNS demyelination: predictors of response. Neurology 2002; 58: 143–146.

180. Keegan M, Konig F, McClelland R et al. Relation between humoral pathological changes in multiple sclerosis and response to therapeutic plasma exchange. Lancet 2005; 366: 579–833.

181. Goto T, Kino T, Hatanaka H et al. Discovery of FK-506, a novel immunosuppressant isolated from Streptomyces tsukubaensis. Transplant Proc 1987; 19(suppl 6): 4–8.

182. Schreiber SL, Crabtree GR. The mechanism of action of cyclosporin A and FK506. Immunol Today 1992; 13: 136–142.

183. Gold BG, Voda J, Yu X et al. FK506 and a nonimmunosuppressive derivative reduce axonal and myelin damage in experimental autoimmune encephalomyelitis: neuroimmunophilin ligand-mediated neuroprotection in a model of multiple sclerosis. J Neurosci Res 2004; 77: 367–377.

184. Gonsette RE. New immunosuppressants with potential implication in multiple sclerosis. J Neurol Sci 2004; 223: 87–93.

185. Kahan BD. Cyclosporine. N Engl J Med 1989; 32: 1725–1738.

186. Khanna A, Li B, Stenzel KH et al. Regulation of new DNA synthesis in mammalian cells by cyclosporine. Demonstration of a transforming growth factor beta-dependent mechanism of inhibition of cell growth. Transplantation 1994; 57: 577–582.

187. Steck AJ, Regli F, Ochsner F et al. Cyclosporine versus azathioprine in the treatment of multiple sclerosis: 12-month clinical and immunological evaluation. Eur Neurol 1990; 30: 224–228.

188. Multiple Sclerosis Study Group. Efficacy and toxicity of cyclosporine in chronic progressive multiple sclerosis: a randomized, double-blinded, placebo-controlled clinical trial. Ann Neurol 1990; 27: 591–605.

189. Jafri S, Pasricha PJ. Agents used in inflammatory bowel disease: section vi – agents used for diarrhea, constipation, and inflammatory bowel disease; agents used for biliary and pancreatic disease. In: Hardman JG, Limbird LE, Goodman Gilman A, eds. Goodman & Gilman's the pharmacological basis of therapeutics 10th ed. New York: McGraw-Hill; 2001: 1037–1059.

190. Noseworthy JH, O'Brien P, Erickson BJ et al. The Mayo Clinic–Canadian Cooperative trial of sulfasalazine in active multiple sclerosis. Neurology 1998; 51: 1342–1352.

191. Moreau T, Coles A, Wing M et al. CAMPATH-IH in multiple sclerosis. Mult Scler 1996; 1: 357–365.

192. Coles AJ, Deans J, Compston A. Campath-1H treatment of multiple sclerosis: lessons from the bedside for the bench. Clin Neurol Neurosurg 2004; 106: 270–274.

193. Coles A, Wing MG, Molyneux P et al. Monoclonal antibody treatment exposes three mechanisms underlying the clinical course of multiple sclerosis. Ann Neurol 1999; 46: 296–304.

194. Coles A, Wing M, Smith S et al. Pulsed monoclonal antibody treatment and autoimmune thyroid disease in multiple sclerosis. Lancet 1999; 354: 1691–1695.

195. Genzyme Press Release. Genzyme and Schering AG announce interim results from trial of Campath for multiple sclerosis. 16 September 2005. Available on line at: http://www.genzyme.co.uk/corp/news/all_news/GENZ%20PR-091605.asp.

196. Rastetter W, Molina A, White CA. Rituximab: expanding role in therapy for lymphomas and autoimmune diseases. Annu Rev Med 2004; 55: 477–503.

197. Reff ME, Carner K, Chambers KS et al. Depletion of B cells in vivo by a chimeric mouse human monoclonal antibody to CD20. Blood 1994; 83: 435–445.

198. Valentine MA, Clark EA, Shu GL et al. Phosphorylation of the CD20 phosphoprotein in resting B lymphocytes. Regulation by protein kinase C. J Biol Chem 1989; 264: 1182–1187.

199. Einfeld DA Brown JP, Valentine MA et al. Molecular cloning of the human B cell CD20 receptor predicts a hydrophobic protein with multiple transmembrane domains. EMBO J 1988; 7: 711–717.

200. Anderson KC, Bates MP, Slaughenhoupt BL et al. Expression of human B cell-associated antigens on leukemias and lymphomas: a model of human B cell differentiation. Blood 1984; 63: 1424–1433.

201. Maloney DG, Grillo-Lopez AJ, White CA et al. IDEC-C2B8 (Rituximab) anti-CD20 monoclonal antibody therapy in patients with relapsed low-grade non-Hodgkin's lymphoma. Blood 1997; 90: 2188–2195.

202. Taji H, Kagami Y, Okada Y et al. Growth inhibition of CD20-positive B lymphoma cell lines by IDEC-C2B8 anti-CD20 monoclonal antibody. Jpn J Cancer Res 1998; 89: 748–756.

203. Clynes RA, Towers TL, Presta LG et al. Inhibitory Fc receptors modulate in vivo cytoxicity against tumor targets. Nat Med 2000; 6: 443–446.

204. Cree B, Lamb S, Chin A et al. Tolerability and effects of rituximab (anti-CD20 antibody) in neuromyelitis optica (NMO) and rapidly worsening multiple sclerosis (MS). AAN 56th Annual Meeting Program. Neurology 2004; 7(suppl 5): A492.

205. Pender MP. The pathogenesis of primary progressive multiple sclerosis: antibody-mediated attack and no repair? J Clin Neurosci 2004; 11: 689–692.

206. Mohrbacher A. B cell non-Hodgkin's lymphoma: rituximab safety experience. Arthritis Res Ther 2005; 7(suppl 3): S19–S25.

207. Coiffier B, Haioun C, Ketterer N et al. Rituximab (anti-CD20 monoclonal antibody) for the treatment of patients with relapsing or refractory aggressive lymphoma: a multicenter phase II study. Blood 1998; 92: 1927–1932.

208. Rose JW, Lorberboum-Galski H, Fitzgerald D et al. Chimeric cytotoxin IL2-PE40 inhibits relapsing experimental allergic encephalomyelitis. J Neuroimmunol 1991; 32: 209–217.

209. Hayosh NS, Silberg DG, Swanborg RH. Autoimmune effector cells. Part 10: Effector cells of autoimmune encephalomyelitis in healthy nonimmune rats. J Immunol 1987; 138: 3771–3775.

210. Englehardt B, Diamantstein T, Wekerle H. Immunotherapy of experimental autoimmune encephalomyelitis (EAE): differential effect of anti-IL-2 receptor antibody therapy on actively induced and T-line mediated EAE of the Lewis rat. J Autoimmun 1989; 2: 61–73.

211. Bielekova B, Richert N, Howard T et al. Humanized anti-CD25 (daclizumab) inhibits disease activity in multiple sclerosis patients failing to respond to interferon beta. Proc Natl Acad Sci USA 2004; 101: 8705–8708.

212. Stone LA, Frank JA, Albert PS et al. Characterization of MRI response to treatment with interferon beta-1b: contrast-enhancing MRI lesion frequency as a primary outcome measure. Neurology 1997; 49: 862–869.

213. Miller DH, Khan OA, Sheremata WA et al. A controlled trial of natalizumab for relapsing multiple sclerosis. N Engl J Med 2003; 348: 15–23.

214. Rose J, Watt HE, White AT et al. Treatment of multiple sclerosis with an anti-interleukin-2 receptor monoclonal antibody. Ann Neurol 2004; 56: 864–867.

215. National Institute of Neurological Disorders and Stroke (NINDS). Zenapax (daclizumab) to treat relapsing remitting multiple sclerosis. Available online at: http://clinicaltrials.

gov/ct/show/NCT00071838?order=3.

216. Fassas A, Anagnostopoulos A, Kazis A et al. Peripheral blood stem cell transplantation in the treatment of progressive multiple sclerosis: first results of a pilot study. Bone Marrow Transplant 1997; 20: 631–638.

217. Karussis D, Vourka-Karussis U, Mizrachi-Koll R et al. Acute/relapsing experimental autoimmune encephalomyelitis: induction of long lasting, antigen-specific tolerance by syngeneic bone marrow transplantation. Mult Scler 1999; 5: 17–21.

218. Fassas A, Passweg JR, Anagnostopoulos A et al. Hematopoietic stem cell transplantation for multiple sclerosis. A retrospective multicenter study. J Neurol 2002; 249: 1088–1097.

219. Burt RK, Fassas A, Snowden J et al. Collection of hematopoietic stem cells from patients with autoimmune diseases. Blood 2001; 28: 1–12.

220. McAllister LD, Beatty PG, Rose J. Allogeneic bone marrow transplant for chronic myelogenous leukemia in a patient with multiple sclerosis. Bone Marrow Transplant 1997; 19: 395–397.

221. Meloni G, Capria S, Salvetti M et al. Autologous peripheral blood stem cell transplantation in a patient with multiple sclerosis and concomitant Ph+ acute leukemia. Haematologica 1999; 84: 665–667.

222. Mandalfino P, Rice G, Smith A et al. Bone marrow transplantation in multiple sclerosis. J Neurol 2000; 247: 691–695.

223. Fassas A, Kazis A. High dose immunosuppression and autologous hematopoietic stem cell rescue for severe multiple sclerosis. J Hematother Stem Cell Res 2003; 12: 707–711.

224. Fassas A, Anagnostopoulos A, Kazis A et al. Autologous stem cell transplantation in progressive multiple sclerosis – an interim analysis of efficacy. J Clin Immunol 2000; 20: 24–30.

225. Openshaw H, Stuve O, Antel JP et al. Multiple sclerosis flares associated with recombinant granulocyte colony-stimulating factor. Neurology 2000; 54: 2147–2150.

226. Kimiskidis VK, Tsimourtou V, Papagiannopoulos S et al. Autologous stem cell transplantation in multiple sclerosis: the MRI study. J Neurol 2002; 249(suppl 1): I/61.

227. Bredesen C, Forman SJ, Horowitz M et al. Conference synopsis: Hematopoietic stem cell therapy in autoimmune diseases, October 2001. Biol Blood Marrow Transplant 2002; 8: 407–411.

228. Hintzen RQ. Stem cell transplantation in multiple sclerosis: multiple choices and multiple challenges. Mult Scler 2002; 8: 155–160.

CHAPTER 23

Novel and promising therapeutic strategies in multiple sclerosis

M. K. Racke and R. Gold

INTRODUCTION

Today only a handful of drugs have been approved for the treatment of multiple sclerosis (MS), and these treatments are only partially effective. These treatments can also have significant side effects. This is true despite the intense efforts to identify factors involved in its pathogenesis and produce new treatments for MS. The National Institutes of Health (NIH) spend more on MS research than on research into asthma, tuberculosis or cervical cancer.[1] Therapeutic strategies in development for MS are attempting to target specific components of the immune response in an attempt to suppress the autoimmune component of the disease process while avoiding the widespread immunosuppression caused by some of the current therapies.

The underlying pathophysiology of MS is not well understood. While B cells and CD8+ T cells are probably involved,[2–7] the inciting cell is postulated to be the CD4+ helper T (Th) cell. One hypothesis for the pathogenesis of MS is that the inflammation occurs in the central nervous system (CNS) as a result of a shift in the peripheral myelin-specific T-cell population from a naive or an anti-inflammatory Th2 cell population to one composed of predominantly Th1-like myelin-specific cells.[4] This imbalance between Th1 and Th2 lymphocytes when recruited to the CNS results in an inflammatory milieu in which other immune cells recruited to the site of inflammation participate in local inflammation and destruction, and a diversification of the immune response occurs in the CNS. In response to this hypothesis, considerable research is being devoted to disrupting one or more parts of the immune response to myelin antigens. If therapies targeted to disrupt these pathogenic immune cells could be discovered, the entire inflammatory process could potentially be circumvented and result in a reduction in damage to various components of the CNS. These novel strategies being developed for MS will be the topic of this chapter.

CURRENT THERAPY

Treatment with interferon (IFN)β or glatiramer acetate has become the mainstay for reducing the frequency of relapses and delaying the progression of MS. IFNβ, which is administered either subcutaneously or intramuscularly, has more clinical and experimental evidence supporting its use than any of the other drugs approved for MS treatment. While IFNβ has been particularly effective in reducing the number of gadolinium-enhancing lesions by magnetic resonance imaging (MRI), drawbacks include injection-site reactions, flu-like symptoms, fatigue and the development of neutralizing antibodies in some patients after long-term treatment.[8] Glatiramer acetate, a mixture of random polypeptides with a similar amino acid composition to myelin basic protein (MBP), is the other commonly used treatment for relapsing–remitting MS (RRMS). Like some formulations of IFNβ, it is given subcutaneously and can induce an injection-site reaction but unlike IFN it does not carry the risk of flu-like symptoms or hepatic toxicity.[9] Both IFNβ and glatiramer acetate are considered first-line drugs for the treatment of MS; however, because their treatment effect is still modest, better treatments for MS are clearly needed. In June 2006, the US Food and Drug Administration (FDA) approved a supplemental Biologics License Application for the use of the anti-VLA-4 mAb natalizumab, which was also approved by the European Commission; however, its role in the management of RRMS is currently evolving.

In addition to IFNβ and glatiramer acetate, several other drugs have been used for patients with progressive RRMS or secondary progressive MS (SPMS). Mitoxantrone is a cytotoxic and immunosuppressive agent with a significant clinical history in the oncological arena. Because of the risk of cumulative dose-dependent cardiotoxicity, the primary use of this drug in patients with MS is for rapidly progressive disease or for patients who deteriorate on established therapy.[10] Other drugs in the category of global immunosuppressants that have been used to treat severe or rapidly progressing MS are cyclophosphamide, azathioprine and methotrexate.[11] None of these immunosuppressive agents is approved by the FDA for the treatment of MS but they are often used in appropriate clinical situations. Several other immunosuppressive agents currently undergoing clinical trials in MS patients include mycophenolate mofetil, sirolimus, fumaric acid esters and paclitaxel.[11] These drugs may become common therapies for various types of MS and will be discussed further below. Pulses of high-dose methylprednisolone (HDMP) have been shown to reduce the severity of relapses and may modify the long-term course of the disease but are often accompanied by the side effects typically associated with glucocorticoid therapy. The role of HDMP as additive therapy for patients who have failed treatment with first-line agents remains unclear.[12] MS patients clearly need more effective therapies capable of regulating specific immune pathways involved in the pathogenesis of MS while avoiding the systemic immunosuppressant effects of the more potent drugs described above.

IMMUNOSUPPRESSIVE/ ANTIPROLIFERATIVE AGENTS

MYCOPHENOLATE

Mycophenolate mofetil (MMF), licensed to prevent the rejection of transplanted organs, has been used in neuroimmunological diseases for the achievement of either symptom stabilization or remission. MMF is a prodrug. It is metabolized to mycophenolic acid, a reversible, selective and non-competitive inhibitor of the inosine monophosphate dehydrogenase (IMPDH) type II (Fig. 23.1). Compared to its activity towards the housekeeping type I isoform, MMF is five times more potent in inhibiting the type II isoform of IMPDH, found in proliferating lymphocytes.[13] Mycophenolic acid is recirculated by an enterohepatic pathway after glucuronidation to an inactive metabolite with renal elimination. In patients with renal insufficiency, MMF doses should not exceed 2 g/d. Controlled studies in rheumatology have shown that, in some patients, MMF is superior to standard azathioprine therapy.[14]

In a retrospective and uncontrolled study, the safety and tolerability of MMF was evaluated in 79 MS patients with either SPMS ($n=61$), RRMS ($n=14$) or primary progressive (PPMS) ($n=4$) disease course.[15] MMF was started at 250 mg daily and successively increased by 250 mg every week up to 1000 mg daily. MMF was administered as monotherapy to 15 patients. The other patients were treated with MMF in combination with either IFNβ ($n=44$) or glatiramer acetate ($n=20$). Clinical status was not systematically evaluated but, according to the authors, 'clinical observation suggested that many of the MMF treated patients exhibited stabilizing effects from treatment'. Eight patients stopped MMF, mainly because of diarrhea.

In an uncontrolled, surveillance trial, seven patients with refractory MS with disease progression in terms of the Expanded Disability Status Scale (EDSS), despite established treatment, were treated with MMF 2 g daily in addition to their standard medication.[16] Two patients did not respond; however, in five patients administration of MMF led to improvement or stopped progression and three patients even felt subjectively improved, although EDSS had not improved. Two patients had fewer lesions on MRI.

In a phase II trial, the safety and efficacy of MMF in combination with IFNβ were examined. Preliminary results indicated that MMF was well tolerated and that it may possibly have beneficial effects with regard to stabilization and reduction of relapse rate. There are currently several studies ongoing: one randomized, placebo-controlled, double-blind study on IFNβ-1a in combination with MMF or placebo in 24 patients, one open-label trial on MMF monotherapy in 42 patients and one double-blind, placebo-controlled study on MMF in active MS despite first-line therapy (http:// www.nmss.org).

Conclusion/comment

Data on MMF therapy in MS are limited. First results indicate that MMF is well tolerated in MS. The efficacy of MMF in this condition is uncertain, pending the completion of larger, better-designed trials.

TACROLIMUS

Tacrolimus is a macrolide immunosuppressant metabolite also known as FK506. It is administered orally in capsules containing a solid dispersion of the substance. Bioavailability after enteral resorption ranges from 10–60%. Tacrolimus is highly bound to plasma proteins. It is metabolized in the intestinal wall and the liver through CYP3A4/cytochrome P450 3A4. Plasma elimination is significantly prolonged in patients with disturbed liver function. It binds preferentially to FKBP 12, an isoform of cytoplasmic immunophilins. The FKBP–tacrolimus complex inhibits the activity of calcineurin and thus disrupts calcium-dependent signal transduction (Fig. 23.1). Subsequently, cytokine gene activation is impaired, curtailing IL2-mediated T-cell proliferation.[17] Some of the effects of tacrolimus may also be mediated via modulation of cellular immune functions such as inhibition of nitric oxide synthetase activation.

In a chronic relapsing experimental autoimmune encephalomyelitis (EAE) model of MS, where female SJL/J mice were

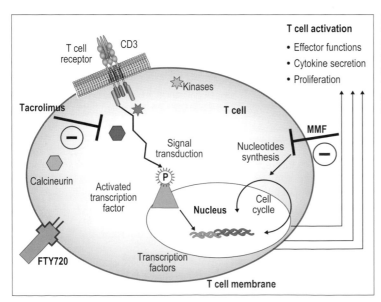

FIG. 23.1. Molecular mechanisms of immunosuppressive drugs on T-cell activation. T-cell-receptor engagement leads to multistep, intracellular signaling cascades. Tacrolimus acts at immunophilins involved in the early stages of T cell activation, while mycophenolate (MMF) blocks nucleotide synthesis required for further cell cycle progression. In contrast, FTY720 exerts agonistic effects at sphingosine receptors and thus modulates T cell homing.

immunized with proteolipid protein 139–151 peptide, daily subcutaneous injections of FK506 reduced the severity of the initial episode of disease and suppressed subsequent relapses.[18] Importantly, in the thoracic spinal cord, FK506 (5 mg/kg) significantly reduced the extent of damage in white matter by 95% compared to controls. A nonimmunosuppressive dose of FK506 (0.2 mg/kg) also significantly ($p < 0.001$) reduced the extent of damage in the spinal cord by up to 45%. Thus, FK506 markedly protected against demyelination and axonal loss in this MS model. Tacrolimus has been used in a small study in MS. In 19 MS patients, no significant effect of tacrolimus on circulating CD4+ T cells expressing CD25 and CD45RA antigens was found.[19] Tacrolimus was well tolerated in this small group of MS patients.

Conclusion/comment

Tacrolimus seems to be safe but no reliable clinical data in MS are presently available.

IMMUNOBIOLOGICALS/MISCELLANEOUS

FUMARATE

Fumaric acid esters influence several aspects of immune function that are thought to be involved in MS. Fumarate therapy has been shown to induce Th2-like cytokines (e.g. interleukin (IL)-4, IL-5, and IL-10) to induce apoptosis in activated T cells and to downregulate intracellular adhesion molecules (ICAM)-1 and vascular cell adhesion molecule (VCAM) expression.[20,21] A reduction in these cellular adhesion molecules may lead to reduced migration of lymphocytes across endothelial barriers into surrounding tissues, considered to be an important event in MS. In experimental models fumarate esters have been shown to be effective in different models of mouse EAE, and were especially active in reducing macrophage inflammation.[22]

Fumaderm (BiogenIdec) is a fumaric acid ester formulation that is approved in Germany for the treatment of severe chronic plaque psoriasis.[23,24] The efficacy and safety of oral fumarate were investigated in a baseline-controlled, open-label pilot study in 10 patients with RRMS by Schimrigk et al.[25] The study consisted of the following four phases: 6-week baseline, 18-week treatment (target dose of 720 mg/d), 4-week washout and a second 48-week treatment phase (target dose of 360 mg/d). Patients with at least one gadolinium-enhancing lesion on T1-weighted MRI brain scan participated in the study. The most common adverse events were gastrointestinal symptoms and flushing; all adverse events were reported as mild and reversible. Fumaric acid esters produced significant reductions from baseline in number ($p < 0.05$) and volume ($p < 0.01$) of gadolinium-enhancing lesions after 18 weeks of treatment; this effect persisted during the second treatment phase at half the target dose after the 4-week washout period. EDSS scores, ambulation index and 9-HPT remained stable or slightly improved from baseline in all patients. Several cytokines were modulated; in particular, circulating tumor necrosis factor (TNF)α was downregulated. Recently, a phase II clinical trial was terminated with a modified fumaric salt BG12, exhibiting far fewer gastroenteric side effects. These promising results have led to initiation of a phase III trial with BG12 in RRMS.

Conclusion/comment

Oral fumaric acid esters are considered to be safe based on more than 30 000 patient years of experience in psoriasis. They may turn out to be an effective oral therapy in RRMS.

TERIFLUNOMIDE

Teriflunomide is the active metabolite of leflunomide, originally called A77 1726. Leflunomide belongs to the group of isoxazole derivatives and has been used for the treatment of rheumatological disorders since the end of the 1990s. Teriflunomide impairs cellular nucleotide metabolism by inhibiting the dihydroorotate dehydrogenase (DHODH), a rate-limiting enzyme of de novo pyrimidine synthesis. Furthermore, it suppresses tyrosine kinases involved in signal transduction pathways. The biological half-life of these compounds is up to 2 weeks, based on enterohepatic recirculation. Leflunomide was successfully used in the animal model of experimental neuritis,[26] where it reduced demyelination and axonal degeneration in the sciatic nerve.

A phase II trial examined the safety and efficacy of oral teriflunomide in 179 patients aged 19–64 years with clinically definite MS and two or more documented relapses in the previous 3 years. Patients were randomized 1:1:1 to receive placebo, 7 mg or 14 mg teriflunomide over 36 weeks in a double-blind, controlled design. A significant (60%) reduction of new active MRI lesions was observed and less EDSS progression was noted in the group receiving 14 mg.[27] Also, a trend towards a reduced relapse rate was noted. Common side effects were headache and nasopharyngitis. Sanofi-Aventis has recently launched a phase III trial in RRMS.

Conclusion/comment

Teriflunomide is derived from a substance already used for treatment of rheumatological diseases and the potential for therapeutic efficacy in RRMS needs to be confirmed in a phase III trial.

LAQUINIMOD

Laquinimod is a novel synthetic quinoline compound with high oral bioavailability that suppresses autoimmune and inflammatory diseases in experimental animal models. It is structurally related to its predecessor, linomide, which had to be discontinued because of undesired inflammatory effects, particularly systemic vasculitis. The mode of action and the molecular targets of laquinimod and linomide are still unknown. It is hypothesized that they alter Th1/Th2 balance, natural killer cell function and inhibited migration of inflammatory cells into nerve tissue.[28,29] Results of a phase II study where doses of 0.1 mg or 0.3 mg laquinimod were compared with placebo over a 6-month period demonstrated its safety and tolerability. A significant reduction of the primary endpoint, gadolinium-enhancing lesions, was observed in 44–52% of patients in the 0.3 mg group. Another phase IIb clinical trial is currently ongoing and will address the efficacy of the higher dose of 0.6 mg laquinimod.

Conclusion/comment

Oral laquinimod is promising for the treatment of RRMS but it has yet to enter phase III trials, so ultimate conclusions regarding its efficacy cannot be made. The new compound, laquinimod, seems to be safe and great care has been taken to avoid the serious side effects observed with linomide.

FTY 720

The novel compound 2-amino-[2-(4-octylphenyl) ethyl]-1,3-propanediol hydrochloride (FTY720) inhibits lymphocyte egress from secondary lymphoid tissues and thymus by agonistic activity at sphingosine 1-phosphate receptors (Fig. 23.1).[30] A striking feature of FTY720 is the induction of a marked decrease in peripheral blood T and B cells. It drives these immune cells into tissues and prevents them from migrating into transplanted organs or autoimmune target organs. FTY720 was studied in Lewis rat EAE[31] and SJL mice.[32] FTY720 treatment almost completely protected the rats against disease and was accompanied by a dramatic reduction in the number of lymphocytes in the spinal cord. Results were further corroborated by mRNA analyses that showed marked expression of Th1 cytokines IL-2, IL-6 and IFNγ in the spinal cord. Through passive transfer EAE studies, FTY720 resulted in the inhibition of encephalitogenic T-cell responses and T-cell migration into the CNS.[31] By MRI-based tracking of macrophages labeled with superparamagnetic iron oxide (USPIO) nanoparticles, these results received further confirmation in acute and chronic EAE.[33]

Initial results of a phase II study in MS (Sponsor: Novartis Pharma) have been presented at the meeting of the European Neurological Society (Vienna, Austria). 281 patients with active, relapsing MS were randomized to receive placebo, 1.25 mg or 5.0 mg FTY720 every day for 6 months. The study demonstrated a 60% reduction in gadolinium-enhancing lesions by MRI and a 50% lower relapse rate. With regard to its side effects, FTY720 may induce reversible bradycardia after the initial dosing and a higher rate of nasopharyngitis.

ANTI-B-CELL THERAPIES

Histopathological studies on MS tissue at the cellular and molecular level led to the classification of actively demyelinating MS plaques into distinct pathological patterns I–IV of MS by Lassmann and colleagues.[34] Of these, pattern II with antibody and complement mediated demyelination covers about 30% of analyzed lesions, and similar findings were obtained in neuromyelitis optica (Devic's disease).[35] Unfortunately, there is no unequivocal surrogate marker that is indicative of or correlates with these lesion patterns. In selected cases, where tumefactive lesions were suggestive of malignant disease, brain biopsies were performed. Deposition of antibody/complement correlated with therapeutic response to plasmapheresis.[36] Thus, we know that B-cell-directed therapies might be effective for acute intervention. Since ectopic B-cell follicles have been identified within the meninges of MS patients, we can anticipate that B-cell-directed approaches may also be of help in long-term therapy. On this background, the following drugs are discussed.

ANTI CD20

Rituximab, an anti-CD20 monoclonal antibody that depletes CD20⁺ B cells, has demonstrated efficacy in peripheral neurological diseases. In humans, CD20 is expressed on most B lymphocytes but not on plasma B cells. It is probable that rituximab depletes B lymphocytes via antibody/complement-dependent cytotoxicity (Fig. 23.2, step 8).[37,38] Whether this efficacy can be translated to neurological diseases of the CNS with possible autoimmune B-cell involvement remains to be determined. In a patient with high disease activity and multiple gadolinium-enhancing MRI lesions, two infusions of rituximab at the standard dosage (375 mg/m² body surface) resulted in significant clinical improvement, reduced inflammatory surrogate markers on MRI and depleted B cells in serum and cerebrospinal fluid (CSF).[39] Similarly, eight patients with worsening neuromyelitis optica were treated with rituximab to achieve B cell depletion. They received the standard dosage of four weekly infusions at 375 mg/m² body surface. Treatment was well tolerated. Six of eight patients were relapse-free and median attack rate declined from 2.6 attacks/patient/year to 0 attacks/patient/year. In addition, seven of eight patients experienced substantial

recovery of neurological function over 1 year of average follow-up.[40]

In contrast to these cases with active disease courses, Monson and colleagues studied the effects of rituximab in four patients with PPMS.[41] Here the B cells in CSF were not as effectively depleted as their peripheral blood counterparts. Rituximab treatment temporarily suppressed the activation state of B cells in CSF. The effect(s) of rituximab on the CSF B-cell compartment was limited in comparison with the effect(s) on the B cells in the periphery. One may speculate whether this finding correlates with the extent of blood–brain barrier damage in PPMS.[41]

Conclusion/comment

Anti-CD20 seems to be a very promising and well tolerated therapy in patients with antibody/complement-mediated MS as defined by pattern II. Unfortunately, the assignment of 'B cell MS' in a routine clinical setting is empirical and lacks reliable surrogate markers in blood or by MRI. Larger controlled studies are needed. Also, the results of an ongoing trial in PPMS are eagerly anticipated.

MITOXANTRONE AND PIXANTRONE

The cytotoxic drug mitoxantrone, introduced into MS by Gonsette in the late 1980s, is a highly effective, immunoactive agent in the treatment of active MS. Despite proven clinical efficacy, there is little data available on its mode of action. In recent ex vivo studies, Chan et al[42] observed a rapid incorporation of mitoxantrone in circulating leukocytes of MS patients. The pronounced suppression of proliferative responses was at least partly mediated by the induction of late apoptotic/necrotic cell death with a preferential susceptibility of B cells.

Pixantrone is less cardiotoxic than and is similarly effective to mitoxantrone as an antineoplastic drug. In acute and chronic relapsing experimental autoimmune encephalomyelitis (EAE) models, pixantrone reduced disease severity.[43] A marked and long-lasting decrease in CD3⁺, CD4⁺, CD8⁺ and CD45RA⁺ blood cells and reduced antimyelin antibody titers were observed with pixantrone, similar to mitoxantrone. Cardiotoxicity was present only in mitoxantrone-treated but not in pixantrone-treated rats. The effectiveness and the favorable safety profile may make pixantrone one of the most promising immunosuppressive agents for severe MS.

Conclusion/comment

It seems as though we retrospectively now understand the superior efficacy of mitoxantrone in view of new data on the role of B cells in active MS. It is relatively economical and convenient, but of course the potentially severe side effects have to be considered, especially when compared with the immunobiological eradication of B cells. The potential cardiotoxicity might be reduced by combination therapy with dexrazoxane, which is even synergistic with mitoxantrone in limiting inflammatory lesions in EAE models.[44] For pixantrone, controlled trials in MS are needed.

BONE MARROW/HEMATOPOIETIC STEM CELL TRANSPLANTATION

Since most available evidence supports the concept of an autoimmune attack in MS pathogenesis, it is reasonable that a 'reset' of the immune system via immunoablation and (autologous) blood stem cell support has been studied in MS, following promising results in experimental animal models. The primary problem is that all these efforts may come too late, after

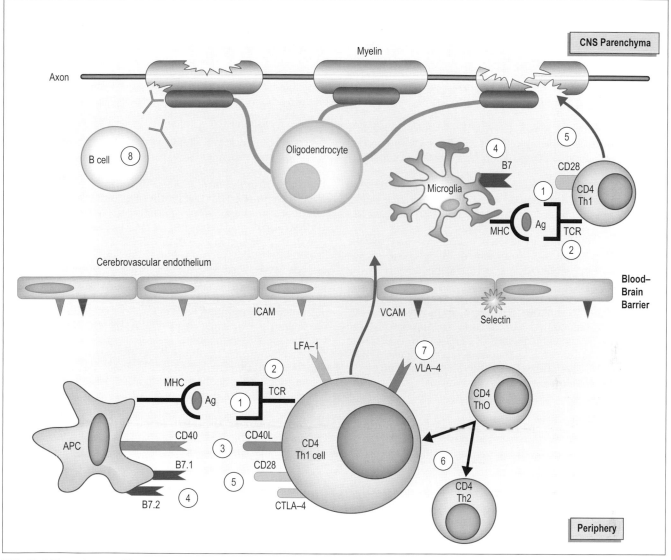

FIG. 23.2 Targeting specific steps in the development of CNS inflammatory, demyelinating disease. The diagram outlines several steps in the activation of autoreactive T cells and their migration to the brain parenchyma, resulting in axon demyelination. Therapeutic strategies acting at each step are: (**1**) DNA vaccine, altered peptide ligands, soluble peptides; (**2**) soluble MHC-peptide, T-cell vaccine; (**3**) anti-CD40/ CD40L antibody; (**4**) CTLA-4-Ig (**5**); anti-CD28 antibody; (**6**) cytokine therapy, nuclear hormone receptor agonists, statins, T-bet siRNA; (**7**) anti-α4-integrin antibody; (**8**) rituximab therapy. Some treatments target many steps but only the primary site of action is shown. Ab, antibody; Ag, antigen; APC, antigen presenting cell; MHC, major histocompatability complex; TCR, T-cell receptor.

inflammation has caused early damage of neuronal elements or if neurodegeneration prevails and has caused permanent disability. Although many MS patients may profit from more powerful immunosuppression, it is often reserved for the advanced stages of MS because of its potential toxicity. Other key variables are the type of immunoablation and the source and form of mobilization of hematopoietic stem cells. Hematopoietic stem cell transplantation as a treatment for MS patients has been initiated worldwide. At this stage, it is impossible to draw general conclusions from the initial data reported and therefore overenthusiastic expectations should be tempered.[45,46] Bone marrow transplantation induces profound qualitative immunological changes that demonstrate a de novo regeneration of the T cell.[47] In the largest published series by Saiz, 14 MS patients with a mean EDSS of less than 6.5 were transplanted but four of them continued to have relapses, raising the question of whether immunoablation was achieved.

Conclusion/comment

The follow-up periods are too short, the groups are too small, the selected patients and protocols too heterogeneous, and publication bias for positive results cannot be excluded. However, there is ample evidence that hematological stem cell transplantation is a technically feasible approach in MS and it does not appear more dangerous than in other hemato-oncological diseases. It is unclear whether the neurodegenerative process that occurs in MS can be stopped merely by halting the immune processes.

SELECTED INNOVATIVE THERAPIES

DNA VACCINES

For several years, researchers have been utilizing DNA vaccines as a means to induce self-tolerance in autoimmune diseases such as EAE. The DNA constructs may be either naked[48,49] or plasmid-encapsulated.[50,51] The DNA product is typically expressed at the injection site, where it is then taken up by antigen presenting cells (APCs) that then migrate to the lymph node (Fig. 23.2, step 1). Two different strategies for treating autoimmunity have been studied. One strategy utilizes DNA that encodes proinflammatory mediators, with the goal of inducing 'beneficial autoimmunity' by producing neutralizing antibodies against these proinflammatory mediators.[49,51,52] The other strategy through which DNA vaccines protect against autoimmunity is by inducing tolerance to the protein encoded by the vaccine, which is expressed on 'self' tissues at the injection site.[48,50]

While both methods have shown some success in treating various EAE models, the method focusing on tolerance induction using DNA encoding encephalitogenic myelin antigens has been the primary approach. DNA vaccines encoding myelin oligodendrocyte glycoprotein (MOG) suppressed EAE in the Lewis rat.[50] Other studies in murine EAE models have shown mixed results. One study showed a time-dependent response to vaccination with DNA encoding proteolipid protein (PLP), another potential myelin self-antigen. Induction of disease within 4 weeks of vaccination resulted in more severe disease, whereas disease induction 10 weeks after vaccination resulted in amelioration of the clinical signs of disease.[48] In contrast to the above study, mice with EAE that were vaccinated with MOG DNA developed worse disease, which was felt to be due to the production of MOG autoantibodies.[53] Interestingly, the increase in disease severity was seen whether MOG or another antigen was used to induce disease. These studies demonstrate some of the important issues in using self-protein-encoding DNA to induce tolerance. Another strategy that has been used successfully to ensure that a protective Th2 immune response occurs instead of activating inflammatory Th1 cells is the simultaneous injection of a DNA vaccine encoding a PLP peptide with naked DNA encoding IL-4. This strategy provided complete protection against the development of EAE due to coexpression of a PLP antigen and IL-4 at the same site, resulting in the PLP-reactive T cells exhibiting almost exclusively a Th2 cytokine profile.[54] Another innovative approach to design DNA vaccines targeted towards specific antigenic epitopes involves the use of protein microarrays.[55] These microarrays have been used to screen the 'myelin proteome' for a wide panel of autoantibody responses in EAE. These responses are then used to design DNA vaccines encoding those myelin epitopes against which autoantibodies are present, providing a targeted therapy specific for each individual. Phase I and II trials using various DNA vaccines are currently under way in human subjects with MS.

Conclusion/comment

While DNA vaccination has shown promising results in EAE models, it remains to be seen whether an antigen-specific strategy will be successful in MS. Thus, this strategy will require success both in the use of this technology and that such a strategy will be beneficial in human MS.

ALTERED PEPTIDE LIGANDS

Altered peptide ligands (APLs) offer another potential mechanism by which pathogenic self-reactive T cells may be altered in their reactivity towards self-antigens. APLs are similar in structure to antigenic peptides except for amino acid substitutions at sites thought to be important for T-cell-receptor (TCR) recognition. Peptides can either be altered in the TCR-binding region or the major histocompatibility complex (MHC)-anchoring region but the end result is that recognition of the peptide is altered when compared to the native peptide. Muta-

tions in the TCR contact region cause different patterns of T-cell activation, whereas mutations in the MHC region of the peptide allow the APL/MHC complex to still bind to the TCR but with altered affinity, thus changing the pattern of TCR signaling and T-cell activation compared to the native ligand (Fig. 23.2, step 1). Studies have demonstrated that differences in MHC binding regions can induce anergy and that differences in binding affinity can ultimately lead to the tolerizing effect of APLs on potentially pathogenic T cells.[56,57] APLs are also capable of causing alterations in the Th1/Th2 phenotype, with the direction of phenotypic alteration and subsequent cytokine production being dependent on the specific amino acid sequence in the TCR-binding region.[58] APLs have been shown to inhibit Th1 differentiation and reduce the encephalitogenicity of activated, myelin-specific T cells through increased production of Th2-type cytokines.[59,60]

Clinical trials utilizing APL in MS patients have focused on a specific MBP sequence, peptide 83–99, which is considered to be an immunodominant epitope for many HLA haplotypes commonly associated with MS. In one study, MS patients treated with an MBP APL resulted in T cells that were capable of responding to both the APL and to the native MBP peptide, but generally responded with a Th2-like cytokine profile.[61] In a phase II trial utilizing this APL in RRMS, the number and volume of MRI-enhancing lesions was decreased with APL treatment and a Th2 response was observed in response to both the APL and the native peptide.[62] This trial was terminated before completion because of a high incidence of hypersensitivity reactions, but another trial utilizing a different dosage regimen with the same APL is currently under way. Another trial conducted at the NIH found no improvement in MRI lesions and noted three patients on therapy with exacerbations of MS.[63] This trial, however, included only eight patients and used a higher dose of the APL in most patients. The immune response to APLs was shown to persist for several years in MS patients, as evidenced by a Th2 cytokine profile in response to stimulation with either MBP APL or native MBP lasting 2–4.5 years after treatment, although some patients also showed a dramatic increase in their response to native peptide.[64] As noted above, current trials will determine whether this strategy will eventually have greater utility in treating MS patients.

Conclusion/comment

The results of the initial APL trials have dampened enthusiasm for this strategy. However, perhaps studies of APL at lower doses will provide more favorable clinical results.

SOLUBLE PEPTIDES

Soluble peptides of autoantigens administered either intranasally, orally or intravenously have been shown to be effective in altering the immune response in several models of autoimmune disease. In EAE models utilizing the Lewis rat, nasal or mucosal administration of MBP_{68-86} resulted in the prevention of EAE but was not successful in treating established disease. However, coadministration of this same peptide along with cytokines that typically promote Th2 differentiation (IL-10 or IL-4) effectively treated EAE.[65,66] Activating the T cell with autoantigen in the presence of Th2-differentiating cytokines has been an effective method for suppressing the inflammatory Th1 cell type (Fig. 23.2, step 1). In another study, EAE in Lewis rats was prevented by a novel technique for administration of MBP and PLP antigens. The investigators constructed recombinant lactobacilli expressing human and guinea pig MBP and PLP. Oral and intranasal administration of the genetically engineered lactobacilli prior to disease induction inhibited clinical signs of EAE in Lewis rats.[67] While treatment of active EAE was not demonstrated, this study provides a novel strategy for delivery of antigens capable of inducing immune tolerance. Multiple intravenous injections of high doses of MBP have also been shown to be effective in treating active EAE through deletion of CD4+ MBP-reactive T cells in an antigen-specific induction of programmed cell death.[68]

In addition to administration of soluble peptides alone by various techniques, another strategy utilized native peptides bound to soluble MHC molecules for tolerance induction (Fig. 23.2, step 2). In this strategy, by having the MHC/peptide complex bind to the TCR in the absence of costimulation, T cells specific for the peptide become anergic. Because susceptibility to MS is associated with HLA-DR2 haplotype, studies were conducted using soluble DR2 bound to an MBP peptide that would target self-reactive CD4+ T cells with a high degree of specificity. Such complexes generate a population of T cells that are subsequently unresponsive when restimulated with APCs pulsed with the same MBP peptide.[69] A double-blind, placebo-controlled phase I trial in 33 MS patients used a soluble DR2 bound to MBP peptide 84–102 and demonstrated no increase in adverse event rates, although larger studies are needed to determine whether this strategy has clinical efficacy.[70]

Conclusion/comment

This strategy also is highly dependent on knowing the specific antigenic targets of the immune response in MS. While the early trials have been well tolerated, there has been little evidence to suggest that targeting a single epitope during MS has much impact on the clinical signs of the disease.

T-CELL VACCINES

The use of T-cell vaccines presents yet another novel therapeutic strategy that targets specific autoreactive clonal T-cell subsets for regulation or deletion. This approach has been applied successfully in the EAE model as well as a host of other autoimmune disease models. The two methods that have been used for T-cell vaccination are immunizing with whole autoreactive T cells that have been inactivated,[71] and immunizing with peptide segments from the TCR of myelin-specific, autoreactive T cells.[72] Both methods ultimately have the same effect; inducing an anti-idiotypic immune response against the T cells or TCRs that are responsible for the initiation of autoimmunity, and thereby deleting or attenuating these autoreactive T cells in the periphery (Fig. 23.2, step 2). There are several components of the immune response likely to be involved in T-cell vaccination, including effects on CD4+ deviation, anti-inflammatory Th2-expressed cytokines, regulatory CD8+ T cells and humoral anti-idiotypic antibody production.[73–75] Vaccination with either TCR peptides or inactivated (irradiated) autoreactive T cells has been shown to induce these types of immune response in MS patients. Using different adjuvants and methods of administration, investigators have been able to induce immune response to TCR peptides in anywhere from 80–100% of MS patients, a significant accomplishment given the deficient response to TCR peptides often observed in MS patients.[72,76]

One possible limitation of these methods is the incorporation of one or only a few clonal TCR reactivities. Many MS patients have T cells reactive to multiple antigens as a result of epitope or determinant spreading. Using irradiated, pooled CD4+ T cells from either CSF[77] or peripheral blood,[78] investigators have generated T-cell vaccines capable of inducing a regulatory immune response in MS patients against a wider array of myelin-reactive TCR idiotypes. While these small phase I safety studies lacked the statistical power to detect significant clinical responses, trends towards clinical improvement were seen in both trials. A larger trial utilized this strategy in 20 patients with aggressive RRMS who were not responding to standard therapy and who were immunized with attenuated MBP- and MOG-reactive T cells. These MS patients experienced a decrease in annual relapse rate, showed stabilization in their neurological disability scores and also demonstrated a decrease in the number and volume of MRI lesions.[79] This trial highlights the therapeutic potential of T-cell vaccination but must be viewed with caution, as it was neither blinded nor placebo-controlled. Another even larger trial studying both RRMS and SPMS patients reached mixed conclusions. Relapse rate was reduced in the relapsing–remitting patients but neurological disability was only minimally reduced in these same patients and increased slightly in the patients with SPMS.[80] Recently, T-cell vaccination has been shown to induce regulatory T-cell responses in patients with MS.[81]

Conclusion/comment

While T-cell vaccination strategies showed early promise in animal models, it must be emphasized that the restricted usage of TCR usage observed in EAE has not been observed in MS. Thus, this strategy may have a fundamental flaw when applied to the outbred human MS population.

COSTIMULATION

The CD40/CD40L and the B7/CD28:CTLA-4 costimulatory pathways are a central component in regulating the immune system. Dysfunction of these costimulatory pathways may contribute to the pathogenesis of immune-mediated diseases such as MS. Targeting the costimulatory molecules that define these pathways may provide novel therapeutic options for regulating the immune response in MS. Strategies targeting various costimulatory receptors are discussed below.

CD40 and CD40L

One of the first costimulatory molecules engaged during T-cell activation occurs between CD40 expressed on the APC and CD154 (CD40L) expressed on the T cell. This receptor–ligand interaction is crucial for successive costimulatory events to occur, and blocking this interaction can severely impair T-cell responses to protein antigens such as those that may be encountered in MS.[82] In addition to its role in T-cell activation, CD40/CD40L has been shown to induce expression of inflammatory cytokines by activated human microglia.[83] These observations have led to the development of monoclonal antibodies directed against CD40L to block this interaction and reduce T-cell-mediated inflammation in MS (Fig. 23.2, step 3). There is substantial evidence to support this approach in mice with EAE.[84,85] Blockade of CD40L during disease activity was shown to reduce frequency, severity and duration of clinical relapses.[84] This treatment appears to work through suppression of encephalitogenic Th1 differentiation and cytokine production without having a significant effect on total T-cell proliferation.[85]

In addition to blocking the CD40L molecule, investigators have also used reagents that target the other half of this pair, CD40, which is expressed on APCs (Fig. 23.2, step 3). Monoclonal antibodies directed against this receptor were able to prevent the induction of EAE in marmoset monkeys and were also shown to prevent epitope spreading.[86] This therapy was effective even when administered after the onset of clinical disease, as confirmed by MRI imaging.[87]

Conclusion/comment Despite the promising results in animal models of MS, interest in the use of CD40 blockade has been dampened by the occurrence of thromboembolic events in patients with lupus nephritis receiving anti-CD40L antibody in an open-label phase II clinical trial.[88]

B7, CD28 and CTLA-4

B7 molecules are a class of cell surface ligands involved in the costimulatory activation of T cells. B7 predominantly consists of two distinct molecules, B7.1 (CD80) and B7.2 (CD86). B7 molecules are expressed on APCs and bind to the CD28 or CTLA-4 (CD152) receptors on T cells, causing up- or down-regulation of the subsequent immune response, respectively. Interaction of B7 with CD28 leads to increased production of IL-2 and productive activation of T cells, even those T cells that are naive. Association of the B7 and CTLA-4 molecules leads to decreased signaling through the TCR and decreased IL-2 production, thereby limiting the immune response.[82] Several studies suggest that engagement of the TCR in the absence of B7/CD28 interaction results in the development of an anergic T-cell population. The importance of this pathway in autoimmune demyelinating disease is evident from studies showing that CD28-deficient mice are resistant to spontaneous EAE[89] whereas transgenic mice constitutively expressing B7.2 (CD86) on microglia are prone to develop spontaneous autoimmune demyelination.[90]

One successful strategy to block B7 from binding to CD28 has been to create a CTLA-4-Ig fusion protein, which can then be administered systemically (Fig. 23.2, step 4). In studies in murine models of EAE, CTLA-4-Ig has been shown to reduce the incidence and severity of disease. This same study showed that using monoclonal antibodies to block B7.1 (CD80) inhibited only the first disease episode, blocking B7.2 (CD86) had no effect, and blocking both B7 molecules simultaneously resulted in disease exacerbation.[91] These results highlight the need for caution in determining whether costimulatory molecules can be safely blocked and whether the outcome will always be to improve clinical outcome. Another study confirmed these beneficial effects and showed histological improvements using CTLA-4 bound to mouse Fc to prevent the induction of EAE and to reduce inflammation and demyelination in the CNS.[92] CTLA-4-Ig has also been shown to reduce disease severity and inflammation in CNS of Lewis rats when administered after the onset of clinical signs of EAE. This was due to suppression of Th1 inflammatory cytokines (IL-2 and IFNγ) while sparing Th2 cytokines (IL-4, IL-10 and IL-13).[93] Strategies to enhance the effectiveness of this approach in EAE have included injecting CTLA-4-Ig directly into the CNS or employing a nonreplicating adenoviral vector to deliver a gene encoding CTLA-4-Ig into the CNS.[94]

Some studies have utilized monoclonal antibodies directed at CD28 to block costimulation without affecting the inhibitory B7/CTLA-4 interaction (Fig. 23.2, step 5). This strategy was able to prevent and treat EAE, reduce TNFα production and significantly inhibit clinical relapses.[95]

At the present time, it is unclear whether these strategies observed in EAE models can be translated in successful treatment for the human disease, MS. There are several factors that could make costimulatory blockade less successful in treating established MS. One important factor is the length of time in which myelin-specific, autoreactive T cells have already been stimulated in patients with MS. Some studies on peripheral blood lymphocytes from humans with MS suggest that the CD4+ T cells can expand and proliferate independent of costimulation as a result of prior in vivo activation.[96] Human studies have also shown that MBP-reactive T cells from healthy individuals or stroke patients are effectively blocked from proliferating by anti-CD28, suggesting that the MBP-specific T cells from these patient subgroups are naive. However, when proliferation was examined in MBP-specific lymphocytes from MS patients, proliferation was only minimally inhibited under the same conditions, suggesting that these T cells had previously been activated or primed in MS patients.[97] Whether costimulatory

blockade can overcome these issues and be a successful therapy for MS remains to be determined, but a preliminary clinical trial utilizing CTLA-4Ig in patients with RMS is currently under way.

A number of significant complications occurred with a humanized superagonistic anti-CD28 monoclonal antibody in phase I. The anti-CD28 antibody directly activates regulatory T cells and had shown promising results in models of MS, neuritis and experimental arthritis. While no significant side effects occurred in any of the preceding animal experiments, including primates, all six healthy volunteers who were exposed to this antibody during a phase I study suffered from immediate, severe and life-threatening allergic reactions (see news.bbc.co.uk/1/hi/england/london/4808836.stm). Fortunately most of the volunteers have made a full recovery.

Conclusion/comment While costimulatory blockade has certain intrinsic advantages, such as not requiring the knowledge of the autoantigens in MS, it remains to be seen whether it will be effective on T cells that have already been primed by autoantigens. As noted above, there are clinical studies underway, and preliminary studies using CTLA-Ig in psoriasis were promising.[98]

REGULATORS OF T-CELL DIFFERENTIATION

Another area of intense research has been identifying factors that may influence the fate of naive, myelin-specific CD4+ T cells, i.e. whether these T cells differentiate into proinflammatory Th1 cells or anti-inflammatory Th2 cells. Th1 cells have traditionally been viewed as the T-cell subtype responsible for inducing the inflammatory lesion characteristic of MS and EAE, while Th2 cells are viewed as being regulatory in nature when it comes to cell-mediated inflammation. While this model oversimplifies the potential mechanisms involved and largely ignores the role of CD8+ T cells and B cells, many potential therapies have developed by targeting this step in T-cell differentiation. Several examples are discussed below.

Cytokines

The utilizing of monoclonal antibodies to neutralize proinflammatory cytokines in Th1-mediated processes such as EAE and potentially MS is perhaps the most straightforward strategy of altering the Th1/Th2 balance (Fig. 23.2, step 6). Examples of antibodies targeting cytokines that have been evaluated in MS or EAE include antibodies against IFNγ, TNFα, IL-2, IL-12 and IL-16.

Neutralizing the effects of TNFα in MS seemed like a logical choice given its potential role in inflammation and demyelination. Unfortunately, clinical trials have shown that attempts to neutralize TNFα actually aggravated symptoms of MS.[99] This sharply contrasts with the therapeutic benefit of anti-TNFα reagents in the treatment of rheumatoid arthritis.

IFNγ is another important inflammatory cytokine with potential for therapeutic intervention. This cytokine also demonstrates how mouse studies and human trials can often yield conflicting results. EAE mice demonstrate improvement in disease with administration of IFNγ but have worsening of clinical signs of disease if anti-IFNγ antibodies are used.[100] Clinical trials in patients with MS have shown contrasting results, with administration of IFNγ leading to increased relapses and worsening of disease[101] while anti-IFNγ therapy led to clinical and MRI improvement.[102] The study that showed a positive effect with anti-IFNγ was a double-blind, placebo-controlled trial in a small sample of 15 patients with SPMS assigned to one of three arms: anti-IFNγ, anti-TNFα or placebo. Only the anti-IFNγ subgroup showed an improvement in this preliminary study.

IL-2 is another potential candidate for T-cell-specific therapy due to its important role in T-cell expansion. Daclizumab is a humanized monoclonal antibody that recognizes the IL-2 receptor α chain and blocks signaling through the IL-2 receptor. Two small, open-label clinical trials, one with 10 MS patients and the other with 19 patients, have shown this drug to be well tolerated and to result in rather dramatic improvement in both clinical and MRI diseases measures.[103,104]

Targeting IL-12, which is important for Th1 CD4+ T-cell differentiation, has also been investigated. Studies conducted in mice[105] and marmoset monkeys[106] have demonstrated that antibodies directed against the p40 subunit of IL-12 are effective in the treatment of EAE. Recent evidence suggests that the p40 subunit is the critical component of IL-12, and perhaps another member of the IL-12 family called IL-23, as mice lacking the p35 subunit of IL-12 are still susceptible to disease.[107] It seems that IL-23, which shares the p40 subunit of IL-12 as well as utilizing its own p19 subunit, is capable of inducing EAE without functional IL-12.

There are also studies that suggest that anti-IL-16 antibodies could be another strategy to be used in autoimmune, demyelinating disease. IL-16 is a T- and B-cell chemoattractant that is thought to be important in recruiting autoreactive immune cells to the CNS in EAE. Administration of monoclonal antibodies that neutralized IL-16 was shown to decrease CNS pathology by CD4+ T cells and, perhaps even more relevant for human disease, reversed paralysis and other clinical signs of disease.[108] This is another example of an anticytokine strategy that could represent a novel therapeutic strategy for the treatment of MS.

Conclusion/comment Strategies that have targeted specific cytokines have been rather disappointing in MS. Some strategies have conflicted rather dramatically with EAE studies, such as TNFα blockade, even though this strategy has proved useful in other suspected autoimmune diseases such as rheumatoid arthritis. These studies have also highlighted the fact that what are traditionally considered proinflammatory cytokines may also initiate important regulatory events that result in the resolution of inflammation.

Nuclear hormone receptors

Nuclear hormone receptors are a large class of intracellular ligand-activated transcription factors. Strategies that target several different nuclear hormone receptors have shown mixed results in reducing the clinical signs of EAE in mice. These therapeutic effects are probably due to a number of different mechanisms but the major pathways include broad anti-inflammatory effects, including effects on CD4+ T-cell differentiation and APC activation (Fig. 23.2, step 6). In general, one observes suppression of Th1 inflammatory cytokines and a corresponding increase in Th2-like cytokine expression.[109–113] Of the several nuclear hormone receptors that have been tried in EAE, those shown to have beneficial effects include the retinoic acid receptor (RAR),[109,110] retinoid X receptor (RXR),[111] peroxisome proliferator-activated receptor (PPAR)-α[112] and PPAR-γ.[111,113] Agonists for each of these receptors individually have demonstrated significant improvement in the clinical signs of EAE in vivo and some have caused Th2 deviation in vitro. Because PPARs and RXR form a heterodimer prior to binding regulatory elements of DNA, studies have also examined the effects of administration of the PPAR-γ agonist 15-deoxy-$\Delta^{12,14}$-prostaglandin J2 (15d-PGJ2) and the RXR agonist 9-cis-retinoic acid together in the EAE model. These nuclear hormone agonists exerted an additive effect in suppressing T-cell proliferation, inhibiting production of inflammatory cytokines and reducing clinical disease in mice with EAE.[111] This suggests that, by targeting both members of the heterodimers mediating the regulatory effect, lower doses of each agonist may be used in combination with the other to achieve the greatest clinical effect with lower risk for adverse side effects.

Interestingly, using microarray technology, we have recently observed that all these receptors demonstrate increased expression in the peripheral blood of MS patients as compared to healthy controls, with PPAR-α showing the greatest upregulation (Muir and Racke, unpublished data). Further studies will be necessary to confirm whether increased expression of these transcription factors will translate into increased sensitivity to their respective agonists in MS. Another attractive feature of the PPAR family of transcription factors as a therapeutic target in MS is the wide availability of these agonists and their extensive history of human use. Agonists for the PPAR-α family of receptors include the fibrate class of lipid-lowering medications, gemfibrozil, fenofibrate and clofibrate. These medications have been in use for many years, have very mild and well defined side effects and are inexpensive and orally available, all features of an ideal treatment for a chronic disease like MS.

Conclusion/comment PPAR agonists offer an attractive alternative to many agents in that they have a long history of human use. Clinical trials with PPAR-γ agonists are under way and the results are eagerly anticipated.

HMG-CoA reductase inhibitors (statins)

The statins are a class of drugs that have also been in wide use for over a decade in the treatment of hypercholesterolemia, particularly in patients at risk for the development of cardiovascular disease. While some of the immunomodulatory effects of statins have been known for a decade, it is only recently that investigators have studied the impact of these drugs in models of demyelinating disease. Statins were shown to reduce EAE severity in Lewis rats and to reduce mononuclear cell infiltrates in the CNS as well.[114] Statins also prevented or reversed clinical signs of EAE in mice and had a persistent therapeutic effect, even after discontinuation of the drug.[115] Like the nuclear hormone receptor agonists, there are a number of potential mechanisms for how statins exert their therapeutic effect, with CD4+ T-cell deviation predominating (Fig. 23.2, step 6). The statins induce Th2 cytokines while reducing Th1 cytokine production in both rat and murine EAE models[114,115] but the statins also appear to have effects on MHC-II expression and costimulatory signaling.[115] One of the statins, simvastatin was shown to reduce MRI burden in a small open-label study in RRMS patients.[116] Recent results highlight the synergistic potential of statin therapy when combined with glatiramer acetate.[117]

Conclusion/comment These animal and human results are particularly exciting, given the oral availability and reasonable safety profile of these agents. The results of larger placebo-controlled trials currently underway will determine whether statins will realize their potential as a treatment strategy for MS.

Transcription factor blockade

Perhaps the most specific method of inducing Th2 deviation would involve manipulation at the level of transcription factors involved in T cell differentiation. Several transcription factors critical in determining the differentiation of a naive T cell have recently been described and transcription factors that are essential to either Th1 or Th2 differentiation have been elucidated. One of these transcription factors is T-bet, the 'master regulator' of Th1, CD4+ T-cell differentiation.[118] If T-bet is critical to Th1 differentiation, then inhibiting its effects would effectively block Th1 differentiation and might be beneficial in Th1-mediated autoimmune diseases such as MS (Fig. 23.2, step 6). One method we have recently used to block gene expression of molecules of interest is through small interfering RNA (siRNA). T-bet-specific siRNA was shown to suppress IFNγ production and STAT1 levels (another important transcription factor in Th1 differentiation) along with suppressed T-bet expression. A more exciting observation was that in vivo administration of T-bet siRNA was able to inhibit clinical signs of EAE.[119] Similar effects were also found using a T-bet antisense oligonucleotide to inhibit T-bet expression. The use of similar strategies to disrupt signaling via T-bet and other transcription factors important in T-cell differentiation may lead to a highly targeted therapy for MS.

Conclusion/comment The manipulation of transcription factors may offer a great deal of insight into the molecular regulation of the immune response. These strategies are clearly just in their infancy in terms of their eventual human application.

CELL ADHESION

The ability of peripheral blood mononuclear cells to exit the bloodstream, cross the blood–brain barrier and migrate into the brain parenchyma is an essential step in the pathogenesis of MS. Cell-surface molecules on the invading lymphocytes involved in this process include α4-integrin (VLA-4) and lymphocyte function-associated antigen (LFA)-1, which must interact with their respective ligands VCAM-1 and ICAM-1 on the surface of endothelial cells.[82] This strategy to ameliorate MS using natalizumab, a monoclonal antibody directed against the VLA-4 molecule (Fig. 23.2, step 7), appeared to be quite successful until the occurrence of progressive multifocal leukoencephalopathy (PML) resulted in its withdrawal from the market.[120-122] It had initially been shown that antibodies directed against VLA-4 were able to inhibit disease activity in EAE mice, and this corresponded with a substantial decrease in the lymphocyte infiltrate in the CNS.[123] One randomized, double-blind, placebo-controlled trial showed that a single dose of natalizumab during acute relapse reduced the volume of MRI lesions, but did not shorten the time for clinical recovery.[124] Another larger randomized double-blind, placebo-controlled trial followed patients with monthly injections of natalizumab for six months. The natalizumab group reported fewer lesions on MRI and fewer relapses during the course of the trial.[125]

Based on these findings, natalizumab was approved for use in the USA in November 2004. However, the sale of natalizumab was suspended in February 2005 after three patients developed PML, two of whom had MS and were involved in MS clinical trials.[120-122] PML is a rapidly progressive and usually fatal demyelinating disease of the CNS. It is caused by the JC virus and is typically only seen in severely immunocompromised patients such as AIDS patients or those patients receiving immunosuppression. In the two cases of PML in MS, patients were taking natalizumab in combination with IFNβ, and the third patient was taking natalizumab for Crohn's disease.

Conclusion/comment

Natalizumab was the first commercially available drug designed to block cell adhesion molecules in autoimmune diseases. As part of its return to the market, a risk management plan is being developed because of the potential risk for the development of PML. A recent study has shown that natalizumab significantly reduces the number of CSF lymphocytes in MS patients who have received the drug.[126] Further studies will need to determine the impact of natalizumab on immune surveillance of the nervous system. Investigators have identified several other cell adhesion molecules that can be disrupted to improve clinical signs of EAE, but the unexpected adverse effects of natalizumab may discourage the use of these drugs in human trials. Natalizumab also serves as a reminder that even highly targeted therapies may have unintended side effects on the ability of the immune system to fulfill its protective role.

A VIEW TO THE FUTURE

The next several years hold great promise for MS patients seeking more effective and less toxic treatments to slow disease progression and improve overall quality of life. It is only within the past decade that every potential treatment discussed above has come under investigation for MS. The next several years will continue to produce new agents that will be tested in clinical trials, and those currently undergoing clinical trials may become available to patients in the near future. As has occurred in the past, some of these agents that showed great promise in EAE studies will yield disappointing results in human studies. Other therapies, such as natalizumab, that showed great initial success in treating MS may ultimately have long-term risks that could ultimately limit their widespread use. As has been the case with cancer chemotherapy, it is also unlikely that any one strategy will emerge as a 'magic bullet' cure for MS in the foreseeable future. Ultimately, it is likely that MS clinicians will employ combinations of drugs to achieve disease suppression greater than would be possible with any of the drugs alone, while simultaneously allowing for lower doses and fewer side effects than one might expect from each individual drug. Perhaps the culmination of research into targeted immunotherapy will be the achievement of antigen-specific treatments tailored to the exact pattern of reactive autoimmune cells present in each individual MS patient. While this scenario is certainly several years away, it is no more unrealistic than many of the therapies currently in clinical trials seemed to be a decade ago.

REFERENCES

1. Johnston RB. Preface. In: Joy JE, Johnston RB, eds. Multiple sclerosis: current status and strategies for the future. Washington, DC: National Academy Press; 2001: vii–viii.
2. Qin Y, Duquette P. B-cell immunity in MS. Int Mult Scler J 2003; 10, 110–120.
3. Crawford MP, Yan SX, Ortega SB et al. High prevalence of autoreactive, neuroantigen-specific CD8+ T cells in multiple sclerosis revealed by novel flow cytometric assay. Blood 2004; 103: 4222–4231.
4. O'Connor KC, Bar-Or A, Hafler DA. The neuroimmunology of multiple sclerosis:

possible roles of T and B lymphocytes in immunopathogenesis. J Clin Immunol 2001; 21: 81–92.
5. Friese MA, Fugger L. Autoreactive CD8+ T cells in multiple sclerosis: a new target for therapy? Brain 2005; 128: 1747–1763.
6. Skulina C, Schmidt S, Dornmair K et al. Multiple sclerosis: brain-infiltrating CD8+ T cells persist as clonal expansions in the cerebrospinal fluid and blood. Proc Natl Acad Sci USA 2004; 101: 2428–2433.
7. Frohman EM, Racke MK, Raine CS. Multiple sclerosis – the plaque and its pathogenesis. N Engl J Med 2006; 354: 942–955.

8. Polman CH, Herndon RM, Pozzilli C. Interferons. In: Rudick RA, Goodkin DE, eds. Multiple sclerosis therapeutics. London: Martin Dunitz; 1999: 243–276.
9. Ford CC. Glatiramer acetate. In: Rudick RA, Goodkin DE, eds. Multiple sclerosis therapeutics. London: Martin Dunitz; 1999: 277–298.
10. Hartung HP, Gonsette R, Morrissey S et al. Mitoxantrone. In: Rudick RA, Goodkin DE, eds. Multiple sclerosis therapeutics. London: Martin Dunitz; 1999: 299–348.
11. Waubant E, Goodkin DE. Emerging disease-modifying therapies. In: Rudick RA, Goodkin DE, eds. Multiple sclerosis

therapeutics. London: Martin Dunitz; 1999: 379–394.

12. Kinkel RP. Methylprednisolone. In: Rudick RA, Goodkin DE, eds. Multiple sclerosis therapeutics. London: Martin Dunitz; 1999: 349–370.

13. Allison AC, Eugui EM. Mycophenolate mofetil and its mechanism of action. Immuopharmacology 2000; 47: 85–118.

14. Chan TN, Li FK, Tang CS et al. Efficacy of mycophenolate mofetil in patients with diffuse proliferative lupus nephritis. Hong Kong–Guangzhou Nephrology Study Group. N Engl J Med 2000; 343: 1156–1162.

15. Frohman EM, Brannon K, Racke MK, Hawker K. Mycophenolate mofetil in multiple sclerosis. Clin Neuropharmacol 2004; 27: 80–83.

16. Ahrens N, Salama A, Haas J. Mycophenolate-mofetil in the treatment of refractory multiple sclerosis. J Neurol 2001; 248: 713–714.

17. Gummert JF, Ikonen T, Morris RE. Newer immunosuppressive drugs: a review. J Am Soc Nephrol 1999; 10: 1366–1380.

18. Gold BG, Voda J, Yu X et al. FK506 and a nonimmunosuppresant derivative reduce axonal and myelin damage in experimental autoimmune encephalomyelitis: neuroimmunophilin ligand-mediated neuroprotection in a model of multiple sclerosis. J Neurosci Res 2004; 77: 367–377.

19. Lemster D, Huang LL, Irioh W et al. Influence of FK506 (tacrolimus) on circulating CD4$^+$ T cells expressing CD25 and CD45RA antigens in 19 patients with chronic progressive multiple sclerosis participating in an open label safety trial. Autoimmunity 1994; 19: 89–98.

20. De Jong R, Bezemer AC, Zomerdijk TP et al. Selective stimulation of T helper 2 cytokine responses by the anti-psoriasis agent monomethylfumarate. Eur J Immunol 1996; 26: 2067–2074.

21. Ockenfels HM, Schultewolter T, Ockenfels G et al. The antipsoriatic agent dimethylfumarate immunomodulates T-cell cytokine secretion and inhibits cytokines of the psoriatic cytokine network. Br J Dermatol 1998; 139: 390–395.

22. Schilling S, Goelz S, Linker R et al. Fumaric acid esters are effective in chronic experimental autoimmune encephalomyelitis and suppress macrophage infiltration. Clin Exp Immunol 2006; 145: 101–107.

23. Altmeyer PJ, Matthes U, Pawlak F et al. Antipsoriatic effect of fumaric acid derivatives. Results of a multicenter double-blind study in 100 patients. J Am Acad Dermatol 1994; 30: 977–981.

24. Mrowietz U, Christophers E, Altmeyer P. Treatment of psoriasis with fumaric acid esters: results of a prospective multicentre study. German Multicentre Study. Br J Dermatol 1998; 138: 456–460.

25. Schimrigk S, Brune N, Hellwig K et al. Oral fumaric acid esters for the treatment of active multiple sclerosis: an open label, baseline-controlled, pilot study. Eur J Neurol 2006; 13: 604–610.

26. Korn T, Toyka K, Hartung H.-P, Jung S. Suppression of experimental autoimmune neuritis by leflunomide. Brain 2001; 124: 1791–1802.

27. O'Connor PW, LI D, Freedman MS et al. A phase II study of the safety and efficacy of teriflunomide in multiple sclerosis with relapses. Neurology 2006; 66: 894–900.

28. Jonsson S, Andersson G, Fex T et al. Synthesis and biological evaluation of new 1,2-dihydro-4-hydroxy-2-oxo-3-quinolinecaboxamides for treatment of autoimmune disorders: structure-activity relationship. J Med Chem 2004; 47: 2075–2088.

29. Polman C, Barkhof F, Sandberg-Wollheim M et al for the Laquinimod in Relapsing MS Study Group. Treatment with laquinimod reduces development of active MRI lesions in relapsing MS. Neurology 2005; 64: 987–991.

30. Cinamon G, Matloubian M, Lesneski MJ et al. Sphingosine 1-phosphate receptor 1 promotes B cell localization in the splenic marginal zone. Nat Immunol 2004; 5: 13–20.

31. Fujino M, Funeshima N, Kitazawa Y et al. Amelioration of experimental autoimmune encephalomyelitis in Lewis rats by FTY720. J Pharmacol Exp Ther 2003; 305: 70–77.

32. Webb M, Tham CS, Lin FF et al. Sphingosine 1-phosphate receptor agonists attenuate relapsing-remitting experimental autoimmune encephalitis in SJL mice. J Neuroimmunol 2004; 153: 108–121.

33. Rausch M, Hiestand P, Foster CA et al. Predictability of FTY720 efficacy in experimental autoimmune encephalomyelitis by in vivo macrophage tracking: clinical implications for ultrasmall superparamagnetic iron oxide-enhanced magnetic resonance imaging. J Magn Reson Imaging 2004; 20: 16–24.

34. Lassmann H, Bruck W, Lucchinetti C. Heterogeneity of multiple sclerosis pathogenesis: implications for diagnosis and therapy. Trends Mol Med 2001; 7: 115–121.

35. Lucchinetti CF, Mandler RN, McGavern D et al. A role for humoral mechanisms in the pathogenesis of Devic's neuromyelitis optica. Brain 2002; 125: 1450–1461.

36. Keegan M, Konig F, McClelland R et al. Relation between humoral pathological changes in multiple sclerosis and response to therapeutic plasma exchange. Lancet 2005; 366: 579–582.

37. Grillo-Lopez AJ, Hedrick E, Rashford M, Benyunes M. Rituximab: ongoing and future clinical development. Semin Oncol 2002; 29(1 suppl 2): 105–112.

38. Martin F, Chan AC. B cell immunobiology in disease: evolving concepts from the clinic. Annu Rev Immunol 2006; 24, 467–496.

39. Stüve O, Cepok S, Elias B et al. Clinical stabilization and effective B-lymphocyte depletion in the cerebrospinal fluid and peripheral blood of a patient with fulminant relapsing-remitting multiple sclerosis. Arch Neurol 2005; 62: 1620–1623.

40. Cree BA, Lamb S, Morgan K et al. An open label study of the effects of rituximab in neuromyelitis optica. Neurology 2005; 64: 1270–1272.

41. Monson NL, Cravens PD, Frohman EM et al. Effect of rituximab on the peripheral blood and cerebrospinal fluid B cells in patients with primary progressive MS. Arch Neurol 2005; 62: 258–264.

42. Chan A, Weilbach FX, Toyka KV, Gold R. Mitoxantrone induces cell death in peripheral blood leucocytes of multiple sclerosis patients. Clin Exp Immunol 2005; 139: 152–158.

43. Cavaletti G, Cavaletti E, Crippal et al. Pixantrone (BBR2778) reduces the severity of experimental allergic encephalomyelitis. J Neuroimmunol 2004; 151: 55–65.

44. Weilbach FK, Chan A, Toyka KV, Gold R. The cardioprotector dexrazoxane augments therapeutic efficacy of mitoxantrone in experimental autoimmune encephalomyelitis. Clin Exp Immunol 2004; 135: 49–55.

45. Saiz A, Blanco Y, Carreras E et al. Clinical and MRI outcome after autologous hematopoietic stem cell transplantation in MS. Neurology 2004; 62: 282–284.

46. Mandalfino P, Rice G, Smith A et al. Bone marrow transplantation in multiple sclerosis. J Neurol 2000; 247: 691–695.

47. Muraro P, Douek D, Packer A et al. Thymic output generates a new and diverse TCR repertoire after autologus stem cell transplantation in multiple sclerosis patients. J Exp Med 2005; 201: 805–816.

48. Selmaj K, Kowal C, Walczak A et al. Naked DNA vaccination differentially modulates autoimmune responses in experimental autoimmune encephalomyelitis. J Neuroimmunol 2000; 111: 34–44.

49. Karin N. Gene therapy for T cell-mediated autoimmunity: teaching the immune system how to restrain its own harmful activities by targeted DNA vaccines. Isr Med Assoc J 2000; 2(suppl): 63–68.

50. Lobell A, Weissert R, Eltayeb S et al. Suppressive DNA vaccination in myelin oligodendrocyte glycoprotein peptide-induced experimental autoimmune encephalomyelitis involves a T1-biased immune response. J Immunol 2003; 170: 1806–1813.

51. Wildbaum G, Netzer N, Karin N. Plasmid DNA encoding IFN-gamma-inducible protein 10 redirects antigen-specific T cell polarization and suppresses experimental autoimmune encephalomyelitis. J Immunol 2002; 168: 5885–5892.

52. Karin N. Induction of protective therapy for autoimmune diseases by targeted DNA vaccines encoding pro-inflammatory cytokines and chemokines. Curr Opin Mol Ther 2004; 6: 27–33.

53. Bourquin C, Iglesias A, Berger T et al. Myelin oligodendrocyte glycoprotein-DNA vaccination induces antibody-mediated autoaggression in experimental autoimmune encephalomyelitis. Eur J Immunol 2000; 30: 3663–3671.

54. Garren H, Ruiz PJ, Watkins TA et al. Combination of gene delivery and DNA vaccination to protect from and reverse Th1 autoimmune disease via deviation to the Th2 pathway. Immunity 2001; 15: 15–22.

55. Robinson WH, Fontoura P, Lee BJ et al. Protein microarrays guide tolerizing DNA vaccine treatment of autoimmune encephalomyelitis. Nat Biotechnol 2003; 21: 1033–1039.

56. Ford ML, Evavold BD. Regulation of polyclonal T cell responses by an MHC anchor-substituted variant of myelin oligodendrocyte glycoprotein 35–55. J Immunol 2003; 171: 1247–1254.

57. McCue D, Ryan KR, Wraith DC, Anderton SM. Activation thresholds determine susceptibility to peptide-induced tolerance in a heterogeneous myelin-reactive T cell repertoire. J Neuroimmunol 2004; 156: 96–106.

58. Singh RA, Zhang JZ. Differential activation of ERK, p38, and JNK required for Th1 and Th2 deviation in myelin-reactive T cells induced by altered peptide ligand. J Immunol 2004; 173: 7299–7307.

59. Fischer FR, Santambrogio L, Luo Y et al. Modulation of experimental autoimmune encephalomyelitis: effect of altered peptide ligand on chemokine and chemokine receptor expression. J Neuroimmunol 2000; 110: 195–208.

60. Young DA, Lowe LD, Booth SS et al. IL-4, IL-10, IL-13, and TGF-beta from an altered peptide ligand-specific Th2 cell clone down-regulate adoptive transfer of experimental autoimmune encephalomyelitis. J Immunol 2000; 164: 3563–3572.

61. Crowe PD, Qin Y, Conlon PJ, Antel JP. NBI-5788, an altered MBP83–99 peptide, induces a T-helper 2-like immune response in multiple sclerosis patients. Ann Neurol 2000; 48: 758–765.

62. Kappos L, Comi G, Panitch H et al. Induction of a non-encephalitogenic type 2 T helper-cell autoimmune response in multiple sclerosis after administration of an altered peptide ligand in a placebo-controlled, randomized phase II trial. The Altered Peptide Ligand in Relapsing MS Study Group. Nat Med 2000; 6: 1176–1182.

63. Bielekova B, Goodwin B, Richert N et al. Encephalitogenic potential of the myelin basic protein peptide (amino acids 83–99) in multiple sclerosis: results of a phase II clinical trial with an altered peptide ligand. Nat Med 2000; 6: 1167–1175.

64. Kim HJ, Antel JP, Duquette P et al. Persistence of immune responses to altered and native myelin antigens in patients with multiple sclerosis treated with altered peptide ligand. Clin Immunol 2002; 104: 105–114.

65. Xu LY, Yang JS, Huang YM et al. Combined nasal administration of encephalitogenic myelin basic protein peptide 68–86 and IL-10 suppressed incipient experimental allergic encephalomyelitis in Lewis rats. Clin Immunol 2000; 96: 205–211.

66. Xu LY, Huang YM, Yang JS et al. Suppression of ongoing experimental allergic encephalomyelitis (EAE) in Lewis rats: synergistic effects of myelin basic protein (MBP) peptide 68–86 and IL-4. Clin Exp Immunol 2000; 120: 526–531.

67. Maassen CB, Laman JD, van Holten-Neelen C et al. Reduced experimental autoimmune encephalomyelitis after intranasal and oral administration of recombinant lactobacilli expressing myelin antigens. Vaccine 2003; 21: 4685–4693.

68. Racke MK, Critchfield JM, Quigley L et al. Intravenous antigen administration as a therapy for autoimmune demyelinating disease. Ann Neurol 1996; 39: 46–56.

69. Appel H, Seth NP, Gauthier L, Wucherpfennig KW. Anergy induction by dimeric TCR ligands. J Immunol 2001; 166: 5279–5285.

70. Goodkin DE, Shulman M, Winkelhake J et al. A phase I trial of solubilized DR2: MBP84–102 (AG284) in multiple sclerosis. Neurology 2000; 54: 1414–1420.

71. Zhang J. T-cell vaccination for autoimmune diseases: immunologic lessons and clinical experience in multiple sclerosis. Expert Rev Vaccines 2002; 1: 285–292.

72. Vandenbark AA. TCR peptide vaccination in multiple sclerosis: boosting a deficient natural regulatory network that may involve TCR-specific CD4+CD25+ Treg cells. Curr Drug Targets Inflamm Allergy 2005; 4: 217–229.

73. Zang YC, Hong J, Tejada-Simon MV et al. Th2 immune regulation induced by T cell vaccination in patients with multiple sclerosis. Eur J Immunol 2000; 30: 908–913.

74. Jiang H, Braunstein NS, Yu B et al. CD8+ T cells control the TH phenotype of MBP-reactive CD4+ T cells in EAE mice. Proc Natl Acad Sci USA 2001; 98: 6301–6306.

75. Hong J, Zang YC, Tejada-Simon MV et al. Reactivity and regulatory properties of human anti-idiotypic antibodies induced by T cell vaccination. J Immunol 2000; 165: 6858–6864.

76. Morgan EE, Nardo CJ, Diveley JP et al. Vaccination with a CDR2 BV6S2/6S5 peptide in adjuvant induces peptide-specific T-cell responses in patients with multiple sclerosis. J Neurosci Res 2001; 64: 298–301.

77. Van der Aa A, Hellings N, Medaer R et al. T cell vaccination in multiple sclerosis patients with autologous CSF-derived activated T cells: results from a pilot study. Clin Exp Immunol 2003; 131: 155–168.

78. Correale J, Lund B, McMillan M et al. T cell vaccination in secondary progressive multiple sclerosis. J Neuroimmunol 2000; 107: 130–139.

79. Achiron A, Lavie G, Kishner I et al. T cell vaccination in multiple sclerosis relapsing-remitting nonresponders patients. Clin Immunol 2004; 113: 155–160.

80. Zhang JZ, Rivera VM, Tejada-Simon MV et al. T cell vaccination in multiple sclerosis: results of a preliminary study. J Neurol 2002; 249: 212–218.

81. Hong J, Zang YC, Nie H, Zhang JZ. CD4+ regulatory T cell responses induced by T cell vaccination in patients with multiple sclerosis. Proc Natl Acad Sci USA 2006; 103: 5024–5029.

82. Benjamini E, Coico R, Sunshine G. Activation and function of T and B cells. In: Immunology: a short course, 4th ed. New York: Wiley-Liss; 2000: 187–209.

83. D'Aversa TG, Weidenheim KM, Berman JW. CD40-CD40L interactions induce chemokine expression by human microglia: implications for human immunodeficiency virus encephalitis and multiple sclerosis. Am J Pathol 2002; 160: 559–567.

84. Howard LM, Dal Canto MC, Miller SD. Transient anti-CD154-mediated immunotherapy of ongoing relapsing experimental autoimmune encephalomyelitis induces long-term inhibition of disease relapses. J Neuroimmunol 2002; 129: 58–65.

85. Howard LM, Miga AJ, Vanderlugt CL et al. Mechanisms of immunotherapeutic intervention by anti-CD40L (CD154) antibody in an animal model of multiple sclerosis. J Clin Invest 1999; 103: 281–290.

86. Boon L, Brok HP, Bauer J et al. Prevention of experimental autoimmune encephalomyelitis in the common marmoset (Callithrix jacchus) using a chimeric antagonist monoclonal antibody against human CD40 is associated with altered B cell responses. J Immunol 2001; 167: 2942–2949.

87. Laman JD, 't Hart BA, Brok H et al. Protection of marmoset monkeys against EAE by treatment with a murine antibody blocking CD40 (mu5D12). Eur J Immunol 2002; 167: 2942–2949.

88. Boumpas DT, Furie R, Manzi S et al. A short course of BG9588 (anti-CD40 ligand antibody) improves serologic activity and decreases hematuria in patients with proliferative lupus glomerulonephritis. Arthritis Rheum 2003; 48: 719–727.

89. Oliveira-dos-Santos AJ, Ho A, Tada Y et al. CD28 costimulation is critical for the development of spontaneous autoimmune encephalomyelitis. J Immunol 1999; 162: 4490–4495.

90. Zehntner SP, Brisebois M, Tran E et al. Constitutive expression of a costimulatory ligand on antigen-presenting cells in the nervous system drives demyelinating disease. FASEB J 2003; 17: 1910–1912.

91. Perrin PJ, Scott D, Davis TA et al. Opposing effects of CTLA4-Ig and anti-CD80 (B7–1) plus anti-CD86 (B7–2) on experimental allergic encephalomyelitis. J Neuroimmunol 1996; 65: 31–39.

92. Cross AH, Girard TJ, Giacoletto KS et al. Long-term inhibition of murine experimental autoimmune encephalomyelitis using CTLA-4-Fc supports a key role for CD28 costimulation. J Clin Invest 1995; 95: 2783–2789.

93. Khoury SJ, Akalin E, Chandraker A et al. CD28-B7 costimulatory blockade by CTLA4Ig prevents actively induced experimental autoimmune encephalomyelitis and inhibits Th1 but spares Th2 cytokines in the central nervous system. J Immunol 1995; 155: 4521–4524.

94. Croxford JL, O'Neill JK, Ali RR et al. Local gene therapy with CTLA4-immunoglobulin fusion protein in experimental allergic encephalomyelitis. Eur J Immunol 1998; 28: 3904–3916.

95. Perrin PJ, June CH, Maldonado JH et al. Blockade of CD28 during in vitro activation of encephalitogenic T cells or after disease onset ameliorates experimental autoimmune encephalomyelitis. J Immunol 1999; 163: 1704–1710.

96. Scholz C, Patton KT, Anderson DE et al. Expansion of autoreactive T cells in multiple sclerosis is independent of exogenous B7 costimulation. J Immunol 1998; 160: 1532–1538.

97. Lovett-Racke AE, Trotter JL, Lauber J et al. Decreased dependence of myelin basic protein-reactive T cells on CD28-mediated costimulation in multiple sclerosis patients: A marker of activated/memory T cells. J Clin Invest 1998; 101: 725–730.

98. Abrams JR, Lebwohl MG, Guzzo C et al. CTLA4Ig-mediated blockade of T-cell costimulation in patients with psoriasis vulgaris. J Clin Invest 1999; 103: 1243–1252.

99. Lenercept Multiple Sclerosis Study Group and University of British Columbia MS/MRI Analysis Group. TNF neutralization in MS: results of a randomized, placebo-controlled multicenter study. Neurology 1999; 53: 457–465.

100. Billiau A. Interferons in multiple sclerosis: warnings from experiences. Neurology 1995; 45(suppl 6): 550–553.

101. Panitch HS, Hirsch RL, Haley AS, Johnson KP. Exacerbations of multiple sclerosis in patients treated with gamma interferon. Lancet 1987; 1: 893–895.

102. Skurkovich S, Boiko A, Beliaeva I et al. Randomized study of antibodies to IFN-gamma and TNF-alpha in secondary progressive multiple sclerosis. Mult Scler 2001; 7: 277–284.

103. Bielekova B, Richert N, Howard T et al. Humanized anti-CD25 (daclizumab) inhibits disease activity in multiple sclerosis patients failing to respond to interferon beta. Proc Natl Acad Sci USA 2004; 101: 8705–8708.

104. Rose JW, Watt HE, White AT, Carlson NG. Treatment of multiple sclerosis with an anti-interleukin-2 receptor monoclonal antibody. Ann Neurol 2004; 56: 864–867.

105. Ichikawa M, Koh CS, Inoue A et al. Anti-IL-12 antibody prevents the development and progression of multiple sclerosis-like relapsing-remitting demyelinating disease in NOD mice induced with myelin oligodendrocyte glycoprotein peptide. J Neuroimmunol 2000; 102: 56–66.

106. Brok HP, van Meurs M, Blezer E et al. Prevention of experimental autoimmune encephalomyelitis in common marmosets using an anti-IL-12p40 monoclonal antibody. J Immunol 2002; 169: 6554–6563.

107. Becher B, Durell BG, Noelle RJ. Experimental autoimmune encephalitis and inflammation in the absence of interleukin-12. J Clin Invest 2002; 110: 493–497.

108. Skundric DS, Dai R, Zakarian VL et al. Anti-IL-16 therapy reduces CD4+ T-cell infiltration and improves paralysis and histopathology of relapsing EAE. J Neurosci Res 2005; 79: 680–693.

109. Racke MK, Burnett D, Pak SH et al. Retinoid treatment of experimental allergic encephalomyelitis: IL-4 production correlates with improved disease course. J Immunol 1995; 154: 450–458.

110. Lovett-Racke AE, Racke MK. Retinoic acid promotes the development of Th2-like human myelin basic protein-reactive T cells. Cell Immunol 2002; 215: 54–60.

111. Diab A, Hussain RZ, Lovett-Racke AE et al. Ligands for the peroxisome proliferator-activated receptor-gamma and the retinoid X receptor exert additive anti-inflammatory effects on experimental autoimmune encephalomyelitis. J Neuroimmunol 2004; 148: 116–126.

112. Lovett-Racke AE, Hussain RZ, Northrop S et al. Peroxisome proliferator-activated receptor alpha agonists as therapy for autoimmune disease. J Immunol 2004; 172: 5790–5798.

113. Diab A, Deng C, Smith JD et al. Peroxisome proliferator-activated receptor-gamma agonist 15-deoxy-Δ(12,14)-prostaglandin J(2) ameliorates experimental autoimmune encephalomyelitis. J Immunol 2002; 168: 2508–2515.

114. Stanislaus R, Singh AK, Singh I. Lovastatin treatment decreases mononuclear cell infiltration into the CNS of Lewis rats with experimental allergic encephalomyelitis. J Neurosci Res 2001; 66: 155–162.

115. Youssef S, Stuve O, Patarroyo JC et al. The HMG-CoA reductase inhibitor, atorvastatin, promotes a Th2 bias and reverses paralysis in central nervous system autoimmune disease. Nature 2002; 420: 78–84.

116. Vollmer T, Key L, Durkalski V et al. Oral simvastatin treatment in relapsing-remitting multiple sclerosis. Lancet 2004; 363: 1607–1608.

117. Stuve O, Youssef S, Weber MS et al. Immunomodulatory synergy by combination of atovastatin and glatiramer acetate in treatment of CNS autoimmunity. J Clin Invest 2006; 116: 1037–1044.

118. Szabo SJ, Kim ST, Costa GL et al. A novel transcription factor, T-bet, directs Th1 lineage commitment. Cell 2000; 100: 655–669.

119. Lovett-Racke AE, Rocchini AE, Choy J et al. Silencing T-bet defines a critical role in the differentiation of autoreactive T lymphocytes. Immunity 2004; 21: 719–731.

120. Van Assche G, Van Ranst M, Sciot R et al. Progressive multifocal leukoencephalopathy after nataluzimab therapy for Crohn's disease. N Engl J Med 2005; 353: 362–368.

121. Kleinschmidt-DeMasters BK, Tyler KL. Progressive multifocal leukoencephalopathy complicating treatment with nataluzimab and interferon beta-1a for multiple sclerosis. N Engl J Med 2005; 353: 369–374.

122. Langer-Gould A, Atlas SW, Bollen AW, Pelletier D. Progressive multiofocal leukoencephalopathy in a patient treated with nataluzimab. N Engl J Med 2005; 353: 375–381.

123. Brocke S, Piercy C, Steinman L et al. Antibodies to CD44 and integrin alpha 4, but not L-selectin, prevent CNS inflammation and experimental encephalomyelitis by blocking secondary leukocyte recruitment. Proc Natl Acad Sci USA 1999; 96: 6896–6901.

124. O'Connor PW, Goodman A, Willmer-Hulme AJ et al. Randomized multicenter trial of natalizumab in acute MS relapses: clinical and MRI effects. Neurology 2004; 62: 2038–2043.

125. Miller DH, Khan OA, Sheremata WA et al. A controlled trial of natalizumab for relapsing multiple sclerosis. N Engl J Med 2003; 348: 15–23.

126. Stuve O, Marra CM, Jerome KR et al. Immune surveillance in multiple sclerosis patients treated with natalizumab. Ann Neurol 2006; 59: 743–747.

CHAPTER 23

Moving towards remyelinating and neuroprotective therapies in multiple sclerosis

N. J. Scolding and M. Dubois-Dalcq

INTRODUCTION

It is now 45 years since Richard and Mary Bunge discovered and reported the phenomenon of spontaneous myelin repair in experimental models of demyelination.[1] Equally importantly, within just a few years the same was found in specimens from patients with multiple sclerosis (Figs 24.1 and 24.2).[2] Almost throughout the past four decades, speculation that new therapies might be developed that augment or enhance spontaneous remyelination in multiple sclerosis (MS) has persisted and indeed steadily grown – and yet still no remotely successful therapies of this nature have emerged despite enormous and concentrated effort. The field of neuroprotection in MS is more recent and promising, although failed efforts in this therapeutic strategy in stroke[3–5] and in degenerative conditions such as motor neuron disease may temper optimism in this approach too.

Why have scientists and clinicians interested in repair and protection in the brain failed to deliver useful treatments for MS? Why does interest yet remain intense? Are there truly grounds for optimism – or is this yet another example of scientific hype and uncritical enthusiasm raising disproportionate hopes in an expectant and vulnerable audience? Here we will attempt to summarize the scientific background to such therapeutic projects, outline progress so far, define the remaining hurdles to be traversed – and, we hope, indicate why both neuroprotection and repair are not only realistic avenues of therapeutic pursuit but are vital for the proper future care of patients with this incurable disease.

RATIONAL AND SCIENTIFIC BACKGROUND TO REMYELINATION AND NEUROPROTECTION IN MULTIPLE SCLEROSIS

Notwithstanding the indisputable description of MS as a demyelinating disease, the key phenomenon of axon loss not only lies at the heart of both neuroprotective and remyelinating treatments but in fact helps to explain why there is good reason to believe MS might have significant advantages over many other central nervous system (CNS) disorders in its inherent eligibility for protective and reparative therapies.

Although axon loss occurs earlier in the course of MS than previously believed,[6,7] neither experimental, imaging nor neuropathological studies have challenged the concept that disease processes in MS are primarily directed against oligodendrocytes and/or myelin: it is indeed a demyelinating disease, and axons are relatively spared until late in its course.[8,9] The first key advantageous implication is that, early in disease, axon pathways remain predominantly intact. Repair therapies therefore 'only' need to reinvest axons with myelin rather than solve the almost overwhelming challenge presented by most other neurological diseases: that of re-establishing connectivity in highly complex but fragmented axonal circuitry.

Axon loss progresses with disease course, however, and represents a principal pathophysiological cause of disability in chronic progressive disease (Fig. 24.2). But the important factor here lies in considering the cause of axon loss. Increasingly it appears that the inflammatory processes driving acute relapse in MS do not represent the principal cause of progression of disability – or, by implication, of progressive axon loss. (This by no means, of course, excludes a role for inflammation in the acute axon fragmentation occurring in acute lesions.) The very similar rates of disease progression in patients with frequent, few or no inflammatory relapses (i.e. primary progressive disease)[10] supports this, as does the failure of even the most intensive immune suppression, or immune modulation that clearly reduces the frequency of inflammatory relapses, to exert significant effects in reducing disease progression. These and other lines of evidence (reviewed by Bjartmar and Trapp,[8] Scolding and Franklin,[11] Rodriguez 2003[12]) have prompted the search for noninflammatory causes of axon loss, and much attention now centers on myelin- and oligodendrocyte-derived support for axons – and its loss in MS. Axonal damage as (at least in part) a consequence of persistent myelin loss is supported by pathological studies showing chronic axon loss not to correlate with either inflammatory cell infiltrate, tumor necrosis factor expression, nitric oxide expression or demyelinating activity, but rather to the overall extent of established myelin loss.[13,14] It is seen in lesions that are demyelinated but exhibit sparse or no inflam-

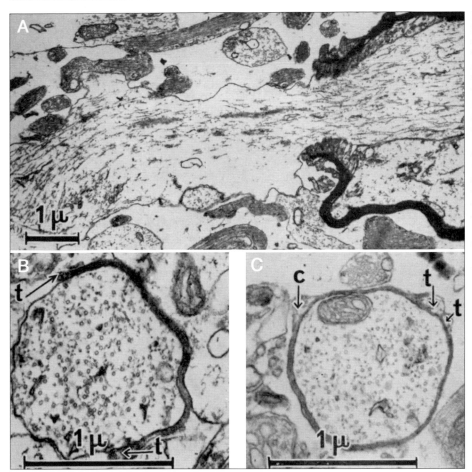

FIG. 24.1 The first electron microscopic images suggestive of remyelination at the edge of a plaque.[2] **A.** A longitudinal section through the ending of a myelin internode with the naked axon continuing without ensheathement into the lesion. ×14 500. **B.** A transversal section through an axon with many well preserved, intact microtubules partially surrounded by a flattened glial process from which most cytoplasm is excluded except at the terminal loops (or tongue t). **C.** Another axon is completely surrounded by a flattened glial process and, on the left, two adjacent compacting membranes closely apposed to the axon suggest an early stage of myelin formation. The apposition of two terminal tongues (t) on the right constitutes the precursor of the future mesaxon. At C, a cytoplasmic loop is detected. **B, C** ×42 000. Reproduced From Perier and Gregoire 1965[2] with permission of Olivier Perier and *Brain*.

mation, but is rare in re-remyelinated lesions.[14] Over the last decades, demyelination-induced axon loss has been shown to occur by a variety of mechanisms such as sustained demyelination-induced conduction block and electrical silence,[15] through increased vulnerability of the exposed axon to injurious agents[16] or directly through the loss of oligodendrocyte-derived trophic support[17–19] and/or the lack of specific myelin proteins.[20,21] The importance of establishing that persistent oligodendrocyte and myelin loss could, at least in part, contribute significantly to progressive axon loss in MS is obvious in terms of repair and protection, and indeed inextricably links the two therapeutic approaches. Replenishment of oligodendrocytes, reinvestment of axons in myelin and the restoration of something approaching a normal glial environment in lesions should not only be useful in its own right as a reparative remyelination therapy, restoring saltatory conduction in axons subject to electrical conduction block, but should represent a major boost to axon survival and a powerful neuroprotective therapy intimately linked to and ameliorating a major cause of axon loss, as also discussed recently.[22] Another positive feature of MS, in terms of developing repair therapies, is found in the clear evidence of spontaneous if partial myelin repair in MS (see Ch. 11). Therefore, to develop promyelinating therapies, one needs to either enhance this spontaneous process by recruiting more endogenous precursor to the lesion site ('endogenous repair') or to provide additional precursors by transplantation (or 'cell therapies'). The now very large body of experimental evidence, employing a wide variety of animal models of demyelination and a range of sources of remyelinating strategies, some summarized in the following, collectively provide proof of the principle: successful remyelination can, without question, be achieved by interventional therapies. How this might be done in patients rather than models must

depend on a better understanding of the clinical biology of the disease: the reasons why endogenous repair is not more successful and how these limitations can be overcome.

NEUROPROTECTION

PHARMACOLOGICAL NEUROPROTECTION TO PREVENT AXON DAMAGE

While the pursuit of neuroprotective therapies in MS is a relatively new approach, only emerging with the past 5 or 6 years' re-emphasis of the pathophysiological significance of axon loss,[23] extraordinary progress has been made.[24] In truth, this is partly because of a large body of research studying the involvement and behavior of axonal ion channels in relation to the disturbed neurophysiological properties of demyelinated axons.[25,26] This, entirely independently of the re-emphasis on axon loss stimulated by neuropathological and neuroimaging studies, had predicted and begun to explore the need for axonal protective therapies using pharmacological approaches targeted upon ion channels.

One recent strategy is based on the elucidation of the precise ion channels redistribution in MS.[3] The Nav1.6 channel can trigger reverse Na^+/Ca^{2+} exchange and both are coexpressed in MS lesions on naked and damaged axons, suggesting that calcium entry may injure demyelinated axons. Interestingly, axonal sodium channel changes in acute lesions and chronic plaques are not identical.[27] Mechanisms of injury related to those of hypoxia, potentially involving NO and consequent intracellular accumulation of calcium ions, provides the link between injury and ion-channel-orientated protective strate-

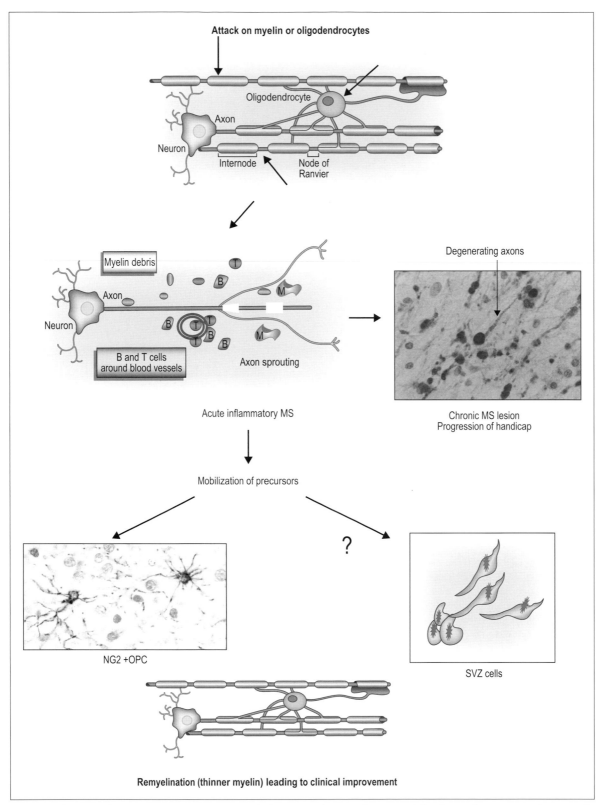

FIG. 24.2 Scheme of cellular events occurring in MS. Demyelination usually occurs following an immune attack on myelin or oligodendrocytes that sustain several myelin internodes. In acute inflammatory lesions, demyelinated axons are surrounded by myelin debris, T and/or B lymphocytes and macrophages (M). One outcome is that demyelination persists and the lesion becomes chronic, resulting in axonal degeneration and progression of the disease. The second outcome is mobilization of oligodendrocyte precursors that migrate into the lesions and, in the best cases, resynthesize thin myelin sheaths, often forming shorter internodes. In periventricular lesions, it is possible that some SVZ precursors are also attracted to the lesions and generate new oligodendrocytes that can remyelinate. Modified from Dubois-Dalcq et al 2005.[22] The NG2-positive OPC picture is from a human MS lesion, courtesy of Ansi Chang and Bruce Trapp. The chronic MS amyloid precursor protein immunostaining of degenerating axons is reproduced from Kornek et al 2000[14] with permission of Hans Lassmann and the *American Journal of Pathology*.

gies.[27,28] Another remarkable recent development is the unraveling of convergent mechanisms for axonal degeneration thanks to the study of the Wallerian degeneration mutant (Wld mouse) and the realization that axon death is occurring through a non-apoptotic death program in several diseases.[29] These mechanisms include alterations in mitochondrial function[30] and anterograde axonal transport together with an increase in axonal calcium concentration. This implies that one specific therapeutic strategy to protect axons might be effective in several diseases. The experience of exploring protection in relation to other neurodegenerative diseases, combined with the rapid demonstration of protection in experimental allergic encephalomyelitis (EAE) models afforded by agents such as phenytoin,[31] flecainide,[32] and lamotrigine,[33] all blockers of sodium channels, has quickly led to trials of comparable agents (e.g. lamotrigine) as protective agents aiming to prevent the accumulation of disability in progressive MS, now under way in the UK and New York, and topiramate (USA). Further dissection of the molecular changes in ion channels in MS[34] is highly likely to present new, more specific therapeutic targets.

Another attractive neuroprotective agent is the AMPA inhibitor NBQX, which, combined with an IGF peptide, ameliorates the clinical course of EAE.[35] AMPA receptors are expressed on both neurons and oligodendrocytes and could be signaled by a glutamate increase in lesions. Such an inhibitor might also attenuate the neuronal damage that can be associated with cortical atrophy in MS.[36] More recent evidence for neuroprotection has emerged in relation to cannabis, in both cell culture paradigms and MS disease models.[37–39] Following the first successfully executed multicenter randomized controlled trial of cannabis in MS,[40] a large-scale study of cannabinoids as protective agents in MS is now under way in the UK (the MRC CUPID trial – Cannabinoid Use in Progressive Inflammatory Disease).

Erythropoietin is another molecule whose neuroprotective properties have only recently come to light;[41] protection is linked to the MAPKs and PI3K pathways, which may lead to AKT activation and neuronal survival.[42] Again, animal model studies have indicated benefit in inflammatory demyelination through inhibition of proinflammatory cytokines.[43,44] In the PNS, erythropoietin released by Schwann cells has been shown to improve symptoms by reducing axonal degeneration, by an as yet unknown mechanism, in a model of diabetic neuropathy.[45] Early trials of erythropoietin in MS have now been reported.[46]

Statins, primarily used as very effective cholesterol-lowering agents, are also now recognized to have unexpectedly potent neuroprotective effects – and in this case, these are also combined with significant immune-modulating actions.[47,48] Protective effects in MS models[49] have been shown, and small-scale studies in patients with MS have already demonstrated partial benefit.[50] Several larger scale studies are under way.

Agents such as tacrolimus (FK506), ciclosporin and rapamycin (sirolimus) are relatively recently introduced immune suppressants. Although structurally varied, they share the action of potently inhibiting calcineurin in the presence of their respective common ligands – the cytoplasmic immunophilins cyclophilin and FK506-binding protein. In fact, immunophilins are expressed in greater quantity in the CNS than in the immune system and, in doses insufficient to suppress the immune system, tacrolimus reduces axon damage in EAE.[51] This class of drug may well have important neuroprotective effects[52,53] – although they are nephrotoxic.

Minocycline, in a comparable way, was first introduced as a tetracycline antibacterial, also having anti-inflammatory activity, but more recently has been shown to have neuroprotective properties in Parkinson's disease, stroke and trauma models of CNS disease.[54] It ameliorates EAE, although this effect may well be through immune deviation rather than neuroprotection;[55,56] a pilot study in MS provides preliminary evidence of a reduction in inflammatory activity.[57]

In addition to these promising experimental studies and early results (Table 24.1), much emphasis, based on the pathophysiological considerations outlined above, also continues to be

TABLE 24.1 Clinical studies of neuroprotective drugs in multiple sclerosis

Agent	EAE	Preliminary studies in patients	Ongoing trials
AMPA/glutamate receptors	✓		
Riluzole	✓	PPMS; 16 patients: no significant effect Mult Scler 2002; 8: 532–533	
Na/Ca exchange blockade/NO	✓		Lamotrigine in SPMS; UK MS Society-funded trial, based at University College, London
Anti-oxidants	✓		
Estrogen (-like)	✓	6 female patients: possible effect Ann Neurol 2002; 52: 421–428.	
Glatiramer	✓	Cochrane Database Systematic Review 2004; PROMISE study – aimed to recruit 900 patients with PPMS; prematurely terminated, interim analysis predicting results would not be able to reach statistical significance (Teva Pharmaceutical Industries Ltd, press release, 11/7/02; Abstract, ECTRIMS 2003) – so far, no clinical evidence to support effect	
Cannabinoids	✓	Extension data from spasticity trial – possible effect Lancet 2003; 362: 1517–1526	CUPID: UK MRC-funded multicenter trial, based in Plymouth
Statins	✓	Open study, 30 patients – possible effect Lancet 2004; 363: 1607–1608	
Erythropoietin	✓	Early trials have now been reported Brain 2007; 130: 2577–2588	Anticipated

CUPI, cannabinoid use in progressive inflammatory disease; EAE, experimental autoimmune encephalomyelitis; PPMS, primary progressive MS; SPMS, secondary progressive MS.

placed on neurotrophic approaches to neuroprotection, and these will be considered next.

NEUROPROTECTION AND GROWTH FACTORS

Such factors should act directly on neurons and their processes to preserve their integrity and prevent axonal degeneration after demyelination. Axonal degeneration results in progressive alteration of axonal transport, loss of appropriate signals for remyelination and, eventually, of synaptic connectivity. A new candidate molecule is vascular endothelial growth factor (VEGF) as it has a neuroprotective effect in acute cerebral ischemia, where it promotes neurogenesis and angiogenesis.[58,59] Remarkably, VEGF intraventricular delivery was recently shown to protect motor neurons and improve motor performance in a rat model of amyotrophic lateral sclerosis (ALS).[60] This is an evolving field that may well have later applications in MS. Neurotrophins have been used in clinical trials of ALS and sensory neuropathies but these trials were stopped because of adverse effects in some patients. Yet neurotrophin (NT)3 and nerve growth factor (NGF) are interesting candidates in MS not only for their neuroprotective effects but also because NT3 enhances oligodendrocyte survival and NGF binding to its low affinity receptor P75 may have a repair function in MS. Indeed, P75 is expressed on some subventricular zone precursors and NG2 expressing oligodendrocyte precursor cells in the vicinity of demyelinating lesions.[61] The three-dimensional resolution of neurotrophins and their receptors is leading to development of small agonists that might be rapidly applicable to neurodegenerative and demyelinating diseases.[62] Three recent observations on unexpected/unpredicted therapeutic ligands in EAE models should promote further studies in MS. First the death ligand TRAIL (tumor necrosis factor-related apoptosis-inducing ligand), which can cause caspase-mediated neuronal death in EAE (induced by transfer of proteolipid-protein-specific T cells), can be inhibited by intracisternal injection of the TRAIL receptor 2 fused to human Fc, resulting in considerable attenuation of the disease.[63] Second, glatiramer acetate (Cop1) administered at the peak of MOG-induced EAE decreased neuronal damage and virtually abolished clinical signs while neurogenesis was enhanced in these mice.[64] Indeed, in patients with multiple sclerosis treated with either glatiramer acetate or interferon-beta 1a, production of brain-derived neurotrophic factor by mononuclear cells is reported.[65] Third, tumor necrosis factor (TNF)α, but not interleukin (IL)-1β, is neuroprotective by rapidly activating microglia in response to acute neurodegeneration and demyelination caused by intracerebral infusion of a nitric oxide donor.[66]

In truth, only a fraction of treatments working in EAE and other models are effective in humans. However, it should be feasible to follow a cohort of patients treated with Cop1 both clinically and by imaging to see whether neuroprotection occurs also in humans.

PROMOTING AXON REGROWTH

Treatments aiming at axon regrowth in spinal cord injury may be beneficial to MS patients where axon transsection has been observed in acute lesions. Myelin contains inhibitors of neurite outgrowth that are released after spinal cord injury and demyelination. The monoclonal antibody IN-1, which binds to NOGO, the first myelin inhibitor to be identified, can locally stimulate sprouting in the lesioned spinal cord[67] and a humanized form of this antibody has been prepared for future clinical trials in spinal cord injury (Martin Schwab, personal communication). Another approach is vaccination with the myelin inhibitor Nogo A, which not only stimulates neurite regrowth but also attenu-

ates EAE.[68] The cloning of the NOGO receptor has led to the engineering of a truncated soluble receptor that also overcomes the myelin inhibition of axonal growth.[69] This is important as there are two other inhibitors of neurite outgrowth in myelin, myelin-associated glycoprotein and oligodendrocyte myelin glycoprotein, and all three inhibitors share the same functional NOGO receptor, which associates with the NGF receptor p75 to activate the signaling cascade.[70] Other partners of the NOGO receptor are Troy, a homolog of P75, and Lingo-1, an inhibitor of oligodendrocyte differentiation.[71] Therefore, another way to counteract the axonal growth inhibition triggered by the NOGO receptor is to interfere with its signaling pathway by blocking the small GTPase Rho or increasing intracellular cyclic adenosine monophosphate (AMP).[72] If drugs blocking all three inhibitors turn out to be active in spinal cord injury, they may well be beneficial in MS patients, where axon survival and regrowth is a prerequisite to remyelination. Another important lesson from studies of spinal cord injury may lie in the early experience of combinatorial treatments. Schwann cell transplants (discussed below), given with local delivery of dibutyryl cyclic AMP (which stimulates neurotrophins and prevents Ca$^+$ influx and apoptosis), induces both motor recovery and extensive remyelination of the regenerating fibers.[73,74]

REMYELINATION

THE BIOLOGY OF MYELIN REPAIR

Spontaneous remyelination is effected by endogenous oligodendrite precursor cells (OPCs). These cells can be isolated from the normal adult human brain and are identified by the expression of transcription factors Olig2 and Nkx2–2 as well as the surface markers platelet-derived growth factor receptor (PDGFR)α and NG2 (Fig. 24.3). These markers are also expressed by OPCs in the MS brain tissues.[75–77] These adult human OPCs become oligodendrocytes and remyelinate when grafted in shiverer myelin-deficient mice.[78] Such precursors would be the most likely to proliferate and migrate toward primary lesions and establish contact with demyelinated axons. Axon–oligodendrocyte interactions are triggered by electrical activity and molecular cues along the axon such as laminin 2, locally-released growth factors and a transmembrane isoform of neuregulin (Nrg)-1 which, in peripheral nerve axons, sends a myelinating signal at a critical density.[79,80] Once the myelination program is turned on, myelin internodes and nodes are synthesized along each demyelinated axon and this should restore fast saltatory conduction and maintain axon integrity. These series of events would be responsible for the myelin repair observed in shadow plaques mentioned above. The new myelin should have the proper molecular structure to maintain its stability. For instance, it should not be enriched in citrullinated myelin basic protein (MBP) isoform – which was found to be increased in MS – as it can compromise the stability of the myelin lipid bilayer.[81]

The recently described properties of the multipotential adult subventricular zone (SVZ) precursors suggest that these cells may also play a role in CNS regeneration and, possibly, remyelination. There are three types of neural precursor in the adult SVZ: the A cells generate neuroblasts going to the olfactory bulb while the B cells express GFAP and generate the 'transit-amplifying C cells', which express the transcription factor DLX2.[82] C cells bear epidermal growth factor (EGF) receptors and respond to EGF by mitosis.[82] The discovery that astrocytes can be stem cells has led to the proposal that a subset of glial cells throughout the brain, outside neurogenic regions, may be 'latent' stem cells.[83] The concept of 'stem cell niches' emerged

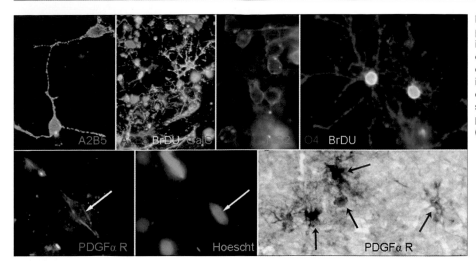

FIG. 24.3 Adult human oligodendrocyte progenitors. The top row shows cells in culture, immunofluorescently stained with various oligodendrocyte cell lineage markers, in some cases double stained with bromodeoxyuridine, indicating proliferation. The bottom row shows central nervous system tissue from multiple sclerosis patients, with oligodendrocyte progenitors immunostained using fluorescent (left) or chromogen (right) techniques.

recently; these are sites where precursors are surrounded by elements favoring neurogenesis such as basement membrane laminin and endothelial cells.[84] Neural stem cells in niches express vascular endothelia growth factor receptor (VEGFR)-2 and release VEGF, which stimulates vessel growth. Endothelial cells, in turn, release soluble factors that favor stem cell renewal in vitro.[85] We will therefore discuss below the growth factors that expand and mobilize both OPCs and SVZ cells.

Growth factors and other molecules to expand and mobilize endogenous precursors

To our knowledge, enhancement of remyelination has not yet been obtained experimentally by systemic injection of a growth factor, and specific promising candidates (such as insulin-like growth factor (IGF)-1) have not produced the anticipated benefit,[86] despite their known role in the process of myelin formation. It is therefore imperative to accelerate drug discovery and find the most appropriate ways to deliver to the CNS candidate factors or their agonists. We will review here experimental evidence for the potential therapeutic value of the morphogen sonic hedgehog (Shh), several growth factors and chemoattractants for SVZ precursors and OPCs, as well as promyelinating factors.

Shh promotes oligodendrocyte fate during CNS development, principally through induction of the Olig transcription factors.[87,88] Importantly, it stimulates mitosis of developing OPCs as well as postnatal and adult SVZ precursors.[89–91] Newly developed Shh agonists, when delivered orally, stimulate mitosis in neural stem cell niches within the SVZ and hippocampus.[92] Shh injected in a spinal cord injury lesion induces significant proliferation of neural precursors around the central canal and this results in an increase in both OPCs and neurons.[93] Furthermore, when OPCs were grafted with and without Shh in such lesion, both groups of rats showed improved motor behavior over untreated animals.[94] Together these observations suggest that Shh or its agonists could be considered in therapeutic approaches to enhance CNS regeneration. Yet its role on remyelination remains to be fully investigated.

A surprising finding is that EGF delivered intraventricularly not only expands 'C' precursors from the SVZ but also stimulates their migration toward white matter tracts where some become oligodendrocytes.[82] Along these lines, overexpression of human EGFR in OPCs was recently found to accelerate remyelination and functional recovery after focal demyelination in corpus callosum.[95] PDGF, on the other hand, has long been known to promote both OPC mitosis and migration.[96] PDGF-responsive precursors were recently isolated from the embryonic basal forebrain and shown to generate OPCs, interneurons and astrocytes.[97] These precursors optimally proliferate in response to

PDGF and fibroblast growth factor (FGF)2 as OPCs do[98] and they depend on Shh for this response.[97] Early OPCs bear polysialyl residues on NCMA, which enhances their migration toward a gradient of PDGF AA in vitro.[99] Of interest is that mimetic peptides of PSA, obtained by selection of a random peptide library, strongly enhance SVZ precursor migration when they express PSA-NCAM.[100] As PDGFRα-expressing precursors have been localized in MS lesions,[77,101] and PSA-positive glial progenitors may migrate to MS lesions from the SVZ.[102] one could envisage locally delivered PSA peptides and PDGF enhancing their migration toward demyelinated lesions. Developmental studies have shown how several other molecules control neural cell migration. In embryonic optic nerve, semaphorins and netrins guide early OPCs, which originate in the diencephalon and enter the optic nerve toward the retina.[103] Of great interest is that chronically dymelinated MS plaques show an increase in Semaphorin 3A, which is repulsive for OPCs, while the OPC attractant, Semaphorin 3F, is increased at the edge of active lesions, suggesting that these molecules may influence whether a plaque is going to be remyelinated or not.[104] While migrating along the nerve, Ephrin-B2-expressing OPCs interact with EphB on axons, resulting in bidirectional signaling that stabilizes OPC.[103] Mouse embryonic striatal precursors and early OPCs, on the other hand, respond by directed migration to the α chemokine CXCL12 binding to g-protein-coupled receptor CXCR4 on their surface.[105] CXCR4 is downregulated when oligodendrocytes differentiate and it is not known whether it can be re-expressed prior to remyelination. In fact, CXCL12 has been detected recently in MS lesions.[106] Fetal human neural precursors also specifically migrate toward a CXCL12 gradient[107,108] and, when grafted in mice with an ischemic lesion, they are attracted by CXCL12 released by endothelia and astrocytes.[109] It might be interesting to test whether existing agonists of CXCR4 signaling induce neural precursor mobilization following demyelination.

Inflammatory lesions may also contain other chemotactic factors for OPCs. In EAE, hepatocyte growth factor (HGF), whose synthesis by microglia/macrophages is induced by the T helper (Th)2 cytokine transforming growth factor (TGF)β, enhances OPC migration and differentiation during the recovery phase of the disease.[110]

Inhibitory molecules in lesions

The presence of OPCs in chronic lesions that are not remyelinated (Fig. 24.4) of course presents a paradox: why, if present in reasonable numbers, have these cells not successfully repaired local myelin? It should always be borne in mind that, in contrast to animal model studies, human MS samples represent only a single 'snapshot': conceivably, lesions containing demonstrable

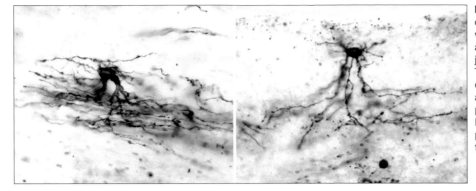

FIG. 24.4 Premyelinating oligodendrocytes in chronic lesions of multiple sclerosis. These were immunostained with proteolipid protein antibodies and were often detected in clusters just beneath the subventricular zone (SVZ). The perikarya of these premyelinating oligodendrocytes were located in an axon-free area of the SVZ and extended processes parallel to the demyelinated axons. Bar=30μm. Reproduced from Chang et al 2002[75] with permission of Ansi Chang and Bruce Trapp and the *New England Journal of Medicine*.

progenitors might have gone on later to benefit from the progenitors' successful remyelinating activity. But this seems unlikely as a major contributing factor. More likely is an alternative temporal aspect of lesions in general and of the axoglial relationship in particular, namely the evolving (and probably diminishing) receptiveness of the demyelinated axon to ensheathing oligodendrocyte processes and myelin formation. Thus while various molecules as mentioned above are able to enhance OPC migration, inhibitory molecules appearing in MS lesions may block the migration or differentiation of OPCs, or their interactions with axons.[75,111,112] Moreover a major inhibitor of remyelination of acute lesions is the accumulation of myelin debris.[113] Thus promoting clearing of myelin debris by macrophages may enhance remyelination.

There are several candidate inhibitory molecules based on experimental work. For instance, while oligodendrocytes can spread on *N*-cadherin made by astrocyte monolayers, this adhesion molecule restricts OPC migration on these cells, a motility that can be restored by treatment with an antibody to *N*-cadherin.[114] Other candidate inhibitors are the glycosaminoglycan hyaluronan, recently found to accumulate in chronic MS lesions, which inhibits oligodendrocyte progenitor maturation[115] and chondroitin sulfate proteoglycan, a component of the glial scar, inhibiting axonal regeneration.[116] In spinal cord injury, chondroitinase can enhance neurite regrowth and remyelination by grafted Schwann cells.[117] On the other hand, the chondroitin sulfate proteoglycan NG2 is expressed by human OPCs in MS[75,76,118] and is necessary for migration of developing OPCs in rodent.[119] As some chronic relapsing MS patients show CSF immunoglobulins binding to NG2, these antibodies might inhibit OPC migration in the lesions.[120] Thus further studies on the role of NG2 in EAE and MS lesions are required to elucidate whether one can maintain NG2 on the oligodendrocyte surface while clearing it from the environment.

Another molecule closely involved in remyelination is polysialyl (PSA) on NCAM. PSA-NCAM expression on the surface of neural precursors has important effects on their migration and on myelination. Expression is downregulated on both the axons and the oligodendrocyte surface before myelination[111,121] and, during development, myelin deposition occurs only on PSA-NCAM-negative axons. In MS, PSA-NCAM is re-expressed by demyelinated axons, while remyelinated axons do not express PSA-NCAM. Re-expression of PSA-NCAM on axons could therefore act as an inhibitor of remyelination.[122]

Hemopoietic cytokines and growth factors

Growth factors Here ciliary neurotrophic factor (CNTF) and leukemia inhibitory factor (LIF) appear promising candidates, first because these cytokines enhance myelination in vitro[123] and second because CNTF promotes remyelination[124] and LIF enhances survival of oligodendrocytes in EAE mice, resulting in attenuation of disease.[125] Similarly, daily administration of LIF

intraperitoneally promotes oligodendrocyte survival after spinal cord injury.[126] In this case LIF acts by increasing IGF-1 synthesis by microglia and macrophages. CNTF, on the other hand, is produced by astrocytes during spontaneous remyelination occurring in mice recovering from a coronavirus-induced demyelinating disease.[127] Surprisingly TNFα, a Th1 cytokine, also promotes OPC mitosis and remyelination by specifically binding to TNF receptor (TNFR)2, as shown in mouse genetic models.[128]

With the aim of enhancing myelination and/or remyelination, two types of transgenic mice were created that overproduce IGF-1 or PDGF. Demyelination was induced by cuprizone in both cases. IGF1 is a promyelinating factor, as mice overexpressing IGF1 under the metallothionein or MBP promoter showed increased oligodendrocyte numbers and rate of myelination and remyelination.[129-131] Along these lines, IGF1 can instruct adult hippocampal precursors to become oligodendrocytes in vitro.[132] Therefore IGF1 could be considered for local delivery in the CNS, possibly in combination with other growth factors. Mice overexpressing PDGFα in astrocytes did not show an increase in ratio of PDGFRα dividing OPCs after demyelination, suggesting that saturation levels of PDGF cannot increase proliferation and remyelination.[133] As PDGF was recently shown to act in synergy with PI3K signaling by α6β1 integrin to stimulate OPC proliferation and survival,[134] enhancement of remyelination might also require increased expression of this integrin. Thus such kinases and components of the integrin signaling pathways might be promising targets for manipulating remyelination.[79]

In relation to the cell therapy approaches discussed below, administration of PDGF, FGF2 or EGF in newborn mice grafted with adult SVZ neural precursors considerably enhances engraftment and generation of myelin-forming cells.[135] This suggests that combining growth factor and cell therapy might be more efficient in enhancing remyelination than either alone.

Immunoglobulins Intriguingly, a recombinant human monoclonal human IgM antibody (rHIg M22) enhances remyelination in Theiler's-virus-infected mice, as detected by magnetic resonance imaging (MRI) and histology.[136] This represents the latest in an extensive series of studies by Moses Rodriguez and his colleagues systematically exploring the promotion of remyelination by immunoglobulins.[137] In experimental animals with CNS demyelination caused by chronic Theiler's virus infection, treatment with systemic whole antiserum, or purified immunoglobulin-G directed against spinal cord homogenate, increased myelin repair.[138,139] Polyclonal immunoglobulins against myelin basic protein also achieved this effect,[140] as did a monoclonal antibody directed against an oligodendrocyte surface antigen.[141] The antibody belongs to the class of 'natural autoantibodies'[142] – naturally occurring polyreactive antibodies of uncertain function and significance.[143] It has been speculated that antibody binding to oligodendrocytes might directly stimulate myelinating function,[144] although in vitro observations suggested that immunoglobulins have no direct effect on oligodendrocyte function.[145-147] It now appears more likely that the immunomodulatory and anti-inflammatory consequences of immunoglobulin treatment are responsible for encouraging remyelination[148,149] – although more recent studies have failed to find evidence of an immune modulatory action.[150,151] rHIg M22 binds to the oligodendrocyte surface, activating calcium flux and antiapoptotic signals, representing an attractive mode of action resolving some of these apparently conflicting experimental data. Most disappointingly, despite the substantial effects in experimental models, the first trials of immunoglobulins delivered intravenously as a putative systemic remyelination therapy in patients with MS have now been completed, unfortunately with negative results.[152,153] However, other trials using the rHIgM22 antibody, so effective in mice demyelinated with infected Theiler's virus, could be considered in the future.

CELL THERAPY AND MULTIPLE SCLEROSIS

Very efficient repair of focal demyelinating lesions in the spinal cord has been observed in rodents after grafting a variety of cell populations.[122,154] Neural precursor transplantation in brain can cause extensive remyelination of dysmyelinating mutants, although correction of the clinical phenotype has not been described.[155] The use of cell therapy raises several questions in MS patients, where immune attack of oligodendrocytes and/or myelin can resume after a relapse. We will therefore divide this discussion in two parts.

Allogenic graft of neural precursors in multiple sclerosis

An important consideration here is to ensure that any donor human cells, whether embryonic or adult, do not carry certain MHC subgroups or other MS susceptibility genes that would render the transplanted cells as vulnerable to the demyelinating process as the patient's own cells. Also, even though grafts in the CNS are not rejected as fast as in other tissues, the possibility of rejection remains a critical issue in the long term.

Human embryonic brain or spinal cord-derived neurospheres Several laboratories have successfully set up this method using legal abortion tissue at about 7–10 weeks postconception.[156-158] In these studies, many more neurons than oligodendrocytes were obtained after adhesion and differentiation of neural precursors from neurospheres. Unlike rodent cells, FGF2-expanded human precursors isolated from both ventral and dorsal spinal cord yielded low numbers of oligodendrocytes in differentiation assays and the few oligodendrocyte lineage cells observed did not proliferate well in response to PDGF and FGF2 in vitro.[159] These results are not so surprising, as the first OPCs emerge ventrally at different levels of the spinal cord between 45 and 60 days postconception[160] and oligodendrogliogenesis does not start till the 20th week in the human fetal brain. Yet human embryo neurospheres transplanted in E16 fetal rat brain in utero can generate not only neurons but also oligodendrocytes, which integrated in the white matter and express myelin proteins at the time of myelination in the postnatal rat brain.[161] Recently, OPCs from human fetal brain obtained at 21–23 weeks postconception were purified by FACS sorting using A2B5 antibodies and their myelination properties were demonstrated in vivo.[78] However, legally obtained tissues at this age are rare; therefore it might be better to choose other approaches, as we will discuss next.

Human embryonic-stem-cell-derived oligodendrocyte precursors This approach was successfully used with mouse embryonic stem cells from which OPCs were derived using lineage selection and specific growth factors followed by FACS sorting. These purified populations of OPCs were shown to myelinate myelin-deficient rats after transplantation.[162,163] Populations enriched in OPCs were also derived from human embryonic stem cells[164,165] and, when grafted, OPCs divided and formed MBP-positive myelin patches in shiverer.[165] Grafting embryonic stem cell-derived OPCs in rats 7 days after spinal cord injury resulted in improved motor recovery and enhanced remyelination in the lesions.[164]

Arguments for and against this approach in humans have been recently reviewed.[166] On the positive side, the protocols established in mice and humans result in cells apparently committed to the oligodendrocyte lineage, a technique that appears so far to avoid tumor formation. Yet this risk has to be eliminated before application to the clinic – careful studies of human ES cells predifferentiated to form dopaminergic neurons prior to rodent transplantation showed a significant proportion of cells still retain tumorigenic potential.[167] Also, one has to exclude contamination with animal products, as most embryonic stem cell lines have been exposed to those and/or expanded on mouse cells. However, human embryonic stem cells are now grown on human feeder layers or without any layer. Furthermore, human cells are being tested in immunodeficient nude mice, assuming that, if these stay free of tumors or infections with human pathogens, the case for transplants in patients would be stronger.

Human multipotential precursors isolated from adult human brain These precursors have been successfully isolated from neurosurgery specimens by FACS sorting with A2B5 antibodies.[168] In this work, transfection with a clone expressing GFP under the control of the CNP oligodendrocyte-specific promoter has been very efficient in purifying human OPC. These precursors were grown as neurospheres and shown to be multipotential, generating neurons and glia in vitro and in vivo after xenografting in the fetal rat brain.[168] The myelinating properties of these precursors sorted from adult human brain were compared to those of human fetal neurospheres: they seemed to carry much more repair potential than human fetal neurospheres after transplantation in shiverer mice.[78] While both populations myelinated well, the fetal cells migrated more, generating astrocytes and oligodendrocytes, but extensive myelination was only seen after 10 weeks. In contrast, adult brain precursors had already achieved widespread myelination at 4 weeks, thus more rapidly then fetal precursors, and each individual adult precursor ensheathed more axons, indicating a remarkable preservation of properties needed to remyelinate adult CNS axons efficiently.

Of course this approach also carries problems, the principal one being the limitation in donor tissue availability and the risk of variability between specimens. To avoid these, one could perform a brain biopsy to obtain and expand the patient's own OPCs, but this is not without risk in an MS patient and may not represent a practical option for any large-scale treatment.

Recent experimental studies with adult SVZ precursors in EAE mice[169,170] suggest another approach in humans that is presently being explored in nonhuman primates (G. Martino, personal communication). It consists of peripheral delivery of these neural precursors grown as neurospheres in the circulation of mice immunized with MOG and treated with cytokines to open the blood–brain barrier. This approach resulted in amelioration of the clinical score due to the penetration of syngenic neural precursors in many places of the affected brain parenchyma. Most recently, authors have analyzed the mechanisms of action of these neural precursors reaching the inflamed CNS in EAE. Using SJL mice with chronic EAE induced by a proteolipid peptide, they found that these cells promote neuroprotection and exert unexpected immune functions.[170] In these mice, neural precursors are capable of crossing the brain endothelia by activating appropriate integrins and chemokine receptors. They then accumulate in perivascular areas where encephalitogenic T cells are present, eventually inducing apoptosis of these T cells, which results in less tissue loss and disability. These intriguing observations raise the hope that peripheral delivery of adult SVZ precursors could one day be attempted in inflammatory demyelinating diseases in humans. However, if these precursors are to be derived from the patient's own adult SVZ, this implies stereotaxic brain biopsy in a fragile environment, a significant practical problem already mentioned. Promoting remyelination by peripheral delivery of more easily obtained bone marrow derived cells[171] (see below) provides further support for the feasibility of intravenous therapies.

In marmosets, when Lac-Z-expressing neurosphere cells from expanded SVZ precursors were grafted in a focal demyelinating lesion in the spinal cord, remyelination was observed[172] but, surprisingly, the majority of the myelin was made by Schwann cells. These were also labeled with Lac Z, indicating that they were derived from the grafted CNS precursors. The generation of Schwann cells by rat developing neural precursors grafted in similar demyelinated lesions has been described[173] and was also observed with human cells grafted in lesioned rat spinal cord.[174]

Non-CNS precursor cells derived from easily accessible sources in humans

This is a priori a much more attractive alternative, as these cells are unlikely to be directly attacked by the disease process taking place in MS. Moreover, it could allow grafting the patient's own cells without the risk of rejection. But are these cells efficient at myelin repair?

Schwann cells Significantly, Schwann cells make a contribution to endogenous myelin repair in MS, particularly in the spinal cord[175–179] – although, as yet, neither the quantitative role of Schwann cells compared to oligodendrocytes in spontaneous remyelination, nor their origin, has been determined. Additionally, experimental models clearly confirm the functionally useful repair of CNS myelin by exogenous implanted Schwann cells (reviewed by Baron-Van Evercooren and Blakemore[154] and Lubetzki et al[122]). Furthermore, methods for preparing cultures of Schwann cells (from adult peripheral nerve biopsies) and for purifying and expanding the cells in vitro to generate large populations of highly enriched Schwann cells have been established.[178,179] When so purified, human Schwann cells successfully lay down new myelin in the mouse[180] and the rat spinal cord.[181,182] In recent nonhuman primate studies, highly successful large-scale remyelination was achieved by autologous transplantation of expanded macaque Schwann cells into the demyelinated macaque spinal cord.[183] Some – but not all – of the key proofs of principle for therapeutic Schwann cell repair in MS are therefore in place. Autologous Schwann cell harvesting from peripheral nerve biopsy, expansion in vitro and transplantation into patients offers the considerable attractions of relative availability and the avoidance of rejection. Furthermore (and by contrast with oligodendrocyte-established new myelin), Schwann cells and their myelin sheaths should be resistant to continuing MS-related immunological attack. Importantly, however, firm evidence is required that expanded implanted human Schwann cells do not form tumors in vivo, a hazard described when rodent Schwann cells immortalized by growth factor expansion were transplanted;[184] unpurified preparations of human peripheral nerve cells result in substantial fibroblast overgrowth with axon destruction,[181] obviously presenting a serious barrier to the clinical application of Schwann cell transplants. The apparent inhibitory effect of astrocytes on Schwann-

cell-mediated CNS remyelination[185–187] represents another potential problem for the use of Schwann cells in remyelination therapy. A further understanding of the molecular mechanisms implicated in Schwann cell migration[188–190] and in Schwann cell:astrocyte interactions[191,192] may allow this problem to be addressed. Recently, rodent Schwann cells engineered to show increased and sustained surface expression of PSA on NCAM have been generated, and these show markedly enhanced migration in vitro.[193] Engineered Schwann cells successfully myelinated cerebellar axons in slice cultures. Modified Schwann cells might therefore be of considerable interest for therapeutic approaches in both CNS and PNS disease.[193] Recently, embryonic Schwann cell precursors were found to survive and migrate through normal CNS tissue and myelinate extensively while intermingling with astrocytes of the retina.[194] One study of intracerebral implantation of autologous noncultured (or purified or expanded) Schwann cells in patients, the first of its kind, has been undertaken in the USA. Some years on, no formal publication of the results has emerged: it is understood that three patients were treated and the study then stopped.

Olfactory ensheathing cells Olfactory ensheathing cells (OECs)[195] represent a special class of PNS glial cells with some features of CNS glia. In vivo and in vitro they can be immunolabeled for P75, the low-affinity NGF receptor, GFAP and with the O4 antibodies. The best mitotic response is to Neu differentiation factor, which is encoded by a spliced form of the Neuregulin 1 gene. OECs can easily be obtained from the patient's first cranial nerve when they traverse the cribriform plate. Although they normally ensheathe thin axons below the threshold diameter necessary for myelination, they can myelinate large axons, but less efficiently than Schwann cells. However, after transplantation they migrate better than Schwann cells in the presence of astrocytes in demyelinating lesions – perhaps through OEC effects on astrocyte expression of chondroitin sulfate proteoglycans.[196,197] Their myelinating potential was optimized by cografting with meningeal cells, which increases the matrix around the PNS myelin made by OECs in the CNS lesions. Further work is necessary to expand the human cells. Of interest is the synthesis of a number of neurotrophic factors by OECs that allow them to promote neurite outgrowth. In rat spinal cord injury, the combination of Schwann cell bridge and OEC grafts allows the regenerating neurites to re-enter the spinal cord[117,198] and the number of myelinated fibers were correlated with improved locomotion in this model. OEC may not only enhance axon regeneration but also provide a permissive matrix and increase the number of Schwann cells invading the damaged spinal cord.[199] Trials of OEC implantation in spinal cord injury are planned in the UK.

Hematopoietic precursors and other cells isolated from bone marrow Hematopoietic stem cell (HSC) plasticity has been the object of many studies and debates over the last years, especially in the field of neuroscience. The stakes are high indeed if a cell population accessible by a bone marrow biopsy could travel to the brain and participate in CNS regeneration. It is well established that precursors of the macrophage lineage can enter the brain and become resident microglial cells but several studies have also suggested that circulating bone marrow cells can home in on brain and transdifferentiate into neural cells, including in humans (reviewed by Crain et al[200]). In favor of this hypothesis are the effects of allogenic bone marrow transplantation in boys affected with adrenoleukodystrophy, a lethal demyelinating, X linked genetic disease caused by a peroxisomal transporter mutation.[201] Over the last 15 years, many affected boys undergoing bone marrow transplantation early in the disease showed clinical stabilization and/or improvement.[202] One interpretation is that wild-type microglia in the brain provide enough normal adreno-leukodystrophy protein to arrest the cascade leading to death of oligodendrocytes carrying the mutation and demyelination;[203] yet another possibility would be that some diseased oligodendrocytes were also replaced. Another genetic disease of myelin is globoid leukodystrophy, whose mouse model, the twitcher, also showed clinical improvement after bone marrow transplantation. In this case, donor cells differentiated in microglia/macrophages but not neurons, astrocytes or oligodendrocytes.[204] Therefore the bone marrow transplantation therapeutic effect in twitcher mice is not mediated by transdifferentiation of bone marrow donor cells in neural cells.

Several studies then examined different cell populations present in the bone marrow for their neurogenic properties and one of these examined their myelinating potential. Embryonic HSCs were chosen for their likely 'plasticity' and purified from the mouse aorta–gonad mesonephros (AGM) region to expose them to the CNS milieu.[205] These precursors are capable of long-term hematopoietic reconstitution and generate colonies containing multipotential HSCs and lymphoid progenies. Intriguingly when cultured in hematopoietic growth conditions, a fraction of CD45+ AGM precursors coexpress nestin, the polysialylated form of neural cell adhesion molecule, the tubulin isoform III, and glial fibrillary acidic protein. When GFP-tagged AGM precursors were cocultured with embryonic striatal precursors into neurospheres, they maintained their hematopoietic phenotype while neural cells differentiated. When grafted into wild-type or newborn shiverer mice, these precursors integrated well into the brain and gave rise to microglia but not neurons or glia, while cografted wild-type embryonic striatal precursors generated oligodendrocytes that synthesized numerous patches of myelin. Thus, in mice, embryonic neural precursors have myelin repair properties not shared by embryonic HSCs. There is, however, converging evidence that HSCs can occasionally generate Purkinje cells, although this event is very rare.[206,207] One recent study using human CD34 HSCs grafted in a chick spinal cord lesion described their frequent differentiation into functionally integrated neurons, without evidence for cell fusion.[208] There is also clinical evidence that adult bone-marrow-derived cells can integrate fully into adult human organs and survive for decades. In these postmortem studies of patients who received sex-mismatched bone marrow transplantation, donor-derived fully-differentiated neurons of a highly complex morphology were found to be established within the host brain[209,210] – many years after intravenous infusion. However, the frequency of this event is rare – 2–5 in 10 000 in one study,[200] 0.1–1% in others.[209,210] So far, no evidence of oligodendrocyte generation by these cells has been reported in grafted human tissues.

Mesenchymal cells (MSCs), another major bone marrow cell type, can transdifferentiate into neural cells including physiologically active neurons in vitro.[211–213] MSC grafting did cause remyelination of a focal chemical lesion but it was initially unclear whether the myelinating cells derived from MSCs and/or the grafted cells enhanced remyelination by endogenous cells.[214] In a later study, when GFP-labeled marrow cells were implanted, GFP-positive myelin profiles and GFP-positive cells colocalized with MBP-positive and P0-positive cellular elements were found, implying that mesenchymal cells can form functional myelin during transplantation into demyelinated spinal cord.[214] One difficulty in comparing different studies is that the antigenic phenotype and the growth properties of mesenchymal stem cells have been much debated.[215]

In two recent studies, MSCs were delivered intravenously in EAE at the time of induction or at the peak of the disease and this improved the clinical scores significantly.[216,217] This was paralleled by decreased inflammatory cell infiltrates and decreased demyelination. MSCs were found in the spleen and brain, either in the subarachnoid space or in the parenchyma, and in one study inhibition of the T cell response was thought to be the major mechanism involved.[217] Injection of MSCs was not compared to other cell types. Therefore the remyelinating potential of well characterized MSC should be further explored. Pilot studies of regenerative bone marrow stem cell treatment in MS patients are now underway.[218]

GENE THERAPY AND MULTIPLE SCLEROSIS

A recent review of gene therapy for autoimmune diseases suggests that it is a possible alternative in MS.[219] The argument here is that systemic delivery of a protein, even at high dose, usually does not allow the desired concentration to be achieved in the brain and therefore a vehicle carrying the active protein to the sites of the lesion would be more efficient and avoid side effects. T cells have been considered an ideal vector of bioactive/therapeutic proteins to the brain, taking advantage of their trafficking across endothelia in neurological immune-mediated disorders.[220,221] In EAE, autoreactive memory Th2 cells have been engineered to produce PDGF upon engagement with self-antigen, leading to tissue repair and amelioration of the clinical phenotype.[220] Yet the viral vectors used to express such genes may have an impact on innate adaptive immunity, sometimes inducing antibodies against a self-antigen.[222]

Local delivery of viral vectors may be a better approach, as it can stimulate regeneration by neural stem cells. For instance, anterior SVZ precursors, which normally give rise to olfactory neurons throughout life in rodents, could be diverted toward an oligodendrocyte fate after being transduced with a retroviral vector containing Olig 2 cDNA following stereotaxic injection into the SVZA.[223] These approaches should be further explored in experimental demyelinating models.

REMAINING HURDLES

MONITORING OF OUTCOME

Whether studying neuroprotection or remyelination, or both, reliable and reproducible means of assessing the therapeutic impact are plainly of paramount importance. At present, the MRI detection of new myelin is not reliably feasible, but new techniques continue to emerge,[224] of which magnetization transfer contrast offers valuable insights:[225] three-dimensional MRI using multiple contrasts is of considerable promise for imaging remyelination,[226] as also is radial diffusivity.[227,228] Magnetic resonance spectroscopy measurement of N-acetyl aspartate levels might offer means of assessing any impact on local neuron/axon survival[229,230] – important both for assessing this anticipated benefit of remyelinating therapies and for non-cell-based approaches to neuroprotection. Tractography,[231] serial imaging to monitor axon loss and/or tissue destruction, and the impact of therapies on these parameters, exploiting techniques such as MRI brain T1 relaxation time (which changes demonstrably in individual MS patients over periods of 12–18 months[232]) are additionally likely to prove useful. Using paramagnetic particles to label cells prior to transplantation, enabling their dispersion to be tracked by MRI,[233–235] has promise, although, from a safety perspective, even the most trivial manipulation of cells prior to implantation would be better avoided. Furthermore, dead cells remain visible using these techniques, so that graft survival and function cannot necessarily be inferred from identifying cells;[233] furthermore, this method not only fails to show new myelin formation but may also impair the ability of other MR modalities to do so. Serial neurophysiology may prove valuable, and monitoring conduction times may provide evidence of returning saltatory conduction in the targeted pathway(s). The optic nerve has particular advantages in this respect but various approaches to more generalized multimodal neurophysiological assessment have been described and may prove useful for any intervention aimed at multifocal or more diffuse myelin repair.[236–238]

Finally, clinical stabilization and improvement, not remyelination per se, is of course the true aim of such therapies. Robust and reproducible methods of clinical assessment and monitoring need to be applied. The difficulties of meaningful, reliable and reproducible quantitative clinical assessment in MS are detailed elsewhere (Ch. 31); for the current purposes it is sufficient to note that specific clinical outcomes measures of function, disability and handicap must be developed, validated, adopted and tailored for each type of intervention. Ultimately, of course, the success or otherwise of these therapies can only be determined using properly designed clinical trials, in which clinical outcomes should be paramount. Considerable advances in clinical scale design have improved physical and functional measurement in MS,[239–241] so that the tools for assessing clinical outcome, on which remyelination therapies must stand or fall, are becoming available.

SITE OF IMPLANTATION

In contrast to the development of neuroprotective or indeed immune-modulating therapies, a key problem in considering cell therapy in MS is the number and distribution of demyelinated lesions. Dozens may be present, in the hemispheres, optic nerves, brainstem and cerebellum and spinal cord – with recent studies re-emphasizing the frequency also of cortical lesions.[36,242] Multiple inoculations of cells into almost innumerable lesions scattered throughout the CNS of patients with MS is of course unrealistic. In contrast, there have been clear advantages in Parkinson's disease of direct, local delivery of neurotrophins (here, glial-cell-derived neurotrophic factor (GDNF)), which avoids the side effects and inefficacy of systemically delivered growth factors.[243,244] In MS, such local delivery of a putative remyelinating growth factor, or indeed cells, might be considered in the case of a large, clinically manifesting lesion. Alternatively, intraventricular delivery of cells has attractions and there is some experimental evidence of efficacy[245] – although, if there are lessons from Parkinson's disease, these mitigate against such means of administration.[246]

What should not be overlooked, however, is that many plaques – perhaps a very significant majority – may be clinically silent, while a much smaller number of critical lesions in eloquent areas often carry responsibility for a disproportionate degree of disability. Thus implantation into a very small number of carefully selected lesions (e.g. the optic nerves, the spinal cord or the superior cerebellar peduncle) could yield a useful therapeutic dividend.[247] As such therapies develop, initial 'proof of principle' clinical studies may justifiably seek to bring about repair in perhaps just a single lesion: redundancy in white matter tracts implies that very partial repair could substantially improve conduction (apart from a hoped-for stabilization of axon numbers) and therefore, it would be argued, a limited but nonetheless valuable improvement in function in the affected pathway or nerve tract.

A more global myelin repair strategy (applicable not only in MS but also for the significantly rarer group of patients with inherited disorders of myelin formation) can be contemplated. One possibility is to bring about wide migration of implanted cells, as occurs during development. Supplementing cellular transplantation with growth factor infusions,[248] grafting remyelinating cells expressing a growth factor[249] and inhibiting molecules that impede migration,[114,191] or other strategies for improving migration as described above, might solve this problem. An alternative approach in MS would exploit the blood–brain barrier disruption present at sites of active inflammation to disseminate cells from the circulation as mentioned earlier for neural stem cells and MSCs.[169,217]

CONTINUING INFLAMMATION

Implanting carefully prepared, possibly engineered cells into inflammatory lesions clearly exposes remyelinating glia and their new myelin to ongoing destructive inflammatory molecules and cells – they might quickly meet a tragic end! Concurrent use of potent immunosuppressive agents would in any case be required with allogeneic transplants to prevent more conventional graft rejection and should help protect exogenous cells; but what of autologous implants?

This question is more complex than it first appears. Perhaps surprisingly, spontaneous remyelination in MS appears to occur maximally in lesions at the time of acute inflammation,[250,251] suggesting a propitious environment. A growing body of evidence suggests that inflammation may paradoxically be an important stimulant of remyelination. Anti-inflammatory drugs[252] or the suppression of inflammation in general[253] may impair myelin regeneration (and this appears be through the effects on immune cells rather than a toxic effect on glia[254]). Inflammatory cells synthesize and release pro-reparative neurotrophins[255] – which may, significantly, also have a neuroprotective effect[256] – while recent studies of experimental remyelination also point to a pro-remyelinating effect of inflammation.[257,258] Nonspecific immune suppression may well therefore have adverse consequences for myelin repair; this is an area requiring much future attention.

HOW CLOSE ARE THESE THERAPIES AND HOW SHOULD THEY BE USED?

The last few decades have seen any number of reviews concerning reparative and/or protective strategies for neurological disease but, as mentioned in the introduction, until recently there has been no immediate prospect of successful repair therapies. How close – or otherwise – are they now? And when in the course of the disease should they be applied?

We have attempted to illustrate what enormous progress there has been and how both reparative and protective therapies are getting closer than ever before. Already neuroprotective agents, despite their more recent emergence in the MS field, seem likely to yield a more rapid therapeutic dividend than cell therapies – helped very significantly by a substantially increasing focus on protection in neurodegenerative disease on the part of the pharmaceutical industry. A small number of trials exploring various promising putative neuroprotectants are, at the time of publication, under way (Table 24.1); more are anticipated. The experience of developing immunotherapy in MS has emphasized that a partial effect is a success, not a failure: while we must of course aim for complete neuroprotection, a significant slowing of the rate of axon damage and progression of disability would be a remarkable achievement, if only a beginning. With a wide range of potentially useful agents – from erythropoietin (and analogues) to cannabinoids, from anti-epileptics to cholesterol-lowering agents – there are surely grounds for real optimism.

Concerning myelin repair therapies, however, it is difficult to be quite as optimistic regarding the imminence of useful therapies. Much progress has indeed been made but almost every aspect – the favored agent (cells or molecules, or both), the means of delivery, the timing, measuring outcome and the question of continuing inflammation – still presents problems and requires more studies in appropriate experimental models for

MS.[22] While the success of bone marrow transplantation in some leukodystrophies offers grounds for optimism,[202] this strategy is based on providing normal donor cells devoid of the gene defect that underlies the disease process and, as discussed before, donor-cell-derived microglia are likely to be responsible for the clinical improvement. This is clearly different from MS, where the initial cause of demyelination is not known and where myelin-forming cells are the most needed. MS patients with rapidly progressive disease who have been treated by myeloablation followed by HSC reconstitution with the patient's own precursors showed complete cessation of inflammation by MRI, progressive reconstitution of a new immune repertoire, prolonged clinical stabilization and, in some cases, improvement.[259] There is so far no reported evidence that this treatment resulted in myelin repair, which is in keeping with evidence that inflammation may in fact encourage repair. Yet, such patients might benefit from neuroprotective treatments in the absence of inflammation.

An increased understanding of the nature of MS disease processes also allows tentative answers to be proposed to the question of the timing of a pro-remyelinating therapy. We have argued elsewhere that, because of the futility of attempting to remyelinate axons long since lost, the now better-understood changes in the cell surface expression of various molecules (e.g. PSA-NCAM[111]) in chronically demyelinated axons actively inhibiting remyelination, the profound inhibitory effect of chronic astrocytosis on remyelinating glia, particularly on migration of OPC,[114,191] and the observations that spontaneous remyelination in MS occurs maximally in acute inflammatory lesions[250,251] and that inflammation may in fact encourage repair, remyelinating interventions should be exhibited early in the course of MS.[260]

The threshold of experimental therapeutic assessment in MS patients of remyelinating treatments by transplantation has been crossed, even if with negative results thus far (as outlined above in the Schwann cell section). A very important point is that safety must remain paramount. MS is a chronic but non-fatal disease, making significant predictable risks of therapies far less acceptable than in, say, cancer treatments. Therefore the potential hazards of tumor formation or infection from expanded embryonic stem-cell-based therapies (as discussed above[261]) serve to reduce the immediate prospects for therapeutic use of these cell types. The case of genetically modified cells enhancing repair[249] can be considered in a more positive light as, despite earlier setbacks in gene therapy,[262] a closer examination of this question concluded that, in most cases, the viral gene has a low risk of causing a deleterious insertional mutagenesis.[263] Thus, while our knowledge of some contenders (e.g. embryonic stem cells) is at present insufficient to allow their use in the near future, some points can be made about which neural cell type to use. First, autologous cells offer clear advantages over 'foreign' transplants. Second, brain or even peripheral nerve biopsy of patients to obtain (and expand) autologous neural stem cells, oligodendrocyte progenitors or Schwann cells is unlikely to represent a realistic, long-term, routinely practicable option. Third, it would be naive to assume there might be only one 'best' cell: different remyelinating cells might be chosen for different purposes – as indeed is beginning to emerge with respect to immune therapy, where success has been correlated with a pathological subtype.[263,264] Cell selection may also depend on the number and location of the lesions. Thus, bearing in mind the apparently greater tendency for spontaneous/endogenous Schwann cell repair in the spinal cord compared to the brain, and the possibility of reduced migration of unmodified Schwann cells toward the lesion, single disabling spinal lesions might be suitable for direct Schwann cell injection or even olfactory glia, although the latter might also be used in the brain because of their better migratory capacity. Cells that have the capacity to 'seek' a lesion might have a higher chance of reaching multiple sites of demyelination, as they can be delivered intravenously and may be drawn from the circulation by chemoattractive factors expressed in lesions; examples are adult neural precursors and mesenchymal cells, as recently shown in EAE.[170,216]

In conclusion, it seems appropriate at present to continue to pursue a broad-based strategy for developing myelin repair therapies and therefore we believe it would be premature to exclude almost any of the putative growth factor or reparative cell approaches. This said, some cells seem presently far less likely to succeed in overcoming the various challenges we have outlined (xenotransplants, for example) while others are rightly seen as particularly promising – endogenous adult human neural precursors and olfactory cells being among these. A multidisciplinary approach is vital, learning from comparable therapeutic endeavors in other neurodegenerative and even non-neurological diseases, and 'cherry-picking' emerging medical and scientific advances in disciplines as diverse as disability monitoring and measurement, neuroimaging, neural stem cell biology and molecular genetics, all converging in intelligently designed clinical trials. A thoughtful, dynamic and watchful approach is required simultaneously to assay the benefit in ongoing trials on neuroprotection and to design safe, efficient promyelinating therapies in MS.

REFERENCES

1. Bunge MB, Bunge RP, Ris H. Ultrastructural study of remyelination in an experimental lesion in the adult cat spinal cord. J Biophys Biochem Cytol 1961; 10: 67–94.

2. Perier O, Gregoire A. Electron microscopic features of multiple sclerosis lesions. Brain 1965; 88: 937–952.

3. Waxman SG, Craner MJ, Black JA. Na+ channel expression along axons in multiple sclerosis and its models. Trends Pharmacol Sci 2004; 25: 584–591.

4. De Keyser J, Sulter G, Luiten PG. Clinical trials with neuroprotective drugs in acute ischaemic stroke: are we doing the right thing? Trends Neurosci 1999; 22: 535–540.

5. Cheng YD, Al-Khoury L, Zivin JA. Neuroprotection for ischemic stroke: two decades of success and failure. NeuroRx 2004; 1: 36–45.

6. Ferguson B, Matyszak MK, Esiri MM, Perry VH. Axonal damage in acute multiple sclerosis lesions. Brain 1997; 120: 393–399.

7. Trapp BD, Peterson J, Ransohoff RM et al. Axon transection in the lesions of multiple sclerosis. N Engl J Med 1998; 338: 278–285.

8. Bjartmar C, Trapp BD. Axonal and neuronal degeneration in multiple sclerosis: mechanisms and functional consequences. Curr Opin Neurol 2001; 14: 271–278.

9. Smith KJ, McDonald WI. The pathophysiology of multiple sclerosis: the mechanisms underlying the production of symptoms and the natural history of the disease. Philos Trans R Soc Lond B Biol Sci 1999; 354: 1649–1673.

10. Confavreux C, Vukusic S, Moreau T, Adeleine P. Relapses and progression of disability in multiple sclerosis. N Engl J Med 2000; 343: 1430–1438.

11. Scolding N, Franklin R. Axon loss in multiple sclerosis. Lancet 1998; 352: 340–341.

12. Rodriguez M. A function of myelin is to protect axons from subsequent injury: implications for deficits in multiple sclerosis. Brain 2003; 126: 751–752.

13. Bitsch A, Schuchardt J, Bunkowski S et al. Acute axonal injury in multiple sclerosis. Correlation with demyelination and inflammation. Brain 2000; 123: 1174–1183.

14. Kornek B, Storch MK, Weissert R et al. Multiple sclerosis and chronic autoimmune encephalomyelitis: a comparative quantitative study of axonal injury in active, inactive, and remyelinated lesions. Am J Pathol 2000; 157: 267–276.

15. Lipton SA. Blockade of electrical-activity promotes the death of mammalian retinal ganglion-cells in culture. Proc Natl Acad Sci USA 1986; 83: 9774–9778.

16. Raine CS, Cross AH. Axonal dystrophy as a consequence of long-term demyelination. Lab Invest 1989; 60: 714–725.

17. Griffiths I, Klugmann M, Anderson T et al. Axonal swellings and degeneration in mice lacking the major proteolipid of myelin. Science 1998; 280: 1610–1613.

18. MeyerFranke A, Kaplan MR, Pfrieger FW, Barres BA. Characterization of the signaling interactions that promote the survival and growth of developing retinal ganglion cells in culture. Neuron 1995; 15: 805–819.

19. Wilkins A, Majed H, Layfield R et al. Oligodendrocytes promote neuronal survival and axonal length by distinct intracellular mechanisms: a novel role for oligodendrocyte-derived glial cell line-derived neurotrophic factor. J Neurosci 2003; 23: 4967–4974.

20. Lappe-Siefke C, Goebbels S, Gravel M et al. Disruption of Cnp1 uncouples oligodendroglial functions in axonal support and myelination. Nat Genet 2003; 33: 366–374.

21. Edgar JM, McLaughlin M, Yool D et al. Oligodendroglial modulation of fast axonal transport in a mouse model of hereditary spastic paraplegia. J Cell Biol 2004; 166: 121–131.

22. Dubois-Dalcq M, Ffrench-Constant C, Franklin RJ. Enhancing central nervous system remyelination in multiple sclerosis. Neuron 2005; 48: 9–12.

23. Waxman SG. Demyelinating diseases – new pathological insights, new therapeutic targets. N Engl J Med 1998; 338: 323–325.

24. Farrell R, Heaney D, Giovannoni G. Emerging therapies in multiple sclerosis. Expert Opin Emerg Drugs 2005; 10: 797–816.

25. Bechtold DA, Smith KJ. Sodium-mediated axonal degeneration in inflammatory demyelinating disease. J Neurol Sci 2005; 233: 27–35.

26. Waxman SG. Sodium channel blockers and axonal protection in neuroinflammatory disease. Brain 2005; 128: 5–6.

27. Black JA, Newcombe J, Trapp BD, Waxman SG. Sodium channel expression within chronic multiple sclerosis plaques. J Neuropathol Exp Neurol 2007; 66: 828–837.

28. Smith KJ, Lassmann H. The role of nitric oxide in multiple sclerosis. Lancet Neurol 2002; 1: 232–241.

29. Coleman M. Axon degeneration mechanisms: commonality amid diversity. Nat Rev Neurosci 2005; 6: 889–898.

30. Dutta R, McDonough J, Yin X et al. Mitochondrial dysfunction as a cause of axonal degeneration in multiple sclerosis patients. Ann Neurol 2006; 59: 478–489.

31. Lo AC, Saab CY, Black JA, Waxman SG. Phenytoin protects spinal cord axons and preserves axonal conduction and neurological function in a model of neuroinflammation in vivo. J Neurophysiol 2003; 90: 3566–3571.

32. Bechtold DA, Kapoor R, Smith KJ. Axonal protection using flecainide in experimental autoimmune encephalomyelitis. Ann Neurol 2004; 55: 607–616.

33. Bechtold DA, Miller SJ, Dawson AC et al. Axonal protection achieved in a model of multiple sclerosis using lamotrigine. J Neurol 2006; 253: 1542–1551.

34. Craner MJ, Newcombe J, Black JA et al. Molecular changes in neurons in multiple sclerosis: altered axonal expression of Nav1.2 and Nav1.6 sodium channels and Na$^+$/Ca2$^+$ exchanger. Proc Natl Acad Sci USA 2004; 101: 8168–8173.

35. Kanwar JR, Kanwar RK, Krissansen GW. Simultaneous neuroprotection and blockade of inflammation reverses autoimmune encephalomyelitis. Brain 2004; 127: 1313–1331.

36. Peterson JW, Bo L, Mork S et al. Transected neurites, apoptotic neurons, and reduced inflammation in cortical multiple sclerosis lesions. Ann Neurol 2001; 50: 389–400.

37. Jackson SJ, Baker D, Cuzner ML, Diemel LT. Cannabinoid-mediated neuroprotection following interferon-gamma treatment in a three-dimensional mouse brain aggregate cell culture. Eur J Neurosci 2004; 20: 2267–2275.

38. Jackson SJ, Diemel LT, Pryce G, Baker D. Cannabinoids and neuroprotection in CNS inflammatory disease. J Neurol Sci 2005; 233: 21–25.

39. Pryce G, Ahmed Z, Hankey DJ et al. Cannabinoids inhibit neurodegeneration in models of multiple sclerosis. Brain 2003; 126: 2191–2202.

40. Zajicek J, Fox P, Sanders H et al. Cannabinoids for treatment of spasticity and other symptoms related to multiple sclerosis (CAMS study): multicentre randomised placebo-controlled trial. Lancet 2003; 362: 1517–1526.

41. Brines M, Cerami A. Emerging biological roles for erythropoietin in the nervous system. Nat Rev Neurosci 2005; 6: 484–494.

42. Bartesaghi S, Marinovich M, Corsini E et al. Erythropoietin: a novel neuroprotective cytokine. Neurotoxicology 2005; 26: 923–928.

43. Sattler MB, Merkler D, Maier K et al. Neuroprotective effects and intracellular signaling pathways of erythropoietin in a rat model of multiple sclerosis. Cell Death Differ 2004; 11(suppl 2): S181–S192.

44. Diem R, Sattler MB, Merkler D et al. Combined therapy with methylprednisolone and erythropoietin in a model of multiple sclerosis. Brain 2005; 128: 375–385.

45. Keswani SC, Buldanlioglu U, Fischer A, Reed N et al. A novel endogenous erythropoietin mediated pathway prevents axonal degeneration. Ann Neurol 2004; 56: 815–826.

46. Ehrenreich H, Fischer B, Norra C et al. Exploring recombinant human erythropoietin in chronic progressive multiple sclerosis. Brain 2007; 130: 2577–2588.

47. Steffens S, Mach F. Anti-inflammatory properties of statins. Semin Vasc Med 2004; 4: 417–422.

48. Stuve O, Prod'homme T, Slavin A et al. Statins and their potential targets in multiple sclerosis therapy. Expert Opin Ther Targets 2003; 7: 613–622.

49. Neuhaus O, Stuve O, Zamvil SS, Hartung HP. Are statins a treatment option for multiple sclerosis? Lancet Neurol 2004; 3: 369–371.

50. Vollmer T, Key L, Durkalski V et al. Oral simvastatin treatment in relapsing-remitting multiple sclerosis. Lancet 2004; 363: 1607–1608.

51. Gold BG, Voda J, Yu X et al. FK506 and a nonimmunosuppressant derivative reduce axonal and myelin damage in experimental autoimmune encephalomyelitis: neuroimmunophilin ligand-mediated neuroprotection in a model of multiple sclerosis. J Neurosci Res 2004; 77: 367–377.

52. Poulter MO, Payne KB, Steiner JP. Neuroimmunophilins: a novel drug therapy for the reversal of neurodegenerative disease? Neuroscience 2004; 128: 1–6.

53. Avramut M, Achim CL. Immunophilins and their ligands: insights into survival and growth of human neurons. Physiol Behav 2002; 77: 463–468.

54. Yong W, Wells J, Giuliani F et al. The promise of minocycline in neurology. Lancet Neurol 2004; 3: 744–751.

55. Giuliani F, Fu SA, Metz LM, Yong VW. Effective combination of minocycline and interferon-beta in a model of multiple sclerosis. J Neuroimmunol 2005; 165: 83–91.

56. Giuliani F, Metz LM, Wilson T et al. Additive effect of the combination of glatiramer acetate and minocycline in a model of MS. J Neuroimmunol 2005; 158: 213–221.

57. Metz LM, Zhang Y, Yeung M et al. Minocycline reduces gadolinium-enhancing magnetic resonance imaging lesions in multiple sclerosis. Ann Neurol 2004; 55: 756.

58. Yano A, Shingo T, Takeuchi A et al. Encapsulated vascular endothelial growth factor-secreting cell grafts have neuroprotective and angiogenic effects on focal cerebral ischemia. J Neurosurg 2005; 103: 104–114.

59. Miki Y, Nonoguchi N, Ikeda N et al. Vascular endothelial growth factor gene-transferred bone marrow stromal cells engineered with a herpes simplex virus type 1 vector can improve neurological deficits and reduce infarction volume in rat brain ischemia. Neurosurgery 2007; 61: 586–594.

60. Storkebaum E, Lambrechts D, Dewerchin M et al. Treatment of motoneuron degeneration by intracerebroventricular delivery of VEGF in a rat model of ALS. Nat Neurosci 2005; 8: 85–92.

61. Petratos S, Gonzales MF, Azari MF et al. Expression of the low-affinity neurotrophin receptor, p75(NTR), is upregulated by oligodendroglial progenitors adjacent to the subventricular zone in response to demyelination. Glia 2004; 48: 64–75.

62. Dawbarn D, Allen SJ. Neurotrophins and neurodegeneration. Neuropathol Appl Neurobiol 2003; 29: 211–230.

63. Aktas O, Smorodchenko A, Brocke S et al. Neuronal damage in autoimmune neuroinflammation mediated by the death ligand TRAIL. Neuron 2005; 46: 421–432.

64. Aharoni R, Arnon R, Eilam R. Neurogenesis and neuroprotection induced by peripheral immunomodulatory treatment of experimental autoimmune encephalomyelitis. J Neurosci 2005; 25: 8217–8228.

65. Sarchielli P, Orlacchio A, Vicinanza F et al. Cytokine secretion and nitric oxide production by mononuclear cells of patients with multiple sclerosis. J Neuroimmunol 1997; 80, 76–86.

66. Turrin NP, Rivest S. Tumor necrosis factor alpha but not interleukin 1β mediates neuroprotection in response to acute nitric oxide excitotoxicity. J Neurosci 2006; 26: 143–151.

67. Bareyre FM, Haudenschild B, Schwab ME. Long-lasting sprouting and gene expression changes induced by the monoclonal antibody IN-1 in the adult spinal cord. J Neurosci 2002; 22: 7097–7110.

68. Karnezis T, Mandemakers W, McQualter JL et al. The neurite outgrowth inhibitor Nogo A is involved in autoimmune-mediated demyelination. Nat Neurosci 2004; 7: 736–744.

69. Fournier AE, Gould GC, Liu BP, Strittmatter SM. Truncated soluble Nogo receptor binds Nogo-66 and blocks inhibition of axon growth by myelin. J Neurosci 2002; 22: 8876–8883.

70. Filbin MT. Myelin-associated inhibitors of axonal regeneration in the adult mammalian CNS. Nat Rev Neurosci 2003; 4: 703–713.

71. Schwab JM, Tuli SK, Failli V. The Nogo receptor complex: confining molecules to molecular mechanisms. Trends Mol Med 2006; 12: 293–297.

72. Domeniconi M, Filbin MT. Overcoming inhibitors in myelin to promote axonal regeneration. J Neurol Sci 2005; 233: 43–47.

73. Pearse DD, Pereira FC, Marcillo AE et al. cAMP and Schwann cells promote axonal growth and functional recovery after spinal cord injury. Nat Med 2004; 10: 610–616.

74. Pearse DD, Sanchez AR, Pereira FC et al. Transplantation of Schwann cells and/or olfactory ensheathing glia into the contused spinal cord: Survival, migration, axon association, and functional recovery. Glia 2007; 55: 976–1000.

75. Chang A, Nishiyama A, Peterson J et al. NG2-positive oligodendrocyte progenitor cells in adult human brain and multiple sclerosis lesions. J Neurosci 2000; 20: 6404–6412.

76. Reynolds R, Dawson M, Papadopoulos D et al. The response of NG2-expressing oligodendrocyte progenitors to demyelination in MOG-EAE and MS. J Neurocytol 2002; 31: 523–536.

77. Scolding NJ, Franklin RJM, Stevens S et al. Oligodendrocyte progenitors are present in the normal adult human CNS and in the lesions of multiple sclerosis. Brain 1998; 121: 2221–2228.

78. Windrem MS, Nunes MC, Rashbaum WK et al. Fetal and adult human oligodendrocyte progenitor cell isolates myelinate the congenitally dysmyelinated brain. Nat Med 2004; 10: 93–97.

79. Colognato H, Ffrench-Constant C. Mechanisms of glial development. Curr Opin Neurobiol 2004; 14: 37–44.

80. Michailov GV, Sereda MW, Brinkmann BG et al. Axonal neuregulin-1 regulates myelin sheath thickness. Science 2004; 304: 700–703.

81. Moscarello MA, Pritzker L, Mastronardi FG, Wood DD. Peptidylarginine deiminase: a candidate factor in demyelinating disease. J Neurochem 2002; 81: 335–343.

82. Doetsch F, Petreanu L, Caille I et al. EGF converts transit-amplifying neurogenic precursors in the adult brain into multipotent stem cells. Neuron 2002; 36: 1021–1034.

83. Doetsch F. A niche for adult neural stem cells. Curr Opin Genet Dev 2003; 13: 543–550.

84. Alvarez-Buylla A, Lim DA. For the long run: maintaining germinal niches in the adult brain. Neuron 2004; 41: 683–686.

85. Shen Q, Goderie SK, Jin L et al. Endothelial cells stimulate self-renewal and expand neurogenesis of neural stem cells. Science 2004; 304: 1338–1340.

86. Cannella B, Pitt D, Capello E, Raine CS. Insulin-like growth factor-1 fails to enhance central nervous system myelin repair during autoimmune demyelination. Am J Pathol 2000; 157: 933–943.

87. Lu QR, Yuk D, Alberta JA et al. Sonic hedgehog–regulated oligodendrocyte lineage genes encoding bHLH proteins in the mammalian central nervous system. Neuron 2000; 25: 317–329.

88. Zhou Q, Wang S, Anderson DJ. Identification of a novel family of oligodendrocyte lineage-specific basic helix-loop-helix transcription factors. Neuron 2000; 25: 331–343.

89. Lai K, Kaspar BK, Gage FH, Schaffer DV. Sonic hedgehog regulates adult neural progenitor proliferation in vitro and in vivo. Nat Neurosci 2003; 6: 21–27.

90. Murray K, Calaora V, Rottkamp C et al. Sonic hedgehog is a potent inducer of rat oligodendrocyte development from cortical precursors in vitro. Mol Cell Neurosci 2002; 19: 320–332.

91. Palma V, Lim DA, Dahmane N et al. Sonic hedgehog controls stem cell behavior in the postnatal and adult brain. Development 2005; 132: 335–344.

92. Machold R, Hayashi S, Rutlin M et al. Sonic hedgehog is required for progenitor cell maintenance in telencephalic stem cell niches. Neuron 2003; 39: 937–950.

93. Bambakidis NC, Wang RZ, Franic L, Miller RH. Sonic hedgehog-induced neural precursor proliferation after adult rodent spinal cord injury. J Neurosurg 2003; 99: 70–75.

94. Bambakidis NC, Miller RH. Transplantation of oligodendrocyte precursors and sonic hedgehog results in improved function and white matter sparing in the spinal cords of adult rats after contusion. Spine J 2004; 4: 16–26.

95. Aguirre A, Dupree JL, Mangin JM, Gallo V. A functional role for EGFR signaling in myelination and remyelination. Nat Neurosci 2007; 10: 990–1002.

96. McKinnon RD, Dubois-Dalcq M. Cytokines and growth factors in the development and regeneration of oligodendrocytes. In: Ransohoff RM, Benveniste EN, eds. Cytokines and the CNS. Boca Raton, FL: CRC Press; 1996: 85–114.

97. Chojnacki A, Weiss S. Isolation of a novel platelet-derived growth factor-responsive precursor from the embryonic ventral forebrain. J Neurosci 2004 24: 10888–10899.

98. McKinnon RD, Matsui T, Dubois-Dalcq M, Aaronson SA. FGF modulates the PDGF-driven pathway of oligodendrocyte development. Neuron 1990; 5: 603–614.

99. Zhang H, Vutskits L, Calaora V et al. A role for the polysialic acid-neural cell adhesion molecule in PDGF-induced chemotaxis of oligodendrocyte precursor cells. J Cell Sci 2004; 117: 93–103.

100. Torregrossa P, Buhl L, Bancila M et al. Selection of poly-alpha 2,8-sialic acid mimotopes from a random phage peptide library and analysis of their bioactivity. J Biol Chem 2004; 279: 30707–30714.

101. Maeda Y, Solanky M, Menonna J et al. Platelet-derived growth factor-alpha receptor-positive oligodendroglia are frequent in multiple sclerosis lesions. Ann Neurol 2001; 49: 776–785.

102. Nait-Oumesmar B, Picard-Riera N, Kerninon C et al. Activation of the subventricular zone in multiple sclerosis: Evidence for early glial progenitors. PNAS 2007; 104: 4694–4699.

103. Le Bras B, Chatzopoulou E, Heydon K et al. Oligodendrocyte development in the embryonic brain: the contribution of the plp lineage. Int J Dev Biol 2005; 49: 209–220.

104. Williams A, Piaton G, Aigrot MS et al. Semaphorin 3A and 3F: key players in myelin repair in multiple sclerosis? Brain. 2007; 130: 2554–2565.

105. Dziembowska M, Tham TN, Lau P et al. A role for CXCR4 signaling in survival and migration of neural and oligodendrocyte precursors. Glia 2005; 50: 258–269.

106. Calderon TM, Eugenin EA, Lopez L et al. A role for CXCL12 (SDF-1alpha) in the pathogenesis of multiple sclerosis: regulation of CXCL12 expression in astrocytes by soluble myelin basic protein. J Neuroimmunol 2006; 177: 27–39.

107. Peng H, Huang Y, Rose J et al. Stromal cell-derived factor 1-mediated CXCR4 signaling in rat and human cortical neural progenitor cells. J Neurosci Res 2004; 76: 35–50.

108. Tran PB, Ren D, Veldhouse TJ, Miller RJ. Chemokine receptors are expressed widely by embryonic and adult neural progenitor cells. J Neurosci Res 2004; 76: 20–34.

109. Imitola J, Raddassi K, Park KI et al. Directed migration of neural stem cells to sites of CNS injury by the stromal cell-derived factor 1α/CXC chemokine receptor 4 pathway. Proc Natl Acad Sci USA 2004; 101: 18117–18122.

110. Lalive PH, Paglinawan R, Biollaz G et al. TGF-beta-treated microglia induce oligodendrocyte precursor cell chemotaxis through the HGF-c-Met pathway. Eur J Immunol 2005; 35: 727–737.

111. Charles P, Hernandez MP, Stankoff B et al. Negative regulation of central nervous system myelination by polysialylated-neural cell adhesion molecule. Proc Natl Acad Sci USA 2000; 97: 7585–7590.

112. Charles P, Reynolds R, Seilhean D et al. Re-expression of PSA-NCAM by demyelinated axons: an inhibitor of remyelination in multiple sclerosis? Brain 2002; 125: 1972–1979.

113. Kotter MR, Li WW, Zhao C, Franklin RJ. Myelin impairs CNS remyelination by inhibiting oligodendrocyte precursor cell differentiation. J Neurosci 2006; 26: 328–332.

114. Schnadelbach O, Blaschuk OW, Symonds M et al. N-cadherin influences migration of oligodendrocytes on astrocyte monolayers. Mol Cell Neurosci 2000; 15: 288–302.

115. Back SA, Tuohy TMF, Chen H et al. Hyaluronan accumulates in demyelinated lesions and inhibits oligodendrocyte progenitor maturation. Nat Med 2005; 11: 966–972.

116. Carulli D, Laabs T, Geller HM, Fawcett JW. Chondroitin sulfate proteoglycans in neural development and regeneration. Curr Opin Neurobiol 2005; 15: 116–120.

117. Fouad K, Schnell L, Bunge MB et al. Combining Schwann cell bridges and olfactory-ensheathing glia grafts with chondroitinase promotes locomotor recovery after complete transection of

the spinal cord. J Neurosci 2005; 25: 1169–1178.

118. Chang A, Tourtellotte WW, Rudick R, Trapp BD. Premyelinating oligodendrocytes in chronic lesions of multiple sclerosis. N Engl J Med 2002; 346: 165–173.

119. Niehaus A, Stegmüller J, Diers-Fenger M, Trotter J. Cell-surface glycoprotein of oligodendrocyte progenitors involved in migration. J Neurosci 1999; 19: 4948–4961.

120. Niehaus A, Shi J, Grzenkowski M et al. Patients with active relapsing-remitting multiple sclerosis synthesize antibodies recognizing oligodendrocyte progenitor cell surface protein: implications for remyelination. Ann Neurol 2000; 48: 362–371.

121. Franceschini I, Vitry S, Padilla F et al. Migrating and myelinating potential of neural precursors engineered to overexpress PSA-NCAM. Mol Cell Neurosci 2004; 27: 151–162.

122. Lubetzki C, Williams A, Stankoff B. Promoting repair in multiple sclerosis: problems and prospects. Curr Opin Neurol 2005; 18: 237–244.

123. Stankoff B, Aigrot MS, Noel F et al. Ciliary neurotrophic factor (CNTF) enhances myelin formation: a novel role for CNTF and CNTF-related molecules. J Neurosci 2002; 22: 9221–9227.

124. Linker RA, Maurer M, Gaupp S et al. CNTF is a major protective factor in demyelinating CNS disease: a neurotrophic cytokine as modulator in neuroinflammation. Nat Med 2002; 8: 620–624.

125. Butzkueven H, Zhang JG, Soilu-Hanninen M et al. LIF receptor signaling limits immune-mediated demyelination by enhancing oligodendrocyte survival. Nat Med 2002; 8: 613–619.

126. Kerr BJ, Patterson PH. Leukemia inhibitory factor promotes oligodendrocyte survival after spinal cord injury. Glia 2005; 51: 73–79.

127. Albrecht PJ, Murtie JC, Ness JK et al. Astrocytes produce CNTF during the remyelination phase of viral-induced spinal cord demyelination to stimulate FGF-2 production. Neurobiol Dis 2003; 13: 89–101.

128. Arnett HA, Mason J, Marino M et al. TNFα promotes proliferation of oligodendrocyte progenitors and remyelination. Nat Neurosci 2001; 4:1116–1122.

129. Luzi P, Zaka M, Rao HZ et al. Generation of transgenic mice expressing insulin-like growth factor-1 under the control of the myelin basic protein promoter: increased myelination and potential for studies on the effects of increased IGF-1 on experimentally and genetically induced demyelination. Neurochem Res 2004; 29: 881–889.

130. Mason JL, Jones JJ, Taniike M et al. Mature oligodendrocyte apoptosis precedes IGF-1 production and oligodendrocyte progenitor accumulation and differentiation during demyelination/remyelination. J Neurosci Res 2000; 61: 251–262.

131. Mason JL, Xuan S, Dragatsis I et al. Insulin-like growth factor (IGF) signaling through type 1 IGF receptor plays an important role in remyelination. J Neurosci 2003; 20;23: 7710–7718.

132. Hsieh J, Aimone JB, Kaspar BK et al. IGF-I instructs multipotent adult neural progenitor cells to become oligodendrocytes. J Cell Biol 2004; 164: 111–122.

133. Woodruff RH, Fruttiger M, Richardson WD, Franklin RJ. Platelet-derived growth factor regulates oligodendrocyte progenitor numbers in adult CNS and their response following CNS demyelination. Mol Cell Neurosci 2004; 25: 252–262.

134. Decker L, Ffrench-Constant C. Lipid rafts and integrin activation regulate oligodendrocyte survival. J Neurosci 2004; 24: 3816–3825.

135. Lachapelle F, Vellana-Adalid V, Nait-Oumesmar B, Baron-Van Evercooren A. Fibroblast growth factor-2 (FGF-2) and platelet-derived growth factor AB (PDGF AB) promote adult SVZ-derived oligodendrogenesis in vivo. Mol Cell Neurosci 2002; 20: 390–403.

136. Pirko I, Ciric B, Gamez J et al. A human antibody that promotes remyelination enters the CNS and decreases lesion load as detected by T2-weighted spinal cord MRI in a virus-induced murine model of MS. FASEB J 2004; 18: 1577–1579.

137. Warrington AE, Bieber AJ, Ciric B et al. Immunoglobulin-mediated CNS repair. J Allergy Clin Immunol 2001; 108: S121–S125.

138. Rodriguez M, Lennon VA, Benveniste EN, Merrill JE. Remyelination stimulated by antiserum to spinal cord. J Neuropathol Exp Neurol 1987; 46: 84–95.

139. Rodriguez M, Lennon VA. Immunoglobulins promote remyelination in the central nervous system. Ann Neurol 1990; 27: 12–17.

140. Rodriguez M, Miller DJ, Lennon VA. Immunoglobulins reactive with myelin basic protein promote CNS remyelination. Neurology 1996; 46: 538–545.

141. Asakura K, Miller DJ, Murray K et al. Monoclonal autoantibody SCH94.03, which promotes central nervous system remyelination, recognizes an antigen on the surface of oligodendrocytes. J Neurosci Res 1996; 43: 273–281.

142. Asakura K, Pogulis RJ, Pease LR, Rodriguez M. A monoclonal autoantibody which promotes central nervous system remyelination is highly polyreactive to multiple known and novel antigens. J Neuroimmunol 1996; 65: 11–19.

143. Coutinho A, Kazatchkine MD, Avrameas S. Natural autoantibodies. Curr Opin Immunol 1995; 7: 812–818.

144. Warrington AE, Asakura K, Bieber AJ et al. Human monoclonal antibodies reactive to oligodendrocytes promote remyelination in a model of multiple sclerosis. Proc Natl Acad Sci USA 2000; 97: 6820–6825.

145. Stangel M, Compston DAS, Scolding NJ. Polyclonal immunoglobulins for intravenous use do not influence the behaviour of cultured oligodendrocytes. J Neuroimmunol 1999; 96: 228–233.

146. Stangel M, Compston A, Scolding NJ. Oligodendroglia are protected from antibody-mediated complement injury by normal immunoglobulins ('IVIg'). J Neuroimmunol 2000; 103: 195–201.

147. Stangel M, Joly E, Scolding NJ, Compston DA. Normal polyclonal immunoglobulins ('IVIg') inhibit microglial phagocytosis in vitro. J Neuroimmunol 2000; 106: 137–144.

148. Miller DJ, RiveraQuinones C, Njenga MK et al. Spontaneous CNS remyelination in β2 microglobulin-deficient mice following virus-induced demyelination. J Neurosci 1995; 15: 8345–8352.

149. Miller DJ, Rodriguez M. A monoclonal autoantibody that promotes central nervous system remyelination in a model of multiple sclerosis is a natural autoantibody encoded by germline immunoglobulin genes. J Immunol 1995; 154: 2460–2469.

150. Ciric B, Howe CL, Paz SM et al. Human monoclonal IgM antibody promotes CNS myelin repair independent of Fc function. Brain Pathol 2003; 13: 608–616.

151. Ciric B, Van Keulen V, Paz Soldan M et al. Antibody-mediated remyelination operates through mechanism independent of immunomodulation. J Neuroimmunol 2004; 146: 153–161.

152. Noseworthy JH, O'Brien PC, Weinshenker BG et al. IV immunoglobulin does not reverse established weakness in MS. Neurology 2000; 55: 1135–1143.

153. Stangel M, Boegner F, Klatt CH et al. Placebo controlled pilot trial to study the remyelinating potential of intravenous immunoglobulins in multiple sclerosis. J Neurol Neurosurg Psychiatr 2000; 68: 89–92.

154. Baron-Van Evercooren A, Blakemore W. Remyelination through engraftment. In: Lazzarini RA, ed. Myelin biology and disorders. Elsevier, New York; 2004: 143–172.

155. Mitome M, Low HP, van Den Pol A et al. Towards the reconstruction of central nervous system white matter using neural precursor cells. Brain 2001; 124: 2147–2161.

156. Murray K, Dubois Dalcq M. Emergence of oligodendrocytes from human neural spheres. J Neurosci Res 1997; 50: 146–156.

157. Vescovi AL, Parati EA, Gritti A et al. Isolation and cloning of multipotential stem cells from the embryonic human CNS and establishment of transplantable human neural stem cell lines by epigenetic stimulation. Exp Neurol 1999; 156: 71–83.

158. Caldwell MA, He X, Wilkie N et al. Growth factors regulate the survival and fate of cells derived from human neurospheres. Nat Biotechnol 2001; 19: 475–479.

159. Chandran S, Compston A, Jauniaux E et al. Differential generation of oligodendrocytes from human and rodent embryonic spinal cord neural precursors. Glia 2004; 47: 314–324.

160. Hajihosseini M, Tham TN, Dubois DM. Origin of oligodendrocytes within the human spinal cord. J Neurosci 1996; 16: 7981–7994.

161. Brustle O, Choudhary K, Karram K et al. Chimeric brains generated by intraventricular transplantation of fetal human brain cells into embryonic rats. Nat Biotechnol 1998; 16: 1040–1044.

162. Brustle O, Jones KN, Learish RD et al. Embryonic stem cell-derived glial precursors: a source of myelinating transplants. Science 1999; 285: 754–756.

163. Glaser T, Perez-Bouza A, Klein K, Brustle O. Generation of purified oligodendrocyte progenitors from embryonic stem cells. FASEB J 2005; 19: 112–114.

164. Keirstead HS, Nistor G, Bernal G et al. Human embryonic stem cell-derived oligodendrocyte progenitor cell transplants remyelinate and restore locomotion after spinal cord injury. J Neurosci 2005; 25: 4694–4705.

165. Nistor GI, Totoiu MO, Haque N et al. Human embryonic stem cells differentiate into oligodendrocytes in high purity and myelinate after spinal cord transplantation. Glia 2005; 49: 385–396.

166. Vogel G. Cell biology. Ready or not? Human ES cells head toward the clinic. Science 2005; 308: 1534–1538.

167. Roy NS, Cleren C, Singh SK et al. Functional engraftment of human ES cell-derived dopaminergic neurons enriched by coculture with telomerase-immortalized midbrain astrocytes. Nat Med 2006; 12: 1259–1268.

168. Nunes MC, Roy NS, Keyoung HM et al. Identification and isolation of multipotential neural progenitor cells from the subcortical white matter of the adult human brain. Nat Med 2003; 9: 439–447.

169. Pluchino S, Quattrini A, Brambilla E et al. Injection of adult neurospheres induces recovery in a chronic model of multiple sclerosis. Nature 2003; 422: 688–694.

170. Pluchino S, Zanotti L, Rossi B et al. Neurosphere-derived multipotent precursors promote neuroprotection by an immunomodulatory mechanism. Nature 2005; 436: 266–271.

171. Sasaki M, Honmou O, Akiyama Y et al. Transplantation of an acutely isolated bone marrow traction repairs demyelinated adult rat spinal cord axons. Glia 2001; 35: 26–34.

172. Oka S, Honmou O, Akiyama Y et al. Autologous transplantation of expanded neural precursor cells into the demyelinated monkey spinal cord. Brain Res 2004; 1030: 94–102.

173. Keirstead HS, Ben Hur T, Rogister B et al. Polysialylated neural cell adhesion molecule-positive CNS precursors generate both oligodendrocytes and Schwann cells to remyelinate the CNS after transplantation. J Neurosci 1999; 19: 7529–7536.

174. Akiyama Y, Honmou O, Kato T et al. Transplantation of clonal neural precursor cells derived from adult human brain establishes functional peripheral myelin in the rat spinal cord. Exp Neurol 2001; 167: 27–39.

175. Itoyama Y, Webster HD, Richardson-EP J, Trapp BD. Schwann cell remyelination of demyelinated axons in spinal cord multiple sclerosis lesions. Ann Neurol 1983; 14: 339–346.

176. Ludwin SK. Remyelination in the central nervous system and the peripheral nervous system. Adv Neurol 1988; 47: 215–254.

177. Ogata J, Feigin I. Schwann cells and regenerated peripheral myelin in multiple sclerosis: an ultrastructural study. Neurology 1975; 25: 713–716.

178. Morrissey TK, Kleitman N, Bunge RP. Human Schwann cells in vitro. II. Myelination of sensory axons following extensive purification and heregulin-induced expansion. J Neurobiol 1995; 28: 190–201.

179. Rutkowski JL, Kirk CJ, Lerner MA, Tennekoon GI. Purification and expansion of human schwann cells in vitro. Nat Med 1995; 1: 80–83.

180. Levi ADO, Bunge RP. Studies of myelin formation after transplantation of human Schwann cells into the severe combined immunodeficient mouse. Exp Neurol 1994; 130: 41–52.

181. Brierley CM, Crang AJ, Iwashita Y et al. Remyelination of demyelinated CNS axons by transplanted human schwann cells: the deleterious effect of contaminating fibroblasts. Cell Transplant 2001; 10: 305–315.

182. Kohama I, Lankford KL, Preiningerova J et al. Transplantation of cryopreserved adult human Schwann cells enhances axonal conduction in demyelinated spinal cord. J Neurosci 2001; 21: 944–950.

183. Bachelin C, Lachapelle F, Girard C et al. Efficient myelin repair in the macaque spinal cord by autologous grafts of Schwann cells. Brain 2005; 128: 540–549.

184. Langford LA, Porter S, Bunge RP. Immortalized rat Schwann cells produce tumours in vivo. J Neurocytol 1988; 17: 521–529.

185. Franklin RJM, Blakemore WF. Requirements for Schwann cell migration within CNS environments: a viewpoint. Int J Dev Neurosci 1993; 11: 641–649.

186. Harrison B. Schwann cell and oligodendrocyte remyelination in lysolecithin-induced lesions in irradiated rat spinal cord. J Neurol Sci 1985; 67: 143–159.

187. Woodruff RH, Franklin RJ. Demyelination and remyelination of the caudal cerebellar peduncle of adult rats following stereotaxic injections of lysolecithin, ethidium bromide, and complement/anti-galactocerebroside: a comparative study. Glia 1999; 25: 216–228.

188. Barber S, Mellor H, Gampel A, Scolding NJ. S1P and LPA trigger Schwann cell actin changes and migration. Eur J Neurosci 2004; 19: 3142–3150.

189. Lai C. Peripheral glia: Schwann cells in motion. Curr Biol 2005; 15: R332–R334.

190. Yamauchi J, Chan JR, Miyamoto Y et al. The neurotrophin-3 receptor TrkC directly phosphorylates and activates the nucleotide exchange factor Dbs to enhance Schwann cell migration. Proc Natl Acad Sci USA 2005; 102: 5198–5203.

191. Fawcett JW, Asher RA. The glial scar and central nervous system repair. Brain Res Bull 1999; 49: 377–391.

192. Fok-Seang J, Mathews GA, Ffrench-Constant C et al. Migration of oligodendrocyte precursors on astrocytes and meningeal cells. Dev Biol 1995; 171: 1–15.

193. Lavdas A, Franceschini I, Dubois-Dalcq M, Matsas R. Schwann cells genetically engineered to express PSA show enhanced migratory potential without impairment of their myelinating ability in vitro. Glia 2006; 53: 868–878.

194. Woodhoo A, Sahni V, Gilson J et al. Schwann cell precursors: a favourable cell for myelin repair in the Central Nervous System. Brain 2007; 130: 2175–2185.

195. Franklin RJ, Barnett SC. Olfactory ensheathing cells. In: Lazzarini RA, ed. Myelin biology and disorders. New York: Elsevier; 2004: 371–384.

196. Lakatos A, Franklin RJ, Barnett SC. Olfactory ensheathing cells and Schwann cells differ in their in vitro interactions with astrocytes. Glia 2000; 32: 214–225.

197. Lakatos A, Barnett SC, Franklin RJ. Olfactory ensheathing cells induce less host astrocyte response and chondroitin sulphate proteoglycan expression than Schwann cells following transplantation into adult CNS white matter. Exp Neurol 2003; 184: 237–246.

198. Raisman G. Olfactory ensheathing cells and repair of brain and spinal cord injuries. Cloning Stem Cells 2004; 6: 364–368.

199. Boyd JG, Doucette R, Kawaja MD. Defining the role of olfactory ensheathing cells in facilitating axon remyelination following damage to the spinal cord. FASEB J 2005; 19: 694–703.

200. Crain BJ, Tran SD, Mezey E. Transplanted human bone marrow cells generate new brain cells. J Neurol Sci 2005; 233: 121–123.

201. Aubourg P, Dubois-Dalcq M. X-linked adrenoleukodystrophy enigma: how does the ALD peroxisomal transporter mutation affect CNS glia? Glia 2000; 29: 186–190.

202. Peters C, Charnas LR, Tan Y et al. Cerebral X-linked adrenoleukodystrophy: the international hematopoietic cell transplantation experience from 1982 to 1999. Blood 2004; 104: 881–888.

203. Feigenbaum V, Gelot A, Casanova P et al. Apoptosis in the central nervous system of cerebral adrenoleukodystrophy patients. Neurobiol Dis 2000; 7: 600–612.

204. Yagi T, McMahon EJ, Takikita S et al. Fate of donor hematopoietic cells in demyelinating mutant mouse, twitcher, following transplantation of GFP+ bone marrow cells. Neurobiol Dis 2004; 16: 98–109.

205. Vitry S, Bertrand JY, Cumano A, Dubois-Dalcq M. Primordial hematopoietic stem cells generate microglia but not myelin-forming cells in a neural environment. J Neurosci 2003; 19: 10724–10731.

206. Priller J, Persons DA, Klett FF et al. Neogenesis of cerebellar Purkinje neurons from gene-marked bone marrow cells in vivo. J Cell Biol 2001; 155: 733–738.

207. Wagers AJ, Sherwood RI, Christensen JL, Weissman IL. Little evidence for developmental plasticity of adult hematopoietic stem cells. Science 2002; 297: 2256–2259.

208. Sigurjonsson OE, Perreault MC, Egeland T, Glover JC. Adult human hematopoietic stem cells produce neurons efficiently in the regenerating chicken embryo spinal cord. Proc Natl Acad Sci USA 2005; 102: 5227–5232.

209. Cogle CR, Yachnis AT, Laywell ED et al. Bone marrow transdifferentiation in brain after transplantation: a retrospective study. Lancet 2004; 363: 1432–1437.

210. Weimann JM, Charlton CA, Brazelton TR et al. Contribution of transplanted bone marrow cells to Purkinje neurons in human adult brains. Proc Natl Acad Sci USA 2003; 100: 2088–2093.

211. Jiang Y, Henderson D, Blackstad M et al. Neuroectodermal differentiation from mouse multipotent adult progenitor cells. Proc Natl Acad Sci USA 2003; 100(suppl 1): 11854–11860.

212. Kohyama J, Abe H, Shimazaki T et al. Brain from bone: efficient 'meta-differentiation' of marrow stroma-derived mature osteoblasts to neurons with Noggin or a demethylating agent. Differentiation 2001; 68: 238–244.

213. Wislet-Gendebien S, Hans G, Leprince P et al. Plasticity of cultured mesenchymal stem cells: switch from nestin-positive to excitable neuron-like phenotype. Stem Cells 2005; 23: 392–402.

214. Akiyama Y, Radtke C, Kocsis JD. Remyelination of the rat spinal cord by transplantation of identified bone marrow stromal cells. J Neurosci 2002; 22: 6623–6630.

215. Rice CM, Scolding NJ. Adult stem cells–reprogramming neurological repair? Lancet 2004; 364: 193–199.

216. Zhang J, Li Y, Chen J et al. Human bone marrow stromal cell treatment improves neurological functional recovery in EAE mice. Exp Neurol 2005; 195: 16–26.

217. Zappia E, Casazza S, Pedemonte E et al. Mesenchymal stem cells ameliorate experimental autoimmune encephalomyelitis inducing T-cell anergy. Blood 2005; 106: 1755–1761.

218. Scolding N, Marks D, Rice C. Autologous mesenchymal bone marrow stem cells: Practical considerations. J Neurol Sci 2007; 265: 111–115.

219. Chernajovsky Y, Gould DJ, Podhajcer OL. Gene therapy for autoimmune diseases: quo vadis? Nat Rev Immunol 2004; 4: 800–811.

220. Mathisen PM, Yu M, Yin L et al. Th2 T cells expressing transgene PDGF-A serve as vectors for gene therapy in autoimmune demyelinating disease. J Autoimmun 1999; 13: 31–38.

221. Muraro PA, Wandinger KP, Bielekova B et al. Molecular tracking of antigen-specific T cell clones in neurological immune-mediated disorders. Brain 2003; 126: 20–31.

222. Goncalves MA. A concise peer into the background, initial thoughts and practices of human gene therapy. Bioessays 2005; 27: 506–517.

223. Hack MA, Saghatelyan A, de Chevigny A et al. Neuronal fate determinants of adult olfactory bulb neurogenesis. Nat Neurosci 2005; 8: 865–872.

224. Barkhof F, Bruck W, De Groot CJ et al. Remyelinated lesions in multiple sclerosis: magnetic resonance image appearance. Arch Neurol 2003; 60: 1073–1081.

225. Deloire-Grassin MS, Brochet B, Quesson B et al. In vivo evaluation of remyelination in rat brain by magnetization transfer imaging. J Neurol Sci 2000; 178: 10–16.

226. Merkler D, Boretius S, Stadelmann C et al. Multicontrast MRI of remyelination in the central nervous system. NMR Biomed 2005; 23: 7710–7718.

227. Song SK, Sun SW, Ramsbottom MJ et al. Dysmyelination revealed through MRI as increased radial (but unchanged axial) diffusion of water. Neuroimage 2002; 17: 1429–1436.

228. Song SK, Yoshino J, Le TQ et al. Demyelination increases radial diffusivity in corpus callosum of mouse brain. Neuroimage 2005; 26: 132–140.

229. Davie CA, Barker GJ, Webb S et al. Persistent functional deficit in multiple sclerosis and autosomal dominant cerebellar ataxia is associated with axon loss. Brain 1995; 118: 1583–1592.

230. De Stefano N, Matthews PM, Antel JP et al. Chemical pathology of acute demyelinating lesions and its correlation with disability. Ann Neurol 1995; 38: 901–909.

231. Behrens TE, Johansen-Berg H, Woolrich MW et al. Non-invasive mapping of connections between human thalamus and cortex using diffusion imaging. Nat Neurosci 2003; 6: 750–757.

232. Parry A, Clare S, Jenkinson M et al. MRI brain T1 relaxation time changes in MS patients increase over time in both the white matter and the cortex. J Neuroimaging 2003; 13: 234–239.

233. Bulte JW, Zhang S, van Gelderen P et al. Neurotransplantation of magnetically labeled oligodendrocyte progenitors: magnetic resonance tracking of cell migration and myelination. Proc Natl Acad Sci USA 1999; 96: 15256–15261.

234. Franklin RJ, Blaschuk KL, Bearchell MC et al. Magnetic resonance imaging of transplanted oligodendrocyte precursors in the rat brain. NeuroReport 1999; 10: 3961–3965.

235. Lewin M, Carlesso N, Tung CH et al. Tat peptide-derivatized magnetic nanoparticles allow in vivo tracking and recovery of progenitor cells. Nat Biotechnol 2000; 18: 410–414.

236. Leocani L, Medaglini S, Comi G. Evoked potentials in monitoring multiple sclerosis. Neurol Sci 2000; 21: S889-S891.

237. Emerson RG. Evoked potentials in clinical trials for multiple sclerosis. J Clin Neurophysiol 1998; 15: 109–116.

238. Filipovic SR, Drulovic J, Stojsavljevic N, Levic Z. The effects of high-dose intravenous methylprednisolone on event-related potentials in patients with multiple sclerosis. J Neurol Sci 1997; 152: 147–153.

239. Hobart JC, Lamping DL, Freeman JA et al. Evidence-based measurement: which disability scale for neurologic rehabilitation? Neurology 2001; 57: 639–644.

240. Hobart J, Kalkers N, Barkhof F et al. Outcome measures for multiple sclerosis clinical trials: relative measurement precision of the Expanded Disability Status Scale and Multiple Sclerosis Functional Composite. Mult Scler 2004; 10: 41–46.

241. Hobart JC, Riazi A, Lamping DL et al. Improving the evaluation of therapeutic interventions in multiple sclerosis: development of a patient-based measure of outcome. Health Technol Assess 2004; 8: iii,1–iii,48.

242. Kidd D, Barkhof F, McConnell R et al. Cortical lesions in multiple sclerosis. Brain 1999; 122: 17–26.

243. Gill SS, Patel NK, Hotton GR et al. Direct brain infusion of glial cell line-derived neurotrophic factor in Parkinson disease. Nat Med 2003; 9: 589–595.

244. Love S, Plaha P, Patel NK et al. Glial cell line-derived neurotrophic factor induces neuronal sprouting in human brain. Nat Med 2005; 11: 703–704.

245. Learish RD, Brustle O, Zhang SC, Duncan ID. Intraventricular transplantation of oligodendrocyte progenitors into a fetal myelin mutant results in widespread formation of myelin. Ann Neurol 1999; 46: 716–722.

246. Nutt JG, Burchiel KJ, Comella CL et al. Randomized, double-blind trial of glial cell line-derived neurotrophic factor (GDNF) in PD. Neurology 2003; 60: 69–73.

247. Compston DAS. Remyelination of the central nervous system. Mult Scler 1996; 1: 388–392.

248. Fricker-Gates RA, Winkler C, Kirik D et al. EGF infusion stimulates the proliferation and migration of embryonic progenitor cells transplanted in the adult rat striatum. Exp Neurol 2000; 165: 237–247.

249. Girard C, Bemelmans AP, Dufour N et al. Grafts of brain-derived neurotrophic factor and neurotrophin 3-transduced primate Schwann cells lead to functional recovery of the demyelinated mouse spinal cord. J Neurosci 2005; 25: 7924–7933.

250. Prineas JW, Barnard RO, Kwon EE et al. Multiple sclerosis: remyelination of nascent lesions. Ann Neurol 1993; 33: 137–151.

251. Raine CS, Wu E. Multiple sclerosis: Remyelination in acute lesions. J Neuropathol Exp Neurol 1993; 52: 199–204.

252. Smith PM, Franklin RJ. The effect of immunosuppressive protocols on spontaneous CNS remyelination following toxin-induced demyelination. J Neuroimmunol 2001; 119: 261–268.

253. Cuzner ML, Loughlin AJ, Mosley K, Woodroofe MN. The role of microglia macrophages in the processes of inflammatory demyelination and remyelination. Neuropathol Appl Neurobiol 1994; 20: 200–201.

254. Halfpenny CA, Scolding NJ. Immune-modifying agents do not impair the survival, migration or proliferation of oligodendrocyte progenitors (CG-4) in vitro. J Neuroimmunol 2003; 139: 9–16.

255. Kerschensteiner M, Gallmeier E, Behrens L et al. Activated human T cells, B cells, and monocytes produce brain-derived neurotrophic factor in vitro and in inflammatory brain lesions: a neuroprotective role of inflammation? J Exp Med 1999; 189: 865–870.

256. Hohlfeld R, Kerschensteiner M, Stadelmann C et al. The neuroprotective effect of inflammation: implications for the therapy of multiple sclerosis. J Neuroimmunol 2000; 107: 161–166.

257. Foote AK, Blakemore WF. Inflammation stimulates remyelination in areas of chronic demyelination. Brain 2005; 128: 528–539.

258. Kotter MR, Setzu A, Sim FJ et al. Macrophage depletion impairs oligodendrocyte remyelination following lysolecithin-induced demyelination. Glia 2001; 35: 204–212.

259. Saccardi R, Mancardi GL, Solari A et al. Autologous HSCT for severe progressive multiple sclerosis in a multicenter trial: impact on disease activity and quality of life. Blood 2005; 105: 2601–2607.

260. Rice CM, Halfpenny C, Scolding NJ. Cell therapy in demyelinating diseases. NeuroRx 2004; 1: 423–415.

261. Braude P, Minger SL, Warwick RM. Stem cell therapy: hope or hype? Br Med J 2005; 330: 1159–1160.

262. Check E. Gene therapy: a tragic setback. Nature 2002; 420: 116–118.

263. Dave UP, Jenkins NA, Copeland NG. Gene therapy insertional mutagenesis insights. Science 2004; 303: 333.

264. Keegan M, Konig F, McClelland R et al. Relation between humoral pathological changes in multiple sclerosis and response to therapeutic plasma exchange. Lancet 2005; 366: 579–582.

R. T. Schapiro

INTRODUCTION

Unpredictability is the hallmark of multiple sclerosis (MS). Persons with MS awake each day unsure of how their bodies will respond. Making MS more predictable and tolerable is the role of the clinician. By controlling the disease with immune modulation, predictability is gained. Managing the symptoms of the disease likewise gives control and improves quality of life. By nature, MS gives multiple symptoms to improve. Even the most minor symptom can appear to be devastating to someone. Symptoms may be interpreted differently by each individual. This requires the management of symptoms to be even more individualized. Clearly some symptoms – weakness, ataxia, tremor and cognitive decline – can portend a more progressive course to the disease and may contribute to the decision-making of disease-modifying treatments.[1–3]

The decision to treat a symptom or not must be based not only on the presence of the symptom but on how bothersome the symptom is to the patient. If every symptom is treated aggressively the likelihood of side effects from the treatments arises. This can be exponential if multiple systems are involved. The goal is to improve function and comfort. The tools to accomplish this purpose include pharmacological (Table 25.1), rehabilitative, surgical, psychological and 'complementary' approaches.

We are in an era of evidence-based medicine. Managing MS should be evidence-based and that includes symptom management. However, useful treatments in MS have all improved with experience. Thus sometimes the 'evidence' behind a symptom treatment is not as rigorous as that of a disease-modifying treatment. Experience becomes an important managing variable. This is particularly true in the rehabilitative management strategies. The clinician must have an empirical bent to be a successful MS clinician.

FATIGUE

Fatigue is one of the more frustrating symptoms to treat because it is so difficult to quantify. In a survey in the UK in 1997 fatigue was the single most common symptom found in MS with 86% of the respondents suffering from a form of fatigue.[4] The patient complains of fatigue but can be suffering from many different facets of what is called 'fatigue' (Table 25.2).

Measuring fatigue is daunting. There are several self-report scales, including: the Fatigue Severity Scale (FSS), Fatigue Impact Scale (FIS), Fatigue Assessment Instrument, Fatigue Rating Scale and Fatigue Descriptive Scale.[5–7] While helpful, all these scales rely on the integrity of the person answering the questions and lose some objectivity.

Normal fatigue afflicts all, MS or not. Clearly, those who have MS can become fatigued simply from working hard. A person with MS is not fragile and becoming fatigued is not necessarily a destructive factor.[8] A person suffering from normal fatigue may want to alter her lifestyle or recognize that hard work brings about fatigue. Fatigue in MS can be differentiated somewhat from normal fatigue because it worsens with heat, prevents sustained physical activity, interferes with physical functioning, comes on easily, interferes with role performance and causes frequent problems.[9] In managing fatigue the first principle is to look for inciting causes and fix them. Some of these may include factors of sleep disturbance, stress, heat, infection, spasticity, concurrent disease, long hours of work, poor nutrition, etc. Occupational therapists can be of considerable assistance in identifying these factors.

A second variation of fatigue is easier to understand. Neuromuscular fatigue is the result of straining a muscle served by a nerve with less than adequate conduction. A conduction block develops, such that the person may feel strong before the fatigue sets in but the activity results in weakness that is described as fatigue.[10] This is measurable, although it may vary in an individual from time to time. Periods of rest interspersed with periods of activity may allow improved function. A graded exercise program with a goal of increasing endurance may be helpful.[11] Studies indicate that strength and fatigue can be improved if the exercise is appropriate for the circumstance and is not in itself fatiguing.[12]

The third variation of fatigue is also easy to understand if recognized. That is the fatigue of deconditioning. It is not

TABLE 25.1 Drugs used in the management of multiple sclerosis

Generic name	Brand name[2]	Use in multiple sclerosis
Alprostadil	Prostin VR	Erectile dysfunction
Alprostadil	Muse	Erectile dysfunction
Amantadine		Fatigue
Amitriptyline	Elavil	Pain (dysesthesias)
Baclofen		Spasticity
Baclofen (intrathecal)	Baclofen Intrathecal	Spasticity
Bisacodyl	Dulcolax	Constipation
Carbamazepine	Tegretol	Pain (trigeminal neuralgia)
Ciprofloxacin	Cipro	Urinary tract infections
Clonazepam	Klonopin (USA) Rivotril (Can)	Tremor; pain; spasticity
Desmopressin	DDAVP	Bladder dysfunction
Desmopressin	DDAVP Nasal Spray	Bladder dysfunction
Dexamethasone	Decadron	Acute exacerbations
Diazepam	Valium	Spasticity (muscle spasms)
Docusate	Colace	Constipation
Docusate	Enemeez Mini Enema	Constipation
Fluoxetine	Prozac	Depression; fatigue
Gabapentin	Neurontin	Pain (dysesthesias; spasticity)
Glatiramer acetate	Copaxone	Disease-modifying agent
Glycerin	Sani-Supp suppository (USA)	Constipation
Imipramine	Tofranil	Bladder dysfunction; pain
Interferon β-1a	Avonex	Disease-modifying agent
Interferon β-1a	Rebif	Disease-modifying agent
Interferon β-1b	Betaseron	Disease-modifying agent
Magnesium hydroxide	Phillips' Milk of Magnesia	Constipation
Meclizine	Antivert (USA); Bonamine (Canada)	Nausea; vomiting; dizziness
Methenamine	Hiprex, Mandelamine (USA); Hip-rex, Mandelamine (Can)	Urinary tract infections (preventative)
Methylprednisolone	Solu-Medrol	Acute exacerbations
Mineral oil		Constipation
Modafinil	Provigil	Fatigue
Nitrofurantoin	Macrodantin	Urinary tract infection
Oxybutynin	Ditropan	Bladder dysfunction
Oxybutynin (extended release formula)	Ditropan XL	Bladder dysfunction
Oxybutynin (transdermal patch)	Oxytrol	Bladder dysfunction
Papaverine	Erectile dysfunction	
Paroxetine	Paxil	Depression; Anxiety
Pemoline	Cylert	Fatigue
Phenazopyridine	Pyridium	Urinary tract infections (symptom relief)
Phenytoin	Dilantin	Pain (parasthesias)
Prednisone	Deltasone	Acute exacerbations
Propantheline bromide	Pro-Banthine	Bladder dysfunction
Psyllium hydrophilic mucilloid	Metamucil	Constipation
Sertraline	Zoloft	Depression; anxiety
Sildenafil	Viagra	Erectile dysfunction
Sodium phosphate	Fleet Enema	Constipation
Sulfamethoxazole	Bactrim; Septra	Urinary tract infections
Tizanidine	Zanaflex	Spasticity
Tolterodine	Detrol (US)	Bladder dysfunction
Topiramate	Topamax	Pain; tremor
Venlafaxine	Effexor	Depression

Source: with permission from Kalb RC, ed. Multiple sclerosis: the questions you have – the answers you need, 3rd ed. New York: Demos Medical, 2004: 471.

SECTION 3

TABLE 25.2 Fatigue types	
1.	Normal
2.	Neuro-muscular
3.	Deconditioning
4.	Depression
5.	Lassitude

unusual for individuals with MS to become deconditioned and with increased activity this becomes obvious. The MS is typically blamed but it is quite possible that this can be remedied using an appropriate exercise program with an emphasis on aerobic exercise.

The fourth fatigue is the result of depression. Many who have MS do not want to recognize the frequent accompaniment of depression. This is discussed later in the chapter, but often with depression comes a feeling of fatigue. Antidepressants that energize are especially helpful in this situation.[13] Recognizing the problem is the first step to managing it.

The fifth variety of fatigue is the most common and the most difficult to understand and treat. It has been called 'lassitude' or 'MS-specific-related' fatigue. It presents as an overwhelming tiredness without signs of depression or relation to activity. Empirically, neurochemicals have been found to be of value.[14] Thus it would appear that this fatigue is probably the result of a neurochemical imbalance within the brain. Amantadine is an antiviral agent with dopaminergic properties often used in the treatment of Parkinson's disease. Its mechanism of action in fatigue is unknown but has been studied with a modicum of effectiveness at a dose of 200 mg/d.[14–17] Side effects are usually minimal and include livo reticularis, decreased concentration and edema of the extremities. Modafinil is an agent developed for the management of narcolepsy and was studied in several small phase II studies.[18] At a dose of 200 mg per day there was an improvement in MS-related fatigue. Side effects include agitation and sleeplessness. On the whole, modafinil was well tolerated. Pemoline is an example of stimulant-appearing medications that have been used for attention deficit syndrome in the young and have potential beneficial effects in fatigue-related problems. It has been plagued with concerns regarding its effects on the liver that have surfaced in its attention deficit disorder indication.[19] The dose is usually 37.5 mg/d and agitation and sleeplessness are potential issues. Monitoring of the blood for abnormal liver function is recommended. 4-aminopyridine is a potassium channel blocker that allows demyelinated nerves to conduct more efficiently. It may improve fatigue in selected individuals but may lower the seizure threshold.[20,21] Doses of 10 mg two to three times/d are often used.

Aerobic exercise, when performed properly for the circumstance, may be an alternative, nonpharmacological approach to MS fatigue.[22] Care must be taken to not overheat and not to continue to the point of actual fatigue induction from the treatment.

This fatigue is very hard to measure and is unrelated to obvious physical disability. A number of fatigue measurements have been developed but they really do not separate the different fatigues of MS well. The Fatigue Impact Scale is a scale that is hard to change despite perceived changes by individuals. Thus changes seen in it are assumed to be significant. To improve the sensitivity of that scale, modifications have been made producing the Modified Fatigue Impact Scale. This scale measures fatigue from several different perspectives and is more sensitive. Simple Likert scales of fatigue may also be helpful but

are open to a lot of subjectivity. Frustration becomes evident from the patient and others because of expectations that seem realistic but become unrealistic with the fatigue.

SPASTICITY

The word 'spasticity' comes from the Greek meaning 'to tug'. This pulling sensation may take the form of stiffness or it may manifest as a spasm. The etiology appears to be demyelination along the regulating, inhibitory pathways of the pyramidal tracts within the brain and spinal cord.[23] This results in uncontrolled excitation – spasticity.

Spasticity is a very common symptom in MS, being found in more than half of a random population of those with MS, and can be an important factor in determining disability.[15]

The presence of spasticity does not by itself necessitate its treatment. Spasticity can preserve muscle tone, decrease blood clot formation in the venous system and be used for transferring and other functions.[24] However, it can also lead to pain, contractures, increased weakness and increased disability. In those circumstances treatment is necessary and essential.

Clearly, pain anywhere within the body will result in an increase of spasticity in those with appropriate central nervous system damage.[25] Decreasing pain can bring about a quick alleviation of the symptoms. This includes irritation from infection such as urinary tract infection or pneumonia. Following a bony fracture, spasticity may increase significantly but temporarily, coinciding with the pain of the break.

Following the removal of noxious stimuli, treatment is begun with an exercise program emphasizing stretching, range of motion and aerobic exercises. These should be instructed professionally by an expert such as a physical therapist but, in the end, the patient should be able to perform them independently if at all possible. If not possible, the assistance of a helper may be necessary. It may be necessary to do the series more than once a day for maximal benefit. Pool therapy can be very helpful, if the water temperature is not too hot or cold, as heat will increase weakness and cold can increase the spasms.

Oral medications are very effective for the majority of spasticity. Baclofen is a γ-aminobutyric acid (GABA) agonist that commonly is used at dosages varying from 5–160 mg/d. Studies done in the 1970s showed the effectiveness of baclofen.[26] Titration appears to be the key. Because of its relatively short half-life, it is often necessary to dose baclofen four times a day. Too high a dose can result in transient weakness.

Tizanidine was studied slightly after the appearance of baclofen in Europe and a decade later in the USA. Tizanidine is an α_2-adrenergic agonist. It appears to have a similar effect on spasticity, with a slightly different side effect profile. As doses of baclofen are increased up to and beyond 80 mg/d, stiffness is traded for weakness. Increased tizanidine dosing tends to trade stiffness for fatigue and dry mouth. Similar to baclofen, the half-life of tizanidine is short (around 4 h).[27] Doses can vary from 1–36 mg/d.

Clonazepam and diazepam are particularly good for nighttime spasms as their sedation can be used to advantage.[28] A disadvantage of these treatments includes potential habituation. Dopaminergic agonists such as pramipexole dihydrochloride and ropinirole hydrochloride are helpful in decreasing spasms.[29] Anticonvulsants, including gabapentin, topiramate and lamotrigine, are similarly of value.[30] Combinations of the various pharmacological agents may be necessary.

Dantrolene sodium has its effect at the level of the muscle. It is one of the oldest spasticity treatments but is also one of the most difficult to use in MS because of a drug-related feeling of weakness that occurs commonly with its use in this disease.[31,32]

385

Cyproheptadine and threonine are occasional adjunctive oral agents that may have some added benefit when combined with other more effective medications.[33]

In situations where the above are either ineffective or not tolerated, the use of phenol or, more commonly now, botulinum toxin injected into specific muscles will decrease the tone of those muscles. Both botulinum toxin A and B have been used to decrease focal muscle spasticity.[34] Care must be taken to not overdo such treatment because of the many large, diverse muscles that are involved in the spasticity. It is possible that toxic doses of this toxin could be unintentionally given in an attempt to control severe spasticity.

The baclofen pump provides baclofen intrathecally and alleviates most situations involving intractable spasticity. It was brought to the forefront in severe spasticity in 1989 in studies involving spinal spasticity from MS and spinal cord injury.[35] Since that time it has achieved relatively common status as an extremely effective treatment.[36,37] There must be a significant amount of education provided to the patient to not have false expectations. A test dose of 50 µg of baclofen is administered intrathecally to give an indication as to the effectiveness of the treatment in a given individual. Implantation involves surgery with placement of an intrathecal catheter with the pump placed in the abdominal area. The two are connected via tunneling beneath the skin. Doses ranging from 50–1000 µg per day may be administered in a variety of combinations.

In extreme situations tendonotomy or rhizotomy may be performed to increase comfort.[38]

The use of cannabinoids for spasticity has generated some controversy. It appears that there is a decrease of spasticity with administration of cannabinoids but whether this outweighs the issues surrounding chronic cannabinoid use is debatable.[39,40] There is also debate as to whether the effects on spasticity are as clinically effective as other available agents.

Spasms are often associated with spasticity. These may be tonic or take the form of clonus. They are often uncomfortable and sometimes very painful. Antiepileptic treatments are beneficial if routine spasticity treatment fails. Gabapentin, carbamazepine, oxazepine topiramate and lamotrigine are among the popular modern treatments borrowed for spasms.[41] Dopamine augmentation with L-dopa or dopaminergic agonists is another management strategy.

Table 25.3 summarizes the management of spasticity.

PAROXYSMAL SPASMS (SYMPTOMS)

Paroxysmal spasms differ from the spasms of spasticity partially by the repetitive quality of the attacks. Some of the 'spasms' are not motor but sensory in nature. The repetitive nature is such that they may come over 20 times a minute in waves. They may manifest as a muscle spasm or a cramping such as is seen with a tonic hand spasm. They can occur as repeating visual blurriness or a pain syndrome in the face – neuralgia (trigeminal). Lhermitte's sign and syndrome, including the electric sensation down the spine into the arms and/or legs, is another example of a paroxysmal symptom.

Treatment with antiepileptic agents as mentioned above in spasticity may dramatically decrease the problem.[42–44]

TREMOR/ATAXIA/DIZZINESS/VERTIGO

Tremor and ataxia are unfortunate symptoms for which management is less than ideal. The nervous system components involving balance, coordination and tremor are numerous and must work together for efficiency. The visual, vestibular, cerebellar, cerebral and spinal systems are involved and thus are easy targets in MS.

The tremor of MS is an action tremor, usually affecting the arms but occasionally involving the legs, head or trunk.[45] It may correlate with other cerebellar symptoms of dysarthria, dysmetria and dysdiadochokinesia. Unfortunately it correlates with increased disability and wheelchair dependence.[46]

Tremor management begins with proper diagnosis and management of associated maladies. Stress will make tremor worse, thus alleviating stress can make the tremor appear less severe.[47] Stress reduction may take the form of relaxation techniques, antianxiety medication (buspirone, clonazepam) or occasionally alternative means such as acupuncture or biofeedback. Occasionally an essential tremor becomes apparent in MS and betablockers such as propranolol or metoprolol are useful.[48,49] Thyroid disease needs recognition and management as that may make an associated tremor appear worse.[50]

Bracing across the wrist joint or weighting with 2.5 kg weights attached to the extremity will occasionally decrease an action tremor. These are simple and safe procedures. As the failure of conservative treatment mounts, the ingenuity of the physician is necessary. Many off-label treatments are popular for this symptom. These include isoniazid, primidone, beta-blockers, ondansetron, acetazolamide and botulinum toxin and others to decrease the amplitude.[51–58] Unfortunately, despite the numerous possibilities, none is very impressive.

Deep brain stimulation has been tried in small numbers with some success but the numbers do not warrant it becoming a popular solution and the risks of creating increased brain damage mitigate against it.[59–61] The cost of this procedure is also a practical issue.

Ataxia is best managed by the development of compensatory techniques. Exercises with the Swiss ball may speed the compensatory process. For some the Balance Master computer system may be helpful at a higher level of sophistication.[62] A specially trained physical therapist is necessary for this type of training.

Dizziness and vertigo are common problems in neurology, not just in MS. Light-headed and vertiginous sensations require some work-up to determine their etiology. Once the determination is that of a symptom of MS, more specific management can be entertained. The use of steroids for the acute problem is common. Both high dose intravenous methylprednisolone and lower doses of oral steroids may be useful acutely. Antihistamines (meclizine) and benzodiazepines (oxazepam, diazepam) can be symptomatically beneficial. The role of vestibular rehabilitation for the more chronic vertiginous sensations cannot be overemphasized.[62] When taught by a knowledgeable physical therapist, this modality can produce amazing results in those thought to be refractory to treatment.

Despite the difficulty in managing balance, coordination and tremor a number of strategies are available to lessen their disabling effects.

TABLE 25.3 **Spasticity management**	
1.	Remove noxious stimuli
2.	Begin physical therapy regimen
3.	Begin oral agents
4.	Consider local injections
5.	Begin intrathecal agents
6.	Cut nerves, tendons

BLADDER

Urinary issues can be a major focal point to those living with MS. These may be the factor that directs quality of life and interferes with living in society. Unfortunately, urinary issues are extremely common!

Some bladders are small and do not store well, while others are large and do not empty well. Some are dyssynergic and want to empty despite the urinary sphincter spasming shut. To make it all the more perplexing, the symptoms for each may be identical – urgency, hesitancy, frequency, incontinence – and they can occur in combination.

Small bladders carry a small residual volume of urine and thus are usually easy to diagnose with a residual urine determination. Anticholinergic medications are plentiful and often successful in slowing the bladder spasms and allowing more time between voidings and more control of emptying.[63] Tolterodine, oxybutynin, solifenacin succinate, trospium chloride and others will modify the urgency and frequency of urination with appropriate dosing.[64] It should be remembered that sweating is a cholinergic function, thus if too aggressive an approach is applied, sweating may become impaired, resulting in an increase in body temperature and decreasing function.

Large bladders carry a large residual volume (>200 ml) of urine. While bethanechol should stimulate emptying, it is often inefficient. Mechanical emptying by catheter techniques can be helpful. Self-catheterization usually brings a decrease in infection rate but requires some coordination skills on the part of the patient.[65] Coordination and sensory capabilities must be kept in mind in the introduction of catheterization techniques. Having a family member perform such catheterizations is frowned upon as it changes the relationships between the family members and usually ends in unhappiness for all. Chronic indwelling (Foley) catheters can be extremely beneficial to quality of life by allowing continence, increased fluid intake and ability to return to society. However they are always accompanied by an increase in bladder infections and sometimes bladder stones, so there is a trade-off.

Dyssynergic bladders are managed by alpha-blockers in combination with catheterization techniques.[66] These are more common in the male and can result in very high bladder pressures with resultant retrograde flow of urine up the ureters toward the kidneys. Thus they are important to recognize via cystometry. Treatment involves catheterization techniques and α-adrenergic blocking agents.

Frequent nocturia can become a major issue keeping a person from having a good nights sleep and adding to the fatigue of the next day. Anti-diuretic hormone (DDAVP) given at a dose of .2 mg at bedtime can successfully decrease urinary output during the night allowing for less toilet trips.[67,68] Care must be taken to watch the serum sodium periodically.

A practical approach toward the bladder includes a check for infection, followed by a check of residual urine and an appropriate strategy based on those results (Table 25.4). If the strategy fails formal evaluation of cystometric parameters may be necessary.

TABLE 25.4 Bladder management	
1.	Check for residual urine
2.	If low: begin anticholinergic regimen
3.	If high: consider catheterization technique depending on hand/eye coordination
4.	If this fails: urodynamic studies

BOWEL

The bowel is less commonly involved than the bladder in the person with MS but when they are involved the results can be catastrophic. Fortunately constipation is more common and is managed by appropriate hydration, bulk forming agents, stool softeners and sometimes laxatives and suppositories. Bowel programs should take advantage of the gastrocolic reflex to time the movement following a meal.

Urgent stools are more of a dilemma. Timing of the bowel movement becomes more essential and scheduling it for regularity is necessary. Thus patients are instructed to try to eliminate around 30 minutes following a meal. Increasing the bulk (fiber) with less liquid will allow for a firmer stool that is easier to control. Care must be taken to avoid dehydration. Judicious use of suppositories at specific times may allow the patient the control necessary to decrease incontinence.[69]

A bowel program managed by a physician or a nurse is a must to avoid embarrassment. Unfortunately the program may have to change from time to time, so follow-up becomes a necessity.

SEXUALITY

The ease of discussing sexual function appears somewhat dependent on the background of the physician. Many physicians are too bound by cultural backgrounds to effectively bring up the topic. Nurses, occupational therapists and psychologists may be necessary contributors to the discussion. It is an important part of virtually every patient's life. Thus it is very essential to break cultural bounds and ask the questions that may lead to treatment of sexual dysfunction.

Sexuality implies relating at many levels. Warm feelings, verbal and nonverbal expressions of caring are important for all, whether MS is present or not. However, when MS is in the picture relationships may change. It is a function of sexuality to maintain warmth and diminish stress between couples.

Erectile dysfunction is a common issue for males with MS at all levels of ability. This may vary from difficulty getting an erection to difficulty maintaining it. Ejaculation may become a problem.[70,71] Manual stimulation is a technique that can provide strong stimulation for both erection and ejaculation. The use of erectile stimulating medications whether by penile injection (alprostadil), penile suppository (alprostadil) or oral administration (sildenafil, vardenafil or tadalafil) is often effective in the male with MS.[72,73] Penile prostheses are available for unresponsive situations.

Female sexual issues often include a change in vagina and clitoral sensation. The judicious use of vibrators and other sexually stimulating instruments (Eros device), along with vaginal lubrication, may be useful.[74] Verbally allowing appropriate conversation opens the possibility of management and should be encouraged.

DEPRESSION

Depression may be situational (exogenous) or neurochemical (endogenous). In the person with MS both are common and both require management. The suicide rate among those with MS is higher than among those with other neurological diseases.[75,76] Demyelination and axonal loss within the brain leads to alteration of neurochemistry, allowing for this increased depression. Management aimed at altering the environmental stresses and also changing the neurochemistry is necessary. Sleep disturbances associated with depression are a significant contributor to fatigue in those with MS. Counseling coupled with antidepressant medication can improve quality of life but often one without the other leaves the situation less than adequately managed.

A unique condition, related to bilateral cerebral damage (pseudobulbar palsy), results in pathological laughing and/or crying. This appears as spontaneous and inappropriate showing of emotions that is uncontrollable. Amitriptyline and other antidepressant and anticonvulsant medications may decrease these outbursts.[77]

PAIN

Discomfort in MS may come from many sources. Open injuries are fairly easy to understand and manage. Psychological pain is more complex and varies greatly from individual to individual. Pain from other organs such as heart or bowels is not eliminated in MS and can play a role in comfort. However most of the pain managed in MS is more mysterious.

Neuropathic pain is better understood in diseases of the peripheral nerves such as diabetes mellitus. It could well be a similar mechanism of action behind the central pain seen as 'neuropathic' in MS.[78] The characteristics are often similar, with a burning, deep quality. It follows no particular neurological distribution. Often, itching, numbness and temperature changes are associated with the pain. The feeling usually is worse at night when the body has less on its conscious mind. There is often a psychological overlay accompanying the situation.

Anticonvulsant therapy has been used for a long time, including phenytoin and carbamazapine. More recently these have been supplanted by gabapentin, topiramate and lamotrigine.[79–81] It is often possible to deliver comfort by dosing and combining pharmaceutical strategies. It seems, however, that the popular use of narcotic agents in this situation is actually not helpful and adds another dimension and complicating factor to the already very complicated situation.

Neuralgias such as trigeminal, glossopharyngeal and other rarer forms present occasionally as severe, lightning-like pain lasting seconds but occurring frequently. After they are recognized the anticonvulsant medications are helpful, and if they fail, surgical procedures may remedy the situation (see Paroxysmal spasms, above).

COGNITION

Demyelination and axonal loss within the brain clearly leads to a subcortical dementia. Transportation of thoughts is interrupted. Problems with memory, planning, foresight and judgment occur in over 50%. These can be the major issue in 10%.[76] While there have been a few promising studies showing that the Alzheimer's disease treatments may be of slight benefit, the pathology is quite different and the pharmacological approaches are less than adequate.[82]

Speech pathologists and neuropsychologists have attempted cognitive rehabilitation, with mixed results. The use of memory devices (computers, hand-held devices) is beneficial if the patient can master them.[83,84]

Depression and sedating medication can amplify the cognitive loss and need to be monitored carefully.

Unfortunately, cognitive changes can occur early in the disease before physical changes in ambulation or upper extremity function are seen. This may bring about a denial of disease progression and may delay the start of disease-modifying treatments. Screening for cognitive problems on a regular basis may sound logical but the means to do so efficiently is lacking. There are neuropsychological tests that profess to be short and efficient but are really not practical in a busy practice situation.

Cognitive dysfunction remains one of the large enigmas of MS management.

WEAKNESS

Weakness is a common symptom in MS. This is because of central conduction problems rather than primary muscle issues. Thus progressive resistive exercises, if done to the point of fatigue, may lead to weakness rather than strengthening.[85] However if there is enough nerve conduction an increase in strength may be found with nonfatiguing strengthening exercises.[86–88] Clearly, disuse must be guarded against. Thus the evaluator must differentiate the type of weakness and determine a rehabilitative program appropriate to the situation. The use of devices to compensate for weakness (canes, crutches, walkers, chairs) will allow for increased mobility and needs to be encouraged in the appropriate situations.

Temperature sensitivity is a common issue in MS. Heat will exaggerate most symptoms, particularly weakness. Air-conditioning may be a medical necessity in such individuals. The use of cooling vests and other cooling garments is another approach.

SWALLOWING

Dysphagia and aspiration can be obvious or silent but lead to medical complications of pneumonia in either case. Bedside and radiological swallowing studies can demonstrate the texture of nutrients that are most likely to be aspirated on an individual basis. Knowing that, a plan involving specific swallowing techniques can be developed, which may include changing the texture of the nutrient.[89,90]

SIDE EFFECTS OF INJECTABLES

The aggressive use of immune-modulating agents to slow down the actual disease process has contributed to the development of a whole new set of symptoms the clinician must recognize and manage.

Interferon initiation often brings about a fever reaction, which may be very disabling to the person with MS. It is often recommended that the interferon be administered in the evening prior to going to bed. This allows for the impact of the fever during the night, when it may be less disabling to activities of living. Antipyretic medications (ibuprofen, acetaminophen/paracetamol) may be administered 4 hours before the infection, at the time of injection and then, if necessary, 4 hours after the injection.

Subcutaneous injections can lead to immune reactions within the skin with inflammation, redness and significant irritation. Good injection technique is essential. This may involve icing or heating the area prior to injecting. A common error is injecting too shallowly. Injection devices have improved techniques and decreased many of these side effects but may contribute to the problem if they are set to deliver the medication too shallowly within the skin rather than beneath it. It is important to allow the air bubble in the syringe to remain to push the medication through the skin and, similarly, it is recommended that the needle be free of lingering medication as it pierces the skin.

Rotation of the injections is an absolute necessity to preserve as much skin area as possible and allow healing between injections. For some, the addition of a cortisone cream or a local anesthetic cream may be helpful.[27]

With some treatments pain can linger after the injection. Applying cooling can offer symptomatic relief. Understanding the issues is often helpful in the development of compensation strategies.

Glatiramer acetate will occasionally induce a 'systemic' reaction. This rare, but real symptom complex presents with a feeling of panic, chest discomfort, shortness of breath and a feeling of doom and gloom. It usually lasts for 20 minutes and then clears rapidly but if panic sets in and an emergency is called the issue may be magnified and complicated. The treatment is to realize that the problem is associated with the medication and requires rest for the duration of the symptoms to allow them to abate on their own. This is not usually a recurrent problem but can occasionally repeat.

REFERENCES

1. Runmarker B, Andersen O. Prognostic factors in a multiple sclerosis incidence cohort with twenty-five years follow-up. Brain 1993; 116: 117–134.

2. Kraft GH, Freal JE, Coryell JK et al. Multiple sclerosis: early prognostic guidelines. Arch Phys Med Rehabil 1981; 62: 54–58.

3. Kurtzke, JF, Beebe GW, Nagler B et al. Studies on the natural history of multiple sclerosis: eight early prognostic features of the later course of the illness. J Chronic Dis 1977; 30: 819–830.

4. Multiple Sclerosis Society. Multiple Sclerosis Society symptom management survey. London: Multiple Sclerosis Society; 1997.

5. Fisk JD, Ritvo PG, Ross L et al. Measuring the functional impact of fatigue: initial validation of the fatigue impact scale. Clin Infect Dis 1994;18(suppl 1): S79–S83.

6. Krupp LB, LaRocca NG, Muir-Nash J, Steinberg AD. The fatigue severity scale: application to patients with multiple sclerosis and systemic lupus erythematosus. Arch Neurol 1989; 46: 1121–1123.

7. Schwartz JF, Jandorf L, Krupp LB. The measurement of fatigue: a new instrument. J Psychosom Res 1993; 37: 753–762.

8. Petajan JH, Gappmaier E, White AT et al. Impact of aerobic training on fitness and quality of life in multiple sclerosis. Ann Neurol 1996; 39: 432–441.

9. Health Technology Assessment 2000; 4: no. 27.

10. Ford H, Trigwell P, Johnson M. The nature of fatigue in multiple sclerosis. J Psychosom Res 1998; 45: 33–38.

11. Schapiro RT. Fatigue. In: Schapiro RT. Managing the symptoms of multiple sclerosis. New York: Demos Publications; 2003: 25–32.

12. Swensson B, Gerdie B. Elert J. Endurance training in patients with multiple sclerosis: five case studies. Phys Ther 1994; 74: 1017–1026.

13. VanOosten BW, Truyen L, Barkof F, Polman CH. Choosing drug therapy for multiple sclerosis. An update. Drugs 1998; 56: 555–569.

14. Cohen RA, Fisher M. Amantadine treatment of fatigue associated with multiple sclerosis. Arch Neurol 1989; 46: 676–680.

15. The Canadian MS Research Group. A randomized controlled trial of amantadine in fatigue associated with multiple sclerosis. Can J Neurol Sci 1987; 14: 273–278.

16. Krupp LB, Coyle PK, Doscher C et al. Fatigue therapy in multiple sclerosis: results of a double blind, randomized, parallel trial of amantadine, pemoline, and placebo. Neurology 1995; 45: 1956–1961.

17. Murray TJ. Amantadine therapy for fatigue in multiple sclerosis. Can J Neurol Sci 1985; 12: 251–254.

18. Rammohan KW, Rosenberg JH, Lynn DJ et al. Efficacy and safety of modafinil (Provigil) for the treatment of fatigue in multiple sclerosis: a two center phase 2 study. J Neurol Neurosurg Psychiatr 2002; 72: 179–183.

19. Weinshenker BG, Penman M, Bass B et al. A double blind, randomized, crossover trial of pemoline in fatigue associated with multiple sclerosis. Neurology 1992; 42: 1468–1471.

20. Sheean GL, Murray NMF, Rothwell JC et al. An open labeled clinical and electrophysiological study of 3,4 diaminopyridine in the treatment of fatigue in multiple sclerosis. Brain 1998; 121: 967–975.

21. Rossigni PM, Pasqualetti P, Pozzilli C et al. Fatigue in progressive multiple sclerosis: results of a randomized, double blind study, placebo-controlled, crossover trial of oral 4-aminopyridine. Mult Scler 2001; 7: 354–358.

22. Mostert S, Kesselring J. Effects of a short-term exercise training program on aerobic fitness, fatigue, health perception and activity level of subjects with multiple sclerosis. Mult Scler 2002; 8: 161–168.

23. Davidoff RA. 1978. Pharmacology of spasticity. Neurology 28: 46–51.

24. Dromerick AW. Clinical features of spasticity and principles of treatment. In: Gelber DA, Jeffery DR, eds. Current clinical neurology: clinical evaluation and management of spasticity. Totowa, NJ: Humana Press; 2002: 13–26.

25. Stenager E, Knudsen L, Jensen K. Acute and chronic pain syndromes in multiple sclerosis. Acta Neurol Scand 1991; 84: 197–200.

26. Sachais BA, Logue JN, Carey MS. Baclofen, a new antispastic drug. A controlled, multicenter trial in patients with multiple sclerosis. Arch Neurol 1977; 34: 422–428.

27. Hoogstraten MC, van der Ploeg RJ, van der Burg W et al. Tizanidine versus baclofen in the treatment of spasticity in multiple sclerosis patients. Acta Neurol Scand 1988; 77: 224–230.

28. Neill RW. Diazepam in the relief of muscle spasm resulting from spinal lesions. Ann Phys Med 1966(suppl): 33–28.

29. Saletu M, Anderer P, Saletu-Zyhlarz G et al. Acute placebo-controlled sleep laboratory studies and clinical follow-up with pramipexole in restless legs syndrome. Eur Arch Psychiatr Clin Neurosci 2002; 252: 185–194.

30. Cutter NC, Scott DD, Johnson JC, Whiteneck G. Gabapentin effect on spasticity in multiple sclerosis: a placebo-controlled, randomized trial. Arch Phys Med Rehabil 2000; 81: 164–169.

31. Gambi D, Rossini PM, Calenda G et al. Dantrolene sodium in the treatment of spasticity caused by multiple sclerosis or degenerative myelopathies: a double blind, crossover study in comparison with placebo. Curr Ther Res Clin Exp 1983; 33: 835–840.

32. Gelenberg AJ, Poskanzer DC. The effect of dantrolene sodium on spasticity in multiple sclerosis. Neurology 1973; 23: 1313–1315.

33. Hauser SL, Doolittle TH, Lopez-Bresnahan M et al. An antispasticity effect of threonine in multiple sclerosis. Arch Neurol 1992; 49: 923–926.

34. Snow BJ, Tsui JK, Bhatt MH et al. Treatment of spasticity with botulinum toxin: a double blind study. Arch Neurol 1990; 28: 512–515.

35. Penn RD, Savoy SM, Corcos D et al. Intrathecal baclofen for severe spinal spasticity. N Engl J Med 1989; 320: 1517–1521.

36. Middel B, Kuipers Upmeijer H, Bouma J et al. Effect of intrathecal baclofen delivered by an implanted programmable pump on health related quality of life in patients with severe spasticity. J Neurol Neurosurg Psychiatr 1997; 63: 204–209.

37. Gianino JM, York MM, Paice JA, Shott S. Quality of life: effect of reduced spasticity from intrathecal baclofen. J Neurosci Nurs 1998; 30: 47–54.

38. Shetter AG. The neurosurgical treatment of spasticity. Neurosurg Q 1996; 6: 194–207.

39. Conroe P, Musty R, Rein J et al. The perceived effects of smoked cannabis on patients with multiple sclerosis. Eur Neurol 1997; 38: 44–48.

40. Killestein J, Hoogervorst El, Reif M et al. Safety, tolerability and efficacy of orally administered cannabinoids in MS. Neurology 2002; 58: 1404–1407.

41. Mueller ME, Gruenthal M, Olson WL, Olson WH. Gabapentin for relief of upper motor neuron symptoms in multiple sclerosis. Arch Phys Med Rehabil 1997; 78: 521–524.

42. Solaro C, Lunardi GL, Capello E et al. An open label trial of gabapentin treatment of paroxysmal symptoms in multiple sclerosis patients. Neurology 1998; 51: 609–611.

43. Matthews WB. Paroxysmal symptoms in multiple sclerosis J Neurol Neurosurg Psychiatr 1975; 38: 618–623.

44. Schapiro R. Management of spasticity, pain, and paroxysmal phenomena in multiple sclerosis. Curr Neurol Neurosci Rep 2001; 1: 299–302.

45. Alusi SH, Worthington J, Glickman S et al. Evaluation of three different ways of assessing tremor in multiple sclerosis. J Neurol Neurosurg Psychiatr 2000; 68: 756–760.

46. McAlpine D, Compston N. Some aspects of the natural history of disseminated

sclerosis: incidence, course, and prognosis; factors affecting onset and course. Q J Med 1952; 21: 135–167.

47. Schapiro R. Managing symptoms of multiple sclerosis. Neurol Clin 2005; 23: 177–187.

48. Findley LJ. Epidemiology and genetics of essential tremor. Neurology 2000; 54(suppl 4): S8–S13.

49. Bain PG, Mally J, Gresty M, Findley LJ. Assessing the impact of essential tremor on upper limb function. J Neurol 1993; 241: 54–61.

50. Alusi SH, Glickman S, Aziz TZ, Bain PG. Tremor in multiple sclerosis. J Neurol Neurosurg Psychiatr 1999; 66: 131–134.

51. Hallett M, Lindsey JW, Adelstein BD, Riley PO. Controlled trial of isoniazid therapy for severe postural cerebellar tremor in multiple sclerosis. Neurology 1985; 35: 1374–1377.

52. Henkin Y, Herishanu YO. Primidone as a treatment for cerebellar tremor in multiple sclerosis. Isr J Med Sci 1989; 25: 720–721.

53. Koller WC. Pharmacologic trials in the treatment of cerebellar tremor. Arch Neurol 1984; 41: 280–281.

54. Rice GP, Lesaux J, Vandervoort P et al. Ondansetron, a 5-HT3 antagonist, improves cerebellar tremor. J Neurol Neurosurg Psychiatr 1997; 62: 282–284.

55. Aisen ML, Holzer M, Rosen M et al. Glutethimide treatment of disabling action tremor in patients with multiple sclerosis and traumatic brain injury. Arch Neurol 1991; 48: 513–515.

56. Alusi SH, Aziz T, Glickman S et al. The efficacy of stereotaxic thalamotomy in the treatment of tremor in multiple sclerosis; a prospective case controlled trial. Mov Disord 2000; 15(suppl 3): 60.

57. Anderson TJ. Spasmodic torticollis. In: Moore P, ed. Handbook of botulinum toxin treatment. Oxford: Blackwell Science; 1995: 103–130.

58. Clifford DB. Tetrahydrocannabinol for tremor in multiple sclerosis. Ann Neurol 1983; 13: 669–671.

59. Geny C, Nguyen JP, Pollin B et al. Improvement of severe postural cerebellar tremor in multiple sclerosis by chronic thalamic stimulation. Mov Disord 1996; 11: 489–494.

60. Haddow LJ, Mumford C, Whittle IR. Stereotactic treatment of tremor due to multiple sclerosis. Neurosurg Q 1997; 7: 23–34.

61. Nguyen JP, Feve A, Cesaro P, Keravel Y. Long term follow-up of patients with multiple sclerosis and action tremor treated by thalamic stimulation. Mov Disord 1998; 13(suppl 2): 132.

62. Schapiro RT. Tremor and balance. In: Schapiro RT. Managing the Symptoms of Multiple Sclerosis. New York; Demos Publications; 2003: 46–48.

63. Haslam C Managing bladder symptoms in people with multiple sclerosis. Nurs Times 2005; 101(2): 48–50.

64. Abrams P, Freeman R, Anderström C, Mattiasson A. Tolterodine, a new antimuscarinic agent: as effective but better tolerated than oxybutinin in patients with an overactive bladder. Br J Urol 1998; 81: 801–810.

65. Glenn J. Restorative nursing bladder training program: recommending a strategy. Rehabil Nurs 2003; 28: 15–22.

66. Gades NM, Jacobson DJ, Girman CJ et al. Prevalence of conditions potentially associated with lower urinary tract symptoms in men. BJU Int 2005; 95: 549–553.

67. Bosma R, Wynia K, Havlikova E et al. Efficacy of desmopressin in patients with multiple sclerosis suffering from bladder dysfunction: a meta-analysis. Acta Neurol Scand 2005; 112: 1–5.

68. Leippold T, Reitz A, Schurch B. Botulinum toxin as a new therapy option for voiding disorders: current state of the art. Eur Urol 2003; 44: 165–174.

69. Schapiro RT. Bowels. In: Schapiro RT. Managing the symptoms of multiple sclerosis. New York: Demos Publications; 2003: 79–87.

70. Zorzon M, Zivadinov R, Bosco A et al. Sexual dysfunction in multiple sclerosis: a case-control study. I. Frequency and comparison of groups. Mult Scler 1999; 5: 418–427.

71. Zivadinov R, Zorzon M, Locatelli L et al. Sexual dysfunction in multiple sclerosis: a MRI, neurophysiological and urodynamic study. J Neurol Sci 2003; 210: 73–76.

72. Goldstein I, Lue TF, Padma-Nathan H et al. Oral sildenafil in the treatment of erectile dysfunction. Sildenafil Study Group. N Engl J Med 1998; 338: 1397–1404.

73. Vidal J, Curcoll L, Roig T, Bagunya J. Intracavernous pharmacotherapy for management of erectile dysfunction in multiple sclerosis patients. Rev Neurol 1995; 23: 269–271.

74. Munarriz R, Maitland S, Garcia SP et al. A prospective duplex Doppler ultrasonographic study in women with sexual arousal disorder to objectively assess genital engorgement induced by EROS therapy. J Sex Marital Ther 2003; 29(suppl 1): 85–94.

75. Siegert RJ, Abernethy DA. Depression in multiple sclerosis: a review. J Neurol Neurosurg Psychiatr 2005; 76: 469–475.

76. Kesselring J, Klement U. Cognitive and affective disturbances in multiple sclerosis. J Neurol 2001; 248: 180–183.

77. Feinstein A, Feinstein K, Gray T, O'Connor P. Prevalence and neuro behavioral correlates of pathological laughing and crying in multiple sclerosis. Arch Neurol 1997; 54: 1116–1121.

78. Moulin DE. Pain in central and peripheral demyelinating disorders. Neurol Clin 1998; 16: 889–898.

79. Khan OA. Gabapentin relieves trigeminal neuralgia in multiple sclerosis patients. Neurology 1998; 51; 611–614.

80. Solaro C, Messmer Uccelli, M, Uccelli A et al. Low dose gabapentin combined with either lomotrigine or carbamazepine can be useful thrapies for trigeminal neuralgia in multiple sclerosis. Eur Neurol 2000; 44: 45–48.

81. Cianchetti C, Zuddas A, Randazzo AP et al. Lamotrigine adjunctive therapy in painful phenomena in MS: preliminary obsevations. Neurology 1999; 53: 433.

82. Krupp LB, Christodoulou C, Melville P et al. Donepezil improved memory in multiple sclerosis in a randomized clinical trial. Neurology 2004; 63(9): 1579–1585.

83. Bagert B, Camplair P, Bourdette D. Cognitive dysfunction in multiple sclerosis: natural history, pathophysiology and management. CNS Drugs 2002; 16: 445–455.

84. Lincoln NB, Dent A, Harding J et al. Evaluation of cognitive assessment and cognitive intervention for people with multiple sclerosis. J Neurol Neurosurg Psychiatry 2002; 72: 93–98.

85. Schapiro RT. Exercise. In: Schapiro RT. Managing the symptoms of multiple sclerosis. New York: Demos Publications; 2003: 125.

86. Brown TR, Kraft GH. Exercise and rehabilitation for individuals with multiple sclerosis. Phys Med Rehabil Clin North Am 2005; 16: 513–555.

87. Surakka J, Romberg A, Ruutiainen J et al. Effects of aerobic and strength exercise on motor fatigue in men and women with multiple sclerosis: a randomized controlled trial. Clin Rehabil 2004; 18: 737–746.

88. White LJ, McCoy SC, Castellano V et al. Resistance training improves strength and functional capacity in persons with multiple sclerosis. Mult Scler 2004; 10: 668–674.

89. Prosiegel M, Schelling A, Wagner-Sonntag E. Dysphagia and multiple sclerosis. Int Mult Scler J 2004; 11: 22–31.

90. DePauw A, Dejaeger E, D'Hoghe B, Carton H. Dysphagia in multiple sclerosis. Clin Neurol Neurosurg 2002; 104: 345–351.

Bladder and sexual dysfunction in multiple sclerosis

V. Kalsi and C. J. Fowler

INTRODUCTION

Estimates of the prevalence of urogenital symptoms in multiple sclerosis (MS) have varied, depending on the populations studied. However, since these problems result mainly from spinal cord involvement, figures that show an occurrence similar to that of lower limb dysfunction seem realistic.[1,2] Thus urogenital symptoms in patients with MS are common and are generally acknowledged to have a very adverse effect on quality of life.[3,4] Fortunately this is an area where therapeutic intervention can be highly effective, as will be outlined in this chapter.

NEURAL CONTROL OF THE BLADDER

Our understanding of the higher processing involved in bladder control such that voiding can be achieved at a socially appropriate time and place has been greatly enhanced by functional brain imaging studies.[5] These have shown that a wide complex of brain networks control the two processes of bladder storage[6,7] and voiding[8,9] but that the final output of these is either activation or inhibition of a center in the dorsal tegmentum of the pons, the pontine micturition center. It is from here that direct pathways project to the sacral segments of the spinal cord (S2–S4) and determine parasympathetic outflow to the detrusor and coordinated activity of the motor units innervating the striated urethral sphincter[10] (Fig. 26.1).

During storage, parasympathetic innervation of the detrusor is inhibited so that the detrusor pressure does not rise as the bladder fills and tonic firing of the motor units of the striated urethral sphincter and pelvic floor maintain the pressure within the urethra at a higher level than within the bladder. At the initiation of micturition there is a relaxation of the striated urethral sphincter and pelvic floor, followed later by a coordinated contraction of the detrusor muscle. This synergistic activity between the sphincter and the detrusor depends on connections with the pontine region. If these are damaged or interrupted, sphincter contraction may occur as the detrusor contracts, a condition known as 'detrusor sphincter dyssynergia' (DSD).[11] The symptoms of abnormal voiding due to the presence of DSD are hesitancy, interrupted flow pattern and complaint of incomplete emptying. Evidence of this is often not the persistent sensation of incomplete emptying but rather having to pass urine again within 5–10 minutes of micturating. Symptomatically, however, the most prominent abnormality that

develops following disconnection from the pontine micturition center is a segmental reflex that causes reflex detrusor contractions in response to bladder distention. It has been shown from animal experiments, and human studies support this, that, following any form of spinal cord lesion, unmyelinated C fibers that were formally quiescent (and therefore known as silent C fibers) become mechanosensitive and respond to bladder stretch.[12] This afferent activity, via synaptic activity in the sacral segment of the intact cord, causes detrusor contractions.[13,14] It is this that is responsible for the emergence of the condition of 'detrusor overactivity', which is the pathophysiology underlying the common complaints of urinary frequency, urgency and urgency incontinence: the overactive bladder syndrome.[15]

From the foregoing account it will be clear why bladder dysfunction may worsen with increasing spinal cord involvement in MS. Imaging studies using magnetic resonance imaging (MRI) have reported a correlation between urological complaints and spinal cord cross-sectional area used as a marker for spinal cord atrophy;[16] however, there is little evidence for the association between urinary symptoms and brain MRI parameters.[17,18] Table 26.1 summarizes the pathophysiological changes that occur and their symptomatic consequences.

MANAGEMENT OF BLADDER SYMPTOMS IN MULTIPLE SCLEROSIS

FIRST-LINE TREATMENTS

Anticholinergic medication

The commonest presenting symptoms are due to detrusor overactivity[19] and can therefore logically be treated with anticholinergic agents. The detrusor muscle expresses mostly M2 muscarinic receptors[20–23] although M3 receptors are the functionally important ones in the detrusor muscle, in conditions of health.[22,23] The benefits of selective blockade of M2 or M3 muscarinic receptors have yet to be translated into clinical effect. Various agents, some of them very recently licensed, are now available to treat symptoms of detrusor overactivity. These are listed in Table 26.2. The formulation of these medications to give a long-acting preparation (extended life 'XL') is a significant advantage for patients who need only take the tablet once a day to provide 24-hour cover for symptoms. Both tolterodine

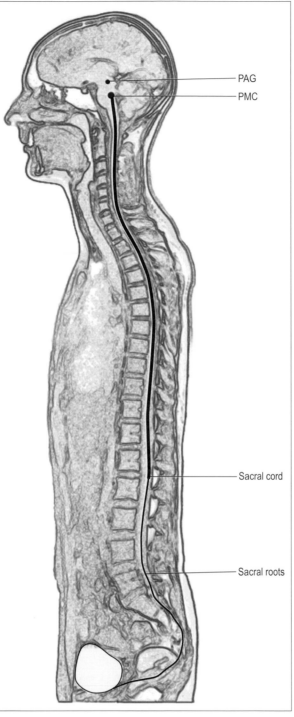

FIG. 26.1 Illustration of the pathways involved in micturition. PAG, periaqueductal gray; PMC, pontine micturition center.

TABLE 26.1 Urinary symptoms from spinal cord lesions
Detrusor overactivity
Detrusor sphincter dyssynergia
Incomplete emptying

and trospium chloride have a chemical structure that renders them less lipophilic and therefore theoretically less likely to cross the blood–brain barrier, possibly conferring the advantage of lesser central side effects.[24,25] This may be important in patients who have cognitive impairment.

Although it might appear desirable to prescribe an anticholinergic for patients complaining of urinary urgency and other symptoms of detrusor overactivity, there is a single crucial measurement to be made first. The postmicturition residual volume should be measured.[26,27] This can now be very conveniently done using a small portable ultrasound device and many specialist nurse continence advisors have access to one, as shown in Figure 26.2. The importance of recognizing incomplete emptying is that any residual volume in the bladder can trigger volume-determined reflex detrusor contractions and thus exacerbate the clinical situation.[28]

It has been demonstrated that patients may not be aware of the extent to which they have incomplete emptying, although those who suspect that they do have this problem are often correct.[19] It is therefore important to ask patients if they either have a sensation of incomplete emptying or if they can void the same amount again as they voided some minutes previously, since these points in the history are strong indicators that a high residual volume must be contributing to their problems.

Figure 26.3 shows a simple algorithm for managing the common symptoms of bladder dysfunction in MS.

Measures to improve bladder emptying

If a raised postmicturition residual volume is demonstrated, some means of reducing this will be necessary to improve symptoms. This can either be by the patient or sometimes their carer, performing clean intermittent catheterization (CISC). CISC is advocated if the postmicturition residual volume is greater than 100 ml. Not all patients will be able to do this and most likely to succeed are those who are well motivated, have preserved cognitive function and adequate manual dexterity. In addition the patient's overall physical status is also an important consideration, as they need to be able to get into a comfortable position to catheterize efficiently, ideally eventually over the toilet. Table 26.3 outlines the processes involved in teaching and a patient embarking on this intervention.

Unfortunately there is little else that improves bladder emptying. Although there have been claims that alpha-blockers can reduce the postmicturition residual volume,[29,30] this has not been confirmed by other studies. Nor is there a strong clinical impression that alpha-blockers are effective in individual patients, which perhaps is not surprising since it is thought the defect of bladder emptying in MS is poorly sustained and coordinate detrusor contraction or an inappropriate contraction of the striated urethral sphincter, a muscle on which alpha-blockers are not thought to be effective.[31]

The only other means of improving bladder emptying, which may benefit some patients, is the application of a suprapubic vibrating stimulus. It was shown many years ago that vibration applied to this region can induce bladder contraction.[32] Although this may not occur in the presence of intact innervation, in those with reflex detrusor overactivity the vibrating stimulus may trigger a detrusor contraction and thus help initiate micturition and possibly improve bladder emptying. Various devices including a small hand-held battery operated vibrator are commercially available and some patients find this helpful for bladder emptying.[33,34]

Other investigations

The first-line treatments therefore consist of oral anticholinergics with or without intermittent self-catheterization depending on the postvoid residual volume. More complex management

TABLE 26.2 Anticholinergic agents used to treat symptoms of detrusor overactivity

Generic name	Trade name	Dose (mg)	Frequency	Receptor subtype selectivity	Molecule type	Elimination half-life of parent drug (h)
Propantheline	Pro-Banthine	15	t.d.s.	Nonselective	Quaternary amine	<2
Tolterodine tartrate	Detrusitol	2	b.d.	Nonselective	Tertiary amine	2.4
Tolterodine tartrate	Detrusitol XL	4	o.d.	Nonselective	Tertiary amine	8.4
Trospium chloride	Regurin	20	b.d.	Nonselective	Quaternary amine	20
Oxybutynin chloride	Ditropan	2.5–5	b.d.–q.d.s.	Nonselective	Tertiary amine	2.3
Oxybutynin chloride XL	Lyrinel XL	5–30	o.d.	Nonselective	Tertiary amine (R and S isomers)	13.2
Propiverine hydrochloride	Detrunorm	15	o.d.–q.d.s.	Nonselective	Ester	4.1
Darifenacin	Emselex	7.5–15	o.d.	Selective muscarinic M3 receptor antagonist	Tertiary amine	3.1
Solifenacin	Vesicare	5–10	o.d.	Selective muscarinic M2 and M3 receptor antagonist	Tertiary amine	40–68

o.d., once daily; b.d., twice daily; t.d.s., three times daily; q.d.s., four times daily; XL, extended life.

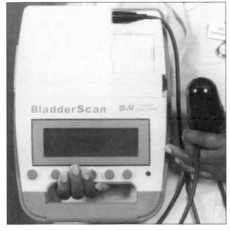

FIG. 26.2 Handheld ultrasound bladder scanner demonstrated by continence advisor.

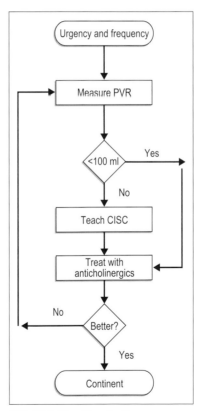

FIG. 26.3 Algorithm for the management of neurogenic incontinence. CISC, clean intermittent self-catheterization. Reproduced with permission from original material by CJ Fowler in Fowler CJ. Investigation of the neurogenic bladder. In: Hughes RAC, ed. Neurological investigations. Oxford: Blackwell Publishing, 1997.

and investigation protocols than that shown in Figure 26.3 have been proposed but, since the treatment options are limited to these two main interventions, the simplicity of that outline has much to recommend it. The place of cystometry and videocystometry in the routine investigation of these patients is highly questionable. It has been argued that it is only through these investigations that detrusor sphincter dyssynergia can be recognized[11,35,36] but, since there is no specific treatment for that disorder other than managing the consequences, i.e. incomplete emptying and raised detrusor pressure, a pragmatic approach is recommended.

The conditions for which other investigations are indicated, and referral to a urologist, are shown in Table 26.4. If patients are performing self-catheterization it is likely that urine specimens sent to the laboratory will grow microorganisms although other criteria by which to recognize a urinary tract infection are not present.[37] However if genuine recurrent urinary tract infections do occur with the expected clinical symptoms of dysuria and change in color and odor of the urine, urological investigations should be carried out to discover if there is a nidus for infection in the urinary tract, such as a calculus. Hematuria is another indication for prompt urological referral. Urine cytology and some form of imaging of the upper urinary tracts, either an ultrasound of the renal tracts or an intravenous urogram (IVU), would then be carried out, and probably a cystoscopy with bladder biopsies.

TABLE 26.3 Advice given to patients for clean intermittent self-catheterization (CISC)

Discussion prior to instruction	Reasons for performing CISC Explanation of pelvic anatomy Importance of personal hygiene (hand washing and perineal hygiene) to avoid any urinary tract infections Discussion of urinary tract infections Process of CISC explained by continence advisor Discussion of different positions
Catheters	Types of catheter and their uses according to dexterity and lifestyle Storage (follow manufacturer's guidelines) Disposal (domestic waste) Supply (prescription, general practitioner, home delivery).
Instruction	CISC carried out by patient under supervision
Follow up	Telephone follow up at 3 days Outpatient appointment with continence advisor at 3 months Annual review with continence advisor Access to continence advisor as MS symptoms change
Other advice	Fluid intake (1.5–2 liters/d unless otherwise advised) Diet (to avoid constipation) Sexual activity

TABLE 26.4 Indications for referral to a urologist

Recurrent urinary tract infections
Hematuria
Evidence of impaired renal function
Pain thought to be arising from the upper or lower urinary tract

DDAVP

The synthetic antidiuretic hormone anti-ADH, DDAVP, was originally licensed to treat the polyuria of diabetes insipidus.[38] Subsequently it became an established treatment for nocturnal enuresis[39] and studies were then carried out to look at its efficacy in women with MS and night-time frequency.[40] A number of small, placebo-controlled trials have shown that it was effective if taken during the day in providing the patients with a period up to 6 hours during which they were not troubled by urinary frequency, without any rebound night-time frequency.[41,42] The patient must, however, be cautioned to use it only once in 24 hours despite the convenience of the effect it has. It should not be given to patients over the age of 65 nor used in those with dependant leg edema through immobility who have night-time frequency when recumbent. In spite of these cautions, a proportion of patients find it may provide additional benefit to that conferred by the combination of anticholinergics and intermittent catheterization, if they are looking to be reliably free of symptoms for a long journey or particular social event.[42]

SECOND-LINE TREATMENTS FOR OVERACTIVE BLADDER

As shown in Figure 26.4 there may be a point in the progression of MS when first-line treatment is insufficient to contain urinary symptoms and yet the patient does not want to have a long-term indwelling catheter. This point in their decline is often reached as their neurological disability, particularly their mobility, is deteriorating and the patient is therefore not in a sufficiently robust state of health to undergo bladder surgery such as a clam cystoplasty. Various new nonsurgical and, at the time of writing, unlicensed treatments are emerging to treat these patients.

Cannabinoids

The illegal use of cannabis by patients with MS had undoubtedly become common in European countries, to the point at which a diagnosis of MS was sometimes argued as an extenuating argument by people found growing *Cannabis sativa*. In 1998 a high-level UK government report argued that the medicinal properties of cannabis should be further explored,[43] giving rise to a number of small-scale open-label studies that examined the effect of medicinal cannabis extracts on patients with chronic pain or various aspects of MS. Included in these was a small, open-label study in patients with advanced MS in whom conventional available treatments had been ineffective and who were therefore facing the prospect of having a long-term indwelling catheter. The results of this pilot study showed a significant decrease in urinary urgency and reduction in the number and volume of incontinence episodes, frequency and nocturia. Significantly decreased too were daily total voided and catheterized urine volumes and urinary incontinence pad weights, while spasticity, quality of sleep and patient self-assessment of pain improved.[44] Subsequently, large, multicenter randomized, placebo-controlled studies were initiated to look at the effect of sublingual sprays of medicinal cannabis extracts on bladder function but at the time of writing the results of these studies are not yet available.

The UK Medical Research Council funded a large, multicenter, placebo-controlled trial to look at the effect of oral nabilone and THC (Δ-tetrahydrocannabinol) on patients with MS (the CAMS study – Cannabis in Multiple Sclerosis). The primary focus of this study was to look at the effect of cannabinoids on spasticity and, although no change was demonstrated on the Ashworth scale, the patients did report subjective improvements of spasticity[45] and further work is still ongoing. A subsidiary study looked at the effect on the bladder and, as recently reported in abstract, it also appears to show a lessening in reduction of urinary urgency and reduced number of episodes of urge incontinence.[46] Whether or not this medication becomes a licensed therapy in the UK for the treatment of specific symptoms in MS such as spasticity and urgency frequency remains to be decided, although so far the medicines licensing authority has not agreed to it on the basis of the existing data.

Intravesical vanilloids

Knowledge of the importance of the emergence of C fiber reflex causing detrusor overactivity following a spinal cord lesion[12] led to the use of intravesical vanilloids to deafferent the bladder. First tried was intravesical capsaicin[47] but, although good evidence was accumulated that this had a significant therapeutic effect,[48] the agent was largely abandoned because of its nonlicensed status and because it caused discomfort on instillation. However, dissolving the capsaicin in glucidic acid was shown to significantly reduce its local irritant effect and makes its administration more acceptable.[49] Intravesical resiniferatoxin, an ultrapotent capsaicinoid,[50] was introduced because it was

SECTION 3

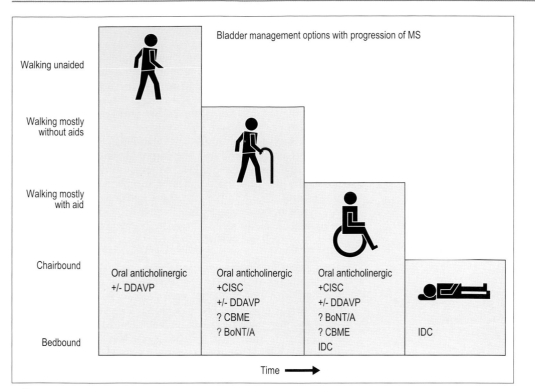

FIG. 26.4 The bladder symptoms in MS becoming increasingly difficult to manage with progression of spinal cord disease. The diagram summarizes the various measures that may be effective at each stage. BoNT/A, botulinum neurotoxin type A; CBME, cannabis-based medical extract; CISC, clean intermittent self-catheterization; DDAVP, desmopressin.)

thought it would have the same neurotoxic effect on the afferents of the bladder[51] but be less pungent.[52] However, a randomized controlled trial comparing the efficacy and tolerance of capsaicin in glucidic acid and a dilute alcoholic resiniferatoxin in patients with neurogenic bladder overactivity, concluded that both formulations are equally well tolerated and efficient in relieving symptoms of detrusor overactivity.[49] Clinical trials with resiniferatoxin were unfortunately marred by an unrecognized effect of the compound's tendency to adhere to plastic. For this reason the number of patients in whom it was effective in treatment trials was small[53] and it is unlikely that a pharmaceutical company will make this medication available in the future. Intravesical capsaicin is still offered as a treatment option in Bordeaux, France.

Detrusor injections of botulinum toxin type A

The discovery by Schürch et al that injection of botulinum toxin A directly into the smooth muscle of the detrusor resulted in a significant improvement in neurogenic bladder dysfunction is having far reaching consequences.[54,55] Originally proposed on the basis that botulinum toxin A would block the presynaptic release of parasympathetic acetylcholine mediating detrusor contraction, the benefits of this treatment appear to exceed those expected from an agent that merely paralyzes the detrusor. It seems likely that botulinum toxin A is also affecting the vesicular release of neurotransmitters involved in the afferent arm of reflex bladder contractions, and work on this is still ongoing.[56] Initial reports were based mostly on patients who had had spinal cord injury, although some patients with MS were included.

In our own studies, a series of 43 patients with MS have received injections of 300 units of botulinum toxin type A using a minimally invasive outpatient technique developed in our

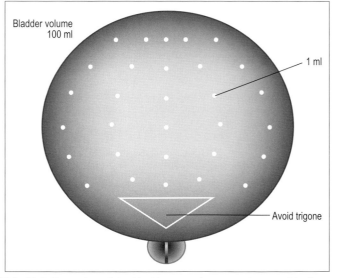

FIG. 26.5 Illustration of the bladder mapping out points used in the minimally invasive technique of intradetrusor injection of botulinum toxin. Reproduced with permission from Kalsi V, Fowler CJ. Therapy insight: bladder dysfunction associated with multiple sclerosis. Nat Clin Pract Urol 2005; 2: 492–501.

department.[57] The patients who received the injections were those in whom oral pharmacotherapy had failed to control symptoms of urinary urgency, frequency and urgency incontinence due to detrusor overactivity. A total of 30 equally spaced points in the bladder, sparing the trigone (Fig. 26.5) are injected using a flexible cystoscope and a superfine needle under local anesthetic. Each injection is comprised of 10 mouse units of Botox© (1 ml). The entire procedure is rapid, taking on average up to 15 minutes, and very well tolerated, with a mean score of 3.6 on a verbal 11-point box scale for discomfort. Voiding diary data show exceptional clinical efficacy with significant improvements in urinary urgency, frequency and incontinence episodes at 4 and 16 weeks postinjection compared to baseline. Urodynamic parameters, i.e. maximum cystometric capacity and detrusor pressures during filling, also show significant and sustained improvement.[58] Initial results of repeated injections demonstrate similar beneficial effects, with duration of action of the treatment being comparable to the first injections.[58,59] Although as yet unlicensed, botulinum toxin type A is now emerging as the preferred second-line treatment of symptoms of the overactive bladder and is increasingly being adopted by many urology, neurology and rehabilitation centers worldwide.

Surgery

The role of surgical interventions in the face of effective noninvasive and minimally invasive treatments for patients with bladder dysfunction due to MS is now diminishing. Results of denervation procedures and sacral nerve neuromodulation may have been good in the short term but are less satisfactory in the long term. The success of augmentation procedures of the bladder, such as a cystoplasty (with or without a catheterizable limb) in patients with MS has been limited.

Long-term indwelling catheter

Despite the advent of these emergent treatments there may be a stage at which a long-term indwelling catheter becomes necessary. This is usually when the patient has become very severely disabled, being unable to stand, certainly chair-bound or even bed-bound. Cognitive impairment, lower limb spasticity and loss of manual dexterity, combined with an ever-increasingly overactive detrusor, mean that intermittent catheterization, even by a carer, is no longer worthwhile. At this stage an indwelling catheter is appropriate and in the first instance a urethral catheter connected to a leg bag will familiarize the patient and their carer with what is involved in the long term. As soon as this is found to be acceptable to all those involved, the urethral catheter should be replaced with a supra pubic catheter,[60] because long-term urethral catheters can cause urethral trauma and erosion.

The suprapubic catheter should be sited by a urological surgeon, who may want to give a general anesthetic so that the bladder can be distended, facilitating suprapubic puncture of the otherwise shrunken bladder. The suprapubic catheter tract must be left to epithelialize for 6–8 weeks before the catheter is changed for the first time. The first change should ideally be performed by the team who performed the operation. Subsequent changes of the catheter will be at intervals of 3 months and may be done by district or practice nurses.

SEXUAL DYSFUNCTION IN MULTIPLE SCLEROSIS

INCIDENCE

Since, like physiological bladder function, sexual function depends on an intact spinal cord, the incidence of dysfunction is comparable to that of bladder complaints. It is interesting that the recognized incidence of sexual dysfunction has increased over the years: recent studies give figures of between 60% and 70%[61,62] of patients being affected, with an overall correlation between general disability and duration of the illness.[63–65]

NATURE OF THE PROBLEM

Men

Much has been learnt about the neural control of sexual function from animal models[66] and clinical observations of human sexual dysfunction resulting from spinal cord lesions.[67] From the studies in men following spinal cord injury, it is clear that the type of dysfunction depends on both the level and the completeness of the lesion.

An erection is achieved by vasodilatation of arterioles of the paired corpora cavernosa and the corpora spongiosa, the erectile bodies of the penis. As the erectile tissue fills with blood, the veins under the tunica albuginea of the penis are compressed, blocking outflow and adding to the turgor of the organ. Cyclic guanosine monophosphate (cGMP) and nitric oxide (NO) are the two main vasodilator neurotransmitters involved in erection.

It is now well established that there are two separate pathways for erection, the reflexive and the psychogenic erection mechanisms.[68,69] Reflex erections that occur following genital stimulation are mediated by sacral segmental pathways and are short-lived and inadequate for penetration. These are preserved in men with suprasacral spinal lesions. The other type of erection is psychogenically driven in response to perceived erotic stimuli and is mediated by the thoracolumbar sympathetic outflow. In men with intact spinal cords these two types of erectile response fuse to produce an adequate and well maintained erection for intercourse. Psychogenic erections may be preserved in men with lumbar cord lesions below the level of the sympathetic outflow, although only if there has not been additional damage to the sacral segments of the cord and the sacral roots. Neural pathways involved in night-time erections have not been fully defined; however, to achieve nocturnal erections of normal quality the preservation of thoracolumbar and sacral neural control is required, as well as spinal connections to higher brain centers responsible for arousal.[70]

In men with MS the commonest complaint is of a failure to maintain an adequate erection for intercourse. Reflex and night-time erections may be preserved but as spinal cord function deteriorates the ability to both initiate and sustain erection worsens. The fact that nocturnal tumescence may continue is probably the explanation for the very low (6%) estimates of early prevalence of ' genuine impotence' in MS,[71] as until recently it was a common tenet of belief among neurologists that, if erections were present at any time but were inadequate for intercourse, the problem was likely to be psychogenic.

Very few men with complete spinal cord injury can ejaculate[72,73] and difficulty with ejaculation may become apparent in men with MS when their erectile dysfunction is successfully treated.

Women

The homologous response of women to erection in men is an increase in vaginal blood flow[74] and vaginal lubrication.[75] This female sexual response is initiated by neurotransmitter-mediated smooth muscle relaxation involving substances such as vasoactive intestinal polypeptide (VIP) and NO, resulting in increased pelvic blood flow, transudative vaginal lubrication and clitoral and labial engorgement. However, the complaints that particularly worry women with MS, are of loss of genital sensation, libido and orgasmic capacity.[76]

TREATMENT

Men

In a double-blind, randomized study of sildenafil citrate for erectile dysfunction in men with MS, significant improvement in erectile function was found in 95% of the 217 participants leading to the ability to engage in satisfactory sexual activity (Fig. 25.6). This improved sexual function was observed to have secondary beneficial effects on several aspects of quality of life, as revealed by assessment of both general and disease specific quality of life outcome measures.[77] Although sildenafil citrate does and can only be expected to improve erectile response, a number of men in the study reported improved orgasmic function. It was thought that this was because they were able to maintain an erection longer to reach this point.

The impact of phosphodiesterase type 5 (PDE5) inhibitors and introduction of sildenafil citrate as an oral treatment of erectile dysfunction resulted in the heightening of patients' expectations[78] and led to the development of more selective PDE5 inhibitors; vardenafil and tadalafil. This family of drugs enhance smooth muscle relaxation within the arteries and arterioles of the corpus cavernosum penis, thereby increasing blood flow and facilitating an erection. These compounds inhibit the breakdown of cGMP and so increase the amount of available NO. Since NO has to be released before any of these agents can function, sexual arousal is necessary for the man to gain an erection. No data specific to patients with MS exists for tadalafil and vardenafil.

Unlike earlier procreation agents, oral PDE5 inhibitors have a low incidence of priapism.[79] Given their pharmacology, these drugs will increase the hypotensive effects of organic nitrates,[80] leading to excessive vasodilation and therefore hypotension, and so are contraindicated in patients receiving nitrates to treat angina.[80,81] Tadalafil is structurally different from both sildenafil and vardenafil[82] and this is reflected by its distinct clinical characteristics. The half-life of tadalafil is much greater than the other two, allowing for a longer period during which erection can be achieved. The dosing regimens, the time to onset of action, elimination half-lives and whether any trials have been conducted studying the efficacy of these drugs in MS patients are shown in Table 26.5.

Unfortunately, impaired ejaculation remains a problem for many men with MS. In a study that looked at neurophysiological abnormalities in men with MS, ejaculation difficulty was found to be more likely in men with severely delayed or absent pudendal evoked responses.[64] This is consistent with the facts as they are known about men with spinal cord lesions, i.e. that few men with a complete spinal cord lesion can ejaculate. There is, as yet, no medical intervention that restores ejaculatory function, although a small proportion of patients report some improvement with yohimbine, an alkaloid derived mainly from the bark of the African tree *Pausinystalia yohimbe* and also found in the South American herb quebracho, *Aspidosperma quebracho-blanco*, that is thought to have some marginal benefit in improving 'erotic sensitivity'.[83] Available as an oral preparation, it is principally a monoamine oxidase inhibitor that stimulates release of norepinephrine; 5–10 mg of yohimbine may be taken on a pro re nata basis, ideally 1–2 hours before intercourse is attempted. Its main side effects include an elevation in blood pressure, a slight anxiogenic action and increased frequency of micturition, all of which may be reversed on discontinuation of therapy.[84] There are, however, no trials specifically investigating the efficacy of this drug in MS patients.

Other pharmacological treatments, less used now since the advent of PDE5 inhibitors, include sublingual and locally (injectable and intraurethrally) administered agents. These are generally used if the patient has had any adverse effects from, or failed oral therapy.

Apomorphine, a dopamine agonist, is a proerectile agent[85] available as a sublingual preparation. This centrally acting drug starts the mechanism of erection. Since intact spinal pathways are required, its efficacy in patients with MS has yet to be proven[86] and on the whole it seems to be less effective than available oral pharmacotherapy.

Intracavernosal injections of prostaglandin E-1, papaverine and phentolamine are known to be an effective treatment for erectile dysfunction,[87] although they are not licensed in the UK for this indication. A synthetic preparation of prostaglandin E-1, alprostadil, is however available. These vasoactive drugs, injected into the corpus cavernosum of the penis, induce erection through smooth muscle relaxation irrespective of sexual arousal. Adverse effects include penile pain, groin pain, hypotension and, less commonly, prolonged erection (priapism) and in some instances long-term penile fibrosis.

Urethral pledgets of alprostadil (medicated urethral system for erection, MUSE) is an alternative route of administration and successful application can produce an erection in about 15 minutes; however, the efficacy rates are only 30–56%[88] and adverse effects include burning and irritation in the urethra, making the therapy unpopular.[89]

Finally there are a variety of nonmedical interventions, which range in degrees of invasiveness and price. Vacuum constriction devices (VCD) are amongst the least invasive and expensive. A

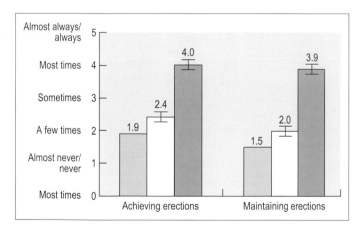

FIG. 26.6 Mean scores (±SE) for IIEF Q 3 (achieving erections) and Q 4 (maintaining erections) are shown at baseline (gray bars) and with placebo (white bars) and sildenafil use (black bars). *$p < 0.0001$ versus placebo. IIEF, International Index of Erectile Function. Reproduced with permission from Fowler et al 2005.[77]

TABLE 26.5 Phosphodiestrase type-5 inhibitors for treatment of erectile dysfunction

Generic name	Trade name	Dose (mg)	Frequency	Time to onset of action (h)	Elimination half-life of parent drug (h)	Trials in multiple sclerosis
Sildenafil	Viagra	25–100	1 dose in 24 h	0.5–1.6	4	Yes
Tadalafil	Cialis	10–20	1 dose in 24 h	0.5–0.75	17.5	No
Vardenafil	Levitra	5–10	1 dose in 24 h	<1	4	No

plastic tube is placed around the penis and the air is pumped out of the chamber, creating a vacuum, thereby drawing blood into the penis, resulting in penile engorgement. Tumescence is maintained by placing one or more tension bands around the base of the turgid penis. These bands may be left in situ for as long as 30 minutes and the device may be used every day. Although some patients may find the device cumbersome to use, the successful use of VCD has been reported in erectile dysfunction of organic and mixed etiology,[90] including patients with spinal injuries.[91] Adverse effects associated include pain, caused either by the vacuum or by the constriction band, decreased sensation caused by the band, bruising and obstructed voiding.

The surgical implantation of penile prostheses is the most invasive of the treatment options available and is offered if oral or locally administered pharmacological therapy is ineffective or contraindicated and if VCDs are unsatisfactory or unacceptable. There are two types of implant: two-piece malleable semi-rigid rods and three-piece inflatable penile prostheses. The implants do not affect libido, ejaculation or orgasm, only providing erection adequate for penetration and intercourse,[92,93] but have very limited application in men with MS, whose neurological condition may deteriorate with worsening bladder function requiring intervention and possible erosion of the prosthesis with increasing sacral sensory loss.

WOMEN

An area of current interest, because of its high prevalence but lack of comprehension or adequate definition, is female sexual dysfunction (FSD). The American Foundation of Urological Disease recently classified FSD into four broad categories:[94] sexual desires disorder, arousal disorder, orgasmic disorder and sexual pain disorders, which were then revised and expanded.[95] The need for accurate definitions of symptoms is because appropriate treatment requires attention to specific individual characteristics and category.

Only a few studies have looked at the nature of sexual dysfunction in women with MS. Lilius et al, in a questionnaire study, identified the most common problem as being loss of orgasm,[62] while Valleroy et al, in a similar study, found it to be fatigue.[61] Table 26.6 summarizes the most frequently encountered symptoms relating to FSD in these studies.

The success of sildenafil citrate in treating sexual dysfunction in men with MS led to a placebo-controlled study of its effects in women.[96] Figure 26.7 shows the baseline sexual function of all the women recruited. Their main motivation for joining (and continuing) with the study was impaired orgasmic function. Unfortunately, neither improvement in this aspect of sexual function nor improvement in quality of life could be shown. The only benefit seemed to be a slight but significant increase in vaginal lubrication response in some women, which may be explained by the pharmacological action of sildenafil causing an increase pelvic blood flow and thereby an increase in lubrication.

As with impaired ejaculation and orgasmic function in men, there is no specific treatment for loss of orgasmic response in women. The best management seems to be to encourage the use of sexual aids: vibrating stimuli in particular are known to be helpful in this respect.

There are, of course, many other aspects of sexual dysfunction in MS besides attempting to treat neurological dysfunction pharmacologically. Both men and women may find that fatigue and depression are having an adverse effect and anxiety about incontinence may exacerbate the situation.[97,98] Furthermore, spasticity and loss of sensation can become dominant features with increasing spinal cord disease. Also, the effect of the onset

TABLE 26.6 Most frequently encountered symptoms of female sexual dysfunction in multiple sclerosis	
Study	Symptoms (in decreasing order of frequency)
Lilius et al 1976[62]	Loss of orgasm Loss of libido Spasticity
Valleroy & Kraft 1984[61]	Fatigue Decreased sensation Decreased libido Decreased frequency or loss of orgasm Difficulty in arousal
Hulter & Lundberg 1995[76]	Sensory dysfunction in the genital area Decreased libido Difficulty in achieving orgasm Decreased vaginal lubrication
Zorzon et al 2001[101]	Loss of orgasm Decreased vaginal lubrication Decreased libido Changes in vaginal sensation
Borello-France et al 2004[98]	Dyspareunia Anorgasmia Lack of enjoyment of sexual activities Lack of arousal

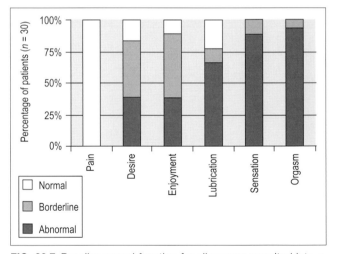

FIG. 26.7 Baseline sexual function for all women recruited into a double blind placebo controlled trial of sildenafil citrate. Reproduced with permission from Dasgupta et al 2004.[96]

of sexual dysfunction on the patient and their partner should also be considered. As a patient with MS becomes more dependent on their partner for care of bodily function, perception of that person as an object of sexual desire may diminish.[99] Sexual difficulties are thought to be a contributing factor to the increased divorce rate among patients with MS.[100]

At MS rehabilitation centers where patients have the opportunity to discuss intimate problems with health-care professionals and one another, psychological support has been shown to be valuable. Many patients are helped by learning how others have overcome or come to live with similar difficulties, and such support is often valuable.

REFERENCES

1. Miller H, Simpson CA, Yeates WK. Bladder dysfunction in multiple sclerosis. Br Med J 1965; 5445: 1265–1269.

2. Kidd D, Thorpe JW, Thompson AJ et al. Spinal cord MRI using multi-array coils and fast spin echo. II. Findings in multiple sclerosis. Neurology 1993; 43: 2632–2637.

3. Nortvedt MW, Riise T, Myhr KM et al. Reduced quality of life among multiple sclerosis patients with sexual disturbance and bladder dysfunction. Mult Scler 2001; 7: 231–235.

4. Fernandez O. Mechanisms and current treatments of urogenital dysfunction in multiple sclerosis. J Neurol 2002; 249: 1–8.

5. Kavia RB, Dasgupta R, Fowler CJ. Functional imaging and the central control of the bladder. J Comp Neurol 2005; 493: 27–32.

6. Athwal BS, Berkley KJ, Hussain I et al. Brain responses to changes in bladder volume and urge to void in healthy men. Brain 2001; 124: 369–377.

7. Matsuura S, Berkley KJ, Hussain I et al. Human brain region response to distention or cold stimulation of the bladder: a positron emission tomography study. J Urol 2002; 168: 2035–2039.

8. Blok BF, Willemsen AT, Holstege G. A PET study on brain control of micturition in humans. Brain 1997; 120: 111–121.

9. Blok BF, Sturms LM, Holstege G. Brain activation during micturition in women. Brain 1998; 121: 2033–2042.

10. Blok BF. Central pathways controlling micturition and urinary continence. Urology 2002; 59(suppl 1): 13–17.

11. Blaivas JG, Barbalias GA. Detrusor-external sphincter dyssynergia in men with multiple sclerosis: an ominous urologic condition. J Urol 1984; 131: 91–94.

12. De Groat WC, Kawatani M, Hisamitsu T et al. Mechanisms underlying the recovery of urinary bladder function following spinal cord injury. J Auton Nerv Syst 1990; 30(suppl): S71–S77.

13. McMahon SB. Sensory-motor integration in urinary bladder function. Prog Brain Res 1986; 67: 245–253.

14. Birder LA, Apodaca G, De Groat WC, Kanai AJ. Adrenergic- and capsaicin-evoked nitric oxide release from urothelium and afferent nerves in urinary bladder. Am J Physiol 1998; 275: F226–F229.

15. Andersson KE, Chapple C, Wein A. The basis for drug treatment of the overactive bladder. World J Urol 2001; 19: 294–298.

16. Nijeholt GJ, van Walderveen MA, Castelijns JA et al. Brain and spinal cord abnormalities in multiple sclerosis. Correlation between MRI parameters, clinical subtypes and symptoms. Brain 1998; 121: 687–697.

17. Kim YH, Goodman C, Omessi E et al. The correlation of urodynamic findings with cranial magnetic resonance imaging findings in multiple sclerosis. J Urol 1998; 159: 972–976.

18. Ukkonen M, Elovaara I, Dastidar P, Tammela TL. Urodynamic findings in primary progressive multiple sclerosis are associated with increased volumes of plaques and atrophy in the central nervous system. Acta Neurol Scand 2004; 109: 100–105.

19. Betts CD, D'Mellow MT, Fowler CJ. Urinary symptoms and the neurological features of bladder dysfunction in multiple sclerosis. J Neurol Neurosurg Psychiatr 1993; 56: 245–250.

20. Yamaguchi O, Shishido K, Tamura K et al. Evaluation of mRNAs encoding muscarinic receptor subtypes in human detrusor muscle. J Urol 1996; 156: 1208–1213.

21. Sigala S, Mirabella G, Peroni A et al. Differential gene expression of cholinergic muscarinic receptor subtypes in male and female normal human urinary bladder. Urology 2002; 60: 719–725.

22. Chess-Williams R, Chapple CR, Yamanishi T et al. The minor population of M3-receptors mediate contraction of human detrusor muscle in vitro. J Auton Pharmacol 2001; 21: 243–248.

23. Harriss DR, Marsh KA, Birmingham AT, Hill SJ. Expression of muscarinic M3-receptors coupled to inositol phospholipid hydrolysis in human detrusor cultured smooth muscle cells. J Urol 1995; 154: 1241–1245.

24. Clemett D, Jarvis B. Tolterodine: a review of its use in the treatment of overactive bladder. Drugs Aging 2001; 18: 277–304.

25. Todorova A, Vonderheid-Guth B, Dimpfel W. Effects of tolterodine, trospium chloride, oxybutynin on the central nervous system. J Clin Pharmacol 2001; 41: 636–644.

26. Kornhuber HH, Schutz A. Efficient treatment of neurogenic bladder disorders in multiple sclerosis with initial intermittent catheterization and ultrasound-controlled training. Eur Neurol 1990; 30: 260–267.

27. Fowler CJ. Investigation of the neurogenic bladder. J Neurol Neurosurg Psychiatr 1996; 60: 6–13.

28. Fowler CJ, van Kerrebroeck PE, Nordenbo A, Van Poppel H. Treatment of lower urinary tract dysfunction in patients with multiple sclerosis. Committee of the European Study Group of SUDIMS (Sexual and Urological Disorders in Multiple Sclerosis). J Neurol Neurosurg Psychiatr 1992; 55: 986–989.

29. Norlen L, Sundin T. α-Adrenolytic treatment in patients with autonomous bladders. Acta Pharmacol Toxicol (Copenh) 1978; 43(suppl 2): 31–34.

30. O'Riordan JI, Doherty C, Javed M et al. Do alpha-blockers have a role in lower urinary tract dysfunction in multiple sclerosis? J Urol 1995; 153: 1114–1146.

31. Schwinn DA. Novel role for alpha1-adrenergic receptor subtypes in lower urinary tract symptoms. BJU Int 2000; 86(suppl 2): 11–20; discussion 20–22.

32. Nathan P. Emptying the paralysed bladder. Lancet 1977; 1: 377.

33. Dasgupta P, Haslam C, Goodwin R, Fowler CJ. The 'Queen Square bladder stimulator': a device for assisting emptying of the neurogenic bladder. Br J Urol 1997; 80: 234–237.

34. Prasad RS, Smith SJ, Wright H. Lower abdominal pressure versus external bladder stimulation to aid bladder emptying in multiple sclerosis: a randomized controlled study. Clin Rehabil 2003; 17: 42–47.

35. Kaplan SA, Chancellor MB, Blaivas JG. Bladder and sphincter behavior in patients with spinal cord lesions. J Urol 1991; 146: 113–117.

36. Barbalias GA, Nikiforidis G, Liatsikos EN. Vesicourethral dysfunction associated with multiple sclerosis: clinical and urodynamic perspectives. J Urol 1998; 160: 106–111.

37. The prevention and management of urinary tract infections among people with spinal cord injuries. National Institute on Disability and Rehabilitation Research consensus statement, January 27–29, 1992. SCI Nurs 1993; 10: 49–61.

38. Kikugawa CA, Cortopassi RF, Ditmer DG, Okamoto WS. Treatment of diabetes insipidus with DDAVP. Am J Hosp Pharm 1977; 34: 1013–1017.

39. Rew DA, Rundle JS. Assessment of the safety of regular DDAVP therapy in primary nocturnal enuresis. Br J Urol 1989; 63: 352–353.

40. Hilton P, Hertogs K, Stanton SL. The use of desmopressin (DDAVP) for nocturia in women with multiple sclerosis. J Neurol Neurosurg Psychiatr 1983; 46: 854–855.

41. Hoverd PA, Fowler CJ. Desmopressin in the treatment of daytime urinary frequency in patients with multiple sclerosis. J Neurol Neurosurg Psychiatr 1998; 65: 778–780.

42. Tubridy N, Addison R, Schon F. Long term use of desmopressin for urinary symptoms in multiple sclerosis. Mult Scler 1999; 5: 416–417.

43. House of Lords Committee on Science and Technology. Cannabis: the scientific and medical evidence (9th report). London: Stationery Office; 1998.

44. Brady CM, DasGupta R, Dalton C et al. An open-label pilot study of cannabis-based extracts for bladder dysfunction in advanced multiple sclerosis. Mult Scler 2004; 10: 425–433.

45. Zajicek J, Fox P, Sanders H et al. Cannabinoids for treatment of spasticity and other symptoms related to multiple sclerosis (CAMS study): multicentre randomised placebo-controlled trial. Lancet 2003; 362: 1517–1526.

46. Freeman R, Adekanmi O, Watfield M et al. The effect of cannabinoids on lower urinary tract symptoms in multiple sclerosis: a randomised placebo controlled trial (CAMS-LUTS study). Neurourol Urodyn 2004; 23: 607 (A149).

47. Fowler CJ, Beck RO, Gerrard S et al. Intravesical capsaicin for treatment of detrusor hyperreflexia. J Neurol Neurosurg Psychiatr 1994; 57: 169–173.

48. De Sèze M, Wiart L, Ferrière J et al. Intravesical instillation of capsaicin in urology: A review of the literature. Eur Urol 1999; 36: 267–277.

49. De Sèze M, Wiart L, de Sèze MP et al. Intravesical capsaicin versus resiniferatoxin for the treatment of detrusor hyperreflexia in spinal cord injured patients: a double-blind, randomized, controlled study. J Urol 2004; 171: 251–255.

50. Appendino G, Szallasi A. Euphorbium: modern research on its active principle, resiniferatoxin, revives an ancient medicine. Life Sci 1997; 60: 681–696.

51. Giannantoni A, Di Stasi SM, Stephen RL et al. Intravesical capsaicin versus resiniferatoxin in patients with detrusor hyperreflexia: a prospective randomized study. J Urol 2002; 167: 1710–1714.

52. Cruz F. Vanilloid receptor and detrusor instability. Urology 2002; 59(suppl 1): 51–60.

399

53. Brady CM, Apostolidis AN, Harper M et al. Parallel changes in bladder suburothelial vanilloid receptor TRPV1 (VR1) and pan-neuronal marker PGP9.5 immunoreactivity in patients with neurogenic detrusor overactivity (NDO) following intravesical resiniferatoxin treatment. BJU Int 2004; 93: 770–776.

54. Schurch B, Stöhrer M, Kramer G, Schmid DM et al. Botulinum-A toxin for treating detrusor hyperreflexia in spinal cord injured patients: a new alternative to anticholinergic drugs? Preliminary results. J Urol 2000; 164: 692–697.

55. Reitz A, Stöhrer M, Kramer G et al. European experience of 200 cases treated with botulinum-A toxin injections into the detrusor muscle for urinary incontinence due to neurogenic detrusor overactivity. Eur Urol 2004; 45: 510–515.

56. Apostolidis A, Dasgupta P, Fowler CJ. Proposed mechanism for the efficacy of injected botulinum toxin in the treatment of human detrusor overactivity. Eur Urol 2006; 49: 644–650.

57. Harper M, Popat RB, Dasgupta R et al. A minimally invasive technique for outpatient local anaesthetic administration of intradetrusor botulinum toxin in intractable detrusor overactivity. BJU Int 2003; 92: 325–326.

58. Kalsi V, Gonzales G, Popat R et al. Botulinum injections for the treatment of bladder symptoms of multiple sclerosis. Ann Neurol 2007; 62: 452–457.

59. Grosse J, Kramer G, Stohrer M. Success of repeat detrusor injections of botulinum a toxin in patients with severe neurogenic detrusor overactivity and incontinence. Eur Urol 2005; 47: 653–959.

60. Barnes DG, Shaw PJ, Timoney AG, Tsokos N. Management of the neuropathic bladder by suprapubic catheterisation. Br J Urol 1993; 72: 169–172.

61. Valleroy ML, Kraft GH. Sexual dysfunction in multiple sclerosis. Arch Phys Med Rehabil 1984; 65: 125–128.

62. Lilius HG, Valtonen EJ, Wikström J. Sexual problems in patients suffering from multiple sclerosis. Scand J Soc Med 1976; 4: 41–44.

63. Kirkeby HJ, Poulsen EU, Petersen T, Dørup J. Erectile dysfunction in multiple sclerosis. Neurology 1988; 38: 1366–1371.

64. Betts CD, Jones SJ, Fowler CG, Fowler CJ. Erectile dysfunction in multiple sclerosis. Associated neurological and neurophysiological deficits, treatment of the condition. Brain 1994; 117: 1303–1310.

65. Bakke A, Myhr KM, Grønning M, Nyland H. Bladder, bowel and sexual dysfunction in patients with multiple sclerosis–a cohort study. Scand J Urol Nephrol Suppl 1996; 179: 61–66.

66. Steers WD, Mallory B, de Groat WC. Electrophysiological study of neural activity in penile nerve of the rat. Am J Physiol 1988; 254: R989–R1000.

67. Courtois FJ, Charvier KF, Leriche A et al. Clinical approach to erectile dysfunction in spinal cord injured men. A review of clinical and experimental data. Paraplegia 1995; 33: 628–635.

68. Sachs BD. Placing erection in context: the reflexogenic-psychogenic dichotomy reconsidered. Neurosci Biobehav Rev 1995; 19: 211–224.

69. Bernabé J, Rampin O, Sachs BD, Giuliano F. Intracavernous pressure during erection in rats: an integrative approach based on telemetric recording. Am J Physiol 1999; 276: R441–R449.

70. Schmid DM, Hauri D, Schurch B. Nocturnal penile tumescence and rigidity (NPTR) findings in spinal cord injured men with erectile dysfunction. Int J Impot Res 2004; 16: 433–440.

71. Muller R. Studies on disseminated multiple sclerosis. Acta Med Scand 1949; 222: 67–71.

72. Vas CJ. Sexual impotence and some autonomic disturbances in men with multiple sclerosis. Acta Neurol Scand 1969; 45: 166–182.

73. Witt MA, Grantmyre JE. Ejaculatory failure. World J Urol 1993; 11: 89–95.

74. Levin RJ. VIP, vagina, clitoral and periurethral glans–an update on human female genital arousal. Exp Clin Endocrinol 1991; 98: 61–69.

75. Mattson D, Petrie M, Srivastava DK, McDermott M. Multiple sclerosis. Sexual dysfunction and its response to medications. Arch Neurol 1995; 52: 862–868.

76. Hulter BM, Lundberg PO. Sexual function in women with advanced multiple sclerosis. J Neurol Neurosurg Psychiatr 1995; 59: 83–86.

77. Fowler C, Miller JR, Sharief MK et al. A double blind, randomised study of sildenafil citrate for erectile dysfunction in men with multiple sclerosis. J Neurol Neurosurg Psychiatry 2005; 76: 700–705.

78. Dinsmore W. Treatment of erectile dysfunction. Int J STD AIDS 2004; 15: 215–221.

79. Rotella DP. Phosphodiesterase 5 inhibitors: current status and potential applications. Nat Rev Drug Discov 2002; 1: 674–682.

80. Webb DJ, Muirhead GJ, Wulff M et al. Sildenafil citrate potentiates the hypotensive effects of nitric oxide donor drugs in male patients with stable angina. J Am Coll Cardiol 2000; 36: 25–31.

81. Rosen RC, McKenna KE. PDE-5 inhibition and sexual response: pharmacological mechanisms and clinical outcomes. Annu Rev Sex Res 2002; 13: 36–88.

82. Gupta M, Kovar A, Meibohm B. The clinical pharmacokinetics of phosphodiesterase-5 inhibitors for erectile dysfunction. J Clin Pharmacol 2005; 45: 987–1003.

83. Riley A, Goodman RE, Kellett JM, Orr R. Double-blind trial of yohimbine hydrochloride in treatment of erectile inadequacy. J Sex Marital Ther 1989; 4: 14–26.

84. Tam SW, Worcel M, Wyllie M. Yohimbine: a clinical review. Pharmacol Ther 2001; 91: 215–243.

85. Altwein JE, Keuler FU. Oral treatment of erectile dysfunction with apomorphine SL. Urol Int 2001; 67: 257–263.

86. DasGupta R, Fowler CJ. Bladder, bowel and sexual dysfunction in multiple sclerosis: management strategies. Drugs 2003; 63: 153–166.

87. Bella AJ, Brock GB. Intracavernous pharmacotherapy for erectile dysfunction. Endocrine 2004; 23: 149–155.

88. Guay AT, Perez JB, Velásquez E et al. Clinical experience with intraurethral alprostadil (MUSE) in the treatment of men with erectile dysfunction. A retrospective study. Medicated urethral system for erection. Eur Urol 2000; 38: 671–676.

89. Fulgham PF, Cochran JS, Denman JL et al. Disappointing initial results with transurethral alprostadil for erectile dysfunction in a urology practice setting. J Urol 1998; 160: 2041–2046.

90. Vrijhof HJ, Delaere KP. Vacuum constriction devices in erectile dysfunction: acceptance and effectiveness in patients with impotence of organic or mixed aetiology. Br J Urol 1994; 74: 102–105.

91. Chancellor MB, Rivas DA, Panzer DE et al. Prospective comparison of topical minoxidil to vacuum constriction device and intracorporeal papaverine injection in treatment of erectile dysfunction due to spinal cord injury. Urology 1994; 43: 365–369.

92. Goldstein I, Newman L, Baum N et al. Safety and efficacy outcome of mentor alpha-1 inflatable penile prosthesis implantation for impotence treatment. J Urol 1997; 157: 833–839.

93. Carson CC. Penile prostheses: are they still relevant? BJU Int 2003; 91: 176–177.

94. Basson R, et al. Report of the international consensus development conference on female sexual dysfunction: definitions and classifications. J Urol 2000; 163: 888–893.

95. Basson R, Berman J, Burnett A et al. Definitions of women's sexual dysfunction reconsidered: advocating expansion and revision. J Psychosom Obstet Gynaecol 2003; 24: 221–229.

96. Dasgupta R, Wiseman OJ, Kanabar G et al. Efficacy of sildenafil in the treatment of female sexual dysfunction due to multiple sclerosis. J Urol 2004; 171: 1189–1193; discussion 1193.

97. Zivadinov R, Zorzon M, Bosco A et al. Sexual dysfunction in multiple sclerosis: II. Correlation analysis. Mult Scler 1999; 5: 428–431.

98. Borello-France D, Leng W, O'Leary M et al. Bladder and sexual function among women with multiple sclerosis. Mult Scler 2004; 10: 455–461.

99. Woollett S, Edelmann R. Marital satisfaction in individuals with multiple sclerosis and their partners; its interactive effect with life satisfaction, social networks and disability. Sex Marital Ther 1988; 3: 191–196.

100. Morales-Gonzalés JM, Benito-León J, Rivera-Navarro J et al. A systematic approach to analyse health-related quality of life in multiple sclerosis: the GEDMA study. Mult Scler 2004; 10: 47–54.

101. Zorzon M, Zivadinov R, Monti Bragadin L et al. Sexual dysfunction in multiple sclerosis: a 2-year follow-up study. J Neurol Sci 2001; 187: 1–5.

Neuropsychological aspects of multiple sclerosis

H. A. Wishart, R. H. B. Benedict and S. M. Rao

INTRODUCTION

Quantitative studies of cognition in multiple sclerosis (MS) emerged in the middle of the 20th century.[1–3] These early investigations set the stage for several decades of research that has yielded a reasonably clear characterization of neuropsychological function associated with the disease. Recent research directions target the neuroimaging, genetics and treatment of cognitive dysfunction. This chapter provides an overview of the neuropsychology of MS.

COGNITION IN MULTIPLE SCLEROSIS

The cognitive abilities most often affected by MS include episodic memory, working memory and speed of processing. These aspects of cognitive functioning are interrelated and neuropsychological tests often assess more than one ability or domain at a time. Abilities that tend to be less affected include attention span, semantic memory and language. The point prevalence of cognitive impairment in MS is estimated to be between 40% and 65%, depending on sampling procedures and other methodological factors.[4–6] However, there is considerable interindividual variation in the neuropsychological presentation of MS patients. For example, the MS Collaborative Research Group identified six distinct cognitive profiles among patients with relapsing MS entering a trial of interferon-β1a.[7] The largest subgroup, which included 34% of the sample, was cognitively intact. Only 2% showed global cognitive impairment across multiple cognitive domains. The remainder showed circumscribed deficits in two or three cognitive domains (Fig. 27.1). Standardized neuropsychological testing is therefore applied routinely in some settings so that an individual's specific impairments can be delineated.[8] Neuropsychological testing in MS predicts activities of daily living such as driving,[9,10] employment,[8,11] success in rehabilitation[12] and social skills.[13–15] It is a potentially useful procedure for early identification of deficits that can affect functional outcomes and for monitoring disease progression.

EPISODIC MEMORY

Episodic memory is defined as memory for events or information acquired in a particular temporal or spatial context.[16] Epi-sodic memory refers to the conscious recollection of previous experiences and is distinct from the recollection of general or semantic knowledge.[17] The neural substrate of episodic memory is thought to include a broadly distributed circuitry of prefrontal and medial temporal regions, including the hippocampus, entorhinal cortex, perirhinal cortex, parahippocampal complex and amygdala.[18,19] Cognitive processes associated with episodic memory include novelty detection, encoding, consolidation and retrieval.

Neuropsychological tests of memory typically involve the presentation of novel stimuli that are recalled by patients via oral or written response. Both the sensory modality (auditory, visual) and processing modality (e.g. verbal, spatial, pictorial, facial) of test stimuli vary across tests. Procedures commonly used to assess learning and memory in MS include verbal list learning tests such as the California Verbal Learning Test II,[20] the Rey Auditory Verbal Learning Test and the Buschke Selective Reminding Test.[21] These tests all involve multiple successive presentations of a relatively lengthy word list, one that is beyond the immediate recall span (i.e. supraspan). Patients are asked to recall the words in any order, and various qualitative aspects of their approach to the task can be measured, along with the overall accuracy of recall and rate of learning. Cueing and recognition formats are used to assess the extent to which difficulties in recall appear to be due to problems encoding the information into memory versus retrieving information once encoded.

Deficits on tests of new learning and recent memory are consistently reported in the MS literature, as summarized in several review articles.[6,22–26] A meta-analytical review showed an overall effect size (d) of 0.705 for long-term episodic memory in MS.[25] This translates to a downward shift of the mean by approximately three-quarters of a standard deviation unit in the MS group. Although useful as estimates of group differences, effect size statistics provide no direct indication of frequencies of impairment of a given severity in MS samples. In a community-based study of 100 patients, 22–31% showed impairment on one or more measures of episodic memory.[4] In this study, impairment was defined as performing below the fifth percentile of the healthy control group. Of the 31 patients who showed deficits in multiple-trial learning, approximately half were

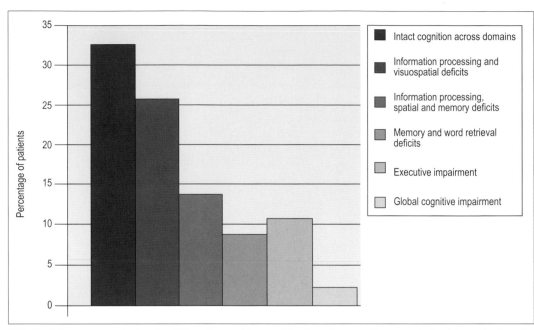

FIG. 27.1 Percentage of relapsing MS patients with cognitive impairments. Data are derived from the baseline neuropsychological assessment of patients entering a clinical trial of interferon β-1a.[7]

impaired on both verbal and visual indices while the remaining patients were impaired on only one. This study highlights the fact that, while episodic memory is often affected in MS, the nature and degree of impairment shows significant interindividual variability.

It is unclear whether the memory deficit in MS arises mainly at the stage of encoding new information into memory or at the retrieval stage, although to some extent this appears to depend on the context or manner in which learning and memory are assessed[25,27–29] One study of new learning in MS demonstrated that patients recalled less information after the first stimulus presentation and benefited less from repeated exposures. However, patients retained information once encoded into memory almost as well as controls.[27] Research has also demonstrated retrieval-based memory deficits in MS.[28] Ongoing research on the issue has potential implications for designing appropriate treatments. For example, studies have demonstrated that use of active learning strategies during encoding improves recall, suggesting a potential avenue for intervention.[30,31]

WORKING MEMORY

Working memory has been defined as a dedicated cognitive system for temporarily maintaining and manipulating a limited amount of information. Working memory supports thought processes by bridging perception, long-term memory and action.[32] It is thought to be fundamental to many human cognitive operations, including language comprehension, problem-solving and long-term memory.[33–35] Current models of working memory include a central executive and an episodic buffer that serve to apportion limited attentional resources to separate verbal and nonverbal processing subsystems.[33,34,36] Working memory is thought to have broadly distributed neural circuitry. Prefrontal, parietal and cingulate regions are prominently involved, possibly with greater left hemispheric representation for verbal processing and greater right hemispheric representation for spatial information processing.[18,37,38]

In Thornton and Raz's meta-analytic review of memory in MS, the overall effect size for working memory was 0.72, similar to the magnitude of effect seen for long-term episodic memory.

The Paced Auditory Serial Addition Test (PASAT),[39] which was included in the working memory domain in the meta-analysis, is part of several recommended batteries for the assessment of patients with MS, including the MS Functional Composite[40] and the Minimal Assessment of Cognitive Function in MS (MACFIMS).[22] The PASAT involves the presentation of a prerecorded series of single-digit numbers that the patient is asked to add together in successive pairs. The task requires constant monitoring and updating of incoming information to guide responding, key aspects of working memory. In the community-based study of patients with MS mentioned above,[4] 22–25% performed below the fifth percentile on the PASAT. Other tests of working memory also showed deficits in a sizeable minority of the sample.[4]

SPEED OF PROCESSING

Slowed cognitive processing is widely recognized as a common deficit in MS. It is thought to be independent of slowed motor responding and may underlie other cognitive impairments.[27,41]

Attempts have been made to determine the extent to which processing speed is related to or separate from other cognitive aspects of the disease. After removing variance in neuropsychological test performance related to demographic variables, fatigue and depression, one study showed that the only neuropsychological variable differentiating patients and controls was speed of processing.[42] Another study indicated that impairment of processing speed was more frequent than impairment of working memory in patients with MS.[43] This study employed the Working Memory and Processing Speed indices of the Wechsler Memory Scale III, which were designed to provide relatively independent measures of these constructs.[44] However, a number of neuropsychological tests assessing processing speed make multiple cognitive demands. A good example is the PASAT, which requires several cognitive processes, including working memory, mathematical skills and auditory-verbal processing, in addition to rapid processing.

A measure of information processing speed commonly used in the assessment of patients with MS is the Symbol Digit Modalities Test.[45] This test starts with the visual presentation

SECTION 3

and explanation of a 'key' that contains a short series of symbols, each of which has a corresponding single-digit number. The patient is then provided with a long series of the same symbols in random order and instructed to supply the digit that corresponds to each symbol by referring to the key. The number of correct responses supplied within the time limit can be compared for written and oral responding, yielding an indication of the extent to which slowed hand motor function affects the results. The oral subtest of the Symbol Digit Modalities Test is recommended for use in the neuropsychological assessment of patients with MS as part of the MACFIMS[22] and correlates well with indices of structural brain involvement, particularly central atrophy, in MS.[46]

EXECUTIVE FUNCTION

Executive function encompasses various facets of goal-directed activities, such as the formulation of goals and hypotheses, and initiation, execution, monitoring and alteration of problem-solving strategies and behaviors. Abstract reasoning and conceptualization are key aspects of higher executive functioning. Executive functions are integral to other cognitive operations, such as using organizational strategies to enhance learning and recall. Frontal cortex and associated cortical and subcortical systems figure prominently in models of the neural basis of executive function and dysfunction.[47–49]

Neuropsychological tests sensitive to executive impairment in MS include the Wisconsin Card Sorting Test, the Stroop Color–Word Interference Test and the Trail-Making Test, among others.[4,21,50] These tests all make demands on mental flexibility in one form or another, e.g. the ability to change behavior in response to feedback, the ability to inhibit a prepotent or over-learned response to a stimulus and substitute a novel response, or the ability to switch between two prepotent response patterns. These tests also make distinct cognitive demands, including concept formation, rapid information processing and verbal processing, and comparisons among tests can yield useful information as to the nature of the underlying cognitive deficit.

The Free Sorting condition of the Sorting Test of the Delis–Kaplan Executive Function System (D-KEFS)[50] is included in the MACFIMS.[22] The Free Sorting condition involves the presentation of a set of six cards displaying a combination of verbal and visuospatial stimuli that the patient is asked to sort into categories with three cards per category. Numerous sorting principles are possible, and the scoring is based on the number of correct sorts obtained as well as other aspects of performance. A Sort Recognition condition is also available that allows the examiner to assess the extent to which the patient can recognize sorting principles s/he may not initiate independently. In a recent study comparing the D-KEFS Free Sorting condition to the Wisconsin Card Sorting Test, both tests were sensitive to MS and both correlated with lesion load and brain atrophy as measured with MRI. The Free Sorting condition was sensitive to MS after controlling for depression, while the Wisconsin Card Sorting Test was not.[51]

VISUAL/SPATIAL PROCESSING

Domains of visual/spatial processing include perceptual, spatial and constructional abilities.[48] Visuoperceptual functions can be divided according to stimulus type, including objects, faces and spatial/motion information. A ventral occipitotemporal pathway is thought to be associated with object recognition, whereas a dorsal occipitoparietal pathway is thought to be associated with processing of spatial information.[18] Perception of faces, like objects, is thought to involve the ventral pathway, but with a more right-hemispheric lateralization.[18]

While assessment of visual perception requires only that the patient make a verbal or gestural response, testing of spatial/constructional ability typically requires manual dexterity. Neuropsychological assessments often include a combination of tests and testing formats to help determine the extent to which perceptual, motor and processing speed requirements contribute to performance on tests of spatial/constructional ability. Neuropsychological tests of visual perceptual, spatial and constructional ability that can be used in the assessment of MS include the Hooper Visual Organization Test,[52] the Judgment of Line Orientation Test,[53] the Perceptual-Organizational subtests of the Wechsler Adult Intelligence Scale III[54] and tests of copying, drawing and three-dimensional construction.[21]

In the community-based sample of patients with MS mentioned above, approximately 12–19% performed below the fifth percentile of controls on tests of visual perceptual ability.[4] Reduced visual/spatial processing ability has been observed independently of basic visual impairment in MS[55] and in patients with mild[56] or mild to moderate disease.[57]

LANGUAGE AND RELATED DOMAINS

Classic aphasias, alexias, agraphias and apraxias, typically seen in the setting of specific focal lesions, are rarely reported in the MS literature.[24] However, aspects of language, semantic memory and related cognitive domains can be affected by the disease.

Tests of word retrieval appear to be more sensitive to MS than naming tests,[26] probably because of the rapid processing and executive demands. Some 22% of patients in the community-based sample showed impairment of controlled oral word association, whereas 9% showed impairment of picture naming; 9% also showed impairment of speech comprehension.[4] Deficits in interhemispheric transfer have been reported in patients with MS[26] and there have been case reports of lateralized deficits in naming, praxis, reading and writing similar to those seen in callosal syndromes.[58,59] Tests commonly used to assess language domains include the Controlled Oral Word Association Test, sometimes referred to as a verbal fluency test,[21,50] the Boston Naming Test[60] and measures of speech comprehension, writing and reading.[21]

Semantic memory refers to general knowledge – or ideas, words and symbols – typically shared by members of a culture. Semantic memory is closely associated with language functioning and is distinguished from episodic memory on the basis of context-dependency. Remembering the meaning of a word or retrieving a fact from semantic memory does not require retrieval of information regarding the context in which that information was learned. Some studies have observed semantic memory to be intact in MS[61,62] but others suggest that it can be affected in terms of storage or retrieval or both.[63–65] Overall, semantic memory has received relatively little research attention in the MS literature compared to more basic naming, word retrieval and speech comprehension functions, and remains an area deserving of further careful investigation.

META-COGNITION AND SELF-REPORTS OF COGNITIVE IMPAIRMENT

Multiple sclerosis patients' self-reports of their memory functioning tend to correlate only modestly with measures of objective memory performance.[66–68] A number of factors may contribute to the discrepancy.[69,70] MS patients with depression, for instance, may underestimate their level of cognitive functioning[66,67,69,71] (but see Marrie et al 2005[72]). Patients with deficits in rapid information processing, attention or other cognitive domains may misattribute their cognitive difficulties to memory impairment. The issue is further complicated as deficits in these other cognitive domains may also affect memory processing.[70] Presumably the changes in brain structure and activity associated with MS can affect patients' ability to appraise their own cognition, although this has received little or no direct investigation. A recent study suggested that the relationship between objective cognitive testing and self-reported cognition may be nonlinear, with either intact or very impaired cognition being associated with fewer cognitive complaints.[72]

One study specifically examined sources of patient/informant discrepancies in reported cognition on the MS Neuropsychological Questionnaire (MSNQ).[73] Patients who overestimated their level of cognitive impairment relative to informants were distinguishable from underestimators on a number of cognitive, personality and neuropsychiatric variables. Those who overestimated their cognition tended to be less depressed and less conscientious, and to have greater cognitive impairment, higher degrees of euphoric behavioral disinhibition and higher frequencies of unemployment relative to those who underestimated their cognition.

A helpful target for intervention may be to assist patients in forming a realistic appraisal of the nature and extent of their cognitive problems. In some cases, collateral reports have been found to equal or exceed patients' self-reports of cognitive functioning in terms of accuracy.[66,67,70,71,74] Overall, assessments of both the patients' and collaterals' impressions are an important part of the neuropsychological assessment. Patient and observer reports of neuropsychological disorders provide a context for test interpretation and treatment planning.

MOOD AND FATIGUE

Emotional problems and fatigue are significantly more common in individuals with MS than in the general population.[75] Neuropsychiatric aspects of MS are covered elsewhere and will be mentioned only briefly in the context of the neuropsychological examination.

Potential effects of mood and fatigue on cognition warrant attention when conducting the neuropsychological evaluation. Depression has been reported to affect cognitive test performance in the areas of rapid information processing, working memory and executive function in MS.[76–78] Subjective reports of fatigue do not necessarily correlate with observable deficits in cognitive function. However, available studies suggest that measurable performance decrements thought to be attributable to fatigue occur during sustained mental effort and after completion of cognitively challenging tasks.[79,80]

While further study is important, it is reasonable to anticipate that patients' performance may be compromised if they are significantly depressed or tired during testing. A more direct and valid assessment of cognition may be obtained if patients can be effectively treated for clinically significant emotional disorders prior to testing. It is important to document effects of fatigue on performance and, when appropriate, simple steps should be taken to minimize fatigue during testing (e.g. scheduling breaks). This may improve the likelihood that patients' maximal cognitive performance is observed.

LONGITUDINAL CHANGE PATTERNS IN COGNITION

Longitudinal change patterns of cognition in MS are not well understood. There are few studies, each with unique methodological aspects, making it difficult to combine findings to construct an overall picture of the trajectory of deficits. The typical duration of follow-up has been short compared to the overall duration of the disease. In addition, many patients take dis-

ease-modifying medications, some of which may affect the course of cognitive deficits.[81] The available literature does suggest, however, that once cognitive impairment manifests in patients with MS, it poses a risk for further cognitive deterioration. In addition, with sufficiently long follow-up periods impairment emerges in some of those unaffected initially.[82–84] Patients in whom cognitive impairment has been detected therefore warrant close clinical follow-up and consideration of treatment options. A care plan that incorporates longitudinal assessment is important whether deficits are manifest at baseline or not.

INDIVIDUAL DIFFERENCES IN COGNITION IN MULTIPLE SCLEROSIS: RELATIONS WITH DEMOGRAPHICS, DISEASE-RELATED VARIABLES AND NEUROIMAGING

DEMOGRAPHIC AND DISEASE-RELATED VARIABLES AND COGNITION

It is unclear whether age and sex help to explain some of the interindividual variance in cognition in patients with MS. A meta-analytic study of neuropsychological research in MS demonstrated a differentially adverse effect of increasing age in patients relative to controls on one measure, the Controlled Oral Word Association Test.[85] Another study showed a differential effect of sex in patients versus controls on tests of memory and visuospatial construction.[86]

Level of neurological disability, as measured with the Expanded Disability Status Scale (EDSS[87]), has generally been found to relate only modestly to cognition in MS (for review, see Feinstein 2005,[88] but see also Lynch et al 2005[89]). This may be due in part to the fact that the EDSS focuses on neurological signs and symptoms rather than cognition. Variations in cognitive performance have been reported as a function of disease subtype,[85,90,91] with several studies demonstrating better cognition in patients with relapsing–remitting MS than with progressive forms of the disease.[92–95] Because disease subtype can be correlated with other demographic and disease variables, specific effects of subtype can be difficult to dissociate, and it has been suggested that it is the underlying brain changes that matter more.[88]

A number of studies have demonstrated no relationship between duration of disease and extent of cognitive impairment[89,96–98] (but see Achiron 2004[99]). Cognitive changes can occur early in the course of the disease[100] and it is possible that some patients experience disease-related cognitive changes prior to the occurrence of a first clinical event that leads to evaluation and diagnosis. The effect of acute exacerbations on cognition has received relatively little research attention. Studies often deliberately exclude patients who are experiencing an exacerbation or taking steroid medication that might influence the test results.

Overall, demographic and disease-related variables appear to be relatively weak or inconsistent predictors of cognition in MS, and differentiating independent effects of these often-related variables can be difficult.

NEUROIMAGING AND COGNITION

Lesion volume

Compared to demographic and disease variables, neuroimaging indices correlate relatively well with cognition in MS. Several studies have demonstrated an inverse relation between cognitive performance and number or volume of lesions on conventional MRI, including T2-weighted or fluid-attenuated inversion recovery (FLAIR) imaging.[101–105] (for review, see Rovaris and Filippi 2000[106]). Lesion number is an imprecise measure: lesions of different size, location and orientation contribute equally to the count. Although more precise, volume measures also do not distinguish confluence, shape and tissue properties of lesions. New quantification techniques are therefore needed to better characterize the effects of lesions on cognition in MS.

Regionally specific relations between lesion volume and cognition have been reported. For example, one study showed specific relations between left frontal lobe involvement and word retrieval, memory and abstract reasoning, and between left parieto-occipital involvement and verbal learning and integration of visuospatial information.[107] Other studies have also demonstrated specific relations, particularly between frontal lesion burden and cognition.[13,106,108,109] However, some of these studies have shown that total lesion volume is at least as good a predictor as the regional measures,[106,108] suggesting that it is the extent and not necessarily the location of damage that affects the nature and severity of cognitive problems in MS.

Although overall lesion volume on conventional imaging correlates at a statistically significant level with cognition, the percentage of variance accounted for is relatively modest. At least two factors may contribute to this: the relative nonspecificity of conventional scanning and its failure to assess changes in nonlesional tissue. Conventional T2-weighted and FLAIR imaging are sensitive to MS lesions but they are fairly nonspecific with respect to underlying pathophysiological processes such as edema, inflammation, demyelination and neuronal loss.[106] Although these different processes may contribute differentially to cognition in MS, they cannot readily be distinguished on the basis of conventional imaging. T1-weighted imaging does add sensitivity and specificity to areas of severe tissue disruption or cell death called black holes, but the relation between T1 hypointensities and cognition remains to be more fully examined.[106,110,111] Changes are known to occur in nonlesional or 'normal-appearing brain tissue' (see below) outside the lesions that can be seen on conventional imaging.[106] Therefore conventional imaging used in isolation gives an incomplete picture of the neural changes in MS and their relationship to cognitive dysfunction.

Brain atrophy

Brain atrophy can be quantified in a number of ways, including measures of whole brain volume and central volume. One common measure of whole brain atrophy is brain parenchymal fraction, which is based on the ratio of the total volume of the gray and white matter compartments to the total volume of the gray, white and cerebrospinal fluid compartments. Various measures of ventricular size are used as indirect indicators of central atrophy. For example, bicaudate ratio can be measured as the minimum intercaudate distance divided by brain width at the same level.[110,112]

Recent studies suggest that measures of central atrophy correlate better with cognition than do measures of global brain atrophy. For example, one study showed a significant relation between a measure of central atrophy and performance on the Symbol Digit Modalities Test, a measure of processing speed and working memory.[110] In a regression model incorporating measures of central atrophy, whole brain atrophy and lesion volume, only bicaudate ratio emerged as a significant predictor of cognition. Another study examined central atrophy, lesion volume and two magnetic resonance spectroscopy (MRS) indices in relation to performance on a brief battery of neuropsychological tests.[113] The strongest predictor of cognition was the measure of central atrophy, accounting for approximately half of the variance in overall cognitive performance. The test bearing the greatest relation to MRI was the Symbol Digit Modalities Test.

A third study examined measures of T1 hypointensities, FLAIR lesion volume, bicaudate ratio, third ventricle width and brain parenchymal fraction in relation to performance on tests from the MACFIMS.[114] Third ventricle width, followed by brain parenchymal fraction, were the top predictors of cognitive performance on measures of speed of information processing and memory. Again, it was the Symbol Digit Modalities Test that was most strongly related to brain imaging. Longitudinal studies have shown a relation between progressive brain atrophy and cognitive changes patterns in MS.[115,116]

Voxel-based measures may contribute to ascertaining effects of regional tissue changes on cognition in MS. Voxel-based morphometry (VBM) uses statistical parametric mapping procedures, similar to those employed for analysis of functional neuroimaging data, to assess regional volume and density of brain tissue compartments on a voxel-by-voxel basis.[117,118] Unlike manual segmentation of selected structures, VBM is a fully automated procedure for examining signal intensities across the entire brain relative to an a priori threshold and therefore provides an unbiased and comprehensive measure. Recent VBM research indicated a specific reduction of gray matter volume in the thalamus bilaterally in patients with mild to moderate relapsing–remitting MS relative to controls. Thalamic atrophy was directly related to processing speed and executive impairment, even after adjusting for intracranial volume, brain parenchymal fraction and FLAIR lesion volume.[119,120]

Recent research also indicates the importance of normalized measures of regional brain atrophy[121] as predictors of cognitive dysfunction in MS. Specific relations have been demonstrated between frontal atrophy and deficits in executive function, working memory and recall consistency, and between lateralized temporal atrophy and verbal and nonverbal memory.[122,123] Tested against regional measures, central and global atrophy measures were the primary predictors of processing speed.[122] Overall, measures of atrophy, including central, regional and whole brain measures, emerge as strong correlates of cognition in MS.[46,119,120,122,123]

Changes within lesions and in normal-appearing brain tissue

Imaging modalities sensitive to changes in the tissue properties within T2-defined lesions and in normal-appearing brain tissue include magnetization transfer imaging (MTI), diffusion tensor imaging (DTI) and MRS.[124–128] Low magnetization transfer ratios, thought to indicate myelin or axonal membrane damage,[129] have been shown to relate to extent of cognitive impairment in MS,[111,130,131] even early in the course of the disease.[100] In one study, MTI appeared to outperform measures of both global and central atrophy in predicting cognition.[100] Decreased axonal integrity, as assessed using N-acetyl-aspartate levels, has also been shown to relate to deficits in cognition, including working memory, episodic memory and executive function.[132–134] MTI, DTI and MRS show promise for elucidating the neural basis of cognitive deficits in MS, including tissue changes in lesional and nonlesional tissue.

Brain activity

Functional MRI (fMRI) shows altered patterns of brain activity in patients with MS relative to healthy controls. Studies have shown altered activation patterns during cognitive, motor, and visual task performance.[135] Regional increases and decreases in signal intensity during task performance have been reported, as well as local spatial expansion of activity and additional proximal and distal activation. The additional activity has been posited to play an adaptive or compensatory role, helping to support a higher level of ability than might otherwise be the case.

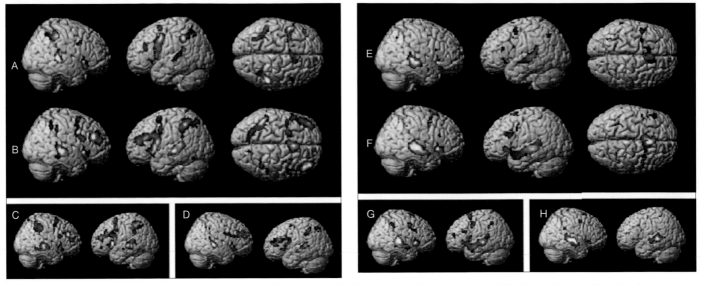

FIG. 27.2 Brain activation patterns associated with working memory (**A–D**) and episodic memory recall (**E–H**) in patients with relapsing–remitting MS. For each cognitive domain, the top panel (**A,E**) shows the brain activation patterns for healthy controls and the middle panel (**B,F**) shows the pattern for the patients as a group. At the bottom, activity in patients with intact fMRI task performance is shown on the left (**C,G**) and in those with abnormal task performance on the right (**D,H**). Note that it is the patients with intact task performance who show additional brain activity relative to controls. Adapted with permission from Mainero et al 2004.[136]

A number of potential confounds that could lead to altered patterns of brain activity have been investigated. One study directly addressed whether differences between patients and controls in accuracy of fMRI task performance could account for altered activation patterns in patients with MS.[136] Patients whose task performance was intact showed additional brain activity during working and episodic memory probes relative to controls, whereas this effect was less apparent in patients with impaired task performance (Fig. 27.2). These results are consistent with the compensatory hypothesis.

Findings from fMRI research in MS have several potential implications. If the additional brain activity serves a compensatory role, fMRI may account for a proportion of the variance in cognition (and other symptoms) not attributable to structural brain involvement on MRI. In addition, the presence of additional brain activity may have prognostic significance[137] and preliminary evidence suggests that it is sensitive to treatment effects in MS[138] and other disorders.[139,140] Further research is needed to determine whether and in what way fMRI will merit a role in the clinical monitoring of patients with MS, and in the evaluation of outcome in clinical trials.

Genetics, cognition and imaging

Research is just beginning on genetic predictors of individual differences in cognition in MS. Apolipoprotein E genotype, an important predictor of brain response to insult,[141,142] has been found to relate to disability and progression in some[143,144] but not all[145] MS studies. Presence of the ε4 allele has been shown to predict cognition[146] and structural neuroimaging variables, including brain atrophy,[147,148] axonal injury[149] and T1 hypointensities in MS.[148] Neuroimaging has good objectivity and sensitivity to neural changes in MS, and may offer new insights into disease-modifying genes.[150] Other potential disease-modifying genes have received less empirical attention in MS, despite the strong likelihood that multiple genes act in concert in this regard.[150,151] Further genetic investigations, including examination of gene–gene and gene–environment interactions, will be important next steps in elucidating mechanisms of cognitive dysfunction, brain structural changes and possible com-

pensatory responses, as well as disease progression and treatment outcome.

Summary

Structural and functional MRI studies are shedding new light on the neural underpinnings of cognitive impairment in MS. Multimodal structural approaches appear promising, especially those that incorporate measures of brain atrophy in addition to volumetric lesion analysis and imaging of tissue properties in lesional and nonlesional tissue. Future work encompassing both structural and functional measures of brain integrity may yield an even closer correspondence between imaging and cognition in this disease and help to refine imaging as a biomarker for MS-related cognitive disorders. Incorporation of genotype data may help to further explain individual differences in cognition. A combined imaging-genetics approach may ultimately be useful for stratifying patients in clinical trials of cognition-enhancing agents in MS and for improving monitoring and prognostic accuracy in clinical practice.

ASSESSMENT OF COGNITION IN MULTIPLE SCLEROSIS

SCREENING FOR NEUROPSYCHOLOGICAL IMPAIRMENT IN MULTIPLE SCLEROSIS

The main purpose of screening tools is to identify, with good sensitivity and specificity, individuals in need of further assessment and treatment for a given problem.[8] Screening tools should be brief and cost-effective so they can be applied broadly in the population in question to identify at-risk individuals. A number of cognitive screening and assessment tools have been designed specifically to identify MS patients at risk for neuropsychological impairment.

The MS Neuropsychological Screening Questionnaire (MSNQ) is a 15-item self- and informant-report inventory designed to provide a cost-effective means of identifying MS patients who would benefit from further cognitive assessment.[66]

TABLE 27.1 MS Neuropsychological Screening Questionnaire: abbreviated descriptions of items[66]

Is easily distracted
Loses focus when listening
Problem-solving is slow
Has trouble describing programs recently watched
Forgets appointments
Forgets what he or she has read
Needs instructions repeated
Needs reminders to do tasks
Forgets errands
Has difficulty answering questions
Has difficulty tracking two things at once
Misses the point of conversations
Has difficulty controlling impulses
Laughs or cries with little cause
Talks excessively

TABLE 27.2 Minimal Assessment of Cognitive Function in MS (MACFIMS) battery[22]

Learning and memory	California Verbal Learning Test, 2nd ed. Brief Visuospatial Memory Test – Revised
Processing speed and working memory	Paced Auditory Serial Addition Test Symbol Digit Modalities Test
Generative verbal fluency	Controlled Oral Word Association Test
Visual/spatial perception	Benton Judgment of Line Orientation Test
Executive function	Delis-Kaplan Executive Function System Sorting Test[22]

The items cover a range of cognitive domains, including attention, memory and language, and are rated on a five-point scale according to the frequency and severity of the problem (Table 27.1). The MSNQ can be administered in conjunction with brief depression screening tests to assess for both cognitive and emotional problems. In one study, elevated scores on the self-report version of the MSNQ were found to occur in the context of depression or cognitive impairment, while elevated scores on the informant version were more specifically indicative of cognitive impairment.[66] These findings underscore the relevance of mood screening and informant ratings to the interpretation of patient ratings on the MSNQ.

MS FUNCTIONAL COMPOSITE

The MS Functional Composite (MSFC) is a measure of MS-related disability designed to remedy some of the short-comings of previously available clinical outcome measures, such as the EDSS.[40] The EDSS has several limitations, one of which is that it weights physical impairment (e.g. ambulation) at the expense of other symptoms.[40] The MSFC includes a measure of ambulation as well as a peg-placing task to assess hand and arm function and the PASAT (described above) as a measure of cognition. One potential disadvantage of the MSFC is that it is vulnerable to practice effects, so improvement in the MSFC score cannot be interpreted directly as an improvement in clinical status.[40,152] This issue could be addressed through the use of reliable change statistics in clinical practice.[153] In clinical trials, relative change in the treatment arms can be compared.

BRIEF NEUROPSYCHOLOGICAL BATTERIES FOR MULTIPLE SCLEROSIS

A number of brief or screening neuropsychological batteries have been designed specifically for the MS population, including the Neuropsychological Screening Battery,[154] the Screening Examination for Cognitive Impairment,[155] the Brief Repeatable Battery and the Neuropsychological Screening Battery for MS.[4]

The MACFIMS[22,156] was designed to cover all major cognitive domains affected in MS in a face-to-face testing time of approximately 90 minutes (Table 27.2). The MACFIMS includes a minimal core battery of tests and recommendations for tests to further assess areas of impairment or answer specific referral questions. Results of the MACFIMS or other brief batteries can be used to guide decisions regarding appropriate follow-up, including comprehensive neuropsychological examination, psychiatric assessment, intervention for cognitive problems, occupational therapy, speech therapy or other medical treatment.[8] Because of its emphasis on psychometric standards and alternate test forms, the MACFIMS is useful for routine monitoring of cognitive function after a baseline examination and for repeat assessments in clinical trials.

COMPREHENSIVE NEUROPSYCHOLOGICAL ASSESSMENT IN MULTIPLE SCLEROSIS

Comprehensive neuropsychological assessment in MS typically entails 3–4 hours of testing, with a focus on domains most often affected by the disease. The assessment can provide detailed baseline and follow-up data as well as information that pertains to complex matters such as differential diagnosis (e.g. MS dementia versus Alzheimer's disease in an elderly patient), guidance for rehabilitation, vocational counseling or other therapies, or determination of disability status. The core flexible battery used at Dartmouth incorporates the MSFC and most of the MACFIMS, as well as additional testing to provide detailed information in specific areas (Table 27.3). Testing is modified as needed to suit individual referral questions and needs. Such a battery facilitates comparisons with the literature and collaboration with other centers.

METHODOLOGICAL FACTORS ASSOCIATED WITH REPEAT NEUROPSYCHOLOGICAL TESTING

Repeat administration of neuropsychological tests may lead to improvements in scores due to familiarity with specific test stimuli or with general test-taking principles and strategies rather than true changes in underlying abilities. Tests particularly vulnerable to practice effects include those with rapid processing demands, unfamiliar stimuli and novel response patterns.[48] These are among the tests most sensitive to MS, and neuropsychologists therefore use various means to minimize practice effects. Alternative forms eliminate practice effects related to repeat exposure to specific stimuli but not those related to general familiarity with testing procedures.[7,48] Reliable change statistics address both, as well as psychometric sources of variability such as statistical regression to the mean. Reliable change statistics, however, require longitudinal normative data on the basis of which to discriminate practice or psychometric changes from actual improvement or decline in cognition.[153] Such data are

TABLE 27.3 Sample comprehensive neuropsychological testing for multiple sclerosis

MS Functional Composite
    Ambulation Index
    Nine Hole Pegboard
    PASAT (3 & 2 second trials; Circle one: Form A or B)

Information & Orientation (WMS III)
Logical Memory I (WMS III)

BVMT-R Trials 1–3 (Form:__)
    D-KEFS Trail-Making Test
    Single Double Simultaneous Stimulation (HRNTB)
    Symbol Digit Modalities Test (Written, Oral)
    Thumb–Finger Sequencing Test

Logical Memory II
BVMT-R Delayed and Recognition (Copy optional)
Beck Depression Inventory II
MS Neuropsychological Questionnaire (Self, MSNQ)
Wechsler Adult Intelligence Scale-III (selected subtests)
CVLT II, Learning, Immediate (Circle One: Form Standard or Alternate)
Finger Tapping Test (HRNTB)
Grooved Pegboard Test
CVLT II, Delayed & Recognition
D-KEFS Verbal Fluency (Circle One: Standard or Alternate)
Boston Naming Test (BDAE)
Sentence Comprehension (BDAE)
WRAT 4 Reading
Wisconsin Card Sorting Test
State-Trait Anxiety Inventory (Form Y)
Perceived Deficits Questionnaire (MSQLI)
Profile of Mood States
Self-report inventories:
Hand Dominance Test
Fatigue Severity Scale
Memory Self-Rating Scale
Background Questionnaire and ADL Scale
Informant inventories:
Perceived Deficits Questionnaire (MSQLI)
MSNQ (Informant Version)

Questionnaires are completed within the week prior to the appointment. References for published tests: Beck Depression Inventory II,[177] Boston Diagnostic Aphasia Examination, 3rd ed. (BDAE),[178] Brief Visuospatial Memory Test – Revised (BVMT-R),[179] California Verbal Learning Test II (CVLT II),[20] Delis-Kaplan Executive Function System (D-KEFS),[50] Fatigue Severity Scale,[180] Grooved Pegboard Test,[21,181] Halstead–Reitan Neuropsychological Test Battery for Adults (HRNTB),[21,182] Memory Self-Rating Scale,[183] MS Functional Composite,[40] MS Neuropsychological Questionnaire (MSNQ),[67] MS Quality of Life Inventory (MSQLI),[184] Profile of Mood States,[185] State–Trait Anxiety Inventory (Form Y),[186] Symbol Digit Modalities Test.[45] Wechsler Adult Intelligence Scale III,[44] Wechsler Memory Scale III (WMS III),[54] Wide Range Achievement Test 4 (WRAT 4),[187] Wisconsin Card Sorting Test.[188,189]

currently available only for a subset of neuropsychological tests and time intervals. Practice effects may differ between patients and controls so, ideally, normative longitudinal data with multiple time points would be available for groups of MS patients stratified by relevant variables. The placebo arms of clinical trials and other longitudinal studies can provide some relevant data. It is essential for the clinician to engage in repeat testing judiciously, employ available alternative forms and reliable change data as appropriate, and be vigilant for differences among tests in susceptibility to practice effects. In clinical trials, statistical comparison between treatment arms provides an effective control for both practice and psychometric changes in test scores, provided baseline cognition does not differ between groups.

TREATMENT OF COGNITIVE PROBLEMS IN MULTIPLE SCLEROSIS

Treatment of cognitive problems in MS has received relatively little clinical or empirical attention in the past. However, recent years have seen the emergence of studies of both pharmacological and nonpharmacological interventions.[157]

Prevention of cognitive impairment in MS is an important target of therapy. Disease-modifying medications have been shown to decrease relapse rates and MRI indicators of disease progression.[158–160] Disease-modifying medications may also have a beneficial effect on cognition, and research is just beginning to assess this.[81,161,162]

Cholinergic enhancement may also help cognition in MS. Early studies of physostigmine indicated limited usefulness because of side effects.[163,164] Donepezil has been tested in two open-label studies.[165,166] More recently, a randomized, placebo-controlled study demonstrated a modest but statistically significant benefit of donepezil on memory test performance in MS.[167] Preliminary fMRI data suggest a normalization of brain activation patterns after a single dose of rivastigmine in MS.[138] These initial findings suggest the promise of further evaluating cholinergic enhancement strategies in the management of cognitive deficits in MS.[157] It may also be helpful to minimize the use of medications with anticholinergic effects, such as bladder-control medications.[168]

Other pharmacological strategies have also been attempted for the treatment of cognitive problems in MS, but with little success.[169] Initial results of trials of 4-aminopyridine,[170] amantadine[171,172] and pemoline[171] were not promising (for reviews see Doraiswamy and Rao 2004[157] and Krupp and Rizvi 2002[173]).

Nonpharmacological treatment for cognitive impairment in MS, variously described as cognitive retraining, cognitive remediation or cognitive rehabilitation, among other labels, includes three main approaches: 1) restorative therapies that aim to improve specific abilities, 2) compensatory approaches that aim to circumvent cognitive problems through the use of cognitive strategies and 3) adaptive approaches that aim to circumvent cognitive problems through the use of external aids and modifications.[161] Compared to other disorders such as traumatic brain injury or stroke, relatively little research has examined nonpharmacological treatment of cognitive problems in MS and the observed outcomes are variable. One problem is that cognitively intact patients have been included in the studies. In future, it will be beneficial to enroll only those patients who have the cognitive problems that the study interventions are designed to treat. Recent studies have begun to assess interventions designed to improve targeted aspects of learning and memory in MS.[30,31,174] It is also important that interventions be designed to improve more than just performance on the training task, and that the generalizability of any improvements be assessed across time, testing method and context.

It is also useful to detect and treat co-morbidities such as depression and fatigue that can influence cognition and quality of life.[161,162,175] Standard pharmacological approaches to the treatment of depression are thought to be effective in MS, especially when combined with psychotherapy.[176] Cognitive–behavioral counseling based in neuropsychological principles has been

SECTION 3

shown to reduce behavioral problems in cognitively impaired patients with MS. An intervention specifically designed to improve insight and social skills, for example, led to a reduction in disinhibition and social aggressiveness compared to standard psychological counseling.[14]

Ultimately, a multidisciplinary approach to the treatment of cognitive problems in MS will probably be maximally effective. Such an approach might ideally incorporate planned systematic longitudinal screening and assessment of cognition and related disorders, informed selection of treatment from an array of pharmacological and nonpharmacological methods, as appropriate, and the use of outcome measurements that allow treatment regimens to be tailored to individual patients' needs, contexts and response to treatment over time.

FUTURE DIRECTIONS

Neuropsychological research over the past 50 years or more has delineated a reasonably clear profile of the cognitive deficits most commonly observed in patients with MS. The domains most often affected include episodic memory, working memory and speed of processing. There is considerable interindividual variability; approximately half of patients show little or no cognitive impairment and other individuals may show deficits in only two or three areas of cognition. Cognitive screening tools and brief batteries have been developed to assist in the detection of deficits in the clinical setting.

A major question for future research is how to prevent and treat the cognitive deficits associated with MS. Improved understanding of their neurobiological basis will assist in this regard, as will development of imaging biomarkers for cognition. Longitudinal studies have shown that the progression of cognitive impairment in MS is variable and that relatively long follow-up periods may be necessary to detect change or response to treatment. Imaging biomarkers, such as fMRI of cognition, could provide an earlier indication of treatment response, although this requires investigation. Widespread adoption of standard cognitive testing and advanced imaging protocols, and development of multicenter treatment studies, would also speed the process of evaluating treatments. Aside from obvious demographic and disease variables, various additional factors deserve consideration for exclusion or stratification in clinical trials for cognitive intervention; these factors include disease-modifying medications, cognition-enhancing drugs and medications with anticholinergic, stimulant, sedative or other psychoactive properties. Patients should be included who have the deficits for which the treatment is designed. Pharmacogenetics may also come to play an important role in the selection of treatment in MS, including interventions for cognitive deficits. An individually tailored, multidisciplinary approach to the treatment of cognitive deficits in MS may ultimately prove most effective.

REFERENCES

1. Canter AH. Direct and indirect measures of psychological deficit in multiple sclerosis. J Gen Psychol 1951; 44: 3–50.
2. Fink SL, Houser HB. An investigation of physical and intellectual changes in multiple sclerosis. Arch Phys Med Rehabil 1966; 47: 56–61.
3. Ivnik RJ. Neuropsychological stability in multiple sclerosis. J Consult Clin Psychol 1978; 46: 913–923.
4. Rao SM, Leo GJ, Bernardin L, Unverzagt F. Cognitive dysfunction in multiple sclerosis. I. Frequency, patterns, and prediction. Neurology 1991; 41: 685–691.
5. Bobholz JA, Rao SM. Cognitive dysfunction in multiple sclerosis: a review of recent developments. Curr Opin Neurol 2003; 16: 283–288.
6. Rao SM. Neuropsychology of multiple sclerosis. Curr Opin Neurol 1995; 8: 216–220.
7. Fischer JS. Assessment of neuropsychological function. In: Rudick RA, Goodkin DE, eds. Multiple sclerosis therapeutics. New York: Martin Dunitz; 1999.
8. Benedict RHB. Integrating cognitive function screening and assessment into the routine care of multiple sclerosis patients. CNS Spectr 2005; 10: 384–391.
9. Schultheis MT, Garay E, DeLuca J. The influence of cognitive impairment on driving performance in multiple sclerosis. Neurology 2001; 56: 1089–1094.
10. Schultheis MT, Garay E, DeLuca J. Motor vehicle crashes and violations among drivers with multiple sclerosis. Arch Phys Med Rehabil 2002; 83: 1175–1178.
11. Rao SM, Leo GJ, Ellington L et al. Cognitive dysfunction in multiple sclerosis. II. Impact on employment and social functioning. Neurology 1991; 41: 692–696.

12. Langdon DW, Thompson AJ. Multiple sclerosis: a preliminary study of selected variables affecting rehabilitation outcome. Mult Scler 1999; 5: 94–100.
13. Arnett PA, Rao SM, Bernardin L et al. Relationship between frontal lobe lesions and Wisconsin Card Sorting Test performance in patients with multiple sclerosis. Neurology 1994; 44: 420–425.
14. Benedict RHB, Shapiro A, Priore R et al. Neuropsychological counseling improves social behavior in cognitively-impaired multiple sclerosis patients. Mult Scler 2000; 6: 391–396.
15. Knight RG, Devereux RC, Godfrey HP. Psychosocial consequences of caring for a spouse with multiple sclerosis. J Clin Exp Neuropsychol 1997; 19: 7–19.
16. Tulving E, Donaldson W. The organization of memory. New York: Academic Press; 1972.
17. Tulving E, Markowitsch HJ. Episodic and declarative memory: role of the hippocampus. Hippocampus 1998; 8: 198–204.
18. Cabeza R, Nyberg L. Imaging cognition II: An empirical review of 275 PET and fMRI studies. J Cogn Neurosci 2000; 12: 1–47.
19. Desgranges B, Baron JC, Eustache F. The functional neuroanatomy of episodic memory: The role of the frontal lobes, the hippocampal formation, and other areas. NeuroImage 1998; 8: 198–213.
20. Delis DC, Kramer JH, Kaplin E, Ober BA. California Verbal Learning Test – second edition: adult version manual. San Antonio, TX: Psychological Corporation; 2000.
21. Spreen O, Strauss E. A compendium of neuropsychological tests: administration, norms, and commentary. New York: Oxford University Press; 1998.
22. Benedict RHB, Fischer JS, Archibald CJ et al. Minimal neuropsychological assessment

of MS patients: a consensus approach. Clin Neuropsychol 2002; 16: 381–397.
23. Brassington JC, Marsh NV. Neuropsychological aspects of multiple sclerosis. Neuropsychol Rev 1998; 8: 43–77.
24. Rao S. Neuropsychology of multiple sclerosis: a critical review. J Clin Exp Neuropsychol 1986; 8: 503–542.
25. Thornton AE, Raz N. Memory impairment in multiple sclerosis: a quantitative review. Neuropsychology 1997; 11: 357–66.
26. Wishart HA, Sharpe D. Neuropsychological aspects of multiple sclerosis: a quantitative review. J Clin Exp Neuropsychol 1997; 19: 810–824.
27. DeLuca J, Barbieri-Berger S, Johnson SK. The nature of memory impairments in multiple sclerosis: acquisition versus retrieval. J Clin Exp Neuropsychol 1994; 16: 183–189.
28. Rao SM, Leo GJ, St Aubin-Faubert P. On the nature of memory disturbance in multiple sclerosis. J Clin Exp Neuropsychol 1989; 11: 699–712.
29. Thornton AE, Raz N, Tucke KA. Memory in multiple sclerosis: contextual encoding deficits. J Int Neuropsychol Soc 2002; 8: 395–409.
30. Chiaravalloti ND, DeLuca J. Self-generation as a means of maximizing learning in multiple sclerosis: an application of the generation effect. Arch Phys Med Rehabil 2002; 83: 1070–1079.
31. Chiaravalloti ND, DeLuca J, Moore NB, Ricker JH. Treating learning impairments improves memory performance in multiple sclerosis: a randomized clinical trial. Mult Scler 2005; 11: 58–68.
32. Baddeley A. Working memory: looking back and looking forward. Nat Rev Neurosci 2003; 4: 829–839.

33. Baddeley A. Working memory. In: Gazzaniga MS, ed. The cognitive neurosciences. Cambridge, MA: MIT Press; 1995.

34. Baddeley A. Recent developments in working memory. Curr Opin Neurobiol 1998; 8: 234–238.

35. Mencl WE, Pugh KR, Shaywitz SE et al. Network analysis of brain activations in working memory: behavior and age relationships. Microsc Res Tech 2000; 51: 64–74.

36. Baddeley AD. Is working memory still working? Am Psychol 2001; 56: 851–64.

37. D'Esposito M, Aguirre GK, Zarahn E et al. Functional MRI studies of spatial and nonspatial working memory. Cogn Brain Res 1998; 7: 1–13.

38. Wager TD, Smith EE. Neuroimaging studies of working memory: a meta-analysis. Cogn Affect Behav Neurosci 2003; 3: 255–274.

39. Rao SM, Leo GJ, Haughton VM et al. Correlation of magnetic resonance imaging with neuropsychological testing in multiple sclerosis. Neurology 1989; 39: 161–166.

40. Fischer JS, Rudick RA, Cutter GR, Reingold SC. The Multiple Sclerosis Functional Composite Measure (MSFC): an integrated approach to MS clinical outcome assessment. National MS Society Clinical Outcomes Assessment Task Force. Mult Scler 1999; 5: 244–250.

41. Rao SM, St Aubin-Faubert P, Leo GJ. Information processing speed in patients with multiple sclerosis. J Clin Exp Neuropsychol 1989; 11: 471–477.

42. Denney DR, Lynch SG, Parmenter BA, Horne N. Cognitive impairment in relapsing and primary progressive multiple sclerosis: mostly a matter of speed. J Int Neuropsychol Soc 2004; 10: 948–956.

43. DeLuca J, Chelune GJ, Tulsky DS et al. Is speed of processing or working memory the primary information processing deficit in multiple sclerosis? J Clin Exp Neuropsychol 2004; 26: 550–562.

44. Wechsler D. Wechsler Adult Intelligence Scale, 3rd ed. Administration and scoring manual. San Antonio, TX: Psychological Corporation; 1997.

45. Smith A. Symbol Digit Modalities Test. Los Angeles, CA: Western Psychological Services; 1991.

46. Benedict RHB, Carone DA, Bakshi R. Correlating brain atrophy with cognitive dysfunction, mood disturbances, and personality disorder in multiple sclerosis. J Neuroimaging 2004; 14(suppl): 36S–45S.

47. Elliott R. Executive functions and their disorders. Br Med Bull 2003; 65: 49–59.

48. Lezak MD. Neuropsychological assessment. New York: Oxford University Press; 1995.

49. Stuss DT, Alexander MP. Executive functions and the frontal lobes: a conceptual view. Psychol Res 2000; 63: 289–298.

50. Delis D, Kaplan E. Delis–Kaplan Executive Function System. San Antonio, TX: Psychological Corporation; 2001.

51. Parmenter B, Zivadinov R, Kerenyi L et al. Validity of the Wisconsin Card Sorting and Delis–Kaplan Executive Function System (DKEFS) Sorting Tests in multiple sclerosis. J Clin Exp Neuropsychol 2007; 29: 215–223.

52. Hooper HE. The Hooper Visual Organization Test. Beverly Hills, CA: Western Psychological Services; 1958.

53. Benton AL et al. Contributions to neuropsychological assessment: a clinical manual. New York: Oxford University Press; 1994.

54. Wechsler D. Wechsler Memory Scale, 3rd ed. WMS-III administration and scoring manual. San Antonio, TX: Psychological Corporation; 1997.

55. Vleugels L, Lafosse C, van Nunen A et al. Visuoperceptual impairment in MS patients: nature and possible neural origins. Mult Scler 2001; 7: 389–401.

56. Van den Burg W, van Zomeren AH, Minderhoud JM et al. Cognitive impairment in patients with multiple sclerosis and mild physical disability. Arch Neurol 1987; 44: 494–501.

57. Ryan L, Clark C, Klonoff H et al. Patterns of cognitive impairment in relapsing-remitting multiple sclerosis and their relationship to neuropathology on magnetic resonance images. Neuropsychology 1996; 10: 176–193.

58. Mao-Draayer Y, Panitch H. Alexia without agraphia in multiple sclerosis: case report with magnetic resonance imaging localization. Mult Scler 2004; 10: 705–707.

59. Okuda B, Tanaka H, Tachibana H et al. Visual form agnosia in multiple sclerosis. Acta Neurol Scand 1996; 94: 38–44.

60. Kaplan E, Goodglass H, Weintraub S. Boston Naming Test. Boston, MA: Lea & Febiger; 1983.

61. Jennekens-Schinkel A, Lanser JB, van der Velde EA, Sanders EA. Performances of multiple sclerosis patients in tasks requiring language and visuoconstruction. Assessment of outpatients in quiescent disease stages. J Neurol Sci 1990; 95: 89–103.

62. Pijpers-Kooiman MJ, van der Velde EA, Jennekens-Schinkel A. Retrieval from semantic memory may be normal in multiple sclerosis patients: a study of free word association. J Neurol Sci 1995; 132: 65–70.

63. Beatty WW, Goodkin DE, Monson N et al. Anterograde and retrograde amnesia in patients with chronic progressive multiple sclerosis. Arch Neurol 1988; 45: 611–619.

64. Beatty WW, Monson N, Goodkin DE. Access to semantic memory in Parkinson's disease and multiple sclerosis. J Geriatr Psychiatr Neurol 1989; 2: 153–162.

65. Laatu S, Hämäläinen P, Revonsuo A et al. Semantic memory deficit in multiple sclerosis; impaired understanding of conceptual meanings. J Neurol Sci 1999; 162: 152–161.

66. Benedict RHB, Cox D, Thompson LL et al. Reliable screening for neuropsychological impairment in multiple sclerosis. Mult Scler 2004; 10: 675–678.

67. Benedict RHB, Munschauer F, Linn R et al. Screening for multiple sclerosis cognitive impairment using a self-administered 15-item questionnaire. Mult Scler 2003; 9: 95–101.

68. Christodoulou C, Melville P, Scherl WF et al. Perceived cognitive dysfunction and observed neuropsychological performance: longitudinal relation in persons with multiple sclerosis. J Int Neuropsychol Soc 2005; 11: 614–619.

69. Randolph JJ, Arnett PA, Freske P. Metamemory in multiple sclerosis: exploring affective and executive contributors. Arch Clin Neuropsychol 2004; 19: 259–279.

70. Randolph JJ, Arnett PA, Higginson CI. Metamemory and tested cognitive functioning in multiple sclerosis. Clin Neuropsychol 2001; 15: 357–368.

71. Benedict RHB, Zivadinov R. Predicting neuropsychological abnormalities in multiple sclerosis. J Neurol Sci 2006; 245: 67–72.

72. Marrie RA, Chelune GJ, Miller DM, Cohen JA. Subjective cognitive complaints relate to mild impairment of cognition in multiple sclerosis. Mult Scler 2005; 11: 69–75.

73. Carone DA, Benedict RH, Munschauer FE et al. Interpreting patient/informant discrepancies of reported cognitive symptoms in MS. J Int Neuropsychol Soc 2005; 11: 574–583.

74. Taylor R. Relationships between cognitive test performance and everyday cognitive difficultues in multiple sclerosis. Br J Clin Psychol 1990; 29: 251–253.

75. Joy JE, Johnston RB. Multiple sclerosis: current status and strategies for the future. Washington, DC: National Academy Press; 2001.

76. Arnett PA, Higginson CI, Voss WD et al. Depression in multiple sclerosis: relationship to working memory capacity. Neuropsychology 1999; 13: 546–556.

77. Arnett PA, Higginson CI, Voss WD et al. Depressed mood in multiple sclerosis: relationship to capacity-demanding memory and attentional functioning. Neuropsychology 1999; 13: 434–446.

78. Arnett PA, Higginson CI, Randolph JJ. Depression in multiple sclerosis: relationship to planning ability. J Int Neuropsychol Soc 2001; 7: 665–674.

79. Krupp LB, Elkins LE. Fatigue and declines in cognitive functioning in multiple sclerosis. Neurology 2000; 55: 934–939.

80. Schwid SR, Tyler CM, Scheid EA et al. Cognitive fatigue during a test requiring sustained attention: a pilot study. Mult Scler 2003; 9: 503–508.

81. Fischer JS, Priore RL, Jacobs LD et al. Neuropsychological effects of interferon beta-1a in relapsing multiple sclerosis. Ann Neurol 2000; 48: 885–892.

82. Amato MP, Ponziani G, Siracusa G, Sorbi S. Cognitive dysfunction in early-onset multiple sclerosis: a reappraisal after 10 years. Arch Neurol 2001; 58: 1602–1606.

83. Camp SJ, Stevenson VL, Thompson AJ et al. A longitudinal study of cognition in primary progressive multiple sclerosis. Brain 2005; 128: 2891–2898.

84. Kujala P, Portin R, Ruutiainen J. The progress of cognitive decline in multiple sclerosis. A controlled 3-year follow-up. Brain 1997; 120: 289–297.

85. Zakzanis KK. Distinct neurocognitive profiles in multiple sclerosis subtypes. Arch Clin Neuropsychol 2000; 15: 115–136.

86. Beatty WW, Aupperle RL. Sex differences in cognitive impairment in multiple sclerosis. Clin Neuropsychol 2002; 16: 472–480.

87. Kurtzke JF. Rating neurologic impairment in multiple sclerosis: An expanded disability status scale (EDSS). Neurology 1983; 33: 1444–1452.

88. Feinstein A. The clinical neuropsychiatry of multiple sclerosis. CNS Spectr 2005; 10: 362.

89. Lynch SG, Parmenter BA, Denney DR. The association between cognitive impairment and physical disability in multiple sclerosis. Mult Scler 2005; 11: 469–476.

90. Comi G, Filippi M, Martinelli V et al. Brain MRI correlates of cognitive impairment in primary and secondary progressive multiple sclerosis. J Neurol Sci 1995; 132: 222–227.

91. Foong J, Rozewicz L, Chong WK et al. A comparison of neuropsychological deficits in primary and secondary progressive multiple sclerosis. J Neurol 2000; 247: 97–101.

92. De Sonneville LM, Boringa JB, Reuling IE et al. Information processing characteristics in subtypes of multiple sclerosis. Neuropsychologia 2002; 40: 1751–1765.

93. Gaudino EA, Chiaravalloti ND, DeLuca J, Diamond BJ. A comparison of memory performance in relapsing-remitting, primary progressive and secondary progressive, multiple sclerosis. Neuropsychiatry Neuropsychol Behav Neurol 2001; 14: 32–44.

94. Heaton RK, Nelson LM, Thompson DS et al. Neuropsychological findings in relapsing–remitting and chronic-progressive multiple sclerosis. J Consult Clin Psychol 1985; 53: 103–110.

95. Rao SM, Hammeke TA, Speech TJ. Wisconsin Card Sorting Test performance in relapsing-remitting and chronic-progressive multiple sclerosis. J Consult Clin Psychol 1987; 55: 263–265.

96. Beatty WW, Goodkin DE, Hertsgaard D, Monson N. Clinical and demographic predictors of cognitive performance in multiple sclerosis. Do diagnostic type, disease duration, and disability matter? Arch Neurol 1990; 47: 305–308.

97. Ivnik RJ. Neuropsychological test performance as a function of the duration of MS-related symptomatology. J Clin Psychiatr 1978; 39: 304–307.

98. Rao SM, Hammeke TA, McQuillen MP et al. Memory disturbance in chronic progressive multiple sclerosis. Arch Neurol 1984; 41: 625–631.

99. Achiron A. Predicting the course of relapsing remitting MS using longitudinal disability curves. J Neurol 2004; 251(suppl 5): V65–V68.

100. Deloire MS, Salort E, Bonnet M et al. Cognitive impairment as marker of diffuse brain abnormalities in early relapsing remitting multiple sclerosis. J Neurol Neurosurg Psychiatr 2005; 76: 519–526.

101. Lazeron RH, Langdon DW, Filippi M et al. Neuropsychological impairment in multiple sclerosis patients: the role of (juxta)cortical lesion on FLAIR. Mult Scler 2000; 6: 280–285.

102. Moriarty DM, Blackshaw AJ, Talbot PR et al. Memory dysfunction in multiple sclerosis corresponds to juxtacortical lesion load on fast fluid-attenuated inversion-recovery MR images. Am J Neuroradiol 1999; 20: 1956–1962.

103. Randolph J, Wishart H, Saykin AJ et al. FLAIR lesion volume in multiple sclerosis: relation to processing speed and verbal memory. J Int Neuropsychol Soc 2005; 11: 205–209.

104. Rao SM, Leo GJ, Haughton VM et al. Correlation of magnetic resonance imaging with neurological testing in multiple sclerosis. Neurology 1989; 39: 161–166.

105. Rovaris M, Filippi M, Minicucci L et al. Cortical/subcortical disease burden and cognitive impairment in patients with multiple sclerosis. Am J Neuroradiol 2000; 21: 402–408.

106. Rovaris M, Filippi M. MRI correlates of cognitive dysfunction in multiple sclerosis patients. J Neurovirol 2000; 6(suppl 2): S172–S175.

107. Swirsky-Sacchetti T, Mitchell DR, Seward J et al. Neuropsychological and structural brain lesions in multiple sclerosis: a regional analysis. Neurology 1992; 42: 1291–1295.

108. Foong J, Rozewicz L, Quaghebeur G et al. Executive function in multiple sclerosis. The role of frontal lobe pathology. Brain 1997; 120: 15–26.

109. Sperling RA, Guttmann CR, Hohol MJ et al. Regional magnetic resonance imaging lesion burden and cognitive function in multiple sclerosis: a longitudinal study. Arch Neurol 2001; 58: 115–121.

110. Bermel RA, Bakshi R, Tjoa C et al. Bicaudate ratio as a magnetic resonance imaging marker of brain atrophy in multiple sclerosis. Arch Neurol 2002; 59: 275–280.

111. Rovaris M, Filippi M, Falautano M et al. Relation between MR abnormalities and patterns of cognitive impairment in multiple sclerosis. Neurology 1998; 50: 1601–1608.

112. Bermel, RA, Bakshi, R. The measurement and clinical relevance of brain atrophy in multiple sclerosis. Lancet Neurol 2006; 5: 158–170.

113. Christodoulou C, Krupp LB, Liang Z et al. Cognitive performance and MR markers of cerebral injury in cognitively impaired MS patients. Neurology 2003; 60: 1793–1798.

114. Benedict RHB, Weinstock-Guttman B, Fishman I et al. Prediction of neuropsychological impairment in multiple sclerosis: comparison of conventional magnetic resonance imaging measures of atrophy and lesion burden. Arch Neurol 2004; 61: 226–230.

115. Hohol MJ, Guttmann CR, Orav J et al. Serial neuropsychological assessment and magnetic resonance imaging analysis in multiple sclerosis. Arch Neurol 1997; 54: 1018–1025.

116. Zivadinov R, Sepcic J, Nasuelli D et al. A longitudinal study of brain atrophy and cognitive disturbances in the early phase of relapsing-remitting multiple sclerosis. J Neurol Neurosurg Psychiatr 2001; 70: 773–780.

117. Ashburner J, Friston KF. Voxel-based morphometry-The methods. NeuroImage 2000; 11: 805–821.

118. Ashburner J, Friston KJ. Why voxel-based morphometry should be used. Neuroimage 2001; 14: 1238–1243.

119. McDonald BC, Wishart HA, et al. Thalamic atrophy predicts cognitive functioning in relapsing-remitting MS. Presented at the 34th Annual Meeting of the International Neuropsychological Society, Boston, MA; 2006.

120. McDonald BC, Wishart HA, Saykin AJ et al. Cognitive impairment in MS is related to thalamic atrophy. 2007; under review.

121. Zivadinov R, Locatelli L, Stival B et al. Normalized regional brain atrophy measurements in multiple sclerosis. Neuroradiology 2003; 45: 793–798.

122. Benedict RHB, Zivadinov R, Carone DA et al. Regional lobar atrophy predicts memory impairment in multiple sclerosis. Am J Neuroradiol 2005; 26: 1824–1831.

123. Locatelli L, Zivadinov R, Grop A, Zorzon M. Frontal parenchymal atrophy measures in multiple sclerosis. Mult Scler 2004; 10: 562–568.

124. Arnold DL, Wolinsky JS, Matthews PM, Falini A. The use of magnetic resonance spectroscopy in the evaluation of the natural history of multiple sclerosis. J Neurol Neurosurg Psychiatr 1998; 64(suppl 1): S94–S101.

125. Bammer R, Augustin M, Strasser-Fuchs S et al. Magnetic resonance diffusion tensor imaging for characterizing diffuse and focal white matter abnormalities in multiple sclerosis. Magn Reson Med 2000; 44: 583–591.

126. Ciccarelli O, Werring DJ, Wheeler-Kingshott CA et al. Investigation of MS normal-appearing brain using diffusion tensor MRI with clinical correlations. Neurology 2001; 56: 926–933.

127. Filippi M, Rocca MA. Magnetization transfer magnetic resonance imaging in the assessment of neurological diseases. J Neuroimaging 2004; 14: 303–313.

128. Werring DJ, Clark CA, Barker GJ et al. Diffusion tensor imaging of lesions and normal-appearing white matter in multiple sclerosis. Neurology 1999; 52: 1626–1632.

129. McGowan JC, Filippi M, Campi A, Grossman RI. Magnetisation transfer imaging: theory and application to multiple sclerosis. J Neurol Neurosurg Psychiatr 1998; 64(suppl): S66–S69.

130. Filippi M, Tortorella C, Rovaris M et al. Changes in the normal appearing brain tissue and cognitive impairment in multiple sclerosis. J Neurol Neurosurg Psychiatr 2000; 68: 157–161.

131. Van Buchem MA, Grossman RI, Armstrong C et al. Correlation of volumetric magnetization transfer imaging with clinical data in MS. Neurology 1998; 50: 1609–1617.

132. Foong J, Rozewicz L, Davie CA et al. Correlates of executive function in multiple sclerosis: the use of magnetic resonance spectroscopy as an index of focal pathology. J Neuropsychiatr Clin Neurosci 1999; 11: 45–50.

133. Pan JW, Krupp LB, Elkins LE, Coyle PK. Cognitive dysfunction lateralizes with NAA in multiple sclerosis. Appl Neuropsychol 2001; 8: 155–160.

134. Staffen W, Zauner H, Mair A et al. Magnetic resonance spectroscopy of memory and frontal brain region in early multiple sclerosis. J Neuropsychiatr Clin Neurosci 2005; 17: 357–363.

135. Filippi M. Linking structural, metabolic and functional changes in multiple sclerosis. Eur J Neurol 2001; 8: 291–297.

136. Mainero C, Caramia F, Pozzilli C et al. fMRI evidence of brain reorganization during attention and memory tasks in multiple sclerosis. NeuroImage 2004; 21: 858–867.

137. Rocca MA, Mezzapesa DM, Ghezzi A et al. A widespread pattern of cortical activations in patients at presentation with clinically isolated symptoms is associated with evolution to definite multiple sclerosis. Am J Neuroradiol 2005; 26: 1136–1139.

CHAPTER 27

138. Parry AM, Scott RB, Palace J et al. Potentially adaptive functional changes in cognitive processing for patients with multiple sclerosis and their acute modulation by rivastigmine. Brain 2003; 126: 2750–2760.

139. Rombouts SA, Barkhof F, Van Meel CS, Scheltens P. Alterations in brain activation during cholinergic enhancement with rivastigmine in Alzheimer's disease. J Neurol Neurosurg Psychiatr 2002; 73: 665–671.

140. Saykin AJ, Wishart HA, Rabin LA et al. Cholinergic enhancement of frontal lobe activity in Mild Cognitive Impairment. Brain 2004; 127: 1574–1583.

141. Waters RJ, Nicoll JA. Genetic influences on outcome following acute neurological insults. Curr Opin Crit Care 2005; 11: 105–110.

142. Wright AF. Neurogenetics II: complex disorders. J Neurol Neurosurg Psychiatr 2005; 76: 623–631.

143. Chapman J, Sylantiev C, Nisipeanu P, Korczyn AD. Preliminary observations on APOE ε4 allele and progression of disability in multiple sclerosis. Arch Neurol 1999; 56: 1484–1487.

144. Chapman J, Vinokurov S, Achiron A et al. APOE genotype is a major predictor of long-term progression of disability in MS. Neurology 2001; 56: 312–316.

145. Zakrzewska-Pniewska B, Styczynska M, Podlecka A et al. Association of apolipoprotein E and myeloperoxidase genotypes to clinical course of familial and sporadic multiple sclerosis. Mult Scler 2004; 10: 266–271.

146. Oliveri RL, Cittadella R, Sibilia G et al. APOE and risk of cognitive impairment in multiple sclerosis. Acta Neurol Scand 1999; 100: 290–295.

147. De Stefano N, Bartolozzi ML, Nacmias B et al. Influence of apolipoprotein E ε4 genotype on brain tissue integrity in relapsing-remitting multiple sclerosis. Arch Neurol 2004; 61: 536–540.

148. Enzinger C, Ropele S, Smith S et al. Accelerated evolution of brain atrophy and 'black holes' in MS patients with APOE-ε4. Ann Neurol 2004; 55: 563–569.

149. Enzinger C, Ropele S, Strasser-Fuchs S et al. Lower levels of N-acetylaspartate in multiple sclerosis patients with the apolipoprotein E ε4 allele. Arch Neurol 2003; 60: 65–70.

150. Kantarci OH, de Andrade M, Weinshenker BG. Identifying disease modifying genes in multiple sclerosis. J Neuroimmunol 2002; 123: 144–159.

151. Wishart H, McDonald B, McAllister T et al. Regional gray matter concentration and brain activity in relapsing-remitting MS: effects of BDNF genotype. European Conference on Treatment and Research in MS, Thessaloniki, Greece; 2005.

152. Cutter GR, Baier ML, Rudick RA et al. Development of a multiple sclerosis functional composite as a clinical trial outcome measure. Brain 1999; 122: 871–882.

153. Chelune GJ. Assessing reliable neuropsychological change. In: Franklin RD, ed. Prediction in forensic and neuropsychology: sound and statistical practices. Mahwah, NJ: Lawrence Erlbaum Associates; 2003: 123–147.

154. Franklin GM, Heaton RK, Nelson LM et al. Correlation of neuropsychological and MRI findings in chronic progressive multiple sclerosis. Neurology 1988; 38: 1826–1829.

155. Beatty WW, Paul RH, Wilbanks SL et al. Identifying multiple sclerosis patients with mild or global cognitive impairment using the Screening Examination for Cognitive Impairment (SEFCI). Neurology 1995; 45: 718–723.

156. Benedict RHB, Cookfair D, Gavett R et al. Validity of the minimal assessment of cognitive function in multiple sclerosis (MACFIMS). J Inter Neuropsychol Soc 2006; 12: 549–558.

157. Doraiswamy PM, Rao SM. Treating cognitive deficits in multiple sclerosis: Are we there yet? Neurology 2004; 63: 1552–1553.

158. Frohman EM, Stüve O, Havrdova E et al. Therapeutic considerations for disease progression in multiple sclerosis: evidence, experience, and future expectations. Arch Neurol 2005; 62: 1519–1530.

159. Lublin F. History of modern multiple sclerosis therapy. J Neurol 2005; 252(suppl 3): iii3–iii9.

160. Tullman MJ, Lublin FD. Combination therapy in multiple sclerosis. Curr Neurol Neurosci Rep 2005; 5: 245–248.

161. Amato MP, Zipoli V. Clinical management of cognitive impairment in multiple sclerosis: a review of current evidence. Int Mult Scler J 2003; 10: 72–83.

162. Bagert B, Camplair P, Bourdette D. Cognitive dysfunction in multiple sclerosis: natural history, pathophysiology and management. CNS Drugs 2002; 16: 445–455.

163. Leo GJ, Rao SM. Effects of intravenous physostigmine and lecithen on memory loss in multiple sclerosis. J Neurol Rehabil 1988; 2: 123–129.

164. Unverzagt FW, Rao SM, Antuono PG. Oral physostigmine in the treatment of memory loss in multiple sclerosis. J Clin Exp Neuropsychol 1991; 131: 74.

165. Greene YM, Tariot PN, Wishart H et al. 12 week open trial of donepezil HCL in multiple sclerosis patients with associated cognitive impairment. J Clin Psychopharmacol 2000; 20: 350–256.

166. Krupp LB, Elkins LE, Schiffer RS et al. Donepezil for the treatment of memory impairment in MS. Neurology 1999; 52: A137.

167. Krupp LB, Christodoulou C, Melville P et al. Donepezil improved memory in multiple sclerosis in a randomized clinical trial. Neurology 2004; 63: 1579–1585.

168. Tsao JW, Heilman KM. Commentary: Donepezil improved memory in multiple sclerosis in a randomized clinical trial. Neurology 2005; 64: 1823–1824.

169 Lovera J, Bagert B, Smoot K et al. Gingko biloba for the improvement of cognitive performance in multiple sclerosis: a randomised, placebo-controlled trial. Mult Scler 2007; 13(3): 376–385.

170. Smits RC, Emmen HH, Bertelsmann FW et al. The effects of 4-aminopyridine on cognitive function in patients with multiple sclerosis: a pilot study. Neurology 1994; 44: 1701–1705.

171. Geisler MW, Sliwinski M, Coyle PK et al. The effects of amantadine and pemoline on cognitive functioning in multiple sclerosis. Arch Neurol 1996; 53: 185–188.

172. Sailer M, Heinze HJ, Schoenfeld MA et al. Amantadine influences cognitive processing in patients with multiple sclerosis. Pharmacopsychiatry 2000; 33: 28–37.

173. Krupp LB, Rizvi SA. Symptomatic therapy for underrecognized manifestations of multiple sclerosis. Neurology 2002; 58(suppl 4): S32–S39.

174. Chiaravalloti ND, Demaree H, Gaudino EA, DeLuca J. Can the repetition effect maximize learning in multiple sclerosis? Clin Rehabil 2003; 17: 58–68.

175. Bakshi R. Fatigue associated with multiple sclerosis: diagnosis, impact and management. Mult Scler 2003; 9: 219–227.

176. Goldman Consensus Group. The Goldman Consensus statement on depression in multiple sclerosis. Mult Scler 2005; 11: 328–337.

177. Beck AT, Steer RA, Brown GK. Beck Depression Inventory-II (BDI-II). San Antonio, TX: Psychological Corporation; 1996.

178. Goodglass H, Kaplan E, Barresi B. Boston Diagnostic Aphasia Examination, 3rd ed. Philadelphia, PA: Lippincott Williams & Wilkins; 2001.

179. Benedict RHB. Brief Visuospatial Memory Test – revised professional manual, Lutz, FL: Psychological Assessment Resources; 1988.

180. Krupp LB, LaRocca NG, Muir-Nash J, Steinberg AD. The Fatigue Severity Scale. Application to patients with multiple sclerosis and systemic lupus erythematosus. Arch Neurol 1989; 46: 1121–1123.

181. Trites RL. Grooved pegboard, Neuropsychological test manual. Ottawa: Royal Ottawa Hospital; 1977.

182. Reitan RM, Wolfson D. The Halstead-Reitan neuropsychological test battery: Theory and clinical interpretation, 2nd ed. Tucson, AZ: Neuropsychology Press; 1993.

183. Squire LR, Wetzel CD, Slater PC. Memory complaints after electroconvulsive therapy: Assessment with a new self-rating instrument. Biol Psychiatr 1979; 14: 791–801.

184. Fischer JS, LaRocca NG, Miller DM et al. Recent developments in the assessment of quality of life in multiple sclerosis (MS). Mult Scler 1999; 5: 251–259.

185. McNair DM, Lorr M, Droppleman LF. Manual for the Profile of Mood States (POMS), revised ed. San Diego, CA: Educational and Industrial Testing Service; 1992.

186. Spielberger CD. State–Trait Anxiety Inventory. Palo Alto, CA: Consulting Psychologists Press; 1983.

187. Wilkinson GS, Robertson GJ. The Wide Range Achievement Test, 4th edn. Odessa, FL: Rsychological Assessment Resources; 2006.

188. Axelrod BN, Goldman RS, Heaton RK et al. Discriminability of the Wisconsin Card Sorting Test using the standardization sample. J Clin Exp Neuropsychol 1996; 18: 338–342.

189. Heaton R, Chelune G, Talley JL et al. Wisconsin Card Sorting Test manual: revised and expanded. Odessa, FL: Psychological Assessment Resources; 1993.

A. J. Thompson

INTRODUCTION

This broad topic has numerous applications throughout the variable and unpredictable course of multiple sclerosis (MS). In this chapter the underlying philosophy and basic principles of rehabilitation will be discussed. This will be followed by a consideration of the rehabilitative approach to each of the four phases of the course of MS.

PHILOSOPHY AND PRINCIPLES

The philosophy of rehabilitation, which emphasizes patient education and self-management, is ideally suited to meet the complex and variable needs of MS. Rehabilitation aims to improve independence and quality of life by maximizing ability and participation. It has been defined by the World Health Organization as 'an active process by which those disabled by injury or disease achieve a full recovery or if a full recovery is not possible realize their optimal physical, mental and social potential and are integrated into their most appropriate environment'. It has also been appropriately described as an educational process that aims to increase ability, participation and autonomy and improve functional independence and quality of life. Reflecting on these definitions, it is clear that the philosophy of rehabilitation is as appropriate to chronic progressive conditions such as MS as it is to the management of the sequelae of acute events affecting the brain, e.g. stroke and traumatic injury, or the spinal cord.[1,2]

Delivering a comprehensive rehabilitation service requires clear structure and process and these should be driven by explicit clinical standards.[3] The essential components of successful rehabilitation, all of which are underpinned by the involvement of the patient include:

* Expert interdisciplinary assessment and problem definition
* Treatment planning (goal-oriented programmes) and delivery
* Evaluation of effectiveness and reassessment (Fig. 28.1).

INTERDISCIPLINARY ASSESSMENT

Patients with complex disability in whom multiple factors affecting functional performance present as a single problem will benefit from comprehensive assessment by a rehabilitation team. The term 'interdisciplinary' implies an integrated approach in which the individual experts work together, often in joint sessions, towards a set of agreed goals. Team members have a fuller understanding of other members' roles and skills and can work together in a holistic way. The advantage of such an assessment is that different disciplines identify different contributory causes and can develop a coordinated plan that addresses all of them. For example, poor mobility in a patient with MS may relate to weakness, spasticity, poor balance, pain and cognitive difficulties, requiring expert input from medical, nursing, physiotherapy, occupational therapy and neuropsychology practitioners.

The necessary structure for such team working is provided by the World Health Organization's International Classification of Impairments, Disabilities and Handicaps (ICIDH), revised in 2001 as the International Classification of Functioning, Disability and Health (ICF).[4] The overall aim of this classification is to provide a unified and standard language and framework for the description of health and health-related states. The ICF classifies functioning at both the level of body/body part and whole person, and emphasizes that disablement and functioning are outcomes of interactions between health conditions and personal and contextual factors (social and physical environment) (Fig. 28.2).

TREATMENT PLANNING

The treatment plan is shaped around goal-setting, a core skill for rehabilitation professionals. There is a small but growing literature on the evidence base for goal-setting. There are a number of key elements to goal-setting, including the goals themselves, which should be SMART (specific, measurable, achievable, relevant and time-limited).[5] The benefits of goal-setting can be moderated by factors such as the individual's commitment to the goal, the importance of the goal to them and their belief that the goal can be attained (self-efficacy). These factors underline the importance of the patients' involvement in the goal-setting and rehabilitation process.[6–8] In a recent study evaluating patient involvement in goal-setting, 201 patients were recruited from an inpatient neurological rehabilitation unit. The study was an AB block design with each block lasting 3 months, over an 18-month period. Patients ($n=100$)

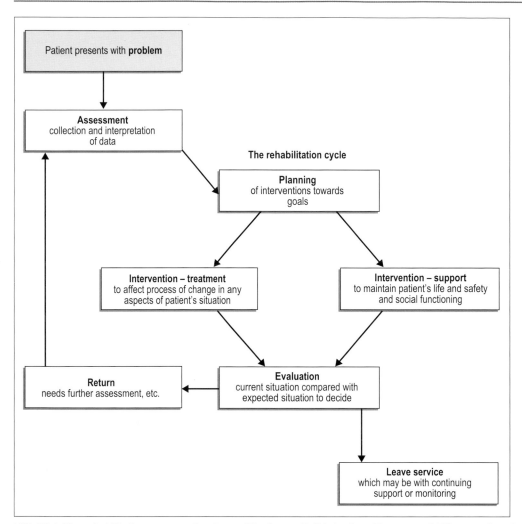

FIG. 28.1 The rehabilitation process. Courtesy of Professor D. Wade, from Thompson 2003, reproduced with permission.[101]

recruited in phase A were involved in standard goal-setting. Patients ($n=101$) recruited in phase B were involved in setting their own goals. Phase B patients were provided with a workbook to help them define and prioritize their own goals. Outcomes included patients' perceptions of the relevance of goal setting, autonomy within the process, functional outcomes and number, type and outcome of goals. Results showed that there were no differences between the two groups in functional outcomes. However, phase B patients reported significantly more participation-related goals, more relevant goals and greater autonomy and satisfaction with goal-setting. Phase B patients also set fewer goals and achieved a higher proportion of those goals.

Recent systematic reviews suggested that goal planning improves patients' adherence to treatment regimes and improves patient performance in some specific situations, although translating this into improved outcomes is inconsistent.[9]

EVALUATION OF EFFECTIVENESS

This can be viewed from several different perspectives including goal achievement, detectable changes on measures of disability, participation and health-related quality of life. However, it is also sobering to appreciate that we may not be able to measure many of the less obvious benefits of rehabilitation which relate to improving the patients' understanding, coping skills and self-efficacy.[10]

Measuring goal effectiveness

In response to the need for goals to be specific and measurable, a variety of goal-based outcome measures have been developed (Table 28.1). The usefulness of these measures depends on how closely they link in to the goal-setting process, although, interestingly, few provide guidance as to how this should be done. Nonetheless they seem to be a sound approach warranting further work to determine their reliability and sensitivity as a measuring tool.[11] Goal achievement may also be audited as part of an integrated care pathway, which has also been shown to be quite effective in the appropriate setting.[12]

Measuring outcome

Evaluating the outcome from interventions at any stage of MS is extremely challenging but also of the greatest importance if there is to be ongoing improvement in the process and impact of rehabilitation.[13] Evaluating the effect on the patient requires the use of outcome measures that are scientifically sound (reliable, valid and responsive) and clinically useful (short, simple, etc.).[14] The measure must be appropriate to the sample under study and the intervention being evaluated. In the case of neurorehabilitation, the potential effects are not expected at the levels of pathology and impairment but rather in improving activity and participation (ICF) and in enhancing the broader, more patient-oriented areas of quality of life, coping skills and self-efficacy. It is particularly important that the perspective of

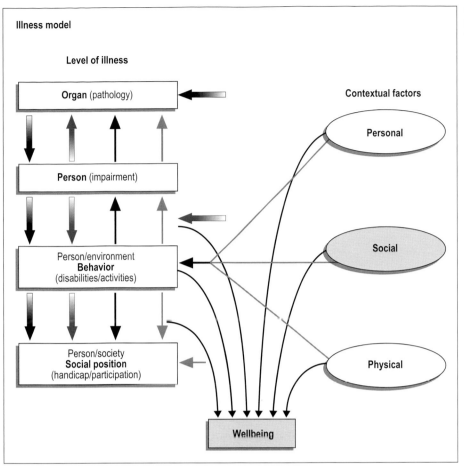

FIG. 28.2 Illness model incorporating levels of impact based on WHO, contextual factors and their complex interactions. Courtesy of Professor D. Wade, from Thompson 2003, reproduced with permission.[101]

TABLE 28.1 Goal-based outcome measures

Outcome measure	Author	Date	Description
Self-Identified Goals Assessment (SIGA)	Melville & Nelson[83]	2001	Developed from research in older people, this is designed for occupational therapists to use with clients in subacute rehabilitation and nursing homes. It is the only goal-based outcome measure that provides a protocol to elicit patient-identified goals, based on an exploratory interview. Each goal is assigned a rating 0 (unable to do) to 10 (can do) on a visual analog scale. Following therapy intervention patients rate their performance and change scores are compared
Goal Attainment Scaling (GAS)	Kirusek et al[84]	1994	A five-point scale. The expected outcome (goal) is assigned the position of 0 on the scale. Better than expected and much better than expected levels of outcome are +1 and +2 respectively. Worse than expected and much worse are –I and –2. A high level of skill on the part of the therapist is needed to quantify various levels of goal achievement. Has been used in a variety of settings, demonstrating acceptable inter-rater reliability and concurrent validity[103]
Canadian Occupational Performance Measure (COPM)	Baptiste et al[85]	1993	Designed for occupational therapists to use with clients to set goals. Standardized instrument with semi-structured interview format that elicits patient-identified goals and quantitative patient ratings of these goals. Change scores between assessment and reassessment are the most meaningful scores derived from this assessment
Self Assessment of Occupational Functioning (SAOF)	Baron & Curtin[86]	1990	Based on the Model of Human Occupation,[104] which promotes collaborative treatment planning between patient and occupational therapist. This instrument elicits written responses to predetermined items
Satisfaction with Performance Questionnaire	Yerxa & Baum[87]	1986	Quantitative scale of satisfaction with performance in daily occupations and community living. The scores highlight areas of decreased satisfaction with performance. Goals are negotiated between the therapist and patient on that basis

Source: courtesy of Dr ED Playford, Institute of Neurology, Queen Square, London, UK.

the patient is incorporated into the measure in a scientifically sound manner.

The standard outcome measure in therapeutic trials in MS, Kurtzke's Expanded Disability Status Scale, is inappropriate for evaluating rehabilitation not only because of its scientific limitations (particularly poor responsiveness) but also because it does not measure many of the relevant areas, such as fatigue and cognition, and does not incorporate the perspective of the patient.[15] Consequently, a number of generic measures of disability/ability (the Barthel Index,[16] Functional Independence Measure (FIM),[17] Functional Independence Measure/Functional Assessment Measure),[18] participation/handicap (the London Handicap Scale (LHS))[19] and health-related quality of life (the Short Form 36 Health Survey Questionnaire (SF-36))[20] have been used in MS rehabilitation (Table 28.2). Generic measures have the advantage of being able to compare outcome across a range of different conditions but may not be able to detect specific aspects of any given condition and may therefore lack responsiveness.

More recently, a number of MS-specific measures have been developed that are currently undergoing evaluation. These address disability (the UK Disability Scale[21]; MS Functional Composite – PASAT, nine-hole peg test and 10 m timed walk), health-related quality of life, which incorporates the patients' perspective (the MS Quality of Life Inventory, Functional Assessment of MS (FAMS), MS QoL 54,[23] Leeds QOL Scale,[24] MS Disease Impact Scale (MSIS) and the MS Walking Scale).[25,26] It is appropriate to focus on the health-related quality of life scales, as these are most relevant to the evaluation of rehabilitation. Those that have received the most attention (and evaluation) include the FAMS, MS QoL 54 and MSIS.[27] Whereas the first two measures are derived from oncology and generic scales respectively, the MSIS was developed along formal psychometric principles. It contains 29 items (20 physical and nine psychologi-

cal) and has been extensively evaluated in a number of MS centers worldwide. It has been shown to be a reliable, valid measure that is responsive to change[28,29] and that compares favorably to the MS Functional Composite.[30] Importantly, it can also be used with proxies of patients with MS in both cross-sectional and longitudinal studies – a valuable attribute in the more severely disabled and cognitively impaired population.[31,32]

CHALLENGES OF MULTIPLE SCLEROSIS

There can be few neurological conditions that pose the range and complexity of problems seen in MS[33] and for which the rehabilitation philosophy is more appropriate.[34] Quite apart from uncertainty about the cause and an incomplete understanding of its pathophysiology, particularly in relation to the development of irreversible disability, medications that can modify the course of the condition are still at a relatively early stage in development. This is a condition that affects people in their early adult years and its hallmarks are those of variability and unpredictability, with the only certainty being that, in time, it will cause moderate to severe disability in the majority of those affected by it. It can, and usually does, affect most parts of the central nervous system, producing a complex array of symptoms that interact with each other to create challenging management issues.

The acute events or relapses, the hallmark of MS, come without warning and result in an unpredictable level of dysfunction and recovery. For most, at some point in the condition, there is an insidious progression that robs them of their mobility, independence and often autonomy. From a social perspective, this condition is associated with high levels of unemployment and results in breakdown in relationships and a high incidence of mood disorders with an increased risk of suicide.

TABLE 28.2 Levels of measurement and examples of generic and MS-specific measures

Term	Definition	Outcome measures	
		Generic	Multiple-sclerosis-specific
Impairment	Clinical signs/symptoms resulting from nervous system damage		Functional system of EDSS[49] MS Functional Composite Scale (T25 FW, 9HP, PASAT)[17]
Disability (ability)	Limitations on activities of daily living from neurological impairment	Barthel Index (BI)[16] Functional Independence Measure[17]/ Functional Assessment Measure (FIM/FAM)[18]	Guy's Neurological Disability Scale (GNDS)[21] MS Impairment Scale (MSIS)[93]
Handicap (participation)	Social and environmental consequences from impairment and disability	London Handicap Scale (LHS)[19]	Environmental Status Scale (ESS)[94]
Health-related quality of life (QoL)	The satisfaction that people have with health-related dimensions of life, from their own perspective	Short Form-36 (SF-36)[20] Nottingham Health Profile[88] Sickness Impact Profile[47,89]	MS Impact Scale, MS Walking Scale,[25,26] MSQoL54*, Functional Assessment of MS QoL Instrument (FAMS)*,[17,22] MS QoL Inventory (MSQLI),* Functional Assessment of MS
Emotional wellbeing		General Health Questionnaire[90]	
Symptoms, e.g. fatigue	Overwhelming sense of tiredness or exhaustion in excess of what might be expected from level of activity	Fatigue Impact Scale[91] Fatigue Severity Scale[48]	MS-Specific Fatigue Scale[95]
Spasticity	Velocity dependent increase in tonic stretch reflexes	Ashworth Scale[92]	MS Spasticity Scale (MSSS-88)[96]

*Developed from existing scales.
Source. with permission from Polman et al 2006,[100] p. 72.

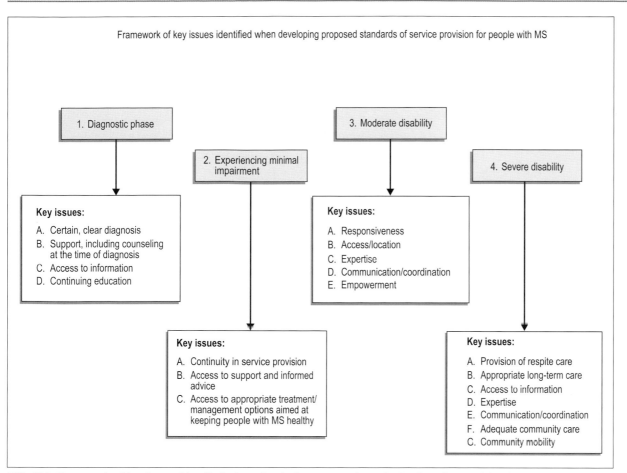

Framework of key issues identified when developing proposed standards of service provision for people with MS

1. Diagnostic phase

2. Experiencing minimal impairment

3. Moderate disability

4. Severe disability

Key issues:

A. Certain, clear diagnosis
B. Support, including counseling at the time of diagnosis
C. Access to information
D. Continuing education

Key issues:

A. Responsiveness
B. Access/location
C. Expertise
D. Communication/coordination
E. Empowerment

Key issues:

A. Continuity in service provision
B. Access to support and informed advice
C. Access to appropriate treatment/management options aimed at keeping people with MS healthy

Key issues:

A. Provision of respite care
B. Appropriate long-term care
C. Access to information
D. Expertise
E. Communication/coordination
F. Adequate community care
C. Community mobility

FIG. 28.3 Framework of key issues identified when developing proposed standards of service provision for people with MS.

While there is no underestimating the challenge of managing such a diverse condition, the rehabilitation philosophy provides a structure that can be useful at every stage of the condition.

SPECIFIC APPLICATIONS

Active management is required throughout the course of MS from initial diagnosis to the later stages when severe disability poses particular challenges (Fig. 28.3). Although there are specific requirements during each of these phases, there are consistent themes that remain relevant throughout the course of the condition. These include:

- Access to up-to-date information
- Availability of appropriate expertise
- Flexibility and accessibility of services
- Good communication
- Empowering the person with MS.

Each of these themes is challenging but perhaps communicating up-to-date information is the most difficult and has certainly been an area of particular focus in recent years.[35]

DIAGNOSTIC PHASE

This is known to be a time of great anxiety and concern and until recently was particularly badly managed. It is clear that the overwhelming majority of patients want to be diagnosed as early as possible and in a straightforward, clear fashion.[36–38] There are now accepted standards outlining the way in which a diagnosis should be made and acceptable timelines contained

within these, laid out in a number of recent documents.[39,40] These incorporate the following key elements:

- Certain, clear diagnosis
- Appropriate support at diagnosis
- Access to information
- Continuing education.

New diagnostic criteria, which have recently been developed and subsequently revised, incorporate more fully the evidence from MRI and allow an earlier diagnosis.[41,42] The process by which the diagnosis is made and communicated to the patient has been greatly enhanced by the introduction of MS nurse specialists and the establishment of diagnostic clinics, which are led by neurologists with an interest in MS and allow relevant investigations, including MRI, to be carried out in a timely fashion. Such an approach minimizes the impact of the diagnosis and has also been shown to be cost-effective and efficient.[43] It also provides an appropriate infrastructure on which to build links with the Multiple Sclerosis Society and ensure the provision of written information, access to a telephone help-line and continuing support and education in the form of regular educational classes.

MINIMAL IMPAIRMENT

Following diagnosis many patients will have a period of a decade or more when they have regular relapses but little or no disability. Many patients in this phase of the condition are taking so-called 'disease-modifying treatments' that reduce the frequency and possibly the severity of relapses. Nonetheless, incomplete recovery from relapse is seen on about 40% of occasions.[44] Patients will have a number of needs during this time, which include access to:

- Advice, support, and information
- Self-management options
- Treatment of relapses including use of disease-modifying agents
- Treatment of other conditions
- Continuing employment.

The main focus should be on self-management, with an emphasis on the concept of wellness incorporating diet, exercise and a healthy lifestyle. A number of studies have been carried out evaluating the role of aerobic exercise, resistive exercise and, more recently, a training program in this early stage of the condition. A recent Cochrane review has indicated that there is a convincing body of evidence to support the benefit of exercise in the management of MS.[45]

The impact of aerobic exercise was evaluated in 46 patients with relatively mild MS.[46] Of these, 21 patients were randomly assigned to a 15-week exercise program while 25 patients had no exercise during that period. There was a wide range of outcome measures, including aerobic capacity, isometric strength, a quality-of-life measure, the Sickness Impact Profile (SIP),[47] the Fatigue Severity Scales (FSS)[48] and the Expanded Disability Status Scale (EDSS).[49] Significant changes from baseline were seen in the exercise group over the 15 weeks in the physiological measures and the physical component of the SIP. There was little sustained change in the psychosocial domain of the SIP and none in the EDSS or FSS.

Recently, the effects of a short-term exercise program on aerobic fitness, fatigue and health perception was evaluated in a group of 26 patients and the results were compared with 26 matched healthy controls.[50] Although compliance was low (65%), benefits were seen in all areas and the regime did not result in symptom exacerbation. Significant benefit was seen in two domains of the SF-36: vitality and social functioning.

Few studies have looked at therapy intervention in the management of MS and the only specific modality examined in some detail has been physiotherapy. A randomized control trial of inpatient physiotherapy (6.5 hours over 2 weeks) was carried out on 45 patients. Outcome measures included the Rivermead Mobility Index, the Barthel ADL Index and a visual analog scale (VAS) of 'mobility-related distress'.[51] The only measure to demonstrate a significant benefit in the treated group was the VAS. A second study went a step further and attempted to compare two forms of physiotherapy. This pilot study involved 23 patients, 20 of whom completed the study. Ten patients received what was described as an impairment-based 'facilitation approach' (e.g. Bobath) while the other group had a more disability-based task orientated approach (e.g. Carr and Shepherd). Patients received a minimum of 15 sessions over 5–7 weeks. The outcome measures were mobility-based and included the 10 m timed walk and the Rivermead Mobility Index. Not surprisingly, given the small numbers studied, no difference was seen between the two small groups, but both improved from baseline ($p < 0.05$).[52]

A randomized, controlled, crossover study evaluated hospital and home-based physiotherapy in 40 MS patients with mobility problems.[53] A very wide range of outcome measures was used but physiotherapy resulted in significant benefit, irrespective of location, on the Rivermead Mobility Index, which was supported by other measures of mobility, gait and balance. There was no difference between treatment at home (the patient's preference) or in hospital, although the latter was less expensive.

Other approaches including yoga, treadmill training and virtual reality cues have been piloted recently in MS. A randomized, controlled trial of yoga and exercise compared yoga and exercise with a wait-list control group. No benefit in cognitive function was seen from either intervention but some positive impact in fact was noted in both treatment groups.[54] A 4-week programme of aerobic treadmill training was piloted in 19 patients with MS.[55] This approach was well tolerated and the treated group showed some short-term improvement. Finally, in a small study of virtual reality cues involving 16 patients some benefit from such cues was seen in gait ataxia, although larger more rigorous studies would be required to confirm this finding.[56]

In keeping with the philosophy of managing people with long-term conditions in the community rather than in hospital, a recent study has compared these two settings in the treatment of acute relapses.[57] Using a newly developed outcome measure of treatment satisfaction,[58] the study showed a significant preference for treatment to be given in the home setting.

In this group of minimally affected patients it is important to remember that, although the majority of relapses resolve completely, up to 40% may leave some residual problems. Therefore, while steroids might hasten recovery from a relapse, there is a role for therapy input and possibly involvement of the multidisciplinary team in those with residual deficit. A recent randomized, controlled trial has shown that, in patients who have not recovered fully following a relapse, there is a significant benefit from therapy input in addition to steroids when compared to steroids alone.[59] Audit data from a neurorehabilitation service also supports the role of rehabilitation in those who have developed severe disability following a relapse.[60]

Vocational rehabilitation

Continuing employment is a major issue at this stage of MS and the much-neglected vocational rehabilitation area has a key role to play. The vast majority of people with MS are in employment at the time of diagnosis but within 10 years between 50% and 80% are unemployed.[61] This high level of unemployment is thought to relate to three factors – the demands imposed by the job, the limitations relating to MS and the barriers and expectations imposed by society. Vocational rehabilitation therefore aims to overcome the barriers that an individual with MS faces in retraining, returning to work or starting work and provides the support needed by both the individual and the employer. Some of the key elements that might be involved in this process include:

- Retraining
- Capacity building
- Graded return to work
- Reasonable adjustments
- Disability awareness
- Symptom management and rehabilitation.

MAJOR DISABILITY

Patients with major mobility problems and a range of other symptoms have greater needs in the management of their increasing disability. These include:

- Rehabilitation and symptomatic management
- Easy access to responsive and coordinated services
- Appropriate level of expertise
- Good communication
- Self-management.

A comprehensive rehabilitation program may be particularly appropriate, although its evaluation may prove challenging. The difficulties of evaluating any intervention within the context of a randomized, double-blind, placebo-controlled trial in a variable and unpredictable condition such as MS are considerable. Evaluating as broad an area as neurorehabilitation, which at the same time has to meet the specific needs of an individual patient, poses additional problems in trial design. Chief among these are a lack of detailed description (e.g. number of disciplines involved, techniques employed, etc.) and inadequate standardization of input, including its duration and location (inpatient, outpatient or community-based). There also is reluctance among therapists to use a control group and limited resources often prohibit the use of independent assessors, which is particularly important when blinding is so difficult and perhaps even impossible. Finally, there is no consensus as to the most appropriate outcome measures and until recently there has been inconsistent use of limited and often inappropriate tools.

Despite these obstacles, it is possible to attempt some degree of evaluation, as has been demonstrated by a number of recent studies, although many more are required. The two key questions that need to be answered are: Is comprehensive rehabilitation effective in improving ability, participation and quality of life (although areas such as coping skills and self-efficacy may be as important) and, if so, do these benefits carry over in the medium to long term?

Evidence for benefit

Most studies have evaluated inpatient rehabilitation, which may be more accessible for study design. The majority of the nine studies of inpatient rehabilitation listed in Table 28.3 suggest potential benefit from rehabilitation in the area of disability; however, all have methodological concerns, with some having a single group design.

The study by Freeman and coworkers was a randomized, wait-list-controlled study of 66 patients with progressive MS.[62] Patients were stratified on entry according to EDSS score and the treatment group received a short period of inpatient rehabilitation (mean 20 days). Measures of disability, the FIM, and handicap, the LHS, were applied on entry into the study and 6 weeks later. The two groups were well matched in relation to age, sex, disease pattern and duration, and the treated group showed a significant benefit in both disability ($p<0.001$) and participation ($p<0.01$) when compared with the control group. No change in the EDSS score was seen in either group.

A randomized, single-blind trial compared a 3-week inpatient rehabilitation program with a home exercise program in 50 less disabled patients who were still ambulatory.[63] Patients were evaluated with the EDSS, FIM and SF-36, a quality-of-life measure, at baseline, 3, 6, 9 and 15 weeks. Significant benefit in disability and some aspects of quality of life (mental not physical) was seen at the end of the 3-week period in the rehabilitation group compared with those doing a home exercise program. This beneficial difference between groups was seen again at 9 weeks but had disappeared by 15 weeks.

A larger study assessed the role of strength and aerobic training, initially as an inpatient for 3 weeks but followed by 23 weeks at home, in patients with MS of mild to moderate severity (EDSS 1.0–1.5).[64] Patients were randomly assigned to an exercise or control group. The primary outcome was walking speed, measured at 7.62 m and 500 m, with secondary outcomes including lower limb strength, upper limb endurance and dexterity, static balance and peak oxygen uptake. Of the 95 patients enrolled, 91 completed the study and were evaluated at baseline and at 6 months.. Benefits in mobility at both distances and upper limb endurance were seen in the intervention group when compared to controls.

More recently, an interesting study assessed the benefit of inpatient rehabilitation in patients whose condition was stable.[65] The study had a randomized, double-blind, parallel group design – the only such study in the literature. A very large battery of outcome measures was used, including two impairment scales (the MS Impairment Scale[66] and the EDSS), a disability scale (Guy's Neurological Disability Scale),[21] measures of upper (nine-hole peg test) and lower (10 m timed walk) limb function and two health-related quality of life measures (FAMS and the Life Appreciation and Satisfaction Questionnaire).[67] Of 233 patients screened only 90 enrolled in the study (the majority of the remaining 143 could not be contacted). Patients received 3–5 weeks in-patient rehabilitation and no difference between the two groups was seen on any of the measures used. It could be argued that these results emphasize the need to select patients carefully for rehabilitation and to ensure that the process is focused on active problems.

Few researchers have attempted to evaluate outpatient-based rehabilitation in MS. One study randomly assigned 45 patients with progressive MS to an active treatment group (20 patients receiving 5 hours of outpatient therapy a week for 1 year) and to a wait-list control group.[68] The range of outcomes used included an MS-related symptoms checklist composite score, a measure of fatigue frequency and items from the Rehabilitation Institute of Chicago's Functional Assessment Scale. A significant reduction in the frequency of MS symptoms and fatigue was seen. A more recent randomized, controlled trial of outpatient rehabilitation involved 111 patients with progressive MS.[69] Those in the treatment arm underwent a 6-week period of treatment. The primary outcome measure was the FIM and moderately significant benefits (effect size greater than 0.4) were seen in the total score and in the sphincter, self-care, transfers and locomotion subscores.

Carry-over

Three studies have attempted to address the question of carry-over of benefit in question; all were restricted to the evaluation of a single group. The first was a retrospective study based on reviewing inpatient records and making subsequent phone contact with 37 patients 6–36 months later.[70] It suggested that gains on the EDSS and FIM documented on discharge were maintained at follow-up. The second study was a prospective evaluation of 47 patients seen 3 months postdischarge and included a measure of handicap (the Environmental Status Scale) along with the EDSS and FIM.[71] No change was seen in the EDSS during or following rehabilitation; gains in the FIM were maintained, while the level of handicap actually improved over the 3-month follow-up period.

The most detailed study involved the prospective longitudinal evaluation of 50 of the patients with progressive MS involved in the randomized, control trial described earlier. This study used a wider range of outcome measures; in addition to the EDSS and FIM there were measures of handicap (LHS), quality of life (SF-36) and emotional well-being (General Health Questionnaire). Patients were evaluated for 12 months at 3-month intervals following discharge, and 12-month data were collected on 48 of the 50 patients (92%). As might be expected, there was great variation between individual patients as well as considerable differences between the outcome measures. Summary measures were used to calculate the time taken to return to baseline. The EDSS deteriorated from a median of 6.8 on discharge to 8.0 at 12-month follow-up. Despite this, the gains in disability were maintained for 6 months before slowly declining. As in the previous study, handicap improved further following discharge but the benefit lessened after 6 months. Quality of life and emotional well-being improved considerably during the rehabilitation period, and this improvement was maintained for

TABLE 28.3 Summary of outcome studies of comprehensive rehabilitation in people with MS

Study	Study design	Sample	Main outcomes/instruments	Time of assessments	Results
Inpatient rehabilitation					
Francabandera et al[97]	Prospective, stratified, randomized study	84	ISS. Need for home assistance (hours)	Admission and at 3-month intervals for 2 years	Preliminary results suggest marginal benefit in inpatient group
Kidd et al[71]	Prospective, single-group, pre- and post-study design	79	DSS, Barthel Index ESS	Admission and discharge	Significant improvement in disability and handicap
Freeman et al[98]	Prospective, single group, longitudinal study design	50 (progressive MS)	EDSS and FS, FIM, LHS, SF-36, GHQ-28	Admission and discharge and at 3-month intervals for 1 year	Benefits in disability, handicap, QoL and emotional wellbeing persist for 6–9 months
Solari et al[63]	Randomized single group study comparing inpatient and home exercise program	50 (ambulatory)	EDSS, FIM, SF-36	Baseline, 3, 9 and 15 weeks	Benefits in disability and some aspects of QoL
Aisen et al[70]	Retrospective, single group, pre- and post-study design	37	EDSS and FS, FIM	Admission, discharge and telephone follow-up (6–36 months post-discharge)	Significant improvement in both FIM and EDSS
Kidd & Thompson[99]	Prospective, single-group, pre- and post-study design	47	EDSS, FIM, ESS	Admission, discharge and 3-month follow-up	Gains in disability maintained at 3 months; handicap improved over study period
Freeman et al[89]	Stratified, randomized, wait-list-controlled study design	66 (progressive MS)	EDSS and FS, FIM, LHS	Baseline and 6 weeks	Significant benefit in disability and handicap
Romberg et al[64]	Ramdomized controlled study	95	Timed walk test (TWT), upper and lower limb strength balance	Baseline and 6 months	Improvement in TWT and upper limb endurance
Storr et al[65]	Randomized, parallel group blinded trial	90	MSIS, EDSS, GNDS, 9HP, TWT	Baseline and 10 weeks	No benefit
Outpatient rehabilitation					
Di Fabio et al[68]	Nonequivalent pre-test, post-test control group design	45 (progressive MS)	MS-related symptoms, RIC-FAS, fatigue frequency	At entry and at 1 year	33 patients completed 1 year. Significant benefit seen in MS-related symptoms, incl. fatigue
Patti et al[69]	Randomized, controlled trial	111	EDSS and FS, FIM, SF-36	Baseline and 6 weeks	Significant improvement in FIM

BUSTOP, Burke Stroke Time-Oriented Profile; CRDS, Computerized Rehabilitation and Data System; DSS, Disability Status Scale; EDSS, Expanded Disability Status Scale; FIM, Functional Independence Measure; FS, Functional Systems; GHQ-28, 28-item General Health Questionnaire; ISS, Incapacity Status Scale; LHS, London Handicap Scale; LORS-II, Revised Level of Rehabilitation Scale; RIC-FAS, Rehabilitation Institute of Chicago Functional Assessment Scale; SF-36, Short Form 36 Health Survey Questionnaire.
Source: with permission from Polman et al 2006,[100] p. 95.

10 and 7 months respectively before beginning to return to baseline. A further finding of this study was that those who made the most gains during the rehabilitation period tended to maintain those gains for a longer time.

A final question is whether we can predict those who have the potential to benefit from neurorehabilitation or perhaps, more importantly, those who will not make gains. From the limited data addressing this issue, severe cognitive impairment and severe ataxia pose a particular challenge and are associated with a poor response.[72]

Although it is difficult to combine the results of all of these studies and there are major methodological differences between them, with few, if any, reaching an adequate scientific level, they all suggest that organized, patient-centered, multidisciplinary rehabilitation is of benefit in MS management. There is also some evidence to suggest that the gains derived from rehabilitation are maintained in the short term, at least in part, in this progressive condition. They emphasize the need for a range of outcome measures to be used and stress the importance of continuity of care.

SEVERE DISABILITY

There have been few, if any, studies evaluating input in those with severe disability. Their needs include:

- Access to information and expertise
- Good communication and coordinated care
- Adequate community care services
- Flexible provision of respite care
- Appropriate long-term care facilities including palliative care.

Palliative care plays a key role at this stage of the condition (Fig. 28.4) and has been the focus of much interest in the last few years. It has been defined as 'an active, holistic care of patients with advanced progressive illness. Management of pain and other symptoms and provision of psychological, social and spiritual care are paramount.'[73] The evaluation of palliative care is quite challenging as most of the measures mentioned earlier are

not sensitive to change in this more disabled population.[74] There is an urgent need for more evaluation and development of services for people with severe disability.

DEVELOPING AND EVALUATING MODELS OF CARE

Evaluating service delivery may be considered the most important and relevant issue in the management of MS because it incorporates acute hospital and neurorehabilitation services together with community-based activities and, in essence, has to bring together medical and social services in a way that meets the complex and ever-changing needs of the person with MS. Ideally, most services should be community-based with supporting expertise from the acute hospital or rehabilitation center at times of particular need (e.g. at diagnosis or at the time of a severe relapse) or complexity (when multiple symptoms interact and intensive inpatient rehabilitation is required). The optimum method of service delivery has not yet been defined, and little work has been done comparing existing services.

A recently published study carried out in Rome compared two forms of service delivery in a randomized controlled trial of 201 patients with MS.[75] One group (133 patients) received what was described as 'hospital' home care, in which patients remained in the community but had immediate access to the hospital-based, multidisciplinary team as and when required, while the other group (68 patients) received routine care. The range of outcomes, which included EDSS, FIM, SF-36 and measures of anxiety and mood, were carried out at baseline and at 12 months. No difference was seen in the level of disability between the two groups but the more intensively treated patients had significantly less depression and improved quality of life.

There continue to be major problems worldwide in delivering a model of care that provides truly coordinated services. There is serious inequity of service provision both within and across countries and an inordinate and unacceptable reliance on family and friends to provide essential care.[76,77] The study by Freeman and Thompson demonstrated that fewer than 50% of people with moderate and severe disability had access to a multidisciplinary team and, perhaps even more worrying, that the situation had not improved over 15 years.

The last few years have seen an outpouring of worthy documents providing guidance, (occasionally evidence-based) on how MS might be best managed. In the UK the National Institute for Clinical Excellence, which has a somewhat notorious reputation following its ruling that disease-modifying treatments were not cost-effective, has redeemed itself to some extent by producing guidelines on the management of MS.[78] These have been followed by a National Service Framework for long-term neurological conditions that contains valuable guidance relating to the management of MS applicable not just to the UK but internationally.[40] This espouses the worthy philosophy of providing choice to people with MS through services planned and delivered around their individual needs, supporting them to live independently and play their full part in society and working towards a partnership between health and social services.

Moving from national to international initiatives, the European MS Platform (EMSP) in conjunction with Rehabilitation in MS (RIMS) has produced a very useful text outlining the key role rehabilitation plays in the management of MS.[79] Taken together, all of these books, along with the many others published in this area, emphasize the importance of minimizing the impact of MS on those affected by the condition and maximizing the quality of life of the person with MS. The latter is the driving force behind a recent publication by the MS

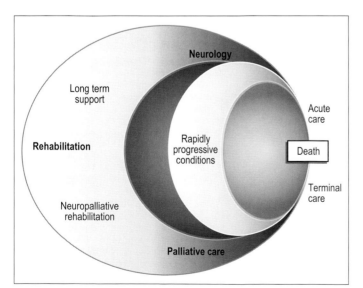

FIG. 28.4 Life circles model. Redrawn with permission from National Council for Palliative Care. Neurological conditions: from diagnosis to death – exploring the interface between palliative care, neurology, and rehabilitation in the management of people with long-term neurological conditions. London: NCPC, 2006, with permission.[102]

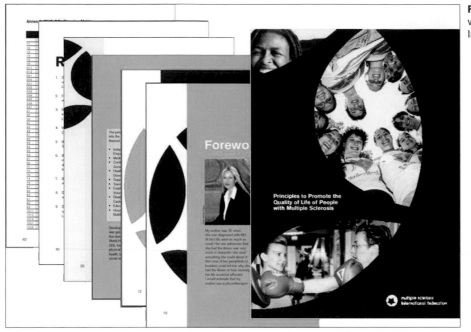

FIG. 28.5 Quality of life principles. Reproduced with permission from the Multiple Sclerosis International Federation.

International Federation entitled Principles to Promote the Quality of Life of People with MS (Fig 28.5).[80,81,82] This document addresses ten key areas which have the potential to have a major impact on the quality of life of those affected by MS.

- Medical care
- Continuing care
- Health promotion and disease prevention
- Independence and patient empowerment
- Support for family members
- Transportation
- Employment and volunteer activities
- Disability benefits and cash assistance
- Education
- Accessibility of housing and buildings in the community.

These principles have been published together with guidelines to help MS societies across the world to apply the principles to their own countries and they have now been used in more than 10 countries, including Canada, the USA, Australia, Germany and Denmark. They have also formed the basis of a program for sharing best practice that is proving very successful.

CONCLUSION

It is difficult to overestimate the importance of rehabilitation in the management of MS. The attempts to evaluate the various approaches are encouraging but this is still at a relatively early stage. This work needs to evolve and develop further. In the meantime, the efforts to raise the standards internationally are encouraging.

REFERENCES

1. Ward CD, Phillips M, Smith A et al. Multidisciplinary approaches in progressive neurological disease: can we do better? J Neurol Neurosurg Psychiatr 2003; 74(suppl 4): iv8–iv12.
2. Thompson AJ. Neurorehabilitation in multiple sclerosis: foundations, facts and fiction. Curr Opin Neurol 2005; 18: 267–271.
3. Turner-Stokes L, Williams H, Abraham R et al. Clinical standards for inpatient specialist rehabilitation services in the UK. Clin Rehab 2000; 14: 468–480.
4. World Health Organization. International classification of functioning, disability and health. Geneva: WHO, 2001. Available on line at: http: //www3.who.int/icf/icftemplate.cfm.
5. Locke EA, Latham GP. Building a practically useful theory of goal setting and task motivation. A 35-year odyssey. Am Psychol 2002; 57: 705–717.
6. Holliday RC, Antoun M, Playford ED. A survey of goal-setting methods used in rehabilitation. Neurorehab Neural Repair 2005; 19: 227–231.

7. Holliday RC, Ballinger C, Playford ED. Goal setting in neurological rehabilitation: patients' perspectives. Disability and Rehabilitation 2007; 29: 389–394.
8. Holliday RC, Cano S, Freeman JA, Playford ED. Should patients participate in clinical decision making? An optimised balance block design controlled study of goal setting in a rehabilitation unit. J Neurol Neurosurg Psychiatr 2007; 78: 576–580.
9. Levack WMM, Taylor K, Siegert RJ et al. Is goal-planning in rehabilitation effective? A systematic review. Clin Rehab 2006; 20: 739–755.
10. Edwards SGM, Playford ED, Hobart JC et al. Comparison of physician outcome measures and patients' perception of benefits of inpatient neurorehabilitation. Br Med J 2002; 324: 1493.
11. Hurn J, Kneebone I, Cropley M. Goal setting as an outcome measure: a systematic review. Clin Rehab 2006; 20: 756–772.
12. Rossiter DA, Edmondson A, Al-Shahi R et al. Integrated care pathways in multiple

sclerosis rehabilitation: completing the audit cycle. Mult Scler 1998; 4: 85–89.
13. Thompson AJ. The effectiveness of neurological rehabilitation in multiple sclerosis. J Rehabil Res Dev 2000; 37: 455–461.
14. Hobart JC, Lamping DL, Thompson AJ. Evaluating neurological outcome measures: the bare essentials. J Neurol Neurosurg Psychiatr 1996; 60: 127–130.
15. Hobart JC, Freeman JA, Thompson AJ. Kurtzke scales revisited: the application of psychometric methods to clinical intuition. Brain 2000; 123: 1027–1040.
16. Mahoney FI, Barthel DW. Functional evaluation: the Barthel Index (BI). Maryland State Med J 1965; 14: 61–65.
17. Granger CV, Cotter AC, Hamilton BB et al. Functional assessment scales: a study of persons with multiple sclerosis. Arch Phys Med Rehabil 1990; 71: 870–875.
18. Van der Putten JJMF, Hobart JC, Freeman JA, Thompson JA. Measuring change in disability after inpatient rehabilitation: comparison of the responsiveness of the Barthel Index and the Functional

Independence Measure. J Neurol Neurosurg Psychiat 1999; 66: 480–485.

19. Harwood RH, Rogers A, Dickinson E et al. Measuring handicap. London handicap scale, a new outcome measure for chronic disease. Qual Health Care 1994; 3: 11–16.

20. Ware JE, Sherbourne CD. The MOS 36-item short form health survey (SF-36). 1. Conceptual framework and item selection. Med Care 1992; 30: 473–483.

21. Sharrack B, Hughes RAC. The Guy's Neurological Disability Scale (GNDS): a new disability measure for multiple sclerosis. Mult Scler 1999; 5: 223–233.

22. Cella DF, Dineen K, Arnason B et al. Validation of the functional assessment of multiple sclerosis quality of life instrument. Neurology 1996; 47: 129–139.

23. Vickrey BG, Hays RD, Harooni R et al. A health-related quality of life measure for multiple sclerosis. Qual Life Res 1995; 187–206.

24. Ford HL, Gerry E, Tennant A et al. Developing a disease specific quality of life measure for people with multiple sclerosis. Clin Rehab 2001; 15: 247–258.

25. Hobart JC, Lamping DL, Fitzpatrick R et al. The Multiple Sclerosis Impact Scale (MSIS-29): a new patient-based outcome measure. Brain 2001; 124: 962–973.

26. Hobart JC, Riazi A, Lamping DL et al. Measuring the impact of MS on walking ability: the 12-item MS Walking Scale (MSWS-12). Neurology 2003; 60: 31–36.

27. Fischer JS, LaRocca NG, Miller DM et al. Recent developments in the assessment of quality of life in Multiple Sclerosis (MS). Multiple Sclerosis 1999; 5: 251–259.

28. McGuigan C, Hutchinson M. The Multiple Sclerosis Impact Scale (MSIS-29) is a reliable and sensible measure. J Neurol Neurosurg Psychiatr 2004; 75: 266–269.

29. Hoogervorst JNP, Jelles B, Polman CH et al. Multiple Sclerosis Impact Scale (MSIS-29): relation to established measures of impairment and disability. Mult Scler 2004; 10: 569–574.

30. Costelloe L, O'Rourke K, Kearney H et al. Does the patient know best? Significant change in the multiple sclerosis impact scale (MSIS-29 physical) over four years. Mult Scler 2006; 12: S86, P328.

31. Van der Linden FAH, Kragt JJ, Klein M et al. Psychometric evaluation of the multiple sclerosis impact scale (MSIS-29) for proxy use. J Neurol Neurosurg Psychiatr 2005; 76: 1677–1681.

32. Van der Linden FAH, Kragt JJ, Hobart JC et al. Longitudinal proxy measurements in multiple sclerosis: agreements between patients and their partners on the impact of MS on daily life over a period of two years. Mult Scler 2006; 12: S86 P330.

33. Kesselring J, Beer S. Symptomatic therapy and neurorehabilitation in multiple sclerosis. Lancet Neurol 2005; 4: 643–652.

34. Thompson AJ. ed. Neurological rehabilitation of multiple sclerosis. Queen Square Neurological Rehabilitation Series. London: Taylor & Francis/Informa Healthcare; 2006.

35. Heesen C, Kasper J, Segal J et al. Decisional role preferences, risk knowledge and information interests in patients with multiple sclerosis. Mult Scler 2004; 10: 643–650.

36. Heesen C, Kolbeck J, Gold SM et al. Delivering the diagnosis of multiple sclerosis. Results of a survey among patients and neurologists. Acta Neurol Scand 2003; 107: 363–368.

37. Janssens ACJW, Boer JBd, Kalkers NF et al. Patients with multiple sclerosis prefer early diagnosis. Eur J Neurol 2004; 11: 335–337.

38. Johnson J. On receiving the diagnosis of multiple sclerosis: managing the transition. Mult Scler 2003; 9: 82–88.

39. National Institute for Clinical Excellence. Multiple sclerosis. National clinical guidelines for diagnosis and management in primary and secondary care. London: The National Collaborating Centre for Chronic Conditions, Royal College of Physicians of London; 2004.

40. Department of Health Long-term Conditions NSF Team. The national service framework for long-term conditions. London: Department of Health; 2005.

41. McDonald WI, Compston A, Edan G et al. Recommended diagnostic criteria for multiple sclerosis: guidelines from the International Panel on the Diagnosis of Multiple Sclerosis. Ann Neurol 2001; 50: 121–127.

42. Polman CH, Reingold SC, Edan G et al. Diagnostic criteria for multiple sclerosis: 2005 revisions to the 'McDonald Criteria'. Ann Neurol 2005; 58: 840–846.

43. Porter B, Keenan E, Record E et al. Diagnosis of MS: a comparison of three different clinical settings. Mult Scler 2003; 9: 431–439.

44. Lublin FD, Baier M, Cutter G. Effect of relapses on the development of residual deficit in multiple sclerosis. Neurology 2003; 61: 1528: 1532.

45. Rietberg MB, Brooks D, Uitdehaag BMJ, Kwakkel G. Exercise therapy for multiple sclerosis. Cochrane Library Issue 4. Chichester: John Wiley; 2006.

46. Petajan JH, Gappmaier E, White AT et al. Impact of aerobic training on fitness and quality of life in multiple sclerosis. Ann Neurol 1996; 432–441.

47. Bergner M, Bobbit RA, Carter WB et al. The Sickness Impact Profile: development and final revision of a health status measure. Med Care 1981; 19: 787–805.

48. Krupp LB, LaRocca NC, Muir-Nash J et al. The fatigue severity scale applied to patients with multiple sclerosis and systemic lupus erythematosus. Arch Neurol 1989; 46: 1121–1123.

49. Kurtzke JF. Rating neurologic impairment in multiple sclerosis: an expanded disability status scale (EDSS). Neurology 1983; 33: 1444–1452.

50. Mostert S, Kesselring J. Effects of short-term exercise training programme on aerobic fitness, fatigue, health perception and activity level of subjects with multiple sclerosis. Mult Scler 2002; 8: 161–168.

51. Fuller KJ, Dawson K, Wiles CM. Physiotherapy in chronic multiple sclerosis: a controlled trial. Clin Rehab 1996; 10: 195–204.

52. Lord SE, Wade DT, Halligan PW. A comparison of two physiotherapy treatment approaches to improve walking in multiple sclerosis: a pilot randomized controlled study. Clin Rehab 1998; 12: 477–486.

53. Wiles CM, Newcombe RG, Fuller KJ et al. A controlled randomized, crossover trial of the effects of physiotherapy on mobility in chronic multiple sclerosis. J Neurol Neurosurg Psychiat 2001; 70: 174–179.

54. Oken BS, Kishiyama S, Zajdel D et al. Randomized controlled trial of yoga and exercise in multiple sclerosis. Neurology 2004; 62: 2058–2064.

55. Van den Berg M, Dawes H, Wade DT et al. Treadmill training for individuals with multiple sclerosis: a pilot randomised trial. J Neurol Neurosurg Psychiatr 2006; 77: 531–533.

56. Baram Y, Miller A. Virtual reality cues for improvement of gait in patients with multiple sclerosis. Neurology 2006; 66: 178–181.

57. Chataway J, Porter B, Riazi A et al. Home versus outpatient administration of intravenous steroids for multiple-sclerosis relapses: a randomised controlled trial. Lancet Neurol 2006; 5: 565–571.

58. Riazi A, Hobart J, Porter B et al. Developing a measure of patients' experiences of relapse management in multiple sclerosis. Mult Scler 2003; 9(suppl 1): S152.

59. Craig J, Young CA, Ennis M et al. A randomised controlled trial comparing rehabilitation against standard therapy in multiple sclerosis patients receiving intravenous steroid treatment. J Neurol Neurosurg Psychiatr 2003; 74: 1225–1230.

60. Liu C, Playford ED, Thompson AJ. Does neurorehabilitation have a role in relapsing remitting multiple sclerosis? J Neurol 2003; 250: 1214–1218.

61. O'Connor RJ, Cano SJ, Torrentà LR et al. Factors influencing work retention for people with multiple sclerosis. Cross-sectional studies using qualitative and quantitative methods. J Neurol 2005; 252: 892–896.

62. Freeman JA, Langdon DW, Hobart JC et al. The impact of patient rehabilitation on progressive multiple sclerosis. Ann Neurol 1997; 42: 236–244.

63. Solari A, Filippini G, Gasco P et al. Physical rehabilitation has a positive effect on disability in multiple sclerosis patients. Neurology 1999; 52: 57–62.

64. Romberg A, Virtanen A, Ruutiainen J et al. Effects of a 6-month exercise program on patients with multiple sclerosis: a randomized study. Neurology 2004; 63: 2034–2038.

65. Storr LK, Sorensen PS, Ravnborg M. The efficacy of multidisciplinary rehabilitation in stable multiple sclerosis patients. Mult Scler 2006; 12: 235–242.

66. Ravnborg M, Blinkenberg M, Sellebjerg F et al. Responsiveness of the Multiple Sclerosis Impairment Scale in comparison with the Expanded Disability Status Scale. Mult Scler 2005; 11: 81–84.

67. Ravnborg M, Storr L, Sorensen PS. Life appreciation and satisfaction questionnaire (LASQ): A conceptual QOL measure complementary to assessments of symptoms, ability and social participation. Mult Scler 2001; 7(suppl 1): P357.

68. Di Fabio RP, Soderberg J, Choi T et al. Extended outpatient rehabilitation: its influence on symptom frequency, fatigue and functional status for persons with progressive multiple sclerosis. Arch Phys Med Rehab 1998; 79: 141–146.

CHAPTER 28

423

69. Patti F, Ciancio MR, Cacopardo M et al. Effects of a short outpatient rehabilitation treatment on disability of multiple sclerosis patients. A randomized controlled trial. J Neurol 2003; 250: 861–866.

70. Aisen ML, Sevilla D, Fox N. Inpatient rehabilitation for multiple sclerosis. J Neurol Rehab 1996; 10: 43–46.

71. Kidd D, Howard RS, Losseff NA et al. The benefit of inpatient neurorehabilitation in multiple sclerosis. Clin Rehab 1995; 9: 198–203.

72. Langdon DW, Thompson AJ. Multiple sclerosis: a preliminary study of selected variables affecting rehabilitation outcome. Mult Scler 1999; 5: 94–100.

73. National Institute for Clinical Excellence. Guidance on cancer services. Improving supportive and palliative care for adults with cancer. London: NICE; 2004.

74. Gruenewald DA, Higginson IJ, Vivat B et al. Quality of life measures for the palliative care of people severely affected by multiple sclerosis: a systematic review. Mult Scler 2004; 10: 690–725.

75. Pozzilli C, Brunetti M, Amicosante AMV et al. Home-based management in multiple sclerosis: results of a randomized controlled trial. J Neurol Neurosurg Psychiatr 2002; 73: 250–255.

76. Carton H, Loos R, Pacolet J et al. Utilisation and cost of professional care and assistance according to disability of patients with multiple sclerosis in Flanders (Belgium). J Neurol Neurosurg Psychiatr 1998; 64: 444–450.

77. Freeman JA, Thompson AJ. Community services in multiple sclerosis: still a matter of chance. J Neurol Neurosurg Psychiatr 2000; 69: 728–732.

78. National Institute for Clinical Excellence. Multiple sclerosis. Management of multiple sclerosis in primary and secondary care. Clinical Guideline 8. London: NICE; 2003.

79. European Multiple Sclerosis Platform, endorsed by Rehabilitation in Multiple Sclerosis. Recommendations on rehabilitation services for persons with multiple sclerosis in Europe. Brussels: EMSP; 2004.

80. Multiple Sclerosis International Foundation (MSIF). Principles to promote the quality of life of people with multiple sclerosis. MSIF, London; 2005.

81. Montalban X, Hartung H-P, for the MSIF International Principles Oversight Group. International principles to promote quality of life for people with multiple sclerosis. Abstract presented at the 23rd Congress of the European Committee for Treatment and Research in Multiple Sclerosis, 6–9 October 2005, Vienna, Austria.

82. Thompson AJ, for the International Principles Oversight Group. Principles to promote the quality of life of people with multiple sclerosis. Mult Scler 2005; 11: S91, P354.

83. Melville L, Nelson D. The Melville–Nelson Occupational Therapy Evaluation System for skilled nursing facilities and sub-acute rehabilitation. Toledo, OH: University of Toledo, 2001. Available on line at hsc. utoledo.edu/healthsciences/ot/melville. html.

84. Kirusek TJ, Smith A, Cardillo JE. Goal attainment scaling: applications theory and measurement Hillsdale, NJ: Lawrence Erlbaum Associates; 1994.

85. Baptiste S, Law M, Pollock N et al. Canadian Occupational Performance Measure (COPM). World Fed Occup Ther Bull 1993; 28: 47–51.

86. Baron KB, Curtin C. A manual for use with the self assessment of occupational functioning. Chicago, IL: University of Illinois at Chicago; 1990.

87. Yerxa E, Baum S. Engagement in daily occupations and life satisfaction among young people with spinal cord injuries. Occup Ther J Res 1986; 6: 272–283.

88. Gladman JR, Lincoln NB, Barer DH. A randomized controlled trial of domiciliary and hospital-based rehabilitation for stroke patients after discharge from hospital. J Neurol Neurosurg Psychiatr 1993; 56: 960–966.

89. Freeman JA, Langdon DW, Hobart JC et al. Health-related quality of life in people with multiple sclerosis undergoing inpatient rehabilitation. J Neurol Rehabil 1996; 10: 185–194.

90. Rabins PV, Brooks BR. Emotional disturbance in multiple sclerosis patients: validity of the General Health Questionnaire (GHQ). Psychol Med 1981; 11: 425–427.

91. Fisk JD, Pontefract A, Ritvo PG et al. The impact of fatigue on patients with multiple sclerosis. Can J Neurol Sci 1994; 21: 9–14.

92. Ashworth B. Preliminary trial of carisoprodal in multiple sclerosis. Practitioner 1964; 192: 540–542.

93. Ravnborg M, Gronbech-Jensen M, Jonsson A. The MS impairment scale: a pragmatic approach to the assessment of impairment in patients with multiple sclerosis. Mult Scler 1997; 3: 31–42.

94. Stewart G, Kidd D, Thompson AJ. The assessment of handicap: an evaluation of the Environmental Status Scale. Disabil Rehabil 1995; 17: 312–316.

95. Krupp LB, Coyle PK, Doscher C et al. Fatigue therapy in multiple sclerosis: results of a double-blind randomized parallel trial of amantadine, pemoline, and placebo. Neurology 1995; 45: 1956–1961.

96. Hobart JC, Riazi A, Thompson AJ et al. Getting the measure of spasticity in multiple sclerosis: the Multiple Sclerosis Spasticity Scale (MSSS-88). Brain 2006; 129: 224–234.

97. Francabandera FL, Holland NJ, Wiesel-Levison P et al. Multiple sclerosis rehabilitation: inpatient versus outpatient. Rehabil Nurs 1988; 13: 251–253.

98. Freeman JA, Langdon DW, Hobart JC et al. Inpatient rehabilitation in multiple sclerosis: Do the benefits carry over into the community? Neurology 1999; 52: 50–56.

99. Kidd D, Thompson AJ. A prospective study of neurorehabilitation in multiple sclerosis (letter). J Neurol Neurosurg Psychiatr 1997; 62: 423–424.

100. Polman CH, Thompson AJ, Murray TJ et al, eds. Multiple sclerosis. The guide to treatment and management, 6th ed. London: Multiple Sclerosis International Foundation; 2006.

101. Thompson AJ. Neurological rehabilitation. In: Fowler TJ, Scadding JW, eds. Clinical neurology. London: Edward Arnold; 2003: 551–556.

102. Turner-Stokes L, Sykes N, Silber E et al. From diagnosis to death: exploring the interface between neurology, rehabilitation and palliative care in the management of people with long-term neurological conditions. Clin Med 2007; 7: 129–136.

103. Emmerson GJ, Neely MA. Two adaptable, valid, and reliable data-collection measures: Goal attainment scaling and the semantic differential. Couns Psychol 1988; 16: 261–271.

104. Kielhofner GA. Model of human occupation: theory and application, 2nd ed. Baltimore, MD: Williams & Wilkins; 1995.

CHAPTER 29

Design and analysis of clinical trials in multiple sclerosis

H. F. McFarland

INTRODUCTION

The most important step when beginning the study of clinical trials is to remember that a clinical trial is an experiment using humans. Consequently, the investigator and the sponsor of a clinical trial must accept the responsibility for conducting a study that is on the one hand scientifically sound and on the other ethically sound, with attention given to the protection of the individuals enrolled in the study. To satisfy both, the study must be designed in a manner to allow the greatest chance of yielding results that, at the end, will provide both patients and physicians with an enhanced understanding of the role of the therapy in treating the disease being studied. A study that puts individuals at risk without a good likelihood of providing useful answers to the question being addressed is not ethical. In contrast, a clinical trial that is well designed will provide valuable information not only on the usefulness of the therapy but also on disease mechanisms. In a disease such as multiple sclerosis (MS), in which the cause is unknown, information from clinical trials is especially helpful.

The history of clinical trials in MS has been variable: examples of extremely well designed and well conducted studies contrast with examples of uncontrolled studies that have been overinterpreted. Without question, MS is one of the more difficult diseases to study clinically. The difficulties include the variability in the course, the relatively poor outcome measures and the probability that the disease processes related to acute clinical disease activity may differ from those related to progression of disability.

The chapter will not attempt to provide the reader with all of the detailed information necessary to design, conduct and analyze a clinical trial. There are a number of very good comprehensive textbooks that accomplish that goal.[1–3] Instead, the chapter will provide a review of the issues that are considered to be central to the design and conduct of a successful clinical trial. Attention to issues relating to clinical trials in MS is particularly timely. The approval of disease-modifying therapies in MS beginning in 1993 has made the conduct of large placebo-controlled trials increasingly difficult. Consequently, attention needs to be given to alternative approaches. Possible alternative trial designs will be discussed.

HISTORY OF CLINICAL TRIALS

Examples of what may now partially fit our definition of a clinical trial or at least an example of evidence-based medicine can be found as far back as the 17th century, when bloodletting was challenged. Van Helmont[4] questioned bloodletting as a treatment for disease and proposed the following experiment:

Let us take out of the Hospitals, out of the Camps, or from elsewhere, 200, or 500 poor People, that have Fevers, Pleurisies, etc. Let us divide them in halfes, let us cast lots that one half of them may fall to my share and the other to your; I will cure them without bloodletting and sensible evacuation; but you do as ye know. . . . We shall see how many Funerals both of us shall have.

Of note, the approach also suggests an effort at randomization and the use of survival analysis as the endpoint.

Some of the most interesting examples of early evidence-based medicine involved scurvy. In 1600 one of four ships sailing for the East India Company was provided with lemons: the number of sailors with scurvy on that ship was far less than the number on the other three ships. In 1747 Sir James Lind took 12 patients with similar disease on board ship and divided these patients into groups of two.[5] Treatment groups included cider, vinegar, sea water and some other interesting remedies. Two patients received two oranges and one lemon a day; these two patients did the best. The results of these experiments, although loosely designed did provide important information on the treatment of a serious disease. Unfortunately, the studies also demonstrate another characteristic of many clinical trials: the results were interpreted in a manner consistent with the interests of the investigator. Because of the expense of citrus fruit, it was not consistently used to prevent scurvy at sea until 1875, when the British navy began to routinely include citrus on ships.

During the late 1800s and early 1900s a number of important advances occurred that provided the foundation for modern clinical trials and evidence-based medicine. In 1865 Sir William Gull and William Sutton reported the importance of placebo in examining treatments for rheumatic fever and emphasized that patients might do better on placebo than on one of the therapies used at the time.[6]

The use of randomization in clinical studies was first well documented in a study by Diehl in a study of treatment for the cold.[7] The study at the University of Minnesota used a double-blind design with randomization to either active therapy or placebo, ushering in the modern clinical trial.

Beginning at about the same time, the development of regulatory aspects for human experimentation also began. A number of landmark events have occurred that have formed the basis of the design, review process and approval processes involved in clinical research. These are discussed below in the section dealing with ethical considerations in clinical research.

HISTORY OF CLINICAL TRIALS IN MULTIPLE SCLEROSIS

As with many diseases, especially those with uncertain causes, many unusual therapies have been applied to MS and often the studies employed less than rigorous experimental designs. In fact, MS may have been even more susceptible to erroneous conclusions being drawn from poorly designed studies than most diseases because of the fluctuating nature of the clinical course. Prior to the 1970s, many clinical trials were uncontrolled and were what would now be called observational studies. Despite the lack of rigor, conclusions were often reached regarding the effectiveness of a particular treatment and often these treatments became part of clinical practice.

The first example of a well thought-out study incorporating what are now considered good design elements was the study of adrenocorticotropic hormone (ACTH) done in 1968.[8] The study was a rigorously controlled study of the effect of ACTH on recovery from acute relapses in MS.

The next important milestone in clinical research in MS was the meeting sponsored by the national Multiple Sclerosis Society (NMSS) held in Grand Island NY.[9] At the time of the meeting a number of small, poorly controlled studies were being conducted. The meeting voiced the need for rigorously designed, well controlled clinical studies. That meeting facilitated the development of a very sophisticated clinical research community interested in MS. The success of the MS research community is evidenced both by the continued focus on methodology seen in a series of workshops dealing with clinical trials and by the success of several phase III clinical studies that have led to the approval of therapies for the illness.

The meeting on clinical trial design held in Charleston, South Carolina in 1995 and again sponsored by the NMSS, began an examination of two issues that remain central to trial design in MS.[10] The first was the choice of outcomes used to measure clinical worsening of MS. Beginning in 1983, the Disability Status Score, developed by John Kurtzke and later revised into the Expanded Disability Status Score (EDSS), was used to measure clinical worsening.[11] Despite its widespread use, many investigators believed that the EDSS had serious flaws. Of the flaws the most important was the almost total focus on ambulation in the higher EDSS scores. Consequently, the EDSS was heavily influenced by a single lesion in the spinal cord and was not sensitive to the overall disease process once some difficulty with ambulation began. An outcome of the Charleston meeting was the creation of a working group charged with the potential development of a measure that would give a more complete assessment of clinical worsening. The outcome was the MS Functional Composite (MSFC), which has now been used in several studies and seems to hold promise for a more comprehensive assessment of disability.[12,13] The working group has continued to evaluate this score and examine the need for refinement such as incorporating a measure of visual function.

A detailed description of these outcome measures is found in Chapter 31.

The second important outcome of the Charleston meeting was the beginning of a formal evaluation of the use of magnetic resonance imaging (MRI) in clinical trials. Prior to that meeting, reports from a number of academic centers indicated that MRI could be a very useful tool in measuring disease activity in MS. Despite the potential usefulness of MRI, careful attention as to how it should be incorporated into clinical trial design was lacking. The report of this second working group began a process of careful assessment of the role of MRI in clinical trials in MS.[14]

The assessment of the use of MRI in clinical trials in MS has continued with a series of meetings beginning with a meeting in Oxford in 1998.[15] A subsequent international meeting, held in Washington, DC and sponsored jointly by NIH and the NMSS, focused specifically on the use of MRI as a surrogate outcome measure in MS.[16] The discussions at that meeting stressed the well-defined criteria needed to establish a measurement as a validated surrogate and concluded that, based on existing data, sufficient evidence did not exist to consider any MRI measure a validated surrogate. However, the participants also concluded that MRI could represent an unvalidated surrogate that could be useful in clinical trials seeking accelerated approval (as defined by the US Food and Drug Administration (FDA)) on the condition that additional safety and efficacy data would be obtained in phase IV studies, which would follow approval. The participants also endorsed the value of MRI in phase II or proof-of-principle studies. These issues are discussed in more detail later in this chapter and in Chapter 6.

The next meeting, again in Washington, DC and sponsored by the NMSS, in 2005 focused on clinical trial design in MS.[17] The impetus for the meeting was, as mentioned in the introduction, the need to begin to consider trial strategies other than placebo-controlled studies. The existence of several approved therapies has raised both ethical and logistical issues about the use of a placebo arm, especially in trials lasting several years. At that meeting a number of approaches to trial design that would lessen the ethical problems with the use of placebo arms were examined. Much of the outcome of that meeting will be incorporated into the discussions of alternative trial design later in this chapter.

CLINICAL TRIAL NOMENCLATURE

The commonly used terminology and the objectives of the various types of studies are shown in Table 29.1.

PHASE 0

Phase 0 studies have recently been introduced by the FDA (www.fda.gov/cder/guidance/6384dft.htm). A phase 0 study uses an exploratory investigation new drug (IND) number to allow some preliminary testing of a new compound. The types of testing that might be done under an exploratory IND include studies of very small doses for preliminary safety information or identification of proof of mechanism. The goal of the phase 0 study is to provide some preliminary data that will be useful in beginning formal drug development in a phase I study.

PHASE I

Phase I studies may be uncontrolled, open-label studies or small, controlled studies. Most importantly, the primary outcome of a phase I study is safety, not efficacy. In most cases a small cohort of patients will be started on experimental therapy at a dose considered to be low. Subsequent patients will

TABLE 29.1 Commonly used terminology and objectives

Type of trial	Alternative terminology	Goals and objectives of study
Phase 0	Exploratory study (exploratory IND)	Proof of mechanism Studies of low doses Compound screening done to obtain preliminary data needed to begin drug development in phase I studies
Phase I	Toxicity/safety or human pharmacology study	Explore dosing Single versus multiple dosing comparison Study pharmacokinetics Obtain preliminary information on outcomes
Phase II	Preliminary or therapeutic exploratory	Proof of principle Preliminary evidence of efficacy – often using biological or surrogate outcome Explore outcome measures Safety
Phase III	Therapeutic confirmatory or registration studies	Well controlled studies to establish efficacy and safety
Phase IV	Postmarketing or therapeutic use	Additional safety Confirmation of efficacy over longer duration Explore additional outcomes

be entered at higher dose levels until some predefined endpoint is reached. Often, pharmacokinetics will be performed after both single and multiple dosing to allow an understanding of drug metabolism. Although little attention has been given to the design of phase I studies, some novel approaches have been reported and will be discussed in the section on study design.

PHASE II STUDIES

Phase II studies (exploratory or preliminary studies) represent one of the most important steps in the development of a new therapy. Not only should the study allow a preliminary assessment of efficacy but it should also provide additional safety information, as well as insights into outcome measures that will be useful for studies of the therapy. Most importantly, the results of the phase II study will provide the information necessary to design the phase III study. Thus, safety and efficacy outcomes, dosing and potential adverse effects should all be addressed. Often, phase II studies will be designed (powered) to provide an answer with respect to efficacy using a surrogate (often unvalidated biomarker) as the primary outcome. The terminology phase IIa and phase IIb is sometimes used. While this distinction is not clearly defined, the intention is that some phase II studies are designed to provide proof of principle and be exploratory, while others are designed to provide more definitive information on efficacy. Often, commercial sponsors will elect to conduct a larger, controlled phase II study in an effort to speed development, since the results can be used to support a new drug application. Doing this means that information that might be obtained from a more preliminary study, such as information on dose–effect relationships, is not available. As with phase I studies, attention to innovative designs for phase II has been limited until the last few years, when some new approaches, including the blending of phase II into phase III and alternatives to conventional randomization, have been described. These designs will be discussed in more detail below.

PHASE III

A phase II trial is done to establish evidence of overall efficacy and safety of the new therapy and to establish the role of the therapy in clinical practice. The evidence evolving from a phase III study should be sufficient to allow a review of efficacy and safety for approval as a new therapy by appropriate regulatory agencies such as the FDA. The essence of a phase III clinical trial is that it is well designed, well controlled and of sufficient size to provide evidence of efficacy. In addition, a phase III study should provide extensive information regarding the safety of the new therapy. To date, most phase III studies done in MS have used a placebo control. As indicated in the introduction and as will be discussed in more detail below, the use of a placebo control, especially in trials involving large numbers of patients in studies lasting several years, has both ethical and logistical difficulties.

PHASE IV

Phase IV or postmarketing studies are usually designed to provide additional safety or efficacy information beyond that available from the phase III study. Phase IV studies will be necessary to provide both types of data when an accelerated approval process has been used to allow clinical use of a new therapy. Since accelerated approval often uses surrogate outcome measures, the studies may not have provided long-term safety and tolerability information. In addition, the effect of the therapy on the conventional clinical outcomes is important. Despite their importance, phase IV studies are often difficult to conduct, since well defined control groups are lacking. In MS one of the great concerns is that the clinical trials of short duration provide, at best, limited information about the long-term effect of the therapy on the disease course. Thus, additional attention to approaches that can be used in a postmarketing environment to obtain reliable long-term efficacy and safety data is very important but has not been forthcoming.

ETHICAL CONSIDERATIONS IN CLINICAL RESEARCH

As stated in the introduction to this chapter, conducting research in humans brings the need for thoughtful attention to the ethical aspects of the research. The investigator must assure that the research is conducted in an ethical manner and that every effort is made to protect the safety and rights of the participants. Beginning in the 1940s a number of guidelines have

TABLE 29.2 Research guidelines

Date	Event	Comment
1931	UK developed regulations for clinical trials	The Medical Research Council establishes a Therapeutic Trials Committee to advise and review properly controlled studies of new treatments
1937	The National Cancer Institute established and US government support for clinical research begins	Regulations for clinical trials developed by the National Institutes of Health
1938	Food and Drug Cosmetic Act	Gives the Food and Drug Administration increased regulatory authority for the approval of new drugs
1964	Declaration of Helsinki[18]	Establishes ethical guidelines for experimentation on humans
1966	Institutional Review Boards established	Provide review process for clinical research
1974	National Research Act	National Commission for the Protection of Human Subjects of Biomedical and Behavioral Research established
1979	Belmont Report[19]	Report from the National Commission establishes three principles for the ethical conduct for clinical research
1981	Title 45	Establishes the Common Rule regulating ethical guidelines for clinical research
2000	Revision of Declaration of Helsinki[20]	Restricts the use of placebo controls in diseases with proven therapies

been presented to assist investigators in assuring that their research is consistent with ethical standards (Table 29.2).

In response to the human experimentation conducted in Germany during World War II, the Nuremberg Code was presented at the conclusion of the Nuremberg Trials in 1949.[21] The code established ten principles for human research and central was the need for participation to be voluntary and for the rights of the subjects to be protected. In 1964, the World Medical Assembly developed guidelines for human experimentation published as the Declaration of Helsinki.[18] An essential part of the Declaration of Helsinki is that an individual participating in clinical research should not be put to a disadvantage with respect to their medical care. In other words, each individual should receive the best available medical treatment. As will be discussed below, the Declaration of Helsinki has recently been revised.[20]

In 1966, a sentinel paper in the *New England Journal of Medicine* by H. Beecher questioned the ethical conduct of a number of published studies.[22] The most notable of these was the Tuskegee syphilis study. The report led to congressional action, resulting in the National Research Act in 1974 and the establishment of the National Commission for Protection of Human Subjects. The Commission produced several reposts dealing with many aspects of clinical research, including the conduct of research in children. Probably the most notable of the reports was the one known as the Belmont Report, which presented basic guidelines for ethical research in humans.[19] The Belmont Report stated that three principles were essential to the ethical conduct of clinical research. These were: 1) respect for persons, 2) beneficence and 3) justice. Essential for respect for persons was that participation in research was based on a considered or educated decision and that self-determination of patients was guarded. A truly informed consent was at the heart of this principle. The essential aspect of beneficence was 'do no harm'. The risk–benefit of a study needed to be carefully assessed and needed to be continually evaluated during the conduct of the study. Justice meant that subjects should be selected fairly and without bias. An important aspect of subject selection was that they should be selected from a population that would benefit from the research. This point addresses the ethics of conducting research in populations who would be unable to receive the benefits of the therapy because of poverty or other reasons even if the new therapy is found to be effective.

The work of the Commission eventually led to federal regulations for the protection of human subjects published as Title

45 and now known as the Common Rule (45CFr46) (www.gpo.gov/nara/cfr/waisidx_00/45cfr46_00.html). The three basic principles needed in assessing the ethical soundness of a study are that 1) the research is important, 2) the research is valid and 3) the rights and welfare of the subjects are protected. The Common Rule forms the basis for review of clinical research by institutional review boards (IRBs) and sets the ethical standards by which clinical research is assessed with respect to protection of human subjects in the USA.

In 2000 the Declaration of Helsinki was revised and two provisions of the revision have resulted in substantive changes.[20] These are: 1) new therapies should be tested against the best current therapy and 2) at the conclusion of a study every patient in the study should be assured of access to the best available therapy. The first part of this revision raises the question of the ethical basis of any use of placebo in a condition for which there is an approved therapy. The Declaration of Helsinki made two exceptions: placebo could be used when there were compelling scientific reasons or when the burden of the medical condition was minor. Some have interpreted the former as meaning that, when a study without a placebo group would be likely to give misleading or uncertain results, a placebo-controlled study would be acceptable. Most IRBs, however, have taken a more restricted interpretation of the revision and have tended not to approve studies with placebo arms when alternative therapies exist, as in relapsing–remitting MS (RRMS).

It is notable that the MS research community has addressed the ethical and practical issues surrounding the use of placebo directly. An international task force was established in 2000 with the specific charge of establishing a position on the use of placebo in clinical trials in MS.[23] That effort resulted in the recommendation that placebo-controlled studies could be carried out but only after patients were given the choice, when appropriate, to consider an approved therapy and that the decision to begin treatment with an approved therapy should be made independently of recruitment for a clinical study. Implementation of these recommendations means that, in RRMS, study participants should be those who have for some reason elected not to go on approved therapy, this election having been made prior to discussion of the research study, or with patients who have failed approved therapies. It is clear that the result would be small numbers of patients and an inherent risk of a patient cohort not being representative of the larger RRMS patient population. Since that report, placebo-controlled studies in MS have continued but with increasing difficulties with respect to both IRB approval and patient recruitment. The guidelines recommended in 2001 have been re-examined by an international working group in 2006 (*Neurology*, in press).

In summary, the ethical guidelines evolving from the Declaration of Helsinki, the Belmont Report and the Common Rule form the basis for judging the ethical aspects of a clinical trial and represent the guidelines that should be used by the investigator and IRBs in reviewing clinical research. An essential part of any clinical protocol is a section addressing the protection of human subjects. While it is common to think that the responsibility for assuring protection of human subjects rests with the IRB, it clearly rests with the investigators: it is the responsibility of each investigator to assure that a research study conforms to the principles regarding the protection of human subjects.

FUNDAMENTAL ISSUES RELATING TO THE DESIGN AND CONDUCT OF A CLINICAL TRIAL

As indicated in the introduction the goal of this chapter is not to provide a comprehensive review of all aspects of clinical trials. Instead, the goal is to provide an introduction to trial design and point out those issues that are critical the design, conduct and analysis of a trial. The basic steps in the design, conduct and analysis of a clinical trial are outlined in Table 29.3.

Although it may seem self-evident, the first fundamental aspect of a clinical trial is to establish what the question is. The question needs both to be clearly stated and to be framed in a manner in which it can be answered. Essential to the development of the trial design is to have the question focused. For example, asking the question 'Does drug X reduce disability in MS?' is not sufficient. An appropriate question might be 'Does drug X decrease the rate of progression in disability compared to placebo in patients with early RRMS over a period of 2 years of treatment?' Once the question is properly framed the design of the trial becomes easier.

Before beginning work on a study, the investigator should ask if the question is relevant and if the question has sufficient merit to expend the resources necessary for the study. It is important to remember that the resources include not only the time of the investigators and the money needed for the study but also the risks and inconvenience imposed on the patients. It is essential that patients be considered as partners in a clinical

study and, before starting a study, the investigator needs to ask if the question has sufficient merit to impose the associated risks and inconveniences on those who will participate.

Finally, the investigator needs to ask if the time is appropriate to address the question. For example therapies often come into use in the clinical community without being based on solid evidence. The result is or should be motivation to conduct an appropriate study to establish whether that therapy is rational and with merit. However, because of uncertainly regarding the use of the therapy it may be appropriate to delay until a trial with optimal use of the therapy can be initiated. The investigator needs to question whether there is sufficient preliminary data to allow the trial to be designed optimally. For example, in MS there has been considerable interest in having a controlled study of hematopoietic stem cell transplantation, since the therapy is being used despite a lack of clear evidence for efficacy. Yet initiating a trial before there is some agreement on the optimal conditioning regimen could result in subjecting individuals to the risk of a study that will not address the most important aspects of the question. The other side of this issue is that the longer one waits to begin a therapy in use in the medical community, the more difficult it will become to conduct the study. For example, a controlled study of the use of corticosteroid treatment of acute relapses would be very difficult today.

A final point for consideration in deciding if a clinical trial should be done is whether there is true uncertainty regarding the effectiveness of the treatment. The term 'equipoise' is often used to express the concept that the investigator is truly uncertain whether the experimental therapy is better than the treatment used in the control group. The issue of equipoise is often difficult and in some instances, some in the medical community may believe that equipoise exists while others do not. For the trial to be successful there needs to be sufficient uncertainty in the community for a successful completion of the study. Investigators should not participate in studies if they do not believe that equipoise exists.

As discussed above, the timing of the study may often be a critical issue in the design of the study. In addition to timing in relation to the optimization of the treatment to be used, the investigator needs to examine the environment in which the study will be conducted. Will sufficient patients be available and is there clear evidence of need for the information that will be provided by the study?

STUDY DESIGN

The design of clinical trials will be examined in more detail in the section on trial design. However, before dealing with the specific aspects of trial design, some general comments are valuable. Probably the most important recommendation is that the inclusion from the earliest planning steps in the team of individuals designing the study of a statistician knowledgeable about clinical trials is essential. The design of a study follows easily if the question for the study is well formulated. The design of a study needs to be one without bias. Although this seems self-evident, it is often easy to incorporate bias into design, especially if equipoise does not truly exist. If an investigator has some bias towards a treatment that is being tested it is not difficult to incorporate design elements that may favor the experimental therapy. For example, a study of a treatment with an expected early treatment effect may be of insufficient duration to establish whether the treatment has durability. An endpoint that might favor a particular class of therapy may be incorporated even though that endpoint is not the one that is the most meaningful to the understanding of the effectiveness of the therapy.

TABLE 29.3 **Steps in the design of a clinical trial**
1. Identify the question
2. Decide if the trial is feasible
3. Establish the trial design a. Identify outcome measures b. Determine sample size c. Establish monitoring plan d. Develop data analysis plan e. Insure that elements of human subject protection are addressed
4. Prepare protocol and/or study manual
5. Develop case report forms
6. Training of staff
7. Develop plan for monitoring quality assurance
8. Adverse event reporting
9. Report results of study

Endpoints

One of the most important choices the investigator needs to make, the choice of endpoints, is examined in detail in Chapter 30. In most cases one single endpoint will be selected as the primary endpoint of the study; the behavior of the endpoint will determine whether the null hypothesis is rejected. As will be discussed later in the chapter, some trials use multiple endpoints or composite endpoints. The important point is that the endpoint must be one that is clinically relevant and also consistent with the proposed mechanism of the treatment being tested.

Three general types of endpoints can be used, dichotomous, continuous and time to failure. The analytical methods will differ depending on the types of outcome variable selected. In addition the choice will influence sample size calculation. Dichotomous variables represent outcomes that can be thought of in terms of yes or no. An example would be the proportion of patients with a relapse over the period of the study. Continuous variables represent measures that can have variable values on a continuum. An example in MS would be relapse rates or the presence of contrast-enhancing lesions. With a continuous variable the question could be proposed for a trial 'Does the treatment produce a 30% reduction in the event rate?' Continuous variables can be measured either just at baseline or at the end of the study or can be measured at various time points in the trial. The final general type of outcome is time to failure or a survival analysis. Most readers will be familiar with survival analyses, since they have been commonly used in trials of new therapies in MS. Examples are time to sustained progression or time to first relapse. Each of these variables has advantages and disadvantages and the reader is referred to several detailed reviews of outcome variables and their strengths and weaknesses. It should be noted that the choice of outcome variables will influence the methods used to calculate the sample size and therefore influence the actual sample size needed for the study.

Efficacy assessment

The statistical methods used for analysis of efficacy are beyond the scope of this chapter. However, some general points can be made.

First, the general approaches will follow the choice of outcome measures selected for the study. Independent of the choice of endpoints, however, is the identification of the patient cohort that will be used for the analysis of the primary outcome. What should be done with patients who have not completed the entire predefined study period or have discontinued in the study before reaching an endpoint if the study uses time for analysis? The most conservative approach and the one usually favored by most regulatory agencies is an intent-to-treat (ITT) analysis. In this, every patient randomized is included in the analysis regardless of the time they remained in the study. Imperative to an ITT analysis is that complete follow-up information on outcomes be obtained on patients who go off study medication before completing the study. If a patient elects to discontinue study medication, an effort needs to be made to insure that study visits specified in the protocol continue. Often patients dropping out of a study will elect not to continue follow-up. In this case an effort to at least get end-of-study evaluation will be helpful.

Investigators often have concerns over ITT analyses, since patients receiving the active study medication for even one dose will be counted as having been on the treatment for the entire study. The argument for ITT is to avoid bias in the analyses. For example, those patients with the worst disease may be the most likely to stop study medication prematurely. Once these patients are eliminated from the analysis the results may provide an incorrect answer as to the value of the therapy. Some studies will incorporate a modified ITT and only include patients in the analysis if they have been on therapy for some specified time. Most regulatory agencies will demand a conservative definition. Commonly the primary analysis will employ an ITT cohort but the analysis plan may also include additional analyses using patients who have remained in their assigned treatment arms for the duration of the study. Regardless of the method, the more complete the follow-up data on the entire cohort the less likely that bias will be a concern as the results of the study are analyzed.

The analytical plan also needs to address how patients dropping out of the study and lost to follow-up will be handled. Various approaches have been used, such as last observation carried forward. None are without problems and the assistance of a statistician is essential in addressing this issue.

The reader will often see references to two general types of statistical approach to data analysis and study design; the frequentist approach and the bayesian approach. It is recommended that the reader consult one of the many comprehensive statistical texts for a complete discussion of these approaches. However in simplest of terms, a frequentist will define a null hypothesis and then test the difference between the groups to determine whether the null hypothesis can be rejected and will establish a level of significance (p value) and confidence limits. A bayesian approach will first establish a set of priors that are thought to reflect the likelihood of the results. The study results will then be used to modify the prior probability. The argument for a bayesian approach is that it will provide a clearer picture of the value of the treatment effect. With the exception of a few statisticians who are closely connected to one or another of these approaches, many analytical plans may incorporate elements of both. Few would design a clinical trial without careful consideration of the previous results with the proposed therapy. However, it is argued that a bayesian approach provides a more rigorous use of this prior information. As will be mentioned in a later section, bayesian approaches may have particular value in the design of phase I and II studies.

Sample size

One of the most important aspects of designing a clinical trial is the determination of the appropriate sample size. The investigator will want to know how many patients will be necessary to identify a difference between the treatment groups with the desired power (the percentage chance of correctly detecting a difference). The investigator must also ask whether that sample size is reasonable with respect to recruitment and, if it is not, what the risks are of a smaller sample size. The investigator must address the risk of both a type I error – a false-positive result – or a type II error – a false-negative result. The probability of a type I error is the statistical significance and is denoted as α in the sample size calculations. In most clinical trials the α is set at 0.01 or 0.05. The type II error is denoted by β and the probability of correctly rejecting the null hypothesis of no difference between the groups is $1-\beta$. $1-\beta$ represents the power of the study and is usually set at 0.80 or 80%. The power will be dependent on α, the sample size and the true difference in the event rates of the two groups. Since the true event rate difference will not be known, it will need to be estimated based on previous data relating to the control group and the expected treatment effect.

Unfortunately, estimated sample sizes are too often lower than what is needed for the study. In an analysis of a large number of published randomized, controlled trials (RCTs) in a variety of diseases, it was found that a large proportion of studies that were reported as failures were underpowered even to identify a relatively common treatment effect.[24] It is essential that a clinical trial has sufficient statistical power to adequately detect differences between the groups. In many cases the preliminary data that can be used to assist in sample size calculations are minimal. In most cases the investigator is left to determine the sample size based on the limited data relating to the expected behavior of the control group and estimates of the magnitude of the treatment effect. Not uncommonly, the control group of large phase III trials will behave differently from what was predicted, leading to an underpowered study. The investigator needs to be conservative in the sample size estimates but must also remember that the larger the sample size the more difficult to recruit the study. The calculations used for establishing the sample size will be determined by the outcome measures being used and by the type of analysis employed in the study.

Data monitoring plan

An essential part of the analytical plan is an approach for monitoring the study. The reader is referred to Chapter 30 for a more detailed discussion of monitoring issues. A couple of points are important enough to repeat here.

A monitoring plan is essential both from the standpoint of protection of subjects and to insure that the study will have the best chance of providing a correct assessment of the value of the experimental treatment; the monitoring should be preformed by individuals independent from the sponsor and investigators and knowledgeable regarding the disease being studied and about trial design and monitoring. In studies that are blinded, a data monitoring committee (DMC) sometimes called a data and safety monitoring committee or board (DSMC or DSMB) will be essential. Even in open-label studies, such as many phase I studies and some phase II studies, a DMC will be helpful to assist the investigator in making decisions regarding the conduct of the study.

Two aspects of the monitoring plan need to be specified in the study protocol. First, the frequency of safety evaluations by the DMC should be specified. Generally the reviews are tagged to some proportion of patients completing some time on study. Second, the extent of the data to be reviewed should be specified. Specifically, if efficacy data is to be monitored as part of the monitoring process, the frequency of 'looks' needs to be defined and the impact of the final analysis of the data with respect to the influence on significance level needs to be determined. If a formal interim analysis of efficacy is specified in the protocol, the impact of that analysis on the final analysis is essential. It is also essential that the group responsible for providing data to the DMC do so in a timely manner. A lag of no more than a few weeks should exist between the generation of the data and its review by the DMC. While this may place demands on the study sponsor, it is essential in order for the DMC to adequately monitor the study.

A number of approaches have been used to monitor efficacy data and the reader is referred to Chapter 30 as well as to several texts that will provide a detailed overview of the subject. Both frequentist and bayesian approaches have been used. Importantly, methods have been established that allow an ongoing assessment of efficacy by the DMC without requiring a large adjustment of the significance level at completion of the study and many studies now employ group sequential methods.25

SPONSORED TRIALS

Clinical trials fall into two general categories: those that are investigator-initiated and funded by a granting agency and those that have corporate sponsors. In the latter case, investigators are generally recruited for the study by the sponsor. The role of investigators in investigator-initiated studies is generally uncomplicated. The investigator, along with a steering committee, is responsible for the conduct of the study. In the case of National Institutes of Health (NIH)-funded studies the granting agency may contribute to or appoint the membership of the steering committee. In some instances the DMC (see Ch. 30) is appointed by the investigators and in other cases by the granting agency.

In the case of cooperate sponsored trials the role of investigators is considerably more complicated. However some general guidelines should be consistently followed. A steering committee should include at least the principal investigator and ideally other investigators. The investigators should have considerable input into the design of the study. Not unexpectedly, corporate sponsors may ask for design elements that differ from what the investigators would prefer. It is important that both parties feel comfortable with the ultimate design. Even more important is the analysis of the data set at the completion of the study. At a minimum, the investigators must have equal access to the complete data set and have the agreement that they can conduct an independent analysis of the data and, following appropriate guidelines allowing the sponsor to review the results, publish the results independently. Unfortunately, an increasingly large number of studies with corporate sponsorship allow the investigators only limited access to the data and study reports consist entirely of results based on the analyses done by the sponsor. In most cases these analyses are performed well but the investigators should always have a role in the analysis and not simply endorse study results provided by the sponsor.

Another important aspect of corporate-sponsored studies is the creation of a DMC. Ideally the DMC should be formed before the study design is finalized. Since the DMC will be responsible for monitoring the safety of the study, it is essential that the DMC members are comfortable with the study design. In addition, issues such as the timing of safety reviews should be specified. Also, if interim analyses are planned, their timing and the nature of the analyses need to be specified. Both the investigators and the members of the DMC should be free of significant conflicts of interest that would compromise their performance or give an appearance of bias.

A final issue with respect to corporate-sponsored studies is the potential conflict surrounding the reimbursement of study centers. Often, funding is based on the number of study visits for each patient. This funding mechanism can produce an inherent conflict with respect to dropping patients from the study. However, the funding mechanism can also represent an incentive to continuing follow-up of patients no longer in one of the treatment arms.

HUMAN SUBJECT PROTECTION

Elements that are central in assuring both the investigator and the IRB that the research has given sufficient attention to the protection of human subjects include evidence that:

- The research plan is scientifically sound and the subject's exposure to risk is minimized
- The selection of subjects is fair and equitable
- The risk to participants is reasonable in relationship to the potential benefit either to the patient or in knowledge relating to the disease
- The appropriate informed consent is obtained from subjects.

The elements of human subject protection that will be incorporated into the study need to be clearly defined in the study protocol. Central to the protection of patients is the informed consent. Unfortunately, too many investigators deal with the informed consent in a pro forma manner. Many investigators also consider the informed consent to be limited to the paper document. While the consent that is signed is essential, a careful description of the study, along with the demands that will be placed on the patients, and with risks, is just as important. In addition, it is very important that conflicts of interest such as financial support for the study and other aspects of the relationship of the investigator to the sponsor be made known to the patient. Finally, many medical centers have competing studies and a part of the informed consent is to share with a patient all the studies for which they may be eligible and to say why one is being recommended over another. Certainly, providing informed consent is much more complicated now than before the expansion of clinical trials in MS and before the approval of disease-modifying therapies.

TRIAL DESIGN

PHASE 0

Since the concept of an exploratory IND is new (www.fda.gov/cder/guidance/6384dft.htm), studies or approaches have not been published. Since the goal is to expose subjects to very low doses and for limited periods in order to gain some insights into the behavior of the therapy, it is expected that the studies will involve very small numbers of patients studied carefully for the behavior of the therapy after a single dose or a small number of doses.

PHASE I

Phase I studies are designed to provide preliminary information on safety and on the highest tolerated dose of an experimental medication. Despite the importance of the phase I study on the ultimate design of phase III studies, little attention has been given to the design of phase I studies until recently. The designs for phase I studies have come largely from the field of oncology and may not be optimal for a disease such as MS. The most common design is to treat patients in small cohorts of three to six patients at each individual dose. Often, the design will involve four or five patients on active medication and one on placebo. Dosing begins at a dose expected to be safe or at the lowest dose considered to have biological activity. The endpoint of a phase I study is most often some predefined level of toxicity such as a proportion of patients experiencing an adverse event thought to be associated with the treatment. After a cohort completes dosing without significant adverse events, the next cohort is started and the dose is escalated. When significant side effects are noted, the design stipulates that the next cohort be treated at the preceding dose. If that dose is free of side effects, some designs may allow rechallenging the next higher dose. The importance of the placebo component is generally small and it is most useful after a number of doses are tested, since the number of placebo patients will then be large enough to provide some guidance regarding the incidence of adverse events occurring independent of active therapy.

Since the goal is to escalate the dose in as short a time as possible, the endpoints are related to safety and can include changes in chemistry, blood counts or general health. Outcomes related to efficacy are generally not included, although worsening of disease is an important outcome in phase I studies in MS. Imaging may also be used as an outcome and some investigators may elect to monitor MRI for evidence of worsening. Special caution needs to be employed if MRI is used as an outcome measure for safety in phase I studies, however. In patients with evidence of active disease on MRI, the level of activity is known to fluctuate or change from month to month. So, unless a long baseline is obtained, the chances of reaching an incorrect conclusion regarding the safety of a new therapy is high.

Phase I studies tend to enroll patients with secondary progressive MS and with more advanced disease because the course is generally less likely to change spontaneously and because worsening of disease due to the experimental medication is thought to be more acceptable in patients who have failed other therapies. Often, patients in this stage of disease have little acute activity on MRI so the appearance of new activity may signal worsening associated with the therapy. However, even in patients with secondary progressive MS, acute activity does occur, so considerable caution needs to be used in using MRI as a safety outcome unless baseline activity in the patient is well understood.

A concern often encountered in phase I studies is the time required to complete a wide dose range. Because corporate sponsors, in particular, often want the testing of new therapies to move as quickly as possible, only a limited number of doses are often tested and in some cases the safety of only a single dose will be tested. While expedient in terms of time, the failure to obtain information on a range of doses and to fully understand the upper dose limits with respect to toxicity will impact on all the clinical studies that follow using that medication.

An aspect of phase I studies that is often ignored is the opportunity to begin to get some biological evidence for proof of principle for the therapy. Based on the proposed mechanism of action of the new therapy, biological testing of patients at the various doses can often be useful in determining the relationship to biological activity versus toxicity.

Some innovative alternatives to the design described have been suggested and some are now being used.[26] A design based on bayesian statistics has been described.[27] The approach first develops a set of prior assumptions regarding both the proposed toxicity and efficacy at the doses to be tested. Small groups are exposed to increasing doses, with an ongoing estimate of the frequency of both toxicity and efficacy as defined in the study until a safe and efficacious dose is found. The investigators argue that the approach will often allow stopping before a study would be stopped using the conventional design. The bayesian design actually incorporates elements of both phase I and phase II studies. While this design has the marked advantage of providing a process for dose finding based on both toxicity and efficacy, it can only be applied to situations where efficacy can be determined over a short time period. Thus the application of this design to MS seems limited, apart from possibly studies using acute changes on MRI as an outcome.

PHASE II

Phase II studies or preliminary studies are designed to provide preliminary evidence of efficacy or proof or principle as well as additional safety information. The most important goal of a phase II study is to provide detailed information that can be used in the design of a phase III study. Since phase III studies are usually extremely costly in both money and human resources, the information from the phase II study on the optimal dose, the best outcome and the appropriate duration of the study will be essential. Although phase II data can also help to decide whether patient characteristics need to be considered in the design, phase II studies are often conducted using patients with very narrow entry characteristics. They are also designed to provide additional safety information at the doses selected for study.

As with phase I studies, only recently has there been much attention to design issues for phase II studies. Many phase II studies resemble a scaled-down phase III, employing randomization to treatment arms and the inclusion of a control group, often placebo-treated. Two of the most common issues faced in the design of a phase II study are the selection of doses to be studied and the choice of outcomes, which, in turn, influences the duration of the study. As mentioned previously, however, a wide range of designs can be used for phase II trials depending on the goals of the study. Some consist of simple crossover studies designed primarily to provide some proof of principle. Examples of this design are those using MRI to examine the effect of a treatment on MRI measures of disease. Examples also exist of phase II studies that use historical controls.

Unless a phase I study has provided some information on the efficacy of various doses, the only thing that will be known as the design of the phase II study begins will be the highest dose that probably has a reasonable safety profile. So, the question will arise as to whether only one dose should be studied; will higher doses have greater efficacy or should some lower doses also be studied, since, if they have efficacy, the safety profile might be better, especially for long-term treatment? Inclusion of multiple arms means that the number of patients needed for the study is greater and will impact on recruitment and cost. If the analytical design requires comparison of each arm with another, the sample size increases considerably. Often, the design will include only a comparison of each dose to the control arm, meaning that the design is really one with multiple trials bundled to use a common placebo group.

The selection of the outcomes for phase II studies is also complicated. In MS one is usually most interested in sustained disability. However, studies designed to measure effect on sustained disability require a long study time and so are not practical for phase II studies. Alternatively, the outcome might be relapse rate or time to relapse but these studies often require either large sample sizes or again a long duration. In most cases the developer of a new therapy has a desire to complete the phase II study in as short a time as possible. Indeed, the effort to shorten the phase II process often means that much of what is needed from the study is not achieved and as a consequence the design of the phase III study is compromised.

Because of the issues discussed above, the use of MRI as an outcome in a phase II study is attractive. Many recent examples of phase II studies have used MRI measures of active disease as the primary outcome. While measures of acute activity on MRI will usually allow a smaller sample size than if a clinical outcome is used, and will also allow a study to be completed in a shorter time, some concerns need to be considered. The first is that the relationship between disease activity on MRI and disability is, at best, unclear.[15,16] A treatment that reduces MRI activity will not necessarily reduce disability. Second, the investigator needs to consider the mechanism of action of the new therapy. If it is one that is expected to target lesion development, then acute disease on MRI as measured by contrast enhancement is a good outcome. However, if the proposed mechanism of the new treatment targets a more distal stage in lesion development, contrast enhancement may not be a sensitive measure of activity.

Because of the difficulties in conducting placebo-controlled studies discussed previously, the design of even small phase II studies that would have normally used a design incorporating randomization to active therapy or placebo are problematic. Several alternative designs have been suggested and will be discussed below under the section on alternative trial designs.

PHASE III

The phase III trial represents the critical step in the development of a new therapy. The RCT has been considered the gold standard. In its purest form the RCT involves randomization of patients to either active therapy or placebo. The study is double-blinded, meaning that neither the patient nor the physician knows the treatment assignment, and patients are entered into the arms of the study in a randomized manner. Analysis of the outcomes is most often done using an ITT cohort and often using a survival analysis type of analysis. A number of modifications can be made to the basic design, including analysis adjusted for covariates or stratification of patients at entry. An interim analysis is often incorporated. The reader is referred to several excellent texts that provide a detailed description of the design and analytical plan used in the RCT.[1–3]

In designing trials in MS today, a more complicated issue is whether the RCT is ethical or practical. An even more fundamental question is whether it is the best design for testing a new therapy. The revision of the Declaration of Helsinki[20] has been discussed and the number of investigators and ethicists who believe that the use of placebo in trials of diseases for which there are approved therapies is wrong is increasing. Some current trials have recruited centers in countries that do not have widespread use of or access to disease-modifying therapies. This practice may be in conflict with the recent revision of the Declaration of Helsinki unless all patients entered into the study are allowed to continue with either the tested therapy if it proves to be effective or an alternative therapy that is known to be effective. Certainly, the expense and logistical difficulties of implementing this policy will be large. A detailed examination of the ethical aspects of this approach is beyond the scope of this chapter and has been discussed at length in relationship to antiretroviral therapies in underdeveloped countries. The approach of using research centers in underdeveloped countries has implications other than the ethical ones, however. Centers may have only limited experience with the conduct of a clinical trial and careful attention needs to be given to the quality of the data collection.

As for the logistical aspects of the RCT in MS, the number of patients eligible for enrollment is increasingly small because of early treatment with disease-modifying therapies. A solution would be to enroll patients who have failed treatment with disease-modifying therapies but this has the risk of providing a very biased patient cohort and one that is not representative of the general MS population. In fact it could represent a population of patients who are less likely to respond to any therapy.

Most important is the question 'Is the RCT the best design for a trial of a new therapy in an environment with several approved therapies?' When new therapies are tested against placebo the results provide little information on the relative value of the new therapy compared to existing therapy. Unless the new therapy yields results dramatically different from those of previous studies the relative value of the new therapy will remain uncertain.

ALTERNATIVE TRIAL DESIGNS

What are the solutions to these problems with the use of the RCT? A recent workshop sponsored by the NMSS addressed this question.[17] Some well documented and well researched approaches exist. In the examples discussed below the reader will see that the effort is most often to minimize the exposure to placebo; in only a few examples is the placebo completely eliminated. In general the approaches minimize the exposure to placebo by reducing the sample size or by shortening the duration of the study and are more applicable to phase II studies. Phase III studies require definitive evidence that efficacy is demonstrated and that the sample size and the duration of the study are sufficient to assess the safety of the treatment. The two approaches that are the most applicable to phase III studies are those using an active control arm – either equivalency- or superiority-type studies – or those using a group sequential type of design. These will be discussed first.

DESIGNS APPLICABLE TO PHASE III TRIALS THAT ELIMINATE A PLACEBO ARM

Add-on designs

One of the easiest solutions to avoiding the use of placebo is to study patients who are on an approved therapy but are only partial responders. These patients are then randomized to either placebo or the study therapy and all patients are kept on the approved therapy. The approach has considerable merit and has been acceptable to regulatory authorities in both the USA and in Europe. Despite the positive aspects of this approach there are also several potential problems. These include: 1) unknown drug interactions, 2) potentially large sample sizes, since the control arm will have a partial treatment effect, and 3) resulting uncertainty about the value of the new therapy as a monotherapy.

The first issue should be addressed in at least a preliminary manner in a phase II study so that patients are not committed to a large phase III study that will fail because of adverse events related to the combined therapy. However, the most important concern is the lack of evidence of efficacy for the new therapy as a monotherapy. Unless there is a compelling objection the design should include a component that includes withdrawal of the approved therapy from the test arm. A recent example of the use of an add-on design is the study of natalizumab in the treatment of RRMS.[28,29] The study enrolled patients under treatment with intramuscular interferon (IFN)β-1a and randomized them to active treatment with natalizumab or placebo. The combination arm showed a highly significant treatment effect. At the same time, a second study was done comparing natalizumab to placebo, and again natalizumab was shown to be effective. The problem with the interpretation of the results is that one does not know whether there is truly an additive treatment effect or whether the results in the first study were simply related to the effectiveness of natalizumab. Inclusion of a subsequent phase of the study that withdrew IFNβ-1a from the active test arm should have provided the answer. It is unfortunate when opportunities to fully explore the value of a new therapy are missed.

Testing against an active comparator as monotherapies

Superiority A superiority study compares a new therapy to an active comparator previously shown to be effective. The design is attractive since it avoids a placebo and provides a true head-to-head comparison of the therapy being tested and an approved therapy. A suggestion has been made that, in a particular disease, one well-studied therapy could be the 'gold standard' against which new therapies are tested.[30] Thus the results are easily translated into clinical practice. However, the design is seldom used, since the samples sizes needed to show a significantly greater treatment effect than one already shown to be effective is often very large. One example of its use in MS was a comparison of two preparations of IFNβ-1a.[31] IFNβ-1a (intramuscularly) was approved in both the USA and Europe while the IFNβ-1a (subcutaneously) was only approved in Europe. The demonstration that the second preparation was superior contributed to the approval of the drug by the FDA in the USA under the provisions of the Orphan Drug Regulations.

Equivalency and noninferiority The object of an equivalency study is to determine whether a new therapy is as good as an active comparator – usually a therapy that has been previously approved for use in the condition being studied. While an equivalency study would seem to be a logical alternative to a placebo-controlled study, especially since it could provide insight into the relative value of the new therapy in comparison to the existing therapy, a number of specific difficulties exist with the design. At a theoretical level, some have argued that an equivalency study has no value, since one can never be sure that the active comparator worked in any particular study if no placebo group is included.[32] If, under the experimental conditions being used, the active comparator was ineffective, the investigators would come to the erroneous conclusion that the new therapy was effective. To overcome this difficulty it is essential that the active comparator has been shown to be effective in a well-designed clinical trial comparing the effectiveness to placebo, that the treatment effect was robust and that the equivalency study is being done under conditions as nearly identical as possible. Thus, the study cohort, outcome measures and duration of treatment must be identical or very similar.

A further difficulty is the analytical plan. Since it is statistically impossible to show that the two therapies are identical in their therapeutic effect (a condition that would require an infinite population), the investigator needs to establish at the beginning the margin of difference between the two treatments that will be considered to reflect a similar treatment effect. The analytical plan for a noninferiority study (looking only at whether the new therapy is worse than the active comparator) can be different from that of an equivalency study (looking at whether the effect of the new study is within certain boundaries – either better or worse – than the active comparator), although the terms are often used interchangeably. Several statistical approaches have been used to address the analysis of equivalency and the involvement of a statistician knowledgeable about clinical trial design is essential in the planning stages and conduct of an equivalency or noninferiority study.

Suboptimal comparator An alternative approach to a study design that avoids a true placebo is to use a dose of the active therapy that is known to be suboptimal. The design of the study is similar to one using a true placebo. Since the control group will be exposed to inadequate therapy, the design does not really avoid the ethical issues surrounding the use of placebo. In fact, the design raises additional ethical issues, since subjects are often not fully informed that the suboptimal group is expected to be no better than a placebo. Thus the approach not only fails to avoid the problems with a placebo but also raises the serious issue of whether the approach is consistent with the elements set forth in the Declaration of Helsinki.[33] The approach has generally been rejected by regulatory authorities in Europe but has been found to be acceptable by the FDA.

Replacing a placebo group with a 'virtual' or natural history control

In theory, as enough natural history data accumulates from large placebo groups it should be possible to extract a cohort matched for the patients recruited to the active arm of a study and avoid a placebo group. In fact this was one of the goals when the Sylvia Lawry Center for MS Research (www.slcmsr.org) was established. To be effective a database would need to include a large cohort in order to match a cohort for the multiple variables that exist. One of the largest problems is that variables will tend to change over time. Placebo groups in studies before the widespread use of disease-modifying therapies may possibly have different characteristics from a group of untreated patients entering a current study. One of the probable advantages of a RCT is that at each site the same investigator is recruiting the patients for the study. Although there may be small differences between centers in a multicenter study, it is likely that the clinical skills of the investigator will result in a relatively homogenous cohort at each site and that these individuals will be distributed between active and placebo or control arms. It is unlikely that a virtual placebo group could ever achieve this level of homogeneity.

DESIGNS APPLICABLE TO PHASE II TRIALS THAT MAY REDUCE EXPOSURE TO PLACEBO

Sequential design

A sequential trial design is really an approach for monitoring accumulating interim data and then using the results to either stop or continue the study or in some designs to modify the enrollment or even modify the randomization scheme.[25] The approaches used most commonly are frequentist-based but approaches based on bayesian statistics have also been used.[34,35] In the most common application a series of interim analyses are used to monitor the study. Boundaries for stopping the study are established prior to starting the study and if the results cross those boundaries the study is stopped, thus reducing both the number of patients exposed to the inactive arm of the study and the duration of exposure to the inactive therapy for those already enrolled. An excellent example of a sequential design is the SERoNE study, which compared carbamazepine to remacemide in the treatment of seizures. The results established the effectiveness of carbamazepine.[36] Of special note, this study combined both the comparison of two active therapies and a sequential design.

The essential aspect of a sequential design is the monitoring plan and sequential methods can be used for monitoring studies that do not incorporate other aspects of a sequential design. One of the most common monitoring procedures is called a group sequential procedure. In the group sequential approach, grouped data from the two arms are considered rather than data from individual patients. The group sequential approach described by O'Brien and Fleming is commonly used by DMCs to monitor clinical trials.[25] The approach has been modified by Lan and DeMets so that the type I error 'spent' by continued monitoring results is known at the onset.[37] The reader is again referred to one of several excellent discussions of the group sequential approach for monitoring clinical studies. Investigators serving on DMCs should, in particular, be familiar with the approach.

Multiple and composite outcomes

In theory, if endpoints could be used that more fully captured the change in disease activity that one is trying to effect with treatment, the sample size for the study could be reduced. As the reader will recall, sample size is related to the proposed difference in the events that are expected to occur in the control group and in the treatment group. If the event rate could be increased and the events reflected the disease process targeted by the treatment, a significant reduction in sample size should follow.

Probably the best example is the MSFC, which is a composite score designed to capture several aspects of the disease process in MS.[12,13] Indeed, evidence suggests that the sample sizes for studies using the MSFC are smaller than are required for the EDSS. The difference in sample size was the basis for one study of IFNβ-1a in SPMS that used the MSFC.[38] The interpretation of the study results is complicated but there was some suggestion that a treatment effect was seen with the MSFC that was not seen with the EDSS. What is not clear is whether the results were related to the use of the MSFC as a composite or to the behavior of one of the components of the MSFC. Regardless of this, the MSFC holds promise as a more informative outcome compared to EDSS.

There is also interest in the use of MRI composite outcomes.[39] One important issue regarding composite outcomes is that the elements in the composite need to be considered independently. Otherwise the outcome tends to measure the same thing twice. Establishing the independence of individual outcomes is often very difficult and this is especially true using MRI measures. When multiple outcomes are used, the investigator must address how the outcomes are weighted. The reader is referred to a discussion of the statistical approaches that can be used in the report of the workshop on Alternative Trial Designs in MS.[17]

Most of the issues relating to composite outcomes also apply to the use of multiple independent outcomes. In theory they can provide increased sensitivity in capturing the events related to disease activity and consequently reduce sample sizes. Multiple outcomes have been used in treatment trials in MS. For example, the study of mitoxantrone used worsening of MS as measured by a multivariate analysis for five clinical variables, EDSS, ambulation index, number of relapses requiring steroid treatment and standard neurological status score.[40] Clearly these were not independent outcomes but they were accepted by the FDA and led to approval of the drug for MS. It is likely that increased attention will focus on the use of multiple and composite endpoints over the next few years.

Surrogate outcomes

A surrogate outcome is a measurement other than the true clinical measurement that predicts the outcome of the true clinical outcome. The use of a surrogate outcome, then, is expected to shorten the duration of the study, since the surrogate outcome will occur in advance of the true clinical outcome such as progression of disability. Over the past years a number of trialists working in various fields have examined the behavior of surrogate outcomes and have developed rules for the validation of a surrogate.[41] In brief, the surrogate needs to be predictive of the clinical outcome and to reflect the disease mechanisms involved in the pathways targeted by various classes of treatments previously approved for the disease. In addition, many of the surrogate outcomes that have been applied in other diseases have often led to erroneous conclusions.[42] The reader is referred to a review of some of the pitfalls in order to appreciate the difficulties encountered in the use of surrogate outcomes.[43,44] Regardless of this, the use of various MRI measures as a surrogate are still thought to have sufficient merit to warrant careful study. Currently, efforts underwritten by the NMSS are under way to examine the potential of the use of contrast-enhancing lesions as a surrogate for relapse rate.

It is important to note that unvalidated surrogates, those that have been shown to correlate with clinical outcomes, can have value in exploratory trials. For example, contrast-enhancing lesion frequency, while not a validated surrogate, can be an effective outcome for early proof-of-principle studies. In addition, unvalidated surrogates can be and have been used to obtain 'conditional approval', with the condition that subsequent follow-up of patients will confirm the value of the treatment with regard to the clinical endpoint. Indeed, this approach was used in the approval of natalizumab.[28] The conditional approval was based on relapse rate determined at 1 year, with the understanding that the study would continue in order to provide data on progression and on safety. As evidenced from this study, one of the concerns about the use of a 'conditional approval' approach is that a treatment may be approved before sufficient safety data exist.

Phase II/phase III

Since both phase II and phase III trials have as an important goal the comparative treatment efficacy of the new therapy, some have examined approaches for moving from phase II to phase III in a single protocol. As mentioned earlier, phase II studies often use an intermediate outcome. This is especially true in MS studies; often the outcome in phase II studies is MRI measures or relapse rates, while the primary outcome in phase II studies is most often a survival analysis of disability. Often the goal of a phase II study is, in addition to providing additional safety data, to establish the optimal dose. Thus an approach combining phase II and phase III is sometimes called 'drop the loser' or sequential weeding.[45] The design has also been applied to phase I studies. Most often, this design has been suggested for studies sponsored by the pharmaceutical industry with the goal of deciding which of several formulations or preparations should go into further testing. A multiple-arm study is started with the goal of allowing the monitoring of preliminary results to elect the best arm and allow that arm, along with the control arm, to continue into phase III. An objection to the study design has been that the phase II study may lack design elements that would exist if the phase II study were completed separately and the results were then used to design a stand-alone phase III study.

Crossover studies

Crossover study designs are most applicable to phase II studies. The design is attractive since all patients will be exposed to the active therapy, eliminating some of the objections to the use of a placebo arm. While the design can have value, there are a number of concerns. The most important of these include the washout period and unblinding. Unless the duration of the treatment effect of the experimental therapy is known (which would be unusual for a new therapy), the duration of the washout period is difficult to determine. If the washout is too short, the sensitivity in determining the treatment effect in the crossover group will be subject to a high type II error. For this reason some crossover designs have based the primary outcome on the first phase of the study and only used the crossover as confirmation. Indeed, several early phase II studies only used a single crossover without a placebo group when MRI measures are used as the outcome measure. This design has been effective in demonstrating proof of principle for new therapies. The second problem with a crossover design is unblinding. Since most therapies have some side effects, patients, and subsequently the investigative team, will be unblinded as patients cross from the active therapy to placebo or from placebo to active therapy. Thus considerable care needs to be given to the influence of unblinding on the study results.

Adaptive randomization

Randomization methods commonly used have one quality in common: individuals have a constant probability of independent assignment to treatment arms. An alternative approach is adaptive randomization, in which the randomization of an individual subject is determined at the time that individual enters the study and is adjusted based on characteristics of individuals previously randomized. The adaptation of the randomization can be based either on some covariate such as a prognostic feature or on a response variable. Adaptive randomization using the response data of previously enrolled subjects[46,47] is often called 'play the winner'. Although this type of design has been considered to present difficulties in analysis, the design is receiving more attention and there are now an increasing number of examples of its use. The design has the advantage of potentially minimizing the number of subjects exposed to placebo or an ineffective therapy. Of interest are designs that incorporate elements of a group sequential design, phase I/phase II study and adaptive randomization.[48]

TRIAL DESIGN FOR STUDIES OF NEUROPROTECTION AND NEUROREPAIR

Although the general principles of trial design apply to any trial regardless of the outcomes used, the trial designs described in this chapter are primarily targeted at testing therapies that will modify acute disease activity. Certainly, a trial of a therapy that is neuroprotective could use similar clinical endpoints such as MSFC, EDSS or ambulation index. However, the potential sample sizes will be large and the duration of the study long. The issues surrounding the design of clinical trials of neuroprotective or reparative strategies were the subject of part of the workshop on trial design held in Washington, DC, in 2005.[17] Clearly the design of strategies for testing protective and reparative treatments is one of the major challenges facing the MS research community. Considerable effort is now being directed at defining the role of unconventional MRI measures and the sample sizes that would be associated with these outcomes. Certainly one of the major hurdles will be to establish an approach that can be used in phase II studies so that only the most promising therapies go into the costly, long clinical studies that will be needed.

SUMMARY

One of the major accomplishments of the MS research community over the past two decades has been the excellence that has evolved with respect to the design and conduct of clinical trials in the disease. Probably few areas of medicine have a clinical research community better practiced as clinical trialists and the record of accomplishments has been impressive. With the successes have come new problems. The success in the MS community with the use of RCTs, which have led to the approval of five therapies for MS, must now be extended to finding alternative approaches that can be used to study new therapies in the presence of approved treatments. Achieving the high ethical standards expected of any clinical trial today and especially the need to safeguard the right of human subjects will need to be addressed, together with the possible alternative designs that will be needed to move the field forward. It is hoped that, as research continues on the use of advanced imaging methods, the MRI will become an even more valuable tool for the assessment of new therapies.

A final point not discussed in this chapter is the importance of tying the clinical testing of new therapies together with laboratory studies designed to examine the mechanisms of the new therapies. Even in studies of failed therapies, a careful examination of the underlying effects on biological responses can provide important insights into the disease process. Conducting clinical studies without providing a means for careful assessment of the related biology is shortsighted. Hopefully funding agencies and corporate sponsors will not neglect the importance of the bed to the bench component of clinical trials.

REFERENCES

1. Meinert CL, Tonascia S. Clinical trials; design, conduct and analysis. Oxford: Oxford University Press; 1986.
2. Friedman ML, Furberg CD, DeMets DL. Fundamentals of clinical trials. New York: Springer; 1998.
3. Chow S, Liu J. Design and analysis of clinical trials. Hoboken, NJ: John Wiley; 2004.
4. Van Helmont JB. Oriatrike, or physick refined. London: Lodowick-Loyd; 1662.
5. Lind JA. A treatise of the scurvy. Edinburgh: Sand, Murray & Cochran; 1753.
6. Sutton HG. Cases of rheumatic fever. Guy's Hosp Rep 1865; 11: 392–428.
7. Diehl HS, Baker AB, Cowan DW. Cold vaccines: an evaluation based on a

controlled study. JAMA 1938; 11: 1168–1173.

8. Rose AS, Kuzma JW, Kurtzke JF et al. Cooperative study in the evaluation of therapy in multiple sclerosis. ACTH vs. placebo – final report. Neurology 1970; 20: 1–59.

9. Herndon R. Proceeding of the International Conference on Therapeutic Trials in Multiple Sclerosis, Grand Island, NY, April 23–24, 1982. Arch Neurol 1983; 40: 663–710.

10. Whitaker JN, McFarland HF, Rudge P et al. Outcomes assessment in multiple sclerosis clinical trials: a critical analysis. Mult Scler 1995; 1: 37–47.

11. Kurtzke JF. Rating neurologic impairment in multiple sclerosis: an expanded disability status scale (EDSS). Neurology 1983; 33: 1444–1452.

12. Cutter GR, Baier ML, Rudick RA et al. Development of a multiple sclerosis functional composite as a clinical trial outcome measure. Brain 1999; 122: 871–882.

13. Rudick RA, Cutter G, Reingold S. The multiple sclerosis functional composite: a new clinical outcome measure for multiple sderosis trials. Mult Scler 2002; 8: 359–365.

14. Filippi M, Horsfield MA, Ader HJ et al. Guidelines for using quantitative measures of brain magnetic resonance imaging abnormalities in monitoring the treatment of multiple sclerosis. Ann Neurol 1998; 43: 499–506.

15. Miller DH, Grossman RI, Reingold SC, McFarland HF. The role of magnetic resonance techniques in understanding and managing multiple sclerosis. Brain 1998; 121: 3–24.

16. McFarland HF, Barkhof F, Antel J, Miller DH. The role of MRI as a surrogate outcome measure in multiple sclerosis. Mult Scler 2002; 8: 40–51.

17. McFarland HF, Reingold SC. The future of multiple sclerosis therapies: redesigning multiple sclerosis clinical trials in a new therapeutic era. Mult Scler 2005; 11: 669–676.

18. World Medical Association Declaration of Helsinki. Recommendations guiding physicians in biomedical research involving human subjects. JAMA 1997; 277: 925–926.

19. National Commission for the Protection of Human Subjects of Biomedical and Behavioral Research. The Belmont Report: Ethical principles and guidelines for the protection of human subjects of research.

Washington, DC: US Government Printing Office; 1979.

20. World Medical Association Declaration of Helsinki. Ethical principles for medical research involving human subjects. JAMA 2000; 284: 3043–3045.

21. Levine RJ. Ethics and regulations in clinical research. Baltimore, MD: Urban & Schwarzenberg; 1981.

22. Beecher HK. Ethics and clinical research. N Engl J Med 1966; 274: 1354–1360.

23. Lublin FD, Reingold SC. Placebo-controlled clinical trials in multiple sclerosis: ethical considerations. National Multiple Sclerosis Society (USA) Task Force on Placebo-Controlled Clinical Trials in MS. Ann Neurol 2001; 49: 677–681.

24. Freiman JA, Chalmers TC, Smith H Jr, Kuebler R. The importance of beta, the type II error and sample size in the design and interpretation of the randomized control trial. Survey of 71 'negative' trials. N Engl J Med 1978; 299: 690–694.

25. O'Brien PC, Fleming TR. A multiple testing procedure for clinical trials. Biometrics 1979; 35: 549–556.

26. Eisenhauer EA, O'Dwyer PJ, Christian M, Humphrey JS. Phase I clinical trial design in cancer drug development. J Clin Oncol 2000; 18: 684–692.

27. Thall PF, Russell KE. A strategy for dose-finding and safety monitoring based on efficacy and adverse outcomes in phase I/II clinical trials. Biometrics 1998; 54: 251–264.

28. Polman CH, O'Connor PW, Havrdova E et al. A randomized, placebo-controlled trial of natalizumab for relapsing multiple sclerosis. N Engl J Med 2006; 354: 899–910.

29. Rudick RA, Stuart WH, Calabresi PA et al. Natalizumab plus interferon beta-1a for relapsing multiple sclerosis. N Engl J Med 2006; 354: 911–923.

30. Brodie MJ, Whitehead J. Active control comparisons: the ideal trial design. Epilepsy Res 2006; 68: 69–73.

31. Panitch H, Goodin DS, Francis G et al. Randomized, comparative study of interferon beta-1a treatment regimens in MS: The EVIDENCE Trial. Neurology 2002; 59: 1496–1506.

32. Leber PD. Hazards of inference: the active control investigation. Epilepsia 1989; 30(suppl 1): S57–S63; discussion S64–S68.

33. Schwabe S. Monotherapy comparative trials: placebos and suboptimal comparators. Epilepsy Res 2001; 45: 93–96; discussion 97–99.

34. Goldman AI. Issues in designing sequential stopping rules for monitoring side effects in clinical trials. Control Clin Trials 1987; 8: 327–337.

35. Freedman LS, Spiegelhalter DJ. Comparison of Bayesian with group sequential methods for monitoring clinical trials. Control Clin Trials 1989; 10: 357–367.

36. Whitehead J. Monotherapy trials: sequential design. Epilepsy Res 2001; 45: 81–87; discussion 89–91.

37. Lan KK, DeMets DL. Changing frequency of interim analysis in sequential monitoring. Biometrics 1989; 45: 1017–1020.

38. Cohen JA, Cutter GR, Fischer JS et al. Benefit of interferon beta-1a on MSFC progression in secondary progressive MS. Neurology 2002; 59: 679–687.

39. Wolinsky JS, Narayana PA, Noseworthy JH et al. Linomide in relapsing and secondary progressive MS: part II: MRI results. MRI Analysis Center of the University of Texas-Houston, Health Science Center, and the North American Linomide Investigators. Neurology 2000; 54: 1734–1741.

40. Hartung HP, Gonsette R, Konig N et al. Mitoxantrone in progressive multiple sclerosis: a placebo-controlled, double-blind, randomised, multicentre trial. Lancet 2002; 360: 2018–2025.

41. Prentice RL. Surrogate endpoints in clinical trials: definition and operational criteria. Stat Med 1989; 8: 431–440.

42. Fleming TR, DeMets DL. Surrogate end points in clinical trials: are we being misled? Ann Intern Med 1996; 125: 605–613.

43. Hughes MD. Evaluating surrogate endpoints. Control Clin Trials 2002; 23: 703–707.

44. Fleming TR. Surrogate endpoints and FDA's accelerated approval process. Health Aff (Millwood) 2005; 24: 67–78.

45. Thall PF, Millikan RE, Sung HG. Evaluating multiple treatment courses in clinical trials. Stat Med 2000; 19: 1011–1028.

46. Chang M, Chow SC. A hybrid Bayesian adaptive design for dose response trials. J Biopharm Stat 2005; 15: 677–691.

47. Thall PF, Wathen JK. Covariate-adjusted adaptive randomization in a sarcoma trial with multi-stage treatments. Stat Med 2005; 24: 1947–1964.

48. Kelly PJ, Stallard N, Todd S. An adaptive group sequential design for phase II/III clinical trials that select a single treatment from several. J Biopharm Stat 2005; 15: 641–658.

The role of data monitoring committees in multiple sclerosis clinical trials

S. C. Reingold

INTRODUCTION

The use of randomized, controlled clinical trials to establish the safety and efficacy of therapeutic interventions is a relatively new concept. For multiple sclerosis (MS), an international meeting in the early 1980s set a 'gold-standard' for such studies[1] that has been followed with appropriate innovations and increasing sophistication since that time. Over the years, recommendations and guidelines have been produced relating to use of placebos[2] and magnetic resonance imaging (MRI)[3,4] in MS trials; revised clinical rating scales have been recommended;[5] issues surrounding interactions with sponsors have been discussed[6] and conduct and interpretation of extension studies have been reviewed.[7] New design and statistical analysis concepts for MS trials in an era of multiple available therapies have been debated.[8]

However, the monitoring of ongoing MS trials to ensure patient safety and quality of trial conduct and to evaluate interim efficacy signals has received little formal attention. Nonetheless, independent committees that undertake these responsibilities, variably called data monitoring committees (DMCs), data safety monitoring boards (DSMBs) or committees (DSMCs), data safety committees (DSCs) or other variants,[9,10] have been in place for all pivotal MS clinical trials that have resulted in regulatory review/approval, and for many earlier-phase clinical trials as well, for nearly two decades. The US Food and Drug Administration (FDA) and National Institutes of Health (NIH) now require such monitoring for all pivotal studies under their jurisdiction. There is a growing literature on the general topic of data and safety monitoring in clinical trials, with over 150 journal articles in the past 20 years, several whole-issue journal volumes devoted to the topic (e.g. *Statistics in Medicine* 1993; 12 and *American Heart Journal* 2001; 141), a number of published monographs[11] and a seminal text[12] that explore the value, specific roles, conduct and controversies of such monitoring groups. Through the late 1990s there were no set procedures for conduct and operation of such monitoring groups for any disease[13] but there have been more recent calls for international standardization of their composition and function.[14]

There is little mention of MS clinical trials in any of these sources and virtually no examples from past MS studies in the wealth of illustrative scenarios that these materials use. However, the general concepts of quality interim trial monitor-

ing and the examples that are provided from trials in other disease areas are broadly applicable to trials for any disease and have informed and guided the structure and conduct of MS clinical trial monitoring as well. The purpose of this chapter is to describe the history, purpose, composition and conduct of clinical trial data monitoring committees (DMCs, to be used hereafter) and to bring the concept closer to the MS clinical investigator community.

WHAT IS THE PURPOSE OF A DATA MONITORING COMMITTEE?

Data monitoring committees have variable roles and responsibilities in clinical trials. At a minimum they are charged with periodically reviewing data from an ongoing clinical trial and advising trial organizers and sponsors about trial continuation and needed modifications.[9] Such monitoring provides an evaluation of the safety and wellbeing of enrolled subjects and of ongoing risk–benefit of the experimental intervention that is independent of sponsors, organizers and investigators. Ongoing assessment of study conduct by a DMC, in addition to assessment of safety and efficacy, can also help to ensure that at the end of the study the integrity of the trial is preserved and data are interpretable and not compromised by avoidable problems in study design or implementation. Such independent oversight can also help to protect sponsors and investigators from allegations of fraud, bias and commercial interests in gathering, analyzing and presenting results.[15]

Nationally and internationally recognized standards for protection of human subjects[16–18] provide the core justification for interim data and safety monitoring in clinical trials. Interim monitoring is advisable for clinical trials independent of the type of disease, intervention or sponsor (commercial, governmental, private). The nature and structure of such monitoring will differ depending on the study in question and can vary from (rarely) a single individual serving as a study monitor in an early exploratory trial or in a trial for an agent intended for purely symptomatic relief to a formally constituted committee with a detailed charter and plan of operations for more complex trials. Cairns et al[10] have suggested that a formal DMC is always needed in large trials where ongoing quantitative evaluation of data can have an impact on assessment of morbidity, mortality or other tangible human (especially disease-specific) outcomes, where the risk of treatment is unknown and especially if early studies indicate a potentially problematic safety profile for the intervention under study.

THE HISTORY OF DATA MONITORING COMMITTEES

Formal interim trial monitoring has been used sporadically at least since the late 1960s, when the US NIH began sponsoring large-scale clinical trials and when a special NIH task force was charged with developing guidelines for conduct of such studies. The resulting Greenberg Report, named after its chair, recommended the use of independent advisors to review study protocols and advise the NIH about study conduct. This report, not published for wide distribution until 1988, also advised creation of a mechanism to terminate studies prematurely if it appeared that a study could not meet its original goals or was determined to be unnecessary because of factors external to the study.[19] US-government-funded studies began to include data and safety monitoring groups in their trials shortly after the Greenberg Report was written. However, the NIH began requiring DMCs in all trials they sponsored only in 1998.[10,20,21]

Guidance from the regulatory sector began to evolve in 1992 when a public meeting between the US FDA and representatives of the pharmaceutical industry evaluated how industry-sponsored trials were then monitored.[22,23] Ongoing discussion and evaluation within the FDA and with its constituencies resulted in formal FDA guidance in 2001 on clinical trial monitoring, albeit still in draft form since its issue.[24] This document reinforces the agency's requirement for monitoring by sponsors of studies for new drugs, biologics and devices and identifies the DMC as a group that can be appointed by a sponsor to evaluate accumulating data. The FDA guidelines charge such groups with advising the sponsor on safety for those currently in a trial and those yet to be recruited and advising the sponsor on the continuing validity and scientific merit of the study. They also provide guidance for a DMC's composition, responsibilities and functions. Regulatory guidance for DMCs has also been produced in draft form by the European Medicines Agency.[25] These provide additional insights into determining the need for a DMC, its functions, responsibilities and composition.

In 2005, the NIH's National Institute of Neurological Disorders and Stroke (NINDS), the agency that oversees most of the MS-specific basic and clinical research supported by the NIH, discussed clinical trials monitoring for the studies it supports. Conwit et al[26] provided the agency's principles for data and safety monitoring, described the NINDS's Data and Safety Monitoring Board program and noted that, as of mid-2005, some 42 NINDS-supported trials and other types of clinical research included such monitoring procedures.

Together, these regulations and guidance documents have led to an increased awareness of the value for DMCs in clinical trials world-wide and have gone far to set standards for their composition and operation.

COMPOSITION OF A DATA MONITORING COMMITTEE

DESIRABLE CHARACTERISTICS OF MEMBERS

The composition of a DMC will vary depending on the nature of the study and special issues surrounding the experimental intervention. All DMC members should demonstrate outstanding qualities in terms of competence (to insure that the appropriate clinical, statistical and safety monitoring expertise is in hand), commitment (to attend all meetings, to follow a study through its entire conduct, to prepare for meetings in advance, to ensure that data are adequately reviewed), confidentiality (to ensure that no information about trial data is made available to study sponsors, investigators, patients or the general public) and independence (to avoid financial, institutional and intellectual conflicts of interest).[9–11,27]

While there is no dictated composition of a DMC, relevant clinical (in this case, in MS), biostatistical and pharmacological (especially related to evaluation of laboratory data that are part of safety monitoring) expertise are essential. For MS clinical trials, where imaging may be an important safety and efficacy outcome in a trial, appropriate expertise from a neuroradiologist or neurologist familiar with the intricacies of MS image collection and analysis is vital. Similarly, in trials where other accepted (e.g. electrophysiological or cerebrospinal fluid analysis) or exploratory (e.g. immune markers as potential surrogates) outcomes are important, relevant expertise should be included on the DMC. Expertise in general conduct of clinical trials is desirable, either in one or more individuals who fulfill other roles or as a separate specialty area, as is epidemiology related to clinical trials and biomedical ethics.[9] For certain trials, DMC members with expertise in one or more aspects of the basic science that underlies the trial hypothesis can be highly desirable (e.g., depending on the experimental intervention in MS trials, immunology, glial cell biology, virology, etc.), especially if such expertise can be found in individuals who also have MS clinical expertise. DMCs may include more than one individual representing each special category of expertise and this is often common practice in large-scale NIH-supported trials.

Representatives of the patient community may also be included on DMCs, even lay people. Such individuals can provide a perspective on the burden of the study for trial participants that is not appreciated by clinicians and scientists. But including such a member on a DMC is an issue of some debate and controversy. To be considered a member, such an individual must have an adequate scientific/clinical background to be a fully contributory participant in deliberations and decision-making, which may be difficult to find in a lay person. As with all DMC members, such representatives must be objective and unbiased in their deliberations,[12] criteria that might be difficult for an individual who is personally affected by, or close to individuals affected by, MS. Retaining the confidentiality of data could additionally be difficult for representatives of the patient community who have personal or organizational interests in a trial, especially in the face of emerging positive or negative data in an ongoing trial. Of course, such issues are not of concern for patient representatives in a DMC alone but apply to all DMC members equally. A DMC is not a place for a 'patient advocate' per se but a DMC will benefit from including a committed patient-focused evaluator who will be able to view study risks/benefits from a unique perspective.

While at the onset of a clinical trial the composition of a DMC might seem to be ideal, during the course of the study unforeseen clinical or safety issues may arise that require additional ad hoc or full voting members to be added or special consultative services to be sought. It should be possible for the DMC to request such additions (and the request should be honored by the sponsor who formally appoints the DMC), or the sponsor may make such strategic DMC membership additions during the course of the trial.

Including members with prior MS DMC experience on a new MS clinical trial DMC is desirable but such individuals are relatively rare and requiring such experience in all members severely limits the available labor pool. Consequently, experienced individuals may often serve on several DMCs simultaneously, requiring special attention to confidentiality, conflicts of interest and scheduling. There is a need for 'new blood' and DMCs may serve as a training ground for inexperienced individuals who will learn 'on the job' from more experienced mentors and be available for future DMC membership and subsequent mentoring. Including motivated 'novices' on DMC membership rosters can add vigor and new perspective and provide much needed education to grow the pool of experienced potential DMC members in the future.[11]

As far as it is possible, it is highly desirable for DMC membership to include individuals who come from the geographical areas in which the study will be conducted (i.e. an international study should be monitored by a group with international representation, preferably from the regions in which trial sites are located but usually not from trial sites themselves). In addition, while often difficult to achieve (or sometimes simply overlooked), DMCs should represent as far as possible some of the key demographic characteristics of the study population.[9,12] For instance, for MS trials, DMCs should include women, since the disease is more prevalent among women. For an MS clinical trial that might focus on aspects of the disease that may affect ethnic or racial groups differentially, DMC membership should ideally include some members who represent the relevant groups themselves.

SIZE

The actual size of a DMC will vary depending on the demands and complexity of a study but should be kept at a minimum to make meetings and deliberations maximally efficient.[12] It is essential, though, that the right expertise is available with relation to the disease, intervention and potential side effect profile, and this consideration is more important than the size of the group. Wherever possible, DMCs should have an odd number of voting members. This will facilitate making recommendations to the sponsor in the event of split decisions. However, in general most DMC decisions will be made by consensus among members and for important issues – premature termination of a study for safety, efficacy or futility for instance – it is desirable, but not essential, that the recommendation of the DMC to the sponsor be unanimous.

IDENTIFICATION OF A CHAIR

Each DMC will have a chair, who will be particularly influential within the group and who, in general, will have a stronger reporting link to the sponsor and other trial committees than other DMC members. This individual should be experienced in clinical trials in MS and in DMC operations and if not expert in, at least very familiar with, statistical and clinical issues surrounding the trial and the disease. The chair must be a strong leader, a demonstrated consensus-builder and particularly impartial.[11]

In addition, the chair should be an individual with a reputation for fairness, for adhering to schedules and for relative availability by phone, e-mail or in-person meetings, since s/he has to work closely with the DMC and the sponsor or its agents throughout the trial, often on time-sensitive issues. As detailed below, the chair will also often have the responsibility for preparing and/or reviewing draft minutes of all meetings, distributing them to other DMC members and maintaining full files of all records, especially closed minutes of each meeting, for submission to the sponsor at the close of the trial. For NIH-supported studies, these responsibilities are often shared with an NIH institute representative who supports the DMC; corpo-

rate sponsors sometimes employ a contract research organization (CRO) to help with these functions. However, because of these additional responsibilities, the tasks for the DMC chair will be generally more time-consuming than for other members and this needs to be kept in mind in identifying a chair and, for the chosen individual, in accepting the responsibility.

The chair normally will be identified and appointed by the sponsor but it is desirable to confirm the appointment with the study Steering Committee (if such a committee is in place) and the rest of the DMC prior to its first meeting, to ensure that the individual has the confidence and support of the entire study group from the onset. While the specific discipline that the chair represents may not be as important as his/her other qualifications, it is typical that chairs are chosen for DMCs who are either clinicians or statisticians.[12] However, the current author, who is neither a clinician nor a statistician, has served as chair of three DMCs.

COMPENSATION AND LIABILITY

Membership of a DMC requires a significant contribution of time and talent from generally busy professionals. Avoiding financial conflicts of interest is essential for DMC members (e.g. investments in sponsoring companies); however, payment of a modest contract-specified consulting fee on a per hour, per meeting or per project basis, along with full reimbursement of travel and associated expenses for meeting attendance, is appropriate and is not considered to be a conflict of interest.[12,26]

An important and often overlooked complication of DMC activity is the potential liability of the DMC or of an individual DMC member for his/her actions in monitoring a clinical trial. This is particularly relevant in the context of trials that may reveal harmful adverse events or unexpected mortality and in which the DMC may draw attention and 'fire' because of its role in interim safety monitoring and in decision-making about continuation of such trials. Typical, contractual agreements between corporate sponsors and DMC members often do not identify the steps that the sponsor will take to indemnify a DMC member from liability that is not due to a member's own negligence or dereliction of responsibilities. Often, such contracts present language that only indemnifies the sponsor from the intentional or unintentional actions of the DMC member! Government-sponsored trials and DMCs often make no mention of liability or indemnification at all.

DMC members are entitled to (and would be wise to insist upon) indemnification by the sponsor for the work they do for all acts other than those due to their own negligence. This is sometimes a stumbling-block in the initial steps of contractual arrangements and charter development for DMCs but needs to be attended to prior to the first functional activity of the group.[28] See relevant sections below regarding appropriate wording that might be included in DMC contracts and charters to cover this important issue.

RELATIONS WITH THE SPONSOR AND OTHER TRIAL COMMITTEES

DATA MONITORING COMMITTEE POWERS

Contemporary clinical trials are complex undertakings and are usually overseen by a variety of advisory groups, including the DMC.[6] These groups are appointed by the sponsor and are advisory to the sponsor. While they can be highly influential in the course of a study, such groups do not have ultimate control, which is in the hands of the sponsor. It is important that the DMC understands that its 'powers' are limited and a DMC must understand clearly its reporting relationship within a given trial.[27] However, it would be difficult to envision a situation where a sponsor or lead investigator would ignore or overturn the recommendations of a thoughtful DMC.[26] The ultimate power, of course, should a sponsor choose to ignore the recommendations of a DMC, is resignation by any or all of the DMC's members. This is not a trivial consideration by any means and has regulatory implications, since regulatory agencies will surely be concerned about any changes in DMC composition or function during the course of a study. While this is an option in an extreme situation, such an act could do much to destroy the integrity of a trial.

REPORTING RELATIONSHIPS FOR A DATA MONITORING COMMITTEE

It is usually the case that DMCs are appointed by and report directly to the sponsor, since this is the government agency or corporate entity that finances the study and has ultimate scientific and regulatory responsibility. Direct reporting is most often to the sponsor's designated medical director for the study in a corporate-sponsored study[27] or an executive secretary and project officer for an NIH-supported study. However, interactions between the DMC and the sponsor are generally limited, at least for industry-sponsored trials.

The sponsor or its designated CRO is usually responsible for all meeting logistics and arrangements. The sponsor's study director and often sponsor staff involved in regulatory affairs, biostatistics and site monitoring will attend open sessions of DMC meetings but not closed sessions (although exceptions to this do exist[12]). If a sponsor uses a CRO to help manage study details, representatives of that organization also usually attend open sessions of DMC meetings and can, along with sponsor staff, provide valuable study update information at each meeting, including group information about enrollment, study subject drop-outs, and adverse event and serious adverse event details (in a blinded fashion). Since sponsor and CRO staff will usually be responsible for implementing protocol and study conduct revisions recommended by the DMC, they are better positioned to understand the rationale for such revisions if they participate fully in open session discussions.

For government-sponsored studies, particularly those at the US NIH, sponsor representatives sometimes have far more involvement in DMC operations and deliberations, and sometimes sit ex officio as full voting members on DMCs. This can raise controversies about intellectual and sometimes even financial conflicts of interest.[12,27] At the NINDS, where many NIH-supported MS trials are sponsored, Institute trials staff will be involved in open session discussions of a DMC, and some may participate in closed DMC deliberations, but they generally do not serve as voting members. Exceptions do occur, however, especially with regard to Institute statisticians, who may be responsible for assessing unblinded data. This is usually a procedural detail that is deliberated and determined before or at the first meeting of a DMC.[26]

In most clinical trials, including those for MS, there is a separate trial steering committee, also appointed by the sponsor, which usually has designed the study, carries shared responsibility with the DMC and the sponsor for overseeing and ensuring study quality and patient safety, and usually (sometimes in association with a publications committee) writes and presents for publication the final study report. DMCs usually have access to the steering committee, or at least its chair, for discussion of critical aspects of the study (most often in a data-blinded fashion only). Often minutes of meetings of the two groups (from the DMC, open session minutes only during the course of the study) are exchanged.

Some trials will also have endpoint adjudication committees, which, in a blinded fashion, determine whether individual patients have met predefined endpoints for primary study outcomes and/or require that they be removed from study drug administration or withdrawn from the study entirely. The DMC usually does not interact directly with such groups, except to know their operating principles and to understand the implications of their decisions on overall trial conduct and outcomes.

Finally, a publication committee is often set up in advance of a trial, composed of members of the steering committee and/or trial investigators. The deliberations of a DMC may be quite relevant to the interpretation of a study once it has been concluded and might be a valuable addition to publication(s) of trial results. These can generally be shared after the completion of a study and after a data-lock and study analysis has occurred. It is not recommended, however, that DMC members serve on a trial publication committee or serve as coauthors on trial publications (although acknowledgment of their role in the study and listing of the DMC members is appropriate), since such direct involvement in publishing results can be seen as compromising the neutrality of the DMC, even once a study has been concluded.

While both DMCs and local institutional review boards (IRBs) share the responsibility of overseeing patient safety in clinical trials, the scope of their responsibilities is different: DMCs have this responsibility for the entire study and often have access to unblinded interim data for the study on a regular basis. IRBs, on the other hand, have responsibility for ensuring safety and study conduct at their individual institutional study sites. They will review the initial study protocol and informed consent documents (and subsequent amendments) to ensure that risks to study subjects are minimized, and an IRB may or may not allow a study to be implemented at its local site based on its review. IRBs also receive and review ongoing trial information – but not generally unblinded safety or efficacy data – during the course of a study and can use that information to determine whether the study should continue at its site. Knowledge that a DMC is constituted for a study and how it functions can help a relatively isolated local IRB understand that the trial is being monitored carefully and globally by a safety and efficacy monitoring 'partner',[12] and most are comfortable entrusting overall study safety monitoring to the DMC. However, perhaps as a consequence of NIH and FDA requirements for DMCs in pivotal trials, increasingly IRBs are requesting a copy of the DMC charter (see below) and a list of DMC members for review prior to accepting a study at their site, and a greater required volume of flow of information to IRBs about DMC actions can be anticipated in the future. However, DMCs do not have direct interaction with any IRB generally but rely upon communication between the sponsor and each IRB for dissemination of key trial information and annual trial summaries.[24]

The primary interaction between governmental regulatory agencies and any given trial is through the trial sponsor, and it is highly unusual for a DMC ever to be in direct contact with regulatory authorities in the course of its work. Investigators and sponsors are required to report serious unexpected adverse reactions to study agents in near-real time, and annually in summarized reports, and regulators may review more comprehensive reports at any time depending on the nature of adverse experiences in the study.[12] In addition, for recommendations from the DMC related to trial conduct – in particular recommendations for early termination for safety or efficacy considerations, or significant protocol changes in the midst of a study – the sponsor will communicate with the regulatory authorities and convey the views of the DMC and other advisory groups prior to implementing such recommendations.[24]

Regulatory authorities generally do not participate in DMC deliberations and do not serve as voting members of any DMC,[22] for the simple reason that such involvement compromises the regulatory agency's ability to undertake a truly independent review of data for products presented for registration. However, direct involvement in DMC discussion by regulators is not unprecedented. Ellenberg et al[12] describe two scenarios related to the US FDA, one from an unnamed study that involved two essentially identical clinical trials, one of which was terminated early upon recommendation of its DMC for 'overwhelming efficacy' while the other was not terminated by its DMC (even with the knowledge that the first trial had been stopped and declared successful). The FDA was faced with difficult decisions regarding its evaluation of the first study in the face of the continuation of the second study. It felt it would benefit from direct discussion with the DMC for the ongoing study to better understand its reasons for continuation. The request to the DMC by the FDA for a direct meeting was made through the study sponsor and, while DMC members approached these requests with great caution, the end-product of these very unusual interactions was useful and productive.

INTERACTIONS WITH SPONSOR-APPOINTED STUDY STATISTICIANS

Since the entire process of data monitoring is, in effect, a statistical exercise interpreted in clinical terms, the role of study statisticians and their interaction with DMCs is critical. A sponsor-employed statistician (sometimes called the primary statistician) will be critical in determining the study's statistical design in the protocol development phase and in monitoring study conduct and quality control during the course of the study. It is preferable that a study statistician who is independent from the sponsor (sometimes called the independent statistician or, if a contract organization is brought in to fulfill this role, an independent statistical center) be responsible for preparing and presenting interim safety and/or efficacy analyses to the DMC and assisting with its interpretation. Since this individual or group usually has access to unblinded data, it is essential that information they have be kept in confidence from the study sponsor, other advisory groups and investigators.[12] In some circumstances, a statistician who is employed by the sponsor can fulfill this role and in NIH-sponsored studies it is typical for an Institute statistician to have this role. But there must be clear firewalls in place to ensure that unblinded data are not available beyond the independent statistician and the DMC, while still allowing the independent statistician to understand enough from the sponsor about how data are collected to identify nuances in analysis and interpretation. In some cases, a CRO might be engaged by a sponsor to assist with DMC logistics and also to provide independent statistical services to the study. Internal firewalls between units within such a CRO are also essential to ensure confidentiality of data during the course of the study. This is an issue for discussion and debate among the DMC and the sponsor in the protocol design stage or at the latest, at the first organizational meeting of a DMC.

The properly constituted DMC will also have at least one experienced biostatistician as a full voting member. Sometimes, sponsors request that this individual takes on the additional responsibilities of an independent statistician of analyzing, interpreting and presenting interim analyses to their peers on the DMC. Beyond the potentially enormous extra burden that this can place on the statistical member(s) of the DMC, this is not an advisable strategy: non-statistician members of the DMC will generally depend heavily upon the independent expertise of their statistical colleagues on the committee in understanding and interpreting the statistical aspects of interim analyses. If the statistical member of the DMC is serving as well as a direct analyst on behalf of the sponsor, this could be seen to compromise her/his independence or limit his/her perspectives on the data analysis.

INTERACTION WITH DATA MONITORING COMMITTEES IN OTHER TRIALS

Occasionally, a clinical trial sponsor will run parallel studies on a given agent in the same patient group (sometimes in different geographical regions) or multiple studies on the same agent but in different patient populations. Where such is the case, and where all the trials have independent monitoring, it may be beneficial for the same DMC to monitor all the relevant studies, or for there to be at least some overlap between DMC membership for the different studies. Advantages can include the ability to have a better and broader understanding of safety across more patients and sometimes different patient groups, and the ability to change monitoring procedures on a given study based on emerging issues in related studies. Disadvantages include a loss of true independence in the monitoring process for individual studies and the potential introduction of biases in interpretation for one study based on outcomes from a related study. Even with overlapping membership, however, routine sharing of information between DMCs is not recommended because of the potential impact of information from one study that may not be relevant to a second study. But there should be a mechanism set up in advance for open communication between DMCs engaged for parallel studies that does not compromise study blinding, should a need arise. This is an issue for resolution early in the study(s) between sponsors and relevant monitoring groups.

DEFINING THE ROLE OF THE DATA MONITORING COMMITTEE IN A CLINICAL TRIAL

The specific role that a DMC will have in a trial is not codified. Since the DMC is usually appointed by the study sponsor, the sponsor almost always sets out the responsibilities of the committee. In the best of situations, these responsibilities will be proposed by the sponsor, discussed between the sponsor and DMC members, and then agreed upon and formalized in one or more documents that clearly define responsibilities and also guarantee independence and relative autonomy of the DMC. Relevant documents – confidentiality agreements, consulting agreements and DMC Charters – are legally binding and DMC members are wise to review them carefully, to raise questions and uncertainties and to consult legal counsel if necessary before signing any such agreements.

CONFIDENTIALITY AGREEMENTS

Usually, as a very first step, a sponsor or its agent (a CRO or intermediary consultant) will contact a potential DMC member with a brief description of the project under consideration and ascertain the interest of the individual in serving on the committee. It is unusual at this initial step for very many of the specific details of the proposed clinical trial to be revealed but in short order a signed confidentiality agreement between the sponsor and a willing potential DMC member will be executed, which will be followed by full details – protocol summary, full protocol, investigator's brochure, etc. – of the proposed trial for the potential member to evaluate. Confidentiality agreements at this stage allow the sponsor to share detailed information about the proposed study with a potential DMC member, who will surely wish to understand the nature of the study to determine if s/he is capable of and interested in performing the required tasks for the sponsor.

Initial confidentiality agreements are relatively standard and familiar to any scientist or clinician who has engaged in consultation or collaboration with sponsors who undertake clinical trials. The legal documentation and language for such agreements are usually more extensive in corporate-sponsored studies than for NIH-sponsored studies. More extensive agreements usually state the parties between which the agreement is made and indicate that, in the conduct of consultation, a potential DMC member will receive information that is confidential, proprietary and/or considered a 'trade secret'. The formal agreement will also usually designate exactly what kinds of information provided to the DMC members will be considered confidential and what kinds will not ('definitions of confidential information') and with whom (usually very restricted) and in what format confidential information might be shared with others ('recipient obligations' and 'permitted disclosures'). The duration of the obligation of confidentiality is specified and is usually for a period that exceeds the normal work responsibilities for the DMC on the trial in question ('duration of obligation'). Confidential information is usually considered the property of the sponsor for a trial and formal agreements also usually set down requirements for retention and/or return or disposal of this information ('return of provider property').

Almost all confidentiality agreements argue the seriousness of breaches of confidentiality and set specific terms for the sponsor to seek restraining orders, injunctions or related legal remedies if such breach occurs or is threatened by a DMC member. In some cases, sponsors may require that a DMC member has adequate liability insurance to cover such breaches and other acts of purposeful negligence. Sometimes confidentiality agreements will set out the terms under which the sponsor indemnifies and holds harmless a DMC member for acts that are not considered to be breaches of confidentiality or acts of negligence. If this is provided in an initial confidentiality agreement, such indemnification clauses should also be part of a formal consulting contract and/or DMC charter (see below) executed later on. There is often a statement about responsibility for legal fees in the case of dispute between the DMC member and the sponsor (usually, the prevailing party is entitled to recover legal fees from the losing party).

Additional sections of a confidentiality agreement may relate to the delegation of responsibilities by a DMC member to another individual (usually not allowed without prior written agreement), severability of the agreement and the legal jurisdiction that governs the terms of the agreement (usually the location of the home base of the sponsor).

At a later stage, once an individual has agreed to serve on the DMC, confidentiality must be insured with relation to the data reviewed during the course of the study. In particular, confidentiality of comparative data between study arms (often reviewed by a DMC in an unblinded fashion) is essential to protect the integrity of a trial.[12,27] Disclosure of information during the course of a study can prematurely and erroneously alter the clinical 'equipoise' of a study in the minds of study subjects, investigators and sponsors and can do irreparable harm to the conduct of the study, affecting accrual and drop out rates, assessment of trial endpoints and even completion of the study.[9,12,27,29,30] Once an individual has agreed to serve on a DMC, it is thus typical that additional confidentiality agreements related to actual committee service are executed, containing much of the information carried over from the original 'exploratory' confidentiality agreement and adding specific information related to DMC functions. Sometimes this second confidentiality agreement is contained within a contractual agreement between the sponsor and a DMC member rather than being a separate agreement, and should also be a key part of a DMC charter that defines the group's responsibilities and functions.

Thus, confidentiality agreements serve two purposes: to protect the trial sponsor and organizer from premature disclosure to the public of information pertinent to the development of a new product while the study is being assembled and during its conduct; and, importantly, to ensure that any data seen during the course of the study by the DMC are kept in confidence by the DMC and not shared with anyone, including staff or other consultants (such as trial steering committees, publications committee, etc.) engaged by the sponsor. In this fashion, studies are more likely to be conducted in a truly blinded fashion, if that is the intent, and premature release of data is avoided prior to the actual conclusion of a study and assessment of full study safety and efficacy data.

THE DATA MONITORING COMMITTEE CONTRACT/CONSULTING AGREEMENT

A second key formal document of agreement between a DMC member and the study sponsor is a service contract. This legally binding document defines the work that is asked of the individual DMC member and can include further details about terms of confidentiality during the course of the trial. Such documents are used routinely in corporate-sponsored trials but are not customary for NIH-supported trials, where more often formal letters of appointment to a DMC, with details of responsibilities of the member, are issued by the director of the NIH. Independent of the nature of the contract or agreement, the scope of service for a DMC is similar in corporate- or government-supported studies.

When formal contracts are used, they are signed by individual DMC members and countersigned by a representative of the trial sponsor – usually the study clinical director or the sponsor's appropriate legal or business representative. Contracts usually define quite closely the nature of the consulting services ('engagement' or 'services' or similar). The timing of meetings throughout the study is usually specified, and whether the meetings will occur face to face or by teleconference is also often noted. This information will also often be found in the DMC charter (see below). Contracts also often specify the individual associated with the trial (study director, etc.) to whom the DMC members individually and as a group are responsible. While DMC members are usually not considered to be sponsor employees (and this is often explicitly stated in an 'independent contractor' clause or similar), some sponsors, particularly corporate sponsors, require that DMC members adhere to the sponsor's own 'code of business conduct' usually applied to employees, which can regulate a range of business behaviors and actions.

Contracts will specify the compensation (honoraria, travel and related expenses) that a DMC member will receive for his/her work, the way in which payment will be made (hourly, per meeting, yearly or for the entire project) and whether the DMC member will be required to submit invoices or will be paid proactively by the sponsor. Usually the sponsor will indicate a specific time range in which payment can be expected after meetings or in response to a member's invoice. In virtually all cases, the sponsor assumes no tax responsibilities for the DMC member for income earned. For US sponsors and USA-based DMC members, a contract will usually specify that a Social Security number or Federal Identification Number (for individuals who consult through incorporated entities) must be provided and US Internal Revenue Service tax forms (usually Form 1099 – 'miscellaneous income') will be sent to the consultant (and filed with the IRS) annually.

Contracts will also specify the term of the agreement – sometimes for the duration of a study, and sometimes for a single year and renewable annually for the duration of the study – and will also contain provision for termination of the agreement by either party with a defined notice period ('term and termination').

With relation to issues of confidentiality, contracts will often restate nondisclosure policies related to data ('nondisclosure'). Return to the sponsor of written information and/or destruction of electronic files at the conclusion of the study or upon termination of the contract is usually specified in the 'term and termination' section of a contract. It is common for a contract to remind the parties that the responsibilities of the member cannot be transferred to another individual ('relationship of parties').

DMC members should not be surprised to see clauses within a proposed contract that indicate that any inventions that the member may conceive related to the consultancy relationship must be assigned to the sponsor ('work product' or 'assignment of inventions' or similar). Sometimes, contracts are less carefully drafted and specify simply that any inventions made during the time of consultancy must be assigned to the sponsor. However, the careful consultant will require that such a clause specify that such inventions must be related to the specific topic of the consulting agreement! Many contracts require that consultants assist the sponsor in pursuit of any resulting patents, copyrights or other proprietary rights. Such 'boilerplate' clauses should be carefully considered by potential DMC members, especially those with primary employment agreements/contracts that place ownership of intellectual property rights in the hands of the individual's primary employer (which is common in academic settings).

Because some academic and commercial institutions restrict the 'outside consulting' that its employees may do, or require that honoraria be paid to the institution (rather than the individual) to compensate the employer for 'lost' time on the job, DMC members are often also required to certify that they are in fact entitled to enter into a contractual relationship on their own. If this is not allowed by the primary employer, a separate consulting contract might be made between a DMC member's employer and the sponsor. Additionally, members may be asked to certify that they are not obligated in any other contractual relationship that would compromise their ability to provide the services agreed upon ('representations' clauses or 'no conflict' clauses). Some contracts attempt to limit a consultant in terms of other consulting opportunities during the course of the trial, and sometimes exceeding the duration of the trial, creating in essence an exclusive relationship between the consultant and the trial sponsor. Potential DMC members should be very cautious about accepting any such restrictions, except as they might apply to a direct conflict of interest with a product or concept that is being explored with the sponsor in question.

As noted above, contracts will often require that the consultant indemnify the sponsor from 'any and all losses' that result from the consultant's breach of the contractual agreement(s) related to the study. This is an appropriate requirement but sometimes such indemnification clauses go further and require that the DMC member indemnify the sponsor for all claims related to the trial, not just those as a consequence of breach of contract, and specify that the sponsor will not be liable for any losses incurred by the member as a consequence of their service. This kind of agreement is inappropriate and places DMC members at considerable potential risk. Reasonable decisions that a DMC may make related to interim safety and efficacy, especially those that might result in early study termination, could be called into question in legal terms in our litigious society. Furthermore, such clauses can potentially alter the behavior of DMC members, who may be reluctant to make difficult decisions if they fear such decisions will put them at legal risk. Wise DMC members will insist that the sponsor indemnify them as individuals and as a group from any and all claims, actions, lawsuits, losses and expenses in the course of their work, except for actions brought because of the willful misconduct, negligence or fraud on the part of the consultant(s). In the USA, for clinical trials sponsored by agencies of the federal government, the liability and indemnification situation is more complicated, and conditions of indemnification may depend on whether a DMC member serves as an unpaid consultant, receives honoraria or is considered a 'special government employee' with relation to his/her work on the committee.[28]

It is important to note that, in cases where 'one-sided' indemnification is stated in a contract that protects only the sponsor, it is most often simply a consequence of a sponsor using 'boilerplate' legal language rather than a purposeful effort to shift liability on to DMC members. In my experience sponsors, when challenged, will usually immediately agree to more appropriate terms of indemnification. DeMets et al[28] provide a valuable contemporary assessment of liability issues involved in DMC membership and also provide useful examples of language that should be considered in contractual relationship related to liability and indemnification. Potential members should carefully evaluate these issues and should be comfortable with the potential liability of service on a DMC before agreeing to join and certainly before signing any legally binding document.

Finally, as with original confidentiality agreements, a formal consulting agreement will include a number of additional clauses and considerations, including an indication of the legal jurisdiction whose laws will dictate the interpretation and enforcement of the contract. Each clause deserves to be reviewed carefully and questioned if there is any uncertainty on behalf of the potential DMC member.

SETTING THE RESPONSIBILITIES AND OPERATIONS OF THE DATA MONITORING COMMITTEE: CHARTER DEVELOPMENT

Separate entirely from confidentiality and consulting agreements is a clear and detailed articulation of what a DMC is charged to do, how it will conduct its business and what the limits on its actions might be. This often comes in the form of a charter for DMC operations. While an overview of the responsibilities of any particular DMC is often contained in the contract that is executed before service begins, that usually includes insufficient detail to be practically useful to a committee or sponsor during the often years-long activities of the group.

Virtually every published paper and governmental guideline that focuses on DMC activities in clinical trials articulates the categories of activities in which a DMC might be engaged.[9–12,24–26] Table 30.1 lists the most common tasks that might be given to a DMC. All these, including interim and final analyses of safety and efficacy, early trial termination (for efficacy, safety or futility reasons), mid-trial recommendations for protocol changes, and recommendations for changes in recruitment and retention strategies, have been undertaken by DMCs monitoring phase II and pivotal phase III MS clinical trials in the past 15 years.

The advantages of a detailed Charter are clear: a priori, all partners (DMC members, sponsors, steering committee members, investigators and regulators) have a precise understanding of the responsibilities and expectations of the DMC and how it will function and interact with other trial advisory committees and groups. This can prevent misunderstandings during the course of a trial, which can effectively derail an

TABLE 30.1 Tasks commonly associated with data monitoring committee functions

General issues of human subjects protection
Monitoring adverse events and drug/device safety
Assessing ongoing risk/benefit of the study
Ensuring ethical conduct of the study

General issues of trial credibility
Adding credibility and certifying the clinical trial process
Avoiding concerns about research fraud
Ensuring the integrity and validity of study inferences

Tasks related to mid-stream changes in a study protocol or conduct
Undertaking interim data review and making recommendations to adapt randomization and statistical power as a result of accumulating data (particularly applicable to potential studies that might include adaptive Bayesian statistical design and analysis[8])
Assessing enrollment/accrual and potential need to alter recruitment and retention strategies and/or increase sample size

Tasks related to interim analyses by protocol
Analyzing safety, blinded or unblinded, at interim study time points and at study conclusion
Analyzing efficacy, blinded or unblinded, at interim study time points and at study conclusion
Recommending study continuation under the original protocol or with revisions, based on analysis of ongoing data and incorporation of information external to the study

Recommending termination of a study prematurely after interim analysis due to:
  Unacceptable safety or tolerability
  Overwhelming early evidence of efficacy
  Negative efficacy trends
  Report of positive or negative results from similar clinical trials (usually on the same agent, in parallel studies)
  Assessment of futility (the inability of the study to definitively answer the trial hypothesis, usually based on incorrect calculations of expected outcomes and powering[12,35]).

Essentially, all these functions have been undertaken by DMCs that have monitored MS clinical trials over the past 15 years.

inseparable. For instance, traditional primary efficacy outcomes for studies of relapsing–remitting MS might include reduction in relapse rate, delay of time to (first or subsequent) relapse and sometimes reduction of relapse severity. Studies of progressive disease are usually designed to evaluate a slowing in progression of disability using standard disability rating scales. And in phase II trials, changes in accumulation of lesions in the central nervous system detected by MRI are often primary outcomes of trials; reduction of MRI parameters can signal a successful preliminary trial and encourage development of a pivotal trial with clinical outcomes. However, a change in the opposite direction in any of these parameters – an increase in relapse rate, progression of disability or number/volume of lesions – can be a signal of toxicity. Thus, DMCs monitoring MS trials often end up monitoring changes in outcomes for safety that have a potential impact on interpretation of efficacy. The line between evaluation of safety and efficacy in MS trials is inherently blurred and it makes most practical sense for an MS trial DMC to be involved in monitoring both kinds of outcome and for this to be taken into account in study design. Otherwise, defining how safety can be monitored at regular intervals without inadvertently exposing efficacy outcomes (which affect study statistical power) is a challenge

- A determination that interim data (in controlled trials) will be reviewed in a blinded or unblinded fashion

  While some argue that reviewing of blinded data by a DMC helps to minimize any data biases that might result in decisions to alter study design, others argue that the best way to assess risk–benefit in an ongoing study is through unblinded data analysis.[12] In many MS trials side effects of interventions are often unblinding and thus a requirement that the DMC review data in a blinded fashion is simply a distraction. At a minimum, blinded data should be reported to a DMC in a consistent fashion on each table and listing so that study arms are the same in each report; many DMC members in MS trials prefer to simplify matters and have access to study arm treatment allocations from the outset

- An agreement as to the nature, frequency and timing of data reports to the DMC by the sponsor or its agents
- An understanding about whether or not the DMC will be involved in a final review of data and risk–benefit assessment at the conclusion of the study, in addition to interim monitoring
- An understanding of the role of the DMC in monitoring postprotocol follow-up for patients previously on study protocol who have completed the study or who are dropped from the study but are part of the 'intent to treat' population
- An agreement about the role of the DMC in monitoring parallel or related trials by the same sponsor
- An agreement about the role of the DMC in monitoring phase IV postmarketing studies of the same agent, if it receives regulatory approval.

While it would seem obvious that an agreed-upon DMC charter would be an absolute part of trial management, charters are a relatively recent concept, at least in most MS clinical trials, and are not yet as common in NIH-supported trials (where DMC functions and operations are guided by general agency guidelines) as they are in corporate-supported trials. When they do exist, charters are usually drafted by the sponsor and/or its designated CRO, or may be drafted by the DMC chair or the DMC as a whole, but should be considered to be a document for discussion, revision and final agreement among the relevant parties.

otherwise excellent monitoring process. Examples of issues that are sometimes overlooked at the onset of a trial in the absence of a detailed charter and that can become controversial midway through a trial are:

- A formal agreement on the details of the protocol
- A clear agreement about the specifics of the study statistical analytic plan
- A clear understanding of whether the DMC responsibilities include only safety monitoring or both safety and efficacy monitoring.

  This is often a point of debate and discussion. DMC members often prefer to have both responsibilities, since they view this as the best way to evaluate risk/benefit, a potential dichotomy that is inherent in the monitoring concept. Sponsors sometimes view efficacy evaluation (and ultimate risk/benefit assessment) as being within their own purview, or perhaps done in association with a study steering committee. In MS trials the issue can be more complex since some measures of safety and efficacy are

At least two 'sample charters' have been published.[12,31] There are no hard and fast rules about what should be in a Charter, but key points that should be considered for inclusion are as follows:

1. A 'table of contents' that outlines what the various sections of the charter cover.
2. An introductory section that states the name, number and other identifiers for the trial.
3. A statement of agreed-upon DMC roles and responsibilities. This can be generally outlined (e.g. 'monitor safety and efficacy at interim points in the study') or, preferably, highly specific, including expectations at each sequential DMC meeting, the role of the DMC in any planned extension studies, details of statistical analysis plans at each interim analysis time point, and even (although I do not recommend this) a statement of the 'allowed decisions' that a DMC can make during the course of its deliberations.

   Some sponsors wish to indicate in advance that a DMC may stop a study prematurely only for safety reasons but that it does not have the 'right' to stop a study early for reasons of overwhelming efficacy or of futility. A DMC may agree in advance that it would be unlikely to stop studies prematurely for efficacy or futility so that there might be more data gathered for scientific purposes, so long as there are no ethical or safety concerns if the study is continued. And, in doing so, the DMC may set very stringent statistical boundaries for termination that would apply in such instances, to make early termination difficult except in the most compelling situations. But it is unwise for a DMC to agree a priori to limits on its decision-making power. It is not possible to predict at the onset of a clinical study where DMC deliberations may lead; to agree in advance to a sponsor's wishes in this regard compromises the DMC's independence.

4. A requirement that the DMC review and comment upon the protocol, and where they exist, manuals of operation or procedure for the study (often created as separate documents in NIH-supported studies).

   This is an important early step – certainly before data begin to be gathered and hopefully even before finalization of the protocol – that is often overlooked, especially when DMCs are constituted after the initiation of a clinical trial or well into the protocol planning stage. Each DMC member and the DMC as a whole must be certain that they agree with the specific elements of the protocol design. If a trial design is for any reason unacceptable to members or to the DMC as a whole, and if suggested protocol revisions cannot be made or are rejected by the sponsor or its other advisors, individuals or the group should decline service for reasons of both principle and ethics. Each DMC member has an ethical obligation in his/her monitoring role and it is difficult to conceive how this can be fulfilled if there are significant disagreements about the protocol details at the beginning of the study. Also, an experienced and independent DMC can bring to the table additional trial design insights, including those related to recruitment, protection from adverse events, power calculations, etc., that might otherwise not be considered.

5. DMC composition is usually stated in the charter, including identifying the chair and other members and providing their affiliations and contact information.

   It is useful to indicate how the chair was chosen (by appointment by the sponsor, by acclamation by the DMC or a combination of the two, for example.) The DMC chair's particular (additional) roles in the DMC and interactions with other advisory groups and the sponsor should be delineated. If other DMC members have very specific functions that might be in addition to 'general membership' it is useful to indicate what those are. For instance, if the DMC statistician has a special role in helping to draft data shells in association with the sponsor statistician for presentation to the DMC, this should be stated. If a DMC member is appointed because of his/her special knowledge of a particular safety (e.g. liver function) or efficacy outcome (e.g. imaging), this also should be indicated.

6. DMC meeting organization and conduct is usually detailed.

   The individuals responsible for meeting logistics (usually sponsor or CRO) are identified; timing for their communication to the DMC prior to each meeting is specified. It should be clearly stated if meetings are to be in person, by teleconference or a mix of both.

   Expected timing of meetings throughout the course of the trial is given, usually starting with the first 'introductory meeting', preferably before protocol finalization or at least before initiation of patient accrual. Timing of the first actual data monitoring meeting is set, sometimes triggered by the accrual of a set number or percentage of patients who have been treated on protocol for a set period of time; subsequent meetings are often simply set at specific timing intervals (often dependent upon the speed with which data are expected to be collected, 'cleaned' and analyzed and the overall trial duration, or sometimes based upon set trial recruitment and on-study milestones, or sometimes simply on set calendar intervals.)

   General operating principles for the DMC are stated, including adherence to confidentiality, avoidance of conflicts of interest and others. Expected meeting formats are clearly laid out.

   – In studies that include a blinded comparison analysis between study arms, it is typical that provision is made for initial open sessions at meetings at which the sponsor or its designee presents important trial update information (site information, accrual/enrollment data, drop-out information, adverse and serious adverse reaction experience, etc.) for the study as a whole, to ensure blinding. Baseline demographic data can be presented in an unblinded fashion according to the treatment arm to allow assessment of compliance with baseline randomization and study arm comparability needs.

   – A closed session is then convened that includes only members of the DMC and its consultants, in which information that might compromise the study blinding is reviewed, analyzed and debated. This is also an opportunity for DMC members to discuss among themselves issues related to study conduct, data presentation and sponsor/contractor performance, and to develop consensus. A formally voted-upon summary statement related to study continuation is prepared, devoid of any revealing rationale or qualifying statement that could potentially be unblinding. The DMCs recommendations are then drafted for presentation to the sponsor in the next open session.

   – A concluding open session, preferably attended by all DMC members as well as the sponsor and its representatives, allows the DMC chair, with input and support from members, to present the committee's conclusion about the study as a consequence of the review, and also to present any questions or issues to the sponsor for immediate response or follow-up within a defined time period, often prior to the next scheduled meeting.

7. DMC operating procedures are outlined in as much as is practical.
   - The nature and frequency of reports that the DMC will receive should be clearly stated, including whether data will be distributed on paper, electronically or both.
   - The requirement for the DMC's agreement to 'shell' tables and charts to be prepared by study statisticians, as well as its right to request additional information or format changes during the course of the study should be stated.
   - Whether or not treatment data will be presented and analyzed in a blinded or unblinded fashion (in controlled studies) is indicated and is often a point of debate, as noted elsewhere.
   - Whether data will be delivered 'cleaned' (meaning that the initial site reports have been queried and are as accurate as possible) or 'uncleaned' needs to be defined at the start of a study. This can drive the accuracy of data and its 'vintage' once it reaches the DMC. Most DMCs prefer to review cleaned data, so long as the data it receives for each review are reasonably up to date, but must consider the time needed to review data prior to meetings, the desire to minimize the time between data-locks and interim analysis meetings, and also the enormous effort it can take for sponsors and statisticians to gather, query, clean, enter and present data for their consideration. The timing of data delivery to members prior to a DMC meeting depends on these factors and is usually set in the Charter; it is the sponsor's responsibility to ensure that this timetable is adhered to as closely as possible.
   - The communication path and timing of reports of serious adverse reactions (SAEs) in the study needs to be specified in advance. Some DMCs prefer near-real-time reporting of SAEs if the sponsor's operating procedures allow for such a rapid turn-around; others are content with monthly summaries. Much depends on the nature of the study and any prior indication of problematic SAEs.
   - Although perhaps trivial, it should be clearly stated what DMC members should do with paper or electronic data after each meeting: retain, discard or return to the sponsor's unblinded agents.

8. DMC charters should also indicate the names and functions of other advisory and consultative groups for the trial and indicate clearly the type of communication that is expected between the DMC and these bodies during the course of the study.

   While it is almost always the case that the DMC reports only to the sponsor and has little if any contact with any group other than the sponsor's designated study statisticians, it is often appropriate for the chair of the steering committee (if any) or his/her designee (usually another member of that committee) to attend open sessions of the DMC and to receive copies of open DMC meeting minutes, and for the DMC to receive copies of steering committee minutes as well (see above). Any other discussions with steering committee members about the trial should not occur.

9. Steps involved in DMC decision making should be stated. The nature of a DMC quorum should be defined. It should be made clear whether decisions should be made by consensus or by vote (some decisions, such as those that might result in early study termination, are perhaps best required to be made by unanimous vote).

   DMC charters often state the kinds of decisions that 'might' be made by a committee: to continue a study with no alterations; to continue a study with stated recommended alternations in protocol or conduct; to terminate a study early for safety, efficacy or futility. All are appropriate. As noted previously, DMCs are not encouraged to accept restrictions on the types of recommendation they can make. However, in the anticipation of possible early study termination for efficacy or futility, a DMC should determine a priori explicit statistical probability and stopping rules. Terminating a study early is risky, both ethically and statistically, since such decisions require an assessment that the clinical equipoise underlying the study has changed[32] and early results on which to make that assessment are relatively unstable. Adoption of group sequential boundary statistical rules can reduce this risk by making early termination more difficult, since such rules set very stringent statistical stopping rules at first and set more relaxed rules at each subsequent interim analysis.[12,33,34] If such rules are adopted, they should be clearly stated in the charter.

10. The means by which reports/minutes of DMC meetings are prepared and distributed is stated.

    It is typical that minutes are drafted by the DMC chair or a designated study scribe. The sponsor should review and edit draft open session minutes to ensure accuracy of the sometimes complex study update information it presents in initial open sessions. All DMC members should then review drafts of open and closed meeting minutes prior to finalization by the chair. Open session minutes are distributed to the sponsor and any individuals it designates; closed session minutes must be retained by the DMC chair, other DMC members and any contract group engaged by the sponsor to work with the DMC until the termination or completion of the study and the data lock and analysis has occurred. At that time, full closed session minutes can be transmitted to the sponsor for its use for regulatory purposes.

11. The role of the DMC at the end of a study should be specified:
    - Will it be involved in reviewing and commenting on final efficacy analysis? DMCs should insure that a final review of all safety data occurs before disbanding, as some events may occur late compared to the majority of early data that the DMC has followed over the course of a trial.
    - Will the DMC see the final sponsor safety reports that are provided to investigators and regulators? This is advisable to ensure their accuracy.
    - Will the DMC have a role in reviewing the manuscript of any publications related to the trial? Will it be asked to support the sponsor at poststudy meetings with regulators in an effort to have the agent registered, if this is called for? It is often the case that DMCs have little or no formal role after a study has concluded and their safety and efficacy analyses are complete. But it is also common that, toward the end of the study, the sponsor and/or DMC feel that additional poststudy roles for the DMC would be useful. As far as possible, all these issues should be considered and agreed upon in advance, and not in the last pressing days of an often years-long clinical trial.

CONCLUSIONS

In a relatively short number of years, DMCs have become commonplace in phase III clinical trials and often in earlier-phase studies, including in those for new therapies for MS. Stimulated by recommendations and requirements of the US NIH, and now part of standard guidelines available from regulatory agencies worldwide, such committees are an important part of public, private and commercially sponsored therapeutic trials. While the details of their operations may differ depending on the nature of the sponsor and the trial, the principles that DMCs uphold and the responsibilities they are asked to undertake are the same: to insure the safety of the patients who give their time and goodwill to the experimental process and to insure the highest possible integrity of the trial process. DMCs thus carry a heavy burden of responsibility in overseeing a trial. They provide an assurance of quality study conduct, can help to encourage enrollment of subjects and ultimately can encourage acceptance of study outcomes by regulators, physicians, patients and the public.

There are relatively few hard rules for the composition, responsibilities or conduct of DMCs but an increasingly comprehensive literature provides recommendations for what should be considered and incorporated into DMC functions. While little guidance specific to MS studies has been written to date, there is also little about a DMC for an MS clinical trial that would differ from a DMC for any other chronic, serious disease. Sponsors and clinical trials investigators for MS trials are recommended to understand the value and central role that a DMC has in any prospective clinical trial.

ACKNOWLEDGMENTS

Thanks are due to Dr Gary Cutter, University of Alabama at Birmingham and Ms Amy Pinette; i3 Research, for their review of this manuscript and for helpful suggestions.

REFERENCES

1. Herndon R. Multiple sclerosis. Proceedings of the International Conference on Therapeutic Trials in Multiple Sclerosis, Grand Island, NY, April 23–24, 1982. Arch Neurol 1983; 40: 663–710.
2. Lublin FD, Reingold SC. Placebo-controlled clinical trials in MS: ethical considerations. Ann Neurol 2001; 49: 677–681.
3. Miller DH, Albert PS, Barkhof F et al. Guidelines for the use of magnetic resonance techniques in monitoring the treatment of multiple sclerosis. Ann Neurol 1996; 39: 6–16.
4. McFarland HF, Barkhof F, Antel J, Miller DH. The role of MRI as a surrogate outcome measure in multiple sclerosis. Mult Scler 2002; 8: 40–51.
5. Rudick R, Antel J, Confvreux C et al. Recommendations from the National Multiple Sclerosis Society Clinical Outcomes Assessment Task Force. Ann Neurol 1997; 42; 379–382.
6. Lublin FD, Reingold SC. Guildelines for clinical trials of new therapeutic agents in multiple sclerosis: relations between study investigators, advisors and sponsors. Neurology 1997; 48: 572–574.
7. Goodkin DE, Reingold SC, Sibley W et al. Guidelines for clinical trials of new therapeutic agents in multiple sclerosis: reporting extended results from phase III clinical trials. Ann Neurol 1999; 46; 132–134.
8. McFarland HF, Reingold SC. The future of multiple sclerosis therapies: redesigning multiple sclerosis clinical trials in a new therapeutic era. Mult Scler 2005; 11: 669–676.
9. Ellenberg SS. Independent data monitoring committees: rationale, operations and controversies. Stat Med 2001; 20: 2573–2583.
10. Cairnes JA, Hallstrom A, Held P. Should all trials have a data safety and monitoring committee? Am Heart J 2001; 141: 156–163.
11. Grant AM, Altman DG, Babiker A et al. Issues in data monitoring and interim analysis of trials. Health Tech Assess 2005; 9: 1–238.
12. Ellenberg SS, Fleming TR, DeMets DL. Data monitoring committees in clinical trials. Chichester, West Sussex: John Wiley; 2002.
13. Wittes J. Behind closed doors: the data monitoring board in randomized clinical trials. Stat Med 1993; 12: 419–424.
14. Califf RM, Morse MA, Wittes, J et al. Toward protecting the safety of participants in clinical trials. Control Clin Trials 2003; 24: 256–271.
15. Sleight P. Where are clinical trials going? Society and clinical trials. J Intern Med 2004; 255: 151–158.
16. Nuremberg Code. Permissible medical experiments. Trials of war criminals before the Nuremberg military tribunals under Control Council Law No. 10, Nuremberg, October 1946–April 1949, vol 2. Washington, DC: US Government Printing Office, 1949: 181–182. Available on line at: www.hhs.gov/ohrp/references/nurcode.htm, accessed 28 June 2007.
17. US Code of Federal Regulations. Title 45; Section 46: Protection of human subjects. Washington, DC: Public Welfare, Department of Health and Human Services; National Institutes of Health, Office for Protection from Research Risks, 1991.
18. Declaration of Helsinki. Adopted by the 18th World Medical Assembly, Helsinki Finland, 1963; amended in Tokyo in 1975, Venice in 1983, Hong Kong in 1989, South Africa in 1996 and Edinburgh in 2002. Available on line at: www.wma.net/e/policy/b3.htm, accessed 27 August 2007.
19. Heart Special Project Committee. Organization, review and administration of cooperative studies (Greenberg Report): a report for the Hearth Special Project Committee to the National Advisory Council, May 1967. Control Clin Trials 1988; 9: 137–148.
20. National Institutes of Health. NIH policy for data and safety monitoring. Release date: June 10, 1998. Available on line at: grants.nih.gov/grants/guide/notice-files/not98–084.html, accessed 27 August 2007.
21. National Institutes of Health. Further guidance on data and safety monitoring for phase I and phase II trials. Bethesda, MD: NIH, 2000. Available on line at: grants.nih.gov/grants/guide/notice-files/NOT-OD-00–038.html, accessed 28 June 2007.
22. O'Neill RT. Some FDA perspectives on data monitoring in clinical trials in drug development. Stat Med 1993; 12: 601–608.
23. O'Neill RT. Regulatory perspectives on data monitoring. Stat Med 2002; 21: 2831–2842.
24. US Department of Health and Human Services, Food and Drug Administration. Guidance for clinical trials sponsors: on the establishment and operation of clinical trial data monitoring committees. Rockville, MD: FDA; 2001. Available on line at: www.fda.gov/cber/gdlns/clindatmon.htm, accessed 28 June 2007.
25. European Medicines Agency. Committee for Medicinal Products for Human Use. Guideline on Data Monitoring Committees. London: EMA; 2005. Available on line at: www.emea.eu.int/pdfs/human/ewp/587203en.pdf, accessed 28 June 2007.
26. Conwit RA, Hart RG, Moy CS, Marler JR. Data and safety monitoring in clinical research: a National Institute of Neurologic Disorders and Stroke Perspective. Ann Emerg Med 2004; 45: 388–392.
27. Packer M, Wittes J, Stump D. Terms of reference for data and safety monitoring committees. Am Heart J 2001; 141: 542–547.
28. DeMets DL, Fleming TR, Rockhold F et al. Liability issues for data monitoring committee members. Clin Trials 2004; 1: 525–531.
29. Fleming TR, Ellenberg S, DeMets DL. Monitoring clinical trials: issues and controversies regarding confidentiality. Stat Med 2002; 21: 2843–2851.
30. Slutzky AS, Lavery JV. Data safety and monitoring boards. N Engl J Med 2004; 350: 1143–1147.
31. Damocles Study Group. A proposed charter for clinical, trial data monitoring committees: helping them to do their job well. Lancet 2005; 365: 711–722.
32. Buchanan D, Miller FG. Principles of early stoping of randomized trials for efficacy: a critique of equipoise and an alternative nonexplotation ethical framework. Kennedy Inst Ethics J 2005; 15: 161–178.
33. O'Brien PC, Fleming TR. A multiple testing procedure for clinical trials. Biometrics 1979; 35: 549–556.
34. Lan KKG, DeMetz DL Discrete sequential boundaries for clinical trials. Biometrika 1983; 659–663.
35. Armitage P. Interim analysis in clinical trials. Stat Med 1991; 10: 925–935.

S. S. Cofield and G. R. Cutter

INTRODUCTION

An argument raged between two colleagues: the internist adamantly stating the issue of aging in the US is a clinical issue and the health behavior researcher just as adamant that aging is a serious public health problem. Who is right? Certainly all aging patients experience changes that ultimately lead to problems at a clinical level supporting the internist's view. Just as certain is the fact that, in the USA, a bolus of late-middle-aged persons are altering our social systems and creating anxiety for services, clearly supporting the health behaviorist. Can it be that both are correct? All of us wear multiple hats representing the different perspectives from which we view problems and outcomes.

This multiple perspective belies the problem for outcome measures in multiple sclerosis (MS). The clinician often sees outcome measures in terms of individual patients. The patient with optic neuritis is evaluated with respect to progress in her eyes, not Kurtzke's Expanded Disability Status Scale (EDSS).[1] However, the outcome measure for a clinical trial may focus on the EDSS and is barely influenced by the optic neuritis. The FDA tries to bridge this gap in perspectives by mandating that outcome measures used in trials be clinically meaningful. But that view also has problems of interpretation, implementation and pre-existing bias.

Thus, what are MS outcomes, how do you measure them and why do you measure them? Like the example above, choosing an MS outcome depends on the perspective. The clinical question of interest is: Who will benefit from this treatment and in particular will this patient benefit? The statistical or clinical trial question is: What characteristics or treatments are useful in predicting who will respond to therapy with high sensitivity and specificity?

The clinician is interested in treating his/her patient and the outcome is improvement in the presenting problem, a short-term objective or outcome. This does not mean that the clinician is unaware of long-term consequences but to address that issue a switch to predicting the future may require different outcome measures, such as disability, cumulative damage or atrophy of the brain measured by magnetic resonance imaging (MRI), etc. The clinical decision moves from ameliorating the immediate problem to asking in a broader context if the current therapeutic approach is failing and, if so, to assess alternative approaches. However, deciding what a treatment failure is and when it occurs is not a well-defined outcome measure. There is no accepted universal definition of MS treatment failure.

In this chapter we will discuss some general concepts of outcome measures and summarize some of the major and not so major outcomes being used. Two specific chapters in this book, Chapters 29 and 30, depend heavily on the concepts of outcome measures and provide some concrete settings where outcome specification is critical.

GOLD STANDARD OUTCOME MEASURES

When one talks about outcome measures in MS, the EDSS immediately comes to mind. It is relied upon by the US Food and Drug Administration (FDA) as the gold standard but it has well-known limitations as an outcome measure of choice. Unlike gold, the EDSS is a semi-precious standard. In cardiovascular disease trials, endpoints such as mortality or myocardial infarction are often used. These endpoints are used by the FDA and practicing clinicians as outcomes and as endpoints. They immediately meet the requirement of the FDA standard – they are clinically relevant and meaningful to the patients. In MS, few practicing clinicians routinely measure the EDSS. If this is not measured by practitioners, is it the real outcome for MS? And if it is not the real outcome, what are the real outcomes in MS? Clearly, a complete neurological examination is the basis of the components of the EDSS but the ordinal clinical summation is often imprecise and highly variable. Over the long term such a system clearly classifies the patients, but time to wheelchair or some objective measure of a declining system might work as well.

You could argue that death, myocardial infarction, etc. are so called 'hard endpoints' and many cardiovascular studies also focus on 'softer' endpoints such as blood pressure and/or cholesterol. The path to establish these softer endpoints as effective or valid endpoints took years of epidemiological and statistical work before they were accepted. What makes these endpoints different from candidate outcome measures in MS is that cardiovascular disease is common compared to MS, enabling more and varied studies by a larger research cadre to collect and evaluate presumptive outcomes, but even with the larger numbers these endpoints took years to validate.

449

IMPAIRMENT AND DISABILITY

Outcome measures in MS are broad-ranging and address the complex world of impairment and disability. Many approaches to measuring impairment and disability exist beyond MS, and the terminology often leads to confusion as to the concept being measured. The World Health Organization (WHO) developed the International Classification of Impairments, Disabilities and Handicaps.[2] In this framework, a patient is classified in terms of disease, impairment, disability and handicap. *Disease* represents the underlying diagnosis or pathological process. *Impairment* is the loss of physical or psychosocial capacities. *Disability* refers to limitations in performing a usual activity of normal life. *Handicap* is a disadvantage resulting from impairment or disability that inhibits or prevents a role that is normal for that person.

The medical model of disability focuses on the individual, specifically their impairment. The goal of treatment is to alleviate consequences of the impairment, to return the individual to normal (or as close to normal as possible). This model requires accurate diagnosis of the impairment and its pathology. The second perspective is the health psychology perspective. This vantage point is heavily focused on coping behaviors and developing strategies to minimize the effects of impairment. The view is that people are disabled not only by their impairment, but also by how they respond to the impairment. From this perspective, an assessment of activities of daily living and how a patient plans to accomplish certain tasks make up the tools for assessing that patient. Both approaches are valid for a patient-centered or clinical approach to therapy and both can lead to valid outcome measures with often different choices of therapies and results.

WHAT DEFINES OUTCOME MEASURES

The National Multiple Sclerosis Society sponsored a seminal meeting on the topic in 1994 (Outcomes Assessment in Multiple Sclerosis Clinical Trials: A Critical Analysis). The report stated:

There is a clear need for the development of new assessment systems, probably based on the best aspects of the EDSS (Kurtzke Expanded Disability Status Scale). Any new system must be multidimensional and quantitative. Preferentially, its scoring should be automated to speed the process and to improve the consistency from assessment to assessment, between raters and among centers. It should have adequate evaluation of cognition for which there are many validated, though not currently practical, systems.[3]

This meeting led to a task force[4] that focused on finding a clinical trials outcome measure meeting explicit properties set out in advance. Key characteristics of this task force were to recommend a clinical outcome assessment tool for future MS clinical trials capable of reflecting the impact of an intervention on the progression of disease. The task force found that the outcome measure needs to:

- Be useful to demonstrate clinical change due to MS
- Be multidimensional to reflect the principal ways MS affects an individual
- Have high reliability and validity
- Be sensitive to change over short intervals of time to permit demonstration of a therapeutic effect
- Be both practical and cost-effective.

The task force found that the measure should be more objective and reliable than the EDSS. To this end, the task force chose the Multiple Sclerosis Functional Composite (MSFC).[5] However, the criteria given by the task force can be used in judging and thinking more generally about other outcome measures in MS.

There is often great debate over the value of an outcome measure of disability in MS. For example, some believe that extensive cognitive testing is essential to characterize a patient's disability, while others are content with a more global assessment. Interventions that seek to effect cure are best measured from the medical model perspective. Interventions designed to ameliorate symptoms should often be approached using the health psychology perspective. We expect that disease-modifying agents in MS require different measurement tools from drugs that are directed at symptom management. Further, the outcome measures for the same condition can thus differ immensely even for clear physical impairments such as walking. A study of a pharmacological treatment aimed at improving walking may conclude that it has failed as a therapeutic agent, but the subject of another trial, a provision for walking aids that does not attempt to improve the clinical condition can be considered successful even though there is no change in the physical condition. In the former study the outcome might be a timed walk, whereas in the latter study the outcome might be distance walked, general mobility or quality of life.

CLASSICAL TYPES OF OUTCOME

Most of this chapter will be concerned with the measurement of impairment or disability from the medical model perspective. This is chosen because the evaluation of new therapies is usually focused from this perspective. There are a wide range of measurement tools for application in multiple sclerosis encompassing everything from fatigue through sleep to bowel and bladder functioning. Another dimension of the problem for outcome assessment is that disease activity is probably subclinical in the early phases of the disease and may be undetectable clinically in later stages. So not only do the outcome measures differ with the perspective (medical versus health psychology versus population perspective), they also differ over time within the same patient.

However, rather than provide a listing of outcome measures that have been used in MS, let us classify them into four classes:[6]

- **Rating scales** are ordered scales requiring human assessment, the most common in MS being Kurtzke's EDSS[7]
- **Performance measures** are standardized procedures for testing human function, such as the 25 foot timed walk[8] or the nine-hole peg test[9]
- **Biological measures** use laboratory methods, such as the presence and amount of neutralizing antibodies, myelin basic protein, serum glutamic pyruvic transaminase, to evaluate liver function, etc.
- **Patient self-report measures** require the individual patient to provide information about his/her condition from his/her own perspective. The Incapacity Status Scale,[10] the Guy's Neurological Disability Scale (GNDS)[11] and the MSQLI[12] are examples of such self-report measures in the MS field.

While these classes represent distinct types of measure, the purposes of the measurements are, however, not restricted by the different classes. In other words, the same research question could be addressed by a laboratory test, a rating scale, a performance measure or a self-reported measure. In clinical medicine, more than one measure, and often many measures, are used to evaluate patient status, check progress, alter the course of therapy or make other recommendations. In a clinical trial, it is generally preferred to identify a single measure as the primary outcome but in addition to use several secondary measures of the patient's wellbeing. There is a natural conflict between a complete clinical assessment of a patient from a physician's perspective and the index measure used in a clinical trial. The primary endpoint by itself is often inadequate in practice. This is because a single measure nearly always aggregates information to an average or otherwise representative value and is usually seen as inadequate for individual patients. Clinicians feel an obligation to understand their patient in as detailed a manner as possible, while the trial outcome measure may ignore entirely important factors of a specific patient's condition. The conflict may not show in the choice of instruments but can and does influence the interpretation of the results.

IMAGING OUTCOMES

In MS one of the more interesting and common outcomes is MRI. It is not easy to classify MRI into one of these four categories. For example, T2-weighted image measurements are likely to be considered biological characteristics, but is N-acetylaspartate a biological measurement or a performance measurement? From a practical perspective, does it matter? It can matter when we think about measures that are the indicators of how a body performs and others that are indicators of the underlying consequences of biological processes. The former are useful in treating a patient to diminish the clinical problem; the latter are useful as predictors or harbingers of things to come. We will return to this thought later when we consider the disconnect many MS researchers have between knowing the MRI is important and having unsatisfying evidence for its long-term predictive validity. Nevertheless, consider contrast-enhancing lesions, which offer great face validity as outcome measures. No one argues that the presence of the lesions on an MRI is OK. Clearly, lesions cannot be a good or meaningless occurrence. Some may argue that their impact is unknown but few would argue they are totally unimportant. Some excess risk of poorer prognosis would seem to emanate from finding lots of these lesions versus none in the brain of a patient. So, many clinical trials today are in fact based on the performance of therapies in reducing the number of gadolinium-enhancing lesions. However, if we take the perspective that outcome measures in MS should be capable of showing impact over the long term (predictive validity), contrast-enhancing lesions will probably fail, since they disappear and tend not to recur as the patient progresses to later stages of the disease. Thus, an outcome measure that disappears with and without treatment can be problematic, unless it has strong predictive properties for the course of the disease. These properties are often associated with a class of outcomes called surrogate outcomes. We will discuss this concept in more detail below.

SINGLE VERSUS MULTIPLE ENDPOINTS

Some instruments, as opposed to biological measures, are used to measure disease-specific functions or conditions. Examples are sexual dysfunction, bladder infections and/or cognitive function. Other instruments aim to measure disease dysfunction in a nonspecific manner, thus enabling comparison across diagnostic conditions. The Adult Functional Independence Measure (FIM)[13] is a generic instrument used to measure impairment in a number of diseases or conditions. There are benefits and disadvantages to both disease-specific and generic instruments. These must be weighed and related to the underlying research question. In the chapters on data and safety monitoring committees and the one on clinical trials, outcome measures are used to assess the safety of the patients participating in the trials and for identifying clinical outcomes assessing the differences of one treatment to another. These aims are often best served by disease-specific measures; whereas generalizability is often served by more global measures since they can be used in cost–benefit assessments and for allocating resources. Another domain where there are differences in preference between disease specific and global measures is quality of life instruments and cognitive evaluations. Clinicians generally prefer disease-specific instruments. In areas of psychosocial evaluation, however, disease-specific approaches are often too narrow, although broad-based assessments tend to be cumbersome or time-consuming. This desire for identifying specific problems and functions versus generalized measures has led to a proliferation of choices and a lack of consensus on measurement. Although attempts have been made to define short batteries in cognitive function, they are by no means universally agreed upon or used.

Another important measurement issue is whether to choose an instrument or measure that explores a single dimension of impairment versus one that addresses a broader spectrum of the patient's condition. For example, measures of ambulation focus almost exclusively on leg function in the MS patient, whereas the EDSS was developed as a composite score capturing nine functional systems, at least at the lower end of the scale. Nevertheless, the EDSS is heavily dominated by walking and while perceived as an integrated measure of neurological status could be problematic when used as an outcome measure because of this heavy dependence on walking. This may be an issue in the paucity of agents for secondary progressive MS (SPMS) and primary progressive MS, although with walking such a central function, it is likely that current agents have had little impact on this function. However, the targeted outcomes may become more important as attempts at designer therapies are developed or in the early development of neuron-protective or neuron-repair agents, where success is more physiologically limited.

For certain clinical trials a highly specific outcome measure may be preferred, while in other trials multiple responses may be important. For example, ambulation may be a key outcome measure in a trial of 4-aminopyridine, where the mechanism of action is thought to speed nerve conduction. A more global outcome such as the GNDS[11] may not offer the specificity desired in such a trial even though the GNDS may measure global assessments very meaningful to patients. The GNDS may be preferable in a long-term trial, because the principal question relates to the overall condition of the patient and not just function disrupted.

Thus, while no single measure is ever likely to be completely adequate to characterize an MS patient, a given clinical trial must choose an endpoint that most appropriately addresses the question being asked. This is equally true for the clinician evaluating the patient and the problem at hand, but the choices are probably not the same. Because it is difficult to characterize impairments and disability associated with MS and because the disease results in multiple clinical manifestations, optimal outcome measures in MS clinical trials are likely to be very specific to a narrow question of treatment in the context of the time frame over which the trial is conducted. Clinically we informally use composite clinical measures for assessing the impact of treatment, a gestalt of benefit versus toxicity. In many other diseases or conditions with gold standards, the progress in outcome measures is moved forward by finding surrogates for the gold standard, which may be easier to measure, less costly or yield information about the effects of treatment in a shorter time period. Surrogate outcomes are measures that represent true outcomes but are antecedent to and occur much earlier and are easier to collect than the true outcome. The surrogate must have predictive validity about disease changes in the future. When there is no gold standard, it is difficult if not impossible to develop a surrogate. However, with commonly accepted conventions, such as benchmark changes in the EDSS, surrogate outcomes can be explored. Unfortunately, it generally takes a long time for a community to accept that these surrogate outcomes are tantamount to longer-term outcomes. We must first understand in more detail just what a surrogate outcome is and how difficult is it to establish?

SURROGATE OUTCOMES

Surrogate outcomes (also called surrogate endpoints, measures or markers) are measured variables used in place of a variable that may be difficult, be too costly or take too long to measure. These variables must have specific properties to be validated as a surrogate marker. Surrogate outcome measures have been studied in a variety of diseases (cancer, heart disease, HIV, etc.) and are measured instead of the biologically definitive or most relevant clinical endpoint, such as death or myocardial infarction. When used to establish the effectiveness of a treatment, the criteria for validation of surrogates is stringent:[14,15]

- The surrogate must predict future clinical disease
- The effect of treatment on clinical disease must be explained by the effect of the treatment on the surrogate; the treatment needs to effect clinical outcome by working through the surrogate
- The surrogate must work over various classes or doses of treatment in the same manner.

Fleming[15] defines a surrogate endpoint statistically as 'a response variable for which a test of the null hypothesis of no relationship to the treatment groups under comparison is also a valid test of the corresponding null hypothesis based on the true endpoint'. Alternatively, the FDA defines a surrogate marker as any nonclinical measure that can reliably predict clinical changes 'within a reasonable amount of time'. A surrogate endpoint needs to be convincingly associated with a definitive clinical outcome so that it can be used as a reliable replacement. A good surrogate endpoint should yield the same inference as the definitive endpoint and should also be responsive to the effects of treatment. A good surrogate endpoint can shorten clinical trials because of its short latency with respect to the natural history of the disease. It is advantageous to use surrogates in cases where the definitive endpoint is inaccessible because of time constraints, difficulty of measurement and/or cost. There are also disadvantages to surrogate endpoints; for example, eligibility criteria for a clinical trial may depend on the surrogate measurement truncating a population, which reduces both the predictive validity of a measure and the correlation with other variables. Furthermore, a weak association between the surrogate and the true outcome may not reflect the effects of treatment, as when the treatment affects the true outcome through a mechanism not involving the surrogate and thus, the surrogate does not predict treatment effects on the definitive endpoints accurately.

The EDSS is not equivalent to the MS disease outcome. Nevertheless, it is the gestalt everyone agrees is the clinical condition of the patient. It does tend to predict future status over reasonable time domains but does not predict who will change and thus is more a classification scale. It has grown to become the outcome measure of choice in MS clinical trials. However, in terms of the formal definitions of surrogate outcomes, the EDSS has not been validated to fulfill the characteristics listed above for a true surrogate. It has long been known

that the EDSS is somewhat unreliable from visit to visit, varying in general by 1 point or more and yielding slightly more than 50% agreement from visit to visit. MS clinical trialists introduced the concept of sustained change to avoid this well-known unreliability of the EDSS. While this does improve the properties of the EDSS by identifying patients who most probably have sustained disability, few data are available to show that the predictive validity of the EDSS and the treatment effects observed are sufficiently enhanced to warrant the label of surrogate.

Gadolinium enhancements on MRI, T2 lesion load and/or other MRI parameters are being investigated and even used as surrogate markers of MS disease states. Lacking a definitive outcome measure, it is extremely important to have a keen understanding of the EDSS as well as other measures of impairment and disability when attempting to define surrogacy.

There has been great disappointment with various parameters of MRI that were thought to be a surrogate. The MS community sees the MRI as a tool that is certainly meaningful and visualizes important data about a patient. However, has it really succeeded as an outcome measure? This is separate from the question of whether it has performed as an outcome measure. We will return to this question later in the chapter and some potential reasons for failure to meet these surrogacy requirements to date, but we now more formally address the general question of outcomes for MS.

OUTCOMES FOR MULTIPLE SCLEROSIS

First, recall the five criteria set forth by the task force regarding an outcome measure. An outcome measure needs to:

1. Be useful to demonstrate clinical change due to MS
2. Be multidimensional to reflect the principal ways MS affects an individual
3. Have high reliability and validity
4. Be sensitive to change over short intervals of time to permit demonstration of a therapeutic effect
5. Be both practical and cost-effective

THE FUNCTIONAL SYSTEM SCORES AND EXPANDED DISABILITY STATUS SCALE

Originally developed in 1955,[1] the EDSS[7] is a composite score based upon seven functional systems and patient ambulation. Each patient is examined according to the seven functional systems, paralleling a thorough neurological examination, and each functional system is scored as follows:

- Cerebral (or mental): 0–5 (Normal to Dementia)
- Optic (visual): 0–6 (Normal to Grade 5 plus maximal visual acuity of better eye ≤20/60)
- Brainstem: 0–5 (Normal to Inability to swallow or speak)
- Pyramidal: 0–6 (Normal to Quadriplegia)
- Sensory: 0–6 (Normal to Sensation essentially lost below the head)
- Cerebellar: 0–5 or 9 (Normal to Unable to perform coordinated movements due to ataxia, or Weakness interferes with testing)
- Bowel and Bladder: 0–6 (Normal to Complete loss of bowel and bladder function).

The patient is then assessed for ambulation, generally consisting of the distance the patient can walk with or without assistance. The functional system scores and the ambulation ability are then combined into the composite score known as the EDSS, a combination of assessment and functional ability. Originally, the EDSS, known as the Disability Status Scale or

DSS, ranged from 0–10 in whole-integer increments; however in 1983 the scale was amended and half point changes were introduced to reflect small changes in disease severity. It is important to note, however, that the EDSS is an ordinal not a linear scale. The physical changes represented are not the same for each increase in the EDSS. That is, a change from a EDSS 1 to a 2 is not the same as a change from a 6 to a 7. These numbers are really labels for stages of disease, not numbers in the sense of averaging. Thus, the FDA criteria of what are meaningful changes really can't be explained in terms of changes in the EDSS; it has merely become convention that an average difference of 0.5 means the patients are worse, but the meaningfulness is merely inferred from our knowledge of the disease step. Once a subject is unable to walk unassisted, regardless of the seven functional system scores, the EDSS will be at least a 6 on the 0–10 scale.

In terms of the five criteria set forth by the task force, the EDSS clearly meets criteria 1 and 2 by including leg, arm, sensory, visual, mental or cognitive, bowel and bladder, and sexual dysfunction. However, criteria 3–5 are only partially met by the EDSS and only under certain circumstances. Criterion 3 calls for the outcome to have high reliability and validity but the EDSS can be highly variable, depending upon several factors: multiple examiners can score the same patient differently; the same examiner can score 'equally impaired' subjects differently; the same patient can score differently on two examinations within a short period of time, even without experiencing a relapse between examinations. As such, the EDSS can measure change in a short period of time (criterion 4) but this change could be random noise or lack of inter-rater reliability. Practicality and cost-effectiveness (criterion 5) depend upon the situation in which the test is being administered. Smaller practices with a large patient : physician ratio may not find the EDSS practical nor cost-effective given the examiner time required to administer it. This examination is usually performed by a physician and is therefore more expensive for the patient, hospital and/or insurance company than an examination that another staff member could administer, such as the MSFC, or a self-administered exam that is completed by the patient.

EXACERBATIONS

As the hallmark of MS is the waxing and waning of relapses, it seems natural that such a measure might be a useful and important outcome measure. Though this outcome is a very reasonable clinical outcome, it becomes quite problematic in clinical trials. The definition of an exacerbation requires a temporal component (onset and duration of symptoms); evaluation by a clinician to validate that changes in a functional system have occurred and often it is required that the EDSS has increased by 1 point or more. Exacerbations have not been well studied from the perspective of reproducibility and accuracy. They require the patient to be cognizant in reporting symptoms and successful in being seen in a timely fashion to ensure that indeed these are new symptoms and related to MS. The consequences of these issues of definition are that, if missed, the events would be the more minor relapses.

The predictive validity of exacerbations has been looked at by a number of authors. Confavreaux et al[16] and Held et al[17] have found that the occurrence of relapses was not predictive of reaching benchmark milestones, especially for patients with an EDSS of more than 3.5. If a stringent definition of an exacerbation is applied, it would seem obvious that a patient might get to EDSS 4 sooner if they experienced relapses, since a study by Lublin et al[18] showed that, on average, about 40% of MS patients who experience a relapse are left with some residual deficit and more would probably lead to increased progression.

It may well be that the failure of relapses to predict progression onward from EDSS 4 is the tarnished gold standard of the EDSS. The EDSS may not be related to these events above 4 as it is mostly a walking scale above 4 and ignores a multiplicity of symptoms. Nevertheless, there may be equally important reasons why relapses are a poor outcome measure for the entire spectrum of MS. They decline naturally with duration of and stage of disease. The reasons for the decline are not known, but an outcome measure that has a variable incidence rate is a complex outcome to use in a clinical trail violating most statistical assumptions used in planning trials (a common similar experience of all that are treated).

THE MULTIPLE SCLEROSIS FUNCTIONAL COMPOSITE

The 1994 meeting cited earlier, Outcomes Assessment in Multiple Sclerosis Clinical Trials,[2] recommended development of an improved clinical outcome measure for MS clinical trials that met the criteria noted above. The task force developed six guiding principles for the composite development and analyses that are reported in this paper and these still apply to the development of any purported outcome measure:

- To use measures that reflect the major clinical dimensions of MS
- To avoid redundancy
- To use simple rather than complex measures
- To improve on the valuable characteristics of the EDSS
- To emphasize measures sensitive to change
- To develop an outcome measure that will be useful in clinical trials (and may or may not be directly useful for clinical care).

The task force identified arm, leg, cognitive and visual function as the major dimensions of MS and established criteria to select candidate component measures including good correlation with the biologically relevant clinical dimensions and good reliability of the measurement (the ability to obtain the same result on repeat testing when no change occurred) and have the ability to show change over time.

Construct validity (the extent to which the measure of interest correlates with other measures in predicted ways, but for which no true criterion exists) was used to reduce the number of candidate measures. This was based on the logic that individual measures within the same clinical dimension should correlate with each other (convergent validity) and not with measures of different clinical dimensions (discriminant validity). Applying these criteria, a subset of candidate measures was selected. Reliability estimates observed from the literature, means and standard deviations of change, and the relationship between changes in these candidate variables and the EDSS were assessed. Both concurrent and predictive validity of the composite measure were evaluated. *Concurrent validity* was defined as change in the composite measure compared with concurrent change in the EDSS over a 1 year period. *Predictive validity* was defined as change in the composite occurring over the first year of follow-up compared with subsequent change in EDSS among those patients with no sustained change in EDSS during the first year. Predictive validity was felt to best illustrate and validate the composite construction. The delineation of the MSFC resulted from a pooled data set of placebo control groups and natural history study databases. Detailed discussion of this process is reported by Cutter et al.[19]

The MSFC is a standardized score similar to a z-score including the combination of results from three performance tests: the nine-hole peg test, the timed 25-foot walk and the 3-second paced auditory serial addition test. These performance tests are combined to form a single score, the MSFC.[20] The MSFC correlates well with the EDSS but suffers from three major limitations: the choice of the population on which to standardize the components, the nonlinearity of the changes as the patient's physical function declines and the clinical meaningfulness of changes. In clinical trials, the combined baseline study population is used as the framework for standardizing but this makes changes relative and only directly comparable within the trial. While most populations have exhibited similar standard deviations of the components, which make the changes more comparable, the problem is still present, especially when a broad range of patients are entered into a trial. It is often stated that the clinical meaning of a standard deviation of 2 is too difficult to interpret because clinical meaning depends on what is being measured: seconds, number correct, etc. This is not truly the case: it is rather a matter of custom and comfort with how things are reported. For example, in medicine we define laboratory abnormalities in this way, marking them as adverse events or critical limits when they are two or three times the upper or lower limit of normal based on the local laboratory standards, but are readily interpretable.

A great deal has been learned about the MSFC. The measure has been shown to be reliable, having intraclass correlation coefficients of 0.93 when used in multinational clinical trials and multiple languages involving 436 patients.[21] The MSFC has a defined learning curve that requires at least three administrations to develop an accurate baseline from whence to measure change.[22] Use of the MSFC without taking into account the learning curve would still work in trials but adds noise to the measure of change. It would also underestimate the amount of decline, because of a lower or poorer performance at baseline than would be possible once the patient becomes experienced with the testing procedures. It is sensitive to the standard population used, and results would vary somewhat from trial to trial if the baseline populations used were different. Several authors have shown that the MSFC correlates with MRI parameters,[23,24] with health-related quality of life measures[25] and with clinical outcomes measured prospectively,[26–28] confirming the predictive validity found in the development of the measure for long-term outcomes.

The problem of nonlinearity does impact the interpretation of change but is not an inherent problem in the measure, rather an illustration of how the disease impacts patients. The consequences of the disease are greatest after a long period of small decrements in function. Nevertheless, this nonlinearity does create problems for detecting changes and nonparametric measures may have to be used in analyses to overcome the skewness induced by the lack of linearity. While the MSFC meets the first five criteria above, the sixth criterion needs more complete testing in the realm of clinical trials and definition of the clinical relevance of these measures.[29] Nevertheless, of particular importance is the ability to show small changes in active arm comparison studies. Without increasingly sensitive measures, progress in the MS field will be constrained by cost and the availability of patients for clinical trials.

MAGNETIC RESONANCE IMAGING OUTCOMES

In 1981, Young et al[30] showed that, relative to computed tomography (CT) scans, MRI could identify an order of magnitude of more abnormalities in the brain. This technology has demonstrated clearly that MS is a disease characterized by multiple focal lesions in the white matter. MRI has been exquisitely sensitive in identifying these and their changes in the brain. Attempts have been made to use this technology to study inflammation,

edema, gliosis, myelin density and/or axonal density, with varying degrees of success. Each of these target outcomes would be extremely important for specific questions. To date many studies have tried to demonstrate that the parameters measured on MRI correlate with and predict the outcomes of the course of MS. Initially gadolinium enhancements or contrast-enhancing lesions (CELs) were thought to be a good outcome measure of disease. Patients who present for MS diagnosis or reporting exacerbations often have more CELs on inspection than patients in the remitting phase of the disease but the correlation is much less than might be expected. Clinical trials demonstrated that these lesions are reduced by agents aimed at reducing inflammation, so another characteristic of an outcome measure has conceivably been met. Sormani et al[31] have presented results suggesting that MRI is a surrogate for exacerbations. However, CELs have not been shown to predict long-term disability with any substantial sensitivity. CELs, like relapses, wane as the patient becomes more and more disabled.

In a 2006 article, Goodin[32] theorizes that the reason for the lack of predictive validity lies in at least one of two major factors. One is that lesions are missed because of the varied nature of their occurrence and the frequency of measurement, and the other is that there are really two kinds of CEL: lethal and nonlethal. Goodin's model shows that, depending on the relative frequency of the occurrence of each type of lesion, correlations will be lowered and in fact would routinely be in the 0.10–0.30 range – consistent with what is observed in most analyses. This perspective is highly informative in that one can argue from this that the very high sensitivity of MRI for detecting CELs could indeed lead one to conclude that MRI is potentially overly sensitive and that this is the reason for its predictive validity failures. An analogy might be the screening tool for colon cancer fecal occult blood testing (FOBT).[33] FOBT has numerous false positives because any source of blood is detected, including dietary sources, and thus is overly sensitive, masking the signal from the lethal blood by too many nonlethal sources of blood. Goodin's argument may hold when MRI is performed infrequently, as in clinical trials or as restricted by insurers to one per year. In such a situation, one is asking a single cross-sectional catch to predict a year-long ongoing process. Thus, these potential problems in demonstrating the predictive validity of MRI should be considered when evaluating this outcome and considering alternative outcomes from MRIs.

Another very rational candidate is T2-weighted MRI lesions. This too has had difficulties in showing predictive validity but has correlated widely not only with the EDSS but also with cognitive measures. However, a recent paper by Li et al[34] suggests that T2 lesions plateau with increasing EDSS, making predictive validity difficult to show. This group's findings are based on samples of combined placebo groups from clinical trials. The plausible nature of their findings that lesions are absorbed or disappear as a result of atrophy and/or axonal loss or other changes in the brain is an important observation. However, if such were the case, the ratio of T2 to the amount of brain parenchyma (adjusting for brain loss) might show an increasing trend in the same direction as EDSS. Again, it is quite possible that defining predictive validity against the EDSS could be the problem. The difference between EDSS 6.0 and EDSS 6.5 can merely be whether a patient is using a walker or a cane. Such potentially personal choices would cause misclassification on the EDSS, leading to an appearance of a plateau unrelated to T2. Other plausible explanations also exist, in that T2 ignores changes in the spinal cord where likely impacts on walking occur and this is neither measured nor correlated with the amount of T2 in the brain.

There are many outcomes now proliferating via MRI and these will not be covered in detail here. Newer measures such as diffusion tensor imaging and functional MRI are measuring more and more specific functions and abnormalities but their success as outcome measures will depend on the rules noted above. That is, ultimately they have to be clinically meaningful and have predictive validity.

With the large number of MRI metrics used to assess patient status and progression, including volumes of various tissues and numbers of lesions (with and without gadolinium enhancement), and cerebrospinal fluid volumes, composite measures attempt to capture the diversity of measures into a so-called total burden of cerebral disease (BOD), which might provide an integrated outcome for use clinically or in trials.

One such measure based on these components is the MRI Z4 and the ranked Z4.[35] The MRI Z4 or ranked Z4 are composite measures similar to the MSFC that can be used to measure change in MRI in reference to a standard or baseline population. MRI outcomes have inherent face validity – blood in the brain is not good, atrophy is obviously bad, black holes are certainly not beneficial to the patient. However, more formal validation of these with regard to clinical outcome is essential to justify the high cost and effort of obtaining these measures. The MRI measures meet the criteria noted above: they seem to avoid redundancy, use measures that reflect the major clinical dimensions of MS, may or may not be considered to use simple rather than complex measures, may improve on the valuable characteristics of the EDSS, have a number of trials showing treatment responses and are seemingly sensitive to change.

CONTRAST LETTER ACUITY

A great deal of work has been conducted on contrast sensitivity. This measure was identified as a significant signal in the Optic Neuritis Treatment Trial[36] and has been explored in a number of investigations and publications. Visual dysfunction occurs in 80% of patients with multiple sclerosis during the course of their disease and is a presenting feature in 50% of patients. Balcer et al[37,38] evaluated several tests of binocular contrast sensitivity and contrast letter acuity testing and concluded that contrast sensitivity using Sloan charts and the Pelli–Robson contrast sensitivity measures provide useful measures for distinguishing MS patients from normal controls and can show change over time within MS patients. Several papers have demonstrated key components of the use of the contrast letter acuity assessed by Sloan letter charts (charts that can be used like Snellen charts to assess the impact of MS on visual function). Balcer et al[39] have shown that these measurements are highly reliable (intraclass correlations in excess of 0.90) and can be made simply in the clinic. These tests have face validity in that the mean score correct declines with decreasing contrast.

Balcer showed that MS patients could be distinguished from disease-free controls in a cross-sectional study of visual outcome measures and that contrast letter acuity and contrast sensitivity best distinguished MS patients from disease-free controls in their cohort.[37] Adjusting for age, the odds of being an MS patient were nearly 2.4:1 based on these contrast letter acuity scores. Correlations of Sloan chart scores with MSFC and EDSS scores in both studies were statistically significant and moderate in magnitude (approximately 0.56), demonstrating that Sloan chart scores reflect visual and neurological dysfunction not entirely captured by the EDSS or MSFC. Sloan chart testing also captures unique aspects of neurological dysfunction not captured by current EDSS or MSFC components, making it a strong candidate for a visual function test for the MSFC.

Baier et al[38] have shown that these charts do not appear to be associated with optic neuritis and can distinguish between relapsing–remitting MS (RRMS) and SPMS patients. The scores are correlated with the MSFC but also appear to contain information not presently contained in the MSFC. When the MSFC was calculated and the odds of being an MS case was compared to a control evaluated in their cohort, the estimated odds of correct classification were 2.9:1. Recomputing the MSFC with contrast letter acuity at 1.25% increased the odds of separation between healthy controls and MS patients to 3.8:1. It similarly improved the separation between RRMS and SPMS patients. More formal evaluation of these potential additions to the MSFC awaits analyses of ongoing clinical trials, which should provide evidence for the value of the addition of a vision component to the MSFC. While visual tests alone are likely to fail to satisfy the criteria for outcome measures, adding these tests to existing measures such as the MSFC can enhance their performance in meeting these criteria.

NUMBERS NEEDED TO TREAT

In this current era of evidence-based medicine, new clinically relevant outcomes are being used. For example, when binary outcomes are used, such as progression on the EDSS, a way to examine the resultant difference in percentages after a study is to consider the number of patients that have to be treated to prevent one outcome event. This is a way to consider the cost effectiveness of the treatment in prevention. A quantity has been developed called the 'number needed to treat' or NNT.[40] The NNT essentially determines how many patients must be treated to prevent one case with the outcome measure. The NNT of a trial is calculated quite simply as 1/difference in proportions between the treatment groups. A large number indicates that there is a small treatment benefit and a small number indicates that there is a large treatment benefit. NNTs can be used to compare studies and gauge the relative impact of the differences. For example, in the original glatiramer acetate Copaxone© registration trial,[41] the 2-year proportion of patients relapse-free was 0.336 (33.6%) in the Copaxone Group compared to 0.270 (27.0%) in the placebo group. The difference in these proportions is 0.066 (0.336–0.270). The NNT would be 1/0.066 or 15.2 patients treated to produce 1 additional relapse-free patient. So a small NNT would be indicative of a large effect, because few patients have to be treated to produce benefits. Similarly, a large effect size (difference between groups) would indicate that a continuous outcome has led to a large effect on patients.

One of the drawbacks of the NNT is that, while it can be interpreted in a trial-independent manner, it is not free of the trial completely. The measure allows anyone to assess under the conditions of this trial how many patients need to be treated to increase the benefit by one patient. However, the incidence of disease in the placebo group and the selection criteria for the study, etc. have a great impact on results. Nevertheless, the NNT captures the fact that a small absolute difference will generally lead to a large NNT and a large difference to a smaller NNT. However, comparing one study with another still requires an understanding of the entrance and exclusion criteria as well as other methodological issues in the design and implementation.

OTHER MEASURES OF IMPAIRMENT AND DISABILITY

The majority of other measures of impairment and disability have been scales rather than functional measures. Several scales have been identified that seem to contain important information about the clinical status of the patient. These include the GNDS,[11] the Short and Graphic Ability Score (SaGAS),[42] the Multiple Sclerosis Impact Scale (MSIS-29),[43] the Scripps

Neurological Rating Scale (SNRS),[44] the Functional Independence Measure (FIM)[13] and the Patient Determined Disease Steps (PDDS).[45]

GUY'S NEUROLOGICAL DISABILITY SCALE

The GNDS[11] has 12 separate categories: cognition, mood, vision, speech, swallowing, upper limb function, lower limb function, bladder function, bowel function, sexual function, fatigue and others. The GNDS was found to be acceptable to neurologists and patients, reliable, responsive and valid as a measure of disability. The scale was also found to be valid when applied by non-neurologists, over the phone or via a postal questionnaire. The GNDS has good correlation with both the EDSS and MSFC but can be attributed mainly to the importance of spinal-cord-related neurological functions in all three scoring systems. In addition, the GNDS shows a marked discrepancy between the assessment of cognition from objective measurements and subjective complaints. Like other patients self-report scales, the GNDS provides a good measure of patient daily function but is not a good measure of cognitive dysfunction.

THE SHORT AND GRAPHIC ABILITY SCORE

Vaney[42] correctly points out that the MSFC is sensitive to the standard population chosen – the broader and more variable the population is at baseline, the more difficult it is to show a change. The reference population in that study ranges from EDSS 1.5 to EDSS 9, which indeed does accentuate this deficiency. The MSFC was developed as a clinical trial outcome measure, whereas Vaney's goal was to develop a tracking tool for the individual clinician. Using a clever transformation, he developed a closely-related measure to the MSFC that offers clinically meaningful results based on percent changes. His SaGAS score provides counts of meaningful changes.

Additional work has been conducted to examine ways to make the MSFC changes more clinically meaningful. As Vaney has done, these new examinations include counting the number of 20% changes, using percentage change in the composite, or inverse changes. To date no single overall better performance has been identified. What has been highlighted that may improve the MSFC substantively is the identification of potential visual components, as discussed above.

THE MULTIPLE SCLEROSIS IMPACT SCALE

A patient-based scale, MSIS-29 is an instrument measuring the physical (20 items) and psychological (nine items) impact of multiple sclerosis.[43] The scale measures the two dimensions and correlates well with other known outcomes, but has been used infrequently.

THE SCRIPPS NEUROLOGICAL RATING SCALE

The SNRS was designed to quantify impairment level as assessed by a traditional neurological examination.[44] Developed in the late 1990s at the Scripps Research Institute, ten systems are numerically scored for level of impairment from normal to severe and the total score (out of 100) is the overall SNRS. While the structure of the SNRS seems similar to the EDSS in that underlying system scores form a composite score, the SNRS and EDSS have not been found to be highly correlated. In addition, the SNRS appears to show more gradual changes over time compared to the EDSS. However, like the EDSS, the SNRS requires physician time and is a subjective examination of the patient.

THE FUNCTIONAL INDEPENDENCE MEASURE

The FIM[13] is an 18-item ordinal scale that can be used across many different diagnoses, which rates the level of assistance required to perform various activities of daily living using a seven-level scoring system. Scores range between 124 (normal status) and 18 (totally dependent). While it is a consistent rating scale with high inter- and intrarater reliability, the FIM is not sensitive to the types of clinical change seen in MS.[43]

THE PATIENT-DETERMINED DISEASE STEPS

Developed by Hohol,[45] the PDDS was designed to be a simple to use scale for assessing patient functionality. It is an ordinal scale based primarily on ambulation, ranging from 0 (normal) to 6 (essentially confined to wheelchair), with a separate category for patients who cannot be classified into one of the six categories. Unlike the EDSS, the PDDS shows a more consistent distribution of scores; however, patients with milder levels of disability from RRMS were more likely to demonstrate change over time compared to more disabled or progressive patients. It has been modified to allow for patient self-administration via a questionnaire found to correlate well with the EDSS.

SUMMARY OF MEASURES

Several of the measures described above have been evaluated, each having pros and cons, proponents and detractors. Each measure meets the criteria noted above to various degrees. The arguments that brew over the plethora of candidates may be summed up with the same advice as with quality of life. What is the question? What is the goal? Do you need a disease-specific outcome or a more generic instrument? Are you focused on symptom evaluation or disability or impairment? The field of MS has not placed much confidence to date in self-administered questionnaires but might benefit from overcoming this general attitude. The GNDS appears to have reasonable properties. The North American Research Consortium on Multiple Sclerosis (NARCOMS) registry has made extensive use of self-assessment scales and has published various validations of these scales.[46,47] More attention to such self-administered scales might be beneficial in reducing the complexity of trials and blinded evaluations by examiners, if self-assessment scales can be shown to be good surrogates for clinical measures.

PROMISING NEW OUTCOME MEASURES

It seems clear from the results of the major clinical trials in MS that reduction and/or elimination of inflammation is not the entire story with regards to treatment consequences. This has reinvigorated the notion that using neuron-protective agents and/or neurorestorative agents could enhance the treatment results currently measured by the outcomes described above. However, what would be an appropriate outcome in a neuron-protection or neurorepair trial is the source of many debates. MRI has been unsuccessful to date at clearly identifying axonal loss or even isolating neurons for measurement. The cost and logistical inconveniences associated with MRI have led some to examine other potential outcome measures.

One promising tool is optical coherence tomography or OCT. OCT is an interesting methodology that measures the thickness of the retinal nerve fiber layer (RNFL). The benefit of the procedure is that it can be done in the office setting at a lower cost than MRI. The technique has been shown to identify differences between MS patients and controls,[48,49] is reportedly highly reproducible but still must demonstrate that it represents a window on MS rather than simply a characterization of the consequence of optic neuritis. It still must meet the criteria set out earlier in this chapter to become an outcome measure of choice but does offer a very useful tool for future MS studies as it may be used to measure axonal loss and/or remyelination if that can be separated from edema, which is reduced with the clearing of inflammation.

SUMMARY

The measurement of impairment and disability requires sharply focusing the question being addressed. Patient-specific clinical care questions may require measures of impairment and disability that are directed at guiding therapy. Therapy failure has not been carefully defined and it is unclear what outcomes constitute such a failure on a patient-to-patient level. It is easier to define failure of therapy in a trial setting because prespecified outcomes have been created. The current clinical approach is usually a measure of the disease, perhaps progression or too much MRI activity. Rarely is it a questionnaire, scale or even quality of life.

When the question to be answered requires a controlled clinical trial, outcome measures of group performance are generally preferred. Continuous measures of impairments and disability are preferred over ordinal scales because they allow more precise measures and smaller sample sizes. These measures may result in therapeutic benefits without obvious clinical benefits but, using such tools as effect sizes and NNT (for binary outcomes), clinical benefits can be inferred. Related studies to explore the clinical meaning of the continuous impairment measures, however, are still important.

The MSFC is a relatively new measure of impairment and disability. It is really a paradigm shift to move to outcomes that are more sensitive to change and capture the major multiple dimensions of MS. Clinical interpretability is likely to improve as more information is collected and published about its use. New and better measures will surely be developed and the concept underlying the MSFC goes beyond the current component measures.

MRI techniques continue to offer better and newer ways to visualize what is occurring with the disease in the brain. The failure to provide correlations with future disability as measured by the EDSS may in part be because our ability to summarize the pictures that seem so clearly representative of the state of the patient is inefficient or even incorrect. Alternatively, some of the valuable information from the MRI outcome measures are being lost because we are relying too heavily on an imperfect standard.

Self report measures have long been sought and have had mixed reviews. For clinical trials, these are important because they may, if valid and reliable, reduce the cost of trials and enable trials to be conducted without the huge investments now required. Newer measures such as OCT need to be thoroughly evaluated in real prospective settings to determine whether the changes reported thus far are limited to optic neuritis, overt and even subclinical, or whether the technique offers an easy window on MS.

Finally, however, sentinel events in the course of progression of MS need to be carefully delineated. These events may be MRI benchmarks, achieving some level of EDSS disability that is reliably assessed or some benchmark defined by functional testing. Once clear benchmarks are established, outcomes and then the search for surrogates to simplify the trials and speed the research in MS will be enhanced.

REFERENCES

1. Kurtzke JF. A new scale for evaluating disability in multiple sclerosis. Neurology 1955; 5: 580–583.
2. International classification of impairments, disabilities, and handicaps. Geneva: World Health Organization; 1980.
3. Whitaker JN, McFarland HF, Rudge P, Reingold SC. Outcomes assessment in multiple sclerosis clinical trials: a critical analysis. Mult Scler 1995; 1: 37–47.
4. Rudick R, Antel J, Confavreux C et al. Clinical outcomes assessment in multiple sclerosis. Ann Neurol 1996; 40: 469–479.
5. Rudick R, Antel J, Confavreux C et al. Recommendations from the National Multiple Sclerosis Society Clinical Outcomes Assessment Task Force. Ann Neurol 1997; 42: 379–382.
6. LaRocca NG. Statistical and methodological consideration in scale construction in quantification of neurologic deficit. Stoneham, MA: Butterworth; 1989.
7. Kurtzke JF. Rating neurologic impairment in multiple sclerosis: an expanded disability status scale (EDSS). Neurology 1983; 33: 1444–1452.
8. Schwid SR, Goodman AD, Mattson DH et al. The measurement of ambulatory impairment in multiple sclerosis. Neurology 1997; 49: 1419–1424.
9. Mathiowetz V, Weber K, Kashman N, Volland G. Adult norms for 9 hole peg test of finger dexterity. Occup Ther J Res 1985; 5: 24–38.
10. MRD minimal record of disability for multiple sclerosis. New York: National Multiple Sclerosis Society; 1985.
11. Sharrack, B, Hughes, RA. The Guy's Neurological Disability Scale (GNDS): a new disability measure for multiple sclerosis. Mult Scler 1999; 5: 223–233.
12. Ritvo PG, Fischer JS, Miller DM et al. Multiple Sclerosis Quality of Life Inventory: a user's manual. New York: National Multiple Sclerosis Society; 1997.
13. Granger CV, Hamilton BB, Keith RA et al. Advances in functional assessment for medical rehabilitation. Top Geriatr Rehabil 1986; 1: 59–74.
14. Prentice RL. Surrogate endpoints in clinical trials: definition and operational criteria. Stat Med 1989; 8: 431–440.
15. Fleming, T. Surrogate markers in AIDS and cancer trials. Stat Med 1994; 13: 13–14.
16. Confavreux C, Vukusic S, Moreau T, Adeleine PC. Relapses and progression of disability in multiple sclerosis. N Engl J Med 2000; 343: 1430–1438.
17. Held U, Heigenhauser L, Shang C et al, the Sylvia Lawry Centre for MS Research. Predictors of relapse rate in MS clinical trials. Neurology 2005; 65: 1769–1773.
18. Lublin FD, Baier ML, Cutter GR. Effect of relapses on development of residual deficit in multiple sclerosis. Neurology 2003; 61: 1528–1532.
19. Cutter GR, Baier ML, Rudick RA et al. Development of a multiple sclerosis functional composite as a clinical trial outcome measure. Brain 1999; 122: 871–882.
20. Fischer JS, Jak AJ, Kniker JE et al. Administration and scoring manual for the multiple sclerosis functional composite measure (MSFC). In: National Multiple Sclerosis Society Manual. New York: Demos; 1999.
21. Cohen JA, Cutter GR, Fischer JS et al. Benefit of interferon beta-1a on MSFC progression in secondary progressive MS. Neurology 2002; 59: 679–687.
22. Cohen JA, Fischer JS, Bolibrush DM et al. Intrarater and interrater reliability of the MS functional composite outcome measure. Neurology 2000; 54: 802–806.
23. Kalkers NF, Bergers L, de Groot V et al. Concurrent validity of the MS functional composite using MRI as a biological disease marker. Neurology 2001; 56: 215–219.
24. Fisher E, Rudick RA, Cutter GR et al. Relationship between brain atrophy and disability: an 8-year follow-up study of multiple sclerosis patients. Mult Scler 2000; 6: 373–377.
25. Miller DM, Rudick RA, Cutter GR et al. Clincal significance of the Multiple Sclerosis Functional Composite: relationship to patient-reported quality of life. Arch Neurol 2000; 57: 1319–1324.
26. Kalkers NF, Bergers E, Castelijns JA et al. Optimizing the association between disability and biological markers in MS. Neurology 2001; 57: 1253–1258.
27. Uitdehaag BM, Ader HJ, Roosma TJ et al. Multiple sclerosis functional composite: impact of reference population and interpretation of changes. Mult Scler 2002; 8: 366–371.
28. Uitdehaag BM, Ader HJ, Kalkers NF, Polman CH. Quantitative functional

measures in MS: what is a reliable change? Neurology 2002; 59: 648–649.

29. Schwid SR, Goodman AD, McDermott MP et al. Quantitative functional measures in MS: what is a reliable change? Neurology 2002; 58: 1294–1296.

30. Young IR, Hall AS, Pallis CA et al. Nuclear magnetic resonance imaging of the brain in multiple sclerosis. Lancet 1981; 2: 1063–1066.

31. Sormani MP, Bruzzi P, Comi G, Filippi M. MRI metrics as surrogate markers for clinical relapse rate in relapsing remitting MS patients. Neurology 2002; 58: 417–421.

32. Goodin DS. Magnetic resonance imaging as a surrogate outcome measure of disability in multiple sclerosis: have we been overly harsh in our assessment? Ann Neurol 2006; 59: 597–605.

33. US Preventive Services Task Force. Screening for colorectal cancer: recommendations and rationale. Rockville, MD: Agency for Healthcare Research and Quality, 2002. Available on line at: www.ahrq.gov/clinic/3rduspstf/colorectal/colorr.htm.

34. Li DK, Held U, Petkau J et al, the Sylvia Lawry Centre for MS Research. MRI T2 lesion burden in multiple sclerosis: a plateauing relationship with clinical disability. Neurology 2006; 66: 1384–1389.

35. Wolinsky JS, Narayana PA, Noseworthy JH et al. Linomide in relapsing and secondary progressive MS: part II: MRI results. MRI Analysis Center of the University of Texas-Houston, Health Science Center, and the North American Linomide Investigators. Neurology 2000; 54: 1716–1717.

36. Optic Neuritis Study Group. Visual function 5 years after optic neuritis: experience of the Optic Neuritis Treatment Trial. Arch Ophthalmol 1997; 115: 1545–1552.

37. Balcer LJ, Baier ML, Cohen JA et al. Contrast letter acuity as a visual component for the Multiple Sclerosis Functional Composite. Neurology 2003; 61: 1367–1373.

38. Baier ML, Cutter GR, Rudick RA et al. Low-contrast letter acuity testing captures visual dysfunction in patients with multiple sclerosis. Neurology 2005; 64: 992–995.

39. Balcer LJ, Baier ML, Pelak VS et al. New low-contrast vision charts: reliability and test characteristics in patients with MS. Mult Scler 2000; 6: 163–171.

40. Mancini GB, Schulzer M. Reporting risks and benefits of therapy by use of the concepts of unqualified success and unmitigated failure: applications to highly cited trials in cardiovascular medicine. Circulation 1999; 99: 377–383.

41. Johnson KP, Brooks BR, Cohen JA et al. Extended use of glatiramer acetate (Copaxone) is well tolerated and maintains its clinical effect on multiple sclerosis relapse rate and degree of disability. Neurology 1998; 50: 701–708.

42. Vaney C, Vaney S, Wade DT. SaGAS, the short graphic ability score: an alternative scoring method for the motor components of the Multiple Sclerosis Functional Composite. Mult Scler 2004; 10: 231–242.

43. Ravnborg M, Gronbech-Jensen M, Jonsson A. The MS Impairment Scale: a pragmatic approach to the assessment of impairment in patients with mulitple sclerosis. Mult Scler 1997; 3: 31–42.

44. Sipe JC, Knobler RL, Braheny SL et al. A neurologic rating scale (NRS) for use in multiple sclerosis. Neurology 1984; 34: 1368–1372.

45. Hohol MJ, Orav EJ, Weiner HL. Disease steps in multiple sclerosis: a longitudinal study comparing disease steps and EDSS to evaluate disease progression. Mult Scler 1999; 5: 349–354.

46. Marrie RA, Cutter G, Tyry T. Validation of the NARCOMS Registry: pain assessment. Mult Scler 2005; 11: 338–342.

47. Marrie RA, Cutter G, Tyry T et al. Validation of the NARCOMS registry: fatigue assessment. Mult Scler 2005; 11: 583–584.

48. Frohman E, Costello F, Zivadinov R et al. Optical coherence tomography in multiple sclerosis. Lancet Neurol 2006; 5: 853–863.

49. Fisher JB, Jacobs DA, Markowitz CE et al. Relation of visual function to retinal nerve fiber layer thickness in multiple sclerosis. Ophthalmology 2006; 113: 324–332.

Index

459